Comprehensive Respiratory Care
A LEARNING SYSTEM

Comprehensive Respiratory Care

A LEARNING SYSTEM

David H. Eubanks, Ed.D., R.R.T.

President
Crestwood Career Academy, Inc.
Tempe, Arizona

Roger C. Bone, M.D., F.C.C.P.

Ralph C. Brown Endowed Chair,
Professor and Chairman, Department of Internal Medicine,
Chief, Section of Pulmonary and Critical Medicine,
Rush Medical College,
Rush-Presbyterian St. Luke's Medical Center,
Chicago, Illinois

SECOND EDITION

with 973 illustrations

The C. V. Mosby Company

ST. LOUIS • BALTIMORE • PHILADELPHIA • TORONTO   1990

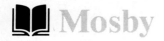

Publisher: David T. Culverwell
Developmental Editor: Christi Mangold
Editorial Assistant: Teena Wolfe
Project Manager: John A. Rogers
Production Editor: Shauna Burnett Sticht
Designer: Susan E. Lane

Cover Photograph: Courtesy Boehringer Ingelheim Pharmaceuticals, Inc.

Illustrations: Medical Media
           Ron Boisvert, M.S.M.I.
           Richard Hall, M.S., A.M.I.

           Top Graphics
           Denise Laposa Dingman
           Craig Hoffmann

SECOND EDITION

Printed in the United States of America

The C.V. Mosby Company
11830 Westline Industrial Drive, St. Louis, Missouri   63146

Library of Congress Cataloging-in-Publication Data

Eubanks, David H., 1937-
    Comprehensive respiratory care: a learning system / David H.
Eubanks, Roger C. Bone.—2nd ed.
      p.   cm.
    Includes bibliographical references.
    ISBN 0-8016-2932-2
    1. Respiratory therapy.   I. Bone, Roger C.   II. Title.
    [DNLM: 1. Respiratory Therapy.   WF 145 E86c]
RC735.I5E93   1990
615.8'36—dc20
DNLM/DLC
for Library of Congress   89-13793
ISBN 0-8016-2932-2   CIP

C/VH/VH 9 8 7 6 5 4 3 2

To
Jacquie, Julie, Jawn, and Katie

Dave

To
my wife Rosemary
and daughters, Mary Katherine and Cynthia

Roger

Preface

Since the early 1950s respiratory therapy, now respiratory care, has changed as a profession from primarily the administration of oxygen to the application and monitoring of advanced life support techniques using sophisticated computerized equipment. Also during this time period respiratory care has grown to a profession involving some 100,000 practitioners and support personnel.

Respiratory care is a specialty that requires more than just a casual encounter with technology and treatment modalities. Information identifying the scope of practice of respiratory care personnel was published in a 1978 study conducted by the American Association for Respiratory Care. Based on this study and other supportive data obtained from its own study, the National Board for Respiratory Care (NBRC) reached the decision that there was a core of knowledge and competencies expected of persons entering the field of respiratory care. This core of knowledge and skills was essentially the same for both respiratory therapy technicians and therapists. On this premise the NBRC developed an entry-level examination. The impact of this examination was to change the way in which students, educators, and employers viewed respiratory care school graduates. In contrast to the previous technician certification examination, graduates now became qualified to sit for the entry-level examination without waiting for postgraduate clinical experience.

This change required schools to reevaluate their curricula and textbooks for practical application of knowledge and skills so that the new graduate would be prepared to enter the work environment almost immmediately as a practitioner with full credentials.

A review of existing texts quickly revealed that no single source provided the information or the sequencing necessary to instruct a person in respiratory care from entry level to advanced practitioner. *Comprehensive Respiratory Care: A Learning System* is a text developed in response to this need.

The format of the book is different from that of other texts. It is divided into modules, with content units instead of chapters and sections. The numbering system correlates the contents to learning objectives so that the book functions as a complete learning system. Learning objectives introduce each module. Each objective is keyed by a numbering system to titles of the units in the module, which helps the reader easily and quickly understand the intended purpose of the material. Where appropriate, clinical procedures are also numerically keyed. Module One functions as a detailed explanation of the book's structure.

The outline format and succinct sentences enable the reader to identify information quickly without reading complex paragraphs. Technical language is defined as it is used, and concepts are developed as they are applied to a situation. Over nine hundred illustrations have been used to provide visual examples of concepts. These numbered illustrations, which are discussed in the text, enable the reader to visually follow gas flow through tubes, the mechanical action of valves, and other dynamics as they appear. This practical and visual approach for presenting information makes the book useful not only as a primary text but also as a bridge to help students better understand the complex information and vocabularies used in other respiratory care texts.

The second edition has been expanded to thirty modules, and all previous modules have been updated to include the most current respiratory care concepts and equipment. Three new modules have been included to cover gerontology and the process and problems of aging, critical care cardiorespiratory monitoring with invasive and non-invasive procedures, and the evaluation and application of computers to mechanical ventilators and patient care. Updated topics include: philosophical and legal aspects of the right-to-die issue, a discussion on mental health and depression, the effects of hepatitus B and AIDS on patients and employees, the most current cardiorespiratory drugs, third generation ventilators and alarm systems, and an expanded module on pulmonary function with illustrations of equipment and case studies to be solved by the reader.

In addition to practical respiratory care information, the text presents in a single source the background sciences and respiratory care knowledge and skills requisite for entry level positions (respiratory therapy technician) to advanced practitioner (respiratory therapist). Material on the background sciences is presented immediately before or in conjunction with respiratory care concepts. Knowledge, theory, and principles are developed so that learning occurs sequentially in steps that progress from the simple to the complex. Throughout the book concepts and principles are applied to practical situations that provide the reader the benefit of the authors' clinical experiences and knowledge of the field.

Questions on the content, which have been keyed to the information in each module, are provided in an Instructor's Manual. This manual also contains recommendations and instructional strategies for teaching topics covered by the book.

David H. Eubanks
Roger C. Bone

Foreword

Certainly the art and practice of respiratory care have evolved in dramatic fashion during the last two decades. Once called inhalational therapy and essentially equated with setting up oxygen tanks at the bedside for use with tents and masks, the field of respiratory care today encompasses a broad area of clinical expertise. Thus a thorough understanding of basic anatomy, physiology, biochemistry, pharmacology, and the physics of gases and a familiarity with a growing number of respiratory care devices are required of the present-day respiratory therapist or technician. In addition, the disease states that necessitate respiratory care procedures must be understood with equal facility. Thus those entering the important health care profession of respiratory care must meet exacting educational standards before they are eligible to provide their services in hospital wards, intensive care units, or the home.

Drs. David Eubanks and Roger Bone have organized and written a highly detailed text that is filled with vital facts for all respiratory therapists and technicians. Learning objectives, detailed anatomic drawings, and physiologic illustrations and tables are packed with a massive amount of information. I congratulate my two friends and colleagues for their efforts on behalf of everyone who would pursue the knowledge necessary for a competent background in today's comprehensive respiratory care. I am sure that all who read this book will be richly rewarded!

Thomas L. Petty, M.D.
Professor of Medicine,
Director, Webb-Waring Lung Institute

Acknowledgments

Special recognition is given to Larry R. House, R.R.T., whose financial and professional support enabled the original Academy for Allied Medical Sciences (AFAMS) program to be developed. A special thanks goes to Warren G. Sanborn, Ph.D., for Module Thirty. His expertise in the ventilation field is respected, and we sincerely thank him for his contribution.

The following persons are recognized for their contributions to the content of the original AFAMS program: William Funderbruk, R.R.T., Karen Shaffran, R.R.T., Stanley Pearson, R.R.T., Robert Demers, R.R.T., Michael Paine, R.R.T., Lee King, R.R.T., and Bruce Ott, R.R.T.

A note of thanks to the following individuals whose assistance helped us complete this book:
Jerry Coursen, Ph.D., *Reviewer*
Barbara Dailey and Terri Salter, *Typists*
Ron Boisvert, M.S., AMI, *Medical illustrator*
Kathi Schirtzinger, C.R.T.T., *Reviewer*
Beth Smith, *Figure coordinator*
Karen Standermieer, R.R.T., *Research assistant*
Kelly Wiehn, R.R.T., *Test item coordinator*

Contents

Understanding the book as a learning system

On completion of this module the reader will be able to:

1.1 Explain terms and concepts used in the book.

2.1 Define "system" by listing the characteristics of a system.

2.2 Explain why the book fits the definition of a system.

3.1 Point out the difference between the format of a traditional book and this modular-unit approach.

3.2 Describe how each module is identified.

4.1 Explain the purpose of the list of learning objectives that introduces each module.

4.2 and **4.3** Discuss how the learning objective correlates to the content in the module.

5.1 Sequentially explain the steps recommended for studying this book as a learning system.

As noted in the Preface, this book is not only a text about respiratory care; it is designed to function as a *learning system* for group or self-instruction. The purpose of this first module is to explain the format of the text and to point out how the reader may gain maximum benefit from its use. It also provides a sample module to familiarize the reader with the format.

The first unit contains terms that are used to describe the philosophy and design of the book.

1.0 GLOSSARY OF TERMS

1.1 Learning module

A *learning module* is an independent grouping of related facts, concepts, and principles about specific topics. A module can stand alone or be joined with other modules to form a complete course of instruction. As previously stated, the book has a total of 30 learning modules.

1.2 Learning unit

Each module is made up of still smaller, more specific, groupings of related information known as learning units. A learning unit presents very specific facts, principles, and/or concepts about a content area. Two or more learning units are combined to form a learning module.

1.3 Learning system

Planned instruction guides the learner's progress through a thought process that results in behavioral changes. Each step in the process is defined with objectives and verified by testing.

1.4 Learning objective

A statement that clearly describes what the reader is expected to learn from the module content. All content in a module, including clinical procedures, is designed to answer and/or evaluate completion of the stated objectives.

1

1.5 Mastery learning

An educational concept defines a learning process whereby the learner does not progress until each stated learning objective is achieved.

2.0 CHARACTERISTICS OF A LEARNING SYSTEM
2.1 Definitions

Webster's New World Dictionary of the American Language (second college edition) defines system as:

1 "A set or arrangement of things so related or connected as to form a unity or organic whole."
2 "A method or plan of classification or arrangement."
3 "An established way of doing something; method; procedure."

2.2 Rationale

This book fits all the definitions in 2.1, because all content is arranged in a modular-unit format with the parts (units) forming the whole (module). The book comprises the 30 collected learning modules. All content is based on specified learning objectives that are cross-referenced to all content, including any special learning activities and questions.

This interdependency of all content to the learning objectives creates an instructional nucleus that causes the reader to learn, to be evaluated, and to experience remediation in a systematic fashion.

The book, if used as suggested in Unit 5.0, provides a systematic approach to mastery learning instead of providing merely a compilation of facts.

3.0 LEARNING MODULES
3.1 Modular-unit approach

This book uses a *modular-unit format* instead of the traditional section and chapter organization of most texts.

3.2 Identification of the module and unit

1 Each module is identified by spelling out the number followed by the module title, for example, "Module One, Understanding the Book as a Learning System."
2 Sections of the module are identified by a unit number (in arabic), followed by a zero, which introduces the topic and functions as a title. Then sequential numbers highlight the details of the unit, for example, "Unit 1.0, Glossary of Terms"; Units 1.1 through 1.5 name the terms.
3 A learning module is made up of two or more learning units.

4.0 LEARNING OBJECTIVES
4.1 Purpose

Each module is introduced by a *list of learning units* with their respective *learning objectives*. These objectives state what the reader is expected to accomplish after studying the module.

4.2 Learning objective 1.1

By reading the learning objectives that introduce the module, the reader is prepared for the first task: "discuss how the learning objective correlates with the content in the module." By referring to the Glossary of Terms in the module content (1.0), the reader quickly identifies the term "learning module" (1.1).

4.3 Correlating objectives with units

This same approach is used to cross-*reference* all the learning objectives to the content in each module. This system enables the reader to constantly keep track of progress toward completion of the stated learning objective(s). In this respect the learning objectives are not just statements of intent but actual guides to the reader's learning.

The benefit of cross-referencing all content to a specific learning objective becomes even more clear as one becomes familiar with the system and uses the objectives to direct the learning process.

5.0 STUDYING THE BOOK
5.1 Sequential steps

The reader is encouraged to use the following steps when studying this book.

1 Read all learning objectives preceding each module to gain an overview of what is presented in the module.
2 Read any introductory material to the module.
3 While reading the units, refer to each stated learning objective. This approach helps the reader focus on the key factors and concepts to be learned from a unit.
   NOTE: The content in a module will flow as a text even though it is preceded by an objective identification number.
4 Complete any learning activities that are suggested in the module.
5 Review the learning objectives and determine your mastery of them. Reread those units that contain material about which you are still uncertain.

Professional growth and interactions

Respiratory care is a new specialty, which has emerged in the past 20 years, to diagnose and treat persons with cardiopulmonary disorders such as asthma, bronchitis, emphysema, and other forms of obstructive and restrictive diseases.

Respiratory care personnel are instrumental in assisting in the diagnosis, treatment, management, control, rehabilitation, and preventive care of patients with cardiopulmonary problems. These patients may be found in the neonatal nursery, surgical and medical wards, the emergency room, the outpatient department, and the critical care unit of the hospital. They may be suffering from a variety of acute and chronic conditions that are either life threatening or disabling.

Disease pathologies most frequently encountered include asthma, bronchitis, emphysema, and other types of chronic and acute restrictive and obstructive respiratory disorders.

Historically, the development and growth of respiratory care as a specialty trace its development back to Hippocrates.

1.0 HISTORICAL DEVELOPMENT AND GROWTH OF RESPIRATORY PHYSIOLOGY AND CARE
1.1 Significant contributors and events

The contributions of those individuals in the following list were instrumental in developing the scientific concepts and techniques that have resulted in the professions of *respiratory physiology*, *cardiopulmonary medicine*, and *respiratory care*. It is not only difficult but unfair to single out specific individual's contributions as more important than others, because without one event the others may not have occurred.

1 Hippocrates (460-377 BC). Influenced modern experts in oxygen therapy by his treatise entitled "On Air, Mineral Waters and Places."

2 Aristotle (384-322 BC). Recorded the first experiment in respiratory physiology. He placed animals in airtight boxes and concluded that their death resulted

3

from their inability to cool themselves. Respiration at this time was considered a means of controlling body temperature.

3 Galen (131-201 AD). Taught that blood left the right ventricle, passed through the "artery-like" vein to the lungs, and mixed with air to form the "Vital Spirits."

4 Da Vinci (1452-1519). Concluded that fire consumed something in air and that animals could not live in an atmosphere that did not support a flame.

5 Harvey (1578-1657). In 1615 he announced his discovery of circulation of the blood and in 1628 published his book, which stated that the heart was responsible for blood circulation. Respiration at this time was considered a means of cooling the blood.

6 Lower and Willis (1631-1691). Were the first to note the difference in the color of arterial and venous blood.

7 Stahl (1660-1734) with Becher. Established *phlogiston theory*. He noted that during combustion something (as gas) was given off, which he called phlogiston. The remaining gas was called "dephlogisticated air." The phlogiston theory seriously hampered progress in chemistry.

8 Boyle (1627-1691)
   a 1666. Demonstrated that without air life is impossible. He later proved that the human blood contained gases in solution.
   b 1670. Determined the reciprocal relation between volume and pressure of air. He surmised from his experiments that lack of oxygen was a destructive factor to the human body.

9 Hooke (1635-1703). Observed that dark blood became red on passing through the lungs and concluded this occurred because it mixed with air.

10 Lower (1631-1691). Established that blood, in passing through the lungs, changes color by deriving something from the air in the lungs. This was termed the "nitro-aereal spirit."

11 Black (1728-1799). Noted that a gas, which was called "fixed air," is given off by the lungs during exhalation. This gas is what we now call carbon dioxide.

12 Priestly (1733-1804). Discovered that plants could "convert vitiated atmosphere" that had proved fatal to animals, rendering the air respirable and capable of supporting life; that is, that plants used carbon dioxide and produced oxygen. Discovered oxygen, which he erroneously called "dephlogisticated air." On August 1, 1774, Priestly concentrated the sun's rays, through a magnifying glass, on some red mercuric oxide and in this manner produced oxygen.

13 Lavoisier (1743-1794)
   a 1775. Duplicated Priestly's experiments of producing oxygen. At first he called the gas "vital air," later called it oxygen, meaning acid-maker.
   b 1780. Laid down the fundamental principles of respiration. He demonstrated that oxygen is absorbed through the lungs, that carbon dioxide and water are given off in exhalation, and that an inert substance, hydrogen, is released. Lavoisier believed respiration

to be a process whereby oxygen combines with other constitutents to form carbon dioxide, water, and heat; the heat being the result of combustion in the body.
   c Lavoisier and Laplace (1780). Showed that the amount of carbon dioxide produced by respiration is nearly equivalent to the oxygen consumed. Lavoisier made one error. He thought that oxidation of carbon occurred in the lungs to form carbon dioxide.

14 Cavendish (1731-1810). Published a paper describing hydrogen as a gas.

15 Scheele (1742-1786). Discovered oxygen at about the same time as Priestly but did not publish anything on it until 1777.

16 Ingenhousz
   a 1779. Showed that it is only the green portion of the plants that can accomplish the conversion of taking up carbon dioxide and giving off oxygen. This is probably the first description of plant respiration.
   b 1781. Devised a rubber face mask for oxygen administration. This was probably the first oxygen mask.
   c Ingenhousz and Fontanta (1890s). Demonstrated that an animal can die from lack of oxygen as well as "fixed air" or what we now call carbon dioxide. Fontanta later worked on the removal of carbon dioxide from air. This is perhaps the first attempt at demonstrating carbon dioxide absorption.

17 Lagrange (1736-1813). Discovered that as the blood containing oxygen passed through the tissues, the oxygen united with carbon and hydrogen.

18 Beddoes (1760-1808). Established a pneumatic institute at Bristol. There he treated heart disease, asthma, opium poisoning, ulcers, paralysis, leprosy, venereal diseases, and dyspnea, using primarily oxygen. Beddoes was the first to recommend the treatment of diseases through the inhalation of gases. He has been referred to as the "father of inhalation therapy." He used oiled silk rags as a means for administering oxygen. He and James Watt were among the first to build an apparatus with unidirectional valves so that no rebreathing occurred.

19 Legallois (1770-1814). Described and established the respiratory center as being located in the medulla.

20 Hickman (1824). Observed that the administration of carbon dioxide produced coma and collapse. This phenomenon was reaffirmed by Simpson (1856) and Bert (1878). Hickman is credited with the discovery of the anesthetic properties of carbon dioxide.

21 Magnus (1837). Demonstrated that both venous and arterial blood contain oxygen as well as carbon dioxide. This was an important fact in tissue respiration.

22 Hoppe-Seyler (1877). First to observe the appearance of gas (nitrogen) in the blood following sharp and sudden fall of atmospheric pressure. This was confirmed by Sir Leonard Hill in 1912. The phenomenon is known as caisson disease.

23 Glaisher and Coxwell (1862). Ascended in a balloon to

29,000 feet and observed the symptoms of oxygen insufficiency. Their work was reaffirmed by Bert in 1878.

24 Janssen (1868). Using a spectroscope, he discovered helium as an element in the sun.

25 Hering and Breuer (1868). Showed that the mechanism of breathing is automatic and self-regulating, the distention and contraction of the lungs being in themselves a normal stimulus of the vagus nerve. They demonstrated that overinflation of the lungs inhibits inspiration and produces expiration and that sharp deflation of the lungs will initiate inspiration.

26 Bert (1878). Demonstrated that "mountain sickness" was caused by a decrease in the partial pressure of oxygen and explained much of what is known today about disturbed physiology at high altitudes.

27 Oertel (1878). Was the first to apply positive pressure. He employed 100 inspirations of air compressed to ⅟₅₀ of an atmosphere positive pressure in treatment of asthma.

28 Rosenthal (1880). Suggested that pulmonary ventilation is controlled by the level of oxygen in arterial blood.

29 Miescher (1885). Showed that addition of carbon dioxide to inhaled air would result in a material increase in respiratory volume. Henderson and Haggard followed this work in 1908 and introduced carbon dioxide–oxygen mixtures for resuscitation.

30 Kayser (1895). Was first to discover helium in the atmosphere. This was done by spectroscopic means. Ramsay and Travers (1899) later separated helium from the atmosphere by fractional distillation. As a result of this work the other rare gases were discovered.

31 Raleigh and Ramsay (1896). Isolated the gas called argon. Until this time it was believed the atmosphere consisted only of oxygen, nitrogen, and carbon dioxide. Since this gas would not go into combination with any other substance, it was named argon, meaning idle.

32 Ramsay
   a 1896. Discovered helium, which he had isolated from the mineral cleveite.
   b Ramsay and Travers (1898). Discovered the last three rare gases: krypton, neon, and xenon. These discoveries were the result of the work on separating helium from the atmosphere.

33 Norton (1897). Treated advanced pulmonary edema caused by carbolic acid poisoning (fumes), using the Fell-O'Dwyer apparatus, which made possible breathing under positive pressure.

34 Lane (1907). Advised that oxygen be administered by nasal catheter.

35 Emerson (1909). Demonstrated that artificial respiration under pressure was capable of abolishing pulmonary edema in rabbits. These results were confirmed and amplified by Auer, Gates, and Johnson in 1917.

36 Winterstein (1911). Suggested ventilation is controlled by the arterial pH (hydrogen ion concentration).

37 Stokes (1917). Reintroduced the method of administering oxygen by nasal catheter.

38 Haldane (1860-1936). In 1917 he developed an oxygen mask for the treatment of pulmonary edema caused by war gas poisoning.

39 Hill (1920). Built the first oxygen tent. It was used to treat a case of edema and chronic ulceration of a leg. This tent had no means for eliminating heat and moisture given off by the patient.

40 Barcroft (1920)
   a Built (in England) the first oxygen chamber.
   b Classified oxygen deficiency into three types: anoxic, anemic, and stagnant anoxia.

41 Peters and Van Slyke (1931). Added the fourth type of anoxia, which is known as histotoxic. This was the first classification of anoxia.

42 Henderson and Haggard (1920). Demonstrated that carbon dioxide was eliminated more swiftly from the blood when ventilation was increased through the use of carbon dioxide–oxygen mixtures.

43 Rost (1921) and Barker (1937). Administered oxygen by injection into infected areas. Rost also injected oxygen into the peritoneal cavity for the treatment of tuberculosis peritonitis.

44 Stadie (1922). Built first oxygen chamber in America (at Rockefeller Institute in New York City).

45 Davies and Gilchrist (1925). Recommended one-way valve systems so that exhaled gases are not rebreathed. This was the beginning of the demand flow type of apparatus.

46 Barach, Binger, and Roth (1926). Undertook the task of improving oxygen tents. Barach eliminated the heat and moisture by using a motor blower to circulate the air, which was passed over ice. Other methods of controlling the temperature in an oxygen tent were thermal circulation (Taylor), liquid oxygen (Hartman), and dry ice (Cohn).

47 Thunberg (1926). Built a chamber that enclosed the patient completely. This he called the "barospirator," and it was used for artificial respiration. The pressure in this chamber was alternately raised and lowered 55 mm Hg 25 times per minute.

48 Sayers and Yant (1926). Demonstrated that helium has a coefficient of solubility in blood approximately one half of nitrogen and diffusibility of two times that of nitrogen.

49 Drinker and Shaw (1929). Built a chamber on the order of Thunberg's except that the patient's head remained out of the chamber. This is what we refer to today as the "iron lung."

50 Waters and Wineland (1931). Introduced nasal catheter oxygen therapy to America. They advocated the oropharyngeal placement of the catheter.

51 Barach
   a 1931. Devised a portable oxygen room for use in the patient's home.
   b 1934. Introduced helium as a therapeutic gas.
   c Barach et al (1941). Developed the meter mask.

Used Poulton's air injector principle for diluting the concentration of oxygen administered.

d 1942. Developed the positive pressure mask for the treatment of pulmonary edema by modifying the principle of the Campbell-Poulton mask.

52 Felson (1931). Injected oxygen into the rectum at a rate of 125 ml/min until 2000 ml were administered. He thought the presence of oxygen not only inhibited the growth of anaerobic bacteria but made the mucous membrane more capable of resisting infection.

53 Burgess et al (1932). Developed the first oxygen hood, which was modified and improved by Burgess in 1934.

54 Henderson (1932). Advocated the administration of carbon dioxide–oxygen mixtures for the treatment of whooping cough.

55 Plesch (1933). Devised an apparatus for treating pulmonary edema. It consisted of a mask fitted with a water manometer and an expiratory valve, exerting a pressure that can be varied by altering the tension of a spring. Through another opening in the mask a blower motor delivers more than enough air for respiration. The tension exerted by the spring on the expiratory valve was usually set so that expiration can only take place at a pressure of 30 cm H_2O.

56 Campbell and Poulton (1934). Developed a positive pressure apparatus. It consisted of a face mask with two openings. One opening was connected to the motor blower and the other to a tube that was lowered beneath the surface of water in a bottle. "Excess of air is supplied to the mask from the blower and bubbles off beneath the water, so that the patient breathes under a positive pressure which can be regulated by altering the depth of the tube beneath the water."* Barach's positive pressure meter mask is a modification of the Campbell-Poulton mask.

57 Fine (1935). Postulated that the administration of high concentrations of oxygen will hasten the removal of nitrogen and hydrogen from the abdominal cavity and thereby reduce abdominal distension. Later (1938), he advocated the use of high concentrations of oxygen for the treatment of postencephalographic headache.

58 Behnke and Yarbhrough (1938). Demonstrated that the ill effects experienced by divers at depths below 100 feet could be eliminated by substituting helium for the nitrogen in the diver's air supply.

59 Boothby et al

a 1938. Devised the Boothby, Lovelace, and Bulbulion (BLB) oxygen mask. Boothby is responsible for establishing the use of oxygen postoperatively, especially in cases of bronchopneumonia.

b Boothby and Evans (1939). Demonstrated that human beings can tolerate pure oxygen without harmful effects from 2 to 4 days.

60 Wiggers (1940). First to use the term "hypoxia," meaning reduced amounts of oxygen. Previously, the term "anoxia" was used.

61 Poulton (1930s). Established the use of oxygen in cerebral thrombosis and rheumatic heart disease.

62 Cournand and Richards (1948). Developed accurate methods for determining lung function in pulmonary emphysema and tuberculosis.

63 Aeromedical Laboratories (1945). Aviation model of Bennett BX-1 developed at Wright's Field, Ohio.

64 Cournand, Motely, et al (1947). Published data outlining criteria for an ideal ventilator.

65 1947. Fifteen cases of pulmonary edema were reported as cured with intermittent positive pressure breathing (IPPB).

66 Motely, Land, and Gordon (1948). First to use IPPB aerosol to treat patients with chronic lung disease and to report arterial blood gas analysis before and after IPPB treatment.

67 Wittenberger (1949). First reported the use of high-frequency ventilation in experiments with panting dogs.

68 1952. Polio epidemic in Denmark resulted in the Swedish development of the Engström, the first volume ventilator.

69 Bird

a 1952. Developed first demand valve as prototype for Bird line.

b 1955. Developed prototype of Bird Mark 7 ventilator.

c 1957: First Bird Mark 8 ventilator.

d 1959: First Bird Mark 10 resuscitator.

e 1972. First Babybird developed.

70 Asbaugh and Petty (1967). The adult respiratory distress syndrome defined and treated with positive end expiratory pressure (PEEP).

71 Bennett (1971). MA-1 series ventilator introduced.

72 Sjöstrand and Eriksson (1980). Increased clinical descriptions of high-frequency ventilation.

2.0 PROFESSIONAL ORGANIZATIONS
2.1 Development, growth, and current roles

The major professional organizations for respiratory therapy are the American Association for Respiratory Care,* National Board For Respiratory Care and Joint Review, Committee For Respiratory Therapy Education.

1 On April 15, 1947, the Inhalational Therapy Association was incorporated in Chicago, Illinois.

2 In 1948 George A. Kneeland was elected president of this new association.

3 On February 27, 1948, the name changed to the *Inhalation Therapy Association*.

4 In 1950 the first Inhalational Therapy Institute was held in Chicago. Although the attendance was not large, attendees representing a wide geographic area supported the need for an association.

5 From 1950 to 1954 activity in the Inhalation Therapy

---

*Saklad M: Inhalation therapy and resuscitation, Springfield, Ill, 1953, Charles C Thomas, Publisher, p 192.

*We wish to acknowledge the historical information about the AART (now AARC) provided by Robert A. Dittmar, RRT, past historian and past president of the Association.

Association was limited to workshops held in Chicago and New York. Participants were awarded certificates of completion, documenting their knowledge and skills in primarily oxygen therapy and intermittent positive pressure breathing.

6 In 1950 the Committee on Public Health Relations of New York Academy of Medicine conducted a survey of the practice of inhalation therapy in hospitals in terms of the available information on equipment and methods and found a severe lag. The Committee's report, "Standards of Effective Administration of Inhalation Therapy" appeared in the Journal of the American Medical Association (JAMA) on September 2, 1950. Using this as a starting point, a joint committee of the New York State Medical Society and the New York State Society of Anesthesiologists began a long investigation into the problems of inhalation therapy.

7 In 1954 several interested technicians, together with members of American Society of Anesthesiologists and the American College of Chest Physicians, met at the Yale Club in New York City to discuss professional sponsorship of the Inhalation Therapy Association by these medical groups.

8 In 1954 the Inhalation Therapy Association officially became the American Association of Inhalation Therapists (AAIT).

9 By 1955 the public relations firm of Carriere and Jobson in New York and Chicago was appointed counsel for the AAIT. The sixth institute (attended by 115 people) was held in November 1955, and Sister M. Borromea was elected the first president.

10 In 1956 the total membership of the AAIT was 400, and Sister Borromea presented a chapter charter to the Illinois Chapter, Florida Chapter, Michigan Chapter, and Greater New York City Chapter.

11 In 1956 the first volume of the AAIT Journal was published, with James Whitacre as editor.

12 In the 1957 September issue of the AAIT journal, an article by Dr. Edwin Emma announced the cosponsorship of the AAIT by the American College of Chest Physicians (ACCP) and the American Society of Anesthesiologists (ASA).

13 In 1958 200 registrants attended the fourth annual meeting in St. Louis, Missouri, with a registration fee of $40 for members and $50 for nonmembers.

14 By March 1959 the AAIT had grown to 16 chapters.

15 In June 1959 the membership statistics were:

Active members	529
Industrial members	99
Service members	57
Associate members	31
Admitted and awaiting dues	67
Being processed	25
TOTAL	808

16 In 1959 at the fifth annual meeting in Philadelphia a new registry, the American Registry of Inhalation Therapists (ARIT), was announced and explained. The ARIT was to be in operation early in 1960 as a *separate corporation* from the AAIT in the State of Illinois. The ARIT Board was to be composed of three members, one each from the American College of Chest Physicians, American Society of Anesthesiologists, and the American Association of Inhalation Therapists. Dr. Vincent Collins said that "ARIT would exist to determine whether or not the aspirant possesses the *minimum* degree of skill and character necessary for the performance of his duties."

17 On November 7, 1960, the American Registry of Inhalation Therapists was incorporated in the State of Illinois.

18 In 1961 the first 33 therapists qualified for registration at the May 1 meeting of the ARIT Board of Trustees.

The new ARIT began to grow with the following number of registered therapists:

Date	Registered therapists
November 1961	68
August 1963	117
June 1965	265
November 1967	516
1968	688
1969	1025
June 1984	21,159

19 In December 1962 the essentials for an *accredited inhalation therapy program* were approved by the American Medical Association (AMA) House of Delegates. With this approval the *Board of Schools* was organized under the Council on Medical Education of the AMA.

20 The Board of Schools officially convened in November 1963, and Vincent Collins, M.D., was appointed chairman.

21 On April 4, 1967, the American Association of Inhalation Therapists became the *American Association for Inhalation Therapy* (AAIT).

22 In 1970 the AAIT administered the first technician certification examination.

23 In 1970 the American Association for Inhalation Therapy Foundation was incorporated.

24 In January 1973 the AAIT changed its name to the *American Association for Respiratory Therapy* (AART).

25 In March 1974 the membership of the AART had grown to 23,101.

26 In 1974 the ARIT changed its name to the National Board for Respiratory Therapy (NBRT) and agreed to assume the responsibilities from the AART for developing and administering examinations to certify technicians.

27 In January 1975 the technician certification credentialing examination was transferred to the NBRT.

28 In 1975 Professional Recognition of Continuing Education Experience and Development (PROCEED), the AART's first continuing education recognition program, was approved by the board of directors.

29 In 1976 the ARIT designation was changed to RRT.

30 In 1977 the AART implemented membership educational sections at its annual meeting.

31 In November 1978 the last oral examination was given by the NBRT at Las Vegas, Nevada.

32 In 1979 the first clinical simulation was given by the NBRT as a replacement for the oral examination.

33 In June 1979 the NBRT Board of Trustees approved development of an entry level examination.

34 In June 1982 the NBRT resolved to move forward for development of a specialty examination for entry level pulmonary function personnel. The first examination was given on July 7, 1984.

35 Since the initiation of the entry level examination for respiratory care on March 12, 1983, all candidates entering the examination system of the NBRC for either certification or registry must take the entry level examination.

36 On January 1, 1983, the National Society for Cardiopulmonary Technology (NSCPT) became an official sponsor of the NBRT.

37 Also on January 1, 1983, the NBRT changed its name to the National Board For Respiratory Care (NBRC).

38 In November of 1984 the professional designation was changed from respiratory therapy to respiratory care.

39 In November 1986, the American Association for Respiratory Therapy became the American Association for Respiratory Care (AARC).

3.0 RESPIRATORY CARE PERSONNEL
3.1 Roles and functions

1 *Respiratory therapist.* Graduate or registered respiratory therapist shall mean a person who is employed in the practice of respiratory care and who has the knowledge and skill necessary to administer respiratory therapy to patients in need of acute and critical care. The therapist is capable of serving as a resource to the physician and health care facility staff in relation to the technical aspects of respiratory care, is able to function in situations of unsupervised patient contact requiring *great individual* judgment, and is capable of *supervising, directing,* or *teaching* less skilled personnel in the practice of respiratory therapy.

  a *Graduate therapist.* One who is a graduate of a respiratory therapist program accredited by the Committee on Allied Health Education and Accreditation (CAHEA).

  b *Registered respiratory therapist.* One who has been registered by the National Board for Respiratory Care (NBRC) (formerly American Registry of Inhalation Therapists—ARIT) and National Board for Respiratory Therapy, Inc. (NBRT).

2 *Respiratory therapy technician.* Respiratory therapy technician or certified respiratory therapy technician shall mean a person who is employed in the practice of respiratory care who administers respiratory care in accordance with the educational preparation that has provided such an individual with a lesser degree of specialized skill, knowledge, education, or training than that required of a respiratory therapist.

  When it is expedient, the respiratory therapy techni-

cian may carry out certain tasks that are normally performed by a therapist provided that these tasks are performed under the supervision of a qualified physician or respiratory therapist.

  a *Graduate technician.* One who is a graduate of a respiratory therapy technician program accredited by the Committee on Allied Health Education and Accreditation (CAHEA).

  b *Certified respiratory therapy technician.* One who has been certified by the National Board for Respiratory Care (NBRC), formerly administered by the Technician Certification Board of the AARC. According to the entry level examination plan all persons wishing to be certified by the NBRC at any level must sit for the entry level examination. Successful completion of this examination qualifies the candidate as a certified respiratory therapy technician (CRTT).

3 *Respiratory therapy assistant.* One who has received on-the-job training in respiratory therapy.

4.0 RESPIRATORY THERAPY GRADUATES
4.1 Roles of members of the health team

The health team approach to patient care is a popular concept because it brings together the talents and experiences of many professionals involved in the care of a specific patient. Also it promotes cooperative working relations among specialty groups and decreases duplication of tasks and costs of patient care.

Each of the following individuals has a specific role as a member of this team:

1 Physician
  a Usually coordinator of the team.
  b Directs development of patient care efforts.
  c Prescribes treatment.
  d Serves as instructor of other team members.
  e Supervises overall patient care.

2 Registered nurse
  a Coordinates patient care efforts among team members.
  b Ensures uniform and quality care.
  c Carries out physician's orders.
  d Assists respiratory therapy personnel, as required, to complete a procedure.

3 Registered respiratory therapist
  a Assists the physician.
  b Assesses patient's need for respiratory care.
  c Coordinates preparation of respiratory equipment.
  d Administers care according to prescription.
  e Evaluates patient's response and modifies care to obtain maximum benefits.
  f Supervises overall respiratory care of patient.
  g Documents treatment rendered and patient response in progress notes. Makes recommendations for modifications in patient's care.

4 Certified respiratory therapy technician
  a Assists respiratory therapist.
  b Assembles and prepares equipment for use.

c Administers care, usually in noncritical care situations.

d Monitors patient and equipment.

e Keeps therapist informed.

f Services, cleans, and repairs equipment.

5 Radiologic technologist

a Takes radiographs of patient's chest and other areas of involvement both at the bedside and in the radiology department.

b Coordinates special procedures requiring radiographic diagnostic equipment.

6 Registered physical therapist

a Plans physical activities for rehabilitation of patient.

b Applies therapy to control pain, spasm, and weakness.

c Cooperates with respiratory therapy personnel in providing breathing exercises and pulmonary drainage procedures.

d In absence of respiratory personnel renders pulmonary clearance and rehabilitation procedures.

7 Medical laboratory technician/technologist

a Obtains cultures, blood samples, and other body substances for laboratory analysis.

b Works with respiratory therapy department for coordination of arterial blood gas analysis.

c Provides team with reports to keep team members assessed of patient's physiologic status.

8 Social worker

a Informs patient, family, and team members of available community health resources.

b Coordinates patient contact with these agencies.

c Assists family in preparing for patient's discharge and care at home.

9 Registered dietitian

a Plans patient's diet.

b Coordinates any special needs related to newer concepts of hyperalimentation.

5.0 ADMINISTRATIVE STRUCTURE
5.1 Protocol in health care facilities

1 Administrative protocol is the agreed-on formal pathway for referring problems or communications within any organization.

2 Although it will vary from hospital to hospital, most facilities have established administrative structures that resemble the organizational chart presented in Fig. 2-1.

3 The hospital chief administrator is responsible for the total operation of the hospital and usually reports to a board of trustees or directors.

4 The associate/assistant administrators usually report to the chief administrator and are usually responsible for management of specific departments or services such as respiratory care.

5 The director of services reports to an associate or assistant administrator and is responsible for management of one or more departments or services within the hospital.

6 The department chairman reports to the associate or as-

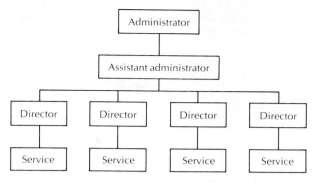

F I G U R E 2 - 1 Typical hospital organizational chart.

sistant administrator and is responsible for the overall daily management of a department.

7 Supervisors usually report to the department chairman and are responsible for completion and quality ensurance of specific clinical functions—for example, supervisor of evening shift in the critical care unit.

8 Generally, the pathway for formal communication with this type of administrative system is as follows:

Technician → Supervisor → Medical and/or Technician director → Assistant administrator → Administrator

9 The organization and operation of departments of respiratory care vary according to the needs and resources of a particular hospital. Recognizing this situation, the *Joint Commission for Accreditation of Hospitals* (JCAH) includes respiratory care services as a part of its hospital accreditation process. Respiratory care personnel at all levels should be familiar with these standards because they establish *minimum* criteria for the operation of a respiratory service in an accredited hospital.

10 The federal government's involvement in reimbursement for services rendered to Medicare patients has resulted in the development and implementation of a *prospective reimbursement system*. This system varies from the former method of *retrospective* payment for services by reimbursing all hospitals according to 475 diagnosis related groups (DRG) of diseases. Simply stated, a Medicare admission is assigned a DRG number that most closely relates to the patient's complaint and admission diagnosis. For example, DRG 89 identifies pneumonia with complications or comorbidity in patients over age 69. This particular DRG accounts for approximately 8.5 hospital days and 3.3% of all Medicare discharges. The respiratory care department is almost always heavily involved in the treatment of these patients. Also, DRGs 474 and 475 identify patients who require mechanical ventilation with a primary respiratory diagnosis. The DRG that is associated with a tracheostomy is more heavily weighted than the one associated with an endotracheal tube.

On the patient's discharge Medicare reimburses the

hospital a *preestablished fee* for treatment of the assigned DRG. If the hospital was able to treat the patient for less than the preestablished fee, it is allowed to retain the difference as an *incentive* (profit). If, on the other hand, the hospital bill was greater than the preestablished fee for the patient's DRG, the hospital would have to absorb any differences as a loss.

In 1988 the federal government passed the health bill that increased payment for prolonged illness. It also provided for demonstration projects for patients requiring chronic ventilator care to be designated in 1989.

The primary objective of this type of reimbursement system is to encourage the hospital to provide more economical care and to enable the federal government to purchase services for Medicare patients at preestablished and uniform rates regardless of where or when the patient may be treated. It was feared that this type of incentive-based health care delivery would restrict the role of respiratory care personnel and probably will result in the emergence of multicompetent professionals who are generalists in providing technical expertise.

Since 1983, this has not been the case. Data collected in 1985 and 1986 by the AARC Task Force on Professional Direction from a survey of acute care hospitals indicate that the number of respiratory-related hospital admissions has in fact increased by 4.5%. More recent data by this Task Force indicate that there is a nationwide shortage of qualified respiratory care personnel, with over 3,000 open job positions.

11 The issuing of credentials is another question that may influence the future scope of practice provided by respiratory care personnel.

In 1985 there were less than six states requiring mandatory licensure for respiratory care personnel. By 1988 more than 20 states required respiratory care personnel to obtain a state credential in order to work.

These licensure bills are primarily directed at ensuring at least minimum levels of competent practice for respiratory care personnel.

A positive feature of most of these bills is that they offer reciprocity for persons having credentials from the National Board For Respiratory Care.

5.2 Specific role of the medical director (advisor)

The role of the medical director of respiratory care will vary from hospital to hospital and from educational program to program. Although the physician's medical specialty will also vary, those specializing in pulmonary medicine, anesthesia, and internal medicine are most frequently employed in the role of medical director.

The Joint Commission for Accreditation of Hospitals' standards for respiratory care services describes the roles of the medical director (advisor) and technical director for a *respiratory care service* in the hospital. The Joint Review Committee For Respiratory Therapy Education (JR-CRTE), in the guidelines to the *Essentials For Accreditation of a Respiratory Therapy Program,* describes the role of the medical director in a school program.

The medical director in a respiratory care (therapy) program shall:
1 In cooperation and collaboration with the program director and director of clinical education, participate in program planning and evaluation of instruction.
2 Actively participate in the didactic and clinical instruction of students.
3 Participate in the instruction and evaluation of the program faculty.

The need for active participation of physicians in a respiratory care (therapy) program has been thoroughly established. For this reason the medical director, by accepting the position, makes a personal commitment to participate actively in the academic and clinical phases of the program. This means that the director must personally teach respiratory care (therapy) students. Assignment of students to sit in on meetings or participate in regular working rounds is recommended but is not by itself considered to be adequate instructional participation by the medical advisor. It is difficult to specify the precise amount of participation that is considered sufficient. However, we and the JRCRTE strongly recommend that, in addition to such activities as scheduled rounds, the medical director meet with students for at least 1 hour each week during the entire course of instruction. This hour may consist of a formal lecture, a bedside discussion, a seminar, a literature review, or any other similar educational activity designed specifically for respiratory therapy students, and it should be a regular part of each week's schedule. In addition, the medical advisor with the school facility should take responsibility for answering questions students may raise as a result of attending conferences and meetings.

Further details concerning the role of the medical director in the hospital setting may be obtained from the National Association of Medical Directors For Respiratory Care (NAMDRC). The primary purpose of this association is to provide its members with educational and political information relative to the practice of pulmonary medicine.

6.0 COMMON MEDICAL/LEGAL TERMS
6.1 Glossary

The ever-expanding role of respiratory care personnel in influencing and providing patient care carries with it increasing moral, professional, and legal liabilities.

No longer can respiratory care personnel claim innocence by hiding behind the license of the physician or hospital authority.

The following terms and definitions address some of the language and medical/legal areas most relevant to respiratory care personnel.

It is incumbent on each respiratory therapist or technician to be informed of federal, state, and hospital legislation and rules governing the practice of respiratory care in a specific state or local geographic area.
1 Abandonment. Termination of a patient's treatment with or without notice while the patient still requires care and previous arrangements have not been agreed on.

2 Accident. An unforeseen event, occurring without the will or design of the person whose act causes it; an unexpected, unusual, or undesigned occurrence.

3 Act of God. A natural happening that occurs without human action.

4 Action. A legal proceeding by one party against another for the protection of a right or the redress of a wrong.

5 Agent. One who represents and acts for another under the contract or relation of agency.

6 Agreement. A verbal or written contract, based on a mutual understanding, binding two parties.

7 Allege. To state positively but without proof; to make an allegation.

8 Appeal. A request for a superior court to review a ruling by a lower court for the purpose of repeal or modification.

9 Appellant. The party who takes an appeal from one court to another.

10 Appellee. The party against whom appeal is taken.

11 Assault and battery. The threat of force to the injury of another person is assault; the use of it is battery, which always includes an assault. Thus the two terms are commonly combined in the term "battery," regardless of its results, and is excusable only when there is express or implied consent by the patient. Merely touching a person or the individual's clothes or anything else attached to the person can be construed as battery.

12 Assistant. A helper; one whose duties include rendering aid to a superior authority to carry out an assigned role.

13 Attractive nuisance. A property owner is liable when all the following circumstances apply.

a A child is injured by an object the child did not recognize as being dangerous.

b The owner of the object knew that it was dangerous and that it was attractive to children.

c The owner of the object knowingly left it exposed in a place liable to be frequented by children.

14 Borrowed servant. An employee who is under the complete control and supervision of an individual other than the employer. Under the doctrine of the "borrowed servant," the person in charge of the employee, e.g., a supervisor, is held accountable for the actions of the employee even though no "master-servant" relationship exists.

15 Breach of contract. Failure without legal excuse to carry out the terms of a legal agreement.

16 Breach of duty. Failure to complete an assignment that is legal and agreed on.

17 "Captain of the ship." This doctrine states that, under certain conditions, the person in charge of a group of persons is responsible for their actions even though no "master-servant" relationship exists (see Borrowed servant).

18 Care, standard of. The expected level of care that would be rendered, under similar circumstances, by any prudent physician or other practitioner.

19 Case law. The aggregate of reported cases as forming a body of jurisprudence, or the law of a particular subject as evidenced or formed by the adjudged cases, in distinction to statutes and other sources of law.

20 Citation. Any legal reference; includes the law book in which the reference is found, the volume number, and the section or page number. Judicial citations refer to court decisions and statutory citations to statutes.

21 Common law. That body of unwritten law, founded on general customs, usage, or common consent and in natural justice or reason; accepted by custom or sanctified by moral usage and judicial decision.

22 Communication, confidential. A class of communication passing between persons who stand in a confidential relationship to each other, which the law will not permit to be divulged or inquired into in a court of justice for the sake of public policy and the good order of society. Examples of such privileged relations would be those between husband and wife, attorney and client, and physician and patient (see Confidential relation).

23 Concealment. To knowingly withhold or hide something that may be relevant to a legal action.

24 Confidential relation. A relation based on or having trust, such as that which exists between patient and physician, attorney and client, parent and child. It covers all forms of relations between parties wherein confidence is held by one in another such that one relies and acts on representation of another.

25 Consent. A concurrence of wills or an act of reason accompanied with deliberation; that is, a voluntary agreement by a person in the possession and exercise of sufficient mentality to make an intelligent choice to do something proposed by another.

26 Consent, implied. Consent by signs, actions, or facts or by inaction or silence that raises a presumption that the consent has been given. For example, it is implicit that when a hospital provides services in another state, it is subject to that state's laws even though it is not incorporated in that state.

27 Contract. A written or verbal agreement establishing promises between two parties to perform or offer up item for exchange.

28 Contractor. One who enters into a legal agreement to perform a service.

29 Contributory negligence. Negligence, when set up as a defense, shows that the plaintiff was guilty of negligence contributing to his or her injury.

30 Credential. A license or other documentation of competence; usually awarded by completion of a set of criteria.

31 Damages. The financial or monetary compensation awarded in court to the person who has suffered injury through the unlawful act, omission, or negligence of another.

32 Defendant. The party against whom relief or recovery is sought in a court action.

33 Diligence, ordinary. Prudent action by persons conforming to the standards of a society.

34 Discretionary powers. Powers or rights to act according to the dictates or conscience of judgment.

35 Due process. The right to be heard and to have an action judged by law.

36 Duty. A legal obligation to perform a service or to act in a particular way.

37 Employee/servant. An individual who works for an employer; one who works for salary or wages.

38 Employer. An individual who employs the services of others; one for whom employees work and who pays their wages and salaries.

39 Error. A mistake based on comparison with facts or expected behavior.

40 Ethical. Actions that conform to a code.

41 Ethics, professional. A general agreement of expert opinions as to necessity of professional standards, such as the AARC Code of Ethics.

42 Evidence. Any documents, tapes, or other proof of innocence or guilt admissible in a legal environment.

43 Factual cause. The obvious, evident, or plainly understood cause of an accident.

44 Foreseeability. The ability to anticipate hazardous situations or potential accident causes; the first test in determining whether or not there was negligence.

45 Governmental immunity. Immunity from tort actions enjoyed by governmental subdivisions in common-law states.

46 In loco parentis. In place of the parent and being charged with some of the parents' rights and responsibilities.

47 Indemnify. To reimburse, to secure against loss or damage; to protect or insure against financial loss.

48 Injury. Any wrong or damage done to another, either in person, rights, reputation, or property.

49 Insurance. A contract by a party to compensate the insured or someone bringing action against the insured after determination of guilt.

50 Interrogatories. Written material developed for the purpose of seeking answers to questions in a legal matter. Persons responding must swear to the accuracy of their response.

51 Intervening cause. The negligent acts of a third party, which serve to break the chain of causation between the accident and the alleged negligence of the defendant.

52 Invitee. One who is at a place on the invitation of another.

53 Judgment. Decision of the court, usually involving the payment of damages.

54 Jurisprudence. A system of laws of a country.

55 Law. That which is laid down, ordained, or established; that which must be obeyed and followed by citizens, or they will be subject to sanctions or legal consequences.

56 Liability. Legal responsibility; the state of one who is bound in law and in justice to do something that may be enforced by action.

57 Liable. Bound or obliged in law or in equity; responsible; chargeable; answerable; compelled to make satisfaction, compensation, or restitution.

58 License. A legal document giving permission by some authority to do some act that without such permission would be illegal.

59 Licensee. A person who is neither a passenger, servant, or trespasser and who does not stand in any contractual relation with the owner of the premises and who is permitted to go thereon for his or her own interest, convenience, or gratification.

60 Limitations, statute of. A specified time period within which legal action must occur if the accused is to be prosecuted.

61 Litigant. One engaged in a lawsuit.

62 Litigation. The act or process of carrying on a lawsuit.

63 Malpractice, medical. Any professional misconduct or unreasonable lack of skill or fidelity in professional duties; negligence. The predominant theory is that of liability. To recover damages for negligent malpractice the injured party must show the dutiful relationship between the professional and patient, that a standard has been violated, that injury has occurred, and that the injury was caused by the violated standard.

64 Maltreatment. In reference to the treatment of a patient by a physician or other professional: any improper or unskillful treatment resulting from ignorance, neglect, or willfulness; not necessarily implying that the conduct of the professional in treatment of the patient is either willfully or grossly careless.

65 Master. A principal who employs another to perform a service in his or her affairs and who controls, or has a right to control, the physical conduct of others in performance of that service.

66 Master and servant. A relationship between individuals in which one individual, for pay or other valuable consideration, enters into the service of another and devotes personal labor for an agreed period. The employer has the right to prescribe, end, and direct the means and methods of doing work.

67 Mental anguish. When connected with a physical injury, it refers to both the resultant mental sensation of pain and the accompanying feelings of distress, fright, and anxiety. In other connections and as a ground for damages or an element of damages, it includes the mental suffering resulting from the excitation of the more poignant and painful emotions such as grief, severe disappointment, indignation, wounded pride, shame, public humiliation, and despair.

68 Ministerial. A definite duty arising under circumstances admitted, required, or imposed by law.

69 Misrepresentation. Any manifestation by words or other conduct by one person to another that, under the circumstances, amounts to an assertion not in accordance with the facts; to represent falsely.

70 Negligence. The omission of doing something that a

reasonable person, guided by those normal considerations which ordinarily regulate human affairs, would do; or the doing of something that a reasonable or prudent person would not do.

71 Negligence, culpable. Failure to perform according to a standard that a person of ordinary prudence in the same situation would not have omitted.

72 Negligence, gross. Intentional failure to perform according to a standard and in disregard to the result of such actions on another.

73 Non compos mentis. Not of sound mind; a general term indicating insanity.

74 Nonfeasance. The neglect or failure to do some act a person ought to do. The term is usually used in reference to a failure to perform a duty toward the public whereby some individual sustains a special damage.

75 Nuisance. That class of wrongs that arise from:
  a The unreasonable, unwarranted, or unlawful use by a person of his or her own property, either real or personal, or
  b An individual's own improper, indecent, or unlawful personal conduct that causes
    • An obstruction or an injury to the right of another or the public.
    • The production of material annoyance, inconvenience, discomfort, or hurt to another or the public.

76 Opinion. The statement of reasons delivered by a judge or court giving the judgment pronounced on a case.

77 Paramedical (also allied health). *Para:* "beside the physician," a term describing persons other than physicians who work with patients.

78 Personal injury. Pain or damage caused to a person or possessions by another.

79 Plaintiff. The person who brings an action; one who sues by filing a complaint.

80 Plea. In law the answer a defendant gives to the plaintiff's charge.

81 Precedent. A judicial decision, a form of proceeding, or a course of action that serves as a rule for future determinations in similar or analogous cases; an authority to be followed in courts of justice.

82 Profession. A vocation, calling, occupation, or employment that involves labor, skill, advanced education, and special knowledge and training. Skills involved are predominantly intellectual rather than physical and manual.

83 Proximate cause. That which, in the natural and continual sequence unbroken by any efficient intervening cause, produces the injury and without which the result would not have occurred.

84 Quasimunicipal corporations. Bodies, political and corporate, created for the sole purpose of performing one or more municipal functions. Public corporations organized for governmental purposes and having for most purposes the status and powers of municipal corporations, but not municipal corporations proper, such as cities and incorporated towns.

85 Record. Written documentation of actions or events that remain as legal evidence of said occurrences.

86 Redress. To make amends as for a loss; to relieve of anything unjust, to make reparation of a wrong.

87 Res ipsa loquitur. The act or thing is self-evident. The occurrence of an injury allows an inference of negligence, provided the nature of the accident and attending circumstances lead reasonably to the belief that in the absence of negligence, the accident would not have occurred and, further, that the situation which caused injury was under the management and control of the alleged wrongdoer.

88 Respondeat superior. Let the master answer. This Latin expression means that the employer is liable in certain cases for the wrongful acts of servants. Under this doctrine the employer is responsible for a servant's carelessness toward those to whom the employer has a duty to render care, provided that failure to give such care occurred in the course of the servant's employment.

89 Risk. The danger or hazard implicit in a procedure or situation or to exposure to the chance of injury or loss.

90 Risk, assumption of. A person who knowingly exposes himself or herself to danger may not recover damages for an injury unless negligence by the defendant is proved.

91 Rule. A written or verbal standard established by authority.

92 Safe-place. Legislative enactments requiring owners to build and maintain buildings, grounds, and equipment safely and holding them responsible if they do not.

93 Save-harmless. Requiring that a body exempts or reserves from harm; specifically, it may require that a school district defend and pay judgments against employees who had been held personally liable for torts committed in connection with their employment.

94 Skill. Knowledge and abilities to perform a specific act according to accepted levels of practice.

95 Stare decisis. To stand by decided cases; to uphold precedents; to maintain former adjudications. Doctrine of stare decisis rests on the principle that the law by which people are governed should be fixed, definite, and known; that when the law is declared by a court of competent jurisdiction authorized to construe it, such declaration, in the absence of palpable mistake or error, is itself evidence of the law until changed by competent authority.

96 Statute. An act of the legislature declaring, demanding, or prohibiting something; particular law enacted and established by the will of the legislative department of government.

97 Statutory law. Those statutes enacted by the legislature of any sovereign state.

98 Subpoena. A legal process for causing an individual to appear and give witness.

99 Subrogation. The substitution of another person in the place of one to whose rights he or she succeeds.

100 Testimony. Evidence given under oath.

101 Tort. Legal wrong committed against the person or property of another, independent of contract.

102 Tort-feasor. A wrongdoer; one who commits or is guilty of a tort.

103 Trespass. Damage done to another person or property by willful and violent action of the defendant.

104 Ultra vires. Acts beyond the scope of authority.

105 Witness. One who sees or otherwise can present evidence that a wrongful act has been committed.

106 Wrongful act. Any action that under ordinary circumstances would infringe on or cause harm to another.

6.2 The legal aspects of respiratory care

The purpose of this unit is to provide the reader with guidelines for a general understanding of the legal aspects of medical and respiratory care practice with particular emphasis on the second. The following presentation provides an outline; for a more comprehensive review, refer to materials available in most public libraries.

1 Law. The term "law" has two applications: abstract and concrete.

  a Abstract denotes a nonspecific use of the term, for example, to "have law and order" or to "live by the law."

  b Concrete deals with a specific law such as "the law of libel," or "the by-laws of the Association."

    • The practitioner is more concerned with the concrete aspects of the law.

2 Law is divided into two distinct types: *criminal law* and *civil law*.

  a Criminal law

    • These laws regulate behavior throughout the land and serve to protect an individual from harm and danger to life and property. A breach of any of these laws is properly called a "criminal offense" and is punishable by imprisonment, fine, or both.

    • Under criminal law, the accuser is the State, and the person prosecuted is the defendant. The United States follows the principles embodied in the British system of law, that is, the defendant is never guilty of the crime until evidence of guilt has been established by the State. Further, the defendant is not required to give evidence that may be self-incriminating. It is the task of the State to search for and produce evidence of guilt.

    • An example of a criminal act that could involve respiratory care personnel under this section is aiding, abetting, or performing a criminal abortion. Another would be involvement in a narcotics offense.

  b Civil law

    • Laws in this category protect the rights and freedom of a citizen. They also prevent one individual from taking unfair and unlawful advantage of another. Whenever the rights and freedom of a citizen

have been interfered with, that citizen may apply for a court hearing of the complaints. The citizen then becomes the plaintiff and the person proceeded against is the defendant. Under civil law the court decides on the restitution to be made or paid by the person who has committed the wrong. Examples of plaintiffs may be:

– A person who has been slandered.

– A person who has been falsely imprisoned.

– A person who has been injured through a negligent act.

  • Civil law is broken down more specifically into branches that are called "torts." One definition of a tort is a branch of civil law under which the plaintiff may proceed against the person(s) who have wronged him or her.

    – Whenever hospitals are proceeded against, by a patient or relatives, such action takes place under civil law and under the specific tort pertaining to the case.

6.3 Common torts affecting hospitals

1 Negligence. This is one of the most common torts under which hospitals are proceeded against. They may be any one or all of the following:

  a Failing to take the correct action.

  b Failing to take any action.

  c Doing the wrong thing altogether.

  d Doing the correct thing at the wrong time.

■ ■ ■

When a person's job or daily work carries with it no responsibility to exercise care and skill, negligence has no legal consequence for that person. An example of this is the laundry worker in the hospital's linen department who uses strong caustic soap. In this instance, the employer (hospital) assumes liability for the wrongs committed by the employee. When there is a duty and responsibility to exercise care and skill, the amount of care to be taken during the performance of a job will depend on the amount of risk to the patient or the amount of damages to the patient's well-being and safety as a result of poor performance of such a job.

All hospital personnel whose work is recognized to be of a *professional nature* have a legal responsibility to exercise care and skill in the performance of their tasks. Nurses and respiratory care personnel fall into this category. For example, if the equipment being used on a patient is not in good repair and some of it breaks and hits the patient, causing fractures or bruises, the practitioner is liable, under the tort of negligence, for that responsibility. Similarly, if an elderly patient being treated by a practitioner falls from the bed because of a lack of adequate supervision, the practitioner and hospital are liable under the tort of negligence.

2 Assault and battery

  a Definition: A "battery" is an act that either intentionally or negligently causes some direct physical contact with a person without having that person's consent or without any lawful justification. Assault is a threat, which is capable of being carried out, to commit battery on another person.

■ ■ ■

In a hospital setting or a clinic, the successful treatment of any patient largely depends on the interference with his or her person by hospital staff members, such as doctors, nurses, and technicians. *Most* of these interferences would constitute batteries were it not that the law presumes *implied consent* on a part of the patient who solicits treatment at the hospital door. Thus for ordinary procedures (blood tests, physical examinations, routine and special respiratory care) the consent of the patient is not sought in writing. The physician usually explains the reason for these tests and therapy and will arrange their sequence. But the law does not presume implied consent on the part of the patient for any unusual, difficult or dangerous, or very painful procedures such as anesthesia, electric shock, or surgery. For all these the patient's written consent must first be obtained. In the case of a mentally incompetent adult, an unconscious adult, a minor, or a child, the permission for such procedures must be obtained from the patient's next of kin or parents.

Usually, a respiratory care practitioner is not liable under this tort except in the instance when a patient complains of having been subjected to undue palpation during the procedure. It is because of this remote possibility that clinicians should *always explain beforehand* their need to touch the patient's body. This is particularly important when (a) examining the lower abdomen or pelvic region and the breasts of a female and (b) when the patient is of a different sex from the practitioner.

3 False imprisonment. This tort refers not only to wrongful confinement but also includes the wrongful conduct of one person that limits the freedom of another. In a hospital the use of restraining devices and bandages, if objected to by the patient and not removed, could result in an action of false imprisonment. For this reason the patient is always asked, on announcing a desire to leave the hospital and forego subsequent treatment, to sign a special form which states that the patient is leaving the hospital against the advice of the physician. Should anything happen to that patient outside the hospital as a result of release, the patient will not have any recourse to any tort against the physician or the hospital.

4 Libel and slander. These are forms of defamation: libel is expressed in writing; slander is expressed orally.

■ ■ ■

In a hospital, unwarranted discussion between a hospital employee and a nonmedical person about the condition, diagnosis, or treatment of a patient is *always* deemed libelous and slanderous. Consequently, department heads should advise practitioners *never* to make statements about any patient's condition or therapy treatment to lay persons

such as the involved patient, relatives, police, or press. This principle is particularly important if the patient is a celebrity, public figure, or other prominent member of the community. But regardless of the patient's status or fame, disclosure of the information that could cause personal or social embarrassment or even loss of employment is reason for action under the tort of libel and slander.

Thus all discussions among members of the medical staff concerning patients should be limited to the sole purpose of either giving or receiving advice, instructions, or imparting knowledge.

5 Invasion of privacy. A hospital patient has the legal right to expect that all information relating to his or her disease or condition or treatment will be kept private.

■ ■ ■

A complex interrelationship exists between invasion of privacy and the libel and slander torts so that, in some instances, both torts are applicable and may result in an action of both. For example, the patient who solicits treatment of a disorder that is socially embarrassing (alcoholism, drug addiction, or venereal disease) and finds that his or her records are being used for display or presentation without consent may bring an action both against the hospital and the person involved.

A practitioner who publishes articles and uses such materials as a patient's chart or treatment procedures for information or who speaks at seminars or gives lectures should (a) first obtain permission from the department head and (b) cover all pertinent information on the records that could reveal the patient's name and address or otherwise identify the individual. A practitioner who is writing a book, article, or thesis and wishes to use sensitive information should avoid reference to the patient's name, address, or other personal identification.

6.4 Medicolegal considerations in the terminal patient

1 Respiratory care personnel, by the very nature of their job descriptions, must work with patients who are terminally ill. Many of these patients may or may not receive "extraordinary" life support.

The decision of if and when to begin and when to terminate life support relates to a broad range of ethical and legal considerations by everyone who may work with these patients providing life support.

Respiratory care personnel sooner or later will experience situations where they question the physician's decision to initiate and to withdraw life support. This is an unavoidable occurrence in a patient care setting, where it is assumed that everyone is concerned about the patient's best interest, yet the practitioners' education and levels of experience are so varied.

The purpose of this unit is to inform respiratory care personnel about some of the issues and the actions that were taken to resolve the legal, moral, ethical, and financial problems encountered whenever extraordinary life support measures have been taken.

2 Historical Case—the decision to withdraw life sup-

port. In 1976 the most widely publicized case in which a decision was made to withdraw life support was that of Karen Quinlan. This patient was admitted to the hospital in coma as a result of a drug overdose complicated by alcohol ingestion.

The patient was placed on a ventilator on April 15, 1975, and life support was continued. The patient's physicians refused to remove the ventilator because they felt the patient would die and they would be held accountable for manslaughter even though all hope for recovery was gone.

The parents sued for relief and in April 1976, the New Jersey Supreme Court ruled that the ventilator *could be* removed.

The patient lived for an additional 10 years, but the court's ruling established precedent for courts to become involved in deciding the legal grounds for beginning and terminating life support.

3 Historical case—a no code order. The Shirley Dinnerstein case, in 1978, was a landmark decision by the Massachusetts Appeals Court that supported the physician's right to enter a no code order for irreversible, incompetent, terminally ill patients.

This precedent mandates that respiratory care personnel will have to carry out an order by a physician not to resuscitate a dying patient. This type of order sometimes has a deep emotional effect on the practitioner who has not personally addressed this issue. The order not to resuscitate (DNR) is a medical order that should be written in the chart by the physician and followed as any other order. Verbal or unwritten DNR orders are both legally and ethically questionable and should not be followed.

4 Baby Doe status. The question of providing or withholding mechanical life support to an infant Baby Doe (a nonviable infant) who has little or no chance of living a quality life has resulted in the federal government's becoming involved. The proposed regulation published through the Department of Health and Human Services states that recipients of government funds to operate a care facility or unit cannot withhold treatment to an infant based on the quality of life criteria. These patients were considered to be handicapped and thus protected under civil rights statutes.

5 Living will. In the past decade the whole question of who decides life support issues has caused patients to take more initiative in deciding the limits of their own medical treatment through legal documents called living wills. A *living will* or advanced directive is a legal document drawn up by a competent person stating what medical measures are to be taken in the event of a terminal illness, coma, or incompetence. This will usually prohibits "extraordinary" life support measures and in many states instructs about donation of organs or a desire for the patient to die at home.

As of 1989, 38 states have recognized some forms of the living will. States have attempted to respond to imperfections in the living will by adopting natural death acts or right to die laws. The purpose of these actions is to protect physicians who honor advanced directives against law suits.

6 Durable power of attorney. A durable power of attorney is still another approach for patients to ensure that their wishes are achieved. This is a legal form that allows an agent to act on an individual's behalf whenever the individual is unable, for whatever reason, to make decisions on his or her own. This agent must be someone in whom the person has complete trust.

With a durable power of attorney the agent can act on a person's behalf in making medical, financial, and other decisions that normally would have been made by the patient. A patient may specify activation of a durable power of attorney document based on his or her own mental or physical competence, or power of attorney may be invoked by a designated relative or trusted friend when that party deems it appropriate to act in the person's behalf.

7 Definition of death legislation. One of the complications associated with the advanced life support technology available today is the question of when death occurs. The absence of a heartbeat or breathing is no longer a valid definition, since both can be artificially sustained.

In an attempt to define death more practically, many states describe death as having occurred "whenever a licensed physician in the state declares that the brain has ceased to function based on ordinary standards of approved medical practice."

Standards defining brain death were established in 1968 by a Harvard Ad Hoc Committee. These Harvard criteria are accepted in many states as the basis for defining death. The concern about decisions of when to initiate and withdraw life support in 1983 resulted in the formation of a President's commission, whose report, entitled "Deciding to Forego Life Sustaining Treatment," recommended that all states accept the Uniform Determination of Death Act, which was developed by the American Medical Association, American Bar Association, and the National Conference of Commissioners on Uniform State Laws. The criteria were similar to those established by the Harvard Ad Hoc Committee.

8 Medical Liability. One need only read or view the daily news to be aware that the frequency and costs of medical liability claims are on the rise. This type of risk is not limited to the physician and hospital but includes all allied health personnel.

In 1971 President Nixon created a Commission on Medical Malpractice. In 1980 the National Association of Insurance Commissions completed a study of 72,000 medical liability claims for cases resolved between July 1975 and December 1978. This study showed that many of the occurrences were preventable. Hospitals have taken steps to minimize situations that can lead to patient injury and possible litigation by establishing departments or offices of risk management.

a Risk management. Medical risk management is a concept that emerged from attempts by industry in the 1960s to lower exposure to possible litigation from product failure or consumer injury related to use of a product. This approach emphasized quality assurance as a preventive measure.

In the medical environment the concept of risk management has been expanded to include quality assurance, as well as oversight review by peer groups. The primary purpose of a peer review or professional review organization is to monitor the progress of the medical facility or practitioners in maintaining quality decisions to begin and provide good medical care according to local and national standards.

9 Euthanasia. Respiratory care personnel, especially those who work with terminally ill patients, are confronted with moral, professional, and ethical issues that may conflict with an individual's feeling of compassion toward human suffering. A patient may plead with the practitioner to terminate his or her life and end the patient's suffering.

The act of taking a patient's life for this purpose is called euthanasia. Euthanasia may be *passive* or *active*. A passive act may involve withholding medications from a patient or respecting a no code order. Active euthanasia usually includes giving a drug to cause death or withdrawing life support without proper authorization. Both types of euthanasia represent legal and moral issues that must still be resolved by society and the courts.

7.0 MEDICAL ETHICS
7.1 General patient care and respiratory care situations

A fundamental purpose of the respiratory care profession is to conserve the life, health, and continued function of the patient. In this role respiratory care personnel receive orders from physicians and are responsible for carrying them out according to standards. Inherent in this responsibility is the moral, professional, and legal responsibility of the respiratory care practitioner not to carry out the order if it is recognized that such action may result in harm to the patient or others.

1 Even though it is important to note that the prescribing physician is legally responsible for the care of his or her patients, it is equally important to note that allied health practitioners, by virtue of their education and professional status, are also legally accountable for any patient mistreatment or malpractice.

An allied health practitioner who refuses to carry out an order must have good reason and should state and document this reason to the physician and in the patient's medical record. If the order is not implemented, the allied health practitioner is potentially guilty of malpractice or negligence, and a court action could ensue with the practitioner as the defendant. Outcome of the case may result in expulsion or suspension, prohibiting the practioner from practicing for an indefinite period of time.

2 Respiratory care personnel probably should *not* work in any institution that does not employ a qualified medical practitioner or specialist. The technician holds in strict confidence any information of a private or personal nature received from either the physician or the patient.

8.0 AARC CODE OF ETHICS*
8.1 Policy statement

As health care professionals engaged in the performance of respiratory care, respiratory therapy practitioners must strive, both individually and collectively, to maintain the highest ethical standards.

The principles set forth in this document define the basic ethical and moral standards to which each member of the American Association for Respiratory Care should conform.

1 The respiratory care practitioner shall practice medically acceptable methods of treatment and shall not endeavor to extend his practice beyond his competence and the authority vested in him by the physician.

2 The respiratory care practitioner shall continually strive to increase and improve his knowledge and skill and render to each patient the full measure of his ability. All services shall be provided with respect for the dignity of the patient, unrestricted by considerations of social or economic status, personal attributes, or the nature of health problems.

3 The respiratory care practitioner shall be responsible for the competent and efficient performance of his assigned duties and shall expose incompetence and illegal or unethical conduct of members of the profession.

4 The respiratory care practitioner shall hold in strict confidence all privileged information concerning the patient and refer all inquiries to the physician in charge of the patient's medical care.

5 The respiratory care practitioner shall not accept gratuities for preferential consideration of the patient. He shall not solicit patients for personal gain and shall guard against conflicts of interest.

6 The respiratory care practitioner shall uphold the dignity and honor of the profession and abide by its ethical principles. He should be familiar with existing state and federal laws governing the practice of respiratory therapy and comply with those laws.

7 The respiratory care practitioner shall cooperate with other health care professionals and participate in activities to promote community and national efforts to meet the health needs of the public.

9.0 AARC MEMBERSHIP
9.1 Membership categories

1 The American Association for Respiratory Care has over 28,000 members who practice or are interested in the practice of respiratory care.

2 The purpose of the Association is described in Article II, Sections 1 through 6—Purpose of the AARC Bylaws, 1979:

---

*AARC Bylaws, article II, sections 1-6, April 15, 1986. Distributed by the American Association for Respiratory Care and reprinted by permission.

a To encourage, develop, and provide educational programs for those persons interested in the field of respiratory therapy.

b To advance the science, technology, ethics, and art of respiratory therapy through institutes, meetings, lectures, publications, and other materials.

c To facilitate cooperation between respiratory therapy personnel and the medical profession, hospitals, service companies, industry, governmental organizations, and other agencies interested in respiratory therapy.

3 The criteria for membership in AARC are stipulated in Article III—Membership of the AARC Bylaws, 1986:

Section 1: classes

The membership of the Association shall include three classes: Active Member, Associate Member, and Special Member.

Section 2: prerequisites

Each applicant for membership shall meet qualifications of ethical practice and suitable moral standards as determined by the membership services committee. Active Members shall be a high school graduate or have evidence of equivalent education.

Section 3: active member

An individual is eligible to be an Active Member if he has had twelve (12) months of consecutive experience or schooling in respiratory therapy and his primary function, within a recognized institution or organization, is directly related to the patient receiving respiratory therapy under medical direction or the education and training of respiratory therapy students. He shall not be an active physician.

Section 4: associate member

An individual is eligible to be an Associate member if he holds a position related to respiratory therapy and does not have the requirements to become an Active Member. Associate Members shall have all of the rights and privileges of the Association except that they shall not be entitled to hold office or vote.

1 Foreign Member. An individual is eligible for Associate membership if he is a resident of any foreign country.

2 Student Member. An individual is eligible for Associate membership as a student while he is enrolled in a formal training program in respiratory therapy not to exceed a maximum period of three (3) months immediately thereafter. Members in student status shall be entitled to wear official Association student shoulder patches or insignia only.

Section 5: special member

1 Life Member. Life Members shall be members who have rendered outstanding service to the Association. Life membership may be conferred by a majority vote of the board of directors, upon recommendation by the house of delegates. They shall pay no dues and shall have all the rights and privileges of an Active Member.

2 Honorary Member. Honorary membership may be conferred upon persons who have rendered distinguished service in the field of respiratory therapy, upon recommendation by the house of delegates, and confirmation by a majority vote of the board of directors. Honorary Members shall have all the rights and privileges of the Association except that they shall not be entitled to hold office, committee chairmanships, or vote; and

they shall be exempt from the payment of dues.

3 Inactive Member. A member is eligible for Inactive membership provided he is an Active or Associate Member in good standing when he applies for Inactive status. Inactive Members shall have all the rights and privileges of the Association except that they shall not be entitled to hold office, committee chairmanship or vote.

Section 6: application for membership

1 An applicant for membership shall submit his completed official application to the national office of the Association.

2 The names and addresses of applicants accepted by the membership services committee shall be submitted by the executive director for publication in the ensuing Association Bulletin.

3 Any member or members may object to approval of an applicant for membership by filing written objection with the chairman of the membership services committee through the national office within thirty (30) days after publication of the applicant's name. If an objection is received, the executive director shall promptly notify the membership services committee. They shall reevaluate the application and make the final decision regarding admission.

9.2 Benefits of belonging to the AARC

The most obvious benefit of belonging to any professional association is becoming a part of a large group of people who share common interests and goals for a profession. This allows the members to participate in determining the destiny of their chosen profession. Other benefits of being a member of the AARC include:

1 Twelve issues of *Respiratory Care,* one of the first journals to publish articles on many innovations in the field of respiratory therapy.

2 Monthly subscriptions to *AARC Times,* a magazine that provides a forum for communications within the Association through articles on more general issues of specific interest to respiratory care personnel, feature stories about people at work in the profession, and regular columns concerning the activities of the Association and its membership.

3 Lifetime participation in the Continuing Respiratory Care Education (CRCE) system, which is the most advanced continuing education credit unit system in the profession.

4 Revenue sharing with the state affiliate. The state affiliate receives a portion of each member's dues from the AARC to keep the state membership charges as low as possible and to offer seminars and special services at the local level.

5 Provision of training institutes to educators and managers.

6 Professional representations to various medical and government groups such as American Medical Association, American College of Chest Physicians, American Society of Anesthesiologists, American Thoracic Society, Department of Health and Human Services, Health Manpower Development, and state legislatures. For example, AARC provides a full-time legislative consultant who follows events in Washington and assists AARC in preparing testimonies before Congress and otherwise informing key legislators about respiratory care.

7 Representation to other allied health professions and organizations such as critical care nurses and cardiopulmonary technicians.

8 Reduced registration fees at state, regional, and national respiratory therapy meetings.

9 Insurance coverage at group rates: group term life, inhospital indemnity, disability income, excess major medical, cancer policy, and professional liability. A dental policy is being investigated.

10 Self-evaluation examinations available by special request or through *Respiratory Care*.

11 Independent study packages available to the membership at a nominal cost.

12 Availability of personnel for planning and salary budgeting.

13 Availability of brochures on a variety of subjects; specifically, position statements on the definition of respiratory therapy, emergency airway management, bronchopulmonary drainage and exercise therapy, medication preparation and administration, pulmonary rehabilitation, blood gas analysis, airway maintenance, physician's assistant and respiratory therapy home care, and research on AARC-related questions.

14 The growth of AARC from a group of 15 people 30 years ago to over 28,000 voices representing the profession.

BIBLIOGRAPHY

AMA Special Task Force on Professional Liability Insurance: Professional Liability in the 80's, Chicago, Reports 1-3, Oct 1984, Nov 1984, March 1985, American Medical Association.

Burton G and Hodgkins J: Respiratory care: a guide to clinical practice, ed 2, Philadelphia, 1984, JB Lippincott Co.

Cataldo BF, Kempin FG, Stockton JM, and Weber CM: Introduction to law and the legal process, ed 3, New York, 1980, John Wiley & Sons, pp 17-19.

Deciding to forego life—sustaining treatment: ethical, medical and legal issues in treatment decisions, President's Commision for the Study of Ethical Problems in Medical and Biomedical and Behavioral Research, Washington, DC, 1983, US Government Printing Office.

In the Matter of Karen Quinlan, 70 N.J. 10, 355 A. 2d 647 (1976).

In the Matter of Shirley Dinnerstein, 380 N.E. 2d 134 (Mass App 1978).

Snider GL: Thirty years of mechanical ventilation: changing inplications, Arch Intern Med 143:745, 1983.

Strain E: The American Academy of Pediatrics comments on the Baby Doe II regulations, N Engl J Med 309:443, 1983.

Medical terminology and communication

On completion of this module the reader will be able to:

1.1 through **1.3** Define and pronounce medical terms using prefixes, roots, and suffixes of words.

2.1 Define medical terms used in the practice of respiratory care.

2.2 Apply medical terms to respiratory care.

3.1 Describe the importance of the medical record as it pertains to the patient and hospital and differentiate among the various formats used for organizing the medical record.

3.2 Distinguish between sections of the medical record.

4.1 Explain general rules for charting.

4.2 Give examples of what is recorded in the nurses' notes and/or therapists' notes.

5.1 Describe the need for correct charting technique and confidentiality of patient information.

6.1 Use correct medical terminology and abbreviations in charting procedures.

6.2 Read the chart according to Procedure 3-1.

7.1 and **7.2** Distinguish between verbal and nonverbal communication.

8.1 and **8.2** Use proper telephone procedures.

9.1 Use a medical dictionary to define and pronounce medical terms.

Medical terminology is the professional language of persons working in the health field. The terms are descriptive and are used to communicate specific conditions, treatments, pathologic conditions, and actions relative to medical care. Most medical terms have Greek and Latin origins, although some are derived from German and French. A peculiarity of medical terminology is that the name of the organ may come from Latin, and the name of the disease affecting the organ may come from Greek. Another peculiarity is that many words come from the personal traits of the individuals coining the terms or even the name of a local fruit or clothing.

1.0 MEDICAL TERMINOLOGY

1.1 Defining medical terms

1 Medical terms are words that have been formed from combining word roots, suffixes, and prefixes.

2 The *word root* is a basic stem word that usually comes from Greek or Latin. It is the basis for forming the medical terms that are used in describing medical sciences, respiratory care procedures, and other aspects of medicine and dentistry.

3 The *prefix* of a word consists of one or two syllables placed before a word to modify its meaning. The root of a word is the main body of the word that the prefix, suffix, or both modify. The *suffix* of a word consists of one or two syllables attached to the end of a word to alter its meaning.*

4 The meaning of a term can be determined by:
   a Identifying and defining the prefix
   b Identifying and defining the word root
   c Identifying and defining the suffix

   EXAMPLE:

neo + natal	= neonatal
(prefix) (root)	= combined form
bronchi + ectasis	= bronchiectasis
(root) (suffix)	= combined form

*For additional information on medical terminology, the reader is directed to LaFleur MW and Starr WK: Exploring medical language, ed 2, St Louis, 1989, The CV Mosby Co.

5 Most students find that correct pronunciation of medical terms is one of the most difficult aspects of mastering the study of medical terminology. This ability comes with experience and use of the language.

6 Applying the following general rules may help the beginner to become more proficient in pronouncing new medical terms.

a Break a term into its parts.

b Using a medical dictionary, become familiar with diacritics, the marks over or under vowels to indicate pronunciation and accent marks. For example, in Mosby's Medical, Nursing & Allied Health Dictionary the following marks are used.

Vowels		*Consonants*	
SYMBOLS	KEY WORDS	SYMBOLS	KEY WORDS
/a/	hat	/b/	book
/ä/	father	/ch/	chew
/ā/	fate	/d/	day
/e/	flesh	/f/	fast
/ē/	she	/g/	good
/er/	air, ferry	/h/	happy
/i/	sit	/j/	gem
/ī/	eye	/k/	keep
/ir/	ear	/l/	late
/o/	proper	/m/	make
/ō/	nose	/n/	no
/ô/	saw	/ng/	sing drink
/oi/	boy	/ng·g/	finger
/o͞o/	move	/p/	pair
/o͝o/	book	/r/	ring
/ou/	out	/s/	set
/u/	cup, love	/sh/	shoe, lotion
/ur/	fur, first	/t/	tone
/ə/	(the neutral vowel, always unstressed, as in) ago, focus	/th/	thin
		/th/	than
		/v/	very
/ər/	teacher, doctor	/w/	work
		/y/	yes
		/z/	zeal
		/zh/	azure, vision

c Have someone who is familar with medical terms to assist you in using pronunciation marks and pronouncing each term properly.

7 The use of a flash cards to familiarize the learner with sight recognition, spelling, and definition of terms along with a tape recorder for review of pronunciation of each term is recommended.

1.2 Medical prefixes

1 Memorize the following medical prefixes.

adeno-	pertains to a gland
arterio-	pertains to an artery
brady-	slow
cardio-	pertains to the heart
cephalo-	pertains to the head
cholecyst-	pertains to the gallbladder
colo-	pertains to the large bowel
cranio-	pertains to the cranium
derma-	pertains to the skin
endo-	within
entero-	pertains to the intestine
gastro-	pertains to the stomach
hepato-	pertains to the liver
hydro-	pertains to water
hyper-	above normal, excessive
hypo-	below normal, under
inter-	between
intra-	within

nephro-	pertains to the kidneys
peri-	around
phlebo-	pertains to the veins
pneumo-	pertains to the lungs
post-	after
pre-	before
pulmono-	pertains to the lungs
pyo-	pus (infection)
reno-	pertains to the kidneys
spleno-	pertains to the spleen
sub-	under
tachy-	rapid
thoraco-	pertains to the chest or thorax
vaso-	pertains to the blood vessels

1.3 Medical suffixes

1 Memorize the following medical suffixes.

-algia	pain
-cele	hernia of
-ectomy	excision of
-emia	blood (condition of)
-genesis	pertains to production of or generation of
-graphy	that which describes or writes
-itis	inflammation of
-lysis	reduction or a loosening of
-ology	science of
-oma	tumorous growth
-orrhaphy	surgical repair or sewing of
-oscopy	inspection of, looking into
-osis	pertains to a disease or morbid process
-ostomy	creation of an opening
-otomy	incision into
-pexy	fixation of
-plasty	repair of
-pnea	pertains to respiration
-pnia	pertains to carbon dioxide

2.0 FREQUENTLY USED TERMS
2.1 Medical terms

Memorize the following list of medical terms used frequently in the care of pulmonary patients.

1 Abscess. Localized collection of pus in a cavity formed by tissue degeneration.

2 Absorption. To soak up; as a sponge.

3 Acapnia. Reduced carbon dioxide tension in the blood; results from increased pulmonary ventilation.

4 Acarbia. Reduced level of carbon dioxide in the blood with a proportional reduction in the alkaline bicarbonate.

5 Acid-base balance. The human body cannot survive if the bloodstream becomes either markedly acid or alkaline; it must remain in a very narrow range of balance between acidity and alkalinity. Normal range is a pH of 7.35 to 7.45, neutral is a pH of 7, so the body normally is slightly alkaline. pH means the inverse of the log of the hydrogen ion concentration in the bloodstream.

6 Acidosis. A condition characterized by the presence of excessive quantities of acids in the blood; used mostly to indicate a decrease in the alkaline reserve below normal levels.

7 Acute. Sharp, severe, occurring suddenly.

8 Adhesive force. The clinging of the walls of the bronchioles of a diseased lung that has sticky secretions as a result of the disease. This tendency of the bronchioles to stick together on expiration results in air trapping inside the lung.

9   Adrenalin (epinephrine). Medication used as a vasoconstrictor and cardiac stimulant in acute circulatory failure; also used as a local vasoconstrictor to relieve hemorrhage and local congestion and to relax the bronchi in asthmatic paroxysms.

10   Aerosol. Liquid droplets suspended in a stream of gas.

11   Air trapping. Abnormal condition in which air cannot be expelled from the alveoli during exhalation as a result of collapse of bronchioles or blockage by tenacious mucus.

12   Airway. The path air travels from the atmosphere to and from the alveoli. In anesthesia or resuscitation, a mechanical device used to keep the passages of the upper respiratory tract open for the passage of air.

13   Alcohol. A colorless, flammable liquid made from the fermentation of carbohydrates by yeast, used primarily for disinfection. In respiratory therapy ethyl alcohol is used to break up bubbles in pulmonary edema by lowering the surface tension of the bubbles.

14   Alkalosis. A condition in which the alkaline (hydroxyl ion concentration) content in the blood increases above normal limits. A term used most often to indicate an increase in alkaline reserve above normal levels.

15   Allergy. A hypersensitive state acquired through exposure to a particular allergen.

16   Alveolar. Pertaining to the alveoli.

17   Alveoli. Air sacs located at the end of the respiratory tract that are microscopic in size. The total number of these sacs has been estimated at 300 million (singular: alveolus).

18   Ambient. Pressure equal to the atmosphere around an organism.

19   Amelioration. Improvement.

20   Anaphylaxis. A rapid, exaggerated, allergic reaction.

21   Anemia. A condition in which blood is deficient in volume or quality of red blood cells.

22   Aneurysm. A weakness in the wall of the artery causing a dilation in that area.

23   Angina. A severe constricting pain; usually related to a heart condition (e.g., angina pectoris).

24   Anoxia. A term that literally means without oxygen. This term is used generally to indicate lack of oxygen in the blood and tissues of the body.

25   Antibiotic. Inhibits the growth of microorganisms and fights infection.

26   Antiseptic. An agent that inhibits the growth of microorganisms.

27   Antitussive. Cough stopping.

28   Aortic. Pertaining to the aorta.

29   Apnea. Complete cessation of respiration from any cause.

30   Apneic. Not breathing.

31   Apneusis. Abnormal respiration characterized by a prolonged inspiration.

32   Aqueous. Watery.

33   Arrested. As this pertains to disease, it means that the course of the disease has been stopped—that the disease is staying in its present condition and not getting worse; the disease is not progressing.

34   Dysrythmia (also known as arythmia). Variation from the normal rhythm, especially of the heart.

35   Arterial. Pertaining to the arteries.

36   Articulate. To unite by joints; to join.

37   Aseptic. Sterile; free from septic or poisonous material.

38   Asphyxia. A condition characterized by interference with oxygenation and carbon dioxide elimination; usually associated with the environment.

39   Aspirate. Inhalation of any foreign matter, such as food, saliva, or stomach contents (as after vomiting), into the airway.

40   Asthma. A disease state characterized with difficult respiration and wheezing on expiration. Wheezes are caused as exhaled air flows past narrowed air passages caused by spasms of circular muscles around bronchi and bronchioles; usually complicated by secretions inside the airway that increase the difficulty in breathing and lead to infection.

41   Atelectasis. An airless area of the lung in which the bronchiole is blocked with secretions and the alveoli have had all residual air absorbed from them by the blood.

42   Atmosphere. Air surrounding the earth's surface. Sea level pressure is approximately 14.7 pounds per square inch (psi) or 760 mm Hg.

43   Atria. Any of the various cavities or chambers, especially the upper chambers of the heart; also the area at the end of a bronchiole in the lung (singular: atrium).

44   Atrophy. Wasting away, as from disease; a part that is withered or nonfunctional.

45   Auscultate. To listen (e.g., as to chest sounds with a stethoscope).

46   Autoregulatory. Self-regulating.

47   Bacteriostatic. Inhibits the growth of bacteria without destroying them.

48   Baffle. A wall or other object placed in the path of an aerosol spray to cause rain-out of the larger droplets.

49   Barbiturate. A hypnotic or sedative drug. Overdoses depress respiration severely.

50   Baroreceptor. Pressoreceptor. A receptor or nerve ending sensitive to changes in pressure (e.g., the Hering-Breuer reflex).

51   Bellows. An instrument that, by expanding and contracting, draws air into an accordian-like chamber and then expels it as its sides are compressed. Refers also to bellows action of rib cage and diaphragm.

52   Bernoulli's law. In a stream flowing through a tube, the pressure is least where the velocity of flow is the greatest. In a tube, this point is along the lateral walls of the tube.

53   Bifurcation. A division into two branches; a fork.

54   Bilateral. Having two sides or pertaining to both sides.

55 Blebs. A blister or bubble pertaining to the lungs. In emphysema, a bleb is a large area in which the alveolar walls have been broken down into each other to form an air sac. Blebs are sometimes large enough to contain several milliliters of trapped air or liquid secretions.

56 Bourdon tube. A flexible, question mark-shaped, coiled metal tube that tends to straighten when pressure is applied to the large open end. This is often used in noncompensating flow indicators.

57 Boyle's law. At a constant temperature, the volume of a dry gas varies inversely with the pressure applied.

58 Bradypnea. A decreased respiratory rate.

59 Bronchi. The air passages of the lungs, beginning with the first bifurcation at the carina, through all their branches, to the smallest tubes at the distal portions of the lungs (singular: bronchus).

60 Bronchiectasis. Chronic dilation of the bronchi and bronchioles with secondary infection and destruction of lung tissue. Characterized by secretions with a repugnant odor.

61 Bronchiole. The smallest conducting airway with cartilage construction in the respiratory tract. The bronchioles connect to the atria and alveoli to complete the lung unit.

62 Bronchodilator. Any of a number of drugs that will enlarge the bronchial air passage either by shrinking the mucous membranes or by relaxing the smooth muscles that constrict the air passages.

63 Bronchogenic. Arising in the bronchi or bronchus.

64 Bronchorrhea. An abnormal condition in which the cells in the walls of the bronchial tubes secrete an excessive amount of mucus.

65 Bronchoscopy. To view inside the trachea and main bronchial tubes by means of a tube and light that are passed through the mouth into the trachea and bronchi.

66 Bullae. Large blebs or blisters inside the lung, as in emphysema.

67 Capillary. The fine blood vessels that feed the tissue cells. These vessels are approximately 8 microns (μg) in diameter.

68 Carbon monoxide (CO). A gas caused by incomplete combustion that, when inhaled, forms a semipermanent bond with the hemoglobin. Death from carbon monoxide poisoning is caused by low oxygen tension in the tissues.

69 Carboxyhemoglobin. Combination of carbon monoxide and hemoglobin. When carbon monoxide is inhaled, it replaces the oxygen in oxyhemoglobin to form carboxyhemoglobin.

70 Carcinoma. Cancer, malignant growth.

71 Cardiac. Pertains to the heart.

72 Cardiac asthma. Wheezing caused by increased airway resistance that occurs in certain heart ailments probably associated with interstitial edema, secondary to heart failure.

73 Cardiopulmonary. Relating to the heart and lungs.

74 Cardiovascular. Pertains to the heart and blood vessel system.

75 Cardiovascular accident (CVA). Stroke, rupture of a blood vessel in the brain.

76 Carina. Bifurcation of the trachea. Area of the tracheobronchial tree where the first two branches leave the trachea.

77 Carotid. The artery on each side of the neck.

78 Carpal pedal spasm. Spasm of the muscles to the fingers and toes and a tingling sensation of the hands and feet, occasionally associated with hyperventilation.

79 Cartilage. A tough elastic tissue found in various parts of the body; in this text it relates to the tissue that forms C-shaped rings around the trachea and larger bronchial tubes to ensure the patency of these organs.

80 Charles' law. If the pressure of the gas is held constant, the volume of a dry gas is directly proportional to the Kelvin (zero base) temperature.

81 Chemoreceptors. Small bodies located in the brain and on the carotid and aortic arteries that are sensitive to changes in blood oxygen and carbon dioxide pressure and that help regulate the rate and depth of respiration.

82 Chemotherapy. Treatment of infectious diseases by chemical substances or drugs.

83 Cheyne-Stokes respirations. Abnormal respirations that are intermittently deep and shallow and then cease temporarily before beginning again.

84 Chronic. Continuing over a long period, as a persistent ailment or sickness.

85 Cilia. Minute, hairlike structures found in the respiratory tract. Using a whiplike motion, they propel foreign matter on a thin layer of mucus toward the pharynx where the mucus is normally swallowed or expectorated.

86 Cohesive force. The force that holds molecules of a substance together.

87 Colloid. A state of matter where small particles that are larger than molecules but smaller than 50 microns are dispersed or suspended in a fluid.

88 Coma. A state of profound unconsciousness from which one cannot be aroused.

89 Comatose. A sleeplike state in which the patient is aroused with great difficulty or not at all.

90 Compliance. A term describing the ability of the lungs, chest wall, and/or healthy tubes to expand when exposed to an internal pressure; expressed as L/cm H_2O.

91 Compressed gas. Gases that are enclosed in some type of container by means of a pressure that is greater than 1 atmosphere (atm).

92 Congenital. Existing at or before birth.

93 Contaminate. Contact with any material that causes loss of purity. In medicine, the loss of sterility or introduction of germs to a germ-free area.

94 Contraindications. Any reason for not giving a treatment or medicine.

95 Convulsion. Involuntary spasm of skeletal muscles characterized by uncontrollable jerking motions of the arms, legs, and head.

96 COPD. Chronic obstructive pulmonary disease.

97 Copious. A lot of; much; an extraordinary amount. Usually used to describe the volume of secretions.

98 Cor pulmonale. Failure of the right side of the heart to empty properly as a result of pulmonary hypertension.

99 Coryza. Common cold.

100 Costal breathing. Respirations produced solely by use of the intercostal muscles.

101 Croup. Disease condition of the larynx that is characterized by harsh, raspy cough, a crowing sound, and difficult respiration.

102 Curarè. A drug (first used as a poison on arrows) that causes paralysis of muscles; it is now used in refined form to control muscle relaxation during anesthesia.

103 Cyanosis. Bluish discoloration of the skin caused by five or more grams (g) of reduced hemoglobin in the bloodstream.

104 Cylindrical plug. Thickened mucus that is coughed or suctioned from the lungs and that has assumed the shape of the inside of the tube in which it was formed.

105 Cyst. An abnormal collection of fluid within a definite sac or wall.

106 Cytolysis. Dissolution of cells in which the cell wall breaks. In the case of the red cell destruction—hemolysis.

107 Dalton's law. The pressure of a mixture of gases equals the sum of the partial pressures of all the gases. So long as no chemical change occurs, each gas in a mixture is absorbed by a given volume in proportion to the partial pressure of the gas.

108 Dead space, anatomic. The air that is always in the tube system of the lungs, normally 150 ml in the normal adult or approximately 1 ml per pound of body weight.

109 Dead space, mechanical. The volume of the apparatus or tubes into and out of which the patient may be forced to breathe and from which carbon dioxide is not effectively removed.

110 Dead space, physiologic. Areas of the lung in which oxygen is not exchanged through the alveolar wall as a result of any interference with ventilation or diffusion of blood supply, such as atelectasis or embolism.

111 Decompensation. Failure of the heart to circulate the blood properly or at a fast enough rate.

112 Defibrillation. Ending the fibrillation (irregular, inefficient contractions of the atria or ventricles) of the heart; usually done with electric shock.

113 Degeneration. Breakdown of tissue.

114 Delirium. Disordered mental state with excitement and delusions.

115 Dermatomyositis. Degenerative changes in skin and muscle that cause weakness and pain, sometimes affects the chest wall.

116 Desquamation. To peel off in layers.

117 Detergents. Drugs, compounds, or solutions used for cleaning.

118 Diagnosis. Determination of the nature of a disease or the disease-producing symptoms.

119 Diaphragm. The dome-shaped muscles that separate the thoracic and abdominal cavities.

120 Diastolic. Rhythmic period of relaxation and dilation of a chamber of the heart during which it fills with blood.

121 Diffuse. Scattered, covering a large area.

122 Diluent. An agent that dilutes the strength of a solution or mixture.

123 Disinfection. Destruction of pathogenic (disease-producing) organisms by use of a chemical agent.

124 Distal. Farthest from point of reference.

125 Distensible. Stretchable.

126 Distilled water. Water that has been evaporated and condensed to remove all minerals and other impurities.

127 Double pneumonia, bilateral. Inflammation of both lungs.

128 Duct. A canal or passage for fluid or gases.

129 Duo Medihaler-Iso. A pressurized vial containing a bronchodilator solution for relief of bronchospasm.

130 Dyspnea. Labored respiration of which the patient is aware.

131 Edema. Accumulation of fluid in the tissues.

132 Elasticity. Ability to stretch.

133 Electrolytes. Particles in the body having an electric charge and having to do with body function and metabolism, mainly sodium, potassium, chloride, and bicarbonate.

134 Embolism. Artery blocked by an embolus.

135 Embolus. A globule of fat, a clot, or gas bubble circulating in the bloodstream that obstructs the blood flow.

136 Emesis. The act of vomiting.

137 Emphysema. Air trapped in lungs or tissue as a result of disease process and/or aging.

138 Empiric. One who does not rely on scientific reasoning or education in practicing medicine; a quack. NOTE: This should not be confused with empirical data, a term that is used to describe data that is derived from observation or experience.

139 Empyema. Presence of pus in a cavity.

140 Endobronchial. Within a bronchus.

141 Endocrine function. Functioning of ductless glands that secrete substances directly into the bloodstream.

142 Endotracheal. Within the trachea, as an endotracheal tube.

143 Enzyme. A chemical produced by the body that acts as a catalyst in the metabolism of food substances.

144 Epiglottis. Elastic cartilage covered by mucous membrane, diverts food from the mouth to the esophagus by closing over the trachea.

145 Epiglottitis. Inflammation of the epiglottis that can cause airway obstruction.

146 Epilepsy. Disorder of the central nervous system that causes convulsions.

147 Erythrocyte. Red blood cells responsible for transportation of oxygen and carbon dioxide.

148 Etiology. Study of a cause or causes of a disease.

149 Eupnea. Normal respiration.

150 Exacerbation. Increase of symptoms and/or activity of disease.

151 Excision. The act of cutting away or taking out.

152 Expectoration. The act of coughing up and spitting out materials from the lungs and trachea. The material so ejected is sputum.

153 Expiration. The act of exhaling or breathing out.

154 Expiratory obstruction. Obstructions in any part of the lung that make exhalation difficult.

155 Expiratory reserve volume (ERV). The amount of air that can be exhaled after a normal resting period, not including residual volume; normally 1200 ml in the adult.

156 External respiration. The exchange of gases between the lungs and the atmosphere.

157 Extracellular. Outside the cell.

158 Exudate. Fluid produced by the lining of a cavity, contains microorganisms and cells.

159 Febrile. Pertains to fever or elevation of body temperature.

160 Fetal. Pertains to the unborn child after the third month of gestation.

161 Fetid. Having a foul odor.

162 Fibrillation. Disorganized contraction of cardiac muscle tissue, resulting in loss of cardiac output.

163 Fibrosis. Abnormal formation of fibrous or scar tissue.

164 Fibrothorax. Fibrous tissue inside the thoracic cavity.

165 Fibrous. Containing or composed of fibers.

166 Fistula. A deep ulcer formed by incomplete closure of a wound or abscess, or an abnormal, tubelike passage within body tissue (e.g., a tracheoesophageal fistula).

167 Flail chest. A condition in which two or more ribs are broken in the anteroposterior aspect of the thorax.

168 Flow rate. The speed at which a substance moves; referred to here as the movement of gases through a registering flowmeter.

169 Foci. Center of a morbid process; plural of focus.

170 Function. The normal or special action of a part.

171 Functional residual capacity (FRC). The amount of air that can be exhaled by force after a normal resting inspiration plus the residual volume (which cannot be exhaled); normally 2400 ml in the adult.

172 Glycerol (glycerin). A colorless syrupy liquid with a sweet taste that mixes easily with water or alcohol and that is incorporated in some aerosol medications to increase the wetting ability of the medicine and to retard evaporation.

173 Guillain-Barré syndrome (polyneuritis). Diffuse infection or irritation of nerves; may affect the respiratory system by causing paralysis of muscles for breathing.

174 Hamman-Rich syndrome. Diffuse interstitial pulmonary fibrosis.

175 Hemithorax. Half or one side of the thorax.

176 Hemoglobin. The red coloring matter of the blood (when oxygenated) in a normal state. The chemical compound found in the red blood cells that combines with oxygen and whose function it is to carry oxygen.

177 Hemoptysis. Spitting or coughing blood or blood-tinged mucus.

178 Hemorrhage. Excessive bleeding.

179 Hemostasis. The stopping of bleeding or stagnation of blood flow.

180 Hemothorax. Blood in the thorax; specifically in the pleural space.

181 Hering-Breuer reflex. Nervous impulses that regulate the rhythm and amplitude of respirations.

182 Histolytic. Referring to the degeneration of tissues.

183 Humidifier. An instrument for adding water vapor to the air.

184 Humidifying. The act of adding water vapor to the air.

185 Humidity. Water vapor in the air.

186 Hydrostatic. Liquids in the state of equilibrium.

187 Hydrothorax. Collection of serous fluids in the pleural sacs.

188 Hygroscopic. Water-seeking substance that absorbs moisture.

189 Hypercapnia. Increased amounts of carbon dioxide in the blood.

190 Hyperinflation. Overdistension of the lungs that could possibly result from careless IPPB treatment.

191 Hyperkalemia. An increase in the concentration of plasma potassium.

192 Hyperpnea. Increased minute volume exchange regardless of cause.

193 Hypertensor. A drug that will elevate the blood pressure.

194 Hypertension. Abnormally high blood pressure.

195 Hyperthyroidism. Abnormal condition brought about by excessive functional activity of the thyroid gland.

196 Hypertonic. Pertaining to increased salt content when compared to body fluid.

197 Hypertrophy. An increase in the size of an organ independent of natural growth as a result of an enlargement or multiplication of its individual cells; usually includes an increase in functional activity and capacity.

198 Hyperventilation. Hyperpnea; forced ventilation; an increase in the quantity of the air breathed as a result of an increase in the rate or depth of ventilation, or both, beyond the metabolic needs of the body; symptoms are tingling of toes or fingers (carpal pedal spasms), light-headedness, and occasionally fainting and muscle spasms.

199 Hypervolemia. Greater than normal blood volume.

200 Hypocapnia. Decreased carbon dioxide in the blood or tissues; alkalosis.

201 Hypostasis. The formation of a sediment, especially settling of the blood in the dependent parts of the body.

202 Hypostatic. As a result of or in the nature of hypostasis.

203 Hypotonic. Below normal strength or decreased salt content when compared to normal body fluid.

204 Hypoventilate. To under aerate the alveoli; to put less air into the lungs than the patient needs for adequate oxygenation as a result of a decrease in rate and/or depth of ventilation.

205 Hypoxemia. Insufficient amounts of oxygen in the blood.

206 Hypoxia, anemic. Hypoxia caused by low hemoglobin or too few red cells.

207 Hypoxia, demand. Increased use of oxygen by the cells; caused by high fever or thyroid dysfunction.

208 Hypoxia, hystotoxic. Inability of cells to use oxygen as a result of poisoning of the cell.

209 Hypoxia, stagnant (ischemic). Hypoxia in the tissue cells that is caused by slow circulation of the blood.

210 Idiopathic. Occurring without known cause.

211 Idiosyncrasy. A mental or physical habit or a peculiar characteristic of an individual's behavior.

212 Impairment. The act of damaging or insulting function.

213 Infarct. An arterial blood clot that occludes a blood vessel, causing a triangular area of tissue being supplied by that artery to die.

214 Infection. Any state of ill health caused by living, growing organisms inside the body.

215 Inflammation. Tissue reaction to injury or infection, usually denoted by redness.

216 Inhalant. Medication given by breathing an aerosol.

217 Inherent. Natural to the organism, a natural part or function of the body.

218 Inspiration. The process of taking air into the lungs.

219 Inspiratory capacity (IC). Maximum amount of air that can be taken into the lungs on forced inspiration from resting expiration; normally 3500 ml in the adult.

220 Inspiratory reserve volume (IRV). The amount of air that can be breathed in after normal resting inspiration; normally 3100 ml in the adult.

221 Inspissated. Thickened secretions usually caused by poor humidity and/or negative fluid balance.

222 Insults. Any effort, disease, or trauma, that adds to any abnormal condition that the patient may already have, for example, pneumonia insults the respiratory ability of the emphysema patient.

223 Intercostal. Located between the ribs.

224 Intermittent positive pressure breathing (IPPB). Pressure on inspiration, followed by a passive exhalation, which usually refers to a short-term breathing treatment; also refers to inspiratory positive pressure breathing.

225 Intermittent positive pressure ventilation (IPPV). See Intermittent positive pressure breathing. Usually refers to continuous mechanical ventilation.

226 Internal respiration. Exchange of gases (oxygen and carbon dioxide) between the tissues and bloodstream.

227 Interstitial. Situated between important parts. In the lungs it refers to the cellular layer between the epithe-lial cells that line the pulmonary capillaries.

228 Intracellular. Inside the cell.

229 Intrathoracic. Inside the rib cage or chest wall.

230 Intratracheal. Inside the trachea.

231 Intubation. The process of passing a tube through the mouth or nose into the trachea.

232 Inundation. Overcome, covered as by a wave.

233 Ion. An atom or group of atoms that by suitable application of energy, such as dissociation of a molecule, has lost or gained one or more orbital electrons and has thus become capable of conducting electricity.

234 Ionization. The dissociation or breaking up of a substance or solution into ions.

235 Ischemia. A decrease in blood supply to a localized area as a result of constriction of blood vessels.

236 Isoproterenol (Isuprel). Medication designed to dilate the bronchial tubes.

237 Isotonic. A solution having the same saline content as that found in intracellular and extracellular fluids.

238 Kyphoscoliosis. Humpback and curvature of the spine to the side and forward.

239 Landry's paralysis. A form of paralysis in which loss of muscle function in the legs and feet gradually extends to the circulatory and respiratory centers. (Another term for Guillain-Barré syndrome.)

240 Laryngitis. Inflammation of the larynx that may obstruct ventilation.

241 Larynx. Organ of the voice; located at the top of the trachea.

242 Lesion. A wound or circumscribed area of tissue damage.

243 Lethargic. A condition of drowsiness.

244 Leukocyte. White blood cell, responsible for fighting infection.

245 Liquefy. To thin by adding fluid or changing the consistency of the solution.

246 Liter (L). 1000 ml or 1.0567 quarts.

247 Liter/minute. Measure of flow; liters per minute, L/min, or lpm.

248 Lobe. A globular part of an organ separated by boundaries, for example, lobes of a lung.

249 Lobectomy. Removal of a lobe of a lung.

250 Lumen. Space within a tube, for example, lobes of a lung.

251 Lung abcess. Enclosed, puss-filled area or cavity inside the lung.

252 Lysing. Loosening, dissolving.

253 Lysis. Destruction or decomposition.

254 Manifestations. Symptoms; the way in which a disease presents itself.

255 Manometer. Device for measuring the pressure of a liquid or gas.

256 Maximally. The most.

257 Maximum ventilatory volume (MVV). Previously called maximum breathing capacity (MBC); the maximum volume of air a patient can move in 1 minute.

258 Mediastinum. The area inside the thoracic cavity directly behind the sternum and between the two lungs, contains the heart, trachea, esophagus, large blood vessels, and nerves.

259 Medihaler. A pressurized chamber that contains medication for inhalation, usually a bronchodilator.

260 Membrane. A thin sheet or layer of pliable tissue that covers a surface, lines a cavity, or divides an organ into sections.

261 Metabolic. Pertaining to the sum of the cellular and tissue changes, physical and chemical, whereby the body functions and energy is produced.

262 Metabolism. Sum total of all chemical activity in the body.

263 Metaplastic. A tissue formed by converting one kind of tissue to another, usually an abnormal type.

264 Miliary. Small, like millet seeds (about 2 mm).

265 Molecule. The smallest form into which a substance can be divided without loss of its character.

266 Moribund. Dying.

267 Mucolysis. The breaking down or loosening up of mucous secretions by chemical means.

268 Mucolytic. Any substance that causes a lysing of mucus, such as acetylcysteine (Mucomyst).

269 Mucopurulent. Mucous secretions containing pus cells.

270 Mucosa. Mucous membrane; the tissue that lines the inside of the nose, mouth, trachea, bronchi, and bronchioles.

271 Mucous plug. Thick, dry pieces of mucus that are of a size to occlude the lumen of a bronchi or bronchiole.

272 Mucoviscidosis. Cystic fibrosis of the pancreas. A disease state characterized by thick, tenacious secretions of the important mucus-secreting glands, especially the respiratory tract.

273 Mucus. Clear, viscid secretions of the mucous membranes (consists of mucin, epithelial cells, white blood cells, and various salts suspended in water).

274 Myasthenia gravis. Disease of the sixth thoracic nerve that causes progressive paralysis of the muscles of breathing.

275 Myocardia. Muscles of the heart.

276 Myocardial failure. Heart failure.

277 Myocardial infarction (MI). Occlusion of a coronary vessel or vessels by a blood clot, causing a triangular area of the heart muscle supplied by that vessel to die; a heart attack.

278 Narcosis. State of unconsciousness.

279 Narcotic. A drug that produces stupor, complete insensibility, or sleep. All types are respiratory depressants.

280 Nebulization. The process of breaking down a fluid into fine particles and suspending them in a gas; this forms a mist called an aerosol.

281 Nebulizer. A device for making a mist (aerosol) of small particles of a solution.

282 Necrosis. Death of a cell or a group of cells in contact with living cells.

283 Negative pressure. Pressure less than ambient.

284 Neonatal. Pertains to the newborn infant.

285 Neoplasm. A new or abnormal formation of growth of tissue.

286 Neoplastic. A new formation of tissue, a tumor.

287 Norepinephrine bitartrate (Levophed). Medication that tends to elevate blood pressure by constricting the small blood vessels.

288 Normal saline. The same saline content as the blood, 0.9%.

289 Obesity. Condition in which excessive fat is stored in the body.

290 Obstruction. Anything that blocks a structure and prevents its normal function.

291 Orifice. Opening.

292 Orthopnea. The inability to breathe except in the sitting or upright position.

293 Oscillation. To vibrate, to swing, or to move regularly but rapidly back and forth.

294 Osmosis. The movement of the molecules of a solvent across a semipermeable membrane until equilibrium occurs.

295 Osmotic pressure. The driving force that causes the molecules of a solution to move through a semipermeable membrane from an area of high concentration to an area of lower concentration until equilibrium is attained.

296 Osteoarthropathy. Clubbing of fingers and toes associated with enlargement of ends of bones; encountered in pulmonary and cardiac disease.

297 Oxyhemoglobin. The combination of oxygen and hemoglobin.

298 Papilledema. Edema of the optic nerve or disc. If severe, it may become a "choked" disc or it may become inflamed; it is associated with pulmonary emphysema and increased intracranial pressure.

299 Paradoxical respiration. The lungs expand on expiration and contract on inspiration.

300 Paranasal. Concerning the nose or approximation to the nose.

301 Parenchyma. The parts of an organ concerned with its function as opposed to its structure.

302 Parenchymatitis. Inflammation of the parenchyma.

303 Parenteral. Introducing a substance into the body by a route other than the intestinal tract.

304 Parietal. Pertaining to or forming the walls of a cavity or organ.

305 Paroxysm. A sudden periodic attack or recurrence of a disease; a seizure of any kind.

306 Partial pressure of carbon dioxide. P_{CO_2}.

307 Particle. Of small mass.

308 Particle size. The overall size (mass) of a particle.

309 Patency. Open.

310 Pathogenic. Disease-producing.

311 Pathology. Study of the nature of the cause of disease.

312 Percussion. Tapping the body lightly but sharply to determine the consistency of underlying structures.

313 Perfusion. Passage of fluids through blood vessels.

314 Peribronchiolar. Around or near the tracheal bronchial tree.

315 Peripheral. Outer parts; parts away from the center.

316 Peristaltic motion. Wavelike muscular motion, for example, motion in the intestine or esophagus.

317 Permeable. Quality of allowing the passage of fluid into or through a structure such as a membrane.

318 pH. A measure of the hydrogen ion concentration of a substance.

319 Phagocytosis. The process of ingestion and digestion by the white blood cells. The substances ingested include other cells, bacteria, bits of necrotic tissue, and foreign particles.

320 Pharyngitis. Inflammation of the pharynx.

321 Pharynx. An area of mucous membrane behind the mouth and nose and above the esophagus and trachea.

322 Phase. Any of the states or forms in a cycle or way in which something may be observed.

323 Physiologic. Concerning normal body function.

324 Pickwickian syndrome. A restrictive disease of the chest that is caused by obesity and that is characterized by somnolence, hypoventilation, and erythrocytosis.

325 Pigeon breast. Malformation of the front of the chest wall causing the sternum to be elevated and pushed forward into a point.

326 Plasma. Fluid portion of the blood.

327 Plethora. Congestion causing overfullness of blood vessels.

328 Pleura. The tissue that lines the inside of the chest walls and the outside of the lungs. These two layers are side by side with only a potential space between them.

329 Pneumoconiosis. A disease of the respiratory tract that results from inhalation of dust particles.

330 Pneumonia. Inflammation of the lungs with fluid in the lung tissue causing consolidation.

331 Pneumonitis. Inflammation of the lungs; often a viral pneumonia.

332 Pneumoparesis. Progressive congestion of the lungs.

333 Pneumothorax. Air leaking into the pleural space from the lung or through the chest wall; if uncorrected will result in a collapsed lung.

334 Poliomyelitis. Inflammation of the gray matter of the spinal cord, sometimes causing paralysis.

335 Polycythemia. Overabundance of red blood cells in the blood.

336 Polymyositis. Inflammation of many muscles, sometimes affects the chest muscles.

337 Postural drainage. Gravitational assistance to the emptying of the secretions from a body cavity by positioning; in respiratory therapy, specifically, the draining of mucus from any part of the lung so that it can be expectorated and/or removed.

338 Precipitation. The process of separating a substance from a solution by action of a reagent causing the substance to fall to the bottom or float on top of the solution.

339 Pressure aerosol. Any liquid under pressure that produces a fog when released, such as spray paint or a metered dose unit.

340 Prognosis. Estimating the probable outcome or course of a disease.

341 Prophylaxis. Preventive treatment.

342 Proteolytic. In the chemistry of enzymes, hastening the lysis of protein.

343 Proximal. Nearest to point of reference.

344 PSI. Pounds per square inch.

345 *Pseudomonas.* A bacterium that produces a blue-green pigment and is infectious.

346 Pulmonary. Pertaining to the lungs.

347 Pulmonary edema. The leakage of fluid from the capillaries into the alveoli as a result of increased pressure inside the capillaries or a leaky capillary wall.

348 Pulmonary emboli. Blood clots in the vessels of the lung that are often fatal.

349 Pulmonary flora. Organisms that normally live inside the lung, trachea, and bronchi; they cause no disease and may often prevent the implantation of other organisms that could produce disease.

350 Pulsating. A rhythmatic throb or movement.

351 Purulent. Containing or forming pus.

352 Pyogenic. Producing pus.

353 Rales. Bubbling sounds heard when mucus or fluid is present in the lumen of the trachea and bronchi.

354 Rate. Speed of movement.

355 Rationale. Explanation based on reason and not on experience alone.

356 Reaction. Extreme physical, emotional, or physiologic response to stimulation, medicine, drugs, or emotional stress.

357 Regurgitation. Casting up of undigested food from the stomach or backflow of blood into the heart as a result of defective valves.

358 Renal failure. Failure of the kidney(s) to function properly.

359 Remission. Abatement of subsidence of symptoms of disease.

360 Restrictive. Any condition that hinders normal motion. In a pulmonary study, any condition that hinders normal chest wall motion or normal expansion of the lungs, such as kyphoscoliosis or cystic fibrosis.

361 Rhinitis. Inflammation of the mucous membranes of the nose.

362 Rhonchi. Abnormal, course sounds heard during auscultation of the chest. These sounds occur in the larger air passages and throat; they may be called dry or sibilant rales.

363 Roentgenogram. Radiogram; an x-ray film.

364 Sclerosis. Abnormal hardening of tissue.

365 Secretions. Liquid drainage, either normal or disease-produced.

366 Segment. A demarcated portion of a whole organ.

367 Septicemia. Infection in the bloodstream.

368 Septum. Dividing wall made of bone or tissue such as in the nose.

369 Sequestration. Dead area in bone or tissue.

370 Shock. Disruption of the circulation, causing a rapid drop in blood pressure; also, a state of profound mental and physical depression as a result of injury or emotional disturbance.

371 Shunt. Bypass.

372 Sigh. Deep breath normally taken about every 10 minutes.

373 Sinusitis. Inflammation of the sinus cavities of the face; if chronic, may be a cause of some pulmonary diseases.

374 Sodium bicarbonate ($NaHco_3$). Used as a mild alkali to relieve hyperacidity in stomach, blood, or urine.

375 Spasm. Involuntary muscular contraction.

376 Spirals. Descending circles.

377 Spirometer. Instrument that measures vital capacity or volume of inhaled and exhaled air.

378 Splanchnic. Pertaining to or supplying the viscera or abdominal organs.

379 Splinting. Procedure used to prevent movement of the chest; failure on the part of the patient to breathe deep or sigh because of pain or trauma; may be conscious or unconscious.

380 Spondylitis. Inflammation and fusing of one or more vertebrae.

381 Spontaneous. Happening by itself without apparent cause.

382 Sputum. Secretions of the lungs, bronchi, trachea, and other secretions coughed or expectorated.

383 Stenosis. Narrowing of a lumen.

384 Sternal. Pertaining to the flat bone in front of the chest wall.

385 Sternum. Breast bone, the bone to which the ribs connect in the front of the chest wall.

386 Stomatitis. Irritation of the inside of the mouth; mouth ulcer.

387 Stretch receptors. Nerve cells inside the lung that react to deep inhalations and cause the chest to rebound to its resting position after inhalation.

388 Stridor. Abnormal, harsh, high-pitched sounds that occur during difficult or obstructed respiration.

389 Stroke volume. Amount of blood put out by ventricles at each heartbeat.

390 Subarachnoid. Beneath arachnoid tissue in brain or spinal cord.

391 Subclinical. Pertaining to a disease in which manifestations are so slight they are unnoticeable.

392 Submucous. Beneath the mucous membrane.

393 Supersaturated. Having more solute than the saturated solution can carry.

394 Suppurative. Formation and discharge of pus.

395 Suppurative bronchitis. Inflammation of the mucous membrane that lines the bronchi; involves the formation of pus.

396 Supraclavicular. Above the clavicle or collar bone.

397 Symptom. Manifestation of a disease.

398 Syncope. Fainting.

399 Syndrome. A collection of symptoms that are associated with a morbid process and that constitute a distinct clinical picture.

400 Systematic. Pertaining to the whole system.

401 Tachycardia. Increased heart rate, usually greater than 100 beats per minute.

402 Tachypnea. Abnormally fast breathing.

403 Therapy. Treatment.

404 Thrombus. A plug or clot that remains at the point of its formation in a blood vessel or at one of the cavities of the heart.

405 Tidal volume (V_T). The amount of air passing in and out of the lung during normal resting respiration.

406 Topical. Application of a medicine to the surface of a tissue or organ; not injected.

407 Total lung capacity (TLC). The total amount of air in a forced maximum inspiration and a forced maximum expiration, including the residual volume; normally 6000 ml in the adult.

408 Toxic. Resembling or caused by poison.

409 TPC. Total pulmonary capacity (see Total lung capacity).

410 Trachea. Conducting passageway that leads to the lungs from the larynx.

411 Tracheal stoma. Minute openings in the tracheal wall for drainage of lymphatic fluids.

412 Tracheitis. Inflammation of the trachea.

413 Tracheitis sicca. Dry inflammation of the trachea.

414 Tracheobronchitis. Inflammation of the trachea and bronchi.

415 Tracheocutaneous fenestrations. Abnormal cavities beneath the mucous membrane of the trachea, often produced by disease.

416 Tracheostomy. An artificial opening in the trachea that facilitates the passage of air or removal of secretions.

417 Tract. A path; an area of greater length than width; for example, the respiratory and digestive tracts.

418 Transudate. A fluid that originates in the blood and lymph vessels and that passes through a membrane.

419 Trauma. A wound or injury; physical damage produced by external force.

420 Trypsin. A digestive enzyme that catalyzes the hydrolysis of most proteins.

421 Tubercle bacillus. A bacteria that causes cavitation in the lungs.

422 Tuberculosis. Disease caused by the tubercle bacillus.

423 Turbulent. Rolling, not smooth or laminar; usually describes flow of air or liquids.

424 Tussigenic reflex. Cough reflex.

425 Tussis. Cough.

426 Tussive. Pertaining to cough.

427 Unresolved. Failing of a diseased area to return to normal.

428 Upper respiratory infection (URI). Any infection that involves primarily the larynx, trachea, and bronchi of the upper respiratory tract, such as the common cold, pharyngitis, laryngitis, bronchitis, etc.

429 Vagal. Pertaining to the vagus nerve.

430 Vagus nerve. The tenth cranial nerve that aids in the control of respiration, most specifically the diaphragm.

431 Vapor. Gaseous state of any substance.

432 Vaporizer. Device for converting liquid into a vapor.

433 Vascular. Pertaining to or composed of blood vessels.

434 Vasoconstriction. Constriction of blood vessels.

435 Vasoconstrictor. A drug that causes constriction of blood vessels.

436 Ventilation. The act of inhaling and exhaling. The movement of gas into and out of the lungs.

437 Venturi system. A method of mixing air into a stream of gas via entrainment.

438 Viscid. Thick, gelatinous, and adhesive or sticky.

439 Viscosity. State of being sticky or gummy; resistant to flow. The tendency of molecules of a fluid to adhere to one another and to the uses of a conducting pathway.

440 Visceral pleura. The membraneous sac that covers the lungs.

441 Vital capacity, forced (FVC). The amount of air in a forced maximum inspiration and a forced maximum expiration; does not include residual volume; normally 4800 ml in the adult.

442 Volume. Term used when measuring pulmonary capacity.

443 Volumetric. Pertaining to the measure of volume.

444 Wet lung. Pathogenic condition in which the lungs have rales and other wet bubbling sounds.

445 Wetting agent. Any agent that liquefies or adds fluid, especially to secretions in the airways.

2.2 Applications to respiratory care (frequently used terms)

1 Large amount of bleeding—hemorrhage.

2 Large volume of secretions—copious.

3 Sticky, stringy secretions—tenacious.

4 Elevated CO_2 levels in the blood—hypercapnia.

5 Air sacs—alveoli.

6 A condition caused by lack of oxygen in the environment—hypoxia, asphyxia.

7 A lack of oxygen in the blood—hypoxemia.

8 Partial collapse of alveoli or lung segments—atelectasis.

9 Decreased respiratory rate—bradypnea.

10 Sickness of long standing—chronic.

11 Blue-gray color of skin associated with oxygen lack—cyanosis.

12 A tube placed within the trachea—endotracheal (tracheal).

13 To expel sputum through the mouth—expectorate.

14 A sleepy, drowsy patient—somnolent, lethargic.

15 Secretions produced by mucous membrane—mucus.

16 Shortness of breath except when in an upright position—orthopnea.

17 A collapsed lung caused by air in the pleural space—pneumothorax.

18 The predicted outcome of a disease—prognosis.

19 To vomit—regurgitate.

20 To exhibit profound physical change to stress or injury—reaction.

21 Fast heart rate—tachycardia.

22 A heart attack resulting from injured heart muscle—myocardial infarction (MI).

3.0 IMPORTANCE OF THE MEDICAL RECORD
3.1 Medical record

1 The medical record is a longitudinal, written report of a patient's history, examinations, tests, diagnosis, prognosis, therapy, and response to therapy. It is started whenever a patient is seen for the first time by a physician and is normally retained by that physician. If a patient is admitted to a hospital, the admitting physician will generate still another medical record that remains on file with the hospital.

2 The chief purpose of a medical record is to provide a written report of the patient's health and previous conditions and treatments.

3 The medical record is the single best source of information about a patient. For this reason it is a legal document admissible as evidence in a court hearing or trial.

4 There are many types of formats that may be used for organizing the medical record. The selection of one method over the other is usually based on the preference of the physician and medical record department.

5 The two most popular methods of organization are the *chronologic/sectional* or *source* method and the *problem-oriented medical record* method (POMR).

6 With the chronologic/sectional (source) method, the record is arranged in chronologic order and is divided into subsections that contain information according to the source. For example, laboratory data are placed in the diagnostic reports section. Other subsections include:

a Medical history

b Physician's notes

c Diagnostic reports

d Correspondence

e Insurance forms

7 The POMR method, also known as the Weed system after its developer, uses the same chronologic approach as the source method. The primary difference between this method and the other is that all information relating to the diagnosis and treatment of the patient is contained in one POMR for the current diagnosis, treatment, or situation.

8 Each POMR includes four different areas: Data base, problems, plans, and progress notes.

9 The *data base* section contains patient history, complaint, physical examination, and laboratory reports. A separate POMR is created each time the patient is seen for a different problem.

10 The *problem list* section lists physical and psychologic conditions related to the presenting problem.

11 The *plan* section contains a detailed description of how the presenting problem will be diagnosed and treated.

12 The *progress notes* section contains a sequential and detailed listing of everything that was done to care for the patient. These notes are best recorded in a logical sequence called SOAP:

S = Subjective data
O = Objective data
A = Assessment
P = Plan of action

13 In the *near future* medical records will be computerized and tied into billing, insurance, and peer review systems. This type of record-keeping system will enable the practitioner to recall any part or all of the medical record instantaneously and will facilitate diagnosis and treatment based on available information on a particular patient and similar cases on record.

14 Under the new prospective payment system the medical record, most importantly the admitting diagnosis, and a precise documentation of the patient's care is used as a basis for reimbursement to the hospital by diagnosis related group (DRG).

3.2 Composition of the medical record

Most medical records are assembled using the following format.

1 *Admission sheet.* Personal data about the patient, i.e., name, address, date of admission, birthdate, admitting physician, sex, marital status, nearest relative, occupation, employer, diagnosis, religion, and record of previous admissions.

Nurse	Therapist	Physician	
MEDICATION PRESCRIBED:		DIAGNOSIS:	
		O_2 % ( ) FREQUENCY OF RX ( )	
		THERAPY ORDERED:	
Date	Time	Patient response (tolerance, side effects, etc.)	Tech.

Patient name _____ Age _____ Equipment _____ Room No _____

F I G U R E 3 - 1 Form for recording respiratory care progress.

2 *Face sheet.* Front sheet in the chart; used to record allergies and history at discharge.

3 *Physician's order sheet.* A record of the physician's orders relative to treatment of the patient. Only physicians should record on this form unless cleared by the physician when giving a verbal order. Any verbal orders should be noted as such and require a cosigning by the physician.

4 *History sheet.* Record of patient's personal and medical history. This sheet is completed by the admitting physician and may be a valuable source of information for the technician or therapist providing subsequent pulmonary care.

5 *Nurses' notes.* A recording of nursing and other therapies the patient has received. These notes usually report treatments, nursing techniques, patient behavior, and response of the patient to treatment. In many hospitals respiratory therapy personnel record their procedures on this sheet. Other hospitals provide a special sheet for recording respiratory care progress (Fig. 3-1).

6 *Special records of laboratory tests and x-ray examinations.* This is a listing of special tests and their results. This section normally contains comments on chest x-ray examinations, arterial blood gas values, sputum reports, and other data useful for respiratory care personnel.

4.0 GENERAL TERMS, CONCEPTS, AND RULES FOR CHARTING
4.1 General charting procedure

Policies regarding charting (recording) in the patient's record vary from hospital to hospital, although the following general guidelines may be applied.

1 An entry in the chart is required for *each* medication given and for *each* treatment administered to a patient.

2 The objectives of this rule are
  a To maintain an exact and sequential record of the patient's condition, illness, and treatment.
  b To aid the physician in making a correct diagnosis and prognosis of the patient's condition.
  c To show daily progress.
  d To provide information on diagnostic tests.
  e When necessary, to be used as legal evidence in court.

3 The chart is a legal document and may be used in court as evidence. For this reason legal action may be taken if a record is falsified or if a person is an accessory to the falsification of a hospital record for any reason, including the following.
  a To conceal the real nature of an incident.
  b To protect one's self, someone else, or the hospital.
  c To deceive insurance companies. (This aspect of the medical record will be even more closely scrutinized as third party insurance carriers move toward a prospective type of reimbursement system.)

4 Accurate checking of medicine and prescriptions is as important as the administration of them.

5 A chart is the property of the hospital. It does *not* belong to the patient or his or her family, and they should *not* be permitted to read it.

6 A chart may be requested in a court proceeding. It may or may not be admitted as evidence by the court.

7 To be accepted as evidence, any notes must be signed, and the individual must be able to recognize his or her handwriting and notes.

8 Charts may be used in case studies for the advancement of science and the education of doctors and nurses. However, if the study is published, the identity of the patient must be concealed.

9 The technician should avoid signing as a witness to legal transactions.

4.2 Nurses'/therapists' notes

1 Many hospitals have the respiratory care personnel record in the nurses' notes portion of the chart. Others have a respiratory care section.

2 When charting, record all dates, times, observations, treatments, and results. Under the new prospective payment system it is extremely important that the practitioner be as specific as possible when describing the results or benefits derived by a patient receiving therapy.

3 Always record the unusual.

4 Learn to observe the patient; learn how to differentiate between symptoms, complaints, reactions, and statements that could be of importance in assessing the patient's condition or in determining the patient's prognosis.

5.0 CORRECT RECORDING AND CONFIDENTIALITY OF INFORMATION
5.1 Importance of correct recording and confidentiality

1 Idle conversation should be limited to a controlled group.

2 Notations on the chart must be neat and clear as to meaning and authenticity.

3 All recordings must be printed in ink; avoid shorthand or abbreviations. Your hospital's procedures for proper ink color should be checked.

4 Signed statements must have first initial and full last name.

5 A series of statements should be signed only once for the series.

6 Recording should be done only after the medication or treatment is given, *not before,* and only after there is a written physician's order to correspond to the medication or treatment.

7 Mistakes should *not* be erased. If an error is made, mark through it with a single line, indicating an error was made. Initial the error, then copy the recorded notation so that it is correct.

8 If the physician was present while the treatment was given, this is recorded.

9 Any *unusual* symptoms or changes in the patient are recorded.

10 *Future tense* should *not* be used when charting the patient's response.

TABLE 3-1 Medical abbreviations

Symbol	Meaning
aa	of each
ac	before meals
ah	every other hour
bid	twice a day
c̄	with
cc	cubic centimeter
C	centigrade
cm	centimeter
F	Fahrenheit
Fr, F	French, reference to catheter size
gtt	drop
Hb	hemoglobin
Hg	mercury
hs	at bedtime
kg	kilogram
L/min l/m, lpm	liter per minute
mg	milligram
ml	milliliter
mm	millimeter
pc	after meals
prn	according to circumstance, as needed
qh	every hour
q2h	every 2 hours (changing the number changes the frequency)
qid	four times per day
sos	if necessary
s̄	without
s̄s̄	half
stat	at once, immediately
tid	three times daily
TPR	temperature, pulse, respiration
Tx	treatment

Reviewing a patient's chart

Locate and become familiar with the following information on the patient's chart.
  1 Name of patient
  2 Age of patient
  3 Admitting diagnosis
  4 Primary complaint
  5 Type of surgery (if any)
  6 Prescription for respiratory therapy
  7 Respiratory therapy treatment record
  8 Vital signs
  9 X-ray examination findings
  10 Blood gas analysis record
  11 Pulmonary function studies
  12 Anesthesia record
  13 ECG report
  14 Medications received
  15 Laboratory reports
  16 History and physical examination

11 A *verbal* and *written* report should be made of any accident involving the patient.

12 Charting should never be done in such a way as to give the impression that you are diagnosing or stating medical conclusion.

EXAMPLE:

Incorrect—patient expectorated sputum that *was* blood-tinged.

Correct—patient expectorated sputum that *appeared* to be blood-tinged.

13 The notation is signed and your job classification should be specified after your signature.

6.0 PROPER CHARTING TECHNIQUES
6.1 Use of medical terms for charting

1 Terminology used in describing the patient's condition should be *brief, accurate,* and *descriptive.* It should reflect only what you saw or did when with the patient and therefore should be stated using the present tense.

2 If you cannot think of an appropriate medical term or phrase, use lay terms to relate the message.

3 Your descriptions should:
  a Record what you *did* for the patient.
  b Record the technique *employed,* or the medication *given* with dosage strength and dilution.
  c Record the *length* of each treatment.

d Record the patient's *response* to your treatment—both desirable and undesirable.

e Record if patient *refuses* treatment, noting reason for refusal.

f Record *results* using concise and descriptive medical terms (if you cannot think of the correct medical term, describe what you observed using layman's terms).

g Note any *special* circumstances or precautions to be observed by the next person treating this patient.

h Record the *date* and *time* you made an entry.

i Use only standardized medical abbreviations such as those presented in Table 3-1.

6.2 Reading the chart

1 Reading the patient's chart is included in Procedure 3-1.

2 A form for systematically reviewing a patient's chart is presented in the box above.

7.0 VERBAL AND NONVERBAL COMMUNICATION TECHNIQUES
7.1 Verbal communication

1 Talking is *not* communication.

2 Communication involves talking (sending), listening (receiving), and comprehension of what was said.

3 What is said is *not* necessarily what was intended to be heard; therefore the listener must learn to ask questions in order to accurately understand the intent of the sender's message.

4 Questions should be used to confirm what was said and to offer the patient or person talking the opportunity to express himself. Questions should be asked in a seeking yet supportive manner. The person questioned should be allowed to respond to each question before another is asked.

5 Proper questioning technique usually relates to who, what, when, where, and for what time.

■ ■ ■

This approach usually provides objective information while allowing the person being questioned to interject subjective feelings.

7.2 Nonverbal communication

1 "I heard what you said but I'm not sure what you meant" can relate to nonverbal communication.
2 *Body language* frequently speaks more clearly of the intent of a statement than the words that were spoken.
3 When speaking, always *look* into the person's eyes. A stunned look or a wayward glance from the person to whom you are speaking frequently suggests that he or she does not understand or is not interested in what is being said.
4 Folded arms, clenched fists, white hands, tightened facial muscles and distended temporal or neck veins frequently express anger, fear, or an unconscious action by the receiver to block communication.
5 For example, the simple act of *pushing away* from a table may be an unconscious act of removing one's self from the discussion.
6 When working with elderly patients be aware of special circumstances such as diminished or loss of hearing and sight and/or mental alertness. These conditions will hinder effective communication unless effective adjustments are made by the communicator.

8.0 TELEPHONE PROCEDURES
8.1 Proper telephone procedure

1 Answer the telephone as quickly as possible.
2 Hold the mouthpiece of the receiver approximately ¼ inch from your mouth and speak in a clear and precise yet natural tone.
3 Identify the service area.
4 Identify yourself.
5 Offer to be of assistance.
6 Record the message as it is given and repeat critical data such as:
  a Spelling of patient's name
  b Location
  c Therapy requested
7 Inquire as to the urgency of the request.
8 Do not allow the caller to hang up until necessary information is complete.
9 If the caller is excited, remain calm and methodically request information.

8.2 Dispatching a phone request

1 Record the message or request on the appropriate form.
2 Contact the appropriate sources and relate the message.
3 If the requested parties are not available, use judgment to contact alternates; otherwise, process the call.

9.0 DEFINING MEDICAL TERMS
9.1 Defining and pronouncing medical terms

1 Use a medical dictionary for the correct definition and pronunciation of each the following terms:
  a Bypass
  b Cathode
  c Fracture
  d Heroin
  e Lymph
  f Intermittent
  g Evacuation
  h Mendel's law
  i Meningitis
  j Reflex
  k Sprain
  l Tympanic
  m Senility

PROCEDURE 3-1

Reading the patient's chart

No.	Steps in performing the procedure
	The practitioner will read the patient's chart before initiating any form of ordered respiratory care and as soon as possible when delivering emergency care.
1	Identify yourself at nursing station.
2	Procure patient's chart.
3	Note patient's admitting diagnosis.
4	Read current physician's orders.
5	Read results of patient's physical examination and history, noting respiratory-related problems.
6	Read physician's progress notes for a minimum of past 2 days.
2	Read nurses' notes for past 2 days (note vital signs).
8	Note any recent surgery (type and time).
9	Read x-ray reports (chest films).
10	Read ECG reports (note major arrythmias).
11	Read laboratory reports (note sputum cultures and CBC, K, Na, Ca, Cl levels.)
12	Read current medications.
13	Read respiratory therapy progress notes.
14	Return chart to appropriate area of nursing station.

BIBLIOGRAPHY

Brunner TF and Berkowitz L: Elements of scientific and specialized terminology, Minneapolis, 1967, Burgess Publishing Co.
Flight M: The credibility of the medical record, Prof Med Assist May/June, 1986.
Gylys B and Wedding M: Medical terminology: a systems approach, ed 2, Philadelphia, 1988, FA Davis Co.
Haskins B and Svanda C: Two ways to sharpen your charting skills, RN Dec 1986.
Mosby's medical, nursing, & allied health dictionary, ed 3, St Louis, 1990, The CV Mosby Co.

General human anatomy and physiology

28.1 Describe coronary circulation.

29.1 Describe blood flow to and from the brain.

30.1 Explain blood flow to and functions of the liver.

31.1 Explain functions of the spleen.

32.1 Describe structure and function of renal circulation.

33.1 Describe structure and function of pulmonary circulation.

33.2 Describe bronchial circulation.

34.1 Differentiate between functions of various structures of the digestive system.

35.1 and **35.2** Differentiate between structures and functions of the kidney.

35.3 Discuss the various causes of renal failure.

35.4 and **35.5** Explain the process of hemodialysis and hemofiltration.

36.1 and **36.2** Differentiate between locations and functions of various glands.

37.1 Explain terms and concepts of the nervous system.

38.1 Describe the structure and function of neurons.

38.2 Explain various types of neurons.

38.3 Give an example of how a nerve impulse is received and transmitted.

38.4 Explain a synapse.

38.5 Demonstrate a reflex action.

38.6 Discuss nerve dynamics as it relates to transmitting impulses.

39.1 through **39.6** Differentiate between various divisions of the brain and their functions.

40.1 Predict physical responses based on dysfunctions of the brain.

41.1 Describe spinal cord structures and their function.

41.2 Explain the source and function of cerebrospinal fluid.

42.1 through **42.5** Discriminate between divisions of the central nervous system and their functions.

43.1 Describe interaction between parasympathetic and sympathetic divisions of the autonomic nervous system.

43.2 Define EEG and briefly discuss its applications.

Anatomy and physiology are the studies of the structures and functions of the body. General knowledge of all parts of the body is necessary for the practitioner to recognize and relate the influence and interplay of the body systems to maintain homeostasis. Specific knowledge of the cardiorespiratory system is required before a clinician begins to assess the patient's condition and administer various treatment modalities. Units 1 through 43 of this module present a general overview of all systems. Because of its importance to respiratory care personnel, the cardiorespiratory system will be presented as a separate module.

Progressing through the module, the reader may wish to refer to *Mosby's Medical, Nursing, and Allied Health Dictionary* for unfamiliar terms and concepts. As anatomic structures are presented, take the time to relate internal organs and structures to external anatomy on yourself or another person. This approach will help you to visualize internal anatomy in its perspective to a human and not just a chart or model.

1.0 ANATOMIC STRUCTURES AND PHYSIOLOGIC ACTIONS

1.1 Glossary of general terms and concepts

1 Active transport. Movement of either water or solute through a cell membrane against a gradient.

2 Anatomy. A study of the structures of the human body.

3 Catalyst. A substance that alters the role of a chemical reaction without itself being permanently affected by the reaction.

4 Concentration gradient. Difference between two concentrations of solutions separated by a membrane. Concentration gradient causes particles in a solution to move from the area of greatest concentration to that of lesser concentration.

5 Conductance. Relative rate of diffusion of an ion through a membrane. For example, the conductance of potassium by the resting membrane is 50 times greater than it is for sodium. Likewise, the chloride ion moves through the membrane with great ease.

6 Diffusion. Scattering or spreading. Movement of solute, solvent, and gas molecules in all directions in a solution or in both directions through a freely permeable (passive) cell membrane.

7 Donnan effect. Unequal distribution of diffusible ions in a solution that is separated by a membrane that blocks the nondiffusible ion. The higher the concentration of nondiffusible ions the greater will be the ionic imbalance between the two sides of the membrane. For example, protein anions do not readily diffuse, causing an ionic imbalance between the inside and outside of the cell.

8 Electrolyte. Substance that produces ions (an electrolyte solution is a solution that will conduct an electric current).

9 Enzyme. A biologic catalyst.

10 Excitability. Property of all living cells to respond to a stimulus.

11 Filtration. Process of blocking or passing molecules of

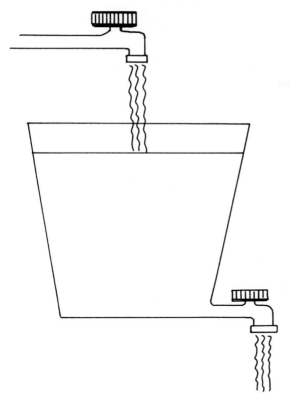

FIGURE 4-1 Figurative representation of principle of homeostasis. Although water is constantly being added to the bucket, the level remains the same because the same amount of water is allowed to drain out.

different sizes as controlled by the size of the opening (pore) in the membrane structure.

12 Homeostasis (Fig. 4-1). Constancy of the internal environment of the body, despite the external influences. It is this tendency for the body to maintain some norm that allows outcomes for specific drugs and treatments to be predicted. In this example a state of homeostasis is presented by the faucet and bucket where as much water is entering the bucket as is leaving it.

13 Hypertonic solution. Solution with higher osmotic potential than another solution to which it is compared.

14 Hypotonic solution. Solution with lower osmotic potential than another solution to which it is compared.

15 Ions. Atoms that have gained a positive or negative charge through loss or gain of electrons during electrovalent compound formation. May exist in dissociated form in aqueous solution as a result of polar nature of water.

16 Isomotic. Two solutions having the same potential osmotic pressure.

17 Isomotic solution. Solution that has same osmotic pressure as another solution to which it is being compared.

18 Metabolism. The process that includes all intracellular activities, such as energy production and use. This process falls into two major categories.

  a Anabolism. Reactions that convert simple substances into more complex molecules (for example, amino acids to tissue proteins).

  b Catabolism. Conversion of complex substances into simple molecules usually for production of energy.

19 Molecule. Unit of matter capable of independent existence.

20 Net diffusion. Movement of more particles in one direction than the other down its own pressure gradient until equilibration occurs (Fig. 4-2). After equilibration, equal diffusion occurs in both directions, and gases diffuse from the alveoli into the blood of the surrounding capillary and vice versa based on differences in concentration (partial pressure) of the gases in the alveoli compared to that of the surrounding capillary.

21 Osmosis (Fig. 4-3). Movement of water (solvent) through a semipermeable or selectively permeable membrane *(1)* (e.g., passes water but not salt molecules from an area of low osmotic pressure [area with the smallest concentration of solute] *[2]*, to one of high osmotic pressure [greatest concentration of solute] *[3]*.)

22 Osmosis, net (Fig. 4-3). The concentration percentages of the solutions equilibrate *(4)* volume/pressure of the originally more concentrated solution, *(3)*, increases *(6)* so that a concentration gradient will always be maintained. When net osmosis occurs, the following changes will occur:

  a Concentrations of the solution equilibrate *(4)*.

  b Volume and pressure of the originally more concentrated solution *(6)* will increase by the same amount as the originally less concentrated solution decreased *(5)*. Osmosis causes water to pass through the walls of living cells which are not freely permeable to all solutes. As an example, the pulmonary capillary membrane normally is not permeable to proteins, and cell membranes are not freely permeable to electrolytes. When these structures become permeable as a result of illness, the patient's lungs may fill with edema (primarily protein), and the heart may become irritable because of the loss of electrolytes from the cell.

23 Partition coefficient. Factors that determine the ability of substance to pass across a cell membrane include:

  a The size of the molecule.

  b The ratio of solubility of the substance in an oil solvent and in water.

24 Physiology. A study of the functions, processes, activities, and phenomena characteristic of living organisms.

25 Resting potential. Electrical difference that exists between the inside and outside of a cell.

  a Polarized membrane. A potential exists.

  b Depolarized membrane. A potential does not exist.

26 Sodium pump. Active movement of Na^+ into and out of a cell by an active force within the cell membrane. The sodium pump constantly moves sodium out of the cell; a potassium pump moves potassium into the cell to maintain an ionic imbalance and membrane potential.

27 Solute. Substance dissolved in the solvent.

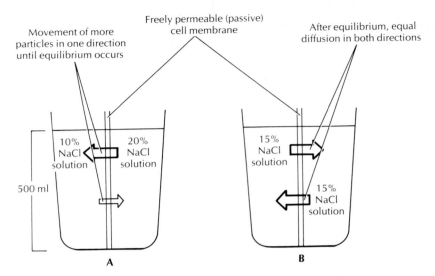

F I G U R E 4 - 2 Principle of diffusion. **A,** Particles move from area of high concentration to area of low concentration until equilibrium is achieved. **B,** After equilibrium, particles diffuse equally in both directions.

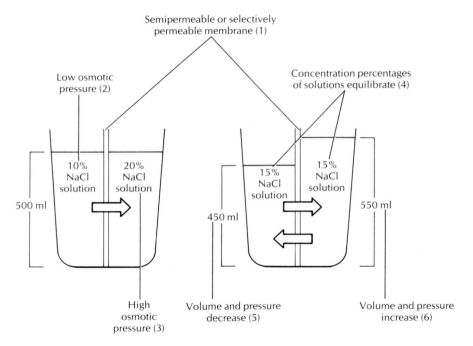

F I G U R E 4 - 3 Principle of osmosis. *Left,* Water moves through semipermeable membrane from area where particles are weakly concentrated to area where they are high concentrated. *Right,* At net osmosis, equilibrium has been achieved so that concentration of particles is equal on both sides of membrane.

28 Solution. Mixture of two or more substances.
29 Solvent. Dissolving agent in a solution.
30 States of matter. Gas, liquid, and solid.

2.0 STRUCTURAL PLANES AND ORGANIZATION OF THE BODY
2.1 Organization of the body

1 The human body is a complex system of bones, tissues, organs, and nerves.
2 The locations of these various structures are described in relationship to the body in an anatomic position (i.e., standing erect facing front with arms extended downward and palms facing outward) (Fig. 4-4).
3 Position of structures within the body or on the body are described in relationship to the following imaginary planes (lines) that pass through the body.
   a Sagittal plane (Fig. 4-4, *A*). A vertical plane passing through the body from front to back dividing the body or any of its parts into right and left sides.
   b Transverse plane (Fig. 4-4, *B*). A horizontal plane passing through the body dividing it or any of its parts into upper and lower parts.

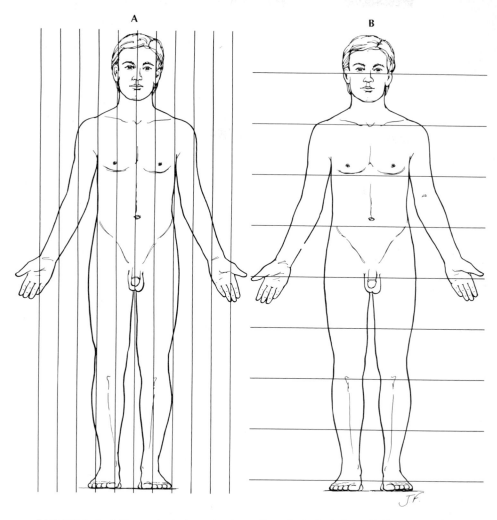

FIGURE 4-4 Human body in anatomic position. **A,** Sagittal plane. **B,** Transverse plane.

c Frontal (coronal) plane (Fig. 4-5). A vertical plane extending from side to side dividing the body or any of its parts into anterior *(1)* and posterior *(2)* sections.

2.2 Terms used to describe the location of structure or objects on or in the body

1 Superior (cranial). Toward the head end of the body.
   EXAMPLE: The larynx is superior to the alveoli.
2 Inferior (caudal). Toward the tail end of the body.
   EXAMPLE: Alveoli are inferior to bronchioles.
3 Anterior (ventral). Front.
   EXAMPLE: The sternum is located on the anterior portion of the chest.
4 Posterior (dorsal). Back.
   EXAMPLE: The spine is located on the posterior portion of the body.
5 Medial. Toward the midline of the structure being compared.
6 Lateral. Away from the midline of the structure being compared.
7 Proximal. Nearest to, toward; nearest the trunk or point of origin or attachment of a structure.

8 Distal. Away from; the most distant point from the trunk or point or origin of a structure.
   EXAMPLE: The alveoli are distal to the bronchi.

2.3 Abdominal structures

1 Structures in the abdominal region can be located according to the ten imaginary regions in Fig. 4-6.
   a Right hypochondriac region *(1)*
   b Right lumbar region *(2)*
   c Right iliac region *(3)*
   d Anterior superior iliac region *(4)*
   e Left hypochondriac region *(5)*
   f Left lumbar region *(6)*
   g Left iliac region *(7)*
   h Epigastric region *(8)*
   i Umbilical region *(9)*
   j Hypogastric region *(10*

2.4 Body cavities

1 The body has two major cavities, the ventral and dorsal cavities, which are subdivided into four smaller cavities that contain specific organs (Fig. 4-7).

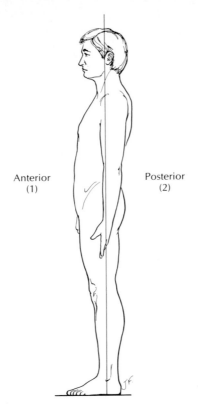

Anterior (1)

Posterior (2)

FIGURE 4-5 Frontal plane.

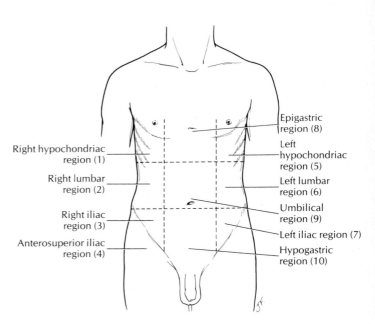

Epigastric region (8)

Right hypochondriac region (1)

Left hypochondriac region (5)

Right lumbar region (2)

Left lumbar region (6)

Right iliac region (3)

Umbilical region (9)

Anterosuperior iliac region (4)

Left iliac region (7)

Hypogastric region (10)

FIGURE 4-6 Regions of the abdominal area.

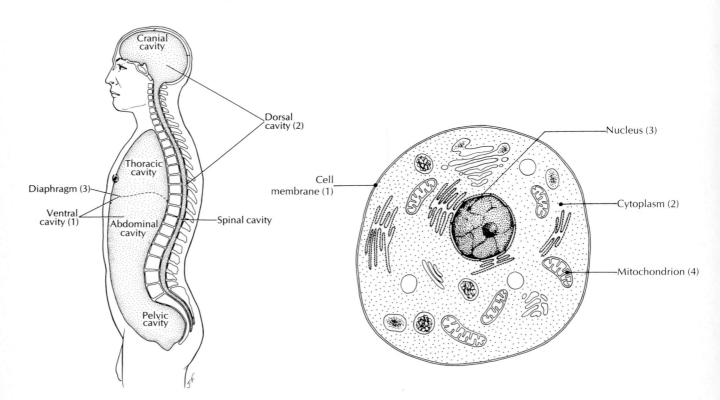

Cranial cavity

Dorsal cavity (2)

Thoracic cavity

Diaphragm (3)

Ventral cavity (1)

Abdominal cavity

Spinal cavity

Pelvic cavity

FIGURE 4-7 Ventral and dorsal cavities of the body.

Nucleus (3)

Cell membrane (1)

Cytoplasm (2)

Mitochondrion (4)

FIGURE 4-8 Typical body cell and its structures.

a Ventral cavity *(1)*. Comprises thoracic cavity and abdominopelvic cavity separated by a diaphragm *(3)*.

b Dorsal cavity *(2)*. Comprises the cranial cavity and spinal cavity.

2 Organs located within each of these cavities will be discussed as anatomic structures are presented.

3.0 CELL STRUCTURE AND FUNCTION
3.1 Structure and function of cells

1 Cells are the building blocks of the body.

2 The human body contains over 60 trillion cells, which are the fundamental units of life.

3 All cells have the same basic plan even though they are united as tissues, organs, and systems for specialized function.

4 Cellular structure includes the following (Fig. 4-8).

a Membrane *(1)*. About 3/10,000,000 of an inch thick, it surrounds the cell like a skin and determines which materials from the outside can enter into the body of the cell by allowing some to pass through the membrane while blocking others.

b Cytoplasm *(2)*. A manufacturing plant that converts materials that enter the cell into a usable form.

c Nucleus *(3)*. Through the interaction of chromosomes, genes are the control center for all processes of growth development.

d Mitochondria *(4)*. The power plants of the cell, generating the energy necessary for the cell to carry on metabolism.

5 All cells are tiny blobs of living matter called protoplasm composed primarily of carbon, oxygen, hydrogen, and nitrogen.

6 The most abundant compound found in cellular protoplasm is water.

3.2 Characteristics of cells

1 Living cells have the following characteristics.

a Irritability (respond to a stimulus)

b Conductivity (able to transmit impulses)

c Contractility (able to contract or move)

d Metabolism (it converts food to produce energy and complex compounds)

e Reproductivity (it is able to continue its existence by reproducing itself)

2 Most cells reproduce by *mitosis,* which is a simple division of the cell into two identical parts.

3 Fig. 4-9 shows the cell in various stages of mitosis. These stages include:

A Interphase. Interphase has the prefix "inter" (between), which implies that the cell has not begun mitosis (cell division).

B Prophase. The centrosome usually contains two centrioles (if there is only one, then it divides); each new centriole moves to opposite sides of the nucleus.

C Metaphase. The chromosomes rest radially on an equatorial axis across the cell between the two asters with each chromosome connected to the spindle fibers.

D Anaphase. The two halved chromosomes move apart, each toward its own pole.

E Telophase. Two independent cells begin to form as the chromosomes end their polar movement. A clear membrane begins to form around each cell. A nucleus is present in each cell and the centriole replicates. When spindle fibers between the two cells disappear and the cell membrane is complete, two daughter cells are created and mitosis is completed.

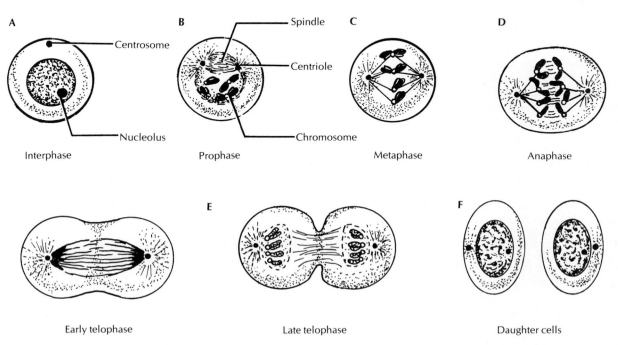

FIGURE 4-9 Cell in stages of mitosis, including **A,** interphase, **B,** prophase, **C,** metaphase, **D,** anaphase, **E,** telophase, and **F,** daughter cells.

TABLE 4-1 Metabolism

Food	Anabolism	Catabolism
Carbohydrates	Temporary excess changed into glycogen by liver cells in presence of insulin; stored in liver and skeletal muscles until needed and then changed back to glucose	Oxidized, in presence of insulin to yield energy (4.1 kcal/g) and wastes (carbon dioxide and water)
	True excess beyond body's energy requirements converted into adipose tissue; stored in various fat depots of body	$C_6H_{12}O_6 \rightarrow$ Energy + 6 CO_2 + 6 H_2O
Fat	Built into adipose tissue; stored in fat depots of body	Fatty acids $\qquad\qquad$ Glycerol
		$\downarrow$ (beta-oxidation) $\qquad$ $\downarrow$ (glycolysis)
		Acetyl-CoA $\leftrightharpoons$ Ketones $\qquad$ Acetyl-CoA
		$\downarrow$ (tissues; citric acid cycle)
		Energy (9.3 kcal/g) + CO_2 + H_2O
Proteins	Temporary excess stored in liver and skeletal muscles	Deaminated by liver forming ammonia (which is converted to urea) and keto acids (which are either oxidized or changed to glucose or fat)
	Synthesized into tissue proteins, blood proteins, enzymes, and hormones	

From Mosby's medical, nursing, and allied health dictionary, ed 3, St Louis, 1990, The CV Mosby Co.

F Daughter cells. Each daughter cell contains the same structure as the original cell and each reverts back to the pattern seen with interphase.

4 Sex cells reproduce by a process called *meiosis*, which is a reduction cell division in which the number of chromosomes is reduced. This process is not discussed here.

5 All cells have mass and are three dimensional. Cells come in various shapes and sizes.

6 Individual cells are like microscopic beings and must have food, water, and oxygen to live.

  a The combined use of these substances is a process known as metabolism.

  b The following definition of metabolism (Table 4-1) is from *Mosby's Medical, Nursing, and Allied Health Dictionary**:

The aggregate of all chemical processes that take place in living organisms, resulting in growth, generation of energy, elimination of wastes, and other bodily functions as they relate to the distribution of nutrients in the blood after digestion. Metabolism takes place in two steps: anabolism, the constructive phase, in which smaller molecules (as amino acids) are converted to larger molecules (as proteins); and catabolism, the destructive phase, in which larger molecules (as glycogen) are converted to smaller molecules (as pyruvic acid). Exercise, elevated body temperature, hormonal activity, and digestion can increase the metabolic rate, which is the rate determined when a person is at complete rest, physically and mentally. The metabolic rate is customarily expressed (in calories) as the heat liberated in the course of metabolism.

■ ■ ■

Respiratory care personnel must be aware that the maintenance of a functional tissue level of oxygen is essential to the overall process of metabolism.

In the hypoxemic patient, tissue levels of oxygen will decrease in a direct relationship to available arterial levels

of oxygen; this is a function of arterial oxygen tension Pao$_2$) and perfusion. As tissue oxygen decreases below physiologic levels, the cell changes from an aerobic to an anaerobic basis in an attempt to continue the metabolic function of the cell. This results in production of excessive carbonic acid, which, if uncorrected, can cause the cell to die. According to Haldane, a recognized physiologist, "Hypoxia not only stops the machine, it destroys the machinery."*

4.0 CELLS AND TISSUES
4.1 Tissues

1 Tissues are organizations of cells that form different structures.

2 Tissues are formed from different types of cells. The type of cell depends on the location and function of the tissue.

3 Table 4-2 shows the type, location, and function of different tissues.

5.0 BODY ORGAN SYSTEMS
5.1 Organ systems

1 An organ is a combination of different kinds of tissue that work together to perform some special function.

2 The combination of different organs to perform a complex function is called a *system*.

3 The body is composed of major body systems that come together to maintain living *homeostasis*. These systems and their functions are presented in Table 4-3.

6.0 BONES
6.1 Structure of bones

1 Bone is defined as[†]:

(1) the dense, hard, and slightly elastic connective tissue, comprising the 206 bones of the human skeleton. It is composed

---

*Mosby's medical, nursing, and allied health dictionary, ed 3, St Louis, 1990, The CV Mosby Co.

*Haldane JS: The therapeutic administration of oxygen, Br Med J 1:181, 1917.

†Mosby's medical, nursing, and allied health dictionary, ed 3, St Louis, 1990, The CV Mosby Co.

TABLE 4-2 Type, location, and function of body tissue

Tissue	Location	Function
1 EPITHELIAL		
Simple squamous	Alveoli	Diffusion of gases
	Lining of vessels	Diffusion/osmosis
Stratified squamous	Surface of mouth, upper esophagus, and skin	Protection
Simple columnar	Stomach, parts of respiratory tract	
Pseudostratified	Bronchi	
Columnar	Trachea	
2 MUSCLE		
Striated voluntary (skeletal)	Eyes, attached to bones	Movement
	Esophagus	Swallowing
Visceral involuntary	Tubular viscera of bronchioles, digestive tract, urinary tract	Movement of substances
Striated involuntary	Heart wall	Pumping (contraction)
3 CONNECTIVE		
Areolar	Between tissues, organs	Connection
Adipose	Under skin	Padding, insulation, food
Dense fibrous	Tendons, ligaments, scars, etc.	Connection
Bone	Skeleton	Support, protection, storage of minerals
Cartilage	Nasal septum	Flexible support
	Bone covering larynx, tracheal, and bronchial rings	
Myeloid	Bone marrow	Red cell production
		Leukocyte production
		Platelet production
		Connective tissue production
		Plasma production
Lymphatic	Lymph nodes, spleen	Monocytes production
	Thymus gland, tonsils	Granular lymphocytes production
		Cell production
Blood	Vessels	Mobility, protection, nourishment
Reticuloendothelial	Lining of spleen, bone marrow, liver	Phagocytosis
4 NERVE	Brain, spinal cord, nerves throughout body	Conduction of nerve impulses

of compact osseous tissue surrounding spongy cancellous tissue permeated by many blood vessels and nerves and enclosed in membranous periosteum. Long bones contain yellow marrow in longitudinal cavities and red marrow in their articular ends. Red marrow also fills the cavities of the flat and the short bones, the bodies of the vertebrae, the cranial diploe, the sternum, and the ribs. Blood cells are produced in active red marrow. Osteocytes form bone tissue in concentric rings around an intricate haversian system of interconnecting canals that accommodates blood vessels, lymphatic vessels, and nerve fibers. (2) any single element of the skeleton, as a rib, the sternum, or the femur.

2 *Connective tissue* is defined by this same source† as:

tissue that supports and binds other body tissue and parts. It derives from the mesoderm of the embryo and is dense, containing large numbers of cells and large amounts of intercellular material. The intercellular material is composed of fibers in a matrix or ground substance which may be liquid, gelatinous, or solid, as in bone and cartilage. Connective tissue fibers may be collagenous or elastic. The matrix or ground material surrounding fibers and cells is not composed of living material, as protoplasm, but is nonetheless a dynamic substance, varying with the general condition of the body, susceptible to its own special diseases, and transporting materials for metabolism, nutrition, and waste

†Mosby's medical, nursing, and allied health dictionary, ed 3, St Louis, 1990, The CV Mosby Co.

TABLE 4-3 Organ systems and related function

System	Function
1 Skeletal	Support, protection, storage of minerals
2 Muscular	Movement
3 Digestive	Reception, preparation of food
4 Circulatory	Transport of blood
5 Respiratory	Exchange of oxygen, carbon dioxide
6 Excretory	Disposal of organic wastes, and excess fluid
7 Endocrine	Regulation of internal processes, adjustment to external environment
8 Nervous and sense organs	Transmission of sensor impulses; coordination of other systems
9 Reproductive	Production of new individuals

elimination. The most common cell in connective tissue is the histiocyte or microphage. Mast cells, plasma cells, and white blood cells are also found in connective tissue throughout different parts of the body. Red blood cells are not usually found in connective tissue unless blood vessels have been injured. Kinds of connective tissue are bone, cartilage, fibrous connective tissue.

3 Bone is formed of living cells, minerals, and calcium salts.

4 Microscopically, bone is composed of less than *six* cylindrical layers of calcified matrix (lamella) like the rings seen in the formation of wood in the trunk of a tree (Fig. 4-10, *1-5*).

5 These rings *(lamella) (1)* enclose a central canal *(haversian canal) (2)* that contains a singel blood vessel.

6 The canal plus the lamella (rings) form a *haversian system (5)*.

7 Living bone cells *(osteocytes)* occupy *lacunae (4)*, which are small spaces between the lamellae.

8 Microscopic canals *(canaliculi) (3)* interconnect the bone cells with haversian canals to provide routes for fluid to reach the cells.

9 The arrangement of lamellae and the distance between haversian units determines the hardness of the bone.

10 Bones are living structures and must have an adequate blood supply to exist.

6.2 Types of bones

1 There are *four* types of bones (Fig. 4-11).

a Long bones. The femur, tibia, fibula, humerus, radius, and ulna are long bones.

b Short bones. The metacarpals, metatarsals, and phalanges are short bones.

c Flat bones. Some cranial bones, ribs, and scapulae are flat bones.

d Irregular bones. The carpals, tarsals, vertebrae, sphenoid, ethmoid (not shown), sacrum, coccyx, and mandible are irregular bones.

7.0 FACTORS DETERMINING MOVEMENTS OF BONES

7.1 Movement of bones

1 Bones that connect with other bones to form a joint are said to articulate. The articulation of a bone and connective tissue forms a joint (Fig. 4-12).

a Joint is defined as*:

Any one of the connections between bones. Each is classified according to structure and movability as fibrous, cartilaginous, or synovial. Fibrous joints are immovable, cartilaginous joints slightly movable, and synovial joints freely movable. Typical immovable joints are those connecting most of the bones of the skull with a sutural ligament. Typical slightly movable joints are those connecting the vertebrae and the pubic bones. Most of the joints in the body are freely movable and allow gliding, circumduction, rotation, and angular movement. Also called articulation.

2 Bones may be fused resulting in a solid immobile structure such as the skull.

3 The ends of bones are capped with cartilage and articulate through joints that usually are held together by bands of tough fibrous materials called *ligaments*.

4 Movement of a joint is accomplished by the contraction (flexion) and relaxation (extension) of muscles attached to the bones as levers.

---

*Mosby's medical, nursing, and allied health dictionary, ed 3, St Louis, 1990, The CV Mosby Co.

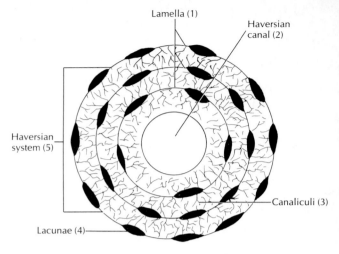

FIGURE 4-10 Microscopic structure of compact bone.

5 The direction of movement of bones is determined by the type of joint, the location and resistance of ligaments, and the location of muscles and tendons.

6 Movement of a bone (joint) beyond its stress limits or in a direction for which it was not structured will result in injury.

8.0 STRUCTURE AND FUNCTION OF BONES OF THE SKULL

8.1 Bones of the skull

1 Eight bones of the skull form a strong, rigid cranium that protects the brain from injury (Fig. 4-13).

2 The rigidity of the cranium may be hazardous in situations that may cause the brain to swell or if intracranial bleeding occurs causing compression and subsequent injury to the brain.

3 The skull is formed by:

a The cranium

b Facial bones

c Ear ossicula

4 The cranium is formed by *eight* bones, the face by *fourteen* bones, and the middle ear by *six* bones.

8.2 Major bones of the skull that form the bony prominence of the head (see Fig. 4-13)

1 The frontal bone forms the forehead.

2 The parietal bone shapes the bulging sides of the cranium.

3 The temporal bone forms the lower sides of the cranium and part of its floor.

4 The zygomatic bone forms the cheek and lateral portion of the orbits.

5 The maxilla serves as the foundation for bones of the face; forms the floor of the orbits, part of the roof of the mouth, and walls of the nose; and holds the teeth of the upper jaw.

6 The nasal bone forms the upper part of the bridge of the nose. Cartilage forms the lower part and part of the nasal septum.

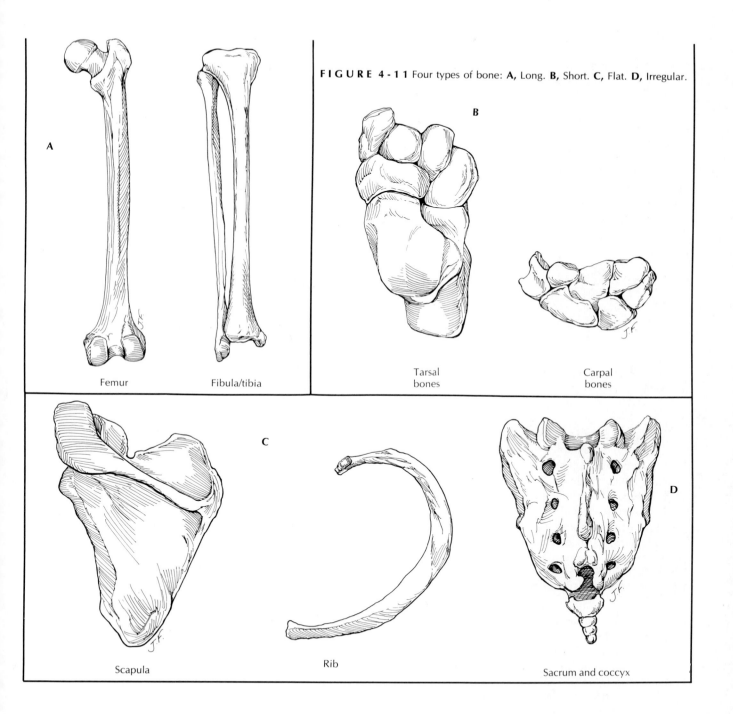

FIGURE 4-11 Four types of bone: **A,** Long. **B,** Short. **C,** Flat. **D,** Irregular.

Femur

Fibula/tibia

Tarsal
bones

Carpal
bones

Scapula

Rib

Sacrum and coccyx

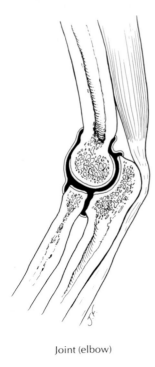

Joint (elbow)

FIGURE 4-12 Joint.

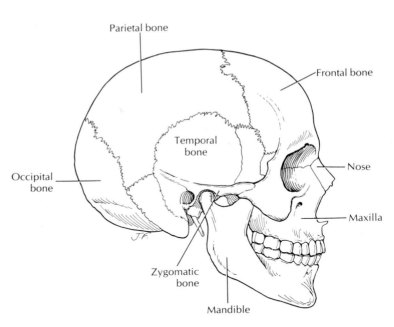

FIGURE 4-13 Bones of the skull.

7 The mandible forms the lower jaw of the face. It articulates with temporal bone and is the strongest bone of the face and the only moveable joint of the skull.

8 The occipital bone forms the lower posterior part of the skull.

8.3 Hyoid bone (Fig. 4-14)

1 The hyoid bone is a U-shaped bone located in the neck between the mandible and upper larynx.

2 It is the only nonsesamoid bone that does not articulate with another bone.

3 It is suspended by ligaments to the styloid process.

4 This bone is usually crushed if a victim is manually choked to death or strikes the steering wheel of a car with his or her neck in an accident.

9.0 THE SPINAL COLUMN

9.1 Bones of the spinal column (Fig. 4-15)

1 The spinal column is composed of 26 irregular bones *(1)* that form a hollow passageway (spinal canal) *(2)*, extending the length of the spine.

2 It extends for the length of the spine as the major supportive structure of the body and protects the spinal cord from injury.

3 The spinous processes *(3)*, which are located on the posterior aspect of the spinal column (dorsal spine), serve as a point for muscle attachment, as does the transverse process *(4)*, which is located on the lateral aspect.

4 Superiorly, the spinal column attaches to the head, forming the posterior aspect of the neck.

5 The spinal column also forms the posterior boundary of the thorax for attachment of ribs *(5)*.

6 The sacrum forms a portion of the pelvic girdle *(6)*.

7 The spine is divided into three major sections.
  a Cervical *(C1-C7)*
  b Thoracic *(T1-T12)*
  c Lumbar *(L1-L5)*

9.2 Bones of the neck

1 The neck (cervical spine) is formed by the first seven vertebrae and is numbered and referred to as *C1 through C7*.

9.3 Bones of the upper back

1 The thoracic vertebrae, which are numbered and referred to as *T1 through T12*, form the upper back and articulate with 12 pairs of ribs.

9.4 Bones of the lower back

1 The lower vertebrae, which are numbered and referred to as *L1 through L5*, form the lower back and do not articulate with any ribs.

2 The sacrum (Fig. 4-15, *7*) articulates with the pelvic girdle via the *sacroiliac* joints.

3 The coccyx *(8)* is formed by the smallest bones of the spine and is fused, in the adult, into a single structure.

■ ■ ■

As an experiment, the reader is requested to locate the seven cervical vertebrae on another person. Have the person flex his or her neck *anteriorly*. The prominent spinal bone (process) observed is C7. If two processes are seen, the superior one is C7 and the inferior one is T1. C1 through C7 are critical vertebrae in that they protect portions of the spinal cord that control breathing.

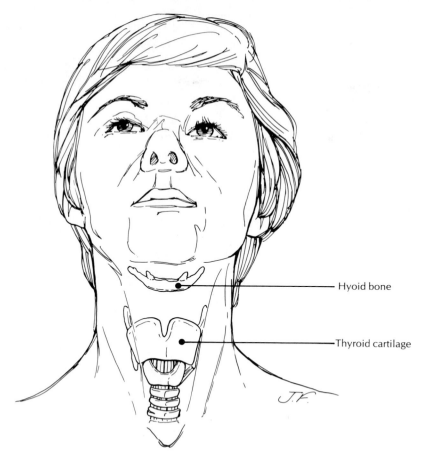

FIGURE 4-14 Hyoid bone.

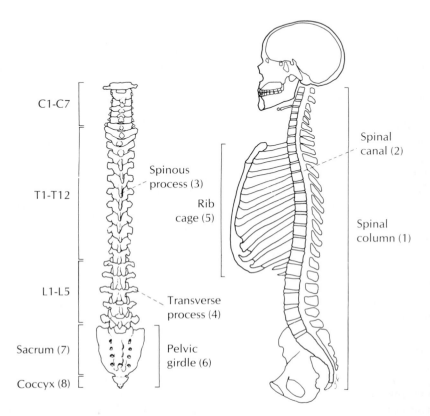

FIGURE 4-15 Bones of the spinal column.

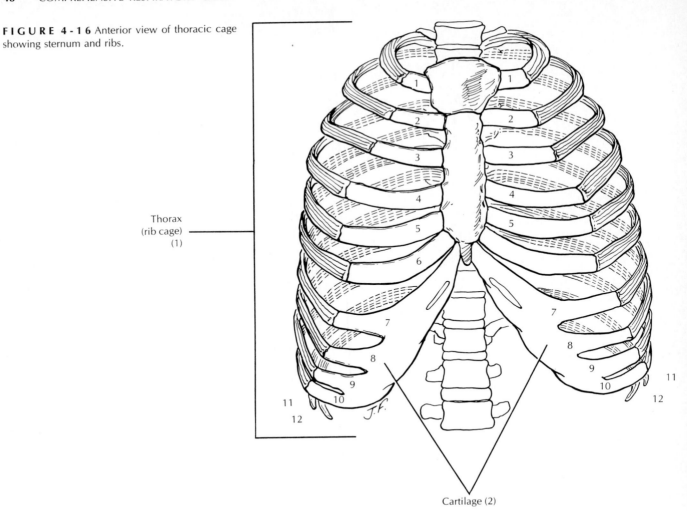

FIGURE 4-16 Anterior view of thoracic cage showing sternum and ribs.

Thorax
(rib cage)
(1)

Cartilage (2)

The diaphragm, a major muscle for breathing, is controlled by the phrenic nerve, which exits the spinal column at C3 to C5.

10.0 BONES OF THE THORAX

10.1 Bones of the thorax

1 The thorax (Fig. 4-16, *1*), or rib cage, is composed of 12 pairs of ribs and cartilages *(2)*, 12 vertebrae, and the sternum (Figs. 4-15 and 4-16).

2 Each rib articulates posteriorly with the vertebral column.

3 The cartilages with the seven upper pair of ribs articulate *directly* with the sternum and are referred to as *true ribs* (see Fig. 4-16).

4 The eighth, ninth, and tenth ribs articulate through their cartilages with the ribs above and are called *false ribs* (see Fig. 4-16).

5 The cartilages of the eleventh and twelfth ribs do not attach even indirectly to the sternum and are called *floating ribs*.

6 All ribs extend outward, forward, and downward from their attachment points with the vertebrae. This formation places the lower seven to ten ribs in a shape that can be likened to a handle that can be raised up and

down from its resting position on the side of a bucket. This movement occurs during breathing (Fig. 4-17). This action causes the chest to become larger then smaller during breathing excursions.

10.2 Sternum (chest bone)

1 The sternum begins at the *suprasternal notch* (Fig. 4-18) and forms the medial part of the chest. It is the point for direct or indirect anterior attachment of 10 ribs.

2 The sternum is dagger-shaped and divided into three bony parts (Fig. 4-19, *1-3*).

  a Manubrium. Thickest part of sternum, located between clavicular notches.

  b Body. Begins at point of attachment of second rib and continues to xiphoid-sternal junction or point of attachment for the ribs.

  c Xiphoid. Tip of the sternum, which usually calcifies during adult life and becomes brittle.

3 During external chest compression for cardiopulmonary resuscitation, the xiphoid is frequently broken and can injure underlying tissue, such as the liver and diaphragm, especially in the infant and child. For practice, the reader is requested to identify the following structures of the thorax on another person.

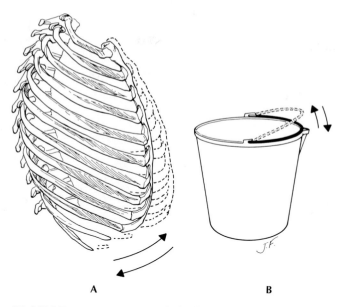

A   **B**

F I G U R E 4 - 1 7 Movement of ribs during breathing is analogous to movement of the handle of a bucket. **A,** End expiration. **B,** Inspiration.

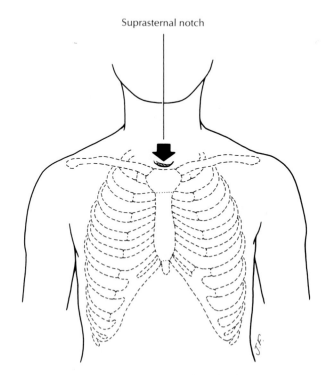

F I G U R E 4 - 1 8 Suprasternal notch of sternum.

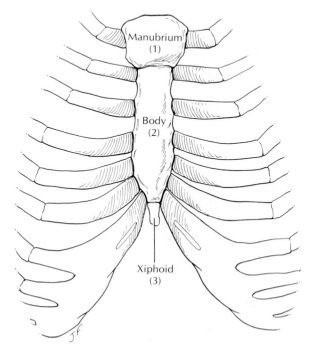

F I G U R E 4 - 1 9 Sternum showing three main parts: manubrium, body, and xiphoid.

a Suprasternal notch
b Manubrium of the sternum
c Body of the sternum
d Xiphoid process of the sternum
e Intercostal spaces

11.0 THE UPPER EXTREMITY

11.1 Structures of the upper extremity (appendicular skeleton) (Fig. 4-20, A-D)

1 The *upper extremity* consists of the shoulder girdle (Fig. 4-20, *A1*), upper arm *(4)*, lower arm *(5 and 6)*, wrist, and hand.

2 The *shoulder girdle* is a bone and muscle ring located at the upper part of the thorax. It serves as a base for attachment of the upper extremity.

3 The shoulder girdle is formed primarily of the scapula (shoulder blade) *(2)* and clavicle (collar bone) *(3)*.

4 The shoulder girdle articulates with the axial skeleton through the sternoclavicular joint between the clavicle and sternum.

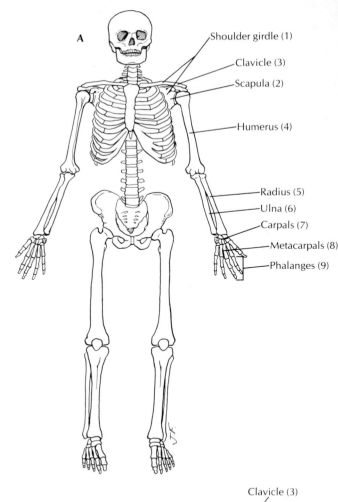

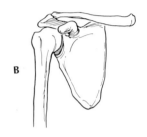

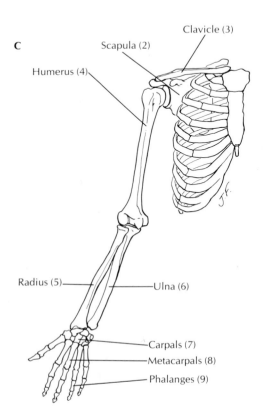

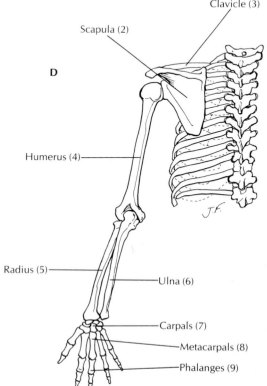

FIGURE 4-20 Bones of the upper extremity. **A,** Anterior view of skeleton, **B,** posterior view of shoulder girdle, **C,** anterior view of upper extremity, and **D,** posterior view of upper extremity.

5 The *clavicle* articulates with the scapula, which articulates with the ribs posteriorly through large muscles.

6 The upper extremity is divided into three parts (Fig. 4-20, *B-D*).

   a Arm (shoulder to elbow)

   b Forearm (elbow to wrist)

   c Hand

7 The humerus *(4)* is the only bone in the upper arm.

8 The humerus articulates proximally with the scapula *(2)* and distally with the radius *(5)* and ulna *(6)*.

9 The forearm has two bones.

   a Radius (on thumb side)

   b Ulna (on little finger side)

10 The radius and ulna articulate proximally with the humerus and distally with the wrist.

11 The hand is composed of three separate groups of bones.

   a Carpals (wrist bones) *(7)*

   b Metacarpals (hand bones) *(8)*

   c Phalanges (fingers) *(9)*

12 The hand articulates proximally with both the radius and ulna through a series of ligaments.

12.0 THE LOWER EXTREMITY
12.1 Pelvis and lower extremities (Fig. 4-21, *A* and *B*)

1 The *lower extremity* is composed of bones of the pelvis hip), thigh, lower leg, ankle, and foot.

2 The *pelvis* is a bony ring formed by the sacrum *(1)* and two *innominate* (hip) bones *(2)*.

3 Each innominate is formed of three separate bones that articulate with the sacrum.

4 The hip is adapted for great strength and support. It contains the socket of two joints that are made up of the union of the bones forming each innominate bone.

5 The lower extremity is divided into three parts.

   a Upper leg (thigh)

   b Lower leg

   c Foot

6 The thigh has only one large bone—the femur *(3)*.

7 The femur is the largest, heaviest, and strongest bone of the body.

8 The head of the femur *(4)* articulates with the hip socket proximally to form a ball and socket (acetabulum) joint.

9 Fractures of the femur are serious and may result in the formation of pulmonary emboli (blood clots that travel and lodge in the pulmonary vessels). A patient can die if these clots block major areas of the pulmonary circulation.

10 Distally the femur articulates with the lower leg, which consists of two bones.

   a The tibia (shin bone) *(5)* forms the bottom half of knee cap *(6)* and most of the proximal portion of the ankle joint.

   b The fibula *(7)* does not connect with the knee joint. It forms the lateral portion of the ankle.

11 The tibia *(5)* forms a majority of the proximal portion of the ankle joint.

12 The distal end of the fibula articulates to form the outer portion (lateral malleolus) of the ankle joint.

13 The medial malleolus (inner ankle) is the end of the tibia.

14 Ligaments connect these bones to the foot at the talus *(8)* and the calcaneus (heel bone) *(9)*.

15 Other bones of the foot include the following.

   a Tarsals (top of foot) *(10)*

   b Metatarsals (proximal joint of toes) *(11)*

   c Phalanges (distal two joints of the toes) *(12)*

■ ■ ■

Point out the location of various bones of the lower extremity on yourself and a fellow student.

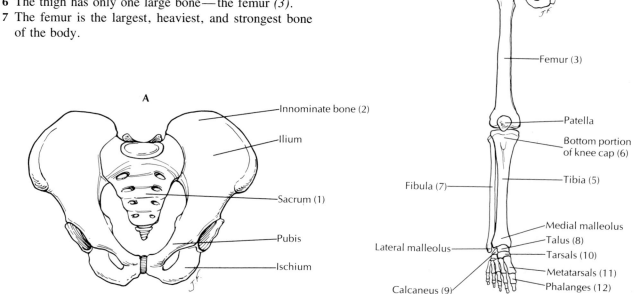

FIGURE 4-21 A, Anterior view of pelvic girdle. **B,** Anterior view of lower extremity.

13.0 MUSCLE TISSUE AND FUNCTION
13.1 Composition of muscles

1 Muscle tissue is extensible (stretches) and responds to nervous stimuli *(irritability)* by contracting to cause motion.
2 Muscle cells produce heat and are responsible for maintaining normal body temperature.
3 Microscopically, muscle cells are long and narrow and are called *muscle fibers.*
4 Muscle cells, like all cells, must have a blood supply for nourishment and gas exchange and nerves to carry action signals from the brain.
5 Muscle tissue is composed of many types of cells among which are *myofibrils* (Fig. 4-22, *1*).
6 Myofibrils run lengthwise through the muscle fiber (cell) and give it alternating light and dark stripes or striations *(2)*.
7 Another name for skeletal muscle is striated or voluntary muscle (Fig. 4-23, *A*).
8 Smooth muscle is made up of spindle-shaped cells each with a single nucleus. This type of muscle is capable of independent or involuntary contraction and is found in the walls of organs, blood vessels, and tracheobronchial tubes (Fig. 4-23, *B*).
9 Cardiac muscle is another type of involuntary muscle unique to the heart. This muscle has striations and central nuclei each capable of independent action (Fig. 4-23, *C*).

13.2 Functions of the muscles

1 Muscles perform two major functions.
  a Contraction
  b Maintenance of posture and production of body heat
2 Functionally, there are two different types of muscles.
  a Voluntary. Muscles that act under conscious will, are attached to bones, and compose a majority of the skeletal muscle.
  b Involuntary. Muscles that act without the conscious will of the individual. These muscles serve all the internal organs and blood vessels except the heart.

14.0 MUSCLE ACTIONS
14.1 Muscle mass

1 The musculoskeletal system is composed of more than 200 voluntary (striated) muscles contributing the principle means of movement.
2 Muscle *mass* accounts for approximately 40% of the weight of an adult.

14.2 Directions of muscle movement

NOTE: Figures illustrating the directions of muscle movement are included in Module Five.
1 Flexion. Bending of joint to approximate the bone it connects.
2 Extension. Straightening a limb.
3 Abduction. Movement of a limb away from the midline of the body or its parts.
4 Adduction. Movement of a limb toward the central axis of the body.
5 Circumduction. Movement of a body part in a circular motion.
6 Internal rotation. Turning of body part inward toward the central axis of the body.
7 Muscles that cause these actions to occur and are named according to the action (e.g., flexors, abductors).

15.0 MUSCLES OF INSPIRATION DURING QUIET, DEEP, AND LABORED BREATHING
15.1 Muscles of inspiration

1 *The diaphragm*
  a The diaphragm is a gentle curving muscle sheet that forms the bottom of the thoracic cavity and separates it from the abdomen (Fig. 4-24). Its structure is such that it is divided into two hemidiaphragms. Although these hemidiaphragms usually work together, under certain conditions one hemisphere (side) may work in opposition to the other.
  b It is attached peripherally to the lateral walls of the thorax causing it to become a closed chamber.
  c It is the principle muscle of inspiration and accounts for 70% of a tidal breath.
  d Contraction of this muscle causes the central tendon domes of the diaphragm to descend (become flattened), increasing the vertical volume of the rib cage.
  e Descent of the diaphragm only 1 cm increases thoracic volume by approximately 270 ml.
  f Descent of the diaphragm 2.5 cm increases the thoracic volume by 700 ml.
  g Fig. 4-25, *A* and *B,* illustrates the proper anatomic position for performing diaphragmatic breathing.
    • Lie on back.
    • Rest left hand across chest *(1)* and right hand on abdomen *(2)*.
    • Inhale deeply through the nose, and let the abdomen rise, raising the hand placed on the abdomen *(3)*.
    • As the abdomen rises, the diaphragm should descend. This increases the size of the thorax and lowers the intrathoracic pressure, causing air to flow into the lungs.
2 *External intercostal muscle* (Fig. 4-26)
  a One of the principle muscles of deep inspiration. It originates from the lower border of the rib above and inserts into the upper border of the rib below.
  b It stretches from the tubercle of the rib to the junction of the rib and costal cartilage.
  c Its fibers pass in a downward and forward direction.
  d The muscle is innervated by the intercostal nerve.
  e Contraction of these muscles results in the ribs being lifted upward and outward, increasing the anteroposterior diameter of the chest.
3 *Pectoralis major* (see Fig. 4-26)
  Deep inspiration.
  a Originates at the medial clavicle and lateral sternum to the seventh costal cartilages.
  b Inserts at crest of the greater tubercle of the humerus.

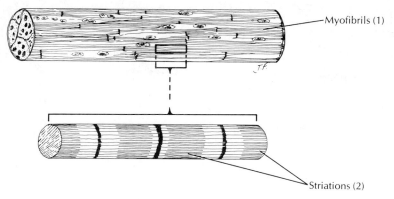

Myofibrils (1)

Striations (2)

FIGURE 4-22 Myofibrils.

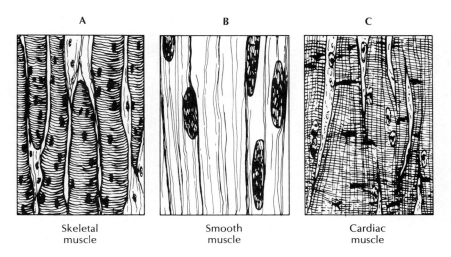

A B C

Skeletal muscle

Smooth muscle

Cardiac muscle

FIGURE 4-23 Cardiac muscle fibers. A, Skeletal muscle, B, smooth muscle, and C, cardiac muscle.

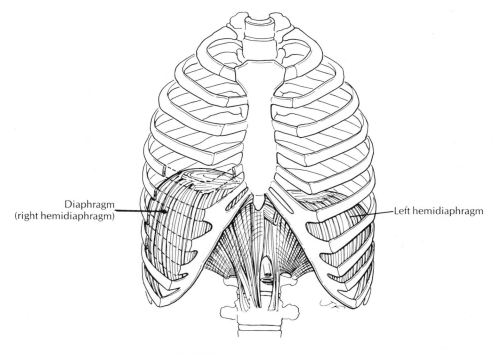

Diaphragm (right hemidiaphragm)

Left hemidiaphragm

FIGURE 4-24 Diaphragm.

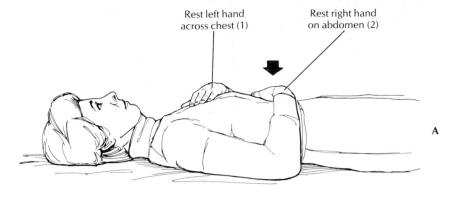

Rest left hand across chest (1)

Rest right hand on abdomen (2)

A

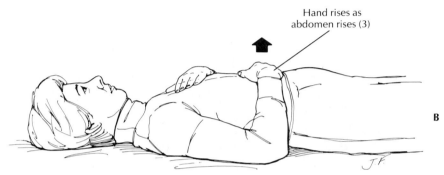

Hand rises as abdomen rises (3)

B

FIGURE 4-25 Proper position for practicing diaphragmatic breathing.

c When the hands are fixed, the pectoralis major is used to raise the chest during inspiration.

4 *Serratus posterior superior* (Fig. 4-27, *A*)
Deep inspiration

a A thin muscle located at the dorsal and cranial part of the thorax.

b It originates from the caudal part of the ligaments nuchae, supraspinal ligament, and spines of vertebrae C7 through T3 superior to the serratus posterior inferior muscle.

c Its insertion begins on upper border of the second through fifth ribs.

d Its action is to raise the ribs during deep respiration.

5 *Levator scapulae* (see Fig. 4-27, *A*)
Deep inspiration

a Located on the dorsal and lateral aspect of the neck.

b It originates from the transverse processes of the atlas and axis and from the transverse processes of C3 and C4.

c It inserts into vertebral border of the scapula and allows the scapula to be fixed causing the upper chest to rise during inspiration.

6 *Sternocleidomastoid* (see Fig. 4-26)
Labored inspiration

a Each sternocleidomastoid muscle extends from the upper sternum and proximal portion of the clavicle to the mastoid process behind the ear.

b These muscles are involved in turning the head, and

they are used in helping to lift the upper chest during labored inspiration.

7 *Levatores costarum* (see Fig. 4-27, *B*)
Labored inspiration

a Twelve small tendons that arise from the ends of the transverse process of C7 and T1 through T11.

b These tendons pass obliquely downward and laterally and are inserted into the outer surface of the rib immediately adjacent to vertebra of its origin.

c Contraction of the levatores costarum increases the volume of the thoracic cage during inspiration.

d Action is to raise the ribs during inspiration.

8 *Pectoralis minor* (see Fig. 4-26)
Labored inspiration

a Originates at upper outer surface of the third through fifth ribs.

b Inserts at coracoid process of the scapula.

c Used to raise ribs of upper chest during labored inspiration.

9 *Trapezius* (see Fig. 4-27, *A*)
Labored inspiration

a Flat triangular muscle that covers upper back and neck.

b It extends from the occipital bone of the skull to the seventh cervical vertebra and to all thoracic vertebrae to the clavicle and spine of the scapula.

c Trapezius muscles are used on shrugging the shoulders, pulling the scapulae downward, drawing the

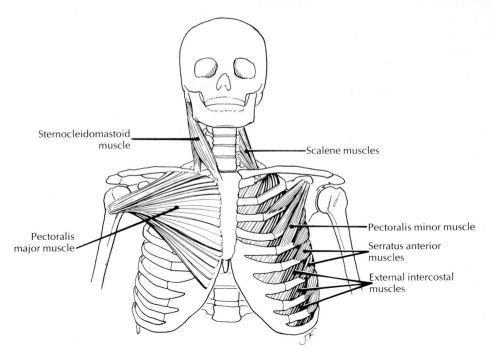

Sternocleidomastoid muscle

Scalene muscles

Pectoralis major muscle

Pectoralis minor muscle

Serratus anterior muscles

External intercostal muscles

FIGURE 4-26 Muscles of inspiration showing pectoralis major, sternocleidomastoid, and external intercostals.

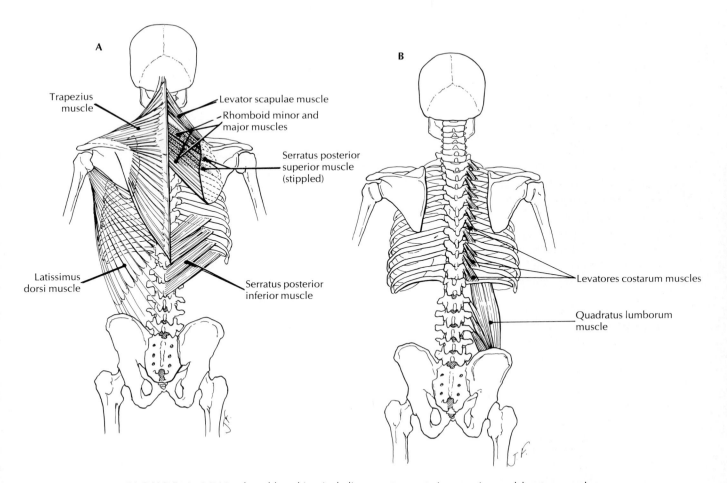

A

Trapezius muscle

Levator scapulae muscle

Rhomboid minor and major muscles

Serratus posterior superior muscle (stippled)

Latissimus dorsi muscle

Serratus posterior inferior muscle

B

Levatores costarum muscles

Quadratus lumborum muscle

FIGURE 4-27 Muscles of breathing including serratus posterior superior, and levator scapulae, trapezius, rhomboid major, rhomboid minor, quadratus lumborum, and serratus posterior inferior.

head from side to side, and lifting the upper chest during forced inspiration.

10 *Rhomboid major* (see Fig. 4-27, *A*)

Labored inspiration

a Arises from the spinous processes of T2 through T5 and supraspinal ligament.

b It inserts into the root of the spine of the scapula.

c When contracted, it raises and fixes the scapula so that pectoral and serratus muscles can raise the ribs.

11 *Rhomoid minor* (see Fig. 4-27, *A*)

Labored inspiration

a Arises from inferior part of ligamentum nuchae and from spinous processes of C7 and T1.

b It also inserts into the root of the spine of the scapulae and allows the scapula to be fixed so that pectoral and serratus muscles can raise the ribs.

12 *Serratus anterior muscle* (see Fig. 4-26)

Labored inspiration

a Originates from outer surfaces and superior borders of upper 8th or 9th rib.

b Inserts into the anterior surface ventricle border of the scapula.

c Its function during inspiration is to pull the shoulder forward—abducts and rotates it upward lifting the superior aspects of the chest.

13 *Scalene muscles* (anterior, medial, posterior) (see Fig. 4-26)

Labored inspiration

a Originate at transverse processes of 2nd to 7th cervical vertebrae.

b Insert at the first two ribs.

c Their function is to raise the first two ribs during labored or deep inspiration.

16.0 MUSCLES OF EXHALATION DURING QUIET, DEEP, AND LABORED BREATHING

16.1 Muscles of exhalation

1 *Abdominal muscles*

a Primary muscles of forced exhalation.

b Includes the external oblique, internal oblique, transversus abdominis.

c Contraction of the obliques increases the intraabdominal pressure forcing the diaphragm upward during a forced exhalation.

d External oblique originates at the lower eight ribs and inserts at the iliac crest and pubis.

e Internal oblique originates at the iliac crest and inguinal ligament and inserts at the lower three ribs.

2 *Internal intercostal muscles* (Fig. 4-28)

Forced exhalation

a Eleven pairs originate from inner surface of the rib and insert into the upper border of the rib below.

b Muscles extend from the sternum to the angles of the rib.

c Action is to lower ribs to compress the thoracic cavity and cause forced expiration.

3 *Quadratus lumborum* (see Fig. 4-27, *B*)

Forced exhalation

a Arises from the iliolumbar ligament and the adjacent portion of iliac crest.

b It inserts into the last rib and into the apices of the transverse process of L1 through L5.

c This muscle fixes the last two ribs during forced exhalation.

4 *Serratus posterior inferior* (see Fig. 4-27, *A*)

Forced exhalation

a A thin muscle located on dorsum of lower thorax.

b Its origin is from the supraspinal ligament and spines of vertebrae T11 through L3.

c Its insertion is on the lower border of the ninth to twelfth ribs lateral to the angles.

d Its action is to lower the ribs during forced exhalation.

16.2 Summary of thoracic structure and movement

1 The shape of the ribs is such that the curve of each rib is greater than the one above it.

2 When the ribs are lifted upward by muscle contraction, the diameter of the chest is increased, resulting in increased volume and decreased pressure in the lung.

3 The first and second rib can be fixed and act as a fulcrum with the sternum so that the entire rib cage lifts upward and outward in forced inspirations.

16.3 Summary of muscles of ventilation

1 Quiet ventilation

a Inspiration. Contraction of diaphragm increases horizontal diameter of the thorax, decreasing intrathoracic pressures.

• External intercostals (third through tenth ribs) raise ribs.

b Exhalation. Exhalation is passive.

2 Deep respiration

a Inspiration. External intercostal, scalene, sternocleidomastoid, levator costarum, serratus anterior, and serratus posterior muscles raise ribs.

b Exhalation. Exhalation is passive.

3 Labored respiration

a Inspiration. All muscles for deep respiration raise ribs.

• The scapulae are *fixed* by contraction of the leavator scapulae, trapezius, and rhomboids so that the pectoral muscles can raise the ribs.

b Exhalation. Exhalation is active and involves quadratus lumborum, internal intercostals, subcostals, transverse thoracic, and serratus posterior inferior muscles, as well as contraction of abdominal muscles to increase intraabdominal pressure and force the diaphragm upward, causing chest volume to be decreased and pressure to be increased.

16.4 Respiratory muscles and related action

As an exercise, the reader is encouraged to observe himself or herself breathing in front of a mirror. Point out various muscles of inspiration and exhalation during simu-

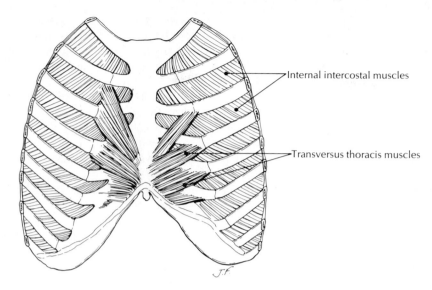

Internal intercostal muscles

Transversus thoracis muscles

FIGURE 4-28 Internal intercostal muscles.

lated breathing patterns (e.g., quiet, deep, labored-forced).

17.0 ROLE OF BLOOD

17.1 The circulatory system

1 Ever since its discovery by William Harvey (1578-1657), circulation has been of great interest to scientists and lay people alike.
2 The circulatory system comprises the heart (pump) and some 60,000 miles of interconnecting tubing (vessels) that carry blood away from and toward the heart.
3 Before studying the structures of the circulatory system, one must understand the fluid itself.

17.2 Blood as a fluid

1 Blood is the transit system of the body.
2 It carries nutrients, oxygen, special cells, and chemicals to the cells, and it carries waste by-products of cellular metabolism away from the cell.
3 Without blood and its constitutents, the cells will quickly die.
4 Blood cells are constantly being produced. It is estimated that in the average adult 8 million cells die every second. These are replaced by new cells, which are produced in the bone marrow, lymph glands, and lymphoid tissues of the tonsils, spleen, thymus, and intestine.
5 Oxygenated blood is bright red and opaque and is 3 to 4 times more viscous (thicker) than water.
6 Viscosity of blood is an extremely important factor in circulation through the many vessels of the system.
7 In the human adult, the total blood volume is approximately 5000 ml or 71.4 ml of blood per kilogram of body weight.

18.0 CONSTITUENTS OF THE BLOOD

18.1 Structure and function of red cells

1 Red cells are referred to as *erythrocytes*.
2 Erythrocytes are biconcave disks of about 7.6 mi-

crometers (μm) in diameter and a thickness of approximately 2.2 μm. About 3000 red cells could be placed side by side in a 1 inch space.
3 Mature cells found in the bloodstream *do not* contain a nucleus. They live for approximately 4 months.
4 There are approximately 25×10^{12} erythrocytes in the total circulatory system. Red cells outnumber white cells by 700 to 1.
5 The function of erythrocytes is primarily to transport *oxygen to* and *carbon dioxide away from* the tissue cells of the body.
6 Originally, erythrocytes were counted using a hemocytometer, a device that allowed red cells to be separated from the blood plasma. Now the red cells are counted following packing by centrifuge.
7 The ratio of the number of red cells to the volume of plasma is the hematocrit. In an adult male the average hematocrit is (47 $\pm$ 7). For an adult female it is (42 $\pm$ 5). Bleeding or any situation that results in a decrease in the number of erythrocytes will cause a *decreased hematocrit*.

18.2 Structure and function of hemoglobin

1 Erythrocytes are composed primarily of hemoglobin (Hb).
2 Hemoglobin is a substance that is synthesized from acetic acid and glycine into a final compound composed of one protein molecule (globin) combined with four molecules of a pigmented compound (heme).
3 Each molecule of heme contains one atom of iron, which results in one Hb molecule having four iron atoms.
4 This structural fact enables one Hb to combine with four oxygen (O_2) molecules to form *oxyhemoglobin* (HbO_2), a reversible reaction.
5 Hemoglobin can also combine with carbon dioxide to form *carbaminohemoglobin,* a reversible reaction. In this reaction, the globin structure makes the combina-

tion possible rather than the heme structure as with oxygen.

6 One gram of Hb can combine with 1.34 ml of oxygen to form HbO_2.

7 The amount of hemoglobin in an adult will vary slightly between a male and a female.

8 In a male, 100 ml of blood will contain 13 to 16 g of hemoglobin. In a female, 100 ml of blood will contain 12 to 14 g of hemoglobin.

9 Any adult with an Hb of less than 12 g/100 ml of blood is *anemic*.

10 Normal disintegration of erythrocytes results in the release of iron molecules. Some are excreted and others are used in the formation of new hemoglobin. The remainder become *biliverdin* and *bilirubin,* which is removed from the blood by the liver and placed into *bile,* which enters the gut and is excreted in feces.

18.3 Structure and function of white cells

1 White cells are called *leukocytes* and are the major defense mechanisms of the body.

2 Leukocytes differ in shape and size from erythrocytes in that they are larger (up to 25 μm) and have nuclei.

3 The normal leukocyte count in a cubic millimeter of blood is 5000 to 10,000 with an average of 7500.

4 There are five types of leukocytes that constitute the total count by percent.
  a Neutrophils = 59%
  b Lymphocytes = 34%
  c Monocytes = 4.0%
  d Eosinophils = 2.5%
  e Basophils = 0.5%

5 *Neutrophils, eosinophils,* and *basophils* are produced in bone marrow.

6 *Lymphocytes* and *monocytes* are formed in the spleen, lymph nodes, and tonsils.

7 The most important function of neutrophils and monocytes is to combat infection by *phagocytosis* (eating foreign substances that invade the body). Once this occurs the leukocytes die, and their remains are seen as pus.

8 Lymphocytes participate in the development of the immunomechanism of the body.

9 Infection causes *leukopoiesis* (formation of white cells), so that within a few hours the white blood cell count may be increased 10% to 20%.

18.4 Structure and function of platelets

1 Platelets are very small structures without a nucleus; they look very much like small plates.

2 The normal platelet count is 250,000 to 500,000 with the average being 300,000 per cubic millimeter of blood.

3 Platelets contain thromboplastin and serotonin both of which are active in the clotting of blood.

4 Platelets are formed in the red blood marrow through fragmentation of very large cells and have a life span of approximately 1 week.

5 When platelets touch the roughened surface of a torn blood vessel, they burst apart, releasing chemicals that cause the formation of fibers that seal the hole by enmeshing red cells and forming a clot.

18.5 Structure and function of plasma

1 Plasma is the fluid portion of the blood.

2 It normally composes 59% to 60% of the total blood volume.

3 Plasma is straw-colored and is composed of 91% water and 9% solids.

4 Protein is the major solid in plasma. Potassium, sodium and chloride ions, iron, and cholesterol compose most of the remaining volume.

5 There are three types of protein in plasma.
  a Albumin, 4.2 g/ml
  b Globulin, 2.5 g/100 ml
  c Fibrinogen, 0.3 g/100 ml

6 The total protein content of blood determines its osmotic pressure and viscosity.

7 Other components in plasma besides ions include glucose, amino acids, lipids, urea, uric acid, creatinine, lactic acid, hormones, enzymes, oxygen, and carbon dioxide.

8 Solutes in plasma less than 1 nanometer (nm) in diameter are called crystalloids (e.g., ions and glucose).

9 Solutes 1 to 100 nanometers in diameter are called colloids (proteins of all types).

10 The maintenance of a proper distribution of plasma components determines the movement of substances in and out of the cell by osmosis.

19.0 ABNORMALITIES OF THE BLOOD
19.1 Abnormal conditions of the blood

1 An adult who has more than 17 g of hemoglobin per 100 ml of blood is *polycythemic*.

2 Anemia is not desirable, because a patient's blood may not be able to carry enough oxygen to the tissues; this results in cellular hypoxia.

3 Polycythemia is also undesirable, because the viscosity of the blood becomes so great that it may increase the work load on the heart and result in decreased blood flow (cardiac output); this also results in cellular hypoxia.

4 Erythrocytes are destroyed when they are placed in a hypotonic solution or are exposed to a hypotonic solution, for example, distilled water. The red blood cell swells until osmotic pressure ruptures the cell wall, liberating hemoglobin. This release of hemoglobin into the plasma is called *hemolysis*. For this reason, it is necessary to make certain that all solutions given intravenously are isotonic to blood plasma.

20.0 THE LYMPHATIC SYSTEM
20.1 Anatomy of lymphatic system (Fig. 4-29)

1 Lymphatics are a network of small vessels that begin as small tubes like capillaries and merge into larger vessels. This network of vessels is spread throughout

the body in a pattern closely resembling the venous system (Fig. 4-29, *1*).

2 Lymph vessels connect with lymph nodes (Fig. 4-29, *2*), which serve as filtering devices for removing bacteria and other foreign matter.

3 Lymph is a fluid that enters the lymphatic system.

4 Lymph serves the circulatory system by acting as a bridge across which oxygen, nutrients, and waste products pass between the body capillaries and cells and by removing proteins and other substances that have leaked or been forced from capillaries as a result of trauma, hypoxemia, and excessive pressure.

5 Fluid that has been forced out of capillaries can be reabsorbed by osmosis. Proteins are too large and accumulate in tissue spaces. Lymphatics remove this protein by transporting it to large ducts into veins, which empty it into the heart and general circulation.

21.0 ANATOMY AND FUNCTION OF MAJOR STRUCTURES OF THE HEART
21.1 Structure and function of the heart

1 The cardiovascular system is composed of a dual-action pump (pumps to and from) and a complex arrangement of conduits (vessels) that pump blood through two interconnected vascular systems.

a The *systemic system* consists of all the vessels of the body except for the pulmonary vessels serving the lungs.

b The pulmonary system (Fig. 4-30) is formed by the pulmonary artery, the pulmonary vein, and all the vessels surrounding the alveoli in the lung. It is differentiated from the systemic circulation because of structural differences that cause blood flowing through it to be at one-sixth the pressure of the systemic pressure.

2 The adult heart, Fig. 4-31, *A*, is a hollow muscular organ weighing about 350 g. It is about the size of an adult's clenched fist.

3 The heart is divided into left *(1)* and right *(2)* sides by a septum wall *(3)*.

4 Each side is further divided into an upper chamber (atrium) *(4)*, which receives blood, and a lower chamber (ventricle) *(5)*, which pumps blood away from the heart.

5 Because of the lower pumping pressure, the walls of the right side of the heart are thinner than those of the left side.

6 There are four valves in the heart. These valves open and close with the heartbeat, causing the blood to flow only in one direction.

a The *tricuspid valve (6)* is located between the right atrium and ventricle.

b The *pulmonary valve (7)* is located between the right ventricle and pulmonary artery *(8)*.

c The *mitral valve (9)* is located between the left atrium and ventricle.

d The *aortic valve (10)* is located between the left ventricle and aorta *(11)*.

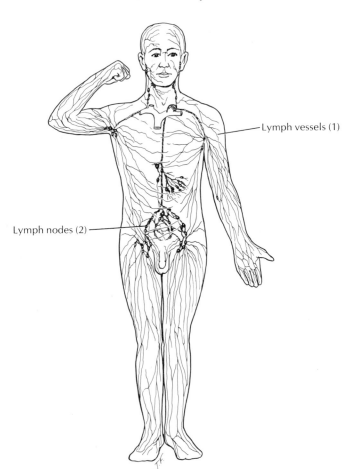

Lymph vessels (1)

Lymph nodes (2)

FIGURE 4-29 Lymphatic system showing lymph vessels and lymph nodes.

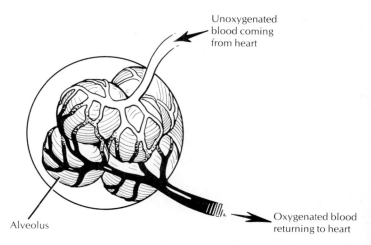

Unoxygenated blood coming from heart

Oxygenated blood returning to heart

Alveolus

FIGURE 4-30 Pulmonary vascular system.

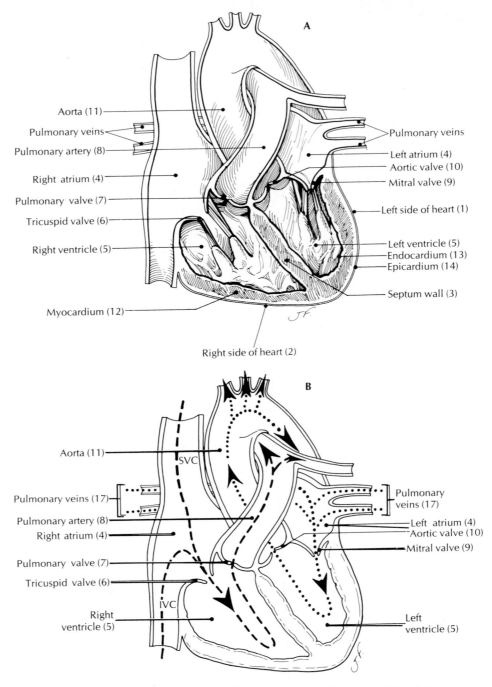

Aorta (11)
Pulmonary veins
Pulmonary artery (8)
Right atrium (4)
Pulmonary valve (7)
Tricuspid valve (6)
Right ventricle (5)
Myocardium (12)

Pulmonary veins
Left atrium (4)
Aortic valve (10)
Mitral valve (9)
Left side of heart (1)
Left ventricle (5)
Endocardium (13)
Epicardium (14)
Septum wall (3)

Right side of heart (2)

Aorta (11)
SVC
Pulmonary veins (17)
Pulmonary artery (8)
Right atrium (4)
Pulmonary valve (7)
Tricuspid valve (6)
IVC
Right ventricle (5)

Pulmonary veins (17)
Left atrium (4)
Aortic valve (10)
Mitral valve (9)
Left ventricle (5)

FIGURE 4-31 A, Internal anatomy of adult human heart. **B,** Sequence of blood flow through heart.

7 All valves have three leaflets with the exception of the mitral valve, which has two. It is also known as the bicuspid valve.

8 The total mass of heart muscle is called the *myocardium (12)* (cardiac muscle). The inner surface of the myocardium is called *endocardium (13)*. A slick, thin layer of tissue called the epicardium *(14)* covers the outer surface of the myocardium so that a very small space containing lubricating fluid between allows the heart muscle to move with minimum friction during heartbeats.

22.0 DYNAMICS OF THE HEART
22.1 Dynamics of the heartbeat

1 The heart beats steadily day and night for 60 to 70 years in most people.

2 Each day it pushes the body's 5 to 6 liters (L) of blood through more than 1000 complete circuits for a total pumping of 5000 to 6000 L of blood each day.

3 Cardiac muscle, unlike skeletal muscle, has the inherent property of *rhythmic* contraction completely independent of any innvervation.

4 There are two phases to a heartbeat.

   a The contraction phase called *systole.*

   b The relaxation phase called *diastole.*

5 Blood flows into and out of the heart in conjunction with these beats.

6 A complete heartbeat (cardiac cycle) is the contraction (systole) and relaxation (diastole) of both atria and of both ventricles.

7 The sequence for a heartbeat involves the following.

   a The simultaneous contraction of both atria and then relaxation.

   b Followed immediately by the contraction of both ventricles and then relaxation.

8 One action flows into another as the electrical impulse causing contraction spreads over the surface of the heart.

9 During diastole, blood flows into all chambers.

10 During systole, blood is pumped from all chambers.

22.2 Blood flow through the heart

1 Blood flows through the heart in the following sequence (Fig. 4-31, *B*).

   a The right atrium *(4)* receives blood from the superior vena cava (SVC) and inferior vena cava (IVC) and from the wall of the heart via coronary sinus and small veins called *venae cordis minimae.* About 70% of this blood flows directly into the ventricles before the atria contract. Any blood remaining is pushed with the contraction of the atrium *(4)* through the tricuspid valve *(6)* and into the right ventricle *(5).*

   b The right ventricle then contracts to propel venous blood to the lungs through the pulmonary valve *(7)* to the pulmonary artery *(8),* which divides into right and left branches (one to each lung).

   c Oxygenated blood returns to the left atrium via the right and left pulmonary veins (two from each lung) *(17).*

   d The left atrium *(4)* receives this blood. As described in *1a* for the right atrium, a large percentage of the blood flows directly into the left ventricle. Any remaining is pumped into the left ventricle *(5)* by way of the mitral valve *(9).*

   e The left ventricle pumps this blood to all parts of the body by way of the aortic valve *(10)* and the aorta *(11).*

   f During diastole blood from the veins enters the atria once again, as previously described, and this cardiac cycle begins anew.

23.0 IDENTIFYING HEART SOUNDS
23.1 Origin of heart sounds

1 The pressure within any chamber represents a ratio between the size of the chamber and the volume of fluid forced into it (Boyle's law).

2 If fluid does not fill the chamber, there is no pressure.

3 Pressure inside the chamber will vary since the size of the chamber becomes larger and smaller during systole and diastole.

4 During diastole, blood flows into the ventricles. This blood is squeezed out during systole.

5 Movement of the valves and blood flowing causes sounds that can be heard with the aid of a stethoscope.

6 Usually, without amplication, two sounds are heard:

   a The onset of systole (closing of atrioventricular valves)

   b Opening of aorta, and pulmonary valves with vibration of ventricles and major vessels

   c Vibration of ventricle walls

24.0 CARDIAC PUMPING ACTION AND CARDIAC OUTPUT
24.1 Cardiac blood flow

1 *Cardiac output* (CO) is the quantity of blood ejected from the heart each minute.

2 Cardiac output depends on:

   a The amount of blood that enters the ventricle during diastole.

   b The force of contraction.

   c The heart rate.

3 In adults, the stroke volume (blood ejected by one side of the heart per beat) is approximately 75 ml and a normal adult heart rate is 70 $\times$ min (stroke volume $\times$ Heart rate = Cardiac output).

4 Normal cardiac output is 5 to 6 L/min.

5 Factors that alter a normal cardiac output are:

   a Heart rate. As the heart rate exceeds 150 beats/min, the filling time is encroached upon and cardiac output begins to drop. At 200 beats/min cardiac output is seriously decreased.

   b Exercise. Increased venous pressure, heart rate; decreased peripheral resistance.

   c Sleep. Cardiac output decreases with demands.

6 *Cardiac index* (CI). Cardiac output varies with body surface area. To compare cardiac output values, one should divide cardiac output (liters) by the body surface area of the patient (square meters). The surface area for an average adult is 1.7 square meters and the cardiac index is 3.34 L/min/m^2.

25.0 ADEQUACY OF BLOOD PRESSURE BASED ON NORMS AND PULSE VARIABLES FOR ADULTS
25.1 Blood pressure (BP)

1 Circulation of blood involves an interrelationship between:

   a Cardiac output. The greater the cardiac output, the greater the pressure.

   b Velocity of blood flow. The more forceful the contraction during systole the greater the BP.

   c Inside diameter of the blood vessels. An application of *Poiseuille's law:* the smaller the inside diameter of a vessel, the greater the pressure needed to pump blood through it.

   d Resistance to flow. Another application of Poiseuille's law: the longer the tube, the greater the pressure required to pump blood through it.

   e Distensibility and elasticity of vessels. A distensible

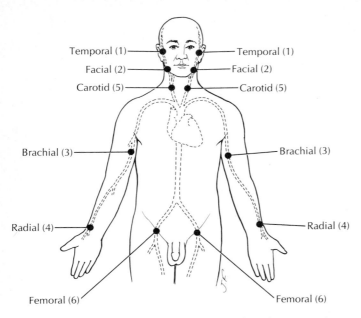

Temporal (1) — Temporal (1)
Facial (2) — Facial (2)
Carotid (5) — Carotid (5)

Brachial (3) — Brachial (3)

Radial (4) — Radial (4)

Femoral (6) — Femoral (6)

F I G U R E 4 - 3 2 Primary pressure points for palpating a pulse.

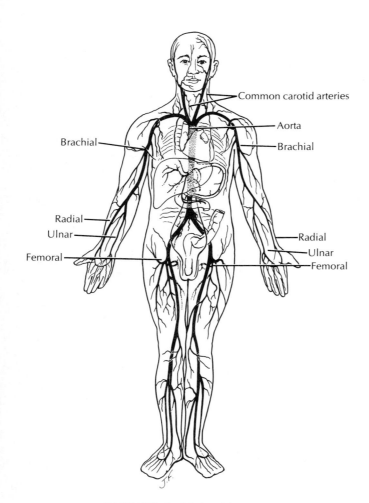

Common carotid arteries
Aorta
Brachial — Brachial
Radial — Radial
Ulnar — Ulnar
Femoral — Femoral

F I G U R E 4 - 3 3 Arterial system.

tube requires a higher stroke volume than a rigid tube.

    f Blood viscosity and volume. A blood volume must be maintained if the ventricles are to be filled and emptied in response to body demands. An increased viscosity will increase blood pressure.

2 During systole, the aortic BP rises during the rapid ejection phase and falls during the reduced ejection phase.

3 The peak pressure heard is systolic BP. The lowest aortic pressure is recorded just before the aortic valve opens and is called the diastolic pressure.

4 Average BP for a young adult is 120/75 to 80 mm Hg.

25.2 Pulse pressure

1 The difference between systolic and diastolic pressure is the *pulse pressure*. This pressure is indicative of the tone of the arterial walls.

2 A systolic BP of less than 80 mm Hg is called *shock*.

3 A normal pulse pressure is approximately 40 mm Hg, e.g., 120 mm Hg − 80 mm Hg = 40 mm Hg.

4 Abnormal pulse pressures can indicate:

    a Aortic stenosis. Pulse pressure is decreased.

    b Aortic regurgitation. Pulse pressure is increased.

    c Arteriosclerosis. Pulse pressure is increased.

    d Circulatory shock. Pulse pressure is low as a result of volume loss; pulse pressure is elevated as a result of vasodilation of blood vessels.

5 Pulse pressure is actually a wave that is generated as the aorta is distended during systole and contracts during diastole. The frequency and force of the wave can be directly related to the cardiac cycle. This wave is transmitted by blood vessels at a speed greater than blood flow. It is the pulsations created by this wave that are counted at pressure points on various parts of the body. The primary pressure (pulse) points, which are shown in Fig. 4-32, are the temporal *(1)*, facial *(2)*, brachial *(3)*, radial *(4)*, carotid *(5)*, and the femoral *(6)* points.

26.0 ARTERIES, VEINS, AND CAPILLARIES
26.1 Vessels of the circulatory system

1 There are three kinds of blood vessels that compose the circulatory system.

    a Arteries (Fig. 4-33). All arteries, with the exception of the pulmonary artery, carry *oxygenated* blood away from the heart. The pulmonary artery carries venous (unoxygenated) blood from the right ventricle to the lungs. Small arteries are called *arterioles*.

    b Veins (Fig. 4-34). Veins are vessels that carry *deoxygenated* blood to the heart, with the exception of the pulmonary vein. The pulmonary vein carries oxygenated blood from the lungs to the left atrium. Small veins are called *venules*.

    c Capillaries. These are microscopic vessels that link arteries and veins via arterioles and venules to carry blood to and from the cells.

2 Capillaries, individually, are very small, but combined

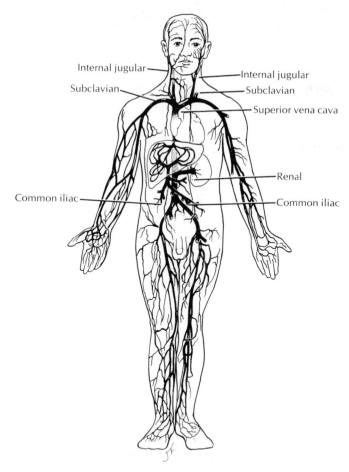

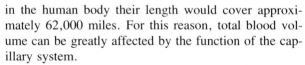

FIGURE 4-34 Venous system.

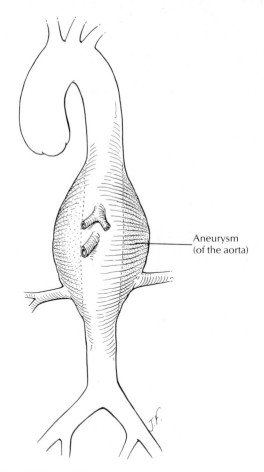

FIGURE 4-35 Formation of an aneurysm in an artery.

in the human body their length would cover approximately 62,000 miles. For this reason, total blood volume can be greatly affected by the function of the capillary system.

3 Capillaries do not have valves and as such serve as connecting conduits. They do have the ability to passively dilate or constrict, thereby allowing more or less blood into their system.

4 Arteries, with the exception of the pulmonary artery, carry *oxygenated* blood away from the heart in reponse to systolic contraction. For this reason, the blood pressure in arteries is greater than that in the veins. The greatest pulse pressure begins in the aorta at approximately 80 to 120 mm Hg to 0 at the entrance to the capillaries, where it becomes smooth rather than pulsating.

5 The walls of arteries and veins are formed of three layers of tissue interwrapped, much like the casing of an automobile tire. Because of greater internal blood pressure, the walls in arteries are much thicker than in veins. If the wall of an artery becomes weakened because of lateral wall pressure, it will cause an *aneurysm* (bulge), causing the cross-sectional area to become greater and the wall thinner (Fig. 4-35). The greater the bulge, the thinner the wall becomes until it

bursts, much like a balloon that has been stretched too thin by overinflation, causing severe bleeding.

6 Veins are *not* exposed to the higher pressure of arteries.

7 In addition to pressure, veins dilate or constrict their internal diameters in response to nervous stimulation, as well as in response to the direct action of various substances (drugs).

8 Constriction is primarily the result of *sympathetic* activity, and dilation results from *inhibition* of sympathetics.

9 In addition to their ability to respond to nervous activity, veins have valves that form chambers. These chambers allow the veins to hold blood as it moves toward the heart, much like the locks in a canal.

10 Venous blood flow is dependent on decreases in intrathoracic pressure and on increases in intraabdominal pressures for its flow back to the chest.

11 The thin walls of the veins cause pressure within the veins to respond to positive and decreased pressure gradients within the thorax and abdomen.

12 A decreased intrathoracic pressure combined with an elevated intraabdominal pressure is conducive to good blood flow back to the heart and vice versa.

13 The effect of gas pressure in the chest on venous return

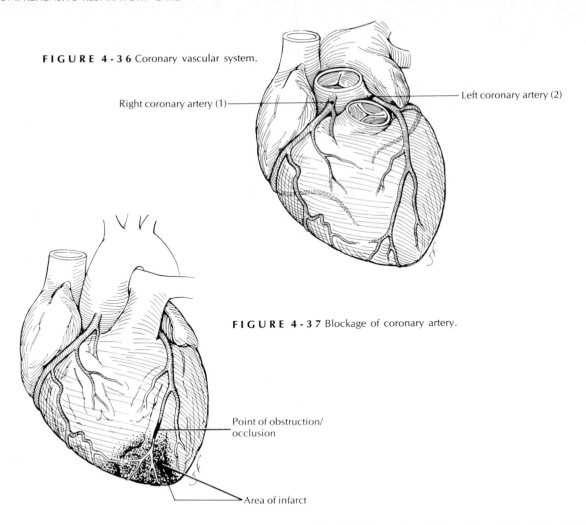

FIGURE 4-36 Coronary vascular system.

Right coronary artery (1)

Left coronary artery (2)

FIGURE 4-37 Blockage of coronary artery.

Point of obstruction/occlusion

Area of infarct

to the heart was studied by Cournand and his group in 1947 and is covered in Module Eight.

26.2 Venous blood pressure

1 The circulatory system is conveniently and functionally divided into an arterial and venous system.
2 It is possible because of this division for very different conditions to prevail in each. For example, a patient may have an arterial systolic pressure of greater than 200 mm Hg and still have a normal venous pressure.
3 The venous pressure varies with body position because of the influence of gravity against a low pressure system.
4 Venous pressure is normally measured with the patient in the *recumbent* position.
5 The technique involves placing a catheter in the median cubital vein and connecting this catheter to a sensitive pressure manometer that is placed at the level of the heart.
6 Venous pressure is useful in determining *blood volume*.
7 A normal venous pressure is approximately 0 to 5 mm Hg.
8 If venous pressure increases above 15 to 20 mm Hg, a patient's neck veins will begin to distend and become quite prominent, as in right-sided heart failure.

27.0 VESSELS AND NERVES OF THE FOREARM AND UPPER EXTREMITY
27.1 Circulation to the extremities

1 Circulation to muscles of the extremities will be presented in conjunction with procedures involving these structures.
2 A practitioner's useful application of knowledge of circulation and muscles of the extremities is limited primarily to identification of puncture sites for drawing of blood for arterial blood gas analysis and in certain exercises in conjunction with pulmonary rehabilitation programs. Functional anatomy will be presented as these units are covered.

28.0 THE CORONARY SYSTEM
28.1 Coronary circulation

1 Living structures *cannot* exist without an adequate flow of blood to nourish the cells and remove wastes.
2 For example, the brain will suffer permanent damage at 37° C after 4 to 6 minutes unless it receives oxygen.
3 The heart will cease to beat unless it is oxygenated after 10 to 12 minutes, and the kidneys will suffer irreversible damage after approximately 30 minutes without oxygen.
4 The heart muscle is nourished by blood supplied by its

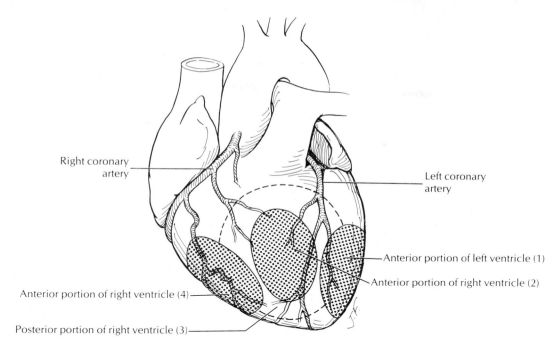

Right coronary artery

Left coronary artery

Anterior portion of left ventricle (1)

Anterior portion of right ventricle (2)

Anterior portion of right ventricle (4)

Posterior portion of right ventricle (3)

F I G U R E 4 - 3 8 Common sites of myocardial infarction.

own specialized circulatory system—the *coronary system* (Fig. 4-36).

5 Two coronary arteries leave the aorta just beyond the aortic valve and branch into right *(1)* and left *(2)* coronary arteries, which then branch into arterioles and capillaries. These are *end* vessels that supply blood to the right and left sides of the heart individually. They do not *anastomose* (connect). If one of them is blocked (Fig. 4-37), the other cannot help, and tissue dies (infarcts) distal to the point of obstruction (Fig. 4-37). The most common sites of myocardial infarct are shown in Fig. 4-38, *1-4*.

6 Venous blood from the coronary circulation is returned through coronary veins to the coronary sinus, which empties blood into the right atrium.

7 Thebesian veins short-circuit (shunt) the deoxygenated blood directly into the ventricles.

8 Anterior cardiac veins return most of the blood from the right coronary artery and ascend the anterior surface of the right ventricle and end in the right atrium.

29.0 CEREBRAL CIRCULATION
29.1 Cerebral blood flow

1 In healthy adults, cerebral blood flow is about 55 ml/100 g of brain per minute or 750 ml/min for an average size brain (Fig. 4-39, *A*).

2 Blood is carried to the brain by the internal carotid *(1)* and vertebral arteries *(2)*.

3 In the brain, the vertebrals *(2)* join to form the single basilar artery (Fig. 4-39, *B3*).

4 The carotid and basilar arteries form the *Circle of Willis.*

5 Venous blood enters dural sinuses and deep veins, which drain from the brain via the internal jugular veins (see Fig. 4-34).

30.0 HEPATIC-PORTAL CIRCULATION
30.1 Structure and function (Fig. 4-40)

1 The liver is the largest internal body organ. It is located in the upper part of the abdomen beneath the dome of the diaphragm.

2 In this location it is vulnerable to compression or penetration injury yet may be overlooked because of its obscured location.

3 It is divided into four lobes, with the right and left side separated by the falciform ligament.

4 Internally the lobules are arranged around a central vein in interconnecting structures called *hepatic laminae.*

5 Circulation through the liver is composed of mixed venous and arterial blood.

6 Arterial blood enters the liver via the hepatic artery.

7 Venous blood enters from the splanchnic areas via the portal vein.

8 Arterial and venous blood meet in the liver lobules to mix in the *sinusoids.*

9 Mixed blood is collected by the hepatic veins, which drain into the *inferior vena cava.*

10 The functions of the liver include:
   a Metabolism. Substances are brought directly from the intestines and mixed with bile which is produced in the liver.
   b Protection. The liver removes digestive products that are not needed.

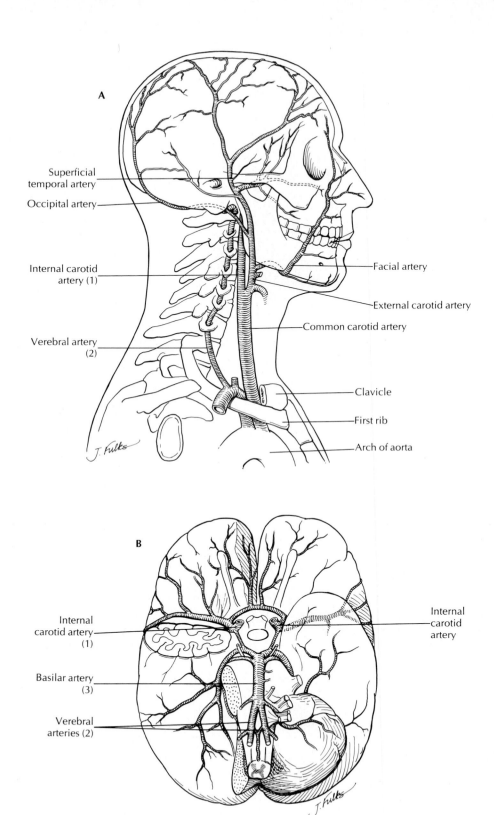

A

Superficial temporal artery

Occipital artery

Internal carotid artery (1)

Verebral artery (2)

Facial artery

External carotid artery

Common carotid artery

Clavicle

First rib

Arch of aorta

J. Fulks

B

Internal carotid artery (1)

Basilar artery (3)

Verebral arteries (2)

Internal carotid artery

J. Fulks

FIGURE 4-39 Cerebral circulation. **A,** Major arteries of head and neck. **B,** Arteries at base of brain.

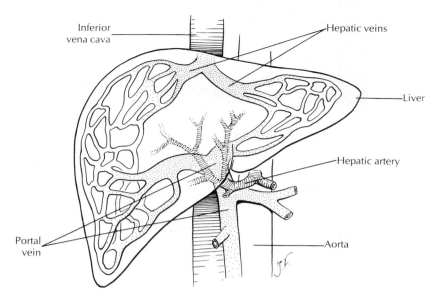

FIGURE 4-40 Hepatic-portal circulatory system.

c Circulation. About ¼ of the total cardiac output passes through the liver. Total blood flow can be altered by altering liver circulation.

d Detoxification. It changes toxic ammonia into less toxic urea and its enzymatic activity inactivates drugs and environmental poisons.

11 One of the most common diseases which destroys the liver is cirrhosis. This disease is most frequently caused by alcoholism. Its pathology includes degeneration of liver cells, inflammation and formation of scar tissue throughout.

31.0 SPLENIC CIRCULATION
31.1 Structure and function (Fig. 4-41)

1 The splenic artery supplies the spleen. In the spleen, the blood flows directly into a capillary bed then to venous sinuses and into the splenic vein, which joins the portal vein.

2 The spleen can serve as a blood reservoir. It normally holds 350 ml of blood but the spleen can hold as much as 500 ml.

3 Two functions of the spleen are:

a Blood reservoir. The spleen holds blood as a buffer against sudden blood loss or excessive body needs like exercise.

b Hematocrit. The spleen traps and holds erythrocytes. The spleen contracts during excessive blood loss to force blood with an elevated hematocrit into the general circulation.

4 In trauma accidents involving the left torso, the spleen is frequently ruptured. This type of injury is critical but may go unnoticed unless one is cognizant of its location in relation to the point of injury.

32.0 RENAL CIRCULATION
32.1 Structure and function (Fig. 4-42)

1 The kidneys are the major excretory organs and play an

important role in circulatory dynamics.

2 Approximately 1300 ml of blood flows through the kidneys per minute because of the low resistance in the renal vessels.

3 Renal vessels are controlled by the sympathetic nervous system, which causes vessels to constrict or dilate as the minute volume of blood flow increases or decreases. The constriction or dilation of renal vessels greatly influences arterial blood pressure.

4 Blood flow through the kidneys is unaffected as long as arterial pressure is between 80 and 250 mm Hg. At 80 mm Hg blood flow decreases and at 250 mm Hg it increases.

5 A more detailed description of the kidney is presented in Unit 35.0, The Excretory System.

33.0 PULMONARY CIRCULATION
33.1 Structure and function (Fig. 4-43)

1 Deoxygenated blood is pumped by the right ventricle into the pulmonary artery. This artery bifurcates (branches) into two main vessels with one going to each lung.

2 Each branch gives off smaller arteries and arterioles connecting with a capillary network that surrounds alveoli.

3 The veins that drain this system converge to empty into the pulmonary veins, which carry oxygenated blood back to the left atrium.

4 Additional details on pulmonary circulation are presented in Module Eight.

33.2 Bronchial circulation (Fig. 4-44)

1 Lung tissue itself is supplied by the bronchial system, which is composed of at least one bronchial artery going to each lung. These arteries arise from either the proximal portion of the thoracic aorta or one of the first two intercostal arteries and follow the course of the

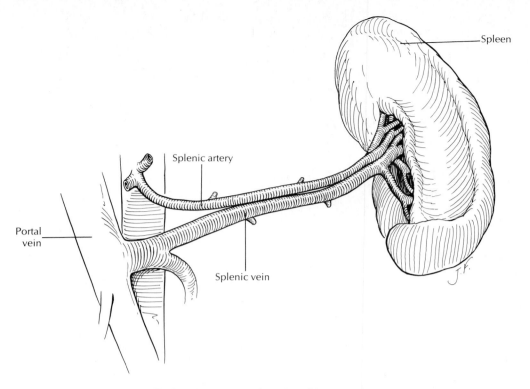

FIGURE 4-41 Splenic circulatory system.

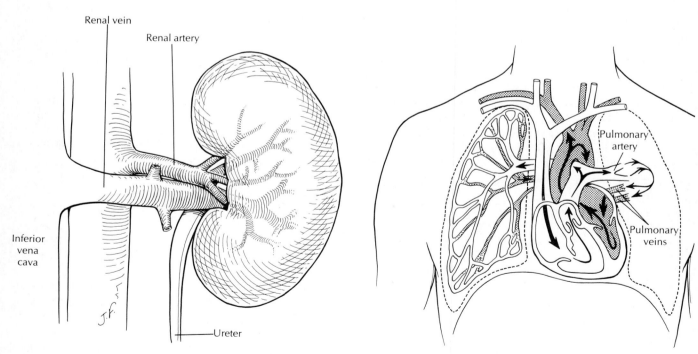

FIGURE 4-42 Renal circulation.

FIGURE 4-43 Pulmonary circulatory system.

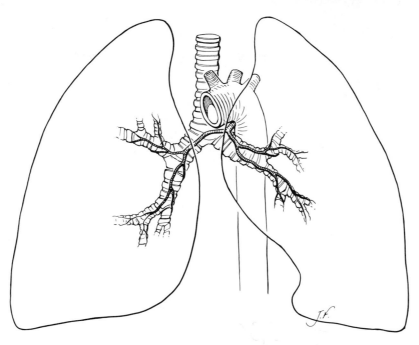

FIGURE 4-44 Bronchial circulation.

bronchial tree into the lung, ending at the terminal bronchioles. Lung structure distal to this point is supplied by blood from the pulmonary arterial system. Veins return blood from the bronchial arteries and empty it into the left atrium of the heart causing a slight mixing of oxygenated and deoxygenated blood.

34.0 THE DIGESTIVE SYSTEM
34.1 Structures and function

1 Digestion is the process of changing foods from complex substances that are eaten to materials that can be used by the cells as nutrients for metabolism.

2 In metabolism, carbohydrates and fats are burned to provide heat and energy; proteins are converted into amino acids used in the growth and repair of tissues.

3 The organs of the digestive system known as the alimentary canal or gastrointestinal tract (Fig. 4-45, *1-7*) are the mouth *(1)*, pharynx *(2)*, esophagus *(3)*, stomach *(4)*, small intestine *(5)*, large intestine *(6)*, and rectum *(7)*.

4 Accessory organs assist the digestive organs in the digestive process. These organs are the tongue *(8)*, salivary glands *(9)*, liver *(10)*, gallbladder *(11)*, pancreas *(12)*, spleen *(13)*, vermiform appendix *(14)*, and teeth *(15)*.

5 The esophagus is a muscular tube about 25 cm long extending from the larynx to the stomach area just below the diaphragm. The esophagus transports food lubricated by saliva from the mouth to the stomach by contraction of muscles that line its walls. This process is called *peristalsis*.

6 The stomach is a bladder-shaped organ that lies in the upper left quadrant of the abdomen inferior to the diaphragm.

7 The stomach is composed of three layers of smooth muscle with fibers running lengthwise around and obliquely in the stomach wall.

8 In the stomach, peristaltic contractions assist in the mixing of food with hydrochloric acid and the enzyme pepsin. This mixture is then propelled down the digestive tract.

9 Food leaves the stomach, where it enters the duodenum, the first 25 cm of the small intestine.

10 The liver and the pancreas neutralize acid from the stomach and complete the digestive process in the duodenum.

11 Food leaves the duodenum and enters the small intestine, where protruding *villi* contact the food, which is now a solution, and transfer it into the blood and lymph systems.

12 That which is not used remains in the large intestine for 10 to 12 hours, where water is absorbed and bacterial action begins to form feces, which are passed to the rectum for excretion from the body.

35.0 THE EXCRETORY SYSTEM
35.1 Structure and function (Fig. 4-46)

1 The excretory system comprises the kidneys *(1)*, ureters *(2)*, urinary bladder *(3)*, and urethra *(4)*.

2 The kidneys are bean-shaped organs (Fig. 4-46, *1*) located on either side of the spine. They are situated high in the posterior portion of the abdominal cavity, extending from T11 or T12 to L2. Other organs close to the kidneys are the liver, spleen, and diaphragm.

3 Each kidney (Fig. 4-47) is 10 to 15 cm long, weighs about 170 g, has an internal structure called a renal medulla *(1)*, and has an external structure called a renal cortex *(2)*.

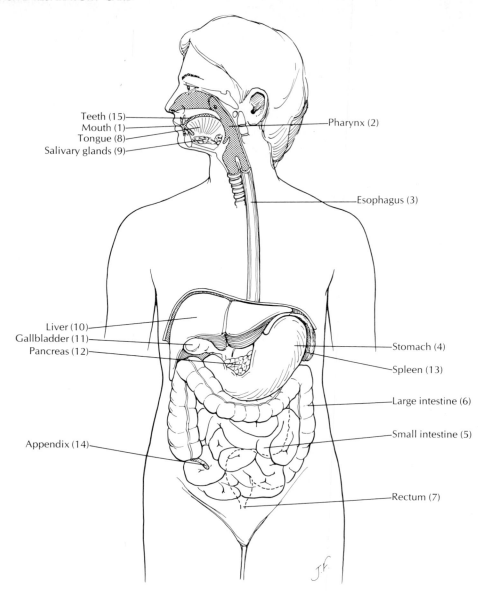

Teeth (15)
Mouth (1)
Tongue (8)
Salivary glands (9)

Pharynx (2)

Esophagus (3)

Liver (10)
Gallbladder (11)
Pancreas (12)

Stomach (4)

Spleen (13)

Large intestine (6)

Small intestine (5)

Appendix (14)

Rectum (7)

FIGURE 4-45 Organs of the digestive system.

4 It is estimated that the kidneys filter approximately 42 gallons of water each day. This volume of water is dealt with by huge numbers of tiny nephrons that function in shifts to selectively reabsorb most of the fluid back into the blood.

5 The functional unit of the kidney is the nephron.

6 It is estimated there are approximately 1 million nephrons in each kidney.

7 The major structures of a nephron (Fig. 4-48, *1-4*) are the glomerulus *(1)*, proximal tubule *(2)*, convoluted loop of Henle *(3)*, and distal tubule *(4)*.

8 The total length of a nephron varies from 20 to 45 mm. The distal tube inside diameter is 0.06 mm and decreases until the thin loop of Henle, which is 0.02 mm, is reached.

35.2 Primary function of the kidneys (see Fig. 4-47)

1 The primary function of the kidneys is to regulate the volume and composition of *extracellular fluid*.

2 Kidneys are essential organs for homeostasis of the body, with an adult voiding some 1000 to 1500 ml/day.

3 Blood flows into this region by a complex system of arteries and veins.

4 In respiratory patients, the kidneys play a major role in regulating arterial blood acid or base content (pH) by excreting or retaining acid and bicarbonate (base).

5 The major artery is the renal artery *(3)*, which branches in interlobar arteries, and finally a ureteral artery.

6 As blood enters the kidneys it is channeled into clusters of arterial capillaries called *glomeruli*.

7 The name glomerulus (a single unit) is from the Latin, meaning a small ball.

8 Each glomerulus has a double membrane that leads into a tubule (little tube).

9 The glomerulus, Bowman's capsule, and the tubule compose the nephron.

10 Kidneys do not just pick up waste. As the blood passes through glomeruli, chemicals and wastes are allowed

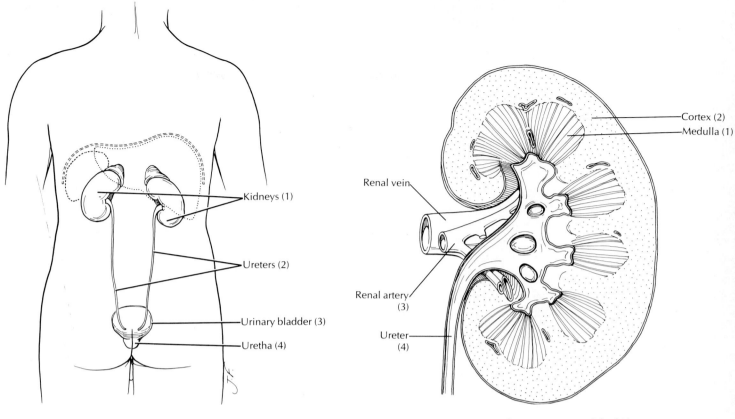

FIGURE 4-46 Excretory system.

FIGURE 4-47 Internal gross anatomy of the kidney.

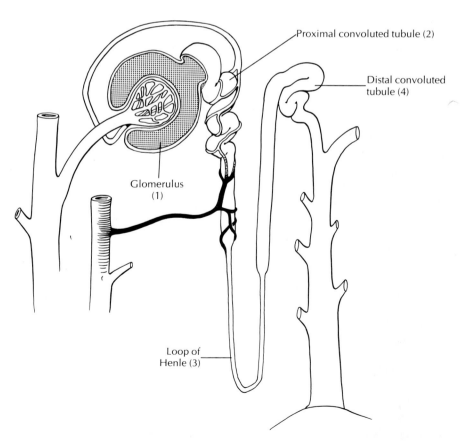

FIGURE 4-48 Structures of the nephron.

to selectively filter out through the membranes.

11 Once fluid has passed the membranes, it flows into the tubules.

12 The tubules select out those materials that are useful and send them back into the blood.

13 Waste products remain trapped inside or are actively secreted into the tubule and are then excreted via the ureter *(4)* to the bladder.

14 This recapturing of useful materials occurs as tubules, which wind away from the glomeruli, come into contact with other capillaries.

15 At this point sugars and salts pass back into the bloodstream by active transport and osmosis.

16 Molecules of water also reenter the blood so that 99% of the fluid that filters out of the glomeruli is reabsorbed. The remaining 1% is formed into urine and excreted.

35.3 Causes of renal failure

1 Renal failure (RF) may be defined as a daily urinary output of less than 400 ml or less than 70 ml/min/m^2 of BSA.

2 RF may be chronic or acute. Tubular necrosis may be suspected in the patient who is in shock or a patient who has ingested a poison that is toxic to the kidney. A serious complication of renal failure is an ever-rising level of blood potassium, which uncontrolled will cause muscular paralysis, cardiac arrhythmias, and death. Young adult patients who have experienced an acute respiratory infection may develop *glomerulonephritis* 10 to 20 days after the episode as a result of an anaphylactic response to the infection. Most of these patients recover without treatment.

3 Acute renal failure (ARF) can be caused by three different actions: prerenal, postrenal, and intrarenal failure.

4 Prerenal failure is the cause of approximately one fourth of all ARF.

5 ARF results from an inadequate volume of blood (for whatever reason) reaching the kidneys.

6 Prerenal failure occurs as a result of blockage to urine flow at the ureters, urethra, or bladder.

7 In 65% of cases, the cause of ARF is intrarenal. Approximately 99% of these cases are the result of renal ischemia, and or renal toxins.

8 Postrenal failure is identified by a complete absence of urine.

35.4 Hemodialysis

1 Hemodialysis is the technique used to remove toxic substances from the blood that are not removed or are not controlled by the kidneys; the device used is called a hemodialyzer.

2 A hemodialyzer (artificial kidney) is a combination of semipermeable membranes that selectively remove toxic substances by osmosis. A pump causes this blood to flow from the patient through an arterial venous cannula. The artificial kidney is appropriately named, because the removal of substances via the membranes

uses the same osmotic principles as the natural kidney. A hemodialysis treatment can reduce toxic substances and return blood urea nitrogen (BUN) and creatinine levels to acceptable levels in 4 to 6 hours. Patients who are completely dependent on hemodialysis usually require three 8-hour sessions weekly.

35.5 Hemofiltration

1 Hemofiltration is the technique of removing toxic substances from the blood by passing it through external filters. This process differs from heodialysis that removes toxins from the blood by osmosis.

36.0 GLANDS AND THEIR FUNCTIONS
36.1 Endocrine system (Fig. 4-49)

1 The endocrine system is composed of glands that secrete hormones into the bloodstream.

2 A *gland,* by definition, is a cell or organ that secretes some substance.

3 The body has two types of glands.
   a *Exocrine gland.* Secretions move outward by way of ducts to some body surface area. They are found in the skin, lining of the digestive tract, and respiratory system.
   b *Endocrine gland.* Secretions move without ducts and are absorbed into the bloodstream. These glands are the chemical regulators of the body.

4 Exocrine glands secrete sweat, mucus, saliva, and milk.

5 Endocrine glands allow the body to adjust its internal process slowly when compared to the nervous system, which provides almost instantaneous responses.

6 Major endocrine glands include the:
   a Pituitary gland *(1).* Located at the base of the brain.
   b Thyroid gland *(2).* Located in the neck on either side of the trachea.
   c Four parathyroid glands *(3).* Located behind the thyroid.
   d Adrenal glands *(4).* Located atop the kidneys.
   e Islets of Langerhans (insulin) *(5).* Located in the pancreas.
   f Ovaries *(6).* Located in the abdomen of the female.
   g Testes *(7).* Located in the scrotum of the male.

NOTE: The brain, liver, and even the placenta function as endocrine glands because they produce and secrete special substances.

36.2 Functions of glands

1 All of the glands play important roles in maintaining the chemical activity of the body. Epinephrine (adrenaline) and norepinephrine hormones, which are secreted by the adrenal glands, are of special interest to respiratory personnel.

2 In time of stress, epinephrine speeds up the respiratory rate, raises the blood pressure, and prepares the body for "fight or flight."

3 Norephinephrine, in response to hypotension, causes an increase in the amount of blood flowing through the

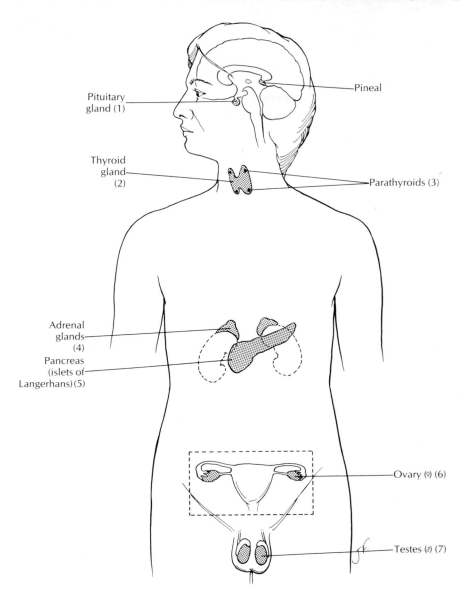

FIGURE 4-49 Endocrine system.

heart and constricts capillaries, causing blood to be shunted (redirected) to major body organs.

4 Hormones produced in the Islets of Langerhans of the pancreas help control sugar balance in the body (insulin). Steroids such as cortisone and aldosterone produced by the adrenal cortex regulate sugar and salt balances.

5 *Steroids* also help to reduce inflammation and relieve pain in many medical conditions.

6 Each endocrine gland is responsible for the production of at least one important *hormone* for the regulation of the body. Some glands, e.g., the pituitary, produce at least nine different types of hormones.

37.0 THE NERVOUS SYSTEM

37.1 Glossary of terms and concepts for the nervous system

1 Action potential. Electrical difference that exists between inside and outside of a nerve cell.

2 Autonomic nervous system. A part of the nervous system that is self-governing; not controlled by consciousness.

3 Conduction. Transmission of an electrical impulse.

4 Innervate. Control with nerves.

5 Multipolar neuron. A type of neuron consisting of a cell body, axons, and several to numerous dendrites.

6 Nerve. A bundle of nerve cell processes joined together by connective tissue.

7 Neuron. Structural and functional unit of the nervous system; a nerve cell.

8 Postganglionic neuron. One that receives impulses from the preganglionic neuron and transmits them to effector sites.

9 Preganglionic neuron. One that terminates in a ganglion of cell bodies that innervates postganglionic neurons.

10 Propagation. Self-generating process of generating and

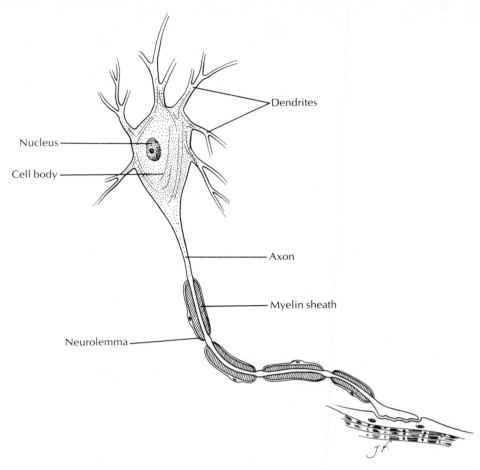

Dendrites

Nucleus

Cell body

Axon

Myelin sheath

Neurolemma

J.F.

F I G U R E   4 - 5 0 Structures of a neuron.

sending an electrical impulse along a nerve (i.e., like an ocean wave).

11 Somatic nervous system. Conscious action.

12 Synapse. Extracellular gap that separates two neurons (nerves).

13 Tract. Pathway of neuron processes in the central nervous system.

14 Transmit. Passing of an impulse across a synapse from one neuron to another.

15 Unipolar neuron. A type of neuron that contains only one process, an axon.

38.0 THE CENTRAL NERVOUS SYSTEM
38.1 Structure and function of neurons

1 The nervous system like other body systems is composed of different structures working together to perform a specialized task.

2 The primary function of the nervous system is to receive and transmit stimuli.

3 The nervous system is composed of the brain, spinal cord, and peripheral nerves, which branch and connect the brain and spinal cord to all parts of the body.

4 The central nervous system (CNS) coordinates all the body's activities in response to external and internal stimuli, which travel at a maximum speed of 322 kilometers per hour (kph) along nerves to and from the brain.

5 As in all body structures, the basic structure for the nervous system is the cell, or neuron. There are three major types of neurons: motor neurons, sensory neurons, and interneurons.

6 Physiologically, nerve cells possess the same mechanisms found in other cells for synthesizing proteins and adenosine 5'-triphosphate (ATP). They are equipped with membranes, nuclei, ribosomes, and mitochondria.

7 Nerve cells do not reproduce or regenerate once destroyed.

8 A typical nerve cell (Fig. 4-50) will have a cell body with a nucleus and a surrounding membrane and at least two processes (fibers) extending from the body of the cell. These processes primarily distinguish a nerve cell from other body cells.

9 One process is the *dendrite*. The dendrite is a thin fiber that spreads from the cell body like a root system on a plant. Dendrites have receptors that pick up impulses and conduct them toward the cell body of the neuron.

10 The *axon* is the thickened single process (fiber) that extends from the cell body.

11 The axon will vary in length from a few thousandths of an inch to 3 feet connecting the toes to the spinal cord.

12 The axon conducts impulses *away from* the cell body.

13 *Neurofibrils* are microscopically fine fibers forming a framework inside the neuron.

14 A *myelin sheath* is segmented, wrapping around a nerve fiber. This myelin sheath plays an essential role in the regeneration and restoration of innervation when two ends of a severed peripheral nerve are surgically reconnected.

38.2 Types of neurons

1 As previously mentioned, neurons are classifed as *sensory* (afferent) neurons, *motor* (efferent) neurons, and interneurons.

2 *Afferent sensory* neurons receive stimuli from the senses and transmit them *toward* the spinal cord or brain.

3 *Efferent motor neurons* transmit stimuli *away from* the brain or spinal cord toward muscle or glandular tissue.

4 *Interneurons* conduct impulses from sensory to motor neurons and represent over 99% of the approximate 10 billion neurons of the nervous system.

5 The structures of a neuron function together in the conduction of impulses.

38.3 Nerve impulse

1 A nerve impulse is defined as a self-propagating wave of electrical activity that travels along the surface of a neuron membrane like an ocean wave.

2 A nerve impulse begins when a stimulus acts on a *sensory receptor,* which is the distal end of a dendrite.

3 If the impulse is strong enough, the receptor membrane potential decreases below its resting level, and an impulse is fired. Once this occurs, the impulse travels the length of the dendrite by way of the membrane or saltatory conduction to the cell body and the axon. Nerve fibers also contain small tubules that provide channels for transporting compounds necessary for the receptor to propagate the signal.

4 The membranous covering of the axon is formed of segments. *Ranvier's nodes,* which are located between the segments, conduct the signal like a wave to a branching of tiny unsheathed fibers called end feet or terminal boutons (buttons), which end in close contact with the dendrites of another neuron.

5 The gap that separates the end feet of the axon of one neuron from the dendrites is called the *synaptic junction.*

38.4 Synapse

1 The electrical impulse will end at this point unless a chemical called a neurotransmitter is released by the end feet at the junction.

2 Once a neurotransmitter is released, the impulse quickly passes to the dendrites of the next neuron to continue the chain of connecting neurons.

3 At the neuromuscular junction, once ACh has been released, a muscle contraction follows. ACh is deactivated by another chemical called *cholinesterase* in approximately 50 microseconds (μs) to prevent undesired transmission.

38.5 Reflex

1 A reflex is a primitive protective stimulus that is generated by sensory neurons. In a reflex arc, the nerve impulses are conducted instantaneously from the point of stimulation to a motor neuron in the spinal cord and hence directly to the reacting organ without passing through the brain.

38.6 Summary of nerve dynamics

1 In summary, there are three types of neurons that send messages through the body.
  a *Sensory neurons* collect information on the external environment and on internal muscle status.
  b *Interneurons* shuttle the signals back and forth between the brain and the spinal cord.
  c *Motor neurons* conduct action signals out to the muscles.

2 Signals that leave the senses and travel toward the brain are conducted by *afferent* neurons.

3 Signals that leave the brain and travel toward the muscle are conducted by *efferent* neurons.

39.0 THE HUMAN BRAIN
39.1 Structure and function

1 The brain plus the spinal cord compose the central nervous system of the body (Fig. 4-51).

2 The brain is the primary controlling organ of the body and is also the center for consciousness and intelligence. These functions include speech, feelings, judgments, emotions, character, appreciation, and other processes that make us human.

3 The brain stops growing at about 20 years of age. The matured brain weighs approximately 3 pounds and is about the size of an acorn squash.

4 The brain is soft, pinkish-gray, and furrowed (convoluted) in appearance, which allows it to fit in a 15 by 20 cm skull. It is 10 cm long and has a 2.5 cm wide central core (brainstem) that extends downward to the spinal cord.

5 The brain is composed of three major divisions forming a *forebrain, midbrain,* and *hindbrain* (Fig. 4-52).

6 The forebrain is formed by the *cerebrum (1)* and *thalamus (2).*

7 The midbrain *(3)* is formed by the *corpora quadrigemina* and by the *cerebral penduncle.* It is just below the thalamus.

8 The hindbrain is formed by the *cerebellum (4), pons (5),* and *medulla oblongata (6).*

39.2 The cerebrum (see Fig. 4-52)

1 The cerebrum *(1)* is the largest division of the brain; it accounts for seven eights of its total weight.

2 The cerebrum is separated into right and left hemispheres by a fissure; the sides of the hemispheres are connected in their lower central portions.

3 Each hemisphere of the cerebrum is further divided into a *frontal, parietal, occipital,* and *temporal lobe.*

4 Each lobe directs specific body functions as identified in the box on p. 77.

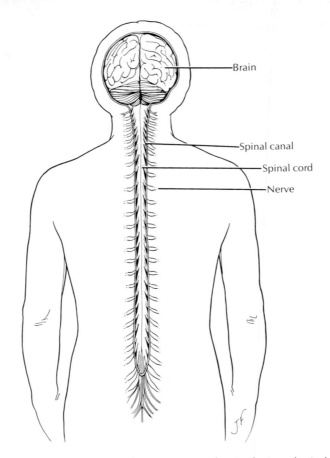

FIGURE 4-51 Central nervous system showing brain and spinal cord.

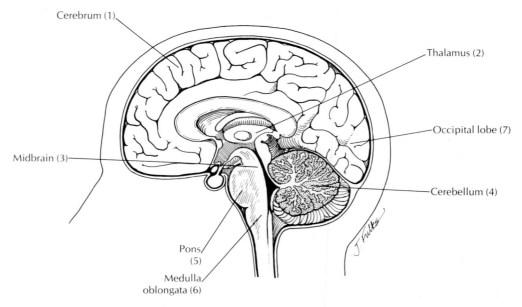

FIGURE 4-52 Structures of the brain.

Function and location of lobes of the cerebrum	
FRONTAL LOBE	**OCCIPITAL LOBE**
Elaboration of thought	Vision
Chief motor functions	
PARIETAL LOBE	**TEMPORAL LOBE**
Hand skills	Memory patterns
Chief sensory area	Hearing, smelling

5 The outer surface (cortex) of the cerebrum is composed of *gray matter* (neurons) and white matter, which are mainly myelinated axons that compose most of the interior of the cerebrum.

6 A network of nerves covers both the internal and external surfaces of the brain.

7 As these nerves descend deep into the interior of the brain they unite to form tracts that conduct impulses toward the brain (ascending) and away from the brain (descending).

8 Within the brain and cord various cells are found in clusters called nuclei.

9 Clusters of nerve cell bodies that are located outside the brain and spinal cord are called *ganglions*.

39.3 The cerebellum (see Fig. 4-52)

1 The cerebellum is the second largest division of the brain and is a part of the hindbrain.

2 It is located under the occipital lobe *(7)* of the cerebrum in the posterior aspect of the skull.

3 The cortex of the cerebellum is mostly gray matter, and the interior is white matter.

4 The primary function of the cerebellum is to coordinate muscle movements and maintenance of body posture.

39.4 The medulla oblongata (see Fig. 4-52)

1 The medulla is the lowest part of the brain and is part of the hindbrain.

2 It is centrally located in the core of the brain and appears to be an extension of the spinal cord itself (spinal bulb).

3 It is the nerve center for many involuntary functions such as heartbeat, diameter of arteries and veins, and respiratory rate.

39.5 Pons (see Fig. 4-52)

1 The pons *(5)*, which is located anterior to the cerebellum between the midbrain *(3)* and medulla *(6)*, is a part of the hindbrain structure.

2 It is a bridgelike structure consisting of white matter linking the various parts of the brain.

3 The pons serves as a relay station between the medulla and higher cortical centers.

39.6 Midbrain (see Fig. 4-52)

1 The midbrain *(3)* is located below the inferior surface of the cerebrum *(1)* and above the pons *(5)*.

2 It consists mainly of white matter with some gray matter around the cerebral aqueduct.

3 The midbrain contains a center for visual reflexes connected to movements of the head. This is important in maintaining posture when the position of the body has been radically disturbed.

40.0 DYSFUNCTIONS RESULTING FROM BRAIN INJURY OR DISEASE
40.1 Physical responses

Dysfunction of brain tissue will cause specific clinical signs, as listed in Fig. 4-53.

41.0 DISTINGUISHING STRUCTURES AND FUNCTIONS OF THE SPINAL CORD AND BRAIN
41.1 Structure and function of the spinal cord

1 The spinal cord (Fig. 4-54, *1*, and Fig. 4-55, *1*) is 46 cm long and is located in a canal formed by the spinal column (see Figs. 4-51 and 4-15). The cord resembles a cable tapered at both ends and extends from the occipital bone to the level of the disk located between the L1 and L2 vertebrae. Here it tapers to a point that branches into nerves extending into the lumbar and sacral regions.

2 Like the brain, the spinal cord contains both gray matter (Fig. 4-54, *2*) and white matter *(3)*. (Refer also to Fig. 4-55, *2* and *3*.) The spinal cord is covered, like the brain, with thin layers of tissue (meninges) called the *pia mater* (Fig. 4-55, *4*), the *arachnoid (5)*, and the *dura mater (6)*. The space between the pia and the arachnoid is called the *subarachnoid space (7)*.

3 The gray matter forms an H-shaped column in the cen-

Cerebral cortex	Frontal lobe	Temporal lobe
Motor paralysis of opposite half of body; positive Babinski reflex	Prefrontal tumor— reverse of personality habits; no concern over disease	Visual hallucinations (light flecks)
Occipital lobe	**Midbrain**	**Cerebellum**
Blindness on nasal half of eye; temporal half of other eye	Abnormal eye movements; paralysis of an upward gaze	Headaches, vomiting, visual disturbance more so than other areas

FIGURE 4-53 Clinical signs of brain dysfunction.

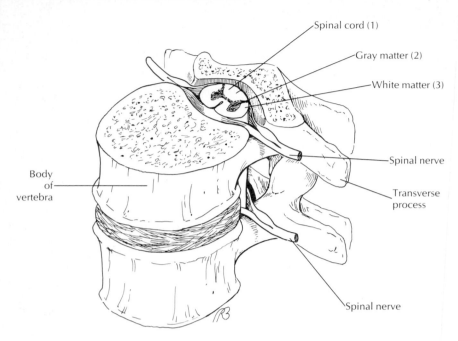

FIGURE 4-54 Spinal cord.

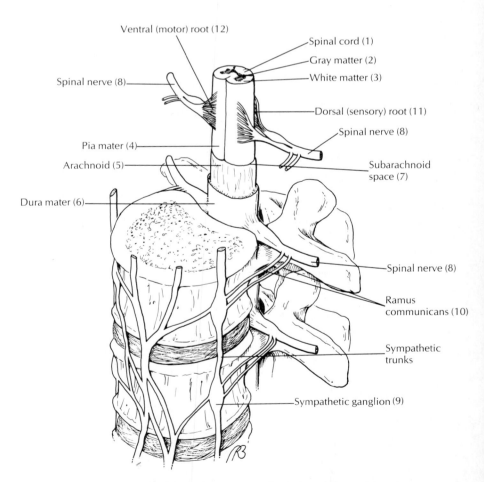

FIGURE 4-55 Cross-section of spinal cord showing its structures.

ter of the cord (Fig. 4-55, 2) and is surrounded by bundles of myelinated fibers of white matter *(3)*.

4 From the white matter originate the spinal nerves (Fig. 4-55, *8*), which form pathways that interconnect and coordinate all body functions.

5 The spinal nerves are connected to the *sympathetic ganglion (9)* by the *ramus communicans (10)*—a branching of nerve fibers.

6 From the spinal cord 31 pairs of spinal nerves pass out between openings between the vertebrae at all levels from top to bottom. These nerves are identified according to the level of the spinal column at which they emerge.

7 From the upper cord, nerves branch to form trunks to control activities of the upper torso, arms, and hands.

8 From the lower cord, nerves branch to form trunks leading to the pelvis, thighs, legs, and feet.

9 Afferent signals travel toward the spinal cord and brain by way of the dorsal or sensory root (Fig. 4-55, *11*), and efferent signals leave the spinal cord by way of the ventral or motor root *(12)*.

41.2 Cerebrospinal fluid

1 The brain and spinal cord are protected externally by bone and internally by the meninges (covering), a cushion of connective tissue, and spinal fluid.

2 As was pointed out previously, the brain is covered by three layers called meninges: the pia mater closest to the brain, the arachnoid, and the dura mater.

3 The space between the pia and arachnoid is the subarachnoid space.

4 This subarachnoid space is continuous and surrounds the length of the cranial and spinal space.

5 Cerebrospinal fluid is a clear fluid that surrounds the spinal cord and fills the subarachnoid space. It cushions and buffers the brain against trauma much as shock absorbers keep the car from bouncing off a bumpy road and jolting the riders inside.

6 Spinal fluid is forced from the choroid plexus in the four brain ventricles by high filtration pressures and circulates until it is returned to venous circulation.

7 The pH of cerebrospinal fluid is 7.32. This changes with alternations in arterial carbon dioxide content and is thought to play a major role in controlling ventilation.

42.0 SYMPATHETIC AND PARASYMPATHETIC ACTIVITY
42.1 Dynamics of the central nervous system

1 Anatomically, the nervous system is divided into two parts.
   a Central nervous system
   b Peripheral nervous system

2 The peripheral nervous system includes all the cranial and the spinal sensory and motor nerves.

3 The central nervous system controls both the voluntary and the *autonomic (automatic)* system that controls nerves to smooth muscle of the walls of blood vessels, the digestive tract, the heart, the lungs, and glandular secretions (Fig. 4-56).

4 The autonomic nervous system differs anatomically from the somatic mechanism in that autonomic neurons that originate in the spinal cord and brain do not directly innervate muscles or glands. Neurons end in a synaptic union with a second neuron that innervates the organ.

42.2 Divisions of the autonomic nervous system

1 The autonomic nervous system is therefore subdivided into *preganglionic* and *postganglionic* neurons.

2 Preganglionic neurons terminate in ganglia and consist of cell bodies that give rise to the postganglionic neurons.

3 The autonomic nervous system is further divided into two divisions, *sympathetic* and *parasympathetic*.

42.3 Sympathetic

1 The sympathetic division (Fig. 4-56) contains two chains (tracts) of ganglia (one on each side of the spine) and fibers that connect ganglia with each other and with all the thoracic and the first three or four lumbar segments of the spinal cord.

2 Other fibers extend from the sympathetic ganglia to the various visceral effectors.

42.4 Parasympathetic

1 The parasympathic nervous system consists of ganglia within viscera. The parasympathetic axons travel from the CNS through the cranial and sacral nerves.

2 These fibers also run from ganglia into viscera and glands.

42.5 Actions of the parasympathetic and sympathetic divisions

1 Parasympathetic
   a Preganglionic neurons and postganglionic parasympathic neurons release *acetylcholine* at the axon ending.
   b Neurons that release acetylcholine are called cholinergic.
   c At the autonomic synapse acetylcholine causes *excitation*.
   d At the effector organ the release of acetylcholine may cause *inhibition* or *excitation*.

2 Sympathetic
   a Postganglionic neurons of the sympathetic division liberate norepinephrine at their axon endings.
   b Neurons that release norepinephrine are called *adrenergic*.
   c An exception is the cholinergic postganglionic sympathetic neurons that innervate sweat glands. Some that innervate blood vessels of skeletal muscle are also cholinergic.

43.0 SYMPATHETIC AND PARASYMPATHETIC INTERACTIONS
43.1 Interactions of parasympathetic/sympathetic divisions

1 Two divisions differ anatomically and physiologically.

2 Most viscera are innervated by both divisions.

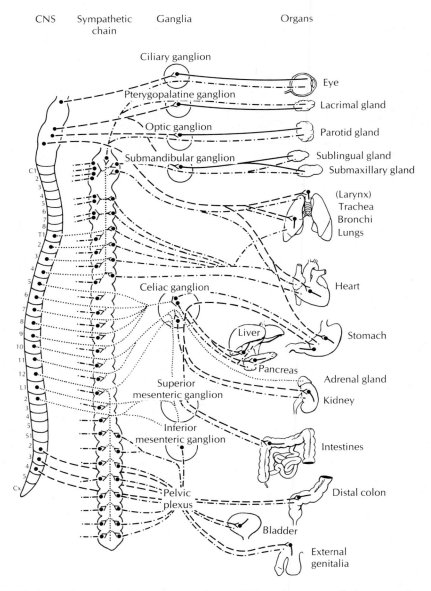

F I G U R E   4 - 5 6 Routes and effector organs of sympathetic and parasympathetic nerves. Preganglionic: parasympathetic (- - - -) and sympathetic (• • • • • • • • • •); postganglionic: parasympathetic (——); and sympathetic (• — • — • — •).

3 Stimulation of one division usually produces effects *opposite* to those noted on stimulation of the other division.

4 This is not always the case, e.g., in the salivary glands, stimulation of either or both divisions will cause production of secretions.

5 Routes and effector organs of sympathetic and parasympathetic nerves are shown in Fig. 4-56. Study these and become familiar with their innervation with the cardio-respiratory system.

43.2 Electroencephalography (EEG)

In some hospitals respiratory care personnel are cross-trained to perform EEG tests. EEG is the recording of electric currents developed in the brain by means of placing electrodes onto the scalp or directly into the brain. The electrodes are connected to an electroencephalograph which consists of a series of amplifiers and pen recorders that work similarly to an ECG machine. The tracings recorded by these instruments reflect patterns that can be identified on the basis of dominant waveform frequency.

For example, the alpha frequency is recorded over the back of the head and is prominent in the quiet, awake adult. The delta frequency appears during slow wave sleep in adults and children. The dominant EEG pattern is unique to each individual but varies with age and state of alertness. The EEG is slowed with theta and delta frequencies dominating in the alert adult with a variety of neurologic and metabolic disorders, including decreased O_2 saturation and/or increased CO_2 levels.

BIBLIOGRAPHY

Anthony CP and Thibodeau GA: Textbook of anatomy and physiology, ed 12, St Louis, 1987, The CV Mosby Co.

Anthony CP and Thibodeau GA: Structure and function of the body, ed 8, St Louis, 1988, The CV Mosby Co.

Brooks, SM and Paynton-Brooks N: The human body: structure and function in health and disease, ed 2, St Louis, 1980, The CV Mosby Co.

Hedemark LL and Kronenberg RS: Chemical regulation of respiration: normal variations and abnormal responses, Chest 82:488, 1982.

McClintic, JR: Human anatomy, St Louis, 1983, The CV Mosby Co.

Mosby's medical, nursing, and allied health dictionary, ed 3, St Louis, 1990, The CV Mosby Co.

Whitcomb ME: The lung; normal and diseased, St Louis, 1982, The CV Mosby Co.

Procedures for the general comfort and safety of the patient

11.4 List potential fire hazards.

11.5 Differentiate among types of fire extinguishers to be used on class A, B, and C fires.

12.1 Adhere to proper procedure for reporting defective equipment.

12.2 Explain correct procedure for reporting defective respiratory therapy equipment.

1.0 GENERAL PHYSICAL COMFORT AND PSYCHOLOGIC WELL-BEING

1.1 Patient's general comfort

1 Definition: Comfort is the enjoyment of physical and mental well-being. It implies absence of pain, anxiety, want, and distress.

2 To a patient, physical comfort means first, absence of pain and, second, a comfortable environment.

3 Module Nineteen, Pulmonary Drainage, presents special techniques for splinting a patient against the pain caused by a cough or unusual body positioning for postural drainage.

4 A patient's environmental comfort can be heightened by proper lighting, room temperature and humidity, arrangement of the bed, and positioning of the patient.

  a Indirect or filtered sunlight is most appropriate if the patient has a window and wishes to look out.

  b Indirect artificial lighting is also desirable except when the patient wishes to read. Then a light that can be directed onto the page without causing a glare will be required.

  c The temperature and humidity of the room is important not only for comfort but for physical well-being. The room temperature should be maintained between 20° to 22° C (68° to 72° F) with a relative humidity of 40% to 60%.

  d The patient's bed should be positioned for the most pleasant view available.

  e Bed covers, pillows, and so on should be placed so the patient is comfortable.

  f Pillows should be placed under the patient's head and arms and at the foot of the bed in case the patient slides down.

  g The patient usually is most comfortable placed in a recumbent position so that the body bends at the hips, *not* at the waist or neck.

  h The patient's position should be changed at least every hour (see Unit 6.1).

  i A cradle should be used to support the weight of any heavy covers or breathing tubes if the patient is connected to a ventilator.

1.2 Glossary of terms

1 Neurosis. A psychologic disorder of the thought processes not related to demonstrable disease involving the central nervous system. This condition usually can be traced to unresolved internal conflicts that cause an uneasy adjustment to life.

2 Psychosis. Those disturbances of such magnitude that there is personality disintegration and loss of contact with reality. Usually characterized by delusions and hallucination; hospitalization is generally required.

3 Paranoia. A condition characterized by systematized delusions.

4 Aberration. A deviation from the normal.

5 Aggression. Unfriendliness or active attack.

6 Amnesia. Loss of memory.

7 Sibling. One of two or more offspring produced by the same parents.

8 Psychosomatic. Pertaining to bodily symptoms that arise from mental status.

9 Hypochondria. Abnormal concern about health with false belief of suffering from some disease.

10 Phobia. Any abnormal fear.

11 Anxiety. A troubled feeling; experiencing a sense of dread or fear, especially of the future, or distress over a real or imagined threat to one's mental or physical well-being.

12 Conversion reactions. A psychoneurotic reaction in which emotional distress is converted into such bodily symptoms as hysteria or paralysis.

13 Adjustment mechanism. A behavior pattern used unconsciously to achieve a more favorable relationship with one's environment.

14 Types of psychologic adjustment mechanisms:

  a Compensation. Covering up an undesirable trait by calling attention to a desirable trait and exaggerating its importance.

  b Identification. Gaining security or prestige by identifying with other persons, groups, or social institutions the individual admires.

  c Projection. Transferring to other people or inanimate objects the causes of one's failures or shortcomings.

  d Rationalization. The use of plausible (believable) and socially acceptable reasons for conduct that is actually the result of unacceptable motives.

  e Regression. The rejection of painful ideas or experiences from levels of consciousness.

  f Sublimation. Substitution of socially approved objectives for unacceptable desires.

  g Substitution. Replacement of an unattainable desire with one that may be obtained.

1.3 Psychologic comfort

A patient's responses are based on psychologic and physical state. For this reason it is important that the practitioner understands the individual wants, desires, needs, and apprehensions of a patient.

It has been shown that a close relationship exists between molecular exchanges and environmental interactions. Specifically, humans react to defend their state of homeostasis (norm). Warm clothing is worn if it is cold; an air conditioner is used if it is hot. Sunshades are used to reduce glare and protect the eyes, ear plugs to guard against loud noises.

Humans are animals of perceptions; their ability to

move, think, and function depends on where they think they are and what they feel their actions should be.

A person depends on the sense of vision for perception; when lying in the supine position in bed, vision becomes distorted, changed.

Restriction of environmental interaction may result in sensory deprivation. For example, psychologically a person functions and lives within territorial boundaries described as the intimate zone, personal distance, solid distance, and public distance.

Health care personnel should be aware that their very presence in a room or around a patient can threaten a patient to a degree closely related to their distance from the patient. Edward Hall, an anthropologist, described human territorial behaviors in terms of four "zones":

1 *Intimate zone:* a distance of 6 to 18 inches or less from the patient. In this zone there normally is little voice contact, usually facial features become distorted, and transmission of a person's body heat, breath, odor, and so on occurs. Patients generally do *not* like strangers in this zone. Therefore health care personnel should always initially identify themselves and be acknowledged before entering this area around the patient.

2 *Personal distance:* a distance of 1½ to 4 feet. In this area visual contact is used and a speaking voice should be moderate. This is the most frequently used distance for talking with a patient.

3 *Solid distance:* a distance of 4 to 12 feet. As distance increases, the psychologic threat to the patient decreases. At this distance, eye contact is maintained and raising one's voice will cause this distance to psychologically shrink to the personal zone. Business is normally conducted at this distance.

4 *Public distance:* a distance of 12 to 25 feet. This is the least threatening distance to the patient. Generally there is impersonal involvement and the voice must be raised or projected to maintain contact when dealing with the patient.

1.4 Other emotional involvement

1 In a hospital a patient establishes new space dimensions—his or her unit, room, bed, and even physician and technician. Therefore it is very important that a clinician understand and use the proper terms, voice levels, and eye contacts when speaking with a patient.

2 Behavior is perceptual, that is, how the patient *sees* and *evaluates* behavior. For this reason health care personnel will find that they more successfully acquire the cooperation and support of some patients even though they use the same approach with all. Thus it is *imperative* to understand the importance of each patient accepting the practitioner's behavior, personality, and techniques.

3 Patients are sick, and their responses may change in direct response to their perception of how well they are doing.

4 Since they are constantly being exposed to change, patients must be kept informed. It is estimated that as many as 47 health team members will visit a patient each day in a critical care unit.

5 Orienting a patient requires awareness of physical position (such as an individual on a stretcher en route to the operating room) as well as the surrounding environment.

6 A hospital has strange odors, sights, and sounds that need to be explained to reduce the patient's apprehensions and to continually develop technician-patient rapport.

2.0 TECHNICIAN'S RESPONSE TO THE PATIENT
2.1 Technician's concept of the patient

1 All health care personnel are individuals who will react differently to a situation based on their own social and cultural background, total life experience, learned reactions, and individual makeup.

2 To be effective in helping patients resolve their feelings, practitioners must first learn to distinguish between their own goals, values, and standards of conduct and those of their patients. To do this they will need to be:
   a Alert to a patient's behavior and interpret it wisely.
   b Sincerely concerned and show interest, sensitivity, and understanding toward the patient.
   c Aware that the patient is a person and requires protection of both identity and dignity.
   d Aware of their own prejudices and work toward meeting each patient with an open mind and a helpful and supportive attitude.
   e Above all, a good listener.

3 Health care personnel must be aware of many situations that will neither change nor disappear and which must be considered from a psychologic point of view:
   a Incurable illness
   b Chronic illness
   c Disfigurement
   d Communicable diseases

2.2 Guide for responding to patients

Guidelines for responding to patients include the following:

1 Be professional, but be yourself. This usually draws a genuine response from others.

2 Let others respond in their own way rather than trying to manipulate them to respond the way you think you would under similar ciircumstances.

3 In unsatisfactory and frustrating situations, ask yourself, "What am *I* doing? Am I really appreciating the values of the patient?"

4 If in doubt, seek assistance from others more qualified to respond to the patient's needs.

2.3 Empathy versus sympathy

1 *Empathy* is the emotional understanding of another person's feelings. For example, since it has probably happened to us, most of us can *emotionally* understand the feelings surrounding the loss of a loved one, even if it was a pet.

2 *Sympathy* is the intellectual understanding of something in another person that is foreign to oneself. For instance, very few of us have ever been told that we have terminal cancer or a defective heart, but *intellectually* we can understand the feelings that the patient must have after being told such staggering news.

3.0 PSYCHOLOGIC RESPONSE TO DEATH AND DYING
3.1 Psychologic stages

Dying and death is a subject about which most Americans hesitate to think or talk about. To many, dying is an awesome event, the last mortal act of a human being. To others it is a sign of weakness and acknowledgment that no one is immortal. Whichever the rationale, most people do not wish to die and therefore are afraid of death and the unknown.

Dr. Elizabeth Kübler-Ross has described the various *psychologic stages* experienced by a patient facing death. She says the stages include:
1 Denial. "It can't be happening to me! There's some mistake."
2 Anger and shock. "Why me? What have I done to deserve this?"
3 Bargaining. "Let me live! I'll do anything!"
4 Depression and grief. "What's the use?"
5 Acceptance. "It's going to happen. I've had a good, full life."

Some terminal patients accept death more rationally than do the practitioners working with them. The feelings about dying and death are very personal, and practitioners must understand their own feelings and how they will deal with them when their patients die.

Practitioners who have concerns for fears about dealing with someone else's death should discuss them with a professional qualified to offer guidance.

3.2 Euthanasia

Euthanasia is the act of inducing a quiet, peaceful death. It is *not* legal and should not be overtly or covertly induced.
1 In some states "brain death" is medically defined as:
  a Patient in coma; totally unresponsive.
  b Patient apneic for 15 minutes.
  c "Flat" EEG for 30 minutes.
  d No cephalic reflexes.
  e Dilated pupils
  f Temperature decreased to 38° C (90° F).
  g No evidence of drug intoxication by history or clinical examination or chemical tests.

3.3 Depression

1 Depression is a mental condition that affects millions of persons of all ages. Psychologists divide depression into two broad categories, endogenous and exogenous. Endogenous (primary) depression usually originates from within the patient, frequently without any traumatic event as its cause. For this reason endogenous depression has been linked to biochemical imbalances. These imbalances can usually be corrected by maintenance dosages of medications called Monoamine Oxi-

dase (MAO) inhibitors, such as Nardil or Parnate. Exogenous (secondary) depression is triggered by an outside event. This condition is best treated with psychotherapy rather than medication.
2 It is estimated by the National Institute of Mental Health that 125,000 Americans are hospitalized each year for treatment of depression, with another 200,000 treated as outpatients. Another 4 to 8 million people are not even aware that they need treatment.
3 Annually in the United States as many as 25,000 to 35,000 suicides of people of all ages are attributed to depression.
4 According to statistics from the Los Angeles Suicide Prevention Center, the rate for suicides among people under 20 years of age has doubled and is the fourth leading cause of death during the teenage years (Committee on Adolescence, 1980).
5 In persons 65 years of age and older it is estimated that 13% have clinically significant depression warranting treatment.
6 In 80-year-old men the prevalence of suicide may be as high as 24%.
7 It is common for physicians to miss a diagnosis of depression in elderly persons; in as many as 75% of patients with depression, the condition goes unrecognized by their primary care physician.
8 The recognition of depression is an important contribution by all health care practitioners. This is especially true of respiratory care personnel who care for the elderly in nursing homes and other alternative care settings.

3.4 Symptoms of depression

Symptoms of depression include:
1 Feeling tired most of the time.
2 Changes in sleep habits with excessive insomnia.
3 Irritability and overreaction to ordinarily insignificant things.
4 Loss of enthusiasm or feeling of enjoyment for normally pleasurable things.
5 Unexplained sadness and crying.
6 Loss of interest in sex.
7 Dull, ever-present headache.
8 Chronic pain in the back or elsewhere.
9 Inability to study, concentrate, or achieve.
10 Chronic indigestion, diarrhea, constipation, and/or changes in eating habits with abnormal weight gain or loss.
11 Feelings of being neglected, wrong, or worthless.
12 Thoughts of suicide.
    NOTE: It is especially important for respiratory care personnel to recognize the symptoms of depression and to be aware that patients receiving certain antidepressant medications, such as monoamine oxidase (MAO) inhibitors, can experience some serious toxic effects if the patient is also given certain respiratory care medications, such as bronchodilators and decongestants. Questions about possible toxic or untoward reactions of giving cardiopulmonary medications to these patients

should be referred to the patient's physician. Before administering treatment, any signs of depression and/or toxic reactions to respiratory care medications in these patients must be reported immediately.

4.0 POSTURE, BODY POSITIONING, AND BODY MECHANICS

4.1 Posture and positioning

1 Posture is the relationship of the parts of the body at rest or in any phase of activity.
2 Most people have heard since childhood the importance of maintaining good posture, primarily for aesthetic reasons. Physiologically, it is important because misalignment of the skeleton places stress on joints and muscles and even the viscera (organs) of the body cavities.
3 Posture is considered good whenever it does not interfere with proper functioning of the body system and poor when *undue* stress is placed at any point.
4 The maintenance of good posture at all times is important. This is especially so when the body is under physical stress such as lifting, pushing, and pulling.
5 Most muscle and joint injuries occur because the individual is not in proper body alignment in preparation for and during the physical activity, or an action is attempted in opposition to a normal range of motion. Examples of normal range of motion for various parts of the body are presented in Fig. 5-1. A more detailed ex-

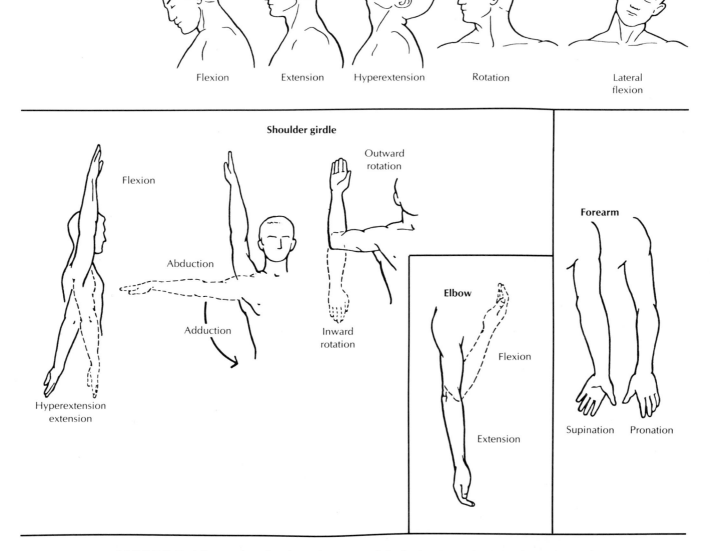

FIGURE 5-1 Range of motion for various parts of the body. (From Phipps WJ, Long BC, and Woods NF: Medical-surgical nursing: concepts and clinical practice, ed 2, St Louis, 1988, The CV Mosby Co.)   *Continued.*

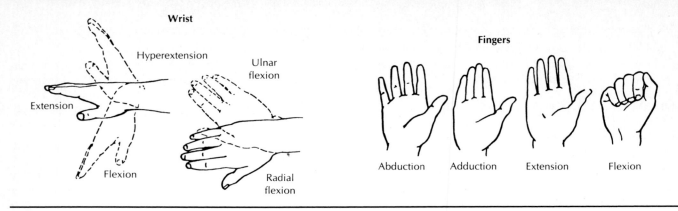

Wrist

Hyperextension

Ulnar flexion

Extension

Flexion

Radial flexion

Fingers

Abduction

Adduction

Extension

Flexion

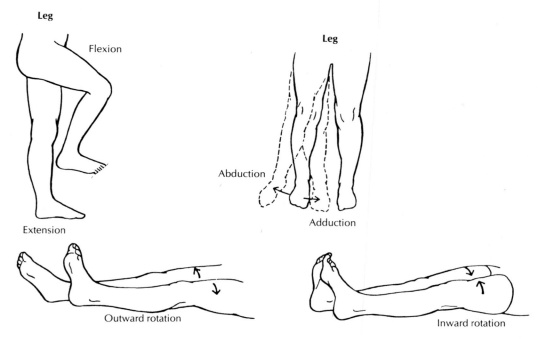

Leg

Flexion

Extension

Outward rotation

Leg

Abduction

Adduction

Inward rotation

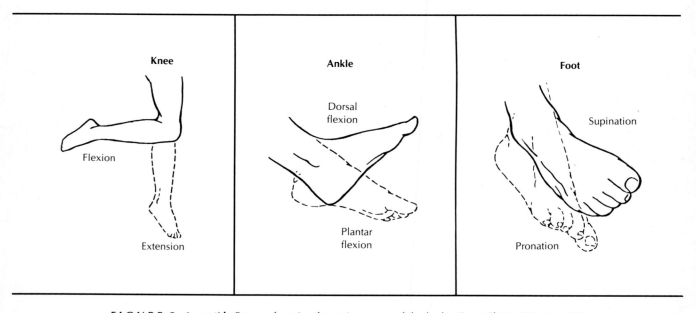

Knee

Flexion

Extension

Ankle

Dorsal flexion

Plantar flexion

Foot

Supination

Pronation

F I G U R E 5 - 1 cont'd. Range of motion for various parts of the body. (From Phipps WJ, Long BC, and Woods NF: Medical-surgical nursing: concepts and clinical practice, ed 2, St Louis, 1988, The CV Mosby Co.)   *Continued.*

Toes

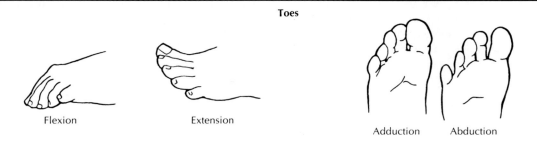

Flexion   Extension   Adduction   Abduction

FIGURE 5-1 cont'd. Range of motion for various parts of the body. (From Phipps WJ, Long BC, and Woods NF: Medical-surgical nursing: concepts and clinical practice, ed 2, St Louis, 1988, The CV Mosby Co.)

planation of range of motion movements and/or exercises may be found in most textbooks on nursing and physical therapy.

6 Muscles work in pairs. When a person is in poor position, unequal stress is placed on one muscle. This can cause muscle strain, a tear, or even breakage of bones. NOTE: Procedure 5-1 is included at the end of this module as an example of how to perform range of motion exercises. This knowledge is useful in preventing the patient from being placed in *adverse* anatomic positions and to prevent practitioners from injuring themselves by moving in an *unorthodox* manner (Fig. 5-2).

7 Instructions for correct posture during various activities are presented in Procedures 5-2 through 5-9 at the end of this module. They should be followed by the practitioner at all times but especially during stressful physical activities.

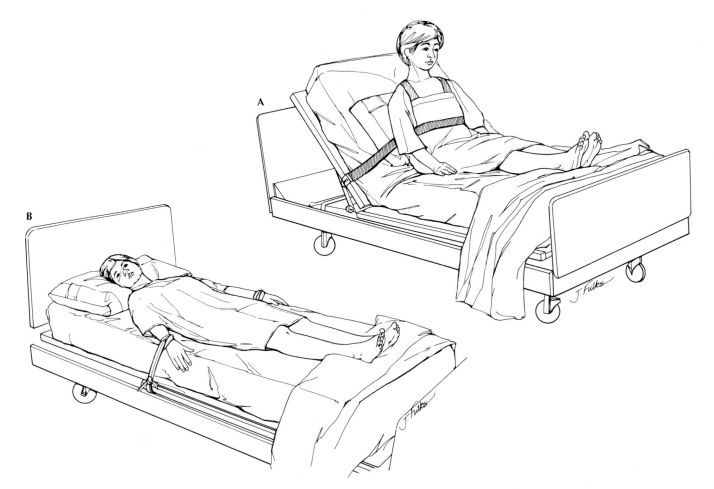

FIGURE 5-2 Material restraints. **A,** Velcro waist restraint. **B,** Posey safety straps.

4.2 Correct posture: standing (see Procedure 5-2)

Procedure 5-2 may be used as a guide for helping a patient stand properly. A correct standing posture is determined by the anatomical position, which is the basis for anatomic direction (Fig. 5-3).

NOTE: In anatomic position, *palms are facing outward* with fingers extended.

4.3 Correct posture: sitting

Procedure 5-3 may be used as a guide for helping a patient sit correctly.

4.4 Correct posture: lying supine

Procedure 5-4 may be used as a guide to assist the patient to achieve correct posture in lying supine (Fig. 5-4).

4.5 Stooping

Procedure 5-5 may be used as a guide to demonstrate correct body mechanics in stooping (Fig. 5-5).

4.6 Lifting and carrying

Procedure 5-6 may be used as a guide for lifting and carrying an object (Fig. 5-6).

4.7 Swing carry (two persons)

Procedure 5-7, a guide for the swing carry, is used to evacuate patients who are able to sit up in an emergency situation (Fig. 5-7).

NOTE: It is not to be used for patients with spinal injury or those who are otherwise restricted to a horizontal position.

4.8 Pivoting

Procedure 5-8 may be used as a guide for pivoting a patient in bed.

4.9 Pushing and pulling

Procedure 5-9 may be used as a guide for pushing and pulling a patient in bed (Fig. 5-8).

5.0 HOSPITAL BED
5.1 Operation of a hospital bed

Because of differences in various models of hospital beds, it would be impossible to cover specific operation of all beds. For this reason it is recommended that the reader visit a hospital or equipment store to receive a demonstration of the various types of beds. The following information pertains to the general operation of beds.

Most modern hospital beds are electrically powered. A control box, which is similar to that used for remote control of television, positions the bed. The height of a hospital bed can be adjusted to enable the practitioner to work with the patient without having to bend over. The bed can also be adjusted to elevate the patient's head or feet. In emergency situations the bed can be positioned in a Trendelenburg's or reverse Trendelenburg's position (see Unit 8.1).

NOTE: Whenever a patient is left unattended in bed, the side rails should be raised to prevent accidental injury from the patient falling out of bed.

6.0 MOVING THE PATIENT WITH AND WITHOUT ASSISTANCE
6.1 Moving and positioning the patient

1 Patients normally assume the most comfortable position. An exception to this is those patients who assume a position for therapeutic reasons, for example, the patient with chronic obstructive pulmonary disease who sits in a chair with arms fixed and shoulders raised with each inspiration. During exhalation this patient purses the lips and blows the air out slowly. The patient assumes this position to use accessory muscles for inspiration. Blowing air out through pursed lips helps to empty air from the chest that otherwise would have been trapped.

2 Patient positions therefore are important not only for comfort but for physiologic therapy. Module Nineteen, Pulmonary Drainage, presents instructions on how to position patients to drain their lungs. General steps for moving and positioning patients in most care situations are described in Procedures 5-10 through 5-18 at the end of this module.

6.2 Moving patient toward head of bed with patient assisting

Procedure 5-10 may be used as a guide for moving the patient toward the head of the bed with the patient's assistance (Fig. 5-9).

6.3 Moving patient to head of bed with assistant

Procedure 5-11 may be used as a guide for moving a patient to the head of the bed using an assistant to help with the procedure.

6.4 Assisting patient to dangle

Procedure 5-12 may be used as a guide for assisting the patient to dangle while sitting on the side of the bed (Fig. 5-10).

6.5 Assisting patient from bed into a chair

Procedure 5-13 may be used as a guide for assisting the patient from the bed onto a chair.

6.6 Moving patient from bed to stretcher with patient assistance

Procedure 5-14 may be used as a guide for assisting the patient from the bed to a stretcher with patient assisting in the move.

6.7 Moving patient from bed to stretcher with two co-workers' assistance

Procedure 5-15 may be used as a guide to move the patient from bed to stretcher with coworkers assistance.

6.8 Assisting patient to walk

Procedure 5-16 may be used as a guide for assisting a patient to walk.

6.9 Safeguarding the falling patient

Procedure 5-17 may be used as a guide to safeguarding the falling patient.

6.10 Turning the patient to right and left sides

Procedure 5-18 may be used as a guide for turning a patient to the right and left sides (Fig. 5-11).

7.0 RESTRAINTS

7.1 Restraining techniques

1 *Physical restraint.* Restraint is employed to prevent a patient from self-harm or from harming the people providing treatment. it is important to explain the purpose of such a device to the patient and family. When using physical restraint, practice the following general rules:

   a Grasp the patient by large bone or tissue areas.

   b Do not restrict circulation or dig your nails into the patient.

   c Do not bruise the patient.

   d Use restraining materials that have some "give" when stressed. Do not restrict the patient's movements *completely* or the patient may fracture bones or pull ligaments by applying contractile leverage against the restraining efforts.

   e *Do not restrict the head or spine* completely unless the restraint is required to maintain spinal alignment in cases of possible neck or spinal injury.

2 *Material restraints.* Materials used for restraints should be soft, strong, and wide enough to prevent damage to tissue or restriction of circulation.

   a Commercially available restraints made of Velcro or other quick-tie techniques can be purchased through hospital supply houses (see Fig. 5-2, *A*).

   b A Posey strap or other soft material can be folded to create 3-inch wide restraints (see Fig. 5-2, *B*).

3 *Securing the restraint.* As previously stated, even if explanation appears useless, the patient should *always* be told of the practitioner's intention and why it is necessary.

   a Place restraint on patient using a no-slip loop. This technique prevents accidental tightening of the restraint (see Fig. 5-2, *B*).

   b Secure restraint to a sturdy base.

   c Secure patient's limb in natural position that will *not* restrict circulation or cause muscle cramps.

   d Restraints should always be applied according to hospital policy. An improperly used restraint can be more dangerous than no restraint.

8.0 SPECIAL POSITIONS

8.1 Placing a patient in special positions

Procedures 5-19 through 5-29 at the end of this module may be used as guides for placing a patient in the following positions:

1 Supine (Fig. 5-12).

2 Prone (Fig. 5-13).

3 Dorsal recumbent (Fig. 5-14).

4 Fowler's (Fig. 5-15, *A*).

5 Semi-Fowler's (Fig. 5-15, *B*).

6 Right side-lying (Fig. 5-16).

7 Left side-lying (Fig. 5-17).

8 Sims' (Fig. 5-18).

9 Legs elevated (Fig. 5-19).

10 Trendelenburg's: a shock position (Fig. 5-20).

11 Reverse Trendelenburg's (Fig. 5-21).

9.0 MICROBES AND THEIR TRANSMISSION (SEE ALSO MODULE NINE)

9.1 Protection against infection

One of the most important principles clinicians must learn is how to protect themselves and their patients against the spread of disease and infection.

Microbes are by definition microscopic and cannot be seen with the unaided eye. Nevertheless, they are ever present and can become especially dangerous to the sick patient whose natural resistance is already lowered or perhaps compromised by antibiotics.

Most microbial diseases are spread by the four *F*s:

1 Fingers

2 Flies

3 Fomites (inanimate objects that are not themselves infected but that transmit microbes)

4 Food

This unit focuses primarily on fingers and hands as primary carriers of infection among patients.

• To prevent this type of cross-contamination, a routine handwashing procedure should be followed before and after each patient contact.

Patients who have known contagious organisms are placed in special rooms and isolated from unauthorized personnel.

• *Isolation* rooms are clearly marked on the outside of the door and should not be entered or left without special precautions.

9.2 Isolation techniques to prevent spread of infection

The clinician follows these guidelines:

1 Wash hands each time the patient receives treatment.

2 If possible, do not carry equipment from room until the patient's therapy has been discontinued.

3 Place all articles leaving the room in a closed container.

4 See that articles too large for a container are washed with detergent and aired for at least 12 hours.

5 Do *not* carry personal items from the room and reuse them until they have been properly decontaminated or cleaned. (This includes such items as watches and stethoscopes.)

6 Procedures 5-30 to 5-35 at the end of this module can be used as guides for isolation precautions:

   a Hand washing (Procedure 5-30).

   b Placement and removal of the face mask (Procedure 5-31).

   c Gowning (Procedure 5-32).

   d Gown removal (Procedure 5-33).

e Gloving and ungloving (Procedure 5-34).

f Removal of contaminated equipment and supplies from an isolation unit (Procedure 5-35).

• Further details on handling equipment and articles that have been exposed to a contaminated patient or area are outlined in Module Nine, Microbiology and Decontamination.

Procedures for entering and leaving isolation areas vary so greatly that a practitioner should refer to a specific hospital procedure manual and to Universal Precautions as recommended by the Center for Disease Control.

10.0 HOSPITAL SAFETY

10.1 Hazards to hospital safety

Hospital accidents are a primary concern to hospital administrators and, in many instances, can be avoided by following simple safety rules.

The following items are primary causes of accidents in the hospital and should be guarded against:

1 Wet floors.
2 Overloaded shelves.
3 Patients left unattended.
4 Bed rails left down.
5 Frayed electrical cords or exposed outlets.
6 Misread prescriptions or instructions.
7 Failure to follow a procedure or orders (e.g., cylinders not properly restrained).
8 Playing.
9 Not paying attention to the task at hand.
10 Thoughtless rushing.
11 Equipment left standing in hallways or other traffic areas.

11.0 DANGER OF FIRE IN HOSPITALS

11.1 Fire safety

Fire can be one of the most dreaded tragedies faced by humans. Since the discovery of fire, humans and animals alike have feared and respected its destructive potential.

Fire in a hospital is especially dangerous because many of the patients are unable to remove themselves and because of the interruption of medical care to the critically ill, which could in itself cause death.

11.2 Initiating the fire plan

Note that the following are *general precautions* and procedures. *Exact* procedures for any given facility should be obtained from a hospital procedure manual.

It is of primary importance in any fire to keep calm, to know and initiate the fire plan, and above all not to interfere with the professional fire fighters.

On discovering a fire (seeing flames or thick smoke):

1 Sound the fire alarm by going to the nearest fire alarm station; *pull* the lever all the way down, and release the lever. If the alarm does not sound after pulling the lever or you cannot locate a fire alarm station, telephone the hospital switchboard operator and state: "I am reporting a fire. This is _____(state your name); the fire is located at _____(describe the location)." *Do*

not ask anyone's permission. Do not hesitate. On seeing flames or thick smoke, sound the fire alarm.

2 Remove persons in immediate danger.
3 Confine the fire.
4 Assist with fighting the fire if needed. Do not become a fire statistic yourself by "playing hero." Most hospitals have a well-informed and trained fire team.

11.3 Fire drill (general rules)

It is important to recognize the audible and visual signals for a fire. When the fire alarm sounds, the following actions are to be taken.

1 *Stop!* Collect your thoughts; *stay calm.*
2 Close all doors.
3 Do *not* use the telephone for routine matters. Do *not* telephone to ask if it is a fire or a drill.
4 Stop people from traveling through the hospital.
  a No patient is to be sent from a nursing unit.
  b Patients in transport are to be taken to the most convenient waiting area.
  c Patients in treatment areas are to be held in the area.
  d Visitors are to stay with the patient being visited or in the dayroom on the floor.
  e Incoming visitors are to be stopped in the main lobby.
5 Supervisors should be prepared to dispatch personnel to render assistance as directed by the fire department, the hospital fire team, or hospital administration.
6 Continue routine duties that do *not* involve travel through the hospital.
  NOTE: Follow a hospital's specific plan for fire drill procedure.

11.4 Potential fire hazards

Fire hazards include:
1 Open gasoline or other flammable agents.
2 Oily rags.
3 Storage areas containing trash.
4 Unchained oxygen or anesthesia gas cylinders.
5 Smoking in areas where oxygen is being stored or used.
6 Oxygen regulators stored in oily and greasy areas.

11.5 Fire control techniques

1 Types of fire
  a Class A fire (wood, paper, cloth)
    • Use water or chemical.
    • Extinguishers may be located on walls, or hoses may be stored in convenient locations ready for use.
  b Class B fire (oil, gas, other liquids)
    • Use carbon dioxide or dry powder extinguishers.
    • *Do not use water.* It will spread the flames and may cause them to flash up into your face.
  c Class C fire (electrical)
    • Use carbon dioxide or dry powder extinguishers.
    • *Do not use water* or other liquid fire extinguisher agents that may conduct an electrical charge.

Procedure 5-36 at the end of this module may be used as a general guide for operating cannister fire extinguishers.

2 Self-protection

a If trapped in a room, keep the door closed between you and the fire.

b If you must vacate a room because of imminent danger, *carefully* feel the door. If it is hot, *do not open it!* The draft will cause the flames behind it to rush into your room much like an explosion.

c If trapped in a smoke-filled room or area:

- Stoop and walk with your face *approximately 2 feet off the floor* toward the closest exit. This level has been shown to have the most breathable air because it is too low for superheated gases above and too high for toxic, heavier-than-air gases at the floor level.
- Because vision will be greatly impaired, listen for voices or other sounds that indicate an exit.
- Follow any fresh air—it will lead to an escape route.
- Above all, do not panic.

12.0 DEFECTIVE EQUIPMENT
12.1 Reporting defective equipment

Recognizing and reporting defective equipment is an ongoing task that all hospital employees must perform to ensure the optimum care for the patient and, frequently, to prevent the expense of having to completely replace an item. The following procedure is general and may be modified according to the needs of a specific hospital.

1 Note that equipment is *not* working properly.

a Appearance—e.g., leaking on floor.

b Sound—e.g., absence of sound or motor making unusual noise.

c Touch—e.g., unit feels too hot or not warm enough.

d Smell—e.g., unit smells hot; burning smell.

e Performance—e.g., unit is not operating according to specifications or desired expectations.

2 Inform supervisors or personnel responsible for area where equipment is being used.

3 If a patient is in *immediate* danger (e.g., fire) remove the patient from equipment, and call for help. *Do not alter or disconnect* equipment unless the patient is in obvious immediate danger.

12.2 Respiratory therapy equipment

1 Note that the equipment is not working.

2 Contact the supervisor of the patient care area and the nurse in charge of the unit in the following order of availability:

a Senior technician or therapist

b Technical director

c Physician or nurse responsible for the patient

3 Remove or alter operation of equipment only if the patient is in obvious immediate danger.

4 If equipment is removed, be sure the patient continues to receive substitute therapy before leaving the area.

5 Return the equipment to the department.

6 Test the equipment in the department and note the operational defect.

a If a major repair is needed, return the equipment to a repair service for correction.

b If minor, and you are *qualified,* effect repair, or refer the equipment to a designated person for service/repair.

7 Always *tag* the equipment as broken, and remove it from active inventory to prevent it from being used on another patient.

8 Always follow your department's procedure for processing defective equipment. *Do not* attempt repair unless you have received instruction and supervised practice with the specific item involved.

PROCEDURE 5-1

Range of motion joints

No.	Steps in performing the procedure
	The practitioner will perform range of motion exercises when they are appropriate for the patient in the clinical facility.
1	Bend patient's fingers and toes forward and backward.
2	Bend each foot forward and backward.
3	Trace an imaginary circle with each hand and foot.
4	Bend and straighten the legs and hips.
5	Move one leg at a time out to the side of the body and bring it back.
6	Bend and straighten each lower arm.
7	Bring each arm forward and backward.
8	With arms forward, turn palms up, then palms down.
9	Move each arm out to the side of the body. Turn palms upward and bring the arm up over the head.
10	Bend the head forward, backward, and from side to side
11	Turn the head from side to side.
12	Bend the trunk forward and backward and from side to side.
13	Turn the trunk from side to side.

PROCEDURE 5-2

Correct posture: standing

No.	Steps in performing the procedure
	The practitioner will, when it is appropriate in the clinical facility, assist the patient in standing properly (Fig. 5-3).
1	Patient's stance is erect.
2	Feet are about 4 inches apart with toes pointing straight ahead.
3	Knees are slightly bent.
4	Pelvis is in line with trunk.
5	Abdomen is tucked in.
6	Chest is up and out.
7	Head is up and chin down.
8	Arms are at the side, with palms facing *inward*.

PROCEDURE 5-3

Correct posture: sitting

No.	Steps in performing the procedure
	The practitioner will, when it is appropriate in the clinical facility, assist the patient in sitting properly.
1	Patient sits all the way back in the chair with spine resting against back of chair.
2	Feet are comfortably apart and resting flat on the floor.
3	Head is up and chin is down.
4	Chest is up and out.
5	Arms should be comfortably resting on the arms of a chair, in patient's lap, or positioned at waist level in front of patient. Shoulders should not be slumped.

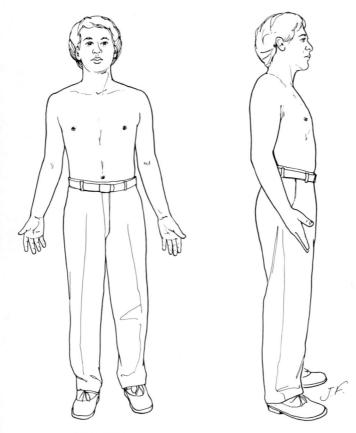

FIGURE 5-3 Correct standing posture.

PROCEDURE 5-4

Correct posture: lying supine

No.	Steps in performing the procedure
1	The practitioner will, when it is appropriate in the clinical facility, assist the patient in achieving the correct posture while lying supine (Fig. 5-4).
	Patient's alignment is the same as for standing (except that the back rests on a firm surface), with support to all the natural curves of the body.

PROCEDURE 5-5

Body mechanics: stooping

No.	Steps in performing the procedure
	The practitioner will demonstrate proper body alignment and movement in performing a stooping activity whenever necessary in the clinical facility (Fig. 5-5).
1	Start action with stable base of support.
2	Keep feet apart, one foot slightly advanced.
3	Keep back and neck straight.
4	Keep knees and hip joints flexed.
5	Lower body to stooped position, using thigh and leg muscles to control action.
6	Prepare to raise self by shifting weight to advance foot and ball of rear foot.
7	Raise body back up to standing position:
	7.1 Initiate upward movement by extending hip and knee joints.
	7.2 Keep back and neck straight.
	7.3 Use extensor muscles to bring body upright.

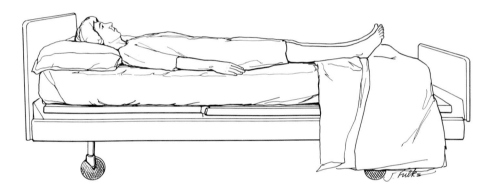

FIGURE 5-4 Correct posture while lying in supine position.

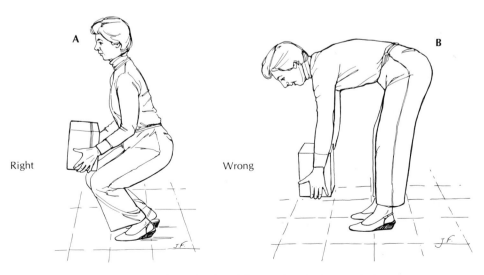

Right

Wrong

FIGURE 5-5 Body mechanics while stooping. **A,** Correct. **B,** Incorrect.

PROCEDURE 5-6

Body mechanics: lifting and carrying

No.	Steps in performing the procedure
	The practitioner will demonstrate proper body alignment and movement, in a safe manner, while lifting and carrying objects (Fig. 5-6) whenever necessary in the clinical facility.
1	Start action with a stable base of support.
2	Demonstrate proper body alignment. **2.1** Legs flexed at knees **2.2** Bend at waist with straight back and neck.
3	Contract abdominal and arm muscles for action.
4	Grasp object (e.g., box) in a manner that balances weight and bulk of object.
5	Lift weight from stooped position, keeping back straight, using leg muscles to rise to standing position.
6	Carry object near midline of body, maintaining proper body alignment (see Fig. 5-6, *B*).

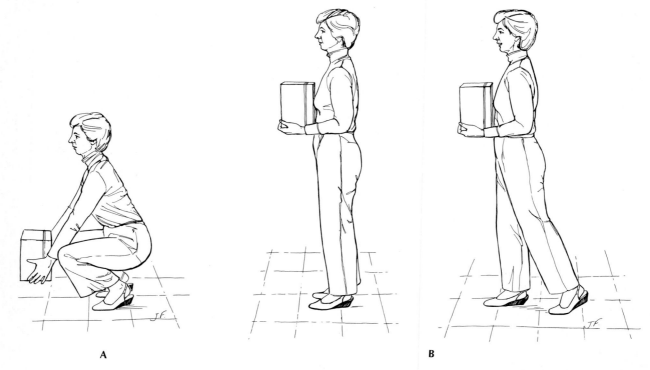

A   **B**

FIGURE 5-6 Correct body mechanics for lifting and carrying an object. **A,** Lifting. **B,** Carrying.

PROCEDURE 5-7

Body mechanics: swing carry (two persons)

No.	Steps in performing the procedure
	The practitioner will perform the proper techniques to swing carry a patient in a safe and comfortable manner in the clinical facility (Fig. 5-7).
1	**BOTH PERSONS** **1.1** Wash hands. **1.2** Greet patient. **1.3** Explain care to be given. **1.4** Bring patient to dangling position.
2	Person no. 1: Stand on the right side of patient; person. Person no. 2: stand on left side of patient. **2.1** Face each other. **2.2** Flex knees and hips.
3	Each person: Take one of patient's wrists, and pull patient's arm around your own neck and down across your own chest.
4	Each person: reach across patient's back and place your free hand on the top of the other.
5	Both: Let go of patient's wrist.
6	Each: Reach under patient's knees and grasp the wrist of the other person (person at right side: palms down; person at left side: palms up).
7	**BOTH PERSONS** **7.1** Extend your knees and thighs to a standing position, pivot, and carry patient to a safe area. **7.2** Wash hands.

PROCEDURE 5-8

Body mechanics: pivoting

No.	Steps in performing the procedure
	The practitioner will demonstrate proper body movement as necessary in administration of patient care in the clinical facility.
1	Stand on a firm base with feet slightly apart, knees slightly flexed, providing stable support for use of leg muscles.
2	Contract trunk and pelvis muscles for action.
3	Contract thigh and leg muscles.
4	Shift weight to ball of each foot, lifting heel slightly.
5	Pivot or make a 90-degree turn on feet.
6	Move body simultaneously with feet so that lower back does not twist.
7	Redistribute weight equally on each foot after turn is completed.

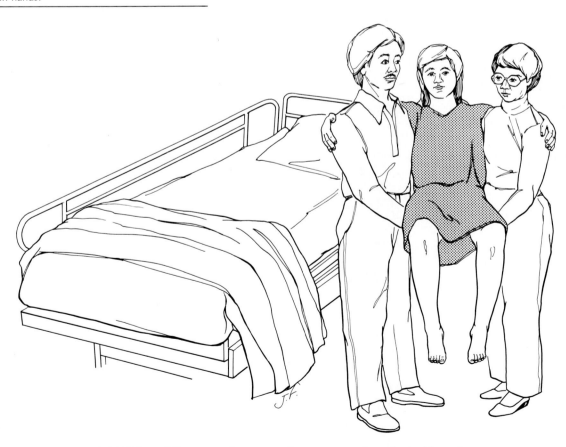

FIGURE 5-7 Proper way for two people to carry a patient who is able to sit up.

PROCEDURE 5-9

Body mechanics: pushing and pulling

No.	Steps in performing the procedure
	The practitioner will, wherever the need arises in the clinical facility, push and pull moveable objects with proper body position and movement. This method of pushing and pulling ensures maximum safety to the practitioner as well as to the object being pushed (Fig. 5-8).
1	Start action with stable base of support.
2	Position feet at least 8 inches apart, with one foot slightly ahead of the other.
3	Position body for appropriate action, observing proper body alignment.
4	Contract trunk and leg muscles.
5	Keep arms flexed at elbows.
6	Lean forward toward object when pushing.
7	Lean backward when pulling.
8	Apply force to move object, using large muscles of legs.
9	Keep back straight and erect when moving.

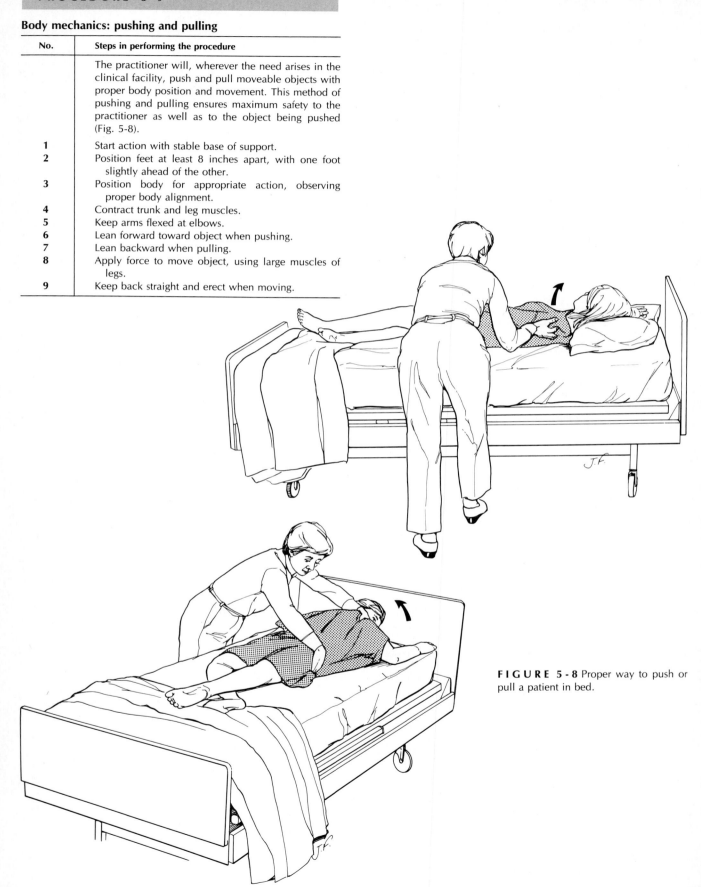

FIGURE 5-8 Proper way to push or pull a patient in bed.

<table>
<tr><td colspan="2">PROCEDURE 5-10</td></tr>
</table>

Body mechanics: movement of patient toward head of bed with patient assisting

No.	Steps in performing the procedure
	The practitioner will, when it is appropriate in the clinical facility, move the patient toward the head of the bed, providing for the safety and comfort of both patient and practitioner (Fig. 5-9).
1	Wash hands.
2	Identify and greet patient.
3	Explain procedure to patient.
4	Lower back rest of bed to horizontal.
5	Adjust bed to working height (waist level).
6	Remove pillow from behind patient's head; place pillow against headboard of bed.
7	Instruct patient on how he or she can assist: 7.1 Flex both knees and place soles of feet on mattress. 7.2 On command, push down with feet.
8	Initiate procedure. 8.1 Place one arm under patient's shoulder. 8.2 Cradle patient's head in bend of your elbow. 8.3 Place other arm under patient's hips.
9	Complete procedure. 9.1 Coordinate own body movement with that of patient. 9.2 On signal, have patient push with feet while simultaneously moving the patient toward the head of the bed.
10	Provide for patient's comfort. 10.1 Adjust patient for good body alignment. 10.2 Replace pillow. 10.3 Return bed to comfortable or prescribed position. 10.4 Place call button within reach. 10.5 Raise side rails (when necessary).
11	Wash hands.

<table>
<tr><td colspan="2">PROCEDURE 5-11</td></tr>
</table>

Body mechanics: moving patient to head of bed with co-worker's assistance

No.	Steps in performing the procedure
	The practitioner will, when appropriate, move the patient to the head of the bed with a co-worker's assistance.
1	Wash hands.
2	Identify and greet patient.
3	Explain care to be given.
4	Lower back rest to horizontal position.
5	Adjust bed to working height (waist level).
6	Remove pillow from behind patient's head; place pillow against headboard of bed.
7	Assistant: Standing on one side of bed, place right arm under shoulder of patient and left arm under hips.
8	Technician: Standing on other side of bed, place left arm under patient's shoulder and right arm under patient's hips.
9	Both health care workers: 9.1 Face head of bed. 9.2 Flex your knees.
10	On signal by assistant, move patient toward head of bed.
11	*Remember to lift* as you move the patient. The patient who slides along the surface of the bed may experience friction burns.
12	Replace pillow under head of patient.
13	Position patient for safety and comfort.
14	Wash hands.

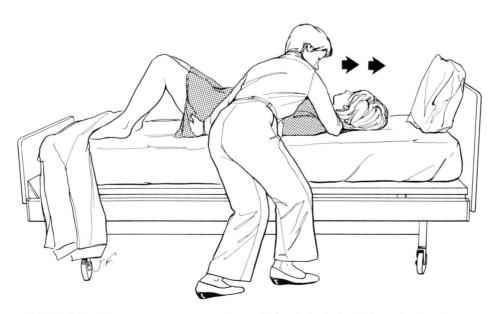

FIGURE 5-9 Proper way to move a patient to the head of a bed with the patient's assistance.

PROCEDURE 5-12

Body mechanics: assisting patient to dangle

No.	Steps in performing the procedure
	The practitioner will assist the patient whenever necessary, in dangling at the bedside in a manner both safe and comfortable to the patient in the clinical facility (Fig. 5-10, *A* and *B*).
1	Wash hands.
2	Identify and greet patient.
3	Explain procedure to patient.
4	Move patient to proximal side of bed.
5	Adjust bed to low position. Raise head of bed to a 45-degree angle (approximately).
6	Place one hand under patient's proximal shoulder and the other hand under patient's distal axilla.
7	Lift patient to a sitting position.
8	Continue to support shoulder while placing other hand under distal knee.
9	Swing patient's legs off bed while pivoting patient's body to a dangling position.
10	Lower bed until patient's feet touch the floor.
11	Maintain principles of good body alignment while completing the motion. Patient's movements should be slow, smooth, and steady.
12	Provide for patient's safety and comfort. **12.1** Dress patient in gown and slippers for comfort and modesty. **12.2** Remove patient's gown and slippers when returning to bed.
13	Return patient to supine position, using one hand on patient's proximal shoulder and the other hand under patient's distal axilla.
14	Provide for patient's comfort. **14.1** Readjust body alignment. **14.2** Readjust bed position. **14.3** Provide call light and stand, and put side rails up (where necessary).
15	Wash hands.

PROCEDURE 5-13

Assisting patient from bed into a chair

No.	Steps in performing the procedure
	The practitioner will assist the patient from bed into a chair in a manner both safe and comfortable to the patient in the clinical facility.
1	Wash hands.
2	Identify and greet patient.
3	Explain care to be given.
4	Place chair at side of bed.
5	Assist patient to sitting position.
6	Assist patient into robe and slippers.
7	Adjust bed to low position.
8	Have patient place his or her hands on your waist.
9	Place your hands on the patient's waist.
10	Flex your knees and bend your trunk forward.
11	Assist patient to rise to a standing position as you straighten your legs and hips.
12	Sidestep with patient to the chair.
13	Have patient feel the back of his or her legs against the front edge of chair.
14	Have patient bend slightly forward and transfer his or her hands from your shoulders to arms of chair.
15	Flex your knees, and bend your trunk as you assist patient into the chair.
16	Position patient for comfort and safety.
17	Wash hands.

PROCEDURE 5-14

Assisting patient from bed to stretcher with patient's assistance

No.	Steps in performing the procedure
	The practitioner will assist the patient from bed to stretcher in a manner both safe and comfortable to the patient in the clinical facility.
1	Wash hands.
2	Identify and greet patient.
3	Explain care to be given.
4	Place a bath towel over the top bedding. (This is for protection of patient's modesty and dignity.)
5	Have patient hold top edge of bath towel.
6	Fold top bedding to foot of bed.
7	Lock wheels on bed.
8	Place stretcher next to side of bed with head of stretcher at head of bed.
9	Lock wheels on the stretcher.
10	Raise bed to level of stretcher
11	Position yourself on the side and in the center of stretcher with your body weight against stretcher to keep it in place.
12	Have patient slide from bed to stretcher. This is often an awkward and difficult maneuver for the patient. Give verbal guidance in bracing and shifting to stretcher.
13	Secure safety straps or rails.
14	Wash hands.

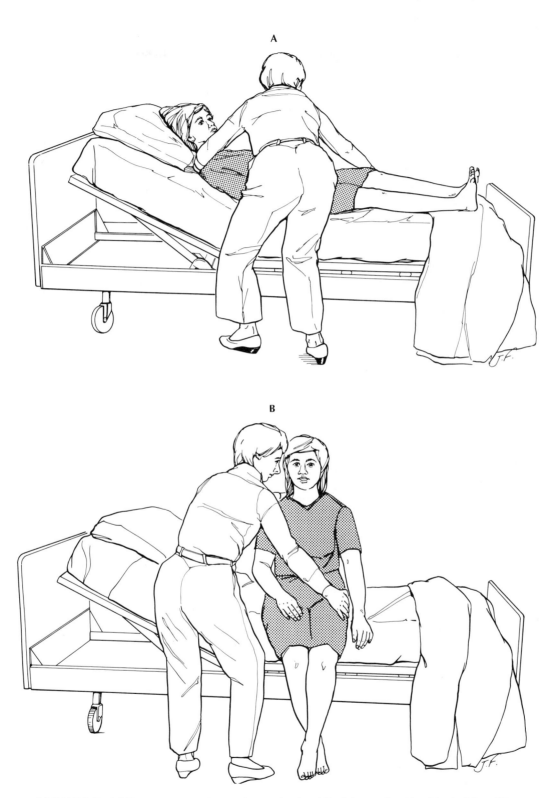

FIGURE 5-10 Proper way to assist a patient to dangle while sitting on the side of the bed **A** and **B**.

PROCEDURE 5-15

Moving patient from bed to stretcher with co-workers' assistance

No.	Steps in performing the procedure
	The practitioner will move the patient from bed to stretcher with co-workers' assistance in a manner both safe and comfortable to the patient in the clinical facility.
1	Wash hands.
2	Identify and greet patient.
3	Explain care to be given.
4	Lock wheels on bed.
5	Loosen draw sheet on each side of bed.
6	Place bath towel over top bedding.
7	Hold bath towel in place.
8	Fold top bedding to foot of bed.
9	Roll ends of both draw sheet and bath towel together until the edges are close to the patient on each side (mummy fashion).
10	Place stretcher next to side of bed, with head of stretcher at head of bed.
11	Lock wheels on stretcher.
12	Raise bed to level of stretcher.
13	Person on stretcher side: **13.1** Stand on the side and in the center of stretcher with your body weight against stretcher. **13.2** Reach over stretcher and grasp the rolled sheet just below patient's shoulder and at the thigh. **13.3** On signal pull patient onto stretcher.
14	Person on opposite side: **14.1** Stand on the side in the center of the bed. **14.2** Grasp rolled sheets at level of patient's shoulders and thigh. **14.3** On signal, lift patient, using sheets, and guide patient toward stretcher.
15	Third person **15.1** Stand on stretcher side near head of stretcher. **15.2** Reach over stretcher, and on signal move patient's head with your body. **15.3** Prevent accidental extubation if a tracheal tube is in place.
16	Secure safety straps.
17	Wash hands.

PROCEDURE 5-16

Body mechanics: assisting the patient to walk

No.	Steps in performing the procedure
	The practitioner will assist a patient to walk, whenever the need arises in the clinical facility, in a manner that is safe and comfortable.
1	Wash hands.
2	Identify and greet patient.
3	Explain procedure to patient.
4	Move patient to proximal side of bed.
5	Adjust bed to low position and wheels to locked position.
6	Raise patient to sitting position with one hand on patient's proximal shoulder and the other hand under patient's distal axilla.
7	Continue to support shoulder while placing other hand under distal knee, slipping legs off bed while pivoting patient's body.
8	Allow patient to dangle for a full minute.
9	Dress patient for comfort and modesty.
10	Assist patient to stand at bedside for a moment, encouraging good body position and posture.
11	Walk with patient, using appropriate support. **11.1** Minimal support: Hold patient's arm. **11.2** Moderate support: Hold patient's left hand in your left hand, with right hand on patient's waist. **11.3** Maximum support: Obtain assistance by having another health worker walk on other side of patient.
12	Wash hands.

PROCEDURE 5-17

Body mechanics: safeguarding the falling patient

No.	Steps in performing the procedure
	The practitioner will safeguard the fall of a patient in a manner safe to both patient and practitioner. The practitioner will provide for the needs of the patient following the fall. This shall be done at any time that the emergency need arises in the clinical facility.
1	Explain rationale for breaking patient's fall rather than catching him or her: **1.1** Injury to patient. **1.2** Injury to self. **1.3** Danger of abrupt change in movement.
2	As patient loses balance and begins to fall, quickly move to rear of patient, attempting to break fall by grasping patient under armpits.
3	Once contact is made, flex legs to lower patient gently to the floor.
4	Fall with patient, supporting his or her head.
5	Maintain patient in a sitting or lying position on the floor.
6	Remain with patient, providing comfort and reassurance.
7	Examine patient for possible injury.
8	Wash hands.
9	Afterward, prepare accident report.

PROCEDURE 5-18

Assisting patient to turn to right and left sides

No.	Steps in performing the procedure
	The practitioner will assist a patient to turn to his or her right or left side, whenever the need arises in the clinical facility, in a manner that is safe and comfortable (Fig. 5-11).
1	Wash hands.
2	Identify and greet patient.
3	Explain care to be given.
4	Lower bed to flat position.
5	Lower side rails near you.
6	Assist patient to side of bed near you.
7	Elevate side rail.
8	Go around to other side of bed.
9	Lower side rail.
10	Have patient cross his or her feet toward the side to be turned.
11	Have patient place an arm over the head on the side to be turned.
12	Have patient place the other arm across his or her chest toward the side to be turned.
13	Place one hand on the patient's hip.
14	Place your other hand on the patient's shoulder.
15	Roll the patient onto his or her side.
16	Position for safety and comfort.
17	Raise side rail.
18	Wash hands.

PROCEDURE 5-19 THROUGH 5-29

General positions

Procedure no.	Steps in performing the procedure
	The practitioner will place the patient in the appropriate position, whenever the need arises in the clinical facility, in a manner that is safe and comfortable.
5-19	**SUPINE** (Fig. 5-12) **1.1** Place patient flat on back with face looking upward.
5-20	**PRONE** (Fig. 5-13) **1.1** Place patient flat on stomach with toes extended over foot end of mattress. **1.2** Turn patient's head to one side.
5-21	**DORSAL RECUMBENT** (Fig. 5-14) **1.1** Place patient on back. **1.2** Place pillow under patient's head and shoulders. **1.3** Flex patient's knees. **1.4** Place soles of patient's feet on bed.

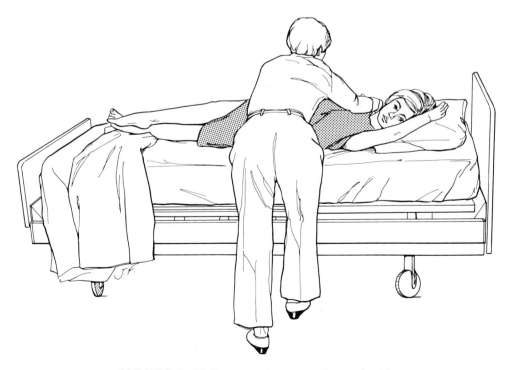

FIGURE 5-11 Proper way to turn a patient to the side.

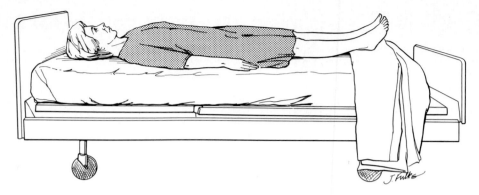

FIGURE 5-12 Supine position.

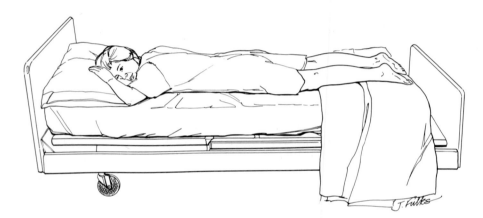

FIGURE 5-13 Prone position.

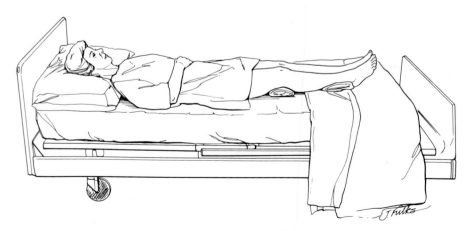

FIGURE 5-14 Dorsal recumbent position.

PROCEDURE 5-19 THROUGH 5-29

General positions— cont'd

Procedure no.	Steps in performing the procedure
5-22	**FOWLER'S** (Fig. 5-15, *A*) **1.1** Place patient on back. **1.2** Place a pillow under patient's head and shoulders. **1.3** Elevate head of bed to about a 45-degree angle. **1.4** Flex patient's knees slightly by raising leg rest of bed (optional).
5-23	**SEMI-FOWLER'S** (Fig. 5-15, *B*) **1.1** Place patient on back. **1.2** Place pillow under patient's head and shoulders. **1.3** Elevate head of bed to about a 20-degree angle. **1.4** Flex patient's knees slightly by raising leg rest of bed (optional).

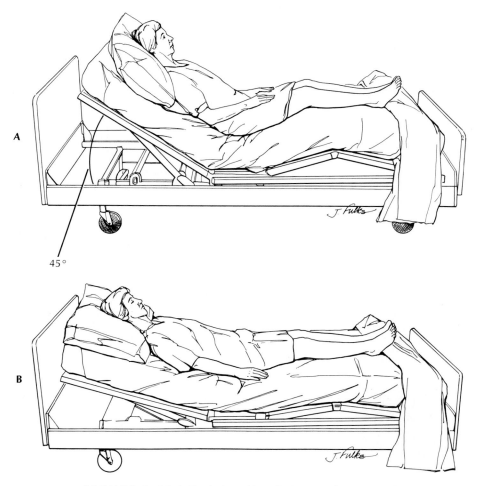

45°

F I G U R E 5 - 1 5 A, Fowler's position. **B,** Semi-Fowler's position.

General positions—cont'd

Procedure no.	Steps in performing the procedure
5-24	**RIGHT SIDE-LYING** (Fig. 5-16) **1.1** Place patient's right arm above his or her head. **1.2** Place patient on his or her right side. **1.3** Place a pillow on bed lengthwise under patient's left arm. **1.4** Flex patient's right knee slightly. **1.5** Flex patient's left knee and thigh over right leg. **1.6** Place a pillow lengthwise on the bed under patient's left thigh and leg.
5-25	**LEFT SIDE-LYING** (Fig. 5-17) **1.1** Reverse of right side-lying position.

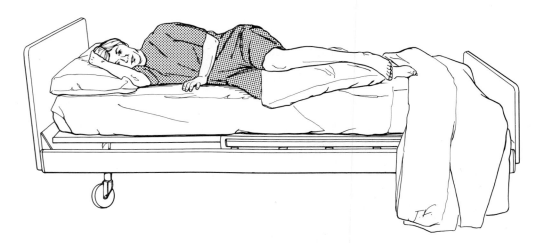

FIGURE 5-16 Right side-lying position.

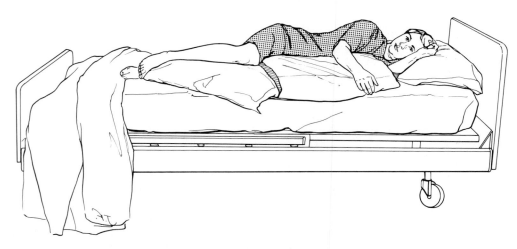

FIGURE 5-17 Left side-lying position.

General positions—cont'd

Procedure no.	Steps in performing the procedure
5-26	**SIMS'** (Fig. 5-18, *A* and *B*) **1.1** Place patient on right side. **1.2** Place patient's right arm behind back. **1.3** Place patient's left arm to the side of his or her head. **1.4** Flex patient's right leg slightly. **1.5** Flex patient's left leg and thigh over right leg.
5-27	**LEGS ELEVATED** (Fig. 5-19) **1.1** Adjust lower section of bed so that patient's legs are slightly elevated at an angle to the trunk.

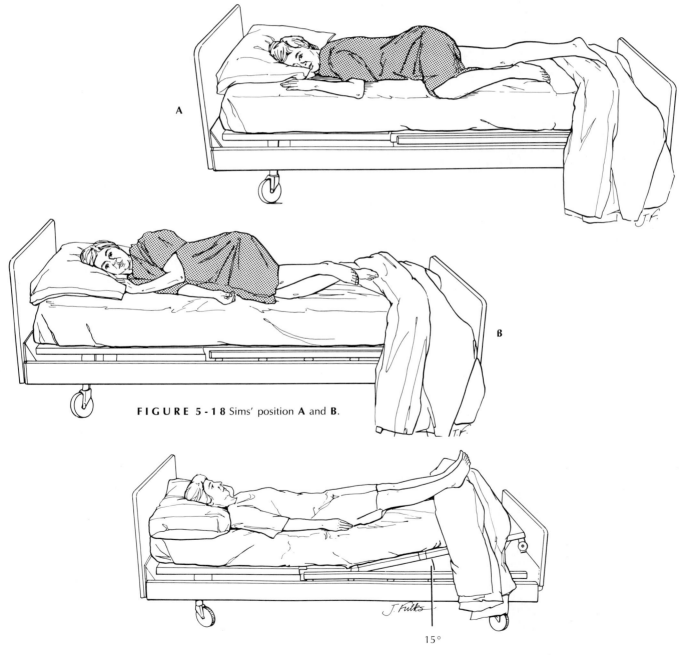

A

B

F I G U R E 5 - 1 8 Sims' position **A** and **B**.

15°

F I G U R E 5 - 1 9 Legs elevated position.

PROCEDURE 5-19 THROUGH 5-29

General positions—cont'd

Procedure no.	Steps in performing the procedure
5-28	**TRENDELENBURG'S (SHOCK POSITION)** (Fig. 5-20) **1.1** Raise complete foot of bed on blocks or by adjustment so that the foot of the entire bed is elevated at least a 20-degree angle to the floor. **1.2** Keep patient's knees straight, trunk horizontal, and head slightly elevated on a pillow.
5-29	**REVERSE TRENDELENBURG'S** (Fig. 5-21) **1.1** Raise complete head of bed on blocks or by adjustment so that the head of the entire bed is elevated at an angle at least 20 degrees to the floor. **1.2** Keep patient's knees straight, trunk horizontal, and head raised slightly on a pillow.

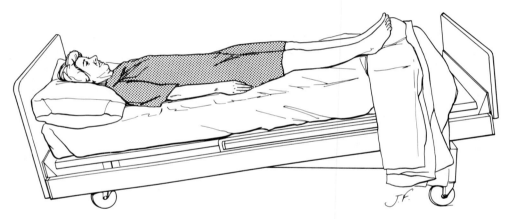

FIGURE 5-20 Trendelenburg's position.

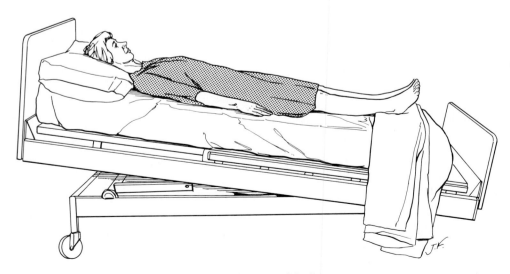

FIGURE 5-21 Reverse Trendelenburg's position.

PROCEDURE 5-30

Handwashing

No.	Steps in performing the procedure
	The practitioner will demonstrate proper aseptic technique in washing hands. This technique shall be used before any contact with patient in the clinical facility.
1	Stand away from sink so as not to place clothing in contact with sink.
2	Remove rings and watch.
3	Turn water on, adjusting to warm temperature. Water is kept running during entire procedure.
4	Wet hands.
5	Apply soap thoroughly, getting under nails and between fingers.
6	Wash palms and backs of hands with strong frictional motion.
7	Wash fingers and spaces between them by interlacing the fingers, rubbing them up and down for 10 seconds.
8	Wash wrists and 3 to 4 inches above wrists, using rotary action.
9	Repeat steps 5 through 8.
10	Rinse well; running water from fingers to wrists.
11	Keeping arms up, dry thoroughly with paper towel from fingertips to wrists.
12	Turn off water with paper towel and discard in receptacle.
13	*If using bar soap:*
	13.1 Turn on water before picking up soap.
	13.2 Hold soap in hand entire time you are washing.
	13.3 After washing procedure, rinse off the soap and put it where it belongs.

PROCEDURE 5-31

Placement and removal of face mask

No.	Steps in performing the procedure
	The practitioner will mask in a manner that provides maximum asepsis, ensuring safety to both patient and practitioner. Following patient care, the practitioner will remove the mask in a similar safe manner. This technique shall be used wherever the need arises in the clinical facility.
	MASK PLACEMENT
1	Wash hands (according to hand washing technique).
2	Obtain clean mask.
3	Unfold mask and place over nose and mouth.
4	Tie top strings (over ears) at back of head, with top edge of mask under glasses (if worn). Bottom strings are tied behind neck.
5	Rewash hands.
	MASK REMOVAL
1	Remove mask by untying lower strings, then top strings.
2	Grasp by strings and discard into proper receptable.
3	Wash hands.

PROCEDURE 5-32

Gowning (isolation area)

No.	Steps in performing the procedure
	The practitioner will demonstrate gowning according to strict aseptic technique. This technique applies anywhere in the clinical facility where the health care member will be required to enter an isolation area.
1	Remove rings and watch.
2	Wash hands according to aseptic hand washing technique.
3	Select gown. Hold gown by neck, and open it away from body.
4	Put arms into sleeves, work up arms, and adjust on shoulders (without touching hands to body).
5	Tie neck tie, close gown, and tie waist ties.

PROCEDURE 5-33

Gown removal (isolation area)

No.	Steps in performing the procedure
	The practitioner will demonstrate proper gown removal following the administration of care to a patient in isolation. This procedure will ensure minimum opportunity for contamination to self or other personnel in or outside of the isolation area.
1	Untie waist tie, and push up sleeves.
2	Wash hands.
3	Untie neck tie.
4	Remove arms from sleeves.
	4.1 Place finger under sleeve cuff, and pull sleeve down over hand.
	4.2 While arm is still in gown, use covered hand to pull other sleeve off.
5	Slip out of gown, turning contaminated side in.
6	Discard gown, making sure not to touch body.
7	Wash hands again before leaving unit or room.

PROCEDURE 5-34

Gloving and ungloving

No.	Steps in performing the procedure
	The practitioner will glove hands, avoiding contact with skin outside gloves. The gloves should fit so that there is minimum opportunity of contamination to self or patient, depending on type of isolation. When the practitioner removes the gloves, this procedure will minimize chance of self-contamination as well as other hospital personnel and patients.
	GLOVING
1	Wash hands according to aseptic handwashing technique.
2	Unfold glove wrapper, taking care not to contaminate gloves in the process.
3	Remove first glove from wrapper at folded edge of cuff, not allowing glove to touch wrapper.
4	Pull glove on hand.
5	With first gloved hand, grasp second glove under loose edge of cuff (sterile surface to sterile surface), and pull glove up on hand.
6	When necessary, adjust gloves over gown cuffs without contaminating gloves or gown.
	GLOVE REMOVAL
1	Remove gloves before removing gown.
2	Pull first glove off without contaminating skin; dispose of glove in appropriate receptacle.
3	Pull second glove off by placing fingers inside cuff of glove, and pull down over hand.
4	Continue with gown removal procedure.

PROCEDURE 5-35

Removal of contaminated equipment and supplies from an isolation unit

No.	Steps in performing the procedure
	The practitioner will handle and process equipment and supplies in a manner that ensures safety, using appropriate techniques whenever the need arises in the clinical facility.
	PERSON NO. 1
1	Place materials to be sterilized in plastic or paper bags. (If items require special handling—e.g., no steam sterilization—place in separate bag, and tag.)
2	Place items to be disposed of in a separate plastic bag labeled "trash only."
3	Tie all bags securely.
4	Call for assistance.
	PERSON NO. 2
1	Stand in doorway of room, and hold appropriate clean bag in which person no. 1 places contaminated bags.
2	Tie bag securely, and label the double-bagged trash, supplies, and equipment.
3	Process per established policy.
	PERSON NO. 1
1	Replace all containers with clean plastic liner.
2	Remove gown.
3	Leave room without touching anything.
4	Wash hands at designated sink.

PROCEDURE 5-36

Operating fire extinguishers

No.	Steps in performing the procedure
	The practitioner will demonstrate correct operation of fire extinguishers, ensuring safety to both patients and practitioners. These techniques shall be used whenever the need arises in the clinical facility.
	OPERATION OF WATER FIRE EXTINGUISHER (TYPE A FIRE)
1	Obtain extinguisher from storage area.
2	Transport to fire.
3	Pistol action type:
	3.1 Place on floor.
	3.2 Remove safety catch pin.
	3.3 Direct water hose at base of fire.
	3.4 Compress handle.
	3.5 To stop flow of water, release handle.
4	Nonpistol action type:
	4.1 Direct hose at base of fire.
	4.2 Invert tank and place on floor.
	4.3 Spray water over base of flame. (There is no way to stop flow of water once activated.)
	OPERATION OF CARBON DIOXIDE FIRE EXTINGUISHER (TYPE B FIRE)
1	Obtain extinguisher from storage area.
2	Transport to site of fire.
3	Place on floor.
	3.1 Remove safety catch pin.
	3.2 Direct nozzle at base of flame.
	3.3 Compress handle (pistol action).
	3.4 Overlay base of flame with blanket of carbon dioxide.
	3.5 Turn off by releasing grasp on handle.
	OPERATION OF DRY CHEMICAL FIRE EXTINGUISHER (TYPE C FIRE)
1	Obtain extinguisher from storage area.
2	Transport to site of fire.
3	Place on floor.
	3.1 Remove safety catch pin.
	3.2 Direct hose at base of flame.
	3.3 Compress handle.
	3.4 Overlay base of flame with dry chemical.
	3.5 Turn off by releasing grasp on handle.

BIBLIOGRAPHY

American Medical Association: Guides to the evaluation of permanent impairment, Chicago, 1977, The Association.

Burns DD: Feeling good—the new mood therapy, New York, 1981, William Morrow & Co Inc.

Ince LP, editor: Behavioral psychology in rehabilitation medicine: clinical applications, Baltimore, 1980, Williams & Wilkins.

Kübler-Ross E: Death: the final stage of growth, Englewood Cliffs, 1975, Prentice Hall, Prentice Hall Press.

McDaniel JW: Physical disability and human behavior, New York, 1976, Pergamon Press Inc.

Stults BM: Preventive health for the elderly in personal health maintenance (special issue), West J Med 141:832, Dec 1984.

Patient observation

On completion of this module the reader will be able to:

1.1 Identify clinical signs that may indicate a patient's general condition.

1.2 Describe the various terms and methods for assessing a patient's level of consciousness.

2.1 Discuss development of the stethoscope and how its principles are applied to current stethoscopes.

2.2 Explain how sound is transmitted through a stethoscope.

2.3 Use a stethoscope.

2.4 Exhibit proper care of and general rules for carrying a stethoscope.

3.1 Discuss measurement of peripheral arterial blood pressure.

3.2 Explain principles involved in indirect measurement of peripheral arterial blood pressure.

3.3 Measure blood pressure by palpation method.

3.4 Measure blood pressure by auscultation method.

3.5 Discuss key points that can affect accuracy of blood pressure determination.

3.6 Use Procedures 6-2 and 6-3 to measure blood pressure by palpatory and auscultatory techniques.

4.1 Explain general concepts related to measurement of vital signs.

4.2 Measure temperature using oral methods.

4.3 Measure pulse using different pulse pressure points on the body.

4.4 Distinguish between normal and abnormal respiration.

4.5 Distinguish respiration by rate, depth, frequency, and patterns.

4.6 Measure peripheral arterial blood pressure and relate it to normal arterial blood pressure.

5.1 Practice observation skills in the clinical situation.

1.0 CLINICAL SIGNS AND PHYSICAL CONDITION RELATED TO A PATIENT'S GENERAL WELL-BEING

1.1 Assessment and observations of a patient's general condition

Observation and *assessment* of a patient are two of the most important skills for all health-related personnel. Practitioners cannot initiate preventive or correct action unless they first recognize that a problem exists. They can frequently use their senses to assess a patient's physical status. The following general observations may be useful.

1 Look. Is the patient alert, stuporous, or restless? Is the skin color natural, pale, blue, or flushed? Are the neck veins normal or distended? Are the respiratory motions normal or exaggerated?

2 Listen. Are the respirations quiet or noisy? Is the patient resting, laughing, talking, or groaning? Does the patient respond to questions and general conversation?

3 Touch. Is the skin warm or cold, wet or clammy, or dry? Is the skin firm, spongy, or flaccid? Is the pulse normal or abnormal?

4 Smell. Does the patient have unusual body odor? Does the patient's breath smell normal or abnormal?

1.2 Assessments of the patient with an altered level of consciousness (ALOC)

1 Altered levels of consciousness are caused by impairment of areas of the brain. Causes may be physical, as with trauma, chemical, as with drug overdose, or pathophysiologic, as with stroke or emboli.

2 The areas of the brain most often involved in ALOC are the frontal lobes and the reticular activating contents of the brainstem.

3 By comparison, a great deal of frontal brain tissue must be involved, whereas involvement of a small amount of midbrain reticular substance will cause ALOC.

4 It is very difficult to determine the subjective level of consciousness. For this reason, observation and assess-

ment of clinical signs and diagnostic tests are used by practitioners.

5 There are two primary components of consciousness:
  a Alertness—patient's ability to respond to stimuli.
  b Cognitive ability—Patient's ability to recognize people, places, and things and to respond to questions about his or her life and environment.

6 Beginning with a level of alertness, the following terms describe decreasing levels of consciousness to coma.

Level of consciousness	Criterion
Alertness	Patient awake and responds to stimuli.
Obtundation and confusion	Patient awake but slow to respond to commands or stimuli with some disorientation.
Lethargy or somnolence	Patient appears unconscious but will awaken with stimulation.
Stupor	Patient unconscious but will awaken temporarily with strong stimulation.
Coma	Patient is unconscious and will not awaken with stimuli.
	The depths of coma will vary and may be categorized as grades 1 through 4, with 4 being deep coma. (Patient does not respond to painful stimuli.)

7 The Glasgow Coma Assessment Scale (Table 6-1) is an attempt to make the description and interpretation of coma more objective. Response is based on eye opening and verbal and psychomotor response. Numeric values 1 to 6 are assigned to levels of response in each category. A patient's score is added, and the sum represents an objective assessment of level of consciousness.

A healthy, alert person would score 14; a patient in deep coma would score 3. This scale is similar to the Silverman and Apgar scales used to assess the respiratory level of newborns (see Module 26).

8 Still another method of determining a patient's mental status is to evaluate his or her response to questions. Areas questioned should include the following:
  a Memory—short-term, long-term, or intermediate
  b Cognition—current events, calculations
  c Feelings—mood
  d Realism—hallucinations

9 To test orientation ask the patient to spell his or her name, give address, date, name of spouse or relatives.

10 To test long-term memory, ask where he or she was born.

11 To test intermediate memory, ask what he or she ate for lunch.

12 To test cognition, ask the patient to perform simple math or describe a current event.

13 To test feelings (affect—outward expression of one's feelings and emotions), note patient's response to being questioned, to changes in light or darkness, or to sudden noise, such as a hand clap.

TABLE 6-1 Glasgow coma scale*

Response	Eye opening	Best verbal	Best motor
6	—	—	Obeys simple commands
5	—	Oriented	Attempts to remove painful stimulus
4	Spontaneous	Confused	Attempts to withdraw from painful stimulus
3	To speech	Inappropriate words	Nonpurposeful elbow flexion
2	To pain	Incomprehensible sounds	Elbow extension, wrist flexion, internal shoulder rotation
1	None	None	None

*Modified from Mosby's medical, nursing & allied health dictionary, ed 3, St Louis, 1990, The CV Mosby Co.

2.0 USE OF THE STETHOSCOPE
2.1 Development of the stethoscope

1 The stethoscope is one of the most valuable devices used by health personnel. Listening (auscultation) to body cavities with a stethoscope will give the practitioner an indication of what is happening inside the patient's body. Areas of the body have normal sounds created by the action of the organs that cause the movement of blood, air, and other substances through the body.

2 Respiratory care personnel must become proficient in the use of the stethoscope. A practitioner must listen for the presence or absence of breath sounds and note the various characteristics.

3 The acoustical stethoscope was invented by René Laënnec, a Frenchman, who was born in Quimper in 1781. He received a doctor's degree in 1804 and began an intensive study of pathologic anatomy.

4 Laënnec's professional appointments included:
  a 1814—physician to Necker Hospital.
  b 1822—appointed physician to Her Royal Highness, the Duchess of Berry; Professor at the College de France; Professor of the Medical Clinic of the Charité.

5 In 1816 he discovered the principle of the stethoscope by observing children playing with long pieces of wood with pins on one end. When struck, the pins would transmit sounds to listeners at the other end of the stick.

6 At Necker Hospital Laënneck took a sheet of paper, rolled it, tied it with a string, and put it to the chest of a patient with a diseased heart and found that the paper amplified heart sounds.

7 He named the device "stethoscope" from the Greek means "chest—to look at." His paper, De L'auscultation Medicate, described much of what we know today about chest diseases.

8 The first production stethoscope was made from a cylinder of wood, either cedar or ebony, 12 inches long and 1¾ inches in diameter with a central canal ¼ inch

in diameter. The cylinder was hinged so that it could be easily carried.

9 George Philip Cammann improved on Laënnec's stethoscope by adding *two* listening tubes *(binaurals)*.

10 Currently, a magnetic stethoscope and electronic stethoscope allow the user to pick up even more faint and distant sounds by amplifying the sounds in the listener's ears.

2.2 Transmission of sounds

1 Sound is transmitted through solids or air by conduction, e.g., as waves or ripples travel away from a splash in a pool of water.

2 Determinants of transmission of sound include:

a Changes in density of the thoracic cage. To be heard, vibrations must be within a certain frequency range and above a minimum intensity.

b Frequency (pitch). Number of cycles of repetition that occur in 1 second, e.g., the pitch of a musical note. Low frequencies with slow rates of repetition produce a low note. High frequencies with high rates of repetition produce a high note. Pitch also depends upon the length and diameter of the tube; i.e., the shorter and narrower the tube, the higher the pitch. This distinction is important because of the succeeding branches of the respiratory tree. Pitch becomes higher in the terminal bronchioles.

NOTE: Sound does not conduct well through clothing or a stethoscope with long conducting tubes. The desired length of a stethoscope's tubing is approximately *16 inches*.

c Intensity. Loudness depends on energy of transmission and frequency. Sound loses intensity if passed from one medium to another, e.g., air-to-water sound vibrations that are cushioned and absorbed at the air/liquid interface.

d Timbre. Character or quality of sound. Depends on relative proportion between the fundamental tone and overtones. Timbre allows one to distinguish between sounds of the same pitch and intensity produced by different instruments.

2.3 Use of the stethoscope

1 The stethoscope is an instrument carried by many but understood by relatively few.

2 It is used by respiratory care personnel to measure blood pressure and to listen to breath sounds.

3 A stethoscope is generally very sensitive to vibrations caused by sounds, provided it is in good working order, properly placed in the user's ears, and properly positioned over the region to be auscultated.

4 The parts of a stethoscope include (Fig. 6-1):

a Diaphragm *(2)*. The large round disk attached to the chest piece *(1)*. The purpose of the diaphragm is to listen for higher-pitched breath sounds.

b Bell (cardiac bell) *(3)*. The bell is used instead of the diaphragm to listen for the lower-pitched cardiac sounds.

NOTE: To obtain sounds, the user must select either the diaphragm or the bell by rotating one or the other around the chest piece *(4)*. The practitioner tests the position by placing the stethoscope in the ears and tapping *very gently* on the diaphragm; if no sound is heard, the user *gently* taps on the bell.

c Plastic tubing *(5)*. A hollow tube conducts sounds from the contact pieces *(2 or 3)* to the binaurals *(6)* and then to the earpieces *(7)*. The tubing should be no longer than 16 inches.

5 It is important that the earpieces fit comfortably yet snugly in the ears. A stethoscope must not leak air because some of the sound transmitted will be lost. To

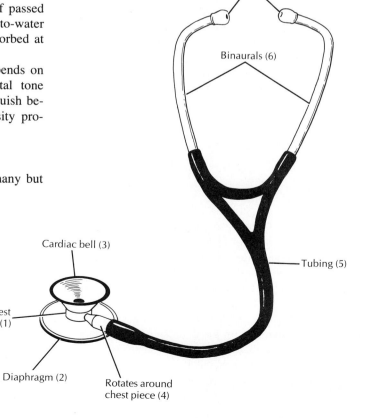

F I G U R E 6 - 1 Parts of stethoscope.

Earpieces (7)

Binaurals (6)

Cardiac bell (3)

Chest piece (1)

Diaphragm (2)

Rotates around chest piece (4)

Tubing (5)

test for air leaks, before placing it in the ears, the practitioner blocks one earpiece and blows in the other. If the air can be moved through the stethoscope, the tubing or diaphragm should be replaced.

6 Earpieces should be positioned to point somewhat forward when placed in the user's ears. This is accomplished by gently bending (shaping) the binaurals (6) until the earpieces are positioned properly.

7 The user places the stethoscope's contact piece, bell or diaphragm side, firmly over the site to be auscultated. The skin, as it is stretched, will serve as a diaphragm and permit better conduction of sound. The tighter the skin is stretched, the better the quality of the sound, especially high-pitched sounds.

NOTE: When listening to a hairy area of the body, the practitioner wets the hair first. The movement of dry hair against the diaphragm will produce sounds similar to those of several lung diseases.

2.4 Proper care and general rules for carrying the stethoscope

1 The stethoscope is a medical instrument and should be treated with proper care.

2 The stethoscope should not be subjected to any stress that will bend the metal work, puncture the diaphragm, or damage the tubing.

3 The diaphragm should be replaced if it is punctured or loses its tension. Some stethoscopes come with extra diaphragms and earpieces.

4 It is not a good practice for practitioners to use one another's stethoscopes. The earpieces should be individually adjusted, since no two people have the same ear placement. Also, using another person's stethoscope can pass infections. If another stethoscope must be used, the earpieces should be wiped with a disinfectant before and after use, just as the chest piece is cleaned after each use.

5 To protect stethoscopes from damage, practitioners should carry them neatly folded in their laboratory coats or jackets.

3.0 MEASURING PERIPHERAL ARTERIAL BLOOD PRESSURE USING BOTH PALPATORY AND AUSCULTATORY METHODS

3.1 Measurement of blood pressure

1 The measurement of peripheral arterial blood pressure is one of the easiest and most valuable means of determining the effectiveness of the cardiovascular system. It is one of the vital signs discussed in Unit 4.0.

2 The peripheral blood pressure is a measurement of the force exerted against the walls of vessels by the blood in response to contraction of the heart. As the heart contracts, a pulse wave is generated that travels like an ocean wave beginning with the opening of the aorta to and eventually involving the entire arterial system. The force of this wave is dependent on cardiac output (blood pumped from the heart in 1 minute), peripheral

resistance of the vessels, and velocity of the arterial blood.

3.2 Principles involved in indirect measurement of blood pressure

1 Occlusion of the arterial wall by direct pressure from an inflated cuff until pressure distal to the occlusion disappears

2 Control of cuff deflation until the blood begins to flow past the occlusion, allowing oscillations (beats) to occur in the artery distal to the cuff

3 Measurement of the oscillation made by using a sphygmomanometer to record oscillations and a stethoscope to determine when the oscillations begin (systolic pressure) and when they disappear (diastolic pressure)

3.3 Blood pressure measurement by palpation (feeling) (Fig. 6-2)

1 With the patient's arm comfortably supported, a cuff (1) with an air bladder inside is snugly wrapped around the upper part of the arm. Position of the air bladder inside the cuff (2) over the brachial artery (3) and the bottom of the cuff should be approximately 2 to 3 cm (1 inch) above the antecubital fossa.

2 The brachial artery is palpated just below the cuff. The cuff is then inflated by turning the control valve (4) completely to the right and slowly squeezing the bulb (5) until the cuff is inflated to 30 mm Hg above the point at which a brachial pulse can no longer be felt.

3 The manometer (6) is read. Air is released from the cuff by slowly opening the control valve to the left until the needle in the pressure manometer drops at 2 to 3 mm Hg per heartbeat.

4 Systolic blood pressure is the pressure at which the brachial pulse can be felt returning to the artery and is then simultaneously read on the manometer.

3.4 Blood pressure measurement by auscultation
(see Fig. 6-2)

1 Determination of blood pressure by auscultation involves the use of the stethoscope placed over the brachial artery (7) so that sounds called *Korotkoff's sounds* can be heard and correlated to readings on the pressure manometer.

2 To determine blood pressure, the practitioner places the cuff around the upper part of the arm so that the cuff is approximately 2 to 3 cm above the antecubital fossa and above the point in which the stethoscope bell will be placed.

3 The brachial artery is palpated and the cuff is inflated at the rate of 12 to 20 mm Hg per second to a peak occlusion pressure of 30 mm Hg greater than the point at which the pulse disappears.

4 The stethoscope is then placed snugly over the brachial artery just below the lower edge of the cuff in the antecubital fossa and the cuff is deflated at the rate of 2 to 3 mm Hg per heartbeat.

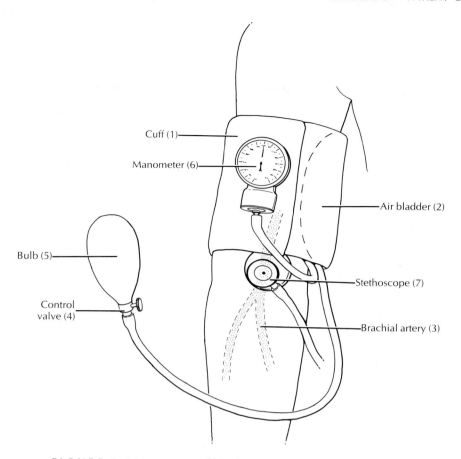

Cuff (1)
Manometer (6)
Air bladder (2)
Bulb (5)
Control valve (4)
Stethoscope (7)
Brachial artery (3)

F I G U R E 6 - 2 Measurement of blood pressure using sphygmomanometer.

5 The pressure is read from the pressure manometer as the needle of the manometer drops and systolic pressure is recorded at the point where Korotkoff's sounds (blood rushing past the cuff) are *first* heard.

6 As air continues to leave the cuff, the indicator on the pressure manometer falls until a *muffling* of Korotkoff's sounds is heard. This point is recorded as *diastolic* pressure.

NOTE: Some procedures require recording diastolic pressure as the point at which the sounds *disappear completely*. This is not as accurate as the point of muffling, because sounds do not disappear in some patients until well below actual diastolic levels.

3.5 Key points that may affect accuracy of a blood pressure measurement

1 The patient should be relaxed and the arm supported.
2 Three readings are taken for accuracy.
3 Between readings *the cuff is completely deflated* and the blood pressure measured in both arms. The practitioner waits 2 minutes between readings.
4 The inflation bladder is placed over the brachial artery.
5 The cuff is inflated until the pressure indicator is approximately 30 mm Hg above the point where the pulse disappears.

6 The cuff is allowed to deflate slowly at a rate of approximately 2 to 3 mm Hg per heartbeat.
7 Artificially high readings may be caused by:
  a A cuff that is too small for the patient's arm
  b A patient who is too tense or excited
8 Artificially low readings may be caused by a cuff that is too large.
  NOTE: A leg cuff may be required to obtain blood pressure in extremely obese patients.
9 Cuffs left in place *must* be completely deflated to prevent interference with circulation.

3.6 Procedures for measuring blood pressure

Procedures 6-2 and 6-3 at the end of this module are examples of how to measure blood pressure using palpatory and auscultatory techniques.

4.0 VITAL SIGNS
4.1 General clinical concepts related to vital signs

1 Vital signs refer to an assessment of *temperature, pulse, respiratory rate,* and *blood pressure*. These functions are closely related to one's ability to maintain life and a state of homeostasis.
2 Vital signs are measurements of a patient's integrated

and unique response to internal and external stimuli and are therefore a good indicator of a patient's physical status.

3 An alteration in one parameter usually results in an accompanying change in another.

4 Changes in vital signs can occur because of the patient's alertness or awareness of external environment that will result in alterations of the internal environment. For example:

a "Fight or flight" syndrome

b Stress responses

c Muscular activity

d Realistic or unrealistic evaluation of states such as fear, anxiety, or loneliness

5 Vital signs are used to determine:

a The patient's response to therapy

b Knowledge of expected results of prescribed medications and treatments

c Evaluation of the influence of environmental factors on vital signs

d A baseline determination of a patient's physical status

6 Meaningful data are provided when vital signs are accurate. Pulse and respirations are determined by using 1 minute as a standardized unit of time.

4.2 Temperature

1 Body temperature reflects the ability of the body to produce, retain, and eliminate heat.

2 Temperature will vary according to time of day (being lowest in the morning) and with the age of the individual (the infant and aged having a higher [by 0.6° C or 1° F] temperature than the young adult).

3 Temperature is measured with a thermometer, which may be manufactured of glass or may be the more modern electronic type.

4 *Oral temperature* can be measured by placing the thermometer under the patient's tongue for a period of 3 to 4 minutes.

5 *Rectal temperature* is accomplished by placing the patient on his or her side and inserting and holding the rectal thermometer (pear-shaped end) 2.5 to 5.0 cm (1 to 2 inches) into the rectum for approximately 2 minutes. Rectal temperature is the most accurate method and is usually *0.6° C (1° F) higher* than an oral temperature reading.

6 *Axillary temperature* is taken by placing the thermometer in the axilla between the inner surface of the patient's arm and the side for 10 minutes. An axillary temperature is normally *0.6° C (1° F) lower* than an oral temperature.

7 Normal temperature values in children, until approximately age 3, are usually greater than 37.2° C (99° F).

8 Normal values for the adult are 33.7° C to 37.8° C (96.5° F to 99.3° F) with an average of 37° C, or 98.6° F.

9 Ranges consistent with life are 24° C (74° F) to 45° C (114° F).

10 Temperature of approximately 29° C (85° F) may cause

a patient's heart rate to slow to the point at which the heart may go into fibrillation, with death following in a matter of minutes.

11 Today many institutions are replacing mercury thermometers with electronic thermometers. A key to proper use of these units is to make sure batteries are active and sensor probes are decontaminated and undamaged.

4.3 Pulse

1 Pulse is the throbbing sensation caused by an artery as it is gently pressed against a bony prominence.

2 Pulse is an indirect measure of cardiac dynamics and cardiac output.

3 A pulse can be measured at any of nine sites on the body. Fig. 4-32 in Module Four shows six of the following:

a Radial. Lateral region of wrist proximal to the thumb.

b Ulnar. Lateral region of wrist distal to the thumb.

c Brachial. Interior lateral region inside the elbow.

d Carotid. Lateral neck.

e Facial. Along the jaw.

f Temporal. Lateral aspect of temporal region.

g Femoral. Anterior aspect of groin.

h Popliteal. Posterior surface of knee.

i Dorsalis pedis. Anterior aspect of top of foot.

4 To measure the pulse, the practitioner should place the index, middle, and fourth fingers gently on the skin at the site where the artery passes next to a bony prominence.

NOTE: the practitioner should never touch a patient with the thumb while taking a pulse. One's own pulse can be felt through the thumb and this may interfere with accuracy.

5 A pulse is counted for 30 seconds and multiplied ×2 if it is regular and 1 full minute if irregular.

6 A pulse is assessed for:

a Rate. Number of beats per minute.

b Rhythm. Pattern of the beats, either regular or irregular.

c Volume. Determination of blood volume can be made by pushing against the walls of the vessels. It is usually described as weak, bounding, feeble, or thready.

7 Normal pulse rates vary with age, activity, and physical condition. The normal rates for different ages are presented in Table 6-2.

4.4 Respiratory rate

1 Respiratory care personnel must be acutely aware of the patient's ability to move air in and out of the lung (ventilation) and the rate at which the patient is breathing.

2 Assessment of respiration includes identification of the *type* of breathing, i.e., abdominal or thoracic, the *rate* of breathing for 1 full minute, and the *pattern* (character) of breathing. When counting respiratory rate, the practitioner *uses either inspiration or exhalation,* not both.

3 The respiratory rate will vary according to age and sex. Table 6-3 presents norms for various age-groups.

4 The character of respirations will vary from normal according to rate, depth, and pattern.

4.5 Types of breathing patterns (Fig. 6-3)

Determine rate and pattern:

1 Eupnea, Normal; 14 to 16 times per minute *(A)*.

2 Hypopnea *(B)*:
   a Shallow respirations; may have some increase in rate
   b Depth about one half normal respirations

3 Hyperpnea *(C)*:
   a Deep respirations with some increase in rate
   b Depth greater than for normal respirations
   c Respirations even and regular

4 Bradypnea. Slow respirations; slow rate *(D)*.

5 Tachypnea *(E)*:
   a Rapid respirations; rapid rate
   b Depth same as for normal respiration

6 Cheyne-Stokes respirations. Waxing and waning with periods of apnea between patterns *(F)*.

7 Biot's respirations. Irregular patterns with periods of apnea *(G)*.

8 Kussmaul breathing *(H)*.
   a Diabetic acidosis with higher blood acidity (arterial blood pH of 7.20 to 6.95)
   b Induces slow, deep respirations

4.6 Blood pressure

1 The measurement of peripheral arterial blood pressure is the quickest and easiest method of evaluating the effectiveness of a patient's cardiovascular system.

2 The technique for measuring a blood pressure is explained in Unit 3.0 of this module.

3 In this unit systolic and diastolic pressures were defined as the arterial pressure at the height of pulsation and at the lowest level of pulsation. These values are

TABLE 6-2 Normal pulse rates according to age

Age	Beats per minute
Birth	70-170
Neonate	120-140
1 year	80-140
2 years	80-130
3 years	80-120
4 years	70-115
Adult	60-100

TABLE 6-3 Normal resting respiratory frequencies

Age (years)	Male	Female
0-1	31 ± 8	30 ± 6
1-2	26 ± 4	27 ± 4
2-3	25 ± 4	25 ± 3
5-6	22 ± 2	21 ± 2
9-10	19 ± 2	19 ± 2
13-14	19 ± 2	18 ± 2
15-16	17 ± 3	18 ± 3
17-18	16 ± 3	17 ± 3
Older	16 ± 3	17 ± 3

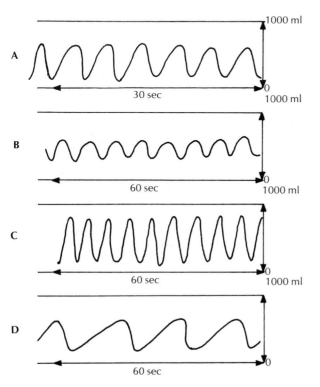

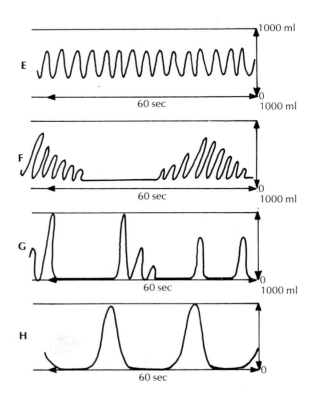

FIGURE 6-3 Breathing patterns. **A,** Eupnea, **B,** Hypopnea, **C,** Hyperpnea, **D,** Bradypnea, **E,** Tachypnea, **F,** Cheyne-Stokes respirations, **G,** Biot's respirations, and **H,** Kussmaul breathing.

recorded as *systolic value over the diastolic value*, e.g., 120/80 mm Hg.

4 The numerical difference between the systolic and diastolic pressure is the *pulse pressure*. This is an indicator of the ability of the vessels to retract as well as of the function of valves. A normal pulse pressure is 80 mm Hg. A discussion on pulse pressure as a clinical indicator is included in Module Four, Unit 25.2.

5 In the adult, normal diastolic pressure is 60 to 90 mm Hg, with 80 mm Hg as average.

6 In the adult, normal systolic pressure is 95 to 140 mm Hg, with 120 mm Hg as average.

7 The systolic pressure in a neonate is 20 to 60 mm Hg.

8 Blood pressure greater than *140/90 mm Hg* is considered hypertension and lower than *95/60 mm Hg*, hypotension.

5.0 THE CLINICAL SITUATION

5.1 Application of patient observation techniques to clinical situations

1 Visual, audible, tactile, and olfactory skills are used to assess a patient's general well-being.

2 Procedure 6-2 included at the end of this module may be used as a guide for measuring peripheral blood pressure by palpation.

3 Procedure 6-3 may be used as a guide for measuring peripheral blood pressure using auscultation. (See Procedure 6-1 for use of stethoscope.)

4 Procedures for monitoring vital signs are included in the following:

a Temperature—Procedures 6-4 and 6-5

b Pulse—Procedure 6-6

c Respiration—Procedure 6-7

d Blood pressure on chronic and acute patients and comparison to normal vital signs (as in nos. 5-8 in Unit 4.6)

PROCEDURE 6-1

Use of a stethoscope

No.	Steps in performing the procedure
1	The practitioner should follows these steps in the proper use of a stethoscope. Identify parts of stethoscope. **1.1** Chest piece **1.2** Disphragm **1.3** Bell **1.4** Plastic tubing (16 inches) **1.5** Binaurals **1.6** Earpieces
2	Rotate head of chest piece to active diaphragm or bell.
3	Place earpieces in ears properly by bending binaurals until earpieces curve forward slightly.
4	With earpieces in place, check operation of chest piece, rotating chest piece to proper position. **4.1** *Gently* tap on diaphragm. **4.2** *Gently* tap on hole of bell.
5	Check stethoscope for leaks by removing from ear and occluding one earpiece with hand while blowing into other. Note and correct any leaks.
6	Explain use of diaphragm.
7	Explain use of bell.
8	Demonstrate positioning of stethoscope on skin by: **8.1** Positioning flat against exposed skin **8.2** Exerting proper amount of pressure
9	Decontaminate stethoscope chest piece after use, using available decontamination agent.
10	Discuss need for stethoscope and how it should be protected and carried.

PROCEDURE 6-2

Blood pressure measurement: indirect—palpation method

No.	Steps in performing the procedure
	The practitioner should implement the following procedure when a noninvasive measurement of systolic blood pressure is desired and sound level of surroundings do not permit auscultation. Systolic pressure only can be obtained by this method.
1	Check assembly equipment. Check that sphygmomanometer is operational.
2	Wash hands.
3	Introduce yourself to patient and verify patient's identity by wrist identity band.
4	Explain procedure as appropriate to patient's condition and familiarity with procedure.
5	Position patient with arm supported. Patient should be relaxed and comfortable.
6	Palpate brachial artery.
7	Place cuff on patient's arm with lower edge of cuff approximately 2 to 3 cm above bend of elbow. Arrow on cuff (appropriate to arm used) should be aligned with brachial artery.
8	Palpate radial pulse.
9	Monitor radial pulse while inflating cuff until meniscus of mercury or dial of aneroid sphygmomanometer is approximately 30 mm Hg above point where radial pulse is no longer felt.
10	Deflate cuff at steady rate of about 2 to 3 mm Hg per heartbeat.
11	Note point at which pulse returns to radial artery (systole).
12	If blood pressure must be rechecked, deflate cuff completely and wait minimum of 15 seconds before repeating procedure.
13	Record systolic pressure on appropriate form. (Blood pressures are always read as even numbers. If reading is between two lines on pressure scale, read it to next highest line.)
14	Remove cuff; reassure and reposition patient. Wash hands.

PROCEDURE 6-3

Blood pressure measurement: indirect—auscultation method

No.	Steps in performing the procedure
	The practitioner should implement the following procedure when a noninvasive measurement of both systolic and diastolic systemic blood pressure is desired. Sound level of surroundings must permit auscultation via stethoscope.
1	Assemble equipment. Check that sphygmomanometer is operational and wipe earpieces and bell of stethoscope with alcohol swab.
2	Wash hands.
3	Introduce yourself to patient and verify patient's identity by wrist identity band.
4	Explain procedure as appropriate to patient's condition and familiarity with procedure.
5	Position patient with arm supported. Patient should be relaxed and comfortable.
6	Palpate brachial artery.
7	Place cuff on patient's arm with lower edge of cuff approximately 2 to 3 cm above bend of elbow. Arrow on cuff (appropriate to arm used) should be aligned with brachial artery.
8	Place earpieces of stethoscope in ears and bell of stethoscope directly over brachial artery.
9	Squeeze bulb rapidly and firmly until meniscus of mercury or dial of aneroid sphygmomanometer is approximately 30 mm Hg above point where sound is no longer heard.
10	Deflate cuff at steady rate of about 2 to 3 mm Hg.
11	Note point at which first beat (systole) is heard and point at which beat can no longer be heard (diastole).
12	If blood pressure must be rechecked, deflate cuff completely and wait minimum of 15 seconds before repeating procedure.
13	Record systolic and diastolic pressures on appropriate form. (Blood pressures are always read as even numbers. If reading is between two lines on pressure scale, read it to next highest line.)
14	Remove cuff; reassure and reposition patient.
15	Wash hands.

PROCEDURE 6-4

Taking oral temperature with glass thermometer

No.	Steps in performing the procedure
	The practitioner should follow these steps in taking an oral temperature with a glass thermometer.
1	Wash hands.
2	Greet patient.
3	Explain care to be given.
4	Obtain equipment.
5	Prepare thermometer for use.
	5.1 If in chemical disinfectant, rinse in cool water and wipe dry.
	5.2 Check level of mercury. Shake to below 35° C (95° F), if necessary, by holding top securely between thumb and forefinger and giving short flipping movement with wrist.
6	Place mercury end of thermometer in patient's mouth under tongue.
	6.1 Request patient to keep mouth closed.
7	Leave thermometer in place for 3 to 4 minutes.
8	Remove thermometer holding end between thumb and index finger, wipe in a spiral manner from top to bulb.
9	Read thermometer.
10	Place thermometer in designated place or holder.
11	Record on appropriate record.
12	Wash hands.

PROCEDURE 6-5

Taking oral temperature with electric thermometer*

No.	Step in performing the procedure
	The practitioner should follow these steps in taking an oral temperature with an electric thermometer.
1	Wash hands.
2	Greet patient.
3	Explain care to be given.
4	Prepare electric thermometer for use.
	4.1 Place clean cover on thermistor.
	4.2 Warm up machine.
5	Place probe under patient's tongue.
	5.1 Ask patient to keep mouth closed.
6	Leave in for 10 to 20 seconds.
7	Remove thermometer; wipe from top to bottom with a tissue.
8	Discard disposable cover and tissue in container.
9	Read temperature on dial indicator.
10	Record reading on appropriate worksheet.
11	Wash hands.

*Optional

PROCEDURE 6-6

Count radial pulse

No.	Steps in performing the procedure
	The practitioner should follow these steps in counting a radial pulse.
1	Wash hands.
2	Greet patient.
3	Explain care to begin.
4	Locate area of radial artery.
5	Place three fingertips over area of radial artery.
6	Press gently to locate pulse.
7	Note sweep of second hand on watch.
8	Count pulse beats for 1 minute.
	8.1 Regular or irregular beats
	8.2 Strong or weak beats
	8.3 Fast or slow beats
9	Record on appropriate record.
10	Report any unusual pulse immediately.
11	Wash hands.

PROCEDURE 6-7

Count respirations

No.	Steps in performing the procedure
	The practitioner should follow these steps in counting respirations.
1	Watch rise and fall of chest or upper abdomen.
2	Note sweep of second hand on watch.
3	Count rise of chest or abdomen for 1 minute.
4	Observe for character and rate.
	4.1 Quiet or noisy
	4.2 Shallow or deep
	4.3 Slow or rapid
5	Record in appropriate record.
6	Report any unusual respirations immediately.

BIBLIOGRAPHY

Brown MS, Bernnenan J, and Walsh K: Student manual of physical examination, Philadelphia, 1977, JB Lippincott Co.

Bruner JMR: Handbook of blood pressure monitoring, Littleton, Calif, 1978, PSG Publishing Co.

Malasanos L, Barkauskas V, and Moss M: Health assessment, ed 4, St Louis, 1990, The CV Mosby Co.

Prior JA, Silbertsein JS, and Stang JM: Physical diagnosis: the history and examination of the patient, ed 6, St Louis, 1981, The CV Mosby Co.

Teasdale G and Jennett B: Assessments of coma and impaired consciousness: a practical scale, Lancet 2:81, 1974.

Thompson JM and Bowers AC: Clinical manual of health assessment, St Louis, 1980, The CV Mosby Co.

Medical gases, production, storage, and control

LEARNING OBJECTIVES

On completion of this module the reader will be able to:

1.1 Discuss the origin and composition of the earth's atmosphere.

1.2 Describe how oxygen is commercially manufactured.

1.3 Explain the physical and chemical properties of oxygen.

1.4 Identify other medical gases that are commercially produced and discuss their physical properties.

2.1 Point out general safety precautions to be observed when using compressed medical gases.

2.2 Compare and contrast methods for manufacturing cylinders.

2.3 Discuss agencies assuring quality control and safety of medical gas cylinders and contents.

2.4 Explain safety precautions for handling and storing compressed medical gas cylinders.

2.5 Demonstrate safe practices by:

  1 Identifying various types and contents of medical gas cylinders.

  2 Moving cylinders of various sizes from one location to another.

  3 Securing cylinders for safe operation and storage.

  4 Checking cylinder for test dates and content labels.

3.1 Discuss agencies and codes regulating cylinder and pipeline connections and fittings.

4.1 Explain operation of a direct-acting valve (needle valve).

5.1 Explain operation of an indirect-acting valve (diaphragm valve).

6.1 Contrast operation of a single stage and multiple stage pressure reducing valve to that of a pressure regulator.

6.2 Discuss potential hazards associated with operation of reducing valves and regulators.

7.1 Differentiate between operation of Thorpe and Bourdon type flowmetering devices.

7.2 Control gas flow at various flow rates using Thorpe and Bourdon flowmeters.

7.3 Check and calibrate a flowmeter.

7.4 Estimate operating time for a cylinder based on cylinder content and gas flow rate.

8.1 Explain functions of component parts of a medical compressed gas manifold system.

8.2 Change cylinders of a bulk medical compressed gas manifold system.

9.1 Explain the function of component parts of a bulk liquid oxygen storage system.

9.2 Monitor operation and volume of a bulk oxygen storage system.

9.3 Point out signs of potential problems when monitoring a bulk oxygen system.

10.1 Describe safe operation of a portable oxygen system.

10.2 Operate a portable oxygen system.

10.3 Operate a Linde or other portable liquid system.

11.1 Explain operation of zone, riser, and main valves related to the flow of oxygen and air in the hospital.

11.2 Explain operation of patient station outlets for delivery of air and oxygen.

11.3 Operate patient station outlets for the delivery of air, oxygen, and suction.

12.1 Explain operation of hospital air production systems.

12.2 Monitor correct operation of a hospital air production system.

12.3 Discuss operation of a hospital vacuum supply system.

13.1 Distinguish between functions and locations of "operating" and "low pressure" alarms used to maintain status of hospital medical gas piping and supply system.

13.2 Locate and test operation of hospital pipeline and gas supply alarms.

13.3 Point out most frequent causes of problems with bulk medical gas systems.

14.1 Explain regulations set forth by the National Fire Prevention Association (NFPA) and other regulations concerning the safe storage, transport, and administration of medical gases.

1.0 ATMOSPHERE AND GASES USED FOR MEDICAL PURPOSES

1.1 Formation of the earth's atmosphere

There are many theories about the formation of the earth and its atmosphere. Following is only one of these theories about the formation and development of this planet:

1 It is speculated that the earth's formation began some 15 to 25 billion years ago.
2 The theory is that all galaxies are moving away from a point of common origin formed from a primordial cloud of dust.
3 As these clouds of primarily hydrogen gas mixed with small amounts of helium and heavier elements and then condensed, rotating spheres of stars and planets were formed.
4 The star formations rapidly consumed most of the primordial gas, setting in motion a birth cycle.
5 Stars were born contracting, condensing, and exploding, creating new generations of stars.
6 As stars contracted and heated, their core temperature reached 100° to 150° million C, causing 150 types of stars to be formed.
7 In this manner, carbon-12, the basic isotope for all of earth's elements, was created.
8 As the earth's mass cooled, a synthesis of elements resulted in the formation of oxygen-16 and all other known elements.
9 Table 7-1 lists by percent the gases currently constituting the earth's atmosphere.
10 Humans are creatures of their environment. This environment is an ocean of air extending upward to some 1200 miles above the earth's surface, where it blends with full space. The gases comprising this ocean of air have mass and therefore are acted on by the downward force of gravity, giving them weight. For example, enough air to fill a 60 × 40 × 8 cubic foot room would weigh over 1500 pounds. The weight of the atmosphere above the earth exerts a downward pressure equal by:
  a 14.69 psi
  b 33.9 feet of water
  c 760 torr (mm Hg)
  d 29.92 in Hg
  e 1014 millibars
  f 1034 g/cm^2
11 A gas can be liquefied when its critical temperature and pressure are reached.
  a Critical temperature. Temperature above which a gas *cannot* be liquefied by the application of pressure.
  b Critical pressure. Force (pressure) required to *liquefy* a gas at its critical temperature.
  c Sublimation. Direct change from solid to vapor state. Heat must be provided to make this change.
12 Specific gases are *separated from the air* by application of critical temperature and pressure.

1.2 Commercial manufacture of oxygen and other gases

1 Most medical gases are produced by a process of *fractional distillation of liquefied air* (Fig. 7-1).

TABLE 7-1 Gases composing the earth's atmosphere

Gas	Percent in atmosphere
Nitrogen (N$_2$)	78.08%
Oxygen (O$_2$)	20.95%
Inert gases	0.93%
Argon	
Neon	
Helium	
Krypton	
Xenon	
Carbon dioxide (CO$_2$)	0.03%
Methane (CH$_4$)	0.01%
Hydrogen (H$_2$)	

2 The fractional distillation process for oxygen, nitrogen, and carbon dioxide (CO$_2$) was developed by Carl Von Linde in 1895. The following steps are involved in this process:
  a Air is compressed *(1)* to 100 atm (see 10 a-f above) and heat is removed *(2)*.
  b Air is compressed to 200 atm and cooled with brine— salt water *(3)*.
  c Air is passed into liquefier—allowed to escape through a throttling valve and expanded to 20 atm *(4)*.
  d Heat is absorbed from the inner coils (incoming air).
  e As the process continues, *each* quantity of air that escapes the valve is *colder* than that which preceded it and the air is liquefied.
  f Later, as the gases are warmed, the more volatile gases escape to the top of the rectifier—separation column *(5)*—and the products are drawn off at the bottom in this order: crude neon gas *(6)*, oxygen gas *(7)*, oxygen liquid *(8)*, and nitrogen liquid *(9)*.
3 The following are separation characteristics of air at 1 atm pressure. As liquefied gas is warmed, each of the elements constituting the atmosphere returns to a gaseous state (boils) and is captured in a container (cylinder).

100° C	H$_2$O boils
0° C	ice melts
−78° C	CO$_2$ sublimes
−183° C	O$_2$ boils
−196° C	N$_2$ boils
−253° C	H boils
−269° C	He boils
−273° C	absolute zero (Kelvin scale)

1.3 Physical and chemical properties of oxygen

The following are properties of oxygen:
1 Physical properties
  a Colorless, odorless, tasteless gas
  b Density = 1.43 g/L at 0° C and 760 mm Hg
  c Density = 1.33 g/L at 20° C and 760 mm Hg
  d Heavier than air:
    • Specific gravity of air = 1.00
    • Specific gravity of O$_2$ = 1.105
    • Critical temperature = −119° C
    • Critical pressure at −119° C = 50 atm

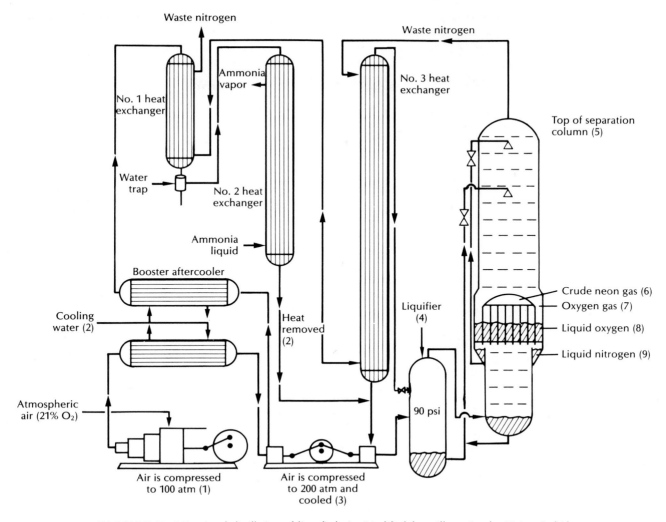

FIGURE 7-1 Fractional distillation of liquefied air. (Modified from illustration by Union Carbide Corp, Linde Division.)

e Will *not* explode but will support combustion of other materials and accelerate their flash point

2 Chemical properties

  a The *atomic number* of oxygen is 8 in the Periodic Table of Elements (has 8 protons in its nucleus).

  b Approximately 99.75% of all O_2 atoms have 8 neutrons in the nucleus. This gives a combined (proton/neutron) *atomic weight* of 16.

  c The remaining 0.25% have either 9 or 10 neutrons in the nucleus, giving them an atomic weight of 17 and 18.

  d Those with 8 neutrons in the nucleus and those that have either 9 or 10 neutrons in the nucleus compose the three isotopes of O_2 80^{16}, 80^{17}, and 80^{18}.

  e Oxygen-16 is the most common form of oxygen.

  f The nucleus of the oxygen atom is surrounded by *four* pairs of orbiting electrons to balance the eight protons in the nucleus.

  g Oxygen *does not* exist uncombined in its atomic form.

  h It combines in a covalent form with two pairs of electrons shared by two oxygen atoms (diatomic—O^2).

Oxygen molecules that are not combined with other elements always pair up.

  i Oxygen then, has a molecular weight of 32 or 2×16 (atomic weight).

  j Oxygen frequently exists with one or more unpaired electrons and is therefore *diatomic-paramagnetic* (attracted to a magnetic field). While two of the three electrons orbit around the nucleus of one of the atoms, the third electron is occupying the corresponding orbit of the other atom. Being unstable in this configuration, oxygen is therefore attracted to a magnetic field. This principle, described by Pauling, is used in the operation of an oxygen analyzer (see Module Thirteen).

NOTE: Nitric oxide also is paramagnetic and can influence the accuracy of this type of analyzer.

1.4 Other medical gases—commercially produced

1 Compressed air. Produced by collection, filtering (cleaning), and compressing air using a water-sealed compressor.

NOTE: Compressors using oil seal rings cannot be used for respiratory purposes because of the danger of injection of harmful oil droplets into the inspired gas. Inhaled oil droplets can cause liquid pneumonia. Oil droplets that may come into contact with equipment that is also used with oxygen are a hazard because oil when pressurized with oxygen will combust, causing a hot fire.

  a Compressed air is used to drive nebulizers or produce mist for patients not needing supplemental oxygen.

  b Compressed air is also used to blend with pure oxygen to obtain specific concentrations between 21% and 100% oxygen.

2 Carbon dioxide and oxygen—carbogen (CO_2/O_2). Clear gas having a sharp, repugnant odor and taste.

  a Mixed with oxygen, carbogen will produce an increase in respiratory rate and depth of breathing in normal people.

  b It is also given as a potent dilator of cerebral blood vessels.

  c Carbogen is stored as a gas in gray and green containers.

  d The usual therapeutic mixture of 95% O_2 and 5% CO_2.

3 Helium (He). Colorless, odorless, and the least dense of all gases besides hydrogen.

  a Helium is nonexplosive.

  b When mixed with oxygen, helium-oxygen (HeO_2), because of its low density, acts as a transport agent to carry oxygen across obstructions in the airway.

  c Helium-oxygen is stored as gas in green and brown cylinders.

  d When helium is inhaled through the larynx, the reduced density of the gas will cause the person to speak with "ducklike" tones.

  e Helium-oxygen mixtures are most useful when used in conjunction with conditions such as status asthmaticus or other situations in which the airway may be partially blocked by secretions or other physical barriers.

4 Nitrous oxide (N_2O). An analgesic gas used in anesthesia.

  a Stored as a liquid in blue cylinders

  b Administered as a gas for relief of pain

2.0 GENERAL SAFETY PRECAUTIONS
2.1 Storage and transport of compressed gas cylinders

1 One of the most important responsibilities of every respiratory care department is enforcing and adhering to the safety rules of the hospital. To carry out this duty, respiratory care personnel should understand the reasons behind the rules.

2 Oxygen is a *potential* hazard if safe practices are not employed. Recognizing these hazards is the responsibility of everyone in the hospital. In the event of a fire, respiratory care personnel *must* know the exact locations of all oxgyen safety shut-off valves throughout the hospital and what rooms these valves control.

3 Although oxygen by itself will not burn, it supports combustion, and anything in the presence of high concentrations of oxygen will burn much more rapidly. It is of utmost importance to stress to all patients that while they are receiving oxygen they are *not to smoke*. NO SMOKING signs should be in conspicuous places to remind patients and their visitors of these rules. If smoking is allowed in the room, the oxygen equipment *must* be completely shut off and removed from the wall before anyone in the room is allowed to smoke. To remove smoking items from a smoker who is receiving oxygen is probably a good idea.

4 Oil and other petroleum-based products should not be used around oxygen. The main hazard of oil is that it will cause an explosion if exposed to oxygen under pressure. Even grease or oil on the hands can be dangerous if one is handling pressure regulators or other oxygen pressure devices. Caution must be taken and hands washed thoroughly before the practitioner handles any of this equipment.

5 Alcohol vapor in the presence of high oxygen concentrations is extremely hazardous and should be avoided inside a tent canopy or other closed chamber. The practitioner should not give alcohol rubs to a patient who is receiving oxygen.

6 Cylinders contain gas under high pressure and should be handled with caution. These cylinders must be stored in a well-ventilated place where the temperature will not become unusually high. They should be stored with the cap covering the valve and chained to something sturdy. The cylinders are to be transported securely strapped on carts specifically made for that purpose and should remain on these carts for easy transport in case of fire.*

7 Administering oxygen in any type of environmental chamber such as an incubator or oxygen tent requires special safety precautions that must be strictly enforced. These rules include:

  a Placing NO SMOKING signs on the environmental chamber to remind patients and visitors of the possible dangers.

  b Not allowing electrical equipment inside the chamber. These articles include telephone, television or radio control, call light cord, electric razors, heating pads, and flashlights.

  c Not allowing friction or battery-operated devices inside the chamber, e.g., children's toys.

  d *Never* using alcohol on a patient in a closed, oxygen-enriched environment. Alcohol and oxygen form an explosive substance.

8 Not placing electroencephologram (EEG) or electrocardiogram (ECG) electrodes or cardiac pacemakers in a chamber. Other methods of administering oxygen

---

*See Bibliography (Standard for bulk oxygen systems at consumer sites) for additional information on nonflammable medical gas systems.

should be used if any of this equipment is necessary.

9 Using electrical devices approved by *Underwriters' Laboratory* for use in oxygen-enriched environments.

10 Not wearing nylon or other clothing that may contain static electricity.

11 Properly grounding equipment used in conjunction with an environmental chamber. Most hospitals have polarized three-prong outlets with a ground wire built in to receive three-prong electric plugs. If equipment does not have a three-prong electrical plug, the proper adapters must be used to ensure safe grounding connections (see Module Eight, Unit 4.0.).

12 Following other considerations when administering medical gases.

a Regardless of mixture combination, inspiratory gases *must contain a minimum of 20.95% oxygen.*

b Oxygen has a low moisture content as it exits from a cylinder or wall outlet and will serve as a *drying agent* to any contacted surface.

c Carbon dioxide is a potent peripheral vascular dilator and can be dangerous if administered to persons having cerebral vascular disease because of increased blood flow to the brain.

2.2 Manufacture of medical gas cylinders*

Most cylinders are produced using one of the three methods described below. The exception is that some manufacturers are producing molded aluminum or fiberglass cylinders. Even though these containers are 25% to 30% lighter than the steel models described below, they are still not accepted (hence refilled) by many dealers as being safe.

1 Steel billet (single-piece construction) (Fig. 7-2, *A*)

a A tube (billet) is punched out of noncorrosive metal materials: high carbon steel; medium manganese steel; heat-treated steel; stainless steel; nickel; aluminum.

b A press *(1)* is forced into a billet of cylinder material *(2)*.

c A tube emerges from the billet *(3)*.

d The bottom of the shell is heated and formed into a cup.

e The top is formed and closed by a hot form.

f The neck of the cylinder is threaded.

g The cylinder is cleaned and hydrostatically tested for safe pressure limits with data imprinted on the collar of cylinder.

NOTE: Hydrostatic testing involves submerging an empty cylinder in a water-filled chamber and filling the cylinder with water under pressure equal to specified safety limits for the cylinder (3000 psi for oxygen). The amount of cylinder expansion is noted based on displacement of the surrounding water. Excessive cylinder expansion and failure to return to

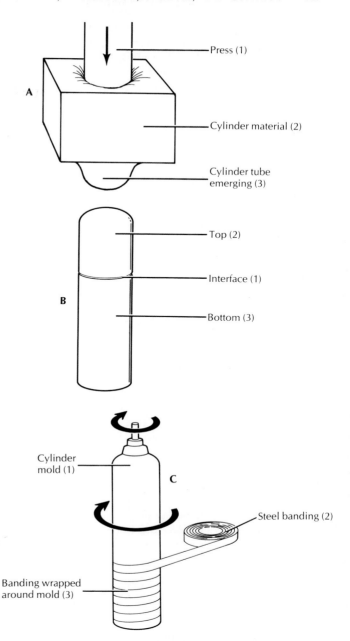

FIGURE 7-2 Formation of a medical gas cylinder. **A,** By forcing press into billet of steel. **B,** From circular steel disks. **C,** By wrapping steel bands around mold.

the original shape after pressure is released indicates possible structural and/or material failure.

h Valve is installed and cylinder is painted to reflect contents.

2 Circular steel disks (two-piece construction) (Fig. 7-2, *B*)

a Circular steel disks are formed into two seamless cups.

b The cups are heat treated and when welded to seamless shells.

c Shells and cups are interlocked *(1)* with one forming the top *(2)* and the other the bottom of the cylinder *(3)*.

---

*Also see the section on cylinders in McPherson listed in the bibliography at the end of this module.

d The cylinder is cleaned and hydrostatically tested.

e The valve is installed.

f The cylinder is painted to reflect the contents.

3 *Spun steel strands* (Fig. 7-2, *C*). The cylinder is formed of treated steel bands wrapped around a mold.

   a The mold is turned *(1)*.

   b Treated banding material of noncorrosive steel is rolled out *(2)*.

   c Steel is coiled onto a mold to be sealed by extreme heat *(3)*.

   d The neck of the cylinder is threaded.

   e The cylinder is cleaned and hydrostatically tested.

   f The valve is installed.

   g The cylinder is painted to indicate the contents.

2.3 Agencies assuring safety and quality control of medical compressed gas cylinders

1 Department of Transportation (DOT). Regulates:

   a Shipping (by air, water, and highways)

   b Filling

   c Marking

   d Labeling

2 Bureau of Medical Devices (Agency of the Food and Drug Administration [FDA]). Regulates:

   a Standards for all medical devices

   b Classification of medical devices

3 Compressed Gas Association (CGA). Regulates:

   a Handling and storage of cylinders

   b Piping and fittings

   c Cylinder markings

4 The FDA (Agency of the Department of Health and Human Services [HHS]). Regulates:

   a Purity, potency, and quality of gas

   • Examples of purity requirements:

Nitrous oxide	95%
Cyclopropane	99%
Ethylene	99%
Oxygen	99%
Carbon dioxide	99%
Helium	95%

   b Identifying labels (tags)

   c Precaution statements

5 American Society of Mechanical Engineers. Concerned with unfilled pressure vessels, e.g., liquid oxygen containers. Regulates:

   a Construction

   b Operating limits

   c Maintenance

   d Safety valves

6 National Fire Protection Association (NFPA). Concerned with all aspects of medical gas safety, storage, identification of cylinders, environment surrounding storage and administration of medical gases, and equipment and techniques for administering medical gas to the patient. Makes recommendations to governmental regulatory bodies.

7 NFPA codes covering medical gas storage and delivery include:

   a NFPA No. 50 (Bulk Oxygen Systems). Standards governing placement, operation, general maintenance, safety valves, and control of bulk oxygen supply systems, both liquid and cylinder.

   b NFPA No. 56F (Nonflammable Medical Gas Systems). Standards governing piped oxygen for therapeutic purposes and piping of oxygen or nitrous oxide and other nonflammable gases to any area of the hospital for medical purposes. Standard includes: Manifold placement and connections, connecting pipelines, and patient station outlets.

   c NFPA No. 56B (Respiratory Therapy). Standards governing use of nonflammable medical gases at normal atmospheric pressure, vapors, and aerosols and the respiratory therapy equipment required for their administration.

8 American Standards Association. Concerned with outlet connections on medical gas cylinders. Developed American Standard Gas Standard Compressed Gas Cylinder Valve Outlet and Inlet Connections to prevent interchange of regulators from cylinders containing one type of gas to another and to prevent accidental administration of the wrong gas to a patient (specific system covered in Units 4.0 through 6.0).

9 Other agencies involved in the development and recommendation of safe practices with medical equipment include:

   a International Standards Organization. An international body for establishing standardization of medical equipment and fittings, terminology, and testing procedures.

   b American National Standards Institute. The Z-79 Committee is best known for the established terminology, fittings, and equipment used to evaluate anesthesia and respiratory care ventilatory devices. The American Association for Respiratory Care (AARC) and other professional organizations sponsor representatives to the above committees.

10 Pin Index Safety System (PISS)

   a The Pin Index Safety System (PISS) was originally described by NFPA in 1952 as a method of preventing accidental attachment of a reducing valve for a specific type of gas to a cylinder with the wrong contents.

   b This system is similar to the *American Standards System* except that it applies to small cylinders with post-type valves, whereas the standard system prevents the same mistake with large cylinders having threaded connections.

   c The PISS is based on a *pin in a hole combination*, allowing a pressure regulator with protruding pins to match with corresponding holes in the post-type cylinder valve. These holes are arranged according to a prearranged numbered position on a scale of 1 to 10 with each medical gas having its own specific arrangement (Fig. 7-3).

   • Fig. 7-3 shows possible pin hole locations for all medical gases.

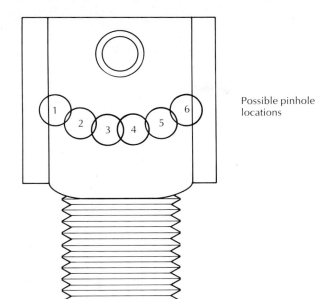

FIGURE 7-3 Possible PISS hole locations.

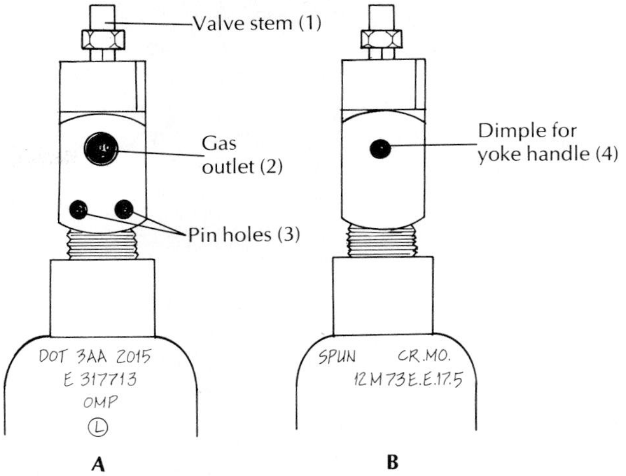

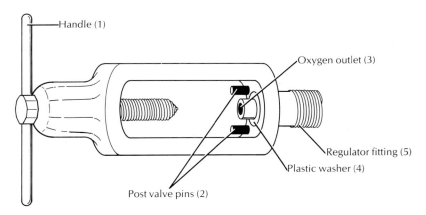

FIGURE 7-4 Components of cylinder post valve. **A,** Anterior view. **B,** Posterior view.

FIGURE 7-5 Yoke connector used to attach regulator to cylinder post valve.

- Fig. 7-4 illustrates a post-type valve in an oxygen cylinder. Illustrated is the valve stem *(1)*, the gas outlet *(2)*, and the two pin holes—in this case a 2-5 position for oxygen *(3)*. On the backside of the valve is a dimple for accepting the yoke-tightening handle *(4)*.
- Fig. 7-5 illustrates a yoke connection showing the tightening handle *(1)*, the two pins that fit in the corresponding holes on the post valve *(2)*, the yoke O_2 outlet *(3)*, which is surrounded with a plastic washer *(4)*, ensuring a tight fit against the post valve. The thread fitting *(5)* is where the yoke fits into a reducing valve (regulator).
- Fig. 7-6 shows eight of ten possible PISS positions for:
  (1) 2-5 oxygen
  (2) 2-6 carbon dioxide/oxygen $\nleftarrow 7\%$ CO_2
  (3) 1-5 compressed air

(4) 1-3 ethylene
(5) 3-5 nitrous oxide
(6) 3-6 cyclopropane
(7) 4-6 helium/oxygen (He >80%)
(8) 1-6 carbon dioxide/oxygen >7% CO_2

11 Diameter Index Safety System (DISS)

The DISS system was developed by the Compressed Gas Association to provide a standard to ensure noninterchangeable connections where removable exposed threaded connections are employed. This standard is used in conjunction with individual gas lines of medical gas administering equipment at pressures of *200 psig or less.* Each connection of diameter-indexing consists of a body and nut (male) and a nipple (female). Except for oxygen, this system is based on having two concentric and specific shoulders on the nipple. To achieve noninterchangeability between different connections, the two diameters on each part vary in

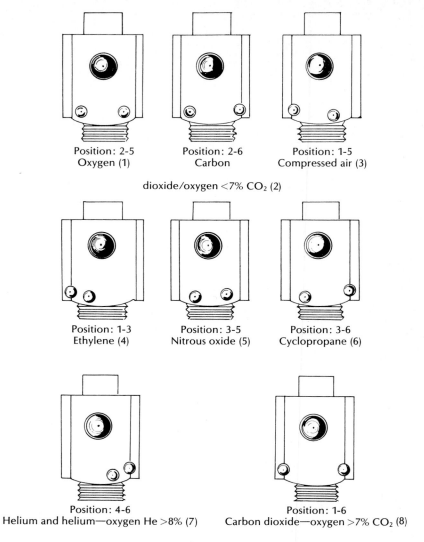

Position: 2-5
Oxygen (1)

Position: 2-6
Carbon

Position: 1-5
Compressed air (3)

dioxide/oxygen <7% CO_2 (2)

Position: 1-3
Ethylene (4)

Position: 3-5
Nitrous oxide (5)

Position: 3-6
Cyclopropane (6)

Position: 4-6
Helium and helium—oxygen He >8% (7)

Position: 1-6
Carbon dioxide—oxygen >7% CO_2 (8)

FIGURE 7-6 Eight possible PISS pin hole positions on post valves.

opposite directions so that as one diameter increases, the other decreases. Diameter indexing is achieved when matched parts fit together to form a union.

Fig. 7-7 shows various combinations of male *(1)* and female *(2)* fittings, which are DISS to form connections. The oxygen blender device has screw-on DISS fittings *(3)* and quick connect DISS fittings *(4)*. The details of the bottom of the blender are shown in *D*.

12 American Standard System

  a As previously discussed, this system prevents the accidental connection of a reducing valve to the wrong type of cylinder valve or one with the wrong gas contents.

  b This system, originally described by the CGA, was subsequently adopted and implemented by the American Standards Association and applies only to cylinders having *threaded gas outlets.* Details regarding American Standard threads may be found in publications distributed by the CGA and by the American Standards Association.

  c The design of the system is such that gas cylinder outlets are matched to regulator inlet connectors. Various combinations include varying the *number, pitch,* and *direction* of threads on the cylinder gas outlet for each type of gas.

  d In addition, the inside diameter and shape of the gas channel of the cylinder outlet is designed so that a size and shape is specific to each medical gas cylinder valve outlet.

  e With this system a reducing valve must have a matched female hexagonal nut and nipple to fit the desired male thread gas outlet on each medical gas cylinder.

  f The specifications for matching cylinder outlets to appropriate fittings are coded by the CGA as a connection number. For example, *No. 540: 0.903-14NGO-RH, EXT. accepting round nipples* describes the fitting for oxygen. *No. 1340: 0.825 in. RH. round nipple* describes the fitting for air. Decoded this means that an oxygen outlet will accept a

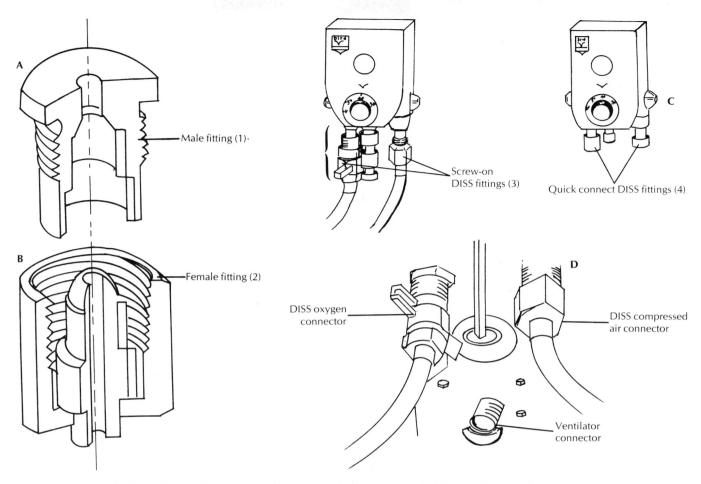

F I G U R E 7 - 7 DISS connector fittings. **A,** Male fitting. **B,** Female fitting. **C,** Screw-on fittings on oxygen blender. **D,** Quick-connect fittings on oxygen blender.

reducing valve or pressure regulator.

g With a female nut that will screw over a male cylinder valve outlet with right-handed threaded external outlet with 14 turns (threads) NGO type 0.903 O.D. Gases classified under the American Standard System have threads that are classified as National Gas Outlet (NGO) type or National Gas Taper (NGT) type.

h Right-handed threads are usually reserved for medical gases and left-handed threads for nonmedical gases such as butane.

2.4 General rules for safe storage and handling of compressed gas cylinders

1 Cylinders should be stored according to gas contents so that flammable agents are stored with nonflammable agents.

2 Cylinders must routinely be inspected for general appearance, tags, valve operation, and inspection test date.

3 Cylinder markings are stamped into the metal when the cylinder is manufactured. The initial hydrostatic pressure test date is stamped in the metal of the cylinder

and updated by 5 years unless the test date is followed by a ★, which indicates a 10-year test cycle.

4 Cylinder markings are controlled by the Department of Transportation (DOT), formerly ICC in the United States, and Ministry of Transport Commission in Canada.

EXAMPLE: See Fig. 7-8 *1* through *10*.

Cylinder markings as stamped on shoulder of cylinder:

DOT3A/2015

174000

ARCO

⊛

a DOT 3A indicates the DOT specifications under which the cylinder was designed and manufactured *(1)*.

b 2015 indicates the working pressure for which the cylinder was designed. Test pressure is $\frac{5}{3}$ greater than working pressure *(2)*.

c 17400 indicates serial number of the cylinder *(3)*.

d ARCO indicates identifying symbol (letters) of the manufacturer, user, or supplier *(4)*.

e ⊛ is symbol of inspecting authority after manufacture *(5)*.

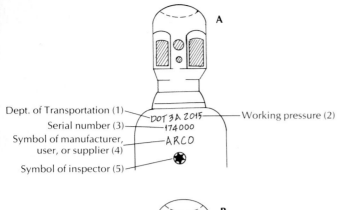

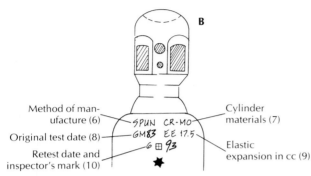

FIGURE 7-8 Cylinder markings. **A,** Anterior view. **B,** Posterior view.

    f SPUN refers to method of manufacture *(6)*.

    g CR-MO indicates materials of manufacture, in this case chromemolybdenum *(7)*.

    h 6M83 indicates date of original test; sixth month 1963 *(8)*.

    i Elastic Expansion is in cubic centimeters (17.5) during original test *(9)*.

    j Retest date and inspector's mark are shown in *10*.

  5 *Danger:* never permit oil, grease, or other readily combustible substances to come into contact with cylinder valves, regulators, gauges, hoses, and fittings. Oil and certain gases such as oxygen or nitrous oxide may combine with explosive violence.

  6 Never lubricate valves, regulators, gauges, or fittings with oil or any other combustible substance.

  7 Do *not* handle cylinders or apparatus with oily hands or gloves. Connections to piping, regulators, and other appliances should always be kept tight to prevent leakage.

  8 Never use an open flame to detect gas leaks, soapy water is generally used.

  9 Prevent sparks or flame from any source from coming into contact with cylinders and equipment.

 10 Never interchange regulators or other appliances used with one gas with similar equipment intended for use with other gases.

 11 Fully open the cylinder valve when cylinder is in use.

 12 Never attempt to mix gases in cylinder. (Mixtures should be obtained already prepared from recognized suppliers.)

 13 Before placing cylinders in service, remove any paper wrappings so that the cylinder label is clearly visible.

 14 Identify gas content by label stencil and/or color on the cylinder before using. If the cylinder is *not* identified to show the gas contained, return the cylinder to the supplier without using it.

 15 Do not deface or remove any markings that are used for identification of contents of cylinder. This applies to labels, decals, tags, stenciled marks, and upper half of shipping tag.

 16 Never subject any part of any cylinder containing a compressed gas to a temperature above 52° C(125° F). A direct flame should never be permitted to come in contact with any part of a compressed gas cylinder.

 17 Never tamper with the safety relief devices in valves or cylinders.

 18 Never attempt to repair or alter cylinders.

 19 Never use cylinders for any purpose other than to contain gas.

 20 Cylinder valves should be closed at all times except when gas is actually being used.

 21 Notify support of cylinder if any condition has occurred that might permit any foreign substance to enter cylinder or valve, giving details and cylinder number.

 22 Do not place cylinders where they might become part of an electric circuit.

 23 Cylinders should be repainted only by the supplier.

 24 Compressed gases should be handled only by experienced and properly instructed persons.

 25 Do not use pressure regulators, pressure reducing valves, pressure gauges, and manifolds provided for use with a particular gas or group of gases with cylinders containing other gases.

 26 Never use medical gases where the cylinder is liable to become contaminated by the feedback of other gases or foreign material unless protected by suitable traps or check valves.

 27 It is important to make sure that the threads on pressure regulator-to-cylinder valve connections or the pin indexing devices on yoke-to-cylinder valve connections are properly mated. Never *force* connections that do not fit.

 28 After attaching pressure regulator, and before cylinder valve is opened, see that the pressure regulator is turned to the "off" position in the case of pressure regulators equipped with a pressure adjusting screw. To turn pressure regulator off, turn the screw counterclockwise until it is free.

 29 Never permit gas to enter the pressure regulating device suddenly. Open the cylinder valve *slowly*.

 30 Before the pressure regulating device and cylinder are disconnected, close the cylinder valve and release all pressure from the device.

 31 General rules for central storage of cylinders:

    a Storage rooms should be dry, cool, and well-ventilated.

    b Rooms should comply with state and local regulations and the hospital procedure manual.

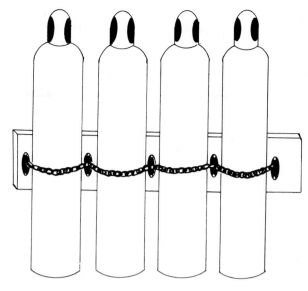

FIGURE 7-9 Chained stands used to secure large gas cylinders.

c As previously stated, cylinders should never be subjected to temperatures above 52° C (125° F).

d Keep cylinders away from steam pipes and radiators (furnace rooms).

e Place large cylinders against a wall for protection from being knocked over (chained stands) (Fig. 7-9).

f Do not store flammable gases in the same room with oxygen.

g The enclosure should not communicate with an area where anesthetic agents are stored, e.g., cyclopropane.

32 Planning a manifold room

a The manifold room should be located on the ground floor at the service entrance of the hospital.

b Adequate cylinder storage space should be provided adjacent to the cylinder room.

NOTE: The area should be divided and marked to show full and empty cylinders.

c Carts with straps or chains for delivery of cylinders should be provided.

d The manifold room should be large enough to accommodate the manifold and additional space for changing cylinders.

e The manifold room should *not* be used to store any other materials. Cylinders should *not* be located near fuel oil pipes, steam pipes, or radiators.

f NO SMOKING signs should be posted and enforced.

g The room must be ventilated according to storage capacity as specified by NFPA.

2.5 Identification of medical gases (Figs. 7-10 and 7-11)

1 Medical compressed gas cylinders can be identified by:

a Color of cylinder

b Dimensions (size of cylinder)

c Labels

d Testing of contents, e.g., analysis of oxygen

e Valve connection, i.e., PISS, American Standard, DISS

2 Movement of cylinder

a The cylinder should be moved using a cart designed for this purpose.

b The cart should have three or four wheels for balance and a chain or other type of restraint (Figs. 7-12 and 7-13).

c A small cylinder should be moved using a small cart carried by hand or laid horizontally, but securely, on a bed.

3 Bedside use of cylinders

a For bedside use, cylinders must be set up in one of the following ways:

• On a cart in three-wheel position

• In an appropriate stand (Fig. 7-13)

• Secured to a stable object—*not the bed*

b A cylinder must not be placed next to sources of heat or in major traffic zones such as aisles.

NOTE: Procedure 7-1 at the end of this module may be used as a guide for moving cylinders.

4 Checking cylinder for test dates

a The cylinder must be retested every 5 to 10 years, depending on original construction.

b 3A indicates high carbon or medium manganese steel.

c 3AA indicates heat-treated steel.

NOTE: Following 3A or 3AA indicates cylinder must be retested every 10 years.

d Procedure 7-2 outlines steps for checking a cylinder.

	Cylinder size	Gallons	Cubic feet	Liters	Approx. weight of lb oz	Valve connector no.	Cylinder color
OXYGEN (O₂) Physical state in cylinder—gas	B	40	5.35	151.40	0—7.08	CGA-870 Pin-indexed	Light green
	D	95	12.70	359.57	1—0.80	CGA-870 Pin-indexed	Light green
	E	165	22.06	624.52	1—13.25	CGA-870 Pin-indexed	Light green
	M	800	106.95	3028.00	8—13.60	CGA-540 .903-14 NGO-RH-ext.	Light green
	G	1400	187.2	5300.00	15—8.00	CGA-540 .903-14 NGO-RH-ext.	Light green
Therapy oxygen—250 cu. ft. cylinder (for information only)		1870	250.00	7080.00	20—11.20	CGA-540 .903-14 NGO-RH-ext.	Light green
NITROUS OXIDE (N₂O) Physical state in cylinder—liquid	B	100	13.37	378.50	1—8.50	CGA-910 Pin-indexed	Blue
	D	250	33.30	946.25	3—13.25	CGA-910 Pin-indexed	Blue
	E	420	56.00	1589.70	6—6.80	CGA-910 Pin-indexed	Blue
	M	2000	266.50	7570.00	30—9.00	CGA-1320	Blue
	G	3655	488.6	13841.00	56—0.00	.825-14 NGO-RH-ext.	Blue
CYCLOPROPANE (C₃H₆) Physical state in cylinder—liquid	A	40	5.34	151.00	0—9.40	CGA-920 Pin-indexed	Orange
	B	100	13.37	378.50	1—7.50	CGA-920 Pin-indexed	Orange
	D	230	30.75	870.00	3—5.50	CGA-920 Pin-indexed	Orange
ETHYLENE (C₂H₄) Physical state in cylinder—gas	B	100	13.37	303	0—15.25	CGA-900 Pin-indexed	Red
	D	200	26.74	757	1—15.50	CGA-900 Pin-indexed	Red
	E	330	44.12	1249	3—3.20	CGA-900 Pin-indexed	Red
	M	1600	214.00	6032	15—8.00	CGA-350 .825-14 NGO-LH-ext.	Red
	G	2800	374.30	10598	27—2.00	CGA-350 .825-14 NGO-LH-ext.	Red
CARBON DIOXIDE (CO₂) Physical state in cylinder—liquid	B	100	13.37	378.50	1—8.45	CGA-940 Pin-indexed	Gray
	D	250	33.35	946.00	3—13.20	CGA-940 Pin-indexed	Gray
	E	420	56.10	1589.70	6—6.70	CGA-940 Pin-indexed	Gray
	M	2000	267.00	7570.00	30—9.00	CGA-320 .825-14 NGO-RH-ext.	Gray
	G	3200	427.40	12112.00	48—15.00	CGA-320 .825-14 NGO-RH-ext.	Gray
HELIUM (He) Physical state in cylinder—gas	B	28	3.74	105.98	0—0.62	CGA-930 Pin-indexed	Brown
	D	80	10.68	302.80	0—1.77	CGA-930 Pin-indexed	Brown
	E	131	17.50	495.83	0—2.89	CGA-930 Pin-indexed	Brown
	G	1100	147.00	4163.50	1—8.31	CGA-350 .825-14 NGO-LH-ext.	Brown
CARBON DIOXIDE AND OXYGEN MIXTURE (CO₂-O₂) Physical state in cylinder—gas	B	40	5.30	151.40	Varies	CO₂ over 7% CGA-320	Light green body Gray shoulder
	D	95	12.70	359.57	Varies	CGA-940	Light green body Gray shoulder
	E	165	22.06	624.52	Varies		Light green body Gray shoulder
	M	800	107.00	3028.00	Varies	CO₂ less than 7% CGA-280	Light green body Gray shoulder
	G	1400	187.20	5300.00	Varies	CGA-880	Light green body Gray shoulder
HELIUM AND OXYGEN MIXTURE (He-O₂) Physical state in cylinder—gas	B	29	3.87	109.76		Helium over 80% CGA-580 or 930	Light green body Brown shoulder
	D	82	10.96	310.37			Light green body Brown shoulder
	E	134	17.91	507.19		Helium less than 80%	Light green body Brown shoulder
	G	1126	150.54	4261.90		CGA-280 or 890	Light green body Brown shoulder

F I G U R E 7 - 1 0 Cylinder specifications for different medical gases.

Type of cylinders and size	Contents (cu. ft.)	Height (inch)	Diameter (inch)	Approximate Weight		Outlet Connection CGA no.	Color
				Full lbs.	Empty lbs.		
Nitrogen K or H	224 at 2200 psi	56	9 1/16	149	132	580	Black
Compressed Air K D	220 at 2200 psi 110 at 2200 psi	56 48	9 1/16 7 1/2	150 123	132 114	400 400	Varies by manufacturer

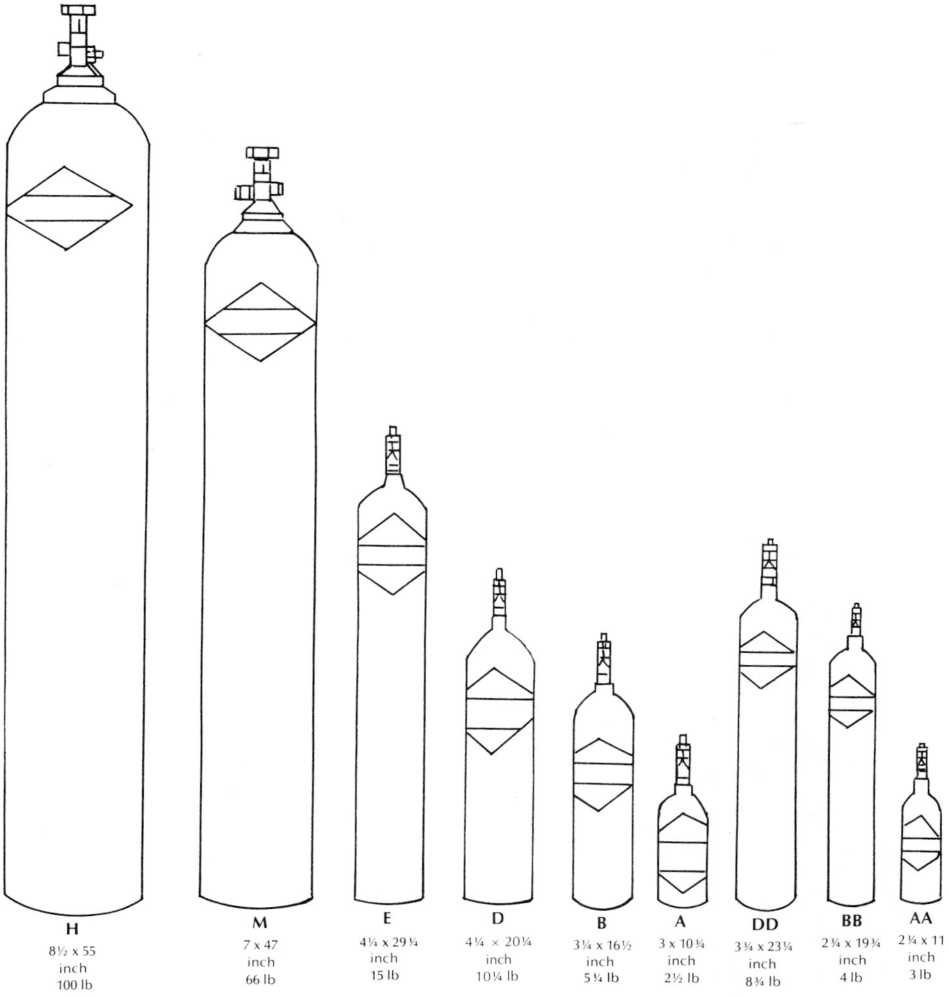
H
8½ x 55 inch 100 lb
M
7 x 47 inch 66 lb
E
4¼ x 29¼ inch 15 lb
D
4¼ × 20¼ inch 10¼ lb
B
3¼ x 16½ inch 5¼ lb
A
3 x 10¾ inch 2½ lb
DD
3¾ x 23¼ inch 8¾ lb
BB
2¾ x 19¾ inch 4 lb
AA
2¾ x 11 inch 3 lb

FIGURE 7-11 Cylinder sizes and colors.

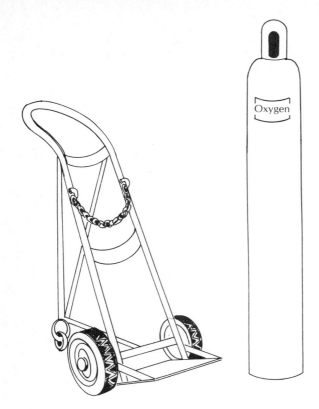

FIGURE 7-12 Three-wheel cylinder transport cart.

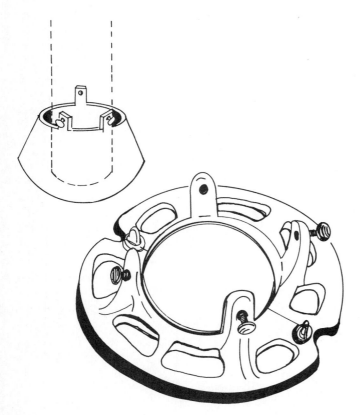

FIGURE 7-13 Two types of cylinder stands.

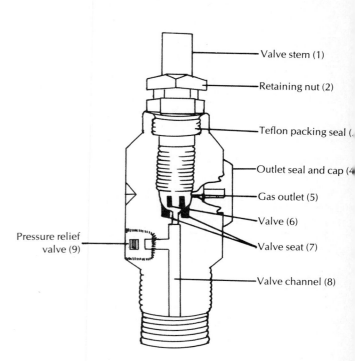

FIGURE 7-14 Components of direct-acting valve as seen in cross section.

3.0 CODES AND STANDARDS FOR CYLINDER AND PIPELINE CONNECTIONS AND FITTINGS

3.1 Agencies and codes dealing with cylinder and pipeline connections and fittings

1 See Unit 2.3, nos. 8, 9, 10, 11.
2 See Unit 2.5, item *1 e.*
3 See Units 4.1, 5.1.

Cylinder valves

The function of valves is to control fluid (gas) flow from one point to another. Cylinder valves are used to start and stop gas exiting from a cylinder. These valves should be *fully opened* when gas is being administered. Points between are not desirable because partially opened valves have a tendency to close themselves off because of gas passing by the valve seat mechanism. Valves used in medical gas cylinders are classified according to their action as *direct* or *indirect* acting.

4.0 DIRECT-ACTING CYLINDER VALVES

4.1 Direct-acting valve

1 Direct-acting valve implies that a turn of the valve stem will result in *direct* movement of the valve in or out of its seat. *Please note* that direct acting valves, also called needle valves, may be either the small cylinder yoke type or the large cylinder American Standard type. For illustration, a yoke-type valve has been chosen, Fig. 7-14.

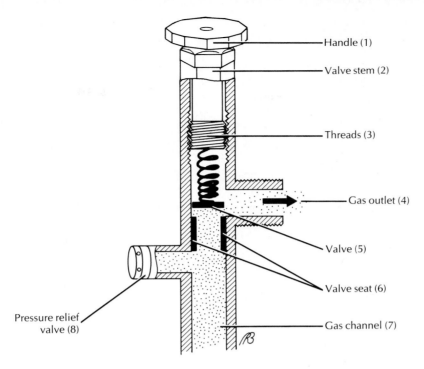

FIGURE 7-15 Components of indirect-acting valve as seen in cross section.

2 Identification of component parts and functions

  a Valve stem *(1)*. Controls gas flow from the valve. Counterclockwise turn will open the valve, allowing gas flow to the patient regulator.

  b Retaining nut *(2)*. Holds valve stem in place. Removal of this part when cylinder is pressurized can result in personal injury as a result of valve stem being blown from its seat.

  c Teflon packing seal *(3)*. Prevents leakage of gas past the valve stem.

  d Outlet seal and cap *(4)*. Placed in outlet of newly filled cylinder to prevent damage to the outlet and dust in the cylinder valve. Must be removed before a cylinder is placed in operation and a fiber or nylon washer used in its place.

  e Gas outlet *(5)*. Exit port for gas leaving the cylinder. Gas pressure at this point is equal to cylinder pressure and should not be administered directly to the patient without reduction.

  f Metal valve *(6)*. Movement of this cylinder-shaped valve in and out of the valve seat *(7)* controls gas flow from the cylinder via the channel *(8)*.

  g Valve seat *(7)*. Teflon or nylon seat works in conjunction with metal valve to control gas flow to valve outlet. More movement of valve away (out of the seat), makes a larger orifice allowing a greater gas flow to pass around the valve to the gas outlet.

  h Valve channel *(8)*. Connects valve to the gas cylinder. Pressure at this point equivalent to pressure in the cylinder.

  i Pressure relief valve ("pop-off valve") *(9)*. Communicates with valve channel. When pressure in cylinder exceeds safe limit of 3200 ± 150 psi, the valve will open allowing gas to escape from the cylinder to the environment. Valve may be spring loaded to allow *only excess* pressure to bleed off or may be plug type (shown) which when ruptured allows all gas in the cylinder to escape.

5.0 INDIRECT-ACTING CYLINDER VALVES

5.1 Indirect-acting cylinder valve*

1 Indirect-acting valve implies that a turn of the valve handle causes another part to move, which acts upon the valve, causing it to move toward or away from its seat. *Please note* that indirect-acting valves, also called diaphragm valves, may be used in either the small-cylinder yoke type or the large-cylinder American Standard type. For illustration, an American Standard type has been chosen (Fig. 7-15).

2 With this valve system the farther the valve is moved away from its seat the greater the gas flow to the valve outlet.

3 Identification of component parts and functions of the valve, Fig. 7-15.

  a Handle *(1)*. Used to turn valve stem *(2)*. Rotation counterclockwise will open the valve *(5)* and cause it to move away from its seat *(6)*.

  b Valve stem *(2)*. Connects handle to valve *(5)* via interfacing mechanisms.

---

*Also see McPherson or Egan in the bibliography at the end of this module.

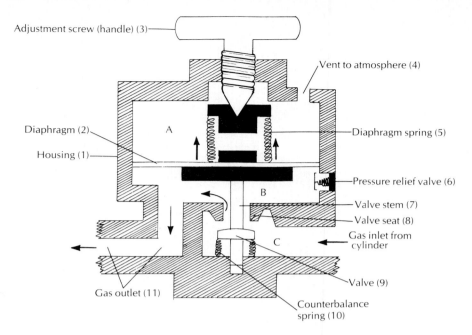

FIGURE 7-16 Components of single-stage reducing valve as seen in cross section.

c Threads *(3)*. Allow valve to move toward or away from seat *(5)* as hand *(1)* is turned clockwise or counterclockwise.

d Gas outlet *(4)*. Threaded outlet American Standard No. 0.903-14 RHT (right-handed thread) for H, K, or M size cylinders:
  • This is used to connect gas reducing valve or regulator to cylinder.
  • Other medical gases would have a different size.
  • American Standard thread connection, e.g., oxygen/carbon dioxide combination would have 0.825-14 RHT.
  • Ethylene cylinders used for welding would have 0.825 LHT (left-handed thread).

e Cylinder valve *(5)*. Usually hard rubber material. Movement toward or away from seat *(6)* will increase or decrease size of valve orifice that determines gas flow past the valve to outlet *(4)*.

f Valve seat *(6)*. Usually highly polished metal or other hard, smooth material. Allows gas flow to be interrupted as valve *(5)* is rested upon it.

g Valve channel to cylinder *(7)*. Communicates cylinder valve with cylinder. Pressure at this point equal to cylinder pressure.

h Pressure relief valve *(8)*. Prevents excessive buildup of pressure in cylinder caused by overfilling or gas expansion (see Fig. 7-14, *9*).
  NOTE: As a rule of thumb, gas pressure in a cylinder will increase 5 psi for each 1° above 21° C (70° F) (its filling temperature) and will decrease 5 psi for each 1° decrease in temperature below 21° C (70° F) (its filling temperature).

6.0 SINGLE AND MULTIPLE STAGE PRESSURE REDUCING VALVES

6.1 Identification and functions of component parts of a single or multiple stage pressure reducing valve and a pressure regulator

1 Purpose of a pressure reducing valve and a pressure regulator.
  NOTE: The distinguishing difference between a pressure reducing valve and a pressure regulator is that the pressure regulator incorporates a flowmeter for setting gas flows in liters per minute (L/min).
  a To reduce cylinder pressure to a useful working level for medical equipment (usually 50 psi ± 5 psi)
  b To provide a uniform gas flow throughout the cylinder's useful pressure range (normally 2200 psi ± 50 psi)

2 Single stage reduction denotes a reduction of cylinder pressure to a workable level (normally 50 psi) in a single operation.

3 For a detailed illustration of the component parts and function of a single stage reducing valve or a pressure regulator, refer to Fig. 7-16.
  a Valve housing *(1)*. Surrounds reducing valve to shield internal mechanism from damage and dirt.
  b Diaphragm *(2)*. A movable partition that separates chamber A from chamber B.
  c Adjustment screw *(3)*. Rotation of screw clockwise will increase tension on diaphragm spring *(5)*. Counterclockwise rotation will decrease tension on diaphragm spring *(5)*.
  d Vent *(4)*. Opens chamber A to the atmosphere, allowing the diaphragm *(2)* to move without causing a compression factor in chamber A.

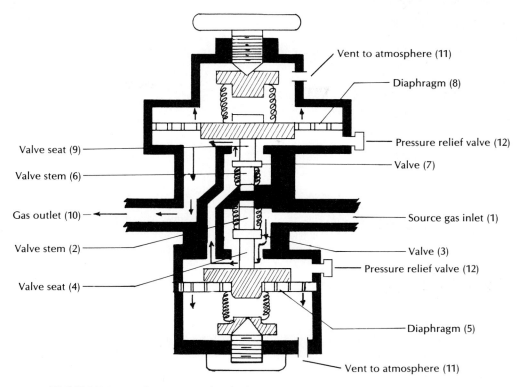

Valve seat (9)

Valve stem (6)

Gas outlet (10)

Valve stem (2)

Valve seat (4)

Vent to atmosphere (11)

Diaphragm (8)

Pressure relief valve (12)

Valve (7)

Source gas inlet (1)

Valve (3)

Pressure relief valve (12)

Diaphragm (5)

Vent to atmosphere (11)

FIGURE 7-17 Components of multiple-stage reducing valve as seen in cross section.

e Diaphragm spring *(5)*. Applies constant tension (force) on diaphragm *(2)* once adjusting screw *(3)* is set.

f Pressure relief valve *(6)*. Spring-loaded valve. Adjusted to open allowing gas to vent to the outside when the pressure in chamber B is 50% greater than the working pressure. When pressure in chamber reaches working level, the relief valve will close, preventing total loss of cylinder pressure.

g Valve stem *(7)*. Connects valve *(9)* to diaphragm *(2)*. As diaphragm moves back and forth, valve must move toward or away from its seat *(8)*.

h Valve seat *(8)*. Works with valve to prevent gas escape from chamber C to B unless valve is pushed away from seat by spring *(5)*.

i Valve *(9)*. Moves toward or away from seat *(8)* to create a space for gas to move from chamber C to B.

j Counterbalance spring *(10)*. Used to balance movement of tension on spring *(5)* as screw *(3)* is adjusted.

k Gas outlet *(11)*. Exit port for gas to leave reducing valve and enter flow administering apparatus such as a flowmeter.

4 Operation of pressure reducing valve or pressure regulator (see Fig. 7-16).

a An opening tension is placed on valve *(9)* by adjustment of screw *(3)*, which causes diaphragm *(2)* separating chamber A from chamber B to move toward B.

b As diaphragm *(2)* moves toward chamber B the valve *(9)* moves "off" its seat *(8)*, allowing gas to leave chamber C to chamber B.

c As gas flows to chamber B, pressure builds until the pressure in B is greater than the open force of the spring *(5)*. When the opening force is exceeded, then diaphragm *(5)* is pushed toward A by the pressure difference between B and A.

d Movement of the diaphragm *(2)* from B toward A causes the valve *(9)* to seat *(8)* closing off the pressure from the cylinder.

e When the pressure in chamber B once again drops because of exit of the gas to the patient *(11)*, the spring *(5)* pushes the diaphragm toward B, causing the valve *(9)* to once again leave its seat, allowing gas to move from chamber C to B.

f When gas is being administered to a patient, this process occurs constantly, causing the pressure in chamber B to remain at the tension determined by the force of the spring *(5)*.

g In most pressure regulators, this spring tension is preset at 50 psi, although in others the valve opening pressure can be adjusted by the operator.

5 The parts and operation of a *multiple stage* pressure reducing valve or regulator (Fig. 7-17) are the same as those for a single stage reducing valve with the exception that:

a The pressure to the regulator outlet is achieved by two-step reducing, i.e., gas passing by two valves instead of one.

b The pressure at the first reduction stage is normally from cylinder pressure to approximately 700 psig.

c Second stage reduction is normally adjusted to 50 psig.

d Multiple stage reducing valves or pressure regulators are single stage devices working together. For this reason the component parts are doubled and the principles established for the single stage reducing valve apply to this device.

e Gas flow can be traced by following steps 1 through 10 as traced on Fig. 7-17. Gas enters at (1) and the pressure is initially reduced at (2) and (4) by the first valve (3) and first diaphragm (5), exactly as in the single stage device. The initially reduced gas then flows to the second valve (7) and diaphragm and is reduced the second time at (6) and (9). The gas leaves the reducing valve or pressure regulator at (10) to a flowmetering or other service device.

f Please note that in a multiple-stage reducing valve there is a vent-to-atmosphere (11) and a pressure relief valve (12) located in the housing for each stage. The purpose of the vent hole is to allow atmospheric gas to escape as the diaphragm moves back and forth. The pressure relief valve prevents excessive gas pressure from building up in the reducing valve by venting any excessive pressure to the outside.

6.2 Potential technical complications related to operation of pressure reducing valves and regulators

1 If the relief valve is improperly adjusted, gas will vent to the outside before working pressure is achieved. This could result in inadequate flow rates being delivered to the therapy apparatus.

2 If the pressure regulator is adjustable, an adjustment pressure that is set too low will result in inadequate flow rates delivered to the therapy apparatus. Pressure adjustment that is too high will result in excessive pressure (flow) delivered to the therapy apparatus and/or cycling of the pressure relief valve.

3 A hole in the reducing valve or pressure regulator diaphragm will result in a constant leak through the atmospheric vent and possible failure of the reducing valve and regulator.

4 A weak adjustment spring will result in a vibrating diaphragm and possibly inadequate flow rate because of premature closing of the inlet valve.

5 Dirt or other foreign particles lodged in the cylinder valve will rupture the reducing valve diaphragm if inadvertently blown into the reducing valve or regulator. This can be avoided by rapidly opening and closing a cylinder valve—"cracking the valve"—before connecting the reducing valve of it. This maneuver should always be performed with the cylinder opening pointed *away* from the practitioner or anyone else.

6 Because of pressure buildup in chambers of a reducing valve or regulator, oil and other petroleum-based products must be avoided. Oil droplets in these chambers will result in closed space combustion and rapid gas expansion, causing an explosive force within the reducing valve housing. Personal injury can occur from flying metal fragments.

7.0 BOURBON AND THORPE FLOWMETERING DEVICES

7.1 Flowmetering devices

Under normal conditions, one cannot see gas movements, only their effects. Flowmeters allow the practitioner to see gas movements by a *flow indicator* and record its rate of movement by a *scale*.

1 Reducing valves or pressure regulators:
  a Reduce cylinder pressure (source gas) to service pressures (45 to 55 psig)
  b Provide an even, steady flow of gas to the therapy apparatus

2 Flowmeters (attached to pressure regulators):
  a *Receive* gas at *service pressure* (50 psig)
  b Further control the gas for patient therapy by altering (metering) the gas to safe working levels
  c Measure liters of gas leaving the device each minute (L/min)

3 Flowmeters may be:
  a Mechanical, such as those used to deliver wall oxygen
  b Electronic, such as those used on ventilators

4 Flowmeters may be:
  a Directly attached to a pressure regulator
  b Indirectly attached via pipeline and wall gas outlets

5 Regardless of the arrangements, flowmeters used for therapy purposes:
  a Are calibrated to operate at 50 ± 5 psig source pressure
  b Must not be exposed to inlet pressures outside this range, if accuracy is required

6 Mechanical flowmeters are classified as:
  a Thorpe type (variable orifice)
  b Bourdon type (fixed orifice)

7 Nomenclature and function of a Thorpe tube type flowmeter (see Fig. 7-18 for detailed illustrations)
  a Flowmeter housing (1). Protects internal mechanism from dirt and damage.
  b Inlet gas connector (adapter) (2). Fits into appropriate wall service outlet to connect flowmeter to available gas source.
  c Internal channel (inlet) to gas connector (3). Pressure at this point is service pressure (50 psig ± 5 psig).
  d Tubing adapter (4). Screws on to flowmeter outlet to allow attachment to small bore gas delivery tube.
  e Gas outlet via tubing adapter (5). Gas exits flowmeter at this point measured as liters per minute flow (L/min).
  f Gas outlet flowmeter (6). Outlet is threaded 9/16-18, allowing attachment of tubing adapters or therapy accessories.
  g Flow indicator (7). Indicates L/min flow as it moves up the transparent tube in response to gas flow. In-

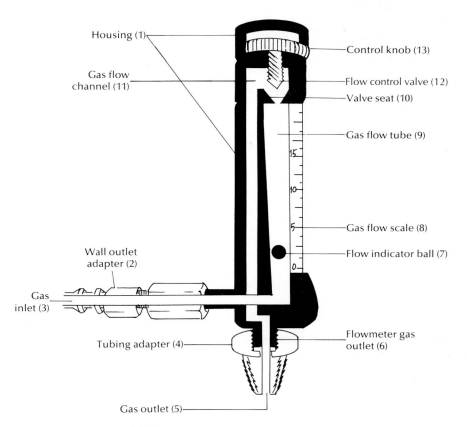

FIGURE 7-18 Thorpe tube flowmeter.

dicators may be balls, rods, or spinning disks. Flow rates should be set using the appropriate point of reference as directed by the manufacturer for each indicator, e.g., top of the ball; center of the ball. The position of the indicator in relation to the scale on the front of the metering device *(8)* indicates gas flow from the outlet of the flowmeter unless the flowmeter is *not* back pressure-compensated. Information regarding the operational characteristics for each flowmeter is imprinted on the front, back, and side of each device.

h Metering scale (L/min). See *(7)* and *(8)* in item *g* above.

i Conical gas flow tube that widens at the top. Position of the indicator ball in this tube in relation to the valve opening determines the space available for gas flow to occur (orifice). As the ball moves toward the top of the tube, the flow across the ball becomes more turbulent with less accuracy *(9)*. (See Fig. 7-19, *A* and *B*). In Fig. 7-19, *A* the position of the ball in the tube determines the amount of space available around the ball for gas flow to occur.

Fig. 7-19, *B* shows the flow tube with the indicator ball at 0, 10, and 30 L/min. The indicator ball has been cut in half with each half resting on a wall of the flow rate tube. As the tube progressively widens toward the top, the halves grow progressively

apart, creating a wider orifice (opening) for gas flow to occur. At low flow rates the weight (mass) of the indicator ball is balanced against the downward pull of gravity by the gas, creating a decreased pressure area across the top surface of the ball, causing lift. The lift effect causes the ball to float, creating a smooth, accurate reading. As the space widens at the top of the flow tube, lift is replaced by velocity of gas flow. This pushing effect results in turbulent flow, causing a buffeting of the indicator ball and metering inaccuracies.

j Valve seat *(1)*. Allows control valve to adjust flow as it is moved in or out of the seat. Prevents gas leakage when flow rate control is in OFF position.

k Gas flow channel *(11)*. Channel through which gas is directed to flow rate control and subsequent exit from the flowmeter. Gas flow at this point is reduced to L/min.

l Flow control valve *(12)*. Permits adjustment of gas flow rate expressed as L/min. Flow rate is determined by turning control knob, which moves needle valve toward or away from the valve seat.

m Control knob *(13)*. Used to adjust gas flow by rotating the control clockwise (OFF) or counterclockwise (ON). This control may be located in different locations in the flowmeter depending upon the particular brand.

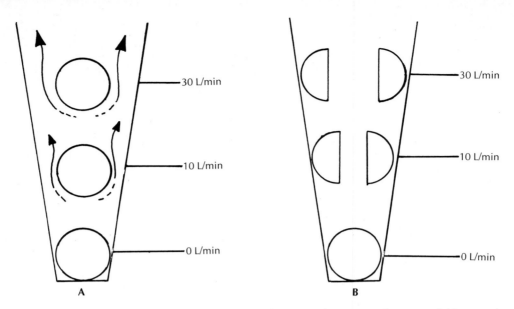

FIGURE 7-19 Position of ball in gas flow tube determines the amount of space available around ball for gas flow to occur.

8 Factors determining accuracy of Thorpe tube flowmeters

a Position. Flow tube must be upright.

b Condition of flow tube. A dirty tube will restrict movement of the indicator.

c Faulty valve seat. A faulty seat will result in a leaking of gas from the OFF flowmeter into the room.

d Pressure compensation. Pressure compensation in any measuring or regulating device normally means that the apparatus has been so designed that anticipated changes in back pressure, caused by tubing or other attachments to the flowmeter outlet, will not affect its accuracy. Medical oxygen flowmeters are commonly used in conjunction with nebulizers, humidifiers, and similar types of equipment. These develop flow restrictions and create a back pressure at the outlet of the flowmeter. The degree of restriction varies with the type of equipment used and the rate of flow.

e Most medical flowmeters are pressure compensated. For this reason, it suffices to point out that the primary difference between a pressure-compensated versus uncompensated flowmeter is the *location of the control valve,* which determines whether the flow tube is calibrated to a 50 psi pressure or to room air.

f The control valve on pressure-compensated flowmeters is located distal to the flow tube such as the one shown in Fig. 7-18 *(12)*. When the control valve is opened, the entire flow tube is exposed to 50 psi pressure. With this system the tube indicator has been calibrated to 50 psi pressure and therefore will not be affected by back pressure that can never exceed 50 psi.

g With a non–pressure-compensated flowmeter the control valve is located proximal to the flow tubes so that the flow tube is calibrated to primarily atmospheric pressure. Back pressure therefore will compress the molecules within the tube, causing the indicator to read lower than the gas flow rate that the patient is actually receiving.

h Gas density and viscosity. An orifice is a channel whose width is greater that its length. Gas flow through an orifice is turbulent and is most influenced by kinetic energy. Since the kinetic energy is proportional to gas density, gases of different densities and viscosities will flow at different rates. Therefore flowmeters that have been designed for use with one gas such as oxygen cannot be accurately used to meter the flow of gases with different densities and viscosities, e.g., oxygen versus heluim. The following is a formula for calculating gas flow through an orifice.

$$\frac{\sqrt{\text{Pressure drop}} \times (\text{Orifice area})}{\sqrt{\text{Gas density}}}$$

9 Nomenclature and function of a Bourdon flowmeter (Fig. 7-20)

Unlike the Thorpe tube type flowmeter, the Bourdon flowmeter is actually a *pressure gauge (1)* calibrated in liters per minute, which operates against a fixed size orifice of a #32 drill bit or an orifice of 0.018 inch inside diameter (I.D.) *(2)*. As the needle valve is opened *(3)*, pressure from a 50 psi source *(4)* is applied to the gauge (giving a liter per minute flow reading), and consequently, more gas passes the fixed orifice *(5)*. The Bourbon flow gauge is normally calibrated on the assumption that the gas passes through the orifice to the atmosphere; there is no restriction distal to the orifice. By restricting the free flow of gas

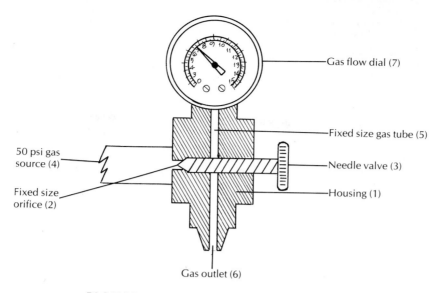

Gas flow dial (7)

Fixed size gas tube (5)

50 psi gas source (4)

Needle valve (3)

Fixed size orifice (2)

Housing (1)

Gas outlet (6)

FIGURE 7-20 Components of a Bourdon flowmeter.

at *(6)*, e.g., with delivery tubing or nebulizers, less gas will flow but a higher reading will still be indicated on the dial, *7*, since it is actuated by pressure rather than flow. A unit of this type will indicate maximum flow even when the outlet is closed off completely since pressure will still be against the gauge. The patient may receive a flow *less* than that indicated on the dial.

10 Fig. 7-21, *1* through *4*, illustrates the nomenclature and function of a *Bourdon pressure gauge only*. This device is used on pressure reducing valves, to indicate flow on Bourdon flowmeters on some ventilators, and in other situations requiring measurements of pressure.

a An external cover protects and shields internal mechanism from dirt and impact *(1)*.

b Question mark–shaped hollow tube *(2)* tends to "straighten" as pressure is applied at *(4)*.

c Geared mechanism *(3)* is attached to the Bourdon tube *(2)* and moves the pressure indicator needle clockwise as the tube tends to "straighten" under pressure.

d Inlet connector *(4)*, for Bourdon gauge, transmits pressure to *(2)*. The primary advantage of a Bourdon gauge over the Thorpe tube type is that it is *not* position dependent and therefore can be used in *any* position.

11 Conditions affecting accuracy of a Bourdon type flow (pressure) meter

a Low flows. Inaccurate with 10% error occurring in range of 1 to 3 L/min. Most accurate in flow range of 3 to 7 L/min.

b Back pressure. *Not pressure compensated.* A restriction of gas flow from the flowmeter outlet will result in a higher reading on the flow gauge than the patient is receiving.

c Enlarging the fixed orifice. Will result in patient re-

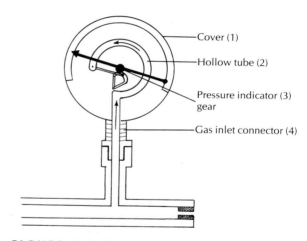

Cover (1)

Hollow tube (2)

Pressure indicator (3) gear

Gas inlet connector (4)

FIGURE 7-21 Components of a Bourdon pressure gauge.

ceiving more gas flow than is indicated on the flowmeter.

d Moisture or other contaminants in flow gauge. Will result in a sticking indicator.

7.2 Operation of Thorpe and Bourdon flowmeters

Typical procedures for operating a flowmeter are included at the end of this module in Procedures 7-4 and 7-5.

7.3 Calibration of flowmeters

Flowmeters are calibrated to operate with 50 psi ± 10 psi source pressure. This pressure may be achieved by using the flowmeter with a reducing valve or wall outlet.

7.4 Estimation of cylinder operating time

1 Practitioners *must* be able to approximate the amount of time a cylinder will operate based on cylinder pres-

TABLE 7-2 Escape factor for various medical gases

Gas	Cylinder size			
	D	E	G	H/K
Air, O_2	0.16	0.28	2.41	3.14
O_2/CO_2	0.20	0.35	2.94	3.84
He/O_2	0.14	0.23	1.93	2.50

sure and flow rate to assure the patient of uninterrupted therapy.

2 According to Boyle's Law, with temperature and pressure held constant, a direct relationship exists between the volume of gas in a container and the pressure measured at any point in the container. Thus, for example, a cylinder fills to 2200 psig at 21° C (70° F) will have half its contents left at 1100 psig. Gas volume leaving a cylinder at a given pressure can be calculated for every psig drop in pressure.

This factor is known as *gas escape factor* and is applied in the following formula for estimating how long a cylinder will continue to operate at a *specific* L/min flow rate. (See Table 7-2 for the escape factor for various medical gases.)

Duration of flow in minutes =

$$\frac{\text{Gauge pressure (psi)} \times \text{Escape factor}}{\text{L/min gas flow}}$$

3 Another way to estimate cylinder operation time is to use a chart (see Table 7-3).

4 Procedure 7-6 included at the end of this module may be used for estimating the operating time for an E cylinder of oxygen.

8.0 COMPRESSED GAS MANIFOLD PIPING SYSTEMS
8.1 Parts and function of a medical compressed gas manifold system

1 Whether oxygen, air, or nitrous oxide, a primary concern for effective medical gas therapy is a continuous gas supply.

2 Medical gases must be free of contaminants such as water, oil, or dust.

3 Gases must be readily accessible to patient care areas.

4 Two systems for providing medical gases for patient care are:
   a Cylinders that are moved to the patient by cart
   b Piping from the wall to each patient bed area

5 Cylinders may be used individually at the bedside or connected together into a manifold system of two or more cylinders.

6 Manifold systems are cylinders connected together with metal tubing and pipes.

7 Component parts that made up a manifold system are illustrated by Fig. 7-22.
   A manifold system normally comprises two or more separate groupings of cylinders called banks A and B. This arrangement allows one bank to be changed

TABLE 7-3 Oxygen flow chart for estimating cylinder service time

	Approximate hours of service remaining in standard oxygen cylinders		
L/min	2200 psig or 244 cu. ft.	1650 psig or 183 cu. ft.	1100 psig or 122 cu. ft.
2	56 hr	42 hr	28 hr
3	37 hr	27 hr	18 hr
4	28 hr	21 hr	14 hr
5	22 hr	16 hr	11 hr
6	18 hr	13 hr	9 hr
7	16 hr	12 hr	8 hr
8	14 hr	10 hr	7 hr
9	12 hr	9 hr	6 hr
10	11 hr	8 hr	5 hr
12	9 hr	6 hr	4 hr
15	7 hr	5 hr	3 hr

while the other is operating. Bank A is normally used first.

8 Component parts (Fig. 7-22). Cylinders normally H or K (244 cubic feet) cylinders with control valves (*1* and *2*).

9 Flexible connecting tubes (*3*). Pigtail-shaped to allow flexibility (movement) as cylinders are changed.

10 Low pressure check valves (*4*). Placed to prevent backflow into a cylinder once it has been emptied. Various forms of check valves (one-way valves) are used extensively in respiratory therapy in ventilator breathing systems and pulmonary function devices to ensure gas movement in one direction only.

11 High pressure header bars. Hollow, elongated pipes (*5*) with threaded inlet connections for attaching cylinders together in a series.

12 High pressure shut-off valve (*6*). Each bank (grouping) of cylinders has a control valve to isolate it from main gas line and other cylinder bank.

13 High pressure regulator (*7*). Each cylinder bank has a pressure reducing valve to reduce the pressure of gas leaving its respective valves.
   a These pressure reducing valves work on the same principle as therapy reducing valves.
   b To ensure that gas flow will only occur from one bank at a time.
   c One pressure reducing valve is set at 60 psig and the other at 50 psig.
   d As long as the primary bank has a pressure greater than 50 psig, the secondary bank will not operate.
   e When the primary bank drops to 50 psig the secondary bank will begin operation.
   f Check valves prevent gas from flowing from the primary bank to the secondary bank (*8*).
   g This arrangement ensures adequate line pressure at all times in that it allows the exhausted cylinder bank to be changed while the other is in operation. The regulator on this bank must now be set at 60 psig and the other pressure reducing valve readjusted to 50 psig.

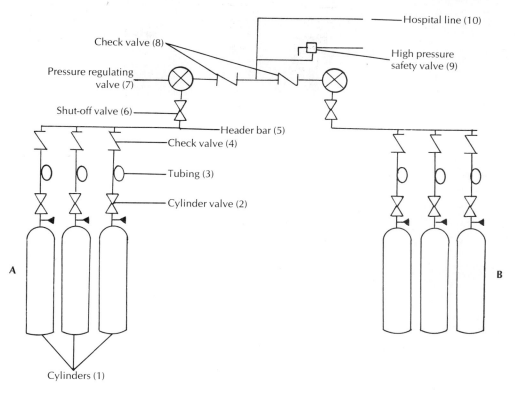

FIGURE 7-22 Components of compressed gas manifold system.

h This procedure must be repeated each time the cylinder bank is changed.

14 Line pressure safety valve *(9)*. A safety relief valve is installed in the main line to prevent excess pressure from being delivered to the piping system. Valve is normally set to vent at 50% above normal pipeline pressure at 50 to 100 psig.

15 Manifold systems. May not be as elaborate as Fig. 7-22. *Two* or *more* cylinders can be interconnected using pigtails and reducing valves when a prolonged continuous gas source is required *away from* the regular main gas supply source.

8.2 Changing a cylinder bank

1 Have a full cylinder on hand.
2 Close cylinder valves on each empty cylinder.
3 Close main control valve for the bank being replaced.
4 Use a wrench of appropriate size.
5 Do not force or overtighten connections.
6 A procedure for changing a cylinder bank is presented at the end of this module in Procedure 7-7.

9.0 LIQUID BULK OXYGEN STORAGE VESSELS.

9.1 Bulk liquid storage system (Fig. 7-23)

1 Shape of liquid storage containers
   a The shape of a pressure vessel has a great deal to do with the transfer of heat into the vessel from the outside, resulting in a loss of useful gas.
   b The heat leakage into a container is greater as the surface area is increased.

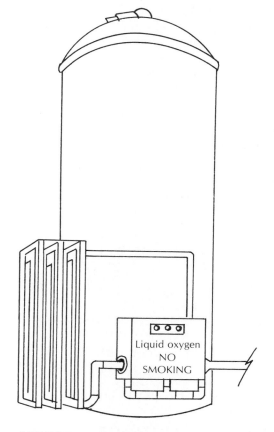

FIGURE 7-23 Bulk liquid gas storage system.

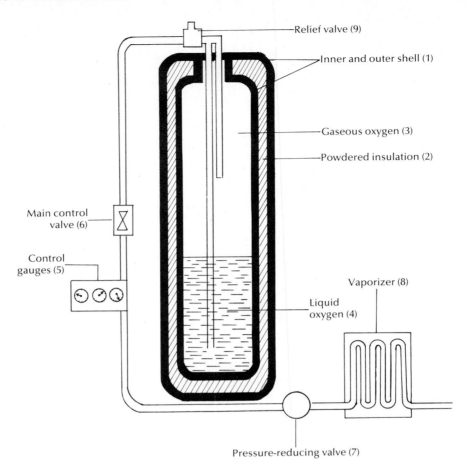

FIGURE 7-24 Cross-sectional view of bulk size liquid oxygen vessel.

c The perfect shape for the storage of liquid gas is a round ball.

d A sphere offers the greatest volume with the least surface area.

e A cylinder with rounded ends is the next best shape.

2 Construction of a bulk liquid container (Fig. 7-23)

a A bulk size liquid oxygen vessel has an inner and outer shell, Fig. 7-24 *(1)*.

b The space between shells contains a dry powdered insulation within a vacuum *(2)* similar to a thermos bottle.

c The outer shell is usually constructed of carbon steel.

d The inner shell is constructed of #304 stainless steel.

e Storage tanks are very rugged; for example, the U.S. Navy tested one by hitting it with a sledge wrecking ball weighing 1½ tons and delivering an impact equal to 130,000 pounds. It took six hits before a bolt loosened.

3 Principles related to operation of liquid gas containers

a Convection. The transfer of heat from one point to another through some medium—air of liquid.

b Radiation. The heat in projected (radiant) form, e.g., electric heater.

c James Dewar. The first man to liquefy a gas. He invented vacuum insulation to prevent evaporation of liquid. A vacuum will not, however, prevent radiation influences. This is prevented by a reflective shield such as those used in thermos bottles.

4 Component parts

a Liquid gas installations. Should be located in secure areas, away from traffic and possible damage.

b The operation of a liquid system usually is not the role of respiratory care personnel.

c However, understanding the basic operation will assist the technician in *monitoring* this type of system.

d Main parts include (Fig. 7-24):

• Storage vessel or container manufactured in various sizes to accommodate usage
  – 25-100 bed hospital—5000 cubic feet of gas
  – 100-250 bed hospital—25,000-100,000 cubic feet of gas
  – 200-500 bed hospital—50,000-300,000 cubic feet of gas
  – 500 + bed hospital—over 300,000 cubic feet of gas

• Control gauges *(5)*. Indicate level of liquid *(4)* in vessel and gas pressure *(3)*. Gauges must be checked daily to determine operational status of the liquid vessel.

- Main control valve *(6)*. Usually painted red. Isolates liquid vessel from hospital main supply line. Closing this valve will *stop* all gas flow to the hospital. Main control valve is never closed without notification of hospital personnel unless there exists an *immediate* and dire danger to the vessel.
- Pressure-reducing (regulating) valve *(7)*. Reduces tank pressure of 200 to 300 psig to hospital line pressure of 50 psig.
- Vaporizer *(8)*. Vertical fins interlaced with hollow pipes that expose liquid gas to a heat source, which causes it to change from liquid back to gas. Vaporizers may be internally, externally, electrically, steam, or ambient heated.
- Relief or vent valve *(9)*. Usually located atop the liquid vessels. Allows excessive gas pressures to vent to the outside. Gas intermittently will vent from this valve if hospital's oxygen usage decreases radically.
- Liquid storage system is usually backed up with a standard high pressure manifold system. In the event of pressure loss from the bulk storage, the manifold automatically maintains 50 psig pressure to the hospital.

9.2 Operation of a bulk oxygen storage system

A guide for monitoring a bulk oxygen storage system is included at the end of this module as Procedure 7-8.

9.3 Potential problems in monitoring a bulk oxygen storage system

When monitoring a bulk oxygen system one should check for signs of potential problems such as those listed in Table 7-4.

10.0 PORTABLE OXYGEN SYSTEMS
10.1 Operation of portable oxygen systems

1. Moving patients who are on oxygen therapy or allowing them to move about on their own is frequently necessary.
2. In these situations, a means must be available to allow patients to take their oxygen with them.
3. The most frequently used method in the hospital is following the patient's wheelchair or stretcher with an E size oxygen cylinder mounted in a small wheeled stand (Fig. 7-25).
   a. With short-term transports or in situations where the gas flow is 4 L/min or less it probably is not necessary to humidify *(1)* the dry oxygen.
   b. The tank should be secured by a tightening screw *(2)*.
   c. As long as the cylinder remains *upright*, the humidifier and Thorpe flowmeter are permissible *(3)*.
   d. Care must be taken *not* to place stress on the connecting tube *(4)* by walking too far behind the patient with the gas source.
   e. As with any cylinder, the cart must not be dropped or allowed to fall to the floor because this can possibly damage the pressure regulator.

TABLE 7-4 Signs of problems in a bulk oxygen system

Problem	Sign
1. Malfunctioning pressure gauge	Gauge does *not* record actual pressure or volume present.
2. Pressure relief valve venting unnecessarily or excessively	There is abnormal gas usage, vapor as cold gas contacts atmosphere, or ice around the valve.
3. Malfunctioning reserve supply	Cylinders do not begin operation when main supply is shut down or begin operation unnecessarily.
4. Leaks around liquid vessel	Ice forms.
5. Alarm malfunction	Alarm activates without cause or does not activate as required.
6. Frozen shut-off or control valves	Valves will not open and close as designed.
7. Low pressure at wall outlets	Equipment will *not* operate properly.
8. Leaking wall outlet	Sound or bubbles occur when outlet is exposed to soapy water.
9. Signs of dirty gas	Contaminants cause low outlet pressure and/or malfunctioning of equipment.
10. Cross connection of lines	Wrong gas comes from outlet.

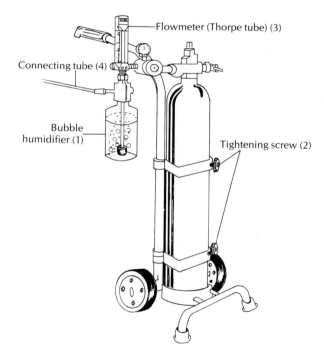

FIGURE 7-25 E-size oxygen cylinder mounted in small wheeled stand.

Flowmeter (Thorpe tube) (3)
Connecting tube (4)
Bubble humidifier (1)
Tightening screw (2)

4. The next most frequently used transport method is placing the cylinder in a special retainer designed for this purpose (Fig. 7-26).
   a. As in item *c* above, a humidifier *(2)* and Thorpe type flowmeter *(1)* may be used (Fig. 7-26, *A*).
   b. However, in the stretcher holder, laying the cylinder on its side is necessary (Fig. 7-26, *B2*), thereby making a humidifier impractical.

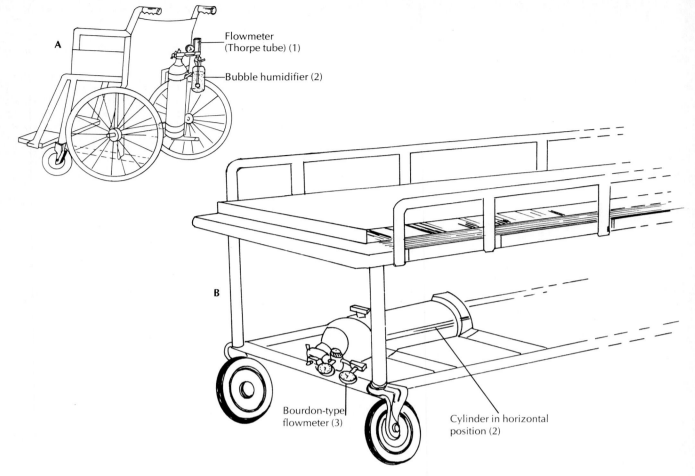

A

Flowmeter
(Thorpe tube) (1)

Bubble humidifier (2)

B

Bourdon-type
flowmeter (3)

Cylinder in horizontal
position (2)

F I G U R E 7 - 2 6 Special retainer for transporting an oxygen cylinder on (**A**) wheelchair, (**B**) on stretcher.

c Because Thorpe flowmeters cannot be read or adjusted on their side, it is necessary to use a Bourdon flow device *(3)* in the horizontal holder.

d If a patient must be on a stretcher for a long period, e.g., for a lung scan, laboratory tests, or x-ray examination, it may be necessary to humidify the oxygen (if the liter flow is greater than 4 L/min) once the patient has arrived at the desired location.

e CAUTION: If it is necessary to transport a patient on a stretcher without a special cylinder holder, it must be accomplished with great care. The cylinder should be *strapped* in place beside the patient, placed between the legs, or carried. If an E cylinder drops and hits the floor at the correct angle, the yoke may break and the tank may become *airborne* as the pressure rushes out.

5 Portable lightweight *liquid oxygen containers* are available to allow mobility to patients receiving supplemental oxygen therapy (Fig. 7-27).

6 Containers weight approximately *11 pounds full* and hold 3 pounds of liquid oxygen to provide approximately 1025 L of gas. Liquid oxygen occupies $\frac{1}{800}$ of the space occupied by an equivalent quantity of gas at atmospheric pressure.

7 Length of useful operation of the portable unit will depend on:

a L/min flow rate being delivered (optimum is 1 to 7 L/min)

b Vent rate (approximately 1 to 5 pounds liquid per day)

c Absence of undesirable leaks

8 Portable units are refilled from large storage containers holding 40 to 75 pounds of liquid (Fig. 7-28).

9 Pressure difference causes transfer of liquid oxygen from storage container *(1)* to portable walker *(2)*.

a Refilling is accomplished by linking two units together with a coupler and a one-way valve system *(3)*.

b Liquid will automatically flow from storage container to walker and will stop when refill is completed (approximately 2 to 4 minutes depending on the unit).

10 Once refilling has been completed, the units should be uncoupled and content level confirmed in the walker. For details, refer to the manufacturer's operator's manual.

11 Possible hazards involved with liquid oxygen:

a Frostbite. Cryogenic gases (liquid) are extremely

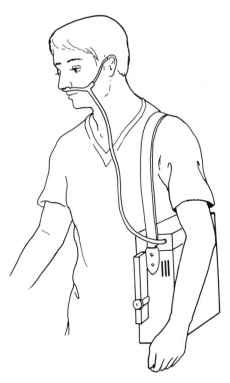

FIGURE 7-27 Person carrying portable, lightweight liquid oxygen container.

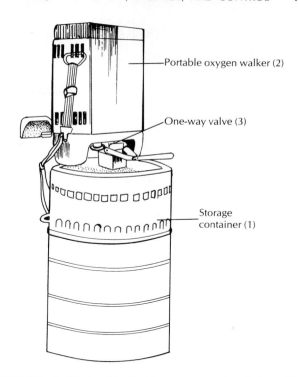

Portable oxygen walker (2)

One-way valve (3)

Storage container (1)

FIGURE 7-28 Portable liquid oxygen container being refilled from large storage container.

cold. Even brief contact may result in burns from frostbite and possible permanent tissue damage.

This type of injury occurs most frequently during transfilling of liquid containers as contact is made with the frost-covered pipes and fittings. Still another example is contact with the liquid oxygen itself that may spill onto the floor if the connecting valve between the storage unit and portable unit freezes open and therefore cannot close once a transfilling operation is completed.

b Fire. Gaseous oxygen will *not* explode, but it *will* support combustion and lower the flash point of certain substances.

Liquid oxygen continues to continuously vent oxygen gas to the environment. For this reason, liquid oxygen units should not be stored in close or poorly vented areas, around electrical fittings, or near sources of heat.

12 Patients traveling with portable oxygen systems should:

a Know the location of dealers or suppliers who can refill spent containers

b Have a medical prescription for oxygen use so that medical suppliers will refill containers

c Be aware of oxygen usage (including venting) per day

d Avoid hazardous situations

e Use personal containers for refill

f Be aware that hospitals, fire departments, and/or public safety units are sources of oxygen should a situation develop where a refill source is not available

g Be aware of regulations regarding the use of oxygen if public transportation is used

10.2 Transporting a patient using a portable oxygen system

A procedure for transporting a patient using a nasal cannula and a portable oxygen system (E cylinder) is included at the end of this module as Procedure 7-9, *A*.

10.3 Operation of a Linde Walker

A guide for filling and operating a Linde Walker is included at the end of this module as Procedure 7-9, *B*.

11.0 PIPELINE, ZONE, AND OTHER CONTROL VALVES
11.1 Hospital piping system

1 Refer to Fig. 7-29 (*1* through *4*)

2 A hospital piping plan usually incorporates:

a Main supply line (*1*). Connects hospital to main gas supply, liquid or cylinders.

b Risers (*2*). Vertical pipes located in hospital to connect subsequent floors with the main supply line.

c Branch lines (*3*). Horizontal pipes that connect various locations on a floor to risers.

d Station outlet pipe (*4*). Pipes that connect branch lines to individual patient station outlets.

e Zones. Piping locations within the hospital that are grouped according to location or function.

3 Valves used to control gas flow

a Main supply valve (*5*). Isolates hospital completely from main gas supply.

b Riser valve (*6*). Isolates all floors attached to riser.

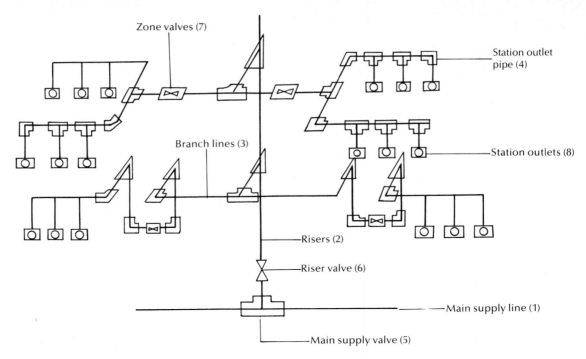

FIGURE 7-29 Hospital gas piping system.

NOTE: More than one riser may service floors above main supply line.

c Zone valves *(7)*. Isolate the branch lines of hospital served by risers.

d Station outlets *(8)*. Individual oxygen, air, and vacuum outlets located at patient stations.

4 Types of valves used with a piping system
  a Needle type (see discussion in Unit 4.1)
  b Ball type. The rotation of a handle closes the channel of a hollow ball, interrupting gas flow (Fig. 7-30, *A* and *B*).
  c Specifications. Shut-off valves shall be full flow, double seal, or ball type with bronze body, Buna-N seals and O-ring packing, and chrome-plated brass ball and designed for working pressures up to 300 psig. Only ¼ turn of the handle shall be required to operate the valve from "open" to "closed" position.

5 Piping materials
  a Must confirm with NFPA No. 56B Standards for Respiratory Therapy and NFPA No. 56F Nonflammable Medical Gas Systems.
  b Gas connections should be of soft metal.
  c Brazing alloys (solder) joining pipes must be silver with a melting point of 540° C (1000° F).
  d Pipe materials must be type K seamless copper—hard temper for exposed locations and soft temper in sheltered locations.

6 Pipe sizes
  a Sizes must be adequate to provide sufficient pressure and flows at all points within the hospital.
  b Pipe sizes vary according to distance served (Table 7-5).

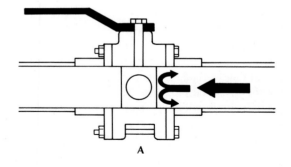

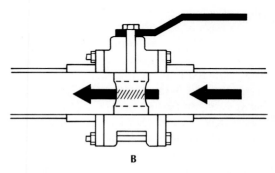

FIGURE 7-30 Ball-type valve used with gas piping system. **A,** Valve closed impedes gas flow. **B,** Valve open to allow gas flow.

c Application of this table clearly shows the effect of the pipe's inside diameter (I.D.) and distance on volume moved. This is a direct application of *Poiseuille's law,* which states that volume of fluid (gas) moved through a smooth, straight tube is directly

T A B L E 7 - 5 Flow capacities of type "K" seamless copper tubing*

Gas	Nominal tubing size (inches)	Distance of tubing far end from supply unit (feet)												
		50	100	150	200	250	300	350	400	450	500	600	800	1000
	¼	100	75	55	50	45	40	40	35	35	30	25	25	20
	⅛	195	145	110	100	85	80	75	70	65	60	55	50	40
Oxygen	½	375	270	220	190	170	150	135	130	125	120	105	90	80
	⅝	580	445	365	310	285	245	225	215	210	195	170	150	135
	¾	885	605	495	460	380	345	320	295	280	260	235	205	180
(supply unit delivery	1	1860	1270	1030	890	800	710	660	630	590	550	500	420	380
pressure: 50 psi)	1¼	3240	2280	1890	1620	1410	1320	1160	1110	1070	1000	890	780	680
	1½	4980	3520	2920	2500	2160	2040	1830	1700	1620	1540	1350	1180	1050
	2	10200	6910	5900	5050	4300	4020	3680	3420	3180	3040	2720	2370	2030
	2½	17050	12050	9950	8550	7440	6970	6150	5850	5560	5330	4690	4260	3600
	3	27700	18900	16200	13400	11650	10940	9840	9400	8920	8420	7580	6400	5770

*Actual liters per minute of oxygen converted to liters per minute (L/min) measured at 14.7 psi and 24° C (70° F) oxygen flow in liters per minute with incoming line pressure at 50 psi.

proportional to the product of the fourth power of the radius of the tube and existing pressure gradient between the ends of the tube. Additionally, the volume moved varies inversely with the product of the length of the tube and the viscosity of the moving fluid (gas).

Application of this law shows that if the length of a tube is increased four times, the driving pressure to maintain a given flow must be increased four times. If the *inside diameter* of the tube is *decreased by one half,* the driving pressure must be *increased 16 times* to maintain original flow.

This law holds true for gas flow through any smooth, straight tube and applies to many other physical and physiologic gas flow situations in patient care such as breathing tubes, ventilator internal circuits, and even tracheal tubes.

$$P = \frac{V}{r_4}$$

or

$$\text{Change in pressure} = \frac{\text{Flow rate}}{\text{Radius}^4}$$

11.2 Patient station outlet

Once medical gas enters the hospital from a bulk supply source, it travels through a piping system to patient rooms and other clinical areas where it dead-ends at a patient station outlet with one or more service outlets. These outlets, usually air, oxygen, and vacuum, are placed in wall locations directly behind or in other locations that are in close proximity to the patient's bed (Fig. 7-31).

Each outlet has one-way check valves that are installed in boxes recessed in the wall (concealed) or attached to the outside wall (exposed) for delivery of air, oxygen, and vacuum to therapy equipment. To facilitate service with minimum leaks, station outlets have two check valves. The proximal one receives the most wear and can be replaced with no loss of gas because of the check action of the second valve (Fig. 7-32, *12*).

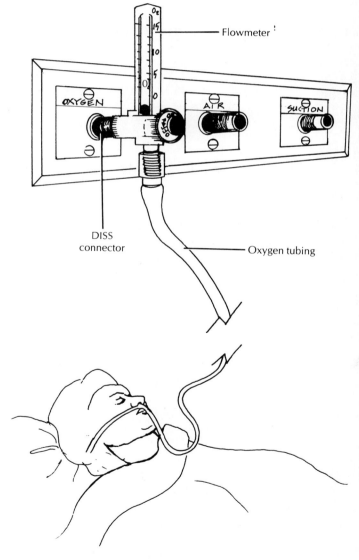

F I G U R E 7 - 3 1 Patient station gas and suction outlets.

1 Two types of patient station outlets
  a DISS
  b Quick connect
2 DISS outlets (receivers)
  a DISS outlets can be used for delivery of oxygen, air, vacuum, and nitrous oxide.
  b They are named this way because the exposed male threaded outlet is DISS for oxygen 9/16-18.
  c Attachment of dispensing equipment is made by screwing apparatus to the outlet.
  d When practitioners attach equipment, they must be careful not to cross-thread, which will strip the outlet threads.
  e Attachment is usually slow and awkward in an emergency situation.

3 Quick connect outlets (receivers)
  a Quick connect outlets are named this way because attachment can be made *quickly* by a single action of pushing an adapter into the corresponding receiver of outlet, such as for air, oxygen, or vacuum.
  b They are not DISS but are based on a similar idea.
  c Geometric shape and size vary for different gas applications according to the manufacturer. In each instance the adapter on the equipment must match the wall outlet receiver before connection can be made.
4 Quick connect adapters
  a A manufacturer will vary size and shape of adapter and receiver (wall outlet) according to the function of the outlet, e.g., air, oxygen, or vacuum.
  b Examples of quick connect geometric adapters are presented in Fig. 7-33.

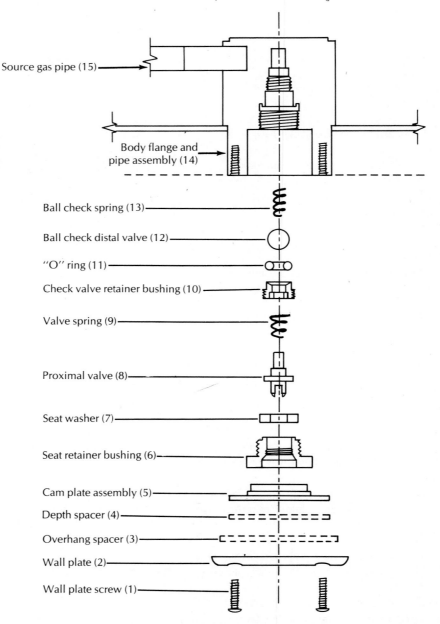

Source gas pipe (15)

Body flange and pipe assembly (14)

Ball check spring (13)

Ball check distal valve (12)

"O" ring (11)

Check valve retainer bushing (10)

Valve spring (9)

Proximal valve (8)

Seat washer (7)

Seat retainer bushing (6)

Cam plate assembly (5)

Depth spacer (4)

Overhang spacer (3)

Wall plate (2)

Wall plate screw (1)

FIGURE 7-32 Component parts of gas station outlet.

c Adapters will have some variation of the following components with shape and size varying according to manufacturer and wall service, i.e., air, oxygen, or vacuum.

NOTE: Gas pressure or vacuum will be at pipeline pressure levels and must be controlled via flowmeter or ventilator before patient attachment.

5 Components of a quick-connect adapter (Fig. 7-33).

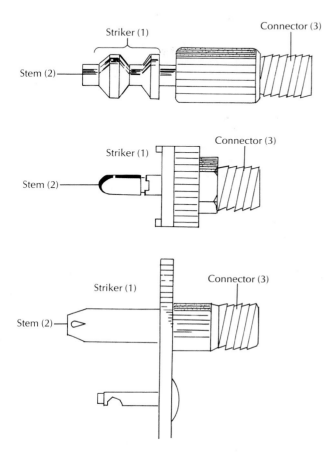

FIGURE 7-33 Quick-connect adapters for attachment of equipment to patient station outlets.

a Striker. Geometrically shaped adapter component that depresses wall outlet (receiver) valve to activate gas flow or vacuum *(1)*.

b Stem. Hollow geometric component that functions with striker to transmit gas or vacuum from wall outlet to therapy attachment *(2)*.

c Threaded connector or nut. Attaches adapter to therapy equipment, e.g., flowmeter or suction regulator *(3)*. Threads and sizes may vary according to National Pipe Taper (NPT) or DISS criteria for each type of gas or service device to be attached.

11.3 Operation of wall outlets

1 Service is activated by attaching the appropriate adapter for air, oxygen, or vacuum to the station outlet.

  a Once the adapter is attached to the wall outlet, pipeline pressures are transmitted through the adapter to service the therapy equipment.

  b If 50 psig is required to operate therapy device, e.g., ventilator, a high pressure hose must be attached from the ventilator to the adapter before attaching it to the wall outlet (Fig. 7-34).

2 Functional characteristics of wall outlet

The following is a sequential explanation of the events that occur in order for one to obtain gas flow or vacuum from a patient station outlet.

  a Stem of adapter is inserted into opening of wall outlet (receiver).

  b Striker portion of adapter depresses plunger of receiver in outlet and removes a check valve from its seat.

  c As long as valve is in place, line service pressure will be available to the attached therapy equipment.

  d Wall service is discontinued by removal of adapter from service unit.

3 Discontinuing service

Manufacturers have designed different mechanisms for *releasing an adapter* (interrupting service). The following actions are used according to varying designs.

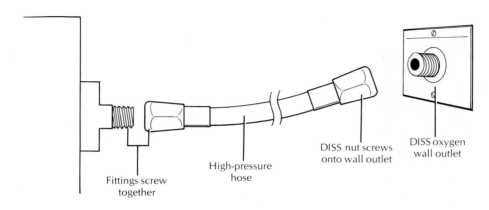

FIGURE 7-34 DISS connector from station outlet to ventilator.

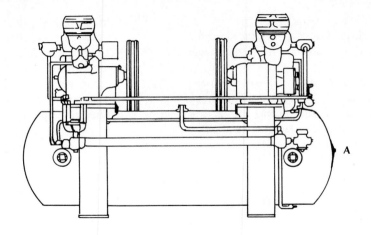

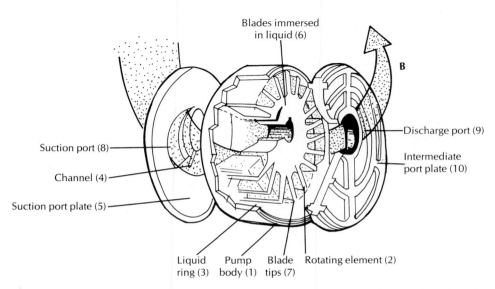

Blades immersed in liquid (6)

Discharge port (9)

Intermediate port plate (10)

Suction port (8)

Channel (4)

Suction port plate (5)

Liquid ring (3) — Pump body (1) — Blade tips (7) — Rotating element (2)

FIGURE 7-35 A, Hospital air compressor system. **B,** Component parts of oil free liquid ring air compressor. (Modified from an illustration of Siemens and Hirsch, Grand Island, NY.)

a Twisting face plate on the adapter
b Pushing release button on cover plate of outlet
c Depressing adapter further into the outlet and then pulling straight back
d Depressing and rotating adapter
e Unscrewing DISS nut from wall outlet

12.0 HOSPITAL AIR PRODUCTION AND VACUUM SYSTEMS

12.1 Hospital air production system

1 An air compressor is a motor-driven device with a storage tank that pulls in room air, compresses it to a preset pressure level, and stores it for subsequent use.
2 Desirable features of medical air compression system
  a Oil free operation. Oil droplets cause lipid pneumonia if inhaled and are detrimental to wound tissue.
  b Provision of clean air. This system provides air free of other contaminants such as dirt, water caused by condensation, or carbon particles produced by compressor wear.

c Pulsation-free operation.
d Adequate distribution line pressure of 50 psig at all station outlets.
  • Pressure drop of gas caused by friction losses of flowing through pipes should not exceed 1 psig/100 feet.
  • Overall pressure drop should not exceed 4 psig between compressor and farthest station outlet.
e Continuous fail-safe operation by incorporating a duplex (double) motor system (Fig. 7-35, A).
  NOTE: Pipes should be of adequate size for required air flow velocity within system (maximum of 4000 feet per minute):
  • Size of riser pipe minimal ⅜ inch I.D.
  • Size of pipes to station outlets minimum ½ inch I.D.
  • Size of main pipe to risers ¾ inch minimum I.D.
3 Functional operation of oil-free liquid ring compressor (Fig. 7-35, B)
In a round pump body (1) a rotating element or shaft is

mounted to impeller *(2)* at a point eccentric to the center line of the pump body. The amount of eccentricity is related to the depth of the liquid ring *(3)*. The liquid ring is formed by introducing service liquid, normally water, via the pump suction casing (not shown) and through the channel *(4)* positioned in the suction port plate *(5)*. The centrifugal action of the rotating impeller forces the liquid toward the periphery of the pump body. Optimum pumping performance will be attained by controlling the amount of service liquid within the pump body so that the impeller blades are completely immersed to their root at one extreme *(6)* and all but their tips are exposed at the other extreme *(7)*. When this pumping action is achieved, the vapor to be handled is induced through the suction port *(8)* when the depth of impeller blade immerson is being decreased. Then as the immersion increases, the vapor is compressed and discharged through the discharge port *(9)* in the intermediate port plate *(10)*. Because there is no metal-to-metal contact between the impeller and the pump body and intermediate plates, the need for lubrication is eliminated and wear is reduced to a minimum.

During the compression cycle, heat is being imparted to the liquid ring. To maintain a temperature below the vapor point, cooling must be applied. This cooling is achieved by continuously adding a cool supply of service liquid to the liquid ring. The amount of coolant added is equal to that discharged through the discharge port *(9)* with the compressed vapor. The mixture of vapor and liquid is then passed to subsequent stages and eventually through the pump discharge for separation.

4 Piping outlets
   a A DISS specification for screw-on air connections
   b If quick connect, geometrically shaped striker for air
5 Flowmeters
   • Calibrated and labeled for metering air flow

12.2 Monitoring hospital air production systems

1 Check station outlets at various locations for adequate working pressure (50 psi ± psi).
2 Low pressure at station outlets may indicate:
   a Leak in the system
   b Failing compressor or storage container
   c Dirty (occluded) line filter at station outlet
      NOTE: This situation may also occur with oxygen and vacuum outlets.
3 If contamination is suspected, remove flowmeter and allow air to blow through a clean 4 × 4 gauze dressing. Note any contamination such as water or dirt.
4 If there is water in the line:
   a Drain collecting tanks on the compressor.
   b Check the operation of compressor dehumidifier (dryer).
5 Note the condition of station outlets and report any leaks or loose connections.
6 Procedure 7-10 may be used as a guide for monitoring an air production system.

12.3 Hospital vacuum supply system

1 Vacuum (suction) in hospitals is produced by motor-driven pumps similar to air compressors with the cycle reversed such that a controlled volume of air is pulled from hospital vacuum pipes instead of from the atmosphere as with air compressors.
2 Adequate vacuum produced at farthest station outlet should be approximately 8 inches Hg minimum (200 mm Hg).
   a 1 inch Hg = 25 mm Hg.
   b Most pipeline medical vacuum units can produce up to 29 inches Hg vacuum or 725 mm Hg at the pump.
3 Like gas piping, vacuum pressure decreases with length and size of piping (see Unit 11.1, no. 6).
   a Riser pipes minimum ½ inch inside diameter (I.D.)
   b Station outlet pipes minimum ¾ I.D.
   c Main pipe minimum 1 inch I.D.
4 Pressure drop resulting from the friction of pipe resistance should not exceed 1 inch Hg per 100 feet or an overall drop of 4 inches Hg between the pump and farthest outlet.
5 Station outlets for vacuum should be DISS threaded and conform with NFPA No. 56B Code for vacuum systems.
6 Factors influencing the operation of vacuum system are as follows.
   a Maintenance of an airtight system
   b Avoidance of aspirants being sucked directly into the pipeline via station outlets
   c Use of adequate suction regulators and connection tubing at station outlets
   d Periodic service of station outlets
7 Vacuum units should *not* be used on patient without an intervening control regulator to limit maximum negative pressure.

13.0 ALARMS FOR MONITORING GAS STORAGE AND DELIVERY

13.1 Functions and locations of operating and low pressure alarms for medical gas hospital piping system

1 Hospital medical gas piping systems. Designed to maintain a predetermined source pressure of gas.
2 Alarms are built into the system to continuously monitor the operational status of piping system.
3 A system of *audible* and *visual* signals includes the following.
   a Normal operation. Light only (indicates switch-over has occurred if cylinder manifold system is in use).
   b Low line presssure. Audible and light signal activated when pressure drops 20% below preset operating level.
   c High line pressure. Audible and light signal activated when line pressure 20% above preset operating level.
   d Loss of reserve supply. Audible and light signal activated when reserve gas supply is lost or when reserve bank drops to 75% of maximum capacity.

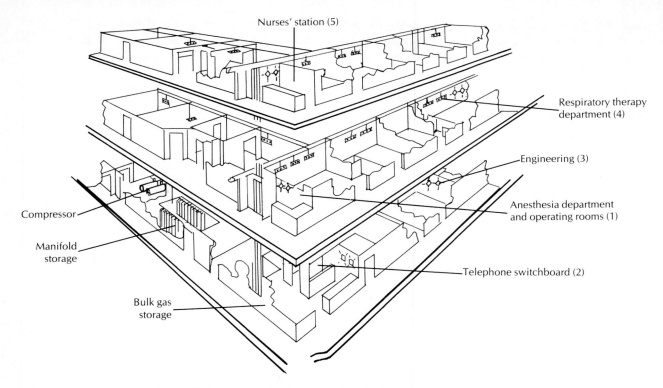

Nurses' station (5)

Respiratory therapy department (4)

Engineering (3)

Anesthesia department and operating rooms (1)

Telephone switchboard (2)

Compressor

Manifold storage

Bulk gas storage

FIGURE 7-36 Typical locations of medical gas piping system alarms.

4 Typical locations of gas alarms include the following (Fig. 7-36).
  a Anesthesia department and operating rooms *(1)*
  b Telephone switchboard *(2)*
  c Engineering *(3)*
  d Respiratory therapy department *(4)*
  e Nurses' station *(5)*

13.2 Testing pipeline alarm system

1 *Do not* shut off gas flow.
2 Press test control to verify light and audible signals.
3 Note operating signal during cylinder bank "switchover" (if used).
4 Conduct other checks according to department policy.

13.3 Causes of failure in bulk gas delivery systems

1 The use of monitors and alarms informs the user that there is a problem with the gas delivery system.
2 Obviously the best and safest procedure is to avoid problems by taking preventive steps.
3 Most frequently occurring causes of problems with medical gas delivery systems are listed in Table 7-6 below.

TABLE 7-6 Frequently occurring problems of medical gas systems

Insufficient gas pressure resulting from low source gas or dirty filters in wall outlets
Excessive gas pressure resulting faulty regulators
Depletion of source gas
Leaks in wall connectors
Cylinders filled with incorrect contents
Leaks in gas pipeline
Explosion of flexible tubing
Frozen regulator resulting from outside exposure
Unannounced system shutdown
Lighting damage to bulk supply
Water in gas pipeline
Control valves inappropriately closed or partially closed

14.0 NATIONAL FIRE PROTECTION CODES (NFPA) AND OTHER REGULATIONS

14.1 National Fire Prevention Association regulations and other codes

1 Refer to NFPA pamphlets #50, #56F, and #56B cited in the Bibliography at the end of this module. Pamphlets are available from local fire officials or usually from the maintenance department.

PROCEDURE 7-1

Transport high pressure cylinders

No.	Steps in performing the procedure
	The practitioner will transport high pressure gas cylinders to and from storage and patient care areas. Great care should be taken to prevent the tanks from falling and presenting a safety hazard.
1	Take a cylinder cart of appropriate size to the cylinder storage area.
2	Check all cylinders to be transported for appropriate levels, color codes, and safety caps.
3	Remove stabilizing apparatus from cylinder being transported.
4	Place cylinder on cart and stabilize.
5	Transport care carefully to area needed.
6	Remove cylinder from cart and stabilize it in area to be used.

PROCEDURE 7-2

Check dates and pressures of high pressure cylinders

No.	Steps in performing the procedure
	The practioner will check dates and pressures of high pressure cylinders whenever placing high pressure cylinders into service.
1	Check code stamped on cylinder for date of last hydrostatic test.
2	Report to vendor expired hydrostatic test dates and place these cylinders apart from serviceable cylinders.
3	Check maximum filling pressure stamped on tank.
4	Compare this with pressure measured on regulator gauge, noting ambient temperatures.
5	Overfilled cylinders should be placed aside and vendor contracted.
6	Underfilled cylinders do not present a safety problem, but if underfilling occurs frequently, it represents purchased gas that is not received and becomes a problem for the purchasing department to handle.

PROCEDURE 7-3

Operating a high pressure regulator

No.	Steps in performing the procedure
	The practitioner will operate the high pressure regulator when deliverying oxygen therapy in those areas of the hospital not serviced by 50 psig wall outlet oxygen.
1	Check regulator for broken parts and gaskets.
2	Remove cylinder cap.
3	Check coded cylinder adapter regulator connector for fit and debris.
4	Turn all valves to "off" position.
5	Turn cylinder valve on gently for 1-2 seconds to clear debris from the valve.
6	Tighten regulator onto cylinder with wrench.
7	Gently open cylinder valve fully with regulator pressure gauges facing away from yourself or others.
8	Observe cylinder pressure.

PROCEDURE 7-4

Checking the Thorpe tube flowmeter

No.	Steps in performing the procedure
	The practitioner will check calibration of flowmeters for routine maintenance of equipment in accordance with department policy and procedures.
1	Collect appropriate apparatus: flowmeter, flowrater*, connecting tubes, adapters, and gas source.
2	Assemble apparatus.
3	Connect flowmeter to gas source cylinder or wall.
4	Turn on flowmeter to be tested to 2, 6, 10, and 12 L/min.
5	Check reading of flowrater to see if it matches flowmeter.
6	If flowmeter is inaccurate (greater than ± 2 L/min), label it as such and place aside to be repaired.

*A flowrater is a device used to accurately measure gas flow. A Wright respirometer or electronic flow measuring device may be used.

PROCEDURE 7-5

Checking a Bourdon type flowmeter

No.	Steps in performing the procedure
	The practitioner will check calibration of flowmeters for routine maintenance of equipment in accordance with department policy and procedures.
1	Collect appropriate apparatus; flowmeter, flowrater,* connecting tubes, adapters, and gas source.
2	Assemble apparatus.
3	Connect flowmeter to gas source cylinder or wall.
4	Turn on flowmeter to be tested to 2, 6, 10, and 12 L/min.
5	Check reading of flowrater to see if it matches the flowmeter.
6	If flowmeter is inaccurate (greater than ± 2 lpm), label it as such and place aside to be repaired.

*A flowrater is a device to accurately measure gas flow. A Wright respirometer or electronic flow measuring device may be used.

PROCEDURE 7-6

Convert cylinder pressure and flow rate to operating time

No.	Steps in performing the procedure
	The practitioner will calculate running time of high pressure cylinders to estimate necessary time for cylinder replacement to provide uninterrupted gas delivery to patient.
1	Calculate or recall conversion factor for specific size cylinder.
2	Multiply conversion factor by cylinder pressure.
3	Divide the answer to No. 2 by the liter flow being used.
4	This quotient equals number of minutes of service remaining.
5	For large tanks, divide number of minutes by 60 to get hours remaining.

PROCEDURE 7-7

Changing a cylinder bank

No.	Steps in performing the procedure
	The practitioner will change high pressure cylinders in bulk cylinder bank when cylinders are depleted in the use of gas supply in accordance with policy and procedure of the hospital.
1	Determine which cylinder bank is in use and which is empty.
2	Turn of valves of all cylinders on empty bank.
3	Exhaust any residual pressure carefully.
4	Disconnect empty cylinders and replace safety caps.
5	Transport full cylinders from storage to empty bank.
6	Remove safety caps and attach to break manifold as if it were a high pressure regulator.
7	Leave newly replaced cylinders open or closed as particular system requires.
8	Remove empty cylinders to storage area.

PROCEDURE 7-8

Monitoring oxygen storage system

No.	Steps in performing the procedure
	The practitioner will monitor oxygen storage systems to determine their capability to supply projected needs of gas. This monitoring can be done on a daily routine basis as part of the respiratory therapy services.
1	Check a standard O_2 outlet to determine pressure within 50-60 psig range.
2	Check for moisture in gas lines.
3	Check various audible and visual alarms throughout hospital.
4	If necessary to shut off bulk supply system and activate emergency oxygen system, notify supervisor.
5	Measure working pressure of emergency system 50-60 psig.
6	Check the quantity of oxygen in the liquid storage system.
7	If quantity is low or zero, notify secretary to contact supplier.
8	If quantity of liquid oxygen is adequate, check for mechanical or electrical malfunction.
9	Monitor emergency supply pressure closely to determine duration of service.
10	When malfunction is repaired, reactivate bulk supply system and refill emergency oxygen source.
11	Check working pressure frequently for several hours.
12	NOTE: Even though no alarm is activated, as in drill above, person must be familiar with procedure in event an alarm situation arises.

PROCEDURE 7-9, A

Using a portable oxygen system to transport a patient using a nasal cannula

No.	Steps in performing the procedure
	The practitioner will prepare an E cylinder with wheeled stand and transport a patient according to the following steps.
1	Verify physicians order.
2	Review patient's progress notes
3	Review respiratory therapy notes.
4	Wash hands.
5	Introduce yourself to patient.
6	Identify patient by identification band.
7	Verify correct L/min flow from flowmeter.
8	Explain transfer procedure to patient.
9	Assist nursing/hospital personnel in moving patient from bed to wheelchair or stretcher.
10	Disconnect humidifier end of oxygen connecting the tube.
11	Turn off patient's flowmeter at wall and disconnect humidifer.
12	Connect humidifier to DISS connector on E cylinder.
13	Reconnect humidifier end of oxygen connecting tubing.
14	Open valve on E cylinder and adjust to correct L/min flow. Note pressure in cylinder.
15	Wash hands.
16	Transport patient to location where appropriate.
17	After returning, assist nursing or other hospital personnel in moving patient back to bed.
18	Turn off E cylinder valve; allow pressure to flow out.
19	Disconnect connecting tubing from humidifier.
20	Disconnect humidifier from cylinder; reconnect on wall flowmeter.
21	Reconnect connecting tubing, turn on correct L/min flow.
22	Check placement of cannula for position and comfort.
23	Question patient as to comfort, remove transport equipment from room.
24	Wash hands.
25	Chart activity.

PROCEDURE 7-9, B

Operation of a Linde Walker

No.	Steps in performing the procedure
	The practitioner will prepare the Linde Walker for use.
1	Collect necessary apparatus: Linde Walker, reservoir, oxygen cannula or mask, electrical source.
2	Fill Linde Walker from reservoir by pressing OFF switch on walker, plug in reservoir and turn on switch, invert walker and attach to couplers on reservoir, latch the latch handle, fill until full light comes on, and disconnect walker from reservoir.
3	Replace coupler seals on walker by pressing down handles.
4	Attach cannula or mask tubing to outlet.
5	Press buttons for appropriate liter flow.
6	Press OFF button to stop flow.
7	Measure contents with spring scale attached to side.
8	Record weight and procedure as appropriate.

PROCEDURE 7-10

Monitoring air production systems

No.	Steps in performing the procedure
	The practitioner will monitor air production systems as directed when performing daily routine respiratory therapy services.
1	With pressure manometer calibrated in psi, check outlet air pressure for 50-60 psig.
2	Check for moisture by allowing gas to flow from outlet rapidly.
3	If pressure is abnormal, check air compressor regulator for proper setting.
4	If there is moisture in air, drain collecting tanks on air compressor or report need to drain to appropriate department.
5	If adjusted air pressure is less than 45 psig, contact preceptor and arrange for air cylinder to be used for apparatus requiring compressed air.

BIBLIOGRAPHY

Bancroft ML, du Moulin GC, and Hedley-Whyte J: Hazards of hospital bulk oxygen delivery systems, Anesthesiology 52:504, June 1980.

Blackman RH: Fire safety of OECO oxygen enricher (pamphlet), Schenectady, NY, Oxygen Enrichment Company, June 3, 1982.

Burton GG and Hodgkin JE, editors: Respiratory care: a guide to clinical practice, ed 2, Philadelphia, 1984, JB Lippincott Co.

CGA Pamphlets G-4, G4:1, P-1, P-2, V-1, Compressed Gas Association, Inc, 1235 Jefferson Davis Hwy, Arlington, Va., 22202.

Chusid E et al: Treatment of hypoxemia with an oxygen enricher, Chest 76:278, 1979.

Hubink DM, editor: Conference report: traveling with oxygen, Respir Care 28:913, 1983.

McDonald GJ: Long-term oxygen therapy delivery systems, Respir Care 28:898, 1983.

McPherson SP and Spearman CB: Respiratory therapy equipment, ed 4, St Louis, 1990, The CV Mosby Co.

Respiratory therapy, NFPA 56 B, Boston, 1973, National Fire Protection Association.

Spearman CB, Sheldon RL, and Egan EF: Egan's fundamentals of respiratory therapy, ed 5, St Louis, 1990, The CV Mosby Co.

Standard for bulk oxygen systems at consumer sites, NFPA 50, Boston, 1974, National Fire Protection Association.

West GA and Primean P: Nonmedical hazards of long-term oxygen therapy, Respir Care 28:906, 1983.

Human respiratory anatomy, physiology, pathology, and applied physics

On completion of this module the reader will be able to:

1.1 Describe anatomic changes that occur in the egg during the weeks after fertilization up to birth of the infant.

1.2 Describe the stages involved in the development of the respiratory system.

1.3 Outline the periods of development of the lung.

2.1 Identify the various microscopic structures of the lung.

2.2 Describe the cellular and tissue formations of the trachea and bronchi.

2.3 Identify the anatomic structures of the gas exchange units of the lung.

2.4 Explain the origin and function of mucus.

2.5 Explain the origin and function of the lymphatic system.

2.6 Differentiate between the two circulatory systems of the lung.

3.1 Point out the general structure and function of the respiratory system.

3.2 Point out the general structure and function of the nose.

3.3 Explain the structure and function of the pharynx.

3.4 Explain the structure and function of the larynx.

3.5 Point out the structure and function of the trachea.

3.6 Point out the structure and function of the bronchi.

3.7 Explain the structure and function of the alveoli and lung surface.

3.8 Identify the structure and function of the thorax.

4.1 Distinguish among the various states of matter.

4.2 Explain the changes that can occur in matter.

4.3 Summarize the kinetic molecular theory.

4.4 Define pressure.

4.5 Define volume.

4.6 Explain the various scales for measuring temperature.

4.7 List the laws that determine the behavior of gases.

4.8 Explain Boyle's law.

4.9 Discuss the kinetic gas theory.

4.10 Describe Charles' law.

4.11 Explain Gay-Lussac's law.

4.12 Identify the combined gas laws.

4.13 Give an example of Dalton's law of partial pressure.

4.14 Distinguish among Graham's law, Henry's law, and the Fick principle.

4.15 Identify the factors determining gas flow.

4.16 Identify the factors determining resistance.

4.17 Give examples of how the laws and principles of electricity may be applied to cardiopulmonary physiology.

4.18 Define the 13 terms contained in the Glossary of Terms.

4.19 Point out the most common causes of electrical shock and electrocution and explain the difference between microshock and macroshock.

4.20 Discuss the physiologic response to accidental exposure of the body to electric shock and differentiate between the most common causes of accidential shock.

4.21 Describe the methods of preventing accidental electric shock.

4.22 Explain how an electrostatic charge is generated and controlled.

4.23 Define the terms relating to temperature and heat.

4.24 Discuss the physiological and physical processes experienced by the body to abnormal temperature.

4.25 Show appreciation for the importance of temperature control in the care of patients by giving examples of the effect of temperature on a patient's hydration and expenditure of energy.

4.26 Differentiate between the various devices used to monitor temperature.

4.27 Identify the Systéme Internationald´ Unitas system and give examples of the seven major SI units.

5.1 Generalize regarding the actions involved in breathing.

5.2 Draw an illustration to explain ventilation.

5.3 Identify the steps involved in breathing.

5.4 Discuss the clinical significance of breathing patterns.

5.5 Draw a diagram to illustrate lung volumes.

5.6 Define the various lung volumes.

5.7 Define the lung capacities.

5.8 Discuss how compliance, elastance, and surfactant influence ventilation.

6.1 Explain how an arterial blood sample is a more reliable indicator of lung function than is a venous sample.

7.1 Define the terms and symbols related to arterial blood gas interpretation and application.

7.2 Distinguish among the symbols used in blood gas physiology.

8.1 Explain how various physical laws and the Fick principle relate to blood gases.

9.1 Define the term "pH."

10.1 Describe how carbon dioxide (CO_2) is transported in the blood.

10.2 Describe how CO_2 production and retention are balanced by other mechanisms in the body.

10.3 Explain how carbon dioxide is produced in the body.

11.1 Using the oxygen dissassociation curve give examples of factors that influence the transportation and release of oxygen to the tissues.

11.2 Explain the factors that can affect oxygen uptake by the tissues.

12.1 Identify the physiologic factors involved in the control of acid-base relationships in the blood.

13.1 Distinguish between acid-base abnormalities.

14.1 Explain how arterial oxygen tension (PaO_2) is calculated.

14.2 Give examples of the various types of hypoxemia and hypoxia.

15.1 Point out the physiologic influences that direct the body's control of blood gases.

16.1 Describe the technique for drawing an arterial blood gas sample.

17.1 Draw an arterial blood gas sample from the radial artery.

18.1 Describe the instruments used to analyze blood gas samples.

19.1 Describe the basic theory of noninvasive oxygen monitoring devices.

20.1 Explain the nature of pathology.

21.1 Define terms related to the study of pathology.

22.1 Explain how pulmonary disease is a worldwide problem that is prevalent in people 65 years of age or older.

23.1 through **23.19** Distinguish among causes, diagnosis, and treatment of the various diseases responsible for pulmonary complications.

23.1 The common cold

23.2 Influenza

23.3 Bronchitis

23.4 Chronic bronchitis

23.5 Acute infectious bronchiolitis

23.6 Bronchiectasis

23.7 Pneumonia

23.8 Tuberculosis

23.9 Fungal infections

23.10 Bronchial asthma

23.11 Pulmonary emphysema

23.12 Restrictive lung disease

23.13 Fibrosis

23.14 Asbestosis

23.15 Silicosis

23.16 Pneumoconioses

23.17 Cystic fibrosis

23.18 Pulmonary disease and heart disease

23.19 Acquired immune deficiency syndrome (AIDS)

24.0 through **24.20** Appreciate the overall impact of adult respiratory distress syndrome (ARDS) by recognizing etiology and by distinguishing modes of treatment and complications.

24.0 ARDS

24.1 Historical description

24.2 Clinical stages of ARDS

24.3 Physiology of ARDS

24.4 Mechanisms of lung injury

24.5 Prostaglandins and the role of cyclooxygenase inhibitors, thromboxane synthetase inhibitors, and corticosteroids

24.6 Polymorphonuclear leukocytes

24.7 Alveolar macrophages in the inflammatory reaction

24.8 Complement

24.9 Platelets in the injury reaction

24.10 Antioxidant agents and therapeutic agents

24.11 Heavy metal chelators as treatment modalities

24.12 Oxygen radical scavengers as treatment modalities

24.13 Niacin

24.14 Surfactant replacement in treatment of neonatal respiratory distress syndrome (RDS)

24.15 Immunizations against *E. coli* endotoxin for septic shock

24.16 Endorphins in endotoxin shock

24.17 Pathophysiology of ARDS

24.18 Pathologic changes in ARDS

24.19 Treatment of ARDS

24.20 Complications of ARDS

1.0 EMBRYOLOGY OF THE LUNG

1.1 Introduction to human development

1 The growth of every human being begins with the development of a fertilized egg, the *ovum*.

2 In 8 weeks an embryo develops from an egg that has increased in length approximately 240 times and in weight over 1 million times.

3 The pattern of the embryo's development is sequenced so that the organic necessities are developed first.

4 By the end of the *second week* of conception the *amniotic fluid*, which serves to cushion the embryo against external shocks and pressures, begins to form.

5 During the *third week fingerlike extensions (villi)*, which begin to form 1 week after conception, form a network including uterine tissues and blood vessels to provide the embryo with food and oxygen and to remove the waste products of metabolism.

6 The lungs begin their earliest embryonic development at approximately *24 days'* gestation. Unlike most systems and organs, the lungs have no actual function during the entire period of gestation. However, the respiratory system must mature to a point that it is able to participate in diffusion of gases and perfusion of alveoli before the embryo is able to survive outside the uterus. Pulmonary capillaries develop about the 20th week of gestation, but they do not move close enough to the alveoli for diffusion to occur until the *26th* to *28th weeks*.

7 By the *fourth week* the embryo has developed a primitive nervous system with a two-lobed brain. A U-shaped heart has been formed that pumps blood through a simple vessel system in the embryo and the placenta (see Module Twenty-six for a description of fetal circulation). Although they are nonfunctioning organs a primitive esophagus and stomach are formed.

8 In the *fifth week* the extremities begin to emerge, with fingers and toes appearing by the end of the eighth week.

9 By the end of the *seventh week* the head has developed, with eyes, ears, nose, and mouth. The brain has developed all five of its major subdivisions, making the embryo more sensitive to stimuli. The stomach begins to secrete gastric juices, the major muscles of the body are completed, and the cartilaginous skeleton begins to change to bone.

10 During the *eighth week* cellular changes are most dramatic, with liver cells, heart cells, and so on, taking on distinguishable characteristics that allow them to specialize.

11 By the *ninth week* the baby is referred to as a *fetus* instead of an embryo.

12 The remaining 24 weeks of gestation are devoted to the development and refinement of function of organs and organ systems. For example, the sex of the fetus becomes more apparent, with primary sex organs forming. By the *16th week* the entire reproductive system is complete, and the fetus begins to kick, the salivary glands function, the kidneys begin to function, and the nervous system is responsive to external stimuli. The fetus is still very small—20 to 25 cm (8 to 10 inches)—and is able to actively change positions within the amniotic sac.

13 A baby born during this period would be called *premature*. Prematurity is based on the baby's *weight* at birth and not length of the mother's pregnancy, although generally there is a close relationship between the two.

14 Most infants weighing *less than 2500 g* at birth, and almost all infants weighing less than *1500 g* are premature (454 g equals 1 lb).

15 Prematurity is the most common cause of infant mortality in the United States. A child born at St. Anne's Hospital in Chicago, who weighed only 340 g (2 ounces) at her birth, is one of the smallest premature babies on record to survive.

1.2 Development of lung structures

1 The lung and other cellular specialization evolves from three distinct groups of cells (germ layers) arranged in a sandwich-type structure called an "embryonic disk" (Fig. 8-1, *A*). In this structure the top layer, ectoderm *(1)*, gives rise to the nervous system and all outer coverings of the body. The middle layer, mesoderm *(2)*,

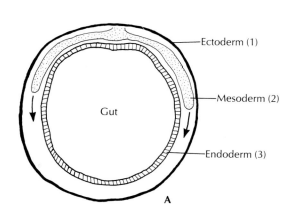

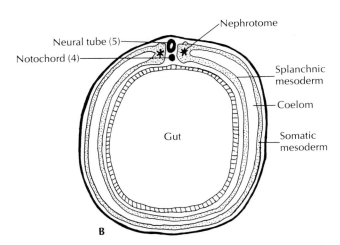

FIGURE 8-1 A, Embryonic disk shows three germ layers. **B,** Development of organs from the germ layers.

will form the musculature, the bones, the heart, veins, and arteries. The lower layer, endoderm *(3),* will form the glands and the lining of internal organs such as the stomach and lungs. These germ layers grow and shift (Fig. 8-1, *B*) so that the cells form rough shapes of early organs around a primitive notochord or spine *(4)* and neural tube *(5).*

2 The respiratory system begins around the fourth week of gestation with development of the *pharyngeal region.* It first appears as rounded ridges resembling gills on each side of a mass that will become the head and neck region of the fetus.

3 The *mouth* appears as a slight depression in the ectoderm (one of the three primary germ layers of the embryo) to form a stomodeum or primitive mouth. This cavity is initially separated from the primitive pharynx by a membrane that ruptures at approximately 24 days' gestation, causing the digestive tract to open into the amniotic cavity.

4 Nasal sacs develop about the same time by growing back and down from the developing brain. Initially these sacs are separated from the oral cavity by the oronasal membrane, which ruptures, bringing the nasal and oral cavities into communication. When the palatine processes (hard and soft palates) connect with each other and the nasal septum, the oral and nasal cavities are again separated. This fusion also separates the nasal cavities from each other, forming nares or nostrils.

5 The *paranasal air sinuses* develop during late fetal life and infancy as a small outpouching of the nasal wall.

During childhood these sinuses will continue to extend into the maxilla, the ethmoid, and the frontal and sphenoid bones; they reach their maximum size around puberty.

6 Development of the lung and its airways is categorized into three main periods: glandular, canalicular, and alveolar.

a The *glandular period* includes the first 14 to 16 weeks of development, during which time the lung resembles an endocrine gland. Fig. 8-2 illustrates lung growth, which begins at approximately the 24th day of gestation *(A).* During this time there is an outpouching of the gut so that by the 26th to 28th day, two main buds (branches) develop into the major bronchi *(B).* The left bud will be slightly smaller than the right and will be directed laterally. The right bud will give rise to two secondary buds. The left bud will give rise to only one secondary bud. Lung buds subsequently develop into three lung lobes on the right side of the chest and two lung lobes on the left side of the chest *(C).* For the next few weeks lung growth consists mainly of continued branching into the surrounding connective tissue that will form the blood vessels and lymph vessels of the pulmonary system *(D).* Between the 10th and 14th weeks of gestation, branching accelerates so that 70% of the number of branching generations occurs during this time. Until the 14th week the right lung may have more branches than the left, with one to five fewer branchings occurring in the left lung. Most

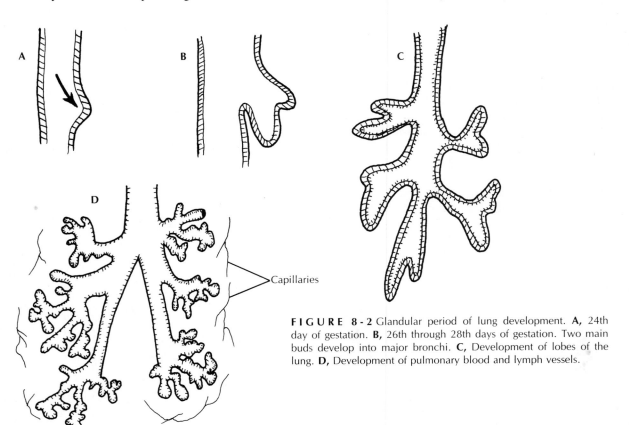

FIGURE 8-2 Glandular period of lung development. **A,** 24th day of gestation. **B,** 26th through 28th days of gestation. Two main buds develop into major bronchi. **C,** Development of lobes of the lung. **D,** Development of pulmonary blood and lymph vessels.

airways are formed by the 16th week, with no additional structures formed after birth.

b The next period of development, the *canalicular period,* includes the 16th through 24th weeks of gestation. This period occupies the middle part of uterine life, during which the airways are still actively dividing. The branching airways are blind at their distal ends, and capillaries following them begin to enter the epithelial tissue. The capillaries will not reach the point where they can carry on sufficient gas exchange until at least the 28th week of gestation.

c Development from the canalicular to the alveolar period involves a change in degree rather than in kind. The *alveolar period* lasts from the 24th week until birth. It is during this time that terminal alveoli appear as outpouchings of the bronchioles. This time frame is quite variable, making it difficult to clearly separate the canalicular and alveolar periods. For example, early areas of developing alveoli often can be seen in a 20-week-old fetus but can still be absent in a 26-week-old stillborn fetus.

• After about 26 to 28 weeks air sacs (alveoli) increase in number to form pouches of a common chamber called an "alveolar duct," which opens to the terminal alveoli. These ducts are shallow and wide-mouthed, and it is not until several months after birth that they assume a characteristic cup-shaped configuration when viewed under the microscope. The growth of the alveoli continues until the child reaches approximately 8 years of age.

• It is also during the *alveolar period* that one of the most important developments in the maturing lung takes place. At approximately the 26th to 28th week of gestation the capillary network, which came about in the 20th week, branches close enough to the developing airways so that gas exchange can take place. It is during this time that the lung becomes the most vascular organ in the body. Before this time the incomplete pulmonary vascular bed would not be able to accommodate the whole of the cardiac output, which primarily is shunted away from the lungs. For this reason an infant would not be able to sustain life until the time when there is sufficient surface area of the lung being perfused to handle a normal cardiac output volume.

7 The production of *cartilage* in the lung starts early in fetal life and continues until around the sixth month of gestation. The first changes in tissue cells indicating the formation of precartilage start in the trachea at approximately the fourth week. At the end of the seventh week distinct rings of cartilage are observable along the trachea.

a Gradually the cartilage spreads toward the periphery so that it reaches the lobar bronchi in the 11th week and the segmented bronchi in the 12th week. This is approximately 6 weeks after airways first appear. Further growth toward the periphery occurs without

a burst of activity like that of the branching bronchial tree. After about the 24th week the cartilage does not spread any further.

b The number of generations that include cartilage remains constant and corresponds to the adult lung. Two systems are used for counting airways. One begins at the top with zero and progresses to the respiratory bronchioles (see Table 8-1). The other starts with the respiratory bronchioles and progresses upward to zero.

8 Mucus in the lung is secreted by *goblet cells* located on the surface of the epithelium and by multicellular tubuloacinar glands under the mucous membranes. Formation of these cells along with cilia begins quite early in gestation and continues in all phases of lung development.

a The first sign of developing mucous cells is seen in the multiplying of base cells of the epithelium, forming small projections or buds. This occurs around the eighth week of fetal life.

b In the bronchi the first buds do not appear until the 13th or 14th week.

c *Cilia* (hairlike structures) arise in the trachea and main bronchi at approximately 10 weeks and reach the end of the branching tree by 13 weeks.

d The larger airways are rich in mucous glands from early development. All of the mucous cells and cilia appear first in the trachea and, like cartilage, extend progressively to the distal parts of the bronchial tree. Goblet cells are not found beyond the cartilage formations of the airway and therefore do not extend to the distally located mucous glands.

T A B L E   8 - 1 Average dimensions of adult airways

Generation (z)	Length (l) in centimeters	Diameter (d) in centimeters	l/d	Area per airway (cm²)	Total area (cm²)
0	12.000	1.800	6.666	2.5447	2.5447
1	4.782	1.219	3.924	1.1689	2.3380
2	1.906	0.825	2.309	0.5436	2.1382
3	0.760	0.564	1.346	0.2498	1.9987
4	1.267	0.372	3.401	0.1087	1.7390
5	1.069	0.324	3.300	0.0845	2.7039
6	0.901	0.260	3.469	0.0531	3.398
7	0.761	0.209	3.647	0.0343	4.391
8	0.462	0.181	3.548	0.0257	6.578
9	0.541	0.143	3.796	0.0161	8.223
10	0.457	0.119	3.834	0.0111	11.389
11	0.385	0.103	3.758	0.0083	17.064
12	0.325	0.087	3.723	0.0060	24.572
13	0.274	0.076	3.611	0.0045	37.159
14	0.231	0.068	3.401	0.0036	59.500
15	0.195	0.060	3.267	0.0025	80.706
16	0.165	0.054	3.046	0.0023	150.647
17	0.139	0.049	2.812	0.0019	251.213
18	0.117	0.046	2.570	0.0016	428.080
19	0.099	0.043	2.302	0.0015	761.370
20	0.083	0.041	2.040	0.0013	1377.82
21	0.070	0.039	1.793	0.0012	2543.84
22	0.059	0.038	1.559	0.00114	4781.50
23	0.050	0.037	1.328	0.00111	9361.68

e The main period of growth for tubuloacinar glands is between the 14th and 28th weeks of gestation. These glands cannot be clearly seen until the 25th or 26th week, when they begin to differentiate into mucous cells containing acid mucopolysaccharides and serous cells producing a serumlike or watery-like substance. Most of these glands change after the 26th week, but this is variable, with some not changing until after birth.

f The *primary function* of the mucous-secreting cells is that of *cleaning* the respiratory system, which is not functionally important in intrauterine life. The fact that mucous secretion in the tracheobronchial tree is only slight in the fetus and increases after birth suggests that the important role of the mucus in fetal life is waterproofing the airways to prevent escape of fetal body fluids to the outside.

9 Another important secretion of the lung is *surfactant*. This surface-active material plays the important role of reducing the surface tension of the alveoli to reduce lung inflation pressures and prevent alveolar collapse. The nature of surfactant makes it difficult to extract from fetal lungs for study, although it is believed that it is produced in the alveolar cells by approximately the 24th week of gestation.

a Surfactant is *not* an important element in fetal life, because the alveoli are not utilized for diffusion. At birth, surfactant plays an important role in maintaining alveolar patency and gas exchange. Recent studies show a direct relationship between the presence of surfactant and survival of the infant, especially premature cases.

b Greater details regarding surfactant and lung function are presented in subsequent units of this module.

1.3 Summary of lung development and growth

1 The lung appears as an outpouching of the gut at 24 days.

2 By the 16th week the lung has its bronchial generations (see Fig. 8-2).

3 From the 16th week to the 24th week a canalicular phase dominates.

4 After the 24th week terminal air spaces begin to appear.

5 After birth, terminal air spaces elongate so that by 6 to 8 weeks after birth, typically shaped alveoli appear

6 Cells appear during all phrases of lung development.

7 Four types of pseudostratified epithelium appear:

a Ciliated cells at the 10th week.

b Goblet cells at the 13th to 14th weeks.

c Brush cells at the 13th to 14th weeks.

d Short basal cells at the 13th to 14th weeks.

8 Alveolar lining cells are last to appear at the 24th to 26th weeks of gestation.

a Type I cell: attenuated epithelial cell.

b Type II cell: a granular cell with many mitochondria, osmiophilic inclusions, Golgi apparatus, and organelles.

c Macrophages are fixed to the cell wall or are free in the lumen. It is these cells that are abundantly found in sputum.

9 The pulmonary artery arises from the aortic arch and nourishes the new lung.

a At the 26th to 28th weeks pulmonary capillaries develop rapidly.

b At the 20th to 24th weeks surfactant is developed.

10 Postnatal lung development continues until about age 8 years, with an increase in alveoli and the dimensions of air spaces.

11 Dimensions of terminal air spaces continue to increase until age 40 years. The average dimensions of adult airways are presented in Table 8-1.

2.0 LUNG STRUCTURE
2.1 Microscopic structures of the lung

Units 1.1 and 1.2 present an overview of certain microscopic structures of the lung during its development.*

Respiratory therapy personnel should understand normal lung structures and functions in order to relate them to abnormal conditions and their treatment.

In the past decade a great deal has been learned about gross and microscopic structures of the lung.

1 Beginning with the trachea, the *airways* can be classified in descending order as they penetrate deeper toward the terminal branching and periphery of each lung, as shown in Table 8-1:

a Cartilaginous: generations 1 through 11

b Membranous: generations 12 through 16

c Gas exchange units: generations 17 through 23

2 *Cartilaginous airways* (Fig. 8-3) include:

a Trachea *(1)*

b Main stem bronchi, left and right *(2)*

c Lobar bronchi going to all lobes *(3)*

d Segmental bronchi going to all segments *(4)*

e Smaller bronchioles—0.1 to 0.3 cm inside diameter (ID)—measured during a maximal inspiration *(5)*

2.2 Trachea and bronchi

1 The *trachea* and main stem *bronchi* (Fig. 8-4) are formed by C-shaped cartilages, opened posteriorly. The interior of these passages is lined with columnar ciliated epithelial tissue and goblet cells *(1),* which produce a thick mucous blanket from mucous and serous glands *(2)* as a transport medium.

2 *Lobar, segmental,* and *smaller bronchi* are formed by helical bands of smooth muscle. Interiorly these airways are lined with columnar ciliated epithelial tissue interspersed with goblet cells (see Fig. 8-4, *3*). These cells produce a mucous blanket that allows foreign particles or lung debris to slide toward the surface as it is propelled by constantly beating cilia. The smooth muscle surrounding these airways is innervated by the sympathetic branch of the autonomic nervous system.

---

*For more detail on basic structure and function of the lung, see Anthony CP and Thibodeau GA: Structure and function of the body, ed 7, St Louis, 1984, The CV Mosby Co.

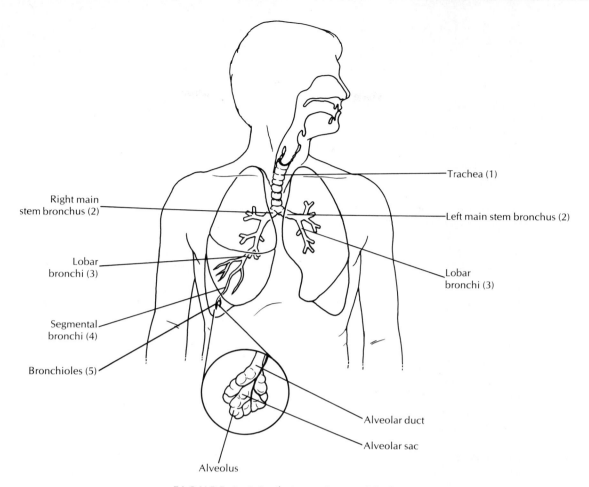

Right main
stem bronchus (2)

Lobar
bronchi (3)

Segmental
bronchi (4)

Bronchioles (5)

Trachea (1)

Left main stem bronchus (2)

Lobar
bronchi (3)

Alveolar duct

Alveolar sac

Alveolus

F I G U R E   8 - 3 Cartilaginous airways of the lung.

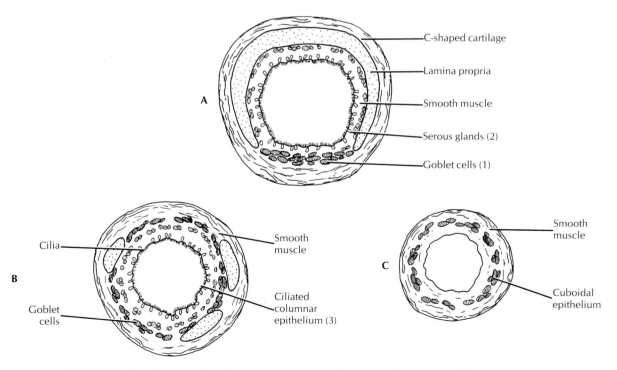

C-shaped cartilage

Lamina propria

Smooth muscle

Serous glands (2)

Goblet cells (1)

A

Cilia

Goblet
cells

B

Smooth
muscle

Ciliated
columnar
epithelium (3)

Smooth
muscle

C

Cuboidal
epithelium

F I G U R E   8 - 4 Anatomy of trachea or main stem bronchi shows cartilage and cellular lining. **A,** Trachea and main stem bronchi. **B,** Lobar, segmental, and smaller bronchi. **C,** Terminal bronchioles.

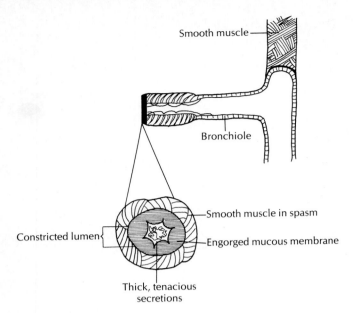

FIGURE 8-5 Constriction of an airway such as occurs in asthma.

Nerve endings located close to the internal surface of the air passages are sensitive to external stimuli and will respond to irritation by causing a cough reflex or by spasm, causing the kind of constriction of the airway that occurs in asthma (Fig. 8-5).

3 *Membranous airways* begin at the level of the terminal bronchioles—12th through 16th generations. At this level cartilage, which is sparse to absent, is replaced by helical bands of smooth muscle. Terminal bronchioles receive their structural support from being directly embedded into the connective tissue of the lung.

4 *Terminal bronchioles* are lined with cuboidal epithelial tissue surrounded by smooth muscle innervated by the sympathetic nervous system. The primary difference between terminal bronchioles and earlier structures is the absence of cartilage and goblet cells. Lubrication of the airway at this level is by a serous (watery), clear substance that gradually picks up mucus as it moves toward the upper airways. Lung disease usually causes a marked increase in the number of goblet cells and in the volume of mucus produced.

2.3 Gas exchange units

1 The *acinus* (Fig. 8-6) begins with the respiratory bronchioles that lead to alveolar sacs, much like grapes bunched on a stem. At this level (17th to 19th generations) the airways are formed of cuboidal to flattened cuboidal tissue, with smooth muscle quickly disappearing and replaced by muscle bands located between alveolar units. In Fig. 8-6 the respiratory bronchiole, with its alveolar buds *(1),* alveolar ducts—passages leading to alveoli *(2)*—and alveoli *(3)* form the terminal respiratory unit where gas exchange occurs. More than 100,000 of these parallel units form the basic gas exchange surface of the lung.

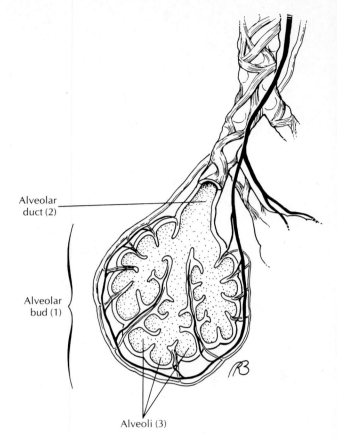

FIGURE 8-6 Components of the acinus.

2 The number of alveoli in an adult is estimated at approximately 250 million from age 8 years to age 30. After age 30, alveoli numbers decrease because of destruction of alveolar walls (septa).

a In an adult, alveoli measure approximately 0.2 mm ($\frac{1}{100}$ of an inch) in diameter and have a total surface area about equivalent to a tennis court, or 70 m^2.

b Alveolar walls are 4 to 8 μm thick and are arranged in a complex three-dimensional structure.

3 Principal cells that cover the major alveolus are *type I cells,* which may have a plasmic connection with the cuboidal cells of the respiratory bronchiole, and *type II cells,* which are more granular and more structurally sophisticated. Both of these cells rest on a basement membrane that surrounds the cell. The type II cell is responsible for secreting *surfactant,* which is vital for maintaining patency of the alveoli during exhalation and reduces inflation pressures during inhalation. An alveolar macrophage (dust cell) migrates from the pulmonary capillaries to remove dust and foreign bodies in the alveoli and carry them to the lymphatic or proximal bronchioles for removal.

4 *Pulmonary capillaries* pass through and around alveolar walls, providing an interface (area) for diffusion of gases to occur.

5 Each capillary-alveolus interface has six structural layers consisting of:

a Capillary endothelium

b Capillary basement membrane
c Connective tissue
d Basement membrane
e Alveolar epithelium
f Fluid
- In a healthy lung the total thickness of this interface is *0.5 μg,* which allows rapid diffusion of respiratory gases back and forth between the alveoli and the blood.

6 Alveolar units that do not open directly to bronchioles exchange gases among other alveoli through small interconnecting holes known as pores of Kohn.

2.4 Mucous system

The submucosa of the airways to the 14th and 15th generations contain tubuloacinar bronchial glands. These glands are innervated by the parasympathetic nervous system and secrete a mucous blanket that lubricates the airway and facilitates ciliary action with removal of foreign particles. Secretions produced by the bronchial glands separate into two layers by the beating of the cilia. The depth of the more fluid bottom layer (sol) is adjusted by the cilia located on the surface of the epithelial cells. The sticky top layer (gel) collects foreign materials and cellular debris and carries them toward the surface.

2.5 Lymphatic system in the lung

1 There are three main groups of lymphatics in the lung.
  a The first group begins in the visceral pleura or in the interlobular septa and drains the periphery of the lung by vessels that follow the pulmonary veins.
  b The second group begins in the alveoli at the alveolar ducts and drains through the peribronchial lymphatics.
  c The third group anastomoses to connect the perivenous and peribronchial lymphatics.
2 Lymphatics reabsorb extravascular fluid and transport it along with any dust or cellular debris to lymph nodes and systemic veins (Fig. 8-7). Therefore interference with lymphatic flow can decrease the reabsorption of lymph and fluid from the lungs, increasing the possibility of pulmonary edema.

2.6 Lung perfusion*

The lung has a double circulatory system: the pulmonary vascular system and the bronchial vascular system.
1 The *pulmonary vascular system* begins with the pulmonary artery as it leaves the right ventricle and ends with the pulmonary veins that empty into the left atrium. Between these two points the blood has passed through the capillaries surrounding the alveoli, exchanged gases, and returned to the pulmonary veins and the heart.
  a The pulmonary artery system carries the same flow of blood as the systemic arterial system but at approximately *one tenth* the pumping pressure and vascular resistance of the systemic circulation.

*Review Module Four, Units 26 and 33.

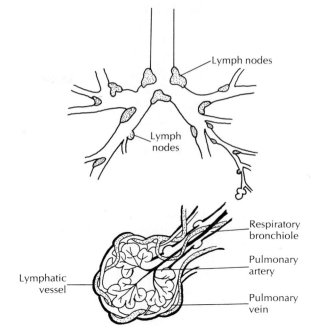

FIGURE 8-7 Lymphatic system of the lung.

  b The large pulmonary arteries are elastic, consisting of smooth muscle fibers bounded by internal and external elastic laminae.
  c The inside diameter of these vessels is small (0.1 to 1.0 mm), and they have thinner walls than arteries of the systemic circulation.
  d Pulmonary arteries branch into arterioles beyond the terminal bronchioles. Arterioles are much smaller than arteries and do not have a muscular coat.
  e Arterioles continue to divide and follow their respective branches of the respiratory tree to the level of the atria. At this point lateral branches are given off to supply the walls of the alveoli and connecting pathways. These arteriole branches further divide to form the capillary network that surrounds the alveoli.
  f Distal to the capillary network, pulmonary venulae arise that empty oxygenated blood into the interlobular septa and finally into four pulmonary veins, which empty into the left atrium of the heart.
2 The *bronchial circulation* provides blood and nutrients to the walls of the tracheobronchial tree and surrounding tissue.
  a The bronchial circulation arises from the aorta, with branches following the airways to the level of the alveoli, where they *anastomose* with vessels of the pulmonary circulation.
  b Alveoli receive their nutrients through the pulmonary circulation.
  c Bronchial veins also anastomose with pulmonary veins and return to the pulmonary artery.
3 Clinically, respiratory therapy personnel should understand the basics of pulmonary circulation because of its major role in determining effective tissue oxygenation.

3.0 FUNCTIONS OF THE LUNG AND CONNECTING AIRWAYS

3.1 General structure and function of the respiratory system

1 The primary function of the respiratory system is to provide oxygen to and remove carbon dioxide from the cells forming the tissues of the body. These cells require approximately 30 times as much surface area for gas diffusion to occur as the entire skin of the body covers. The lungs provide this area, even though they weigh only 1.1 kg (2½ lb) in the adult.

2 In addition to the exchange of gases, the lungs work with the kidneys to regulate the acid-base balance of the blood. This balance is so intricate that most humans will not survive outside a pH range of 6.8 to 7.8, with the normal pH of arterial blood being 7.35 to 7.45.

3 The heart, although it is not an actual part of the respiratory system, is so important to the lung's function that the two are often referred to as the cardiopulmonary system. The heart must pump blood through the vessels of the pulmonary system for continuous gas exchange to occur between the hemoglobin of the red blood cells and the alveoli. This system is so effective that blood is exposed to the alveoli for only 0.75 sec as it passes through the pulmonary capillary surrounding its alveolar unit. The heart then continuously pumps this oxygenated blood to all parts of the body.

4 Specific organs of the respiratory system include the nose, pharynx, larynx, trachea, bronchi, and lungs.

3.2 Structure and function of the nose

1 The nose consists of *external* and *internal* parts. The external portion located on the face is formed by bone and cartilage, which prevent its collapse during a rapid, forced inhalation.

2 The interior of the nose is a hollow cavity that is separated into right and left sides (cavities) by the *nasal septum*. Externally the openings to each nasal cavity are formed by the anterior *nares*. This opening continues to form the posterior nares (conchae) at the back of the nose anterior to the nasopharynx.

3 Internally each nasal cavity is divided into three passageways—the *superior, middle,* and *inferior meatus*—by the projection of *turbinates (conchae)* from the lateral walls of the cavity.

4 The palatine bones form the top and bottom portions of the nose. Sometimes at birth this bone is not completely formed, causing an opening to exist between the mouth and the nasal cavity. This is a condition known as a *cleft palate,* which causes difficulty in swallowing as well as possible aspiration of food into the pulmonary system.

5 The *sinuses* are hollow cavities located above and around the nasal cavity. There are four pairs of sinuses located in the forehead (Fig. 8-8): the frontal *(1)*, ethmoids *(2)*, sphenoids *(3)*, and the maxillary *(4)*. All may be involved in allergic or respiratory infections. Fluid collecting in these sinuses drains through openings *(5)* into the upper nasal passages. If this drainage occurs during sleep, it may be aspirated into the respiratory tract, causing an infection. If the sinuses fail to drain, pressure will build, causing pain in the region of the sinus and, frequently, a headache.

6 The internal surface of the nose is lined with mucosa formed by squamous nonciliated mucous cells with serous and mucous glands. The mucosa is heavily perfused by blood vessels located near the surface. This

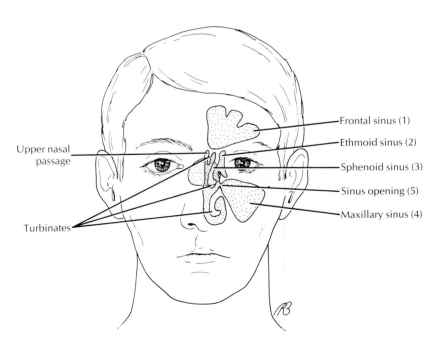

Upper nasal passage

Turbinates

Frontal sinus (1)

Ethmoid sinus (2)

Sphenoid sinus (3)

Sinus opening (5)

Maxillary sinus (4)

F I G U R E 8 - 8 Locations of the sinuses.

combination of moisture and heat from the capillary beds makes the nose an excellent *heat* and *moisture exchanger* (humidifier), as well as a *filter* to trap any small particles carried by gas flow against the curving passageways formed by the turbinates. Inhaled air passing through the nose is warmed by 37° C (98.6° F) at 80% relative humidity. Resistance of air flow through the nose is approximately twice that of gas entering the mouth. For this reason people experiencing dyspnea will breathe through their mouths as well as their noses.

7 Clinically, respiratory care personnel must be aware of the importance the nose plays in the process of breathing. Tubes passed through the nose bypass natural humidification and can cause bleeding from trauma to the capillary beds. Tubes left in the nose longer than 8 hours at a time have a tendency to become encrusted by mucus and cause trauma when they are removed. Free oxygen flowing into the nose from a nasal cannula will dry the mucosa and can cause bleeding and patient discomfort if the rate of flow exceeds 8 L/min or if the oxygen is not properly humidified. Recent data indicate that a humidifier is *not* needed if the oxygen flow rate is not greater than 4 L/min.

3.3 Structure and function of the pharynx

1 The *pharynx* is the upper portion of the throat and begins at the opening of the posterior nares (conchae). The pharynx is a 5-inch-long hollow tube formed by muscle and lined with mucous membrane. It serves as a passageway for food and respiratory gases. For identification it is subdivided into the nasopharynx, oropharynx, and laryngopharynx.

2 The *nasopharynx* is located between the soft palate and the tongue. It is lined with ciliated pseudostratified ep-

ithelium and serves to filter and humidify air. The adenoids (Fig. 8-9, *1*) are located in the posterior portion of the nose at the beginning of the nasopharynx. These tissues frequently become enlarged, along with the tonsils *(2)*, which are located at the level of the tongue at the back of the throat. When this occurs the patient may experience a fever and obstructed breathing. Frequently this condition requires surgical removal of both these tissues. The right and left eustachian tubes (Fig. 8-10, *1*) also open into the nasopharynx. Infection or closure of these tubes will prevent a person from equalizing any pressure that may build in the middle ear. This causes discomfort because the eardrum *(2)* is involved. This situation is most frequently experienced during ascent in an airplane or diving beneath the water. A lack of humidity also causes the custachian tube to block, resulting in an earache, especially if oxygen is being administered.

3 The *oropharynx* is located below the nasopharynx, forming the posterior region of the mouth. The uvula protruding from the roof of the posterior portion of the mouth, and the tonsils can be seen when the mouth is opened. The oropharynx is lined with nonciliated mucosa and extends to the hypopharyngeal (laryngeal) region. Care must be taken when passing a nasotracheal tube, orotracheal tube, or esophageal airway not to lacerate the soft tissue of the oropharynx that covers the cervical vertebrae. The tongue is formed by skeletal muscle covered by mucous membrane. Muscles originating on the skull insert into the tongue, giving it movement. A fold of mucous membrane (frenum) forms the undersurface of the tongue, anchoring it to the floor of the mouth. When the frenum is too short a person is referred to as "tongue-tied." When a patient is unconscious the base of the tongue and soft palate of

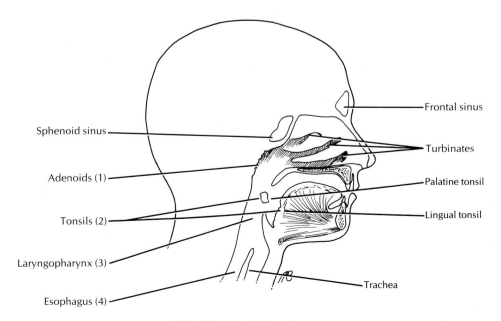

FIGURE 8-9 Nasopharynx.

Sphenoid sinus

Adenoids (1)

Tonsils (2)

Laryngopharynx (3)

Esophagus (4)

Frontal sinus

Turbinates

Palatine tonsil

Lingual tonsil

Trachea

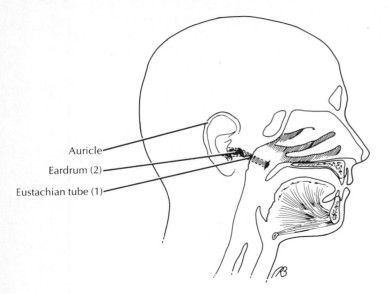

FIGURE 8-10 Communication of the organs of the ear with the nasopharynx.

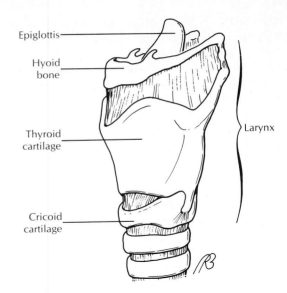

FIGURE 8-11 Skeletal formations of the larynx, thyroid, and cricoid cartilages and the hyoid bone.

the hypopharyngeal region can move into the airway causing a partial or complete obstruction. This can be eliminated by lifting the jaw upward and forward or by inserting an oropharyngeal airway.

4 The *hypopharyngeal region* (laryngopharynx) (see Fig. 8-9, *3*) is located below the oropharynx. It contains the arytenoid cartilages, aryepiglottic folds, and the epiglottis, covering the opening to the larynx and the esophagus *(4)*. Secretions raised from the distal airways during sleep pool in the hypopharyngeal region where they are swallowed or expectorated if the patient awakes.

3.4 Structure and function of the larynx

The *larynx* or voice box is located below the pharynx and at the upper end of the trachea. It connects the pharynx with the trachea and serves as the structural foundation for the vocal cords and upper portion of the trachea.

The larynx consists of nine pieces of cartilage that are joined to form a boxlike structure.

1 Fig. 8-11 identifies the primary skeletal formations of the larynx (voice box): the *thyroid* and *cricoid* cartilages and the *hyoid bone*. These structures can be felt in the anterior portion of the neck.

a The thyroid cartilage is the large triangular-shaped cartilage that forms the Adam's apple. When palpated a V notch can be identified on the midline of the anterior and superior portion of this structure.

b The cricoid cartilage is located along the lower border of the thyroid cartilage. It has the shape of a signet ring and is the only cartilage that *completely encircles* the airway in the upper respiratory tract. The first cartilaginous tracheal ring is attached to the cricoid by a ligament.

c The thyroid cartilage is attached superiorly to the hyoid bone by the thyrohyoid membrane and is at-

tached inferiorly to the cricoid by the cricothyroid membrane.

• The thyrohyoid membrane may be punctured for an emergency airway in a procedure known as a *cricothyroid stab*. This membrane can be identified by placing the head back, extending the neck forward, and by feeling for the transverse indentation that is located about ½ inch below the Adam's apple. The incision is made through the membrane identified as the soft indentation.

2 Two other important structures of the larynx are the epiglottic cartilage and the arytenoid cartilage.

a The *epiglottis* (see Fig. 8-11) is a leaf-shaped cartilaginous structure that is covered with mucous membrane. The upper portion is not attached and moves freely to cover the opening to the esophagus during breathing and the larynx during swallowing. The lateral borders attach to arytenoid cartilages below, causing the posterior portion to be fixed. Current thought is that it is a vestigial structure more related to phonation than the prevention of aspiration. During positive pressure ventilation with a mask, airway pressure *greater than 25 cm H_2O* may cause the esophagus to open in an adult, inflating the stomach with air. This is not only undesirable but potentially dangerous as it may cause the patient to vomit, rupture the stomach, or restrict effective ventilation. Insertion of oropharyngeal airways that are too large also is a problem in that they can push the tip of the epiglottis into the glottis (opening) (see Fig. 20-15).

b The *arytenoid* cartilages are pyramidal shaped and articulate with the posterior portions of the cricoid. The fine muscles of voice control are attached to these two cartilages. The vocal cords attach from the arytenoid cartilage to the thyroid cartilage. Movement of the laryngeal muscles causes a change in the size of the opening between the cords.

3 The *true vocal cords* consist of muscle, ligaments, submucosal soft tissue, and mucous membrane. They stretch between the arytenoid cartilages posteriorly and the thyroid cartilage anteriorly, forming a triangular opening called the *rima glottidis* (glottis). This space is the narrowest point in the adult's airway and consequently experiences the greatest air flow during a forced exhalation.

  a It is this principle of causing a large gas volume—that is, pressure—to be generated by compressing the epigastrium that causes the *Heimlich maneuver* to be effective as an airway clearance mechanism.

  b *False vocal cords,* similar in appearance to the true cords, are located above the laryngeal ventricles. These cords are not as fully developed as the true cords and are nonfunctional for voice production. They do serve as the last protective mechanism for the trachea by contracting and closing the airway against foreign objects. Aspirated food frequently lodges above the larynx or between these cords.

4 The larynx is innervated by the *vagus nerve* located on each side of the neck. Injury to this nerve will cause a loss of speech and protective functions of the larynx.

Respiratory care personnel must be familiar with all structures of the larynx because of its function in guarding the airway and as a route for passing tracheal tubes.

Details regarding tracheal intubation are presented in Module Twenty, Airway Management Techniques.

3.5 Structure and function of the trachea

The *trachea* begins in the neck at the cricoid cartilage (Fig. 8-12, *1*), which maintains patency of the upper portion of the airway. It descends in the midline of the neck to the level of the fifth or sixth vertebra, where it bifurcates into the right *(2)* and left bronchus *(3)*.

1 In the adult the trachea is approximately ⅗ inch in diameter and 4 inches long to the point of bifurcation *(4)*. Internally this bifurcation is called the *carina*.

  • A rough estimate of the inside diameter of an average adult's trachea can be made by looking at the outer diameter of the fifth finger.

2 The walls of the trachea are formed by 20 C-shaped rings of cartilage *(5)* that are closed by cartilage anteriorly and by soft muscle tissue (trachealis) posteriorly.

3 Internally the trachea is lined with a ciliated mucous membrane whose hairlike processes propel mucus and other tracheal contents toward the larynx.

4 Major blood vessels located in close proximity to the trachea are the anterior jugular veins, inferior thyroid veins, innominate artery, internal jugular veins, and the carotid arteries.

3.6 Structure and function of the bronchi

1 The trachea ends at the carina or bifurcation where the upper airway divides into a right (see Fig. 8-12, *2*) and left main stem bronchus *(3)*.

  a The bifurcation *(4)* is positioned slightly to the right

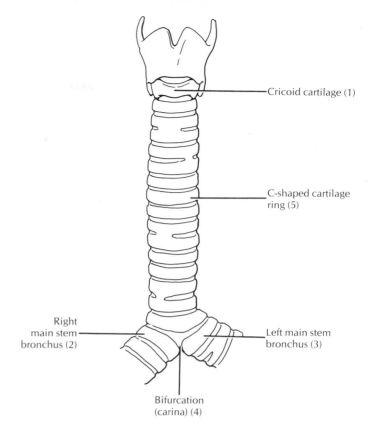

FIGURE 8-12 Gross anatomy of the trachea and main stem bronchi.

so that the angle of the right bronchus is less acute, causing a more direct vertical passage than the left. Clinically this is especially significant because tracheal tubes frequently *are placed into the right bronchus*, instead of being properly positioned 2 to 3 cm (about an inch) above the bifurcation or 4 cm (1½ inches) beyond the glottis.

  b Because of its more direct passage, foreign objects such as aspirated peanuts and pins also are more frequently lodged in the right main stem bronchus than the left.

2 The main stem bronchi divide and subdivide into subsequently smaller bronchi, which serve the lungs and their various lobes and lung segments (Fig. 8-13).

  a The right lung has *three lobes* (see Fig. 8-16, *3-5*). Each lobe is connected with its respective main stem bronchus and segmental bronchi (Fig. 8-13, *1-10*).

  • The right bronchus divides into the *upper lobe bronchus, which subsequently divides into the middle and lower lobe bronchi.*

  • The left lung has *two lobes*, which communicate with their main stem bronchus (see Fig. 8-16, *1* and *2*).

    – The left bronchus divides into *upper* and *lower bronchi*, with the lower part of the upper lobe serving the lingular segment (Fig. 8-13).

  b The upper, middle, and lower lobe bronchi of the

The labels on the figure read: Cricoid cartilage (1); C-shaped cartilage ring (5); Right main stem bronchus (2); Left main stem bronchus (3); Bifurcation (carina) (4).

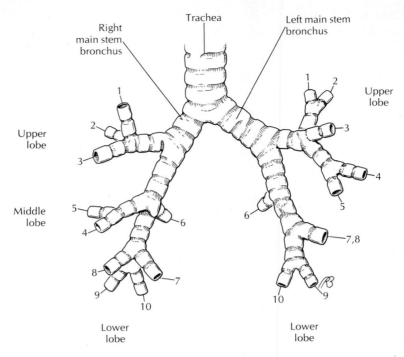

FIGURE 8-13 Tracheobronchial tree.

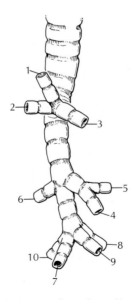

FIGURE 8-14 Position and numbers of segmental bronchi of right lung for anteroposterior and lateral views.

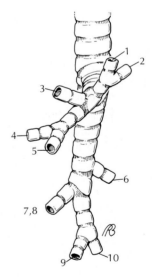

FIGURE 8-15 Position and numbers of segmental bronchi of the left lung for anteroposterior and lateral views.

right lung subdivide to form *10 bronchopulmonary segments in the right lung* and *10 in the left lung* (Fig. 8-13).*

- The position and numbers of segmental bronchi of the right and left lungs for anteroposterior and lateral views are shown in Figs. 8-13 through 8-15. The position of each segment is that of a person *standing*. Table 8-2 identifies and aligns the corresponding bronchi of the right and left lung segments.

3 Topographically the lobes of each lung and their segments can be identified by approximating the location of underlying lobes to external anatomy.

4 Fig. 8-16 represents a view of the anterior thorax.

a The upper lobe of the left lung *(1)* and the lower lobe of the left lung *(2)* can be approximated by comparing their location with the nipple and lower boundaries of the ribs. The right lung with its three lobes, upper *(3)*, middle *(4)*, and lower *(5)*, can be identified using the same topographic landmarks.

b Fig. 8-17 represents a posterior view of the thorax. In this position only the upper and lower lobes of both the right *(1)* and left *(2)* lungs can be seen.

c Fig. 8-18 shows a lateral view of the right thorax. In this position the upper *(1)*, middle *(2)*, and lower *(3)* lobes of the right lung can be seen.

d Fig. 8-19 shows a lateral view of the left thorax. In this position both the upper *(1)* and lower *(2)* lobes of the left lung can be seen.

5 Clinically it is extremely important that the clinician learn the bronchopulmonary segments by *number* and by *location*. This understanding will be applied to identification of mucus and/or disease in specific locations and for positioning the patient to achieve pulmonary drainage.

a A practical method of visualizing internal lung segment to external anatomy is to use water-soluble pens to *locate* and *draw* the position of the lobes of

---

*Depending on the classification system, some anatomists believe the left lung has eight segments.

TABLE 8-2 Names and corresponding numbers of segments

Right lung segment and bronchus	Left lung segment and bronchus
Upper lobe	*Upper lobe*
1. Apical	1. Apical
2. Posterior	2. Posterior
3. Anterior	3. Anterior
Middle lobe	*Lingula*
4. Lateral	4. Superior
5. Medial	5. Inferior
Lower lobe	*Lower lobe*
6. Superior	6. Superior
7. Medial basal	7/8. Anteromedial
8. Anterior basal	
9. Lateral basal	9. Lateral basal
10. Posterior basal	10. Posterior basal

The divisions of the right and left lungs are very similar although some texts show the left lung to have eight segments. In this case the apical-posterior is numbered 1 and the anteromedial segment is numbered 6.

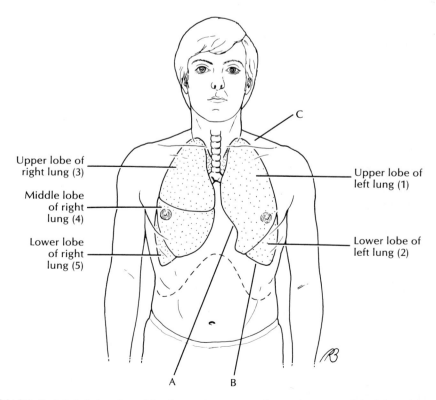

Upper lobe of right lung (3)

Middle lobe of right lung (4)

Lower lobe of right lung (5)

Upper lobe of left lung (1)

Lower lobe of left lung (2)

C

A   B

FIGURE 8-16 Anterior view of the thorax shows approximate placement of the lobes of the lung.

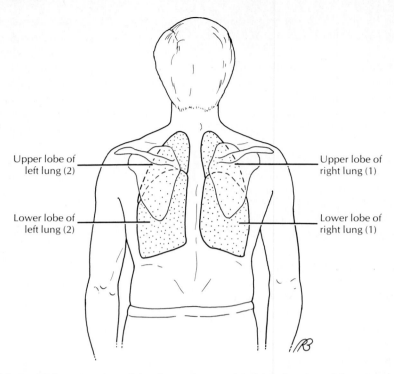

Upper lobe of left lung (2)

Lower lobe of left lung (2)

Upper lobe of right lung (1)

Lower lobe of right lung (1)

FIGURE 8-17 Posterior view of the thorax shows approximate location of the upper and lower lobes of the right and left lungs.

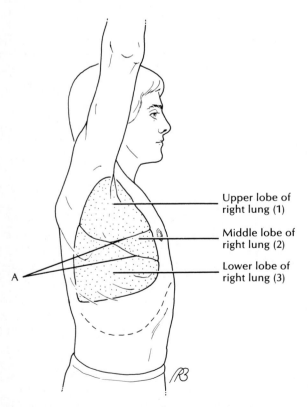

Upper lobe of right lung (1)

Middle lobe of right lung (2)

Lower lobe of right lung (3)

A

FIGURE 8-18 Lateral view of the right thorax shows the approximate location of the upper, middle, and lower lobes of the right lung.

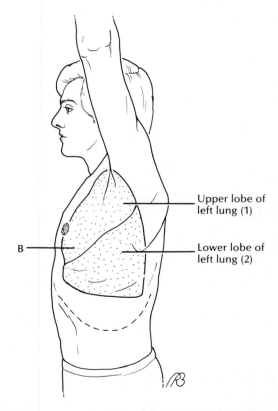

Upper lobe of left lung (1)

Lower lobe of left lung (2)

B

FIGURE 8-19 Lateral view of the left thorax shows the approximate location of the upper and lower lobes of the left lung.

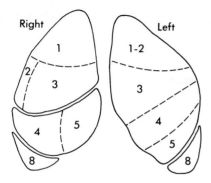

FIGURE 8-20 Bronchopulmonary segments identified by number and location for anterior view of right and left lungs. (From Scanlan CL, Spearman CB, and Sheldon RL: Egan's fundamentals of respiratory care, ed 5, St Louis, 1990, The CV Mosby Co.)

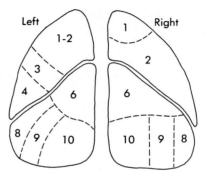

FIGURE 8-21 Bronchopulmonary segments identified by number and location for posterior view of right and left lungs. (From Scanlan CL, Spearman, CB, and Sheldon RL: Egan's fundamentals of respiratory care, ed 5, St Louis, 1990, The CV Mosby Co.)

each lung on another person: Have the person in standing, sitting, and various recumbent positions, and notice corresponding changes in each lobe.

   b Using the same water-soluble pens, the clinician locates and draws in the segments of each lobe, placing his or her partner in the positions listed in *5a* and noticing changes in lung segments. See also Figs. 8-20 through 8-22.

The reader is encouraged to memorize lung segments relative to topographic landmarks and various body positions.

3.7 Structure and function of the alveoli and lung surface

The microscopic structure of alveoli is presented in Unit 2.1 of this module.

1 Conceptually, alveoli are the terminal units of the pharynx, trachea, bronchi, and bronchioles, which form the continuous air passages used for ventilation (that is, the process of gas flowing into and out of the lungs).

2 The periphery of the lungs is formed by the walls of alveoli clusters. Topographically, as detailed in Module Four, the lungs appear as cone-shaped organs that completely fill the thoracic cavity.

3 The medial (interior middle) surface of each lung has cavities to hold the mediastinal structures and the heart (Fig. 8-16, *A*).

   • Because of the position of the heart, a greater portion of the left lung is involved than the right.

4 The main stem bronchi and pulmonary blood vessels form the *root* of the lung. These structures enter the lung through a slit in the medial surface of the lung known as the *hilum.*

5 The bottom portion of the lung toward the diaphragm is the *base* and the upper portion, toward the neck, the *apex* of the lungs (Fig. 8-16, *B* and *C*).

6 The lungs are subdivided into lobes by fissures (Figs. 8-18 and 9-19, *A* and *B*).

   a The right lung has two fissures dividing the lung into *upper, middle,* and *lower* lobes with related bronchi (Fig. 8-18, *A*).

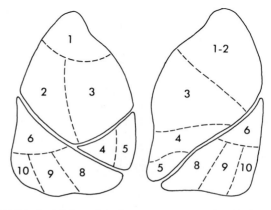

·FIGURE 8-22 Bronchopulmonary segments identified by number and location for lateral view of right and left lungs. (From Scanlan CL, Spearman CB, and Sheldon RL: Egan's fundamentals of respiratory care, ed 5, St Louis, 1990, The CV Mosby Co.)

   b The left lung has one fissure dividing the lung into two lobes (Fig. 8-19, *B*).

      • Each lobe of both lungs further subdivides into segments with related bronchi.

7 The right lung has *10* segments. The left lung has *10* segments.

8 The entire *outer surface of the lung* is wrapped in a covering known as the *visceral pleura.* It consists of a thin layer of connective tissue covered by a single layer of mesothelial cells.

9 The entire *inner surface of the thorax* also is covered with a separate lining known as the *parietal pleura.* These two individual linings, one on the surface of the lung and the other on the inner chest wall, are continuous but form a potential space known as the *intrapleural space.* An actual space does not exist because air is blocked from the inner thorax by the skin and tissues covering the external chest wall. A very thin film of serous fluid fills the intrapleural space and serves to lubricate the surface of the pleurae, allowing them to move freely during breathing.

a The pleurae are richly endowed with a network of blood vessels and lymphatics and numerous nerve endings. For this reason injury to or inflammation of the pleurae is extremely painful and can inhibit effective ventilation because of the patient splinting against chest movement.

b Air or fluids such as blood in the intrapleural space will cause the lung to collapse in the area of contact. A large volume of air in this space can cause the entire lung to collapse (pneumothorax).

c The *parietal* pleura can be easily stripped away from the chest wall during a specific surgical procedure called a "pleurectomy." The visceral pleura, however, is more closely connected to the lung surface and cannot be easily removed.

3.8 Structure and function of the thorax*

1 The thorax (chest) is the region of the body extending from the root of the neck, C-7 vertebra, to the diaphragm, separating the chest from the abdominal cavity.

a Externally the thorax is formed by the sternum, ribs, and vertebrae (Module Four, Units 9.0 and 10.0) and by the tissue covering these structures.

b Internally the thorax is subdivided by partitions of pleurae into the pleural, pericardial, and mediastinal cavities (divisions).

2 The *pleural cavity* is only a potential space formed by the parietal and visceral pleurae. Each of these pleurae is continuous, forming the right and left pleurae, each entirely separate from the other. Clinically this fact is very important, because whenever a hole develops in one lung or chest wall, it does not allow air to enter the other side. The pleural cavity formed by the surrounding pleurae is filled by the lungs.

3 The *pericardial cavity* is the area occupied by the heart and its sac.

4 The *mediastinal cavity* is that part of the thorax between the lungs. It is bordered on either side by the parietal pleura and the lungs, anteriorly by the sternum, posteriorly by the ribs, superiorly by the thoracic inlet, and inferiorly by the diaphragm. It contains the heart and thoracic aorta and its branches; vena cavae; azygos and innominate vein; thoracic duct; lymph nodes; esophagus; trachea; thymus; and the vagus, phrenic, intercostal, and sympathetic nerves. It is important to recognize the viscera of the mediastinum because of the influence that breathing, especially positive pressure ventilation, has on these structures. For example, an alteration in the relative volume of the lungs causes a shift in the mediastinum from its normal midline position.

5 The function of the thorax is to protect the viscera and to work as a bellows, causing air to move in and out of the lungs. Specifics of chest mechanics are presented in subsequent units on physiology.

One of the most difficult aspects of learning respiratory care is the application of physical and chemical principles to the processes that maintain homeostasis in the human organism. These processes are studied as the science of human physiology. The following units present components of physics and chemistry with applications to ventilation and arterial blood gases. Application of these components can assist the reader in understanding subsequent clinical situations and treatment of the patient.

4.0 GAS PRESSURE, FLOW, AND VOLUME
4.1 States of matter

Matter is anything that occupies space and has weight. In most instances matter can be detected by the use of one's senses.

The three states of matter are solid, liquid, and gas.

1 A *solid* has a definite shape and volume, resists compression, and may have any number of free surfaces exposed to the air. On the molecular level molecules of a solid are held in fixed positions with movement limited to a rapid atomic vibration about a fixed point.

2 *Liquids* standing alone have no definite shape. When placed in a container, liquids will assume the shape of the container. On the molecular level molecules move aimlessly throughout the boundaries of the liquid by slipping and sliding over, under, and around each other. Molecules in a liquid actually move from one point to another as can be demonstrated by putting a drop of ink into a glass of water and watching it spread throughout the glass. As molecules in a liquid change position in the liquid, they also spin about a fixed imaginary axis (line) passing through the molecule itself much like a top spins on its point.

3 *Gases*, like liquids, have no definite shape when standing alone and also assume the shape of a container. They have no free surfaces, expand to fill the inside volume of the container, and are easily compressed. Most pure gases cannot be seen or smelled unless colored or scented by a chemical agent.

4.2 Changes in states of matter

1 Matter does not always appear in the same state. For example, a liquid or a gas may be frozen and become a solid. A liquid can be heated and become a vapor (gas). A vapor containing water may be cooled and form small droplets called *condensate*. Condensate in the air forms cloud formations or fog. On the ground, condensate is deposited as dew when the air temperature is above freezing and as frost when the temperature is below freezing.

2 The application or removal of heat can cause the molecules of matter to speed up or slow down.

a *Boiling* of a liquid occurs when the water vapor pressure at the surface of a liquid becomes greater than the atmospheric pressure above the liquid. This causes molecules to leave the surface of the liquid as

---

*Review specific muscles of the thorax and of respiration in Module Four, Units 15.0 and 16.0.

a vapor. The tendency of the molecules to escape is accelerated as the heat is increased, causing the bubbling known as boiling.

b Gas containing water molecules, when cooled, will reach its *dewpoint*, causing the vapor molecules to slow down and combine as *condensate*. This is seen as one exhales on a cold day or as water collects in a ventilator circuit. Water as a vapor cannot be seen.

4.3 The kinetic molecular theory

In 1738 Daniel Bernoulli, a Swiss scientist, explained the phenomenon of molecular movement by the *kinetic molecular theory*.

1 Gases are composed of molecules, which are in constant motion. This is demonstrated by the fact that gases mix or penetrate into every part of a containing vessel.

2 Collisions of the molecules with each other and with the walls of the vessel are frequent. This can be demonstrated by observing that diffusion of a gas into a vacuum is much more rapid than diffusion into a space that is already occupied by a gas; intermolecular collisions retard diffusion in the latter case.

3 Under ordinary conditions the molecules of a gas are so far apart that their mass is negligible; a gas sample is virtually empty space. This property is manifested by the compressibility of gases. One *mole* of any gas occupies 22.4 L at standard temperature and pressure. A mole is a standard measure containing *Avogadro's number* (6.023×10^{23}) of molecules, atoms, or ions.

4 Molecules of gas move in all directions with an average velocity determined by temperature. Individual molecules may possess a velocity that differs markedly from the average. This property is illustrated by the fact that water vapor will remain in a *stable (dynamic) equilibrium* with liquid water in a closed vessel, the water vapor pressure being dependent on temperature alone. In this situation, as many molecules are reentering the liquid as are leaving it. In a mixture of different gases the average kinetic energy of the molecules of all gases will be equal. Molecules with a low mass will travel at higher velocities than molecules with a high mass. At room temperature a hydrogen molecule travels with an average velocity of 1 mile per second! On the average, however, it travels only 2 millionths of a centimeter between collisions with other molecules!

5 Molecular collisions are prefectly elastic. Energy transfers may take place between molecules, but no energy is lost by conversion to heat, light, sound, or the like. This is demonstrated by the observation that the temperature of the gas is constant on standing and by the fact that the molecules do not settle out to the bottom of the container, even if left indefinitely. To understand this theory one must assume that molecules neither attract nor repel each other.

a In a container, molecules of gas travel at rapid rates

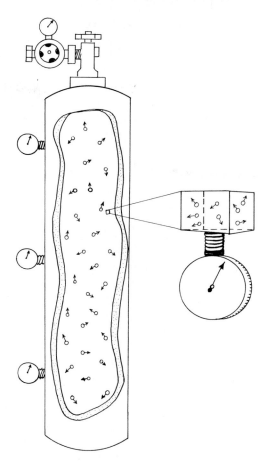

FIGURE 8-23 Measurement of the rebounding of gas molecules (pressure) in a closed container.

and constantly collide with each other and with the walls of the vessel.

b The collisions are elastic, causing the molecules to rebound, striking other molecules. This rapid movement causes gas molecules to move randomly throughout a container.

c In the atmosphere, relatively large spaces exist between gas molecules. When drawn into a container (compressed) the existing space between the molecules is reduced, and the molecules rebound against each other more frequently.

d This rebounding can be measured by inserting a gauge through the walls of the container at *any* point (Fig. 8-23). This gauge will measure the force caused by the rebounding gas molecules per square inch of exposed surface, hence the term "pounds per square inch of pressure."

6 If the volume and temperature of gases in the container are constant and the size of the container is decreased, the molecules will be forced closer together, and the number of molecules striking each other and the wall will increase, causing the recorded pressure to increase. This phenomenon was described by Robert Boyle in 1660 as one of the gas laws. It is based on the relationship that exists between pressure and volume.

A detailed description of the gas laws is presented later in this module.

4.4 Pressure

The following facts relate to understanding the concept of pressure and its applications to physiology. All these terms can be used to express pressure and should be understood in order to convert one value to another.

1 Gases have *mass* and therefore *weight* as caused by the pull of gravity. For example, 1 quart of air weighs approximately 1.3 g.

2 Because air has weight, it exerts a force on a surface called *pressure*.

   Pressure is defined in terms of force per unit area. The metric units for pressure are *newtons per square meter* or *dynes per square centimeter*. The British units are pounds per square inch (PSI) or pounds per square inch gauge (PSIG), the standard most frequently used to express pressure in a gas cylinder.

   a Atmospheric pressure is equal to 14.7 PSI at sea level. This pressure decreases as one ascends above sea level.

   b Pressure can also be expressed directly in *atmospheres* (atm), wherein the actual pressure is expressed as a fraction or multiple of 1 atm.

   c Pressure may also be expressed in terms of millimeters of mercury *(mm Hg)* or *torr* (a unit named after Torricelli who first measured atmospheric pressure). Torr may be used in physiology in lieu of mm Hg. "Centimeter of water" (cm H_2O) is another term used to describe smaller units where mm Hg would not be reflected as accurately.

   d Pressure is also expressed as kPa (kilopascals); 1 kPa = 10.2 cm H_2O or 7.5 mm Hg.

3 Mercury is 13.6 times as dense as water; therefore atmospheric pressure in cm H_2O equals 760 mm Hg × 1.36 cm H_2O = 1033.6 cm H_2O. Thus a column of water 1033.6 cm (or 33.9 feet) high can be supported by the atmosphere.

4 Pressure changes can occur to a human as a result of diving below the surface of the water, causing pressure to *increase 1 atm for every 33.9 feet descent*. At a depth of 34 feet the pressure on the body is atmospheric pressure + 1 atm (depth) or *twice* that felt on the surface of the water.

5 Pressure *decreases* as one ascends in altitude above sea level. This decrease in pressure means that the gas molecules comprising the atmosphere are further apart, hence, less molecules per given cubic liter of gas as compared to sea level.

6 It is important to note that even though there are fewer molecules per given cubic liter of air, the concentration of the gases is the same at an altitude of approximately 70,000 feet as it is at sea level. Table 8-3 summarizes changes in pressure that occur with ascent above sea level.

7 Clinically it is important that respiratory care personnel understand the effect of altitude on breathing. For ex-

TABLE 8-3 Altitude pressure table

Altitude	Pressure (mm Hg/PSI)	Ratio (in atm)
Sea level	760-14.7	1
5,000 ft	633-12.2	
10,000 ft	522-10.1	
15,000 ft	429-8.3	
18,000 ft	380-6.7	$\frac{1}{2}$
20,000 ft	350-6.7	
25,000 ft	282-5.5	
27,000 ft	252-4.9	$\frac{1}{3}$
30,000 ft	226-4.4	
33,000 ft	196-3.8	
35,000 ft	179-3.5	$\frac{1}{4}$
40,000 ft	141-2.7	

ample, a patient who rides in a commercial airliner is exposed to an altitude equivalent to 10,000 feet or a partial pressure of 522 mm Hg, as compared to 760 mm Hg at sea level. This could cause acute hypoxia in patients who are already borderline hypoxemic at sea level. Again, the cause of hypoxia is *not* a decrease in oxygen concentration but in the number of molecules of oxygen available in each breath.

8 Pressure also changes as a result of storm (low pressure) activity. Clear weather is associated with an increase in the pressure of air. Bad weather is associated with a decrease in air pressure. Hospitals frequently note an increase or decrease in the number of pulmonary patients admitted related to changes in the weather, which cause changes in the barometric pressure. These weather highs and lows affect gas molecules the same as ascent or descent in an airplane, by altering the number of oxygen molecules that are present in a given volume of inhaled air.

9 The pressure, or volume of air, can be measured using a device called a *barometer*.

   a Barometers simply measure the *weight* of the air extending upward from the location of the barometer, whether it be at sea level or on a mountain, extending to the upper limits of the atmosphere called the *exosphere*, some 540 miles high.

   • For example, a simple mercurial barometer measures the weight of a column of air 1 inch on each side, extending from the surface of the mercury in the reservoir of the barometer all the way to the exosphere.

   b The weight (pressure) of the atmosphere pushes down on the reservoir of mercury and forces mercury up a calibrated glass tube.

   c The height that the mercury is forced up into the tube depends on the weight of the air pressing down on the reservoir and is expressed as inches of mercury or mm Hg.

   • If this column of air were placed on a scale at sea level, it would take 14.7 lb to balance it (Fig. 8-24), or it would push mercury up a column to a height of 760 mm.

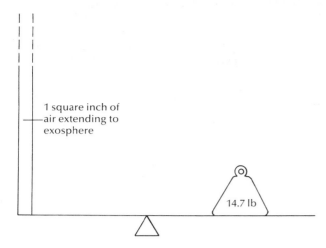

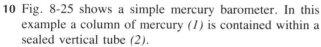

FIGURE 8-24 At sea level a column of air extending through the atmosphere would weight 14.7 lb.

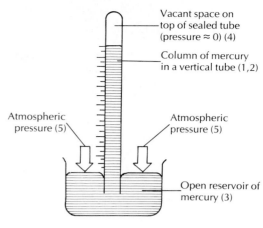

FIGURE 8-25 Mercury barometer.

10 Fig. 8-25 shows a simple mercury barometer. In this example a column of mercury *(1)* is contained within a sealed vertical tube *(2)*.

a This mercury is in communication with more mercury held in an open reservoir *(3)*.

b The vacant space in the uppermost portion of the sealed tube *(4)* contains only mercury vapor, and because mercury for all practical purposes does not vaporize at room temperature, the gas pressure in this space is virtually zero.

c The surface of the mercury in the open reservoir, however, is exposed to the atmosphere *(5)*, and the imbalance between the pressures bearing on the mercury in the tube and that in the exposed reservoir supports the weight of the mercury column within the sealed tube.

d An increase in the ambient atmospheric pressure will create more weight on the surface of the mercury in the reservoir *(5)*, which will cause the mercury column in the tube to rise and the level in the reservoir outside the tube to fall.

e On the other hand, a reduction in the ambient atmospheric pressure no longer supports the weight of the mercury in the tube. Some of the mercury will fall out of the sealed tube and back into the reservoir.

• This summarizes the operation principle of a barometer, wherein variations in the height of a mercury column in response to changes in atmospheric pressure are read directly from a linear scale.

11 Water could be substituted for mercury as the fluid in the construction of a crude barometer, but since mercury is 13.6 times as heavy as an equal volume of water, the height of a water column that could be supported by normal atmospheric pressure is 760 mm × 13.6 = 10,336 mm H_2O, or 33.9 feet in height. This size device could not be used indoors; hence smaller devices with mercurial columns are used when measuring barometric pressure. The *centimeter of water* is a

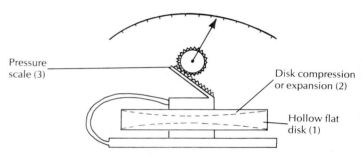

FIGURE 8-26 Aneroid pressure manometer.

convenient unit of pressure, however, when dealing with the characteristically *small* variations in pressure commonly encountered by the respiratory physiologist.

12 The conversion from millimeters of mercury to centimeters of water is based on the differences of the relative densities of the two fluids:

1 mm Hg = (13.6 mm H_2O) × (1 cm/10 mm) = 1.36 H_2O

EXAMPLE: 55 mm Hg = 55 × 1.36 or 74.8 cm H_2O

13 Pressure measurements can also be taken using an *aneroid* type of device such as the one shown in Fig. 8-26.

a Aneroid pressure manometers are activated by atmospheric pressure squeezing a hollow, flat disk *(1)* that has had most of its air removed.

• Compression or expansion of the disk in response to atmospheric pressure changes *(2)* moves a geared level connected to a needle that points to a pressure reading on a scale calibrated in mm Hg or cm H_2O *(3)*.

b These mechanical pressure sensors are used in aneroid barometers, blood pressure cuffs, and in ventilators to record cycling pressures.

14 Whenever a pressure reading is taken, that reading must relate to some point of reference. In the case of a

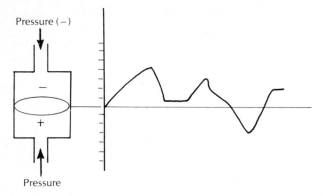

Pressure (–)

–

+

Pressure

FIGURE 8-27 Pressure reading as measured by a bidirectional differential pressure transducer.

mercury barometer reading, the atmospheric pressure that one measures is opposed by a virtual vacuum, because the mercury vapor present in the sealed end of the tube exerts negligible pressure. The pressure that is read therefore will be an *absolute pressure* (that is, the observed pressure compared with zero pressure).

15 Electronically differential pressures (difference in pressure between two points) can be measured with a device called a *bidirectional differential pressure transducer*. This device utilizes a single pressure-sensing element (diaphragm) sealed in a chamber.

a Each side of the diaphragm is exposed to a gas pressure. The diaphragm is pushed away from the side with the greatest pressure.

b This movement creates an electrical signal that is boosted by a preamplifier unit and transmits it to a CRT (cathode ray tube) scope or graph paper for a recording.

c This recording appears as an upward or downward movement of an *x-y* coordinate, as illustrated by Fig. 8-27, depending on the direction of the signal at the transducer.

d A strain gauge is a variation to the differential pressure transducer. It utilizes a wire resistor that becomes thinner when it is stretched by pressure. The stretched wire offers more electrical resistance compared to when it was not stretched. This difference is amplified and displayed on a meter as pressure.

4.5 Volume

Volume measurements are frequently used by respiratory therapy personnel to express the amount of gas in the lungs during various phases of breathing.

These lung volumes are expressed in liters or fractions of a liter. Medications and other solutions also must be measured to specific amounts, by means of units of volume.

1 The *liter* is the *standard* unit of volume used in the metric system. A liter is defined as the volume occupied by 1 kg of water at its point of maximum density (4° C).

$$1 \text{ L} = 10^3 \text{ ml} = 1000 \text{ ml or } 10 \times 10 \times 10 \text{ ml}$$

a Although 1 ml is slightly larger than a cubic centimeter (1.000028 cc to 1000 cc), clinically 1 ml can be equated to 1 cc.

b To convert milliliters to equivalents of a liter, use the following formula:

$$\frac{\text{ml}}{1000 \text{ ml}}$$

Or move the decimal three places to the left.
• For example, 800.0 ml = 0.800 or 0.8 L.
• With this formula the following volumetric conversions may be completed:

$$1 \text{ L} = 1000 \text{ ml}$$
$$5000 \text{ ml} = 5.0 \text{ L}$$
$$526 \text{ ml} = 0.526 \text{ L}$$
$$25 \text{ ml} = 0.025 \text{ L}$$

2 Volume therefore can be defined as the space occupied or displaced by matter, expressed in cubic units. The metric system uses cubic meters, cubic centimeters, or liters. Volume units in the British system are cubic inches, cubic feet, and gallons or quarts. For purposes of comparison, it is useful to remember that a liter is about equal to a quart: 1 L = 1.06 quarts. In subsequent units, additional opportunity will be given for the reader to work with volume conversions.

3 Volumes can be measured simply by:

a Filling a container with a liquid and then measuring the volume of that liquid by pouring it out into a measuring container (volumetric displacement).

b Measuring the change in the size of a movable container after a volume has been inserted.

c Measuring the movement (flow) of a known value for a given period of time (Volume × Time = Total volume after a second of flow, a minute of flow, etc.).

• For example, air moving at a rate of 50 ml/sec for 60 sec will result in a *minute volume* of 3000 ml. This volume determination is frequently used by respiratory care personnel to describe the breathing ability of a patient.

4 This type of reasoning can be used to calculate gas flow in and out of the lungs. When determining gas flow of the lungs, volumes are best calculated by use of *exhaled* volumes, since they are a more accurate indicator of air that was actually contained within the lung. In pulmonary function testing, mechanical and electronic devices are used to measure gas volumes and flows of the lungs.

4.6 Temperature

1 Temperature is defined as the extent to which heat is present in a system.

2 The *Celsius or centrigrade* temperature scale is based on empirically determined phenomena (i.e., the freezing [0° C] and boiling [100° C] points of water).

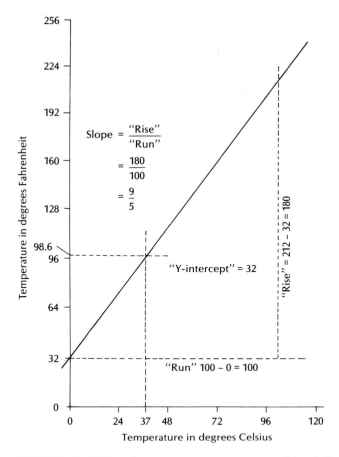

FIGURE 8-28 Coordinate system used to compare Fahrenheit and Celsius temperature systems.

3 A rectangular coordinate system can be used to compare the Fahrenheit and Celsius temperature systems (Fig. 8-28).

4 When points of identical temperature (such as the boiling point and freezing point of water, and normal body temperature) are plotted on this system, a straight line is generated. This line represents the formula:

$$F = \tfrac{9}{5} + 32$$

This formula can be used to convert *Celsius* temperature readings to their corresponding readings on the *Fahrenheit* temperature scale. Algebraic rearrangement yields:

$$C = \tfrac{5}{9} \times (F - 32)$$

which can be used to convert Fahrenheit to *Celsius* temperature readings.

5 It must be noted that heat and temperature are *not* the same.

Heat is a primary entity; it is related to the *number of molecules* (the size of the system), as well as the motion of the molecules. For example, a bathtub full of warm water possesses more heat than a teacup of scalding hot water. In calculations involving the gas laws, temperature *must* be expressed in absolute degrees.

6 *Absolute temperature* = Celsius or centigrade temperature + 273.
 a The value 273 is derived from the experiment that demonstrates when 273 ml of gas at 0° is warmed to 1°, its volume will increase by 1 ml to 274 ml.
  • In other words, a volume of gas at 0° increases 1/273 of its volume for each degree increase in the Celsius or centigrade scale and vice versa for cooling.
   – If cooling is continued from 0° to −273°, the gas should have *no* volume at −273°. This is known as *absolute zero* on the *Kelvin temperature scale* or K. At this theoretical temperature, *all molecular motion ceases,* and all known elements become solids.
 b The concept of gas volumes increasing or decreasing with temperatures is important to accurately calculate lung volumes that have been warmed or cooled.
7 By applying these formulas the following temperature conversions are easily made:
 a Convert Celsius temperature of 78.5° to Fahrenheit using the formula:

$$F = \tfrac{9}{5} C + 32$$

$$78.5° C = 273.3° F$$

 b Convert a Fahrenheit temperature of 50° to Celsius using the formula:

$$C = \tfrac{5}{9} (F - 32)$$

$$50° F = 10° C$$

 c Convert 25° C to Kelvin using the formula:

$$K = C + 273$$

$$25° C = 298° K$$

4.7 Determining the behavior of gases

The behavior of gases under changing conditions of volume, pressure, and temperature can be demonstrated and explained by application of a series of physical laws that deal with gases. These laws include:
1 Boyle's law: relationship of volume to pressure.
2 Bernoulli's kinetic gas theory: interrelationship of gases to pressure.
3 Charles' law: relationship of volume to temperature.
4 Gay-Lussac's law: relationship of pressure to temperature.
5 Dalton's law: the total pressure of a mixture of gases.
6 Graham's law: the diffusion of gases.
7 Henry's law: dissolving gases into solution.

4.8 Boyle's law

Robert Boyle first observed the variability of pressure and volume at a constant temperature. He found that pressure and volume (V) were inversely proportional. This means that as one value is increased, the other value decreases, or the *volume* of a gas varies inversely with the pressure if the temperature remains constant (Fig. 8-29).

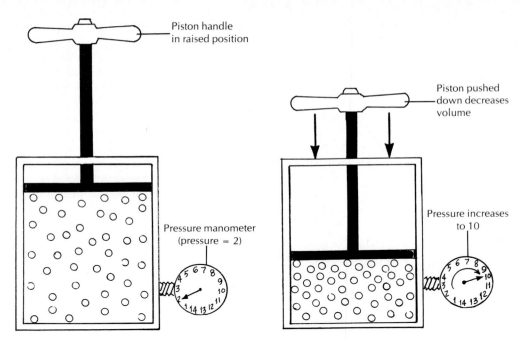

FIGURE 8-29 Illustration of Boyle's law. Volume of a gas varies inversely with the pressure if the temperature remains constant.

1 Mathematically this can be shown as:

$$P \approx \frac{1}{V}$$

a To render the proportion as an equation, one needs only to insert the appropriate constant, K_b:

$$P = \frac{K_b}{V}$$

or

$$PV = K_b$$

b It may be alternately stated:

$$P_1V_1 = P_2V_2$$

4.9 The kinetic gas theory

The kinetic-molecular theory clarifies Boyle's law on the molecular level. This can be illustrated by a piston within a cylinder wherein *temperature* is kept *constant* (Fig. 8-29).

1 If the volume of the cylinder is decreased, the area exposed to molecular collisions will be decreased, because the force exerted per molecule per collision is constant if the temperature is the same. Therefore the force per area (PSI) must increase.

2 The compressibility of gases within a ventilator and its tubing system provides a clinical example of Boyle's law. As the tubing system is cyclically pressurized and depressurized during each breathing cycle, gases are distributed and compressed within the ventilator tubing system and the humidifier.

• This compressed volume is known as the *ventilator compliance* (C_V) (that is, the volume of air compressed, divided by cycling pressure as reflected on the manometer on the panel of the ventilator). For example, for the Bennett MA-1 ventilator, $C_V = 3$ ml/cm H_2O. This means that for every centimeter of water pressure increment observed during the inflation phase, 3 ml of gas will be absorbed by the tubing system because of compression.

3 *Valsalva's maneuver* is a physiologic example of Boyle's law. Valsalva's maneuver can be easily performed by taking a deep breath and attempting to breathe out against a closed glottis. During this maneuver thoracic gas volume is compressed and intrapulmonary pressure increases as one strains to exhale against the closed glottis. This increase in intrathoracic pressure is transmitted from the lungs to the vessels and soft tissue surrounding the lungs, causing it to be compressed. Compression of the superior/inferior vena cavae *reduces blood flow* to the heart and, ultimately, cardiac output.

• The reader is encouraged to perform a Valsalva's maneuver.

   – Note the rate and strength of your pulse; also note the light-headed feeling and feeling of increased thoracic pressure.

4.10 Charles' law

Charles examined the variability between volume (V) and temperature (T) at *constant pressure* (K_C). He found that volume and temperature were *directly* related so that the expansion of a gas is directly proportional to the rise in temperature (absolute) if the pressure remains constant; or stated mathematically:

$$V \simeq T$$

or

$$V \simeq K_C \times T$$

which may be alternately stated:

$$\frac{V_1}{T_1} = \frac{V_2}{V_1 T_2 = V_2 T_1}$$

Charles' law was derived based on experience and, like Boyle's law, is merely descriptive. To understand the law one must refer to the kinetic-molecular theory.

1 Consider a frictionless piston within a cylinder (Fig. 8-30). The piston *(1)* is free to move within its cylinder. If the gas is heated *(2)*, the velocity of gas molecules will increase *(3)*, and the force they exert on the piston per collision will rise. The piston will rise *(4)*, affording more area for increased molecular collisions. When the area exposed to collisions enlarges in direct proportion to the increase in molecular velocity, the position of the piston will stabilize, and the volume will be observed to have increased. There is no increase in pressure because the volume of the cylinder increased as a result of the increased molecular activity.

2 This same type of thermal expansion occurs in inspired gases and provides a clinical demonstration of Charles' law. As gases are drawn into the respiratory system by the patient, they are warmed and expanded.

3 In addition, another gas (water vapor) is added by the body's humidifier. Therefore, when one exhales into a container such as a spirometer that is maintained at a temperature lower than body temperature, the expired volume, which was expanded by heat and the addition of water vapor, contracts as it cools and water vapor "rains out" (condenses).

• This concept is especially important when calculating a patient's exhaled tidal volume.

• For this reason may spirometers correct gas volumes to standard temperature and pressure (STP).

4.11 Gay-Lussac's law

Gay-Lussac investigated the variability between pressure (P) and temperature (T) at *constant volume* (K_G) and found that they were *directly* related so that the pressure of a gas is directly proportional to the absolute temperature if the volume remains constant; or stated mathematically:

$$P \simeq T$$

or, in equation form:

$$P = K_G \times T$$

This law may be stated in the following form also:

$$\frac{P_1}{T_1} = \frac{P_2}{T_2} \left(= \frac{P_3}{T_3} = -- = K_G \right)$$

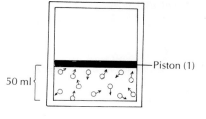

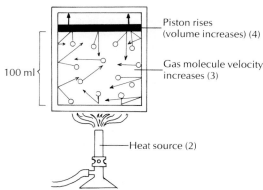

FIGURE 8-30 Illustration of Charles' law. Volume increases proportionately to temperature increases when pressure remains constant.

Like Boyle's and Charles' laws, Gay-Lussac's law is merely descriptive of what happens to pressure as the temperature of a gas is raised or lowered.

1 An example is a closed vessel, such as a cylinder, containing a gas. If the vessel is heated, the velocity and kinetic energy of the molecules will increase, causing an increase in the force of molecular collision.

a Because the velocity of the molecules increases, the *number* of collisions will increase, as well as the force exerted by the molecules per collision.

• This will be reflected on a pressure gauge as an increase in pressure (Fig. 8-31).

b Gay-Lussac's law is demonstrated clinically by the variations in pressure observed in cylinder gas secondary to changes in ambient temperature. Consequently cylinders are usually stored in a cool place.

• It has been estimated that pressure in a gas cylinder will increase *5 PSI* for every *1°* increase in Fahrenheit temperature at which a cylinder is filled (70° F).

– This is an important consideration when storing gases or calculating how long a cylinder will last in abnormal temperatures.

4.12 The combined gas law

1 In certain clinical situations the interplay of pressure, volume, and temperature on a patient's ventilation must be considered by applying the *combined gas laws* of Boyle and Charles, which are expressed as:

$$\frac{PV}{T} = K$$

where K is a constant that depends on the identity and mass of the given gas.

2 The new equation combining the gas laws may be stated in the following form:

$$\frac{P_1 V_1}{T_1} = \frac{P_2 V_2}{T_2} = \frac{P_3 V_3}{T_3} = \underline{\quad} = K$$

EXAMPLE: A gas occupies a volume of 433 cm^3 at 721 torr and 30° C. How much volume would the gas occupy if the temperature were decreased to 0° C and the pressure to 510 torr?

Solution:

Using the formula: $\frac{P_1 V_1}{T_1} = \frac{P_2 V_2}{T_2}$

a Solve for V_2: $\frac{P_1 V_1 T_2}{P_2 T_1}$

b $V_2 = \dfrac{(721 \text{ torr})(433 \text{ cm}_3)(273° \text{ K})}{(510 \text{ torr})(303° \text{ K})}$

c $V_2 = \dfrac{(721)(433 \text{ cm}^3)(273)}{(510)(303°)} = 551.5 \text{ cm}^3$

4.13 Dalton's law of partial pressure

In 1880 John Dalton, an English chemist and physicist, presented his work on the atomic theory. From this work he formulated theories relating to the behavior of gases.

1 Dalton's law predicts that each gas in a mixture of gases will exert pressure as though it occupied the space *alone* in relation to the amount of the gas present. Symbolically stated:

$$P = P_1 + P_2 + P_3 + \underline{\quad} + P_n$$

a Stated another way, the *total pressure* of gases in a mixture is merely the sum of the partial pressures of all the gases (Fig. 8-32).

b Partial pressure is symbolically written as capital *P* followed by the chemical symbol of the gas being described.

• For example, the partial pressure of oxygen is abbreviated as Po_2.

• Similarly the symbol for the partial pressure of carbon dioxide is Pco_2.

1 The partial pressure of a gas is calculated by applying the following formula:

Partial pressure (P) = Barometric pressure (PB) ×
Decimal equivalent of the gas percentage in a mixture

Clinically it is more useful to calculate the partial pressure of the inspired (I) gas. This is accompanied by substituting *P* into the general formula for calculating the atmospheric partial pressure of a gas.

EXAMPLE: Find the partial pressure (PIo_2) of inspired oxygen (21%) at sea level.

Solution: $PIo_2 = PB \times$ Decimal equivalent of gas inhaled (FIo_2)

a Decimal equivalent of oxygen-percentage = 21.0 ÷ 100 = 0.21.

b PB at sea level = 760 torr

c 760 torr × 0.21 = 159.6 torr

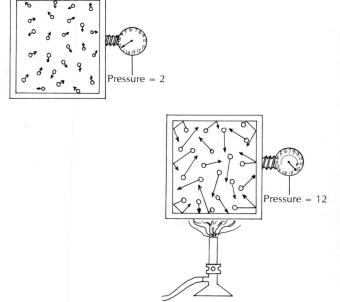

FIGURE 8-31 Illustration of Gay-Lussac's law. As temperature increases in closed container (volume is constant), there will be a proportionate increase in pressure.

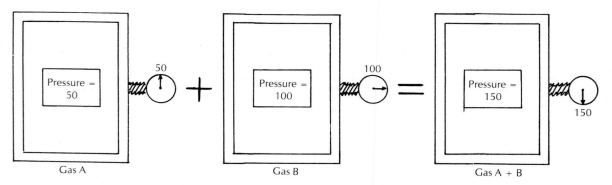

FIGURE 8-32 Illustration of Dalton's law of partial pressure. The total pressure of a mixture of gases is equal to the sum of the partial pressures of each gas.

- Calculated with this formula, the partial pressures of gases at sea level are presented in Table 8-4.
- The formula in the example and the following columnar material may be used to calculate the partial barometric pressures of nitrogen, oxygen, and carbon dioxide at various altitudes:

Altitude (feet)	PB (mm·Hg)
Seal level	760
2000	707
4000	656
6000	609
8000	564
10,000	523

3 Once atmospheric gas is inhaled, it is humidified, and water vapor is added. This gas exerts a pressure like any other gas and must be considered (subtracted) when computing the partial pressure of alveolar gas. Remember, the absolute humidity of gas in the respiratory tract is held at a constant 100% and 37° C. For this reason a standard water vapor pressure of 47 mm Hg can be used when calculating alveolar partial pressures.

a A simplified but useful formula for calculating the partial pressure of alveolar oxygen is:

$$PAo_2 = PIo_2 - \frac{Paco_2}{0.8}$$

or

$$PAo_2 = PIo_2 - (Paco_2 \times 1.25)$$

where:

PAo_2 = Partial pressure of alveolar oxygen,
PIo_2 = Partial pressure of inspired oxygen,
$Paco_2$ = Partial pressure of CO_2 in the lung,
0.8 = Respiratory quotient, and
1.25 = Respiratory quotient expressed differently

b Respiratory quotient is a ratio of carbon dioxide produced to the volume of oxygen consumed during a period of time.

   This is an important consideration when calculating alveolar oxygen or carbon dioxide because of the constant movement (diffusion) of gases from the alveoli capillaries into the alveoli and vice versa.

4 Given the partial pressure of a gas, the percent of the gas can be calculated by the following formula:

$$\% \text{ Gas} = \frac{P}{(PB - H_2O \text{ vapor pressure})} \times 100$$

TABLE 8-4 Percent of major gases of the atmosphere

Gas	Symbol	Percent	Partial pressure (mm Hg)
Nitrogen	N_2	78.084	593.43
Oxygen	O_2	20.95	159.22
Argon	Ar	0.934	7.09
Carbon dioxide	CO_2	0.0314	0.23

For example:

$$\% H_2O = \frac{47}{760} \times 100 = 6.2\%$$

With this formula calculate the percentage of O_2 and CO_2 in the alveoli (that is, PAo_2 and $PAco_2$) with a patient breathing room air at sea level.

a $\% O_2 =$ ___ $PAo_2 = 100$ mm Hg
b $\% CO_2 =$ ___ $PAco_2 = 40$ mm Hg
Solution:
a
$$\% O_2 = \frac{100}{760\text{-}47} = \frac{100}{713} \times 100$$
$$\% O_2 = 0.14 \times 100 = 14\%$$
b
$$\% CO_2 = \frac{40}{713} = 5.6\%$$

4.14 Graham's and Henry's laws and Fick's principle

1 Graham's law and Fick's principle describe the diffusion of gas through a membrane. Henry's law describes the diffusion of a gas into a solution.

2 A combination of Henry's and Graham's laws establishes the scientific explanation for uniting gas and liquid (i.e., the alveolar and blood interface).

3 Graham's law states that the diffusion of gas through a membrane is inversely proportional to the square root of densities of the gas.

4 Henry's law states that the quantity of a soluble gas that dissolves in a liquid at a given temperature is closely related to the partial pressure of that gas in the gas phase.

a For example, the solubility of O_2 dissolved in plasma is 0.003 vol %/mm Hg, and CO_2 is 0.063 vol %/mm Hg. This means that 20 times more CO_2 than O_2 diffuses across the alveolar-capillary (blood) interface during the same time period and at the same partial pressure.

b Clinically this is significant because it means that hyperventilation can reduce CO_2 levels even though some lung units are nonfunctional. Because of the comparative slowness of O_2 diffusion, hyperventilation does not significantly increase the O_2 levels in patients with nonfunctioning lung units.

4.15 Factors determining gas flow

1 Flow is the length of time it takes a given volume of gas or liquid to move from one point to another.
a Symbolically, flow is represented as $\dot{V}$ or volume moved per unit of time and expressed as liters per minute or liters per second.
b *Pressure gradient* is the force generated to cause movement (flow) to occur. A pressure gradient is the difference in pressure existing between two points. Without a gradient, flow does not occur. As previously stated, this is simply explained by the fact that water flows downhill because of the gradient created by the action of gravity on a mass. Gases also flow down a pressure gradient (i.e., from an area of high pressure to one of lower pressure). Both areas can be

a positive pressure, but one will have to exert more positive force than the other if flow is to occur.

c Flow can be dynamic, such as the movement of a large river, or subtle, such as diffusion across the alveolar membrane.

d Flow always occurs within some physical boundary. In physiology, flows occur within tubes and across orifices.

- A tube is a pathway in which the length is greater than its internal diameter.
- An orifice is a pathway in which the internal diameter exceeds the length.

e Flows are described as *laminar* or *turbulent*.

- In laminar flows the molecules move parallel along the walls of the tube. This type of flow is most desirable because less energy is required to move a given volume of gas. In health, gas flow within the airways is primarily laminar.
- Turbulent flow occurs when the molecules move in irregular lines, creating eddy formations and other aerodynamic obstructions. This type of flow is undesirable in the airways, because it requires a great deal of energy to move volumes comparable to that that could be moved with laminar flows. Diseased lungs or reactive airways in spasm create obstructions that cause turbulent gas flows.

f Gas flow is affected by the number and degree of obstructions, the gradient, viscosity (tendency of gas molecules to stick to each other and the walls), gas density, and the inside diameter and the length of the conducting system.

2 In 1882 *Osborne Reynolds* published a series of papers describing the behavior of water flowing in glass tubes. He discussed how, under certain conditions of velocity and tube internal diameter, dyed water would flow in a line parallel to the tube. Yet under different conditions the color would resolve into curls or eddy formations. Reynolds determined from these experiments that critical velocities existed for a given set of conditions that would change laminar to turbulent flow. The conditions were directly proportional to the diameter of the tube. Reynolds calculated the point at which gas flow would change from laminar to turbulent and assigned it a number of 2000. This number, referred to as *Reynolds' number,* is expressed by the formula:

$$\text{Reynolds' no.} = \frac{bpr}{n}$$

where

b = Linear velocity of the fluid,
p = Density,
r = Tube radius, and
n = Fluid viscosity.

3 Gas density (mass per unit volume) has little effect on laminar gas flows. In turbulent flows the lighter the gas, the greater will be its volume flow rate for any given pressure difference. For example, the viscosity

of O_2 and helium (He) is similar—20:19—but the density is different—32:4. This means that three times more helium will flow through an orifice, in a given period of time and pressure gradient, than will oxygen. Clinically this may be significant in situations of severe airway obstruction where oxygen itself cannot easily cross the obstruction, but a He/O_2 mixture may.

4 *Poiseuille* (1846), a French physician, discovered that in *laminar flow* the driving pressure is directly proportional to the viscosity of the fluid. He also found that any variation in the tube would affect the flow or that the pressure to produce a certain flow varies directly with the length of the tube and inversely with the fourth power of the radius. In other words, if the length of the tube is doubled, the pressure must also be doubled to maintain a constant flow, or if the tube internal diameter is halved, pressure must be increased 16 times! For gas to flow through an orifice the molecules must be accelerated, which requires a pressure in proportion to the density of the gas and the square of its velocity.

5 Gas flow is an important consideration clinically, because respiratory therapy personnel can be effective in providing gas delivery systems (tubing) that provide maximum inside diameter and that are short, without sharp turns or angles to create turbulent flow situations. NOTE: In a situation requiring mechanical ventilation, the ventilator will do the work of delivering the gas *during inspiration,* but *the patient must do the work of forcing the gas out on exhalation.* Both are equally important and must be considered in all situations where a mechanical ventilator is used or the patient has an artificial airway in place.

6 Gas flows can be measured with mechanical and/or electric devices called flowmeters, flow raters, or pneumotachographs. These devices may incorporate a ball raised in a chamber that is calibrated in liters per minute, a turbine that spins in response to gas flows, or an electronic pneumotachograph that measures pressure drop as gas flows across a heated screen. These devices and the measurement of gas flow are presented in more detail in Modules Twenty-Three, Mechanical Ventilation, and Twenty-Four, Pulmonary Function.

4.16 Factors determining resistance

1 In everyday terms, resistance means opposition to movement. In physiology, resistance is defined as the pressure differential required for a unit flow change and is expressed as cm H_2O/L/sec.

- This means the amount of pressure in centimeters of water required to move 1 L of gas in 1 sec.

2 Resistance is important as a clinical variable.

a In sick patients flow resistance is probably the factor most responsible for diminished gas flows and increased work of breathing.

b A normal airway resistance in adults is 0.6 to 2.4 cm H_2O/L/sec, measured with a body plethysmograph during rapid, shallow breathing of 0.5 L/sec. An increase in gas flow would cause an increase in resistance.

3 To measure resistance, pressure and flow measured under dynamic (flowing) conditions must be considered.
- Resistance can be calculated mathematically with the following formula:

$$R = \frac{\Delta^* \text{ pressure (cm H}_2\text{O)}}{\Delta \text{ Flow (L/sec)}}$$

4 Diseases causing increased resistance to flow are asthma, emphysema, bronchitis, bronchiectasis during infectious periods, and tissue disorders that infringe on the airway.

5 Mechanically, resistance is increased by artificial airways that are too small and/or too long, bends or kinks in breathing tubes, mucus or other secretions in the tubes or airways, and inspiratory flow rates that are excessive.

  a Increased airway resistance can be visualized by observing the work of breathing by the movement of a patient's muscles of inspiration and exhalation, a sudden rise in a pressure manometer on a ventilator panel, audible noises (such as wheezing), or even panic on the patient's face.

  b Clinical effects of airway resistance are discussed in Module Twenty, Airway Management Techniques.

4.17 Correlation of physiology to electricity

Many of the principles for the movement of electrons apply to respiratory physiology.

As was explained in the previous unit, many physical factors influence the process of gas flow. Resistance is a significant factor not only in determining gas flow but also in calculating blood flow through pulmonary vasculature.

1 The primary components for determining blood flow resistance at a given rate of flow are density and viscosity (see Unit 4.15).

2 Resistance, stated another way, is the impedance to blood flow through a given area.

3 In contrast to air flow resistance, blood flow resistance decreases as flow rate is increased, because the conducting vessels are dilated by the increased internal pressure.

4 Blood flow resistance can be calculated by comparing it to Ohm's law, which describes current flow through an electric circuit.

4.18 Glossary of terms

The following terms and definitions will be useful in understanding electricity and current flow.

1 Ohm's law. Current flow from an area of high potential to an area of lower potential in a *complete* circuit. Current flow through a complete circuit will be directly proportional to voltage and inversely proportional to circuit resistance.

2 Amperes. Unit of current *flow* past some point; analogous to liters per second in a fluid.

3 Voltage. Driving pressure required to push electrons through a circuit (i.e., the potential difference that produces a current of 1 A when 1 W of energy is used); the electromotive force (EMF).

4 Watt. Measurement of power. One watt of power is produced by 1 A of current with a potential of 1 V.

5 Capacitor. Electric conductor separated by nonconducting gaps.

6 Conductor. Any element that will carry (transmit) an electric charge.

7 Impedance. Opposition to electron movement in an alternating-current circuit.

8 AC circuit. Alternating-current circuit where the flow of electrons moves first in one direction and then in the opposite direction as compared to direct current. Most wall outlets are AC.

9 DC circuit. Direct-current circuit where the flow of electrons moves in a steady flow in *one* direction only. A battery is an example of a DC circuit.

10 Ground-earth. Return of an electric current to the earth. This is compared to an ungrounded system that, left undetected, may result in an electric arc (sparking) and possible fire.

11 Ground-redundant. A double grounding system.

12 Ground-equipotential. A local grounding of equipment, instruments, or the like in order to reduce electric potential between the power source and the user should a fault occur.

13 Ground bus. Also called "reference point grounding." A single point used to ground equipment connected to a patient or within reach of the patient.

4.19 Causes of electric shock and electrocution

1 An electric shock occurs whenever current escapes or is allowed to travel where it is not intended to go. Remember the following basic principles:
  a Current will flow only in a completed circuit.
  b The amount of current is a result of applied voltage and resistance to its flow.
  c AC may travel in a circuit even though it is not complete because of capacitive coupling between conductors.

2 Electric current applied to the body causes a depolarization. Current flow across the heart will depolarize it. As a treatment for fibrillation this is a desired outcome; however, accidental exposure of the heart to sufficient current density and frequency will cause fibrillation.

3 The body's exposure to shock may be defined as *macroshock* if sufficient current is applied to the skin to cause fibrillation or sustained cardiac contraction.

4 Microshock is electrocution caused by exposing the heart directly to sufficient current to induce fibrillation or standstill.

4.20 Effects and sources of accidental shock

1 When conducted through the skin, current exposure above 10 mA may cause sustained involuntary muscle

---

*Δ, Changing or dynamic.

contraction and above 100 mA, death by ventricular fibrillation.

2 Accidental shock can occur whenever any of the following events take place:

a Victim accidentally touches a prong of an electric plug when inserting it into an outlet (two-conductor contact). See Fig. 8-33.

b A frayed cord resulting in current flow from the power source to equipment through the victim to the ground and back to the power source (live-to-ground contact). See Fig. 8-34

c An escape of current by a loose connection, frayed insulation, or the like from the power source to the chasis (Fig. 3-34). This leakage of current may be sufficient to cause microshock to a grounded patient. In some cases this may be sufficient to induce cardiac fibrillation or standstill. According to BS5724

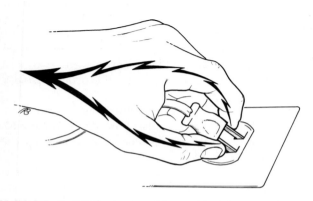

FIGURE 8-33 Shock caused by accidentally contacting two conductors on an electric plug. Current flows from one prong to the other.

Standards, safe limits for current leakage for permanently installed equipment is *1 mA* in the earth wire.

d For portable equipment with one earth wire the maximum safe limit is *0.5 mA*.

For portable equipment with two earth wires the maximum leakage allowed is *5 mA*.

3 Additional details on electric shock and grounding of equipment may be obtained by contacting the biomedical department of a hospital.

4.21 Prevention of accidental electric shock

1 The *best* of all solutions is to routinely check all electric equipment for proper operation and condition of wires and fittings. Leakage checks should be made routinely and recorded.

2 A *second* preventive step is to ensure that all equipment is properly grounded before it is put into operation.

3 A *third* step is to install line monitors in permanently installed systems. Equipment, not patients, should be grounded! These monitors will warn the operator of an electric fault whenever it occurs and, it is hoped, will prevent an accident. Remember electricity is a necessary good and evil in today's modern world. If you are unfamiliar with electric circuits, it would be educational to meet with your biomedical technician or electrician for some basic instruction.

4.22 Electrostatic charge (static electricity)

1 An electrostatic charge occurs when an object is insulated from its surroundings.

2 Electric charges can be accumulated on or wiped off objects that are rubbed with other objects. One example is an electric potential that is built up as a traveler

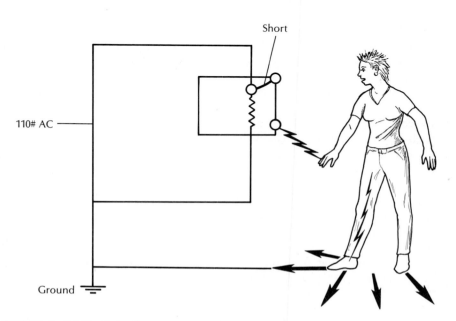

FIGURE 8-34 Shock by live wire to equipment through a short caused by a frayed cord. Grounded victim touches equipment and completes circuit through his body.

rubs his feet across the carpet; on touching the door handle or shaking hands with a friend, an electric charge is passed through the person to the ground, creating a spark.

3 In an explosive environment, such as an oxygen-enriched hyperbaric chamber, this spark could cause combustion.

4 For years operating suites have used conductive floors, have grounded equipment and people, and have raised humidity to prevent such electrostatic occurrences.

5 Hyperbaric chambers use non static producing material and depend on a complete grounding system for safety.

4.23 Temperature/heat: Terms and definitions

The following terms and definitions may be applied to understanding temperature and heat and its application clinically.

1 Heat. A form of energy that can be transferred from a hot form to a colder one.

2 Temperature. A degree of hotness or coldness measured on a definite scale; thermal condition of a substance that determines whether it can transfer or receive heat.

3 Hypothermia. Lowering body temperature below 35° C.

4 Hyperthermia. Raising body temperature above 35° C.

5 Krause/Ruffini thermoreceptors. Senses temperature changes at the skin and transmits signal to the hypothalamus to cause actions that will raise or lower body temperature (see following explanation).

4.24 Importance to clinical practice

1 The relationship between heat loss and gain and temperature is extremely important in the management of patients.

2 Humans are homothermic, and body core temperature should be maintained at 37° ± 0.5° C regardless of environmental constraints that may alter the temperature of the body's surface from 32° to 35° C.

3 A body's primary response to radical changes in its *core* temperature includes:
a Reflex changes in vascular tone.
b Shivering.
c Sweating.
d Vasodilation of skin vessels.
e Loss of consciousness.
f Convulsions.
g Ventricular fibrillation.
h Stimulation of endocrines.

4 A person loses body heat by the following processes:

Method	Approximate loss of heat (%)
a Evaporation	30
b Radiation	30
c Convection	30
d Respiration	10

NOTE: At a core temperature of 30° C or lower the heart becomes very irritable and may begin fibrillation. At a

core temperature of 42° C or higher the brain loses its ability to regulate temperature and convulsion follows.

4.25 Application of heat/temperature to respiratory care

1 The control of heat loss or gain is a major concern in critically ill patients for the following reasons:
a *Dehydration.* A great deal of the patient's energy can be used in humidifying dry inhaled gases. This needless use of energy may overwork an already stressed body system and result in increased oxygen demand.
b *Temperature.* In infants the process of heating and humidifying inspired gases can result in hypothermia and dehydration. Should shivering occur the patient will needlessly use energy and oxygen in a reflex attempt to warm the body. In environmental chambers, care must be taken to monitor the patient's body temperature, since high humidity will interfere with the body's ability to cool itself by evaporation.

4.26 Measurement of temperature

1 The application of heat and cold to a substance may change the characteristics of the substance.

2 For example, heating a wire will increase its resistance to current flow.

3 Some of the effects of radical changes in a patient's temperature have already been discussed. For this reason it is important to be able to accurately measure temperature.

4 The following devices are available for use in clinical practice:

Device	Theory
a Mercury and alcohol thermometers	Heat causes the mercury or alcohol to expand and rise up the numbered scale.
b Dial thermometer	Expansion of a bimetallic metal strip causes a coil to tighten and move a needle along a temperature scale.
c Electric resistance	Resistance to current flow occurs across a wire as the temperature rises. The charge in electron flow is compared to a scale and read as temperature.
d Thermistor probe	A small bead of *metal oxide* or other substance is used to complete an electric circuit. Unlike other metal, the resistance of the bead *decreases* as the temperature rises. Changes in current flow across the thermistor are measured and correlated to read on a scale as temperature. NOTE: Some thermistors also use a bead that has an increase in resistance as the temperature increases.

4.27 Système International d'Unités (SI system)

1 The Système International d'Unités was introduced in 1960 as a universal standard of measurement.

2 Today its acceptance varies, although the American Medical Association has a committee to study use of

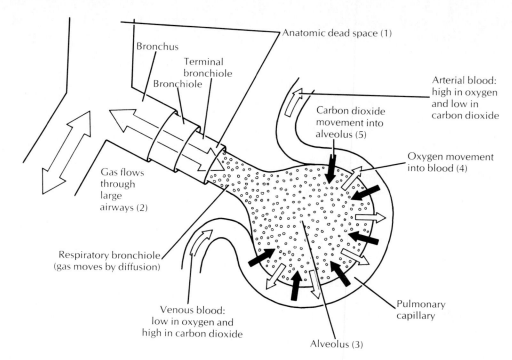

FIGURE 8-35 Inspired gas fills the airway of the lungs.

this system in its scientific literature. Application of this system may be found in the literature published by the International Standards Organization for "Standard Specifications for Breathing Machines for Medical Use."

3 The SI system is comprised of seven major units with multiple subunits.

4 The seven major SI units are presented below:

Application	Unit	Symbol
a Length	Meter	m
b Mass	Kilogram	kg
c Time	Second	s
d Current	Ampere	A
e Temperature	Kelvin	K
f Luminous intensity	Candela	cd
g Amount of substance	Mole	mol

5 Some examples of subunits include:

a Pressure	Pascal	Pa
b Pressure	Bar	Bar
c Power	Watt	w
d Frequency	Hertz	H
e Volume	Cubic meter	H[<]m³
f Volume	Liter	*l*

5.0 THE BREATHING PROCESS
5.1 Breathing

Breathing is a physiologic process that begins with birth and continues until death. In health it is spontaneous and therefore not directly controlled by a conscious level of awareness. It is not until breathing is interfered with or changed by disease or circumstance that one becomes aware of its relationship to the quality and longevity of life.

The lung performs two major functions: provides gas and blood flow to the alveoli and provides the exchange of gases between the alveoli and the blood.

In the following units these functions are studied separately, even though they occur *simultaneously and constantly* in the lung. Table 8-5 presents a brief overview of lung function as a total process and places in perspective the many events that are involved in breathing and how they interrelate as they are studied separately. In the table, although a single alveolus is used as an example, the same process is occurring in more than 250 million alveoli. Clinically the practitioner must picture these events and decide whether a patient's symptoms are gas flow, diffusion, and/or perfusion related. The reader is encouraged to frequently refer to this table for orientation in progressing through the module and becoming involved in units that deal with the specifics of lung physiology.

5.2 Breathing (ventilation)

The process of breathing is complicated and involves a great deal more than the seemingly simple process of rhythmically moving air into and out of the chest. This unit presents the mechanics of breathing (i.e., the interplay of forces and structures that causes the chest to move and gas to flow).

1 To reiterate, gas, like water, flows "downhill." In this example of gas flow the "steepness' of the grade of the hill is called the *pressure gradient*. This means that gas, like water, flows from a point of high pressure to a *relative point* of lower pressure.

2 Gas flow into and out of the lungs can be demonstrated by a model (Fig. 8-36, *A-D*) of two balloons *(A, 1)*

TABLE 8-5 Summary of lung function

Action	Cause
1. The chest enlarges by muscle retraction, causing a pressure gradient.	1. Air flows from the atmosphere to the lung until the gradient is equalized (inspiration).
2. Inspired gas is warmed/humidified/filtered.	2. Heat/humidity are added by the upper airway and mucosa of descending airways. Air is filtered by nose; dust and debris impacted on mucosa is removed by ciliary action.
3. Inspired gas fills the airways (Fig. 8-35).	3. Part of each breath does not reach the alveoli but fills the passageways/partitions formed by the anatomic structures of the lungs (dead space) *(1)*. this is estimated to be 1 ml/lb of a patient's body weight.
4. At the level of the respirataory bronchioles, gas movement is primarily by **diffusion.**	4. The mass flow of gas *(2)* caused by inhalation in the narrow upper airways suddenly drops to zero as the airways widen out into the cross-sectionally large area of millions of partitioned spaces known as alveoli *(3)*. NOTE: Even though alveoli are illustrated as round-shaped, they are not. Alveoli more closely resemble an octagon or octahedron.
5. In the alveoli the final millimeter of gas exchange between the alveolus and the surrounding capillaries is by diffusion only.	5. Gas exchange between the alveoli/capillaries is constant and occurs whether or not air is moving in and out of the upper airways, as long as a diffusive gradient exists between the bases in the alveoli and those in the blood.
6. The diffusion process continues, causing CO_2 to diffuse across the alveolar compartment until it reaches the zone where it is removed by the mass movement of gas caused by breathing. An airway obstruction increases the distance CO_2 must diffuse before it is removed.	6. Constant diffusion occurs, causing O_2 to move across the alveoli-capillary membrane *(4)* into the venous blood that enters the alveolar capillary. Simultaneously, CO_2 moves from the venous blood into the alveoli *(5)*. This diffusion occurs from a constantly gas-filled area of the alveolus as the residual volume. This area never empties of gas, and together with the expiratory reserve volume forms the functional residual capacity, which is the volume of gas that remains in the lung at the end of expiration. It is this volume (compartment) that can be increased or decreased by the addition or removal of positive end-expiratory pressure (PEEP). Changes in this compartment change the constant volume available for gas exchange to occur and will control O_2 and CO_2 levels in the blood.
7. Blood flowing around the alveoli carries the freshly oxygenated blood to all the tissues of the body where diffusion again occurs, with venous blood returning for O_2 renewal and CO_2 elimination. Because alveoli empty and fill at different rates and times, the total ventilation and perfusion may be shared equally or unequally by all compartments. A balance must occur between ventilation and perfusion. This balance is expessed as the ventilation-perfusion ratio ($\dot{V}A/\dot{Q}$), which is approximately *one (1)* in the healthy lung.*	7. Diffusion of gases into and out of oxygenated blood is immediate as the alveoli themselves obtain nutrients from the pulmonary capillaries. In the diseased or traumatized lung, blood may bypass (shunt) alveolar units. When this occurs venous blood ultimately mixes with blood that was oxygenated. This mixture lowers the O_2 percentage of blood going to the body's tissues.

*In the diseased, traumatized, and aged lung, the balance between ventilation and perfusion is altered, causing tissue hypoxia, carbon dioxide retention, and other abnormalities referred to as *respiratory failure*. The following units cover normal lung function and altered lung function. It is the practitioner's job to subsequently relate this knowledge to the symptoms that are occurring in the patient as respiratory support and therapy are being provided.

connected by a Y piece and housed in a bell jar *(2)* that is open to the atmosphere on one end *(3)* and closed by a rubber diaphragm on the other end *(4)*.

a As the diaphragm *(4)* is pulled down *(B)* the space inside the bell jar becomes larger. As the space becomes larger around the balloons the gas molecules become less compacted and the pressure per square inch is less (−) than the air in the balloons that are opened to the atmosphere.

b Applying the concept that gas moves from an area of higher pressure *(5)* to lower pressure, the air in the balloons will attempt to move toward the decreased pressure area surrounding the balloons (−). The walls of the balloon will prevent relocation of the molecules from within the balloons to the area outside the balloons but will expand in response to molecular movement.

• This movement causes the pressure to be decreased within the balloons, resulting in more air flowing in

from the atmosphere into the balloons (high to low) *(6)*.

• This movement will continue, and the balloons will fill until the pressure within the balloons *(C, 7)* and that outside the balloons equalizes with the atmosphere *(8)*. This once again compacts the air molecules and decreases the volume outside the balloons *(9)*.

• When this occurs gas movement stops and the balloons remain inflated. Consequently the more the rubber diaphragm is pulled down, the greater the volume created around the balloons and the greater the tendency for gas molecules in the balloon to move toward the decreased pressure zone, causing more atmospheric air to flow into the balloons.

– This example can be equated to inspiration when the ribs are elevated and the diaphragm moves down, enlarging the volume of the chest.

3 During inspiration the trachea is open to the atmo-

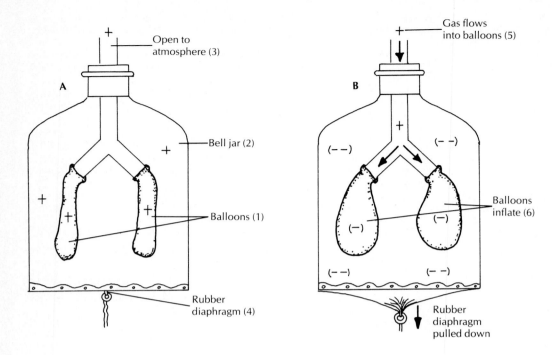

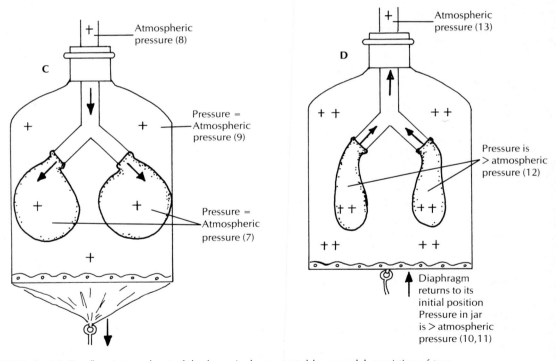

FIGURE 8-36 Gas flow into and out of the lungs is demonstrated by a model consisting of two balloons connected by a Y piece and housed in a bell jar that is closed on the bottom by a rubber diaphragm. The balloons communicate with the atmosphere at the top through the opening in the Y piece. **A,** System at rest (end expiration). **B** and **C,** Diaphragm is pulled down, causing an increased volume and decreased pressure around balloons. Gas enters balloons from atmosphere via the Y piece (inspiration). **D,** When the diaphragm is released, pressure around the balloons increases. Gas exists balloons to atmosphere (expiration).

sphere (Y tube), and air moves from the atmosphere (area of high pressure) to the lung (area of lower pressure) until the pressure within the lung and around the outside of the lungs becomes almost equal. It is important to note that in health the chest is closed to the atmosphere and there is *no* air outside the lungs or in the chest cavity, as is true in the bell jar. Only a potential space exists outside the lungs, which responds by pressure change to the movement of the chest as did the balloons in the bell jar. To cause air to leave the expanded balloons in the bell jar *(10)*, the diaphragm is released.

 a When this occurs the elasticity of the stretched diaphragm causes it to retract and to assume its initial position *(11)*. In this position the volume (space) inside the bell jar is reduced compared to the stretched position of the diaphragm, and the gas pressure both inside and outside the balloons is increased *(12)* compared to the gas pressure of the atmosphere *(13)*.

 b The increased external pressure around the balloons causes the molecules inside the balloons to be compressed. When this occurs the gas pressure within the balloons *(12)* becomes greater than the atmosphere *(13)*, and the gas flows out of the balloons into the atmosphere (high to low). This flow continues until the pressure within the balloons *equals* the atmosphere. At this point gas flow ceases (end of exhalation).

4 Exhalation of gas from the lungs can be related to the example of the bell jar model (see Fig. 8-36, *D*)

 As the ribs are pulled downward and inward by the elastic retraction of the muscles that have been stretched during inspiration and the diaphragm moves back to its passive position, the pressure within the chest but outside the lungs (intrapleural pressure) rises, causing the lungs to deflate as gas moves from the increased pressure within the lungs to the atmosphere.

5 This process of increasing and decreasing the size of the chest by active contraction of inspiratory muscles followed by passive retraction of these muscles causes gas to move in and out of the lungs in response to increased and decreased pressure gradients.

6 This movement of gas to and from the alveoli is most accurately called *ventilation*, although it is frequently referred to as external respiration or breathing.

5.3 Steps involved in breathing

1 The muscles of inspiration cause the chest cavity to enlarge in three dimensions.

2 The visceral pleura lining the surface of the lungs is in contact with the parietal pleura that lines the inner walls of the chest cavity.

3 The pleurae remain in contact as the chest enlarges and the lungs move with the pleurae.

4 The lung volume increases and the pressure within the lungs decreases.

5 Air moves from the atmosphere through an open glottis in the larynx and down the existing pressure gradient

until pressure in the lungs equals that of the atmosphere.

6 Gas pressure within the lungs becomes equal to the atmosphere at the end of inspiration and at the end of expiration, causing gas flow to cease.

7 When gas flow ceases at the end of inspiration, exhalation normally is passive and occurs as the stretched chest muscles recoil back to a normal relaxed position.

8 The pressure changes that occur within the lung are dynamic and occur during the breathing process.

 a Intrapulmonary pressure. Generated within the lungs themselves during the breathing cycle.

 b Intrapleural pressure. Changes within the pleural space during breathing.

 c Transthoracic pressure. Changes to inflate or deflate the lungs and chest wall together.

 d Transmural pressure. Changes during inflation and deflation of the lungs. Difference between intrapleural and esophageal pressure.

 • The dynamic changes that occur between intrapulmonary and intrapleural pressures during breathing are presented in Table 8-6.

 • Pressure changes during the breathing cycle are illustrated in Fig. 8-37.

9 It is important to realize that pressure generated within the airways is transmitted throughout the thorax as intrathoracic pressure. For example, a positive pressure created by performing a Valsalva's maneuver greater than 100 torr held for 15 seconds or longer will cause the positive pressure in the lungs to be transmitted into the intrathoracic space surrounding the great vessels returning blood to the heart.

 a When the external force on these vessels exceeds the internal pressure of the blood, the vessels will collapse inward, cardiac output will be interrupted, cerebral blood flow will cease, and unconsciousness will occur (syncope).

 b Clinically this same situation will occur if a mechanical ventilator delivers a breath under high positive airway pressure with a prolonged inspiratory time and/or if inspiration is held or retarded within the chest.

 c Note in Table 8-6 the difference that exists in pressures between the inside (intrapulmonic) and outside of the lung (intrapleural) during breathing and at the end of inspiration and exhalation. There always ex-

T A B L E 8 - 6 Intrapleural/intrapulmonic pressures

Stage	Intrapleural pressure (mm Hg)—torr	Intrapulmonary pressure (mm Hg)—torr
During inspiration	−8	−3
During exhalation	−2	+3
End of exhalation	−4	+4
End of inspiration	−6	−2
Mean pressure	−5	0

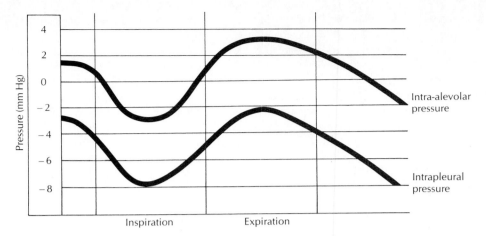

FIGURE 8-37 Pressure changes during the breathing cycle.

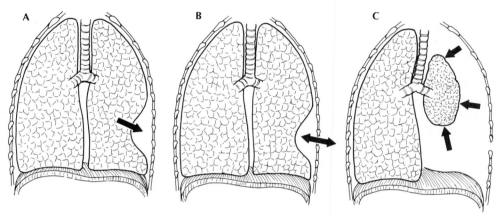

FIGURE 8-38 Pneumothorax. **A,** Closed or tension pneumothorax. Air leaks into intrapleural space from a hole within the lung. **B,** Open pneumothorax. Air enters intrapleural space from outside. **C,** An untreated tension pneumothorax. Lung collapses, and great vessels are pushed to the opposite side.

ists a pressure drop between the inside and outside of the lungs as a result of the resistance of tissue to movement. This is also true of the pressure generated at the mouth as compared to the distal airways.

- This pressure drop occurs because of the physical law that states that there is a gas pressure drop across an orifice. The lung is comprised of passages forming countless orifices and tubes, which cause the gas pressure to decrease drastically between the mouth (proximal airway) and the distal lung units.
- Note also that intrapleural pressure is normally below atmospheric pressure at all times. Even at rest the intrapleural pressure is about −5 torr below the atmosphere. One reason for this is that the rib cage is larger than the lungs; therefore the lungs even at rest are stretched, causing a pressure gradient to exist.

10 As a result of this constant negative pressure, if a hole were to occur in the chest wall and the pleura, atmo-spheric air would rush into the space to neutralize the gradient. This would cause the lung to collapse in the area exposed to the atmosphere. This situation is a medical *emergency* and is called a *pneumothorax*.

In Fig. 8-38 note that a pneumothorax may be of the closed type caused by air leaking from a hole within the lung *(A)* or of the open type with air coming into the chest from the outside *(B)*. A closed pneumothorax is also referred to as a *tension* pneumothorax, because if the air leak continues, it will fill the chest cavity and eventually cause the lung to collapse and push the great vessels toward the opposite side *(C)*. A tension pneumothorax can also occur with an open pneumothorax if the hole acts as a check valve by letting air in during inspiration but closing during exhalation, trapping each successively greater volume of air in the chest.

11 Ventilation occurs as a result of chest movement. This movement has been identified and named so that normal versus abnormal movement can be identified.

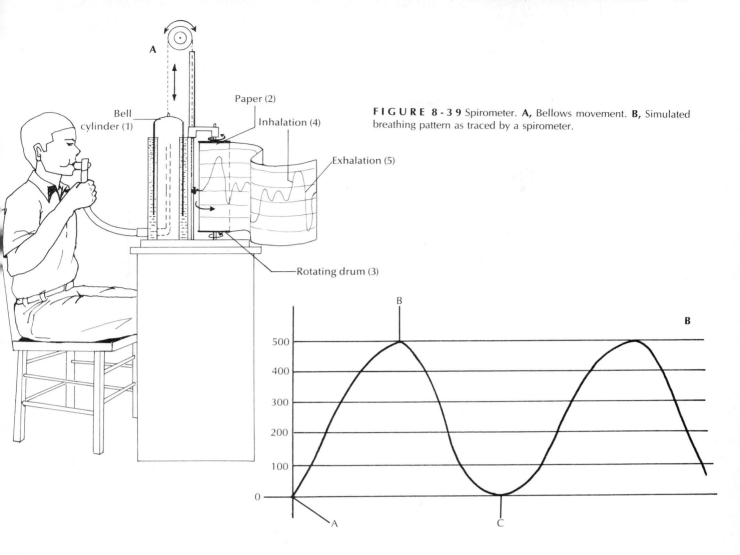

FIGURE 8-39 Spirometer. **A,** Bellows movement. **B,** Simulated breathing pattern as traced by a spirometer.

5.4 Breathing patterns

1 The movement of air into and out of the lungs establishes breathing patterns. These patterns can be used by alert and informed respiratory care personnel as indicators of the patient's progress.

2 Unusual breathing patterns are *not* normal and may represent the first clinical sign that the patient is going into respiratory failure. In many instances the change in the patient's breathing pattern is so subtle that even the patient may not have recognized it until severe dyspnea begins.

5.5 Lung volumes

1 The lung, as previously described, is an anatomic container enclosed by the chest, a second container.

2 As is true with containers, the lung can hold only a certain volume of gas at any given time. However, because the lung is a *flexible* container and because the volume constantly changes with the breathing cycle, physiologists have given names and values to the volume contained within the lung at different levels of inflation (inspiration) and deflation (exhalation).

a Note the boxed material on p. 198 on lung volumes and capacities.*

b Changes in these volumes can be used to reflect the effects of cardiopulmonary diseases.

3 Lung volumes and lung dynamics can be measured by pulmonary function testing. A detailed description of pulmonary function tests is presented in Module Twenty-four.

a Lung volumes can be emasured by having the patient exhale from different inspiratory levels and according to different expiratory efforts into a device known as a spirometer (Fig. 8-39).

• In Fig. 8-39, *A,* as the patient inhales and exhales, a bellows or a bell *(1)* moves up and down, drawing a pattern of the patient's breathing efforts *(2)* on a sheet of paper that is attached to a rotating drum *(3)*. This causes a breathing pattern to be drawn, much like a heart beat causes an ECG to be traced *(b)*.

---

*Additional explanation of the various lung compartments is presented in Units 5.6 and 5.7.

Lung volumes and capacities in milliliters			
TLC 6000	VC 4800	IC 3600	IRV 3100
			TV 500
		FRC 2400	ERV 1200
	RV 1200		RV 1200

TLC, total lung capacity: the sum total of all air in the lung (volumes and capacities).

VC, Vital capacity: maximum exhalation after a maximal inhalation.

RV, Residual volume: air that remains in the lung even after a forced exhalation.

IC, Inspiratory capacity: a maximum inspiration from a resting level.

FRC, Functional residual capacity: air that remains in the lung after a normal exhalation.

IRV, Inspiratory reserve volume: inspiration in addition to normal inspiration.

TV, Tidal volume: a normal inspiration and exhalation.

ERV, Expiratory reserve volume: air that can be forced out following a resting (normal) exhalation.

> – *Normally the tracing will swing upward for inhalation (4) and* downward *(5) for exhalation, although in some instances this may be reversed.*

b The reader is encouraged to follow instructions for the accompanying exercise. This exercise will help clarify the meaning of lung volumes and how they are traced. In this exercise the reader needs a pencil to be able to manually trace what a spirometer pen would be recording if the reader were attached to a spirometer (see Fig. 8-39, *B*).

c Place your pencil at point *A*. Take in a normal breath. As you breathe in, move your pencil slowly toward point *B* with the movement of your chest. When you have taken a normal breath, hold your breath and stop your pencil at point *B*. Now, slowly exhale and move your pencil from point *B* to point *C*. Repeat the exercise, this time without stopping at point *B*. You have just completed what is known as a tidal breath or tidal volume. If you did this for 1 minute, you would complete a minute volume. Also note that your tracing was on a grid that allows you to calculate the amount of air you inhaled; in this case, 500 ml. This same type of exercise is performed by your patient with a spirometer, which records the volume of air moved. Instructions to the patient would vary in order to get the patient to breathe deeper and/or faster or "blow out" harder. The air moved in and out during breathing, in both normal and labored states, can be measured and constitutes what is called *lung volumes*. There obviously exists a direct relationship between these volumes

and the position of the chest; hence the amount of air that is in the lung at any given time.

5.6 Lung volumes—Defined

1 During normal breathing, air moves to and fro, into and out of the lungs. This movement of air has been likened to the ebb and flow of the tides; thus the volume of gas moved during a normal breath has been termed the *tidal volume* (TV or V_T).

2 In precise terms the gas expelled from the lungs during an exhalation will have a different volume than the gas that entered the lung during the preceding inhalation.

a This inequality results from the fact that CO_2 production and O_2 consumption are slightly different: O_2 consumption (250 ml/min) exceeds CO_2 production (200 ml/min). Therefore the *tidal volume* is strictly defined as the *volume of air exhaled during one respiratory cycle*.

b The subject who exerts a maximum muscular effort from the resting end-expiratory level can forcefully expel a volume of air termed the *expiratory reserve volume* (ERV).

c The *residual volume* (RV) is defined as the volume of gas that remains in the lungs at the end of this maximum expiration.

d On the other hand, a subject could be instructed to hold his or her breath after a normal inspiration and then inspire further as deeply as possible. This maximum amount of gas that can be inspired from the end-inspiratory position is termed the *inspiratory reserve volume* (IRV).

• These four lung volumes are depicted in the boxed material in Unit 5.5.

5.7 Lung capacities

1 There are four lung capacities that are various *combinations of two or more of the lung volumes* discussed in the previous unit. The *functional residual capacity* (FRC) consists of the gas that resides in the lungs at the end of a normal, passive exhalation. As such, the functional residual capacity is equal to the sum of the expiratory reserve volume and the residual volume *(ERV + RV = FRC.)*

2 The *inspiratory capacity* (IC) coincides with the amount of air that can be inhaled from the resting expiratory level. Accordingly, the inspiratory capacity is the sum of the tidal volume and the inspiratory reserve volume *(TV + IRV = IC)*.

3 The vital capacity (VC) is defined as the maximum amount of air that a subject can exhale after a maximum inspiration. Therefore the vital capacity is equal to the sum of the expiratory reserve volume, the tidal volume, and the inspiratory reserve volume *(ERV + TV + IRV = VC)*.

4 The total lung capacity (TLC), as its name implies, consists of the total amount of air contained in the lung at the end of a maximum inspiration. Consequently the total lung capacity is equal to the sum of the residual volume, expiratory reserve volume, tidal volume, and inspiratory reserve volume *(RV + ERV + TV + IRV = TLC)*.

- Other details regarding flow rates and time/volume tests are covered in Module Twenty-four or as applicable to a physiologic or pathologic concept in this module.

5.8 Other forces influencing ventilation

There is a size change in the lungs (volume) for each unit of pressure change caused by the expanding chest. The pressure differences between alveolar pressure and intra-pleural pressure are called "intrapulmonary pressures."

1 This change is known as the *compliance* (C) and is used to evaluate the relative elasticity of the lung in response to inflating pressures.

   a Compliance is expressed in liters per centimeter of H_2O pressure and can be calculated with the following formula, which is based on transpulmonary pressure:

   $$C = \frac{\Delta V}{\Delta P},$$

with C meaning compliance and $\Delta V/\Delta P$ meaning changing volume and pressure.

   b Compliance volumes are expressed in terms of liters per centimeter of water.

   - During normal quiet breathing, lung compliance is approximately 0.2 L/cm H_2O. This figure is useful only when the chest is open, such as during surgery. Under normal conditions the lungs are contained with a closed chest cavity, which requires that a compliance value for both the chest wall and the lung be regulated simultaneously.
   - For this reason the clinician normally calculates *total* lung compliance, which assumes that both the chest and lungs are intact.
     - Total lung compliance is approximately one half the value derived for either chest wall or lung compliance individually, or 0.1 L/cm H_2O. This means that for each cm/H_2O pressure change in the lungs, there is a 0.1 L change in lung volume.

   c Clinically compliance can be a useful measure of how well a patient's pulmonary system is responding to treatment. Bronchopulmonary diseases cause *lung* compliance to increase, whereas diseases of nerves, muscles, bones, and even restrictive bandages or obesity cause *chest wall* compliance to decrease.

   d The compliance value decreases as the patient becomes sicker. This is indicated by the fact that it takes more airway pressure to move a given volume of air into the lungs. This can be determined in a closed system such as a ventilator by briefly blocking the expiratory valve at the end of inspiration and quickly noting the amount of pressure showing on the ventilator's pressure manometer. The expiratory valve is then unobstructed, and the patient is allowed

to exhale into a spirometer and the volume is recorded. Some ventilators have separate controls that block the exhalation valve causing plateau pressures.

   e If the patient's compliance improves, the amount of pressure necessary to deliver the same volume of gas will be decreased and vice versa. This can be calculated using the formula in *1a* of this unit.

   f It should be kept in mind that this technique renders, at best, a rough estimate of whether or not the patient's lungs are becoming "stiffer" (less compliant) or more elastic (compliant).

   g Compliance determination is a useful measurement provided one recognizes the fact that it depends on the:
   - Initial volume in the lungs at the time of measurement
   - Time allowed for the volume change to occur

   h It must be remembered therefore that a normal adult compliance measured *under dynamic (gas flow) conditions is independent of the time taken for each volume to be reached*. This is based on the theory that the time constants of the many paralleled airways *are essentially equal*, and therefore the lungs may be treated as a *single lung unit*.

   i In lung disease caused by airway plugging and other variables, these time constants cannot be equal, and the distribution of inspired and expired volumes will change with the time taken for inflation and deflation (i.e., respiratory frequency) to occur.

   j Consequently, if adequate time is *not* allowed for exhalation, gas will be *trapped*, with the total volume dependent on the initial expiratory volume, the degree of compliance (or elastance), and the respiratory rate. This trapped gas causes an elevation in the patient's functional residual capacity, which will alter compliance figures.
   - *Functional residual capacity* (FRC) is the volume of the respiratory system when the respiratory muscles are relaxed and no external forces are applied. It is the volume at which the inward recoil of the lung is exactly balanced by the outward recoil of the chest wall.
     - FRC is the breathing compartment within the lungs that most directly determines the volume of air constantly available for diffusion into the pulmonary capillaries.
     - In certain types of lung disease or trauma the FRC is decreased from normal. This situation is not desirable, because it causes a decrease in lung compliance and in the amount of gas available for diffusion.
     - Current therapy techniques such as *positive end-expiratory pressure* (PEEP) and *constant positive airway pressure* (CPAP) allow one to correct the FRC toward normal. This correction should result in improved arterial blood gases and increased compliance.

   k Note that certain diseases of the lung and chest may

increase or decrease compliance. An increase in lung compliance above normal may not be desirable, because an increased compliance reduces transpulmonary pressure, the stabilizing force that holds small airways open. Without this force, small noncartilaginous airways will collapse toward the end of expiration, causing gas trapping, airway plugging, and subsequent disease processes and alveolar destruction. Patients with chronic pulmonary disease are examples of this situation. Compliance determinations as subsequent judgments must be made relative to the clinical situation.

2 *Elastance* (E) is a term describing the transpulmonary pressure change necessary to produce a unit of change in lung volume. Stated another way, it increases with an increase in the lungs' intraactive force. For example, a transpulmonary pressure change of 5 cm H_2O normally produces a 1 L change in lung volume. Lung elastance is calculated by the formula:

$$E = \frac{\Delta P}{\Delta V},$$

which renders an elastance of 5 cm H_2O/L—a *reciprocal* of lung compliance.

  a Like lung compliance, total elastance is calculated by adding the sum of the individual elastances of the lung and chest wall, for a total of 10 cm H_2O/L.

  b As compliance increases, elastance decreases and vice versa. Clinically a patient whose condition is deteriorating will usually have a decrease in chest/lung compliance and an increase in elastance. Mechanically this will require increasing levels of pressure to move a normal tidal volume.

  c A primary factor that influences compliance is lung surface tension, which is the tendency of the molecules in a liquid to contract toward the center. Surface tension occurs at the liquid-gas interface of the alveoli and plays a major role in preventing collapse of the alveoli during exhalation.

3 Surface tension of the lung is controlled by a microscopic layer of fluid that has the qualitative chemical composition of interstitial fluid plus a component called *pulmonary surfactant*.

  a Pulmonary surfactant is thought to be excreted by alveolar type II cells. It consists of both a protein and a lipid combination.

   • The major portion of this *lipoprotein* combination is dipalmityl lecithin (DPL), which has unique qualities. If it is added to saline or serum, the surface tension is reduced, and if the surface area of the solution is decreased, the surface tension also decreases. Conversely, if the surface area of the DPL solution increases, the surface tension also increases.

    – This unique characteristic of varying surface tension in relation to surface area keeps the surface tension pressure of the alveoli stable, regardless of whether or not they are inflated during inspiration or deflated during exhalation.

  b Without surfactant the surface tension of the alveoli would increase as the alveoli empty during exhalation. This situation would cause air in the small alveoli with increased surface tension to move into the more inflated alveoli with lower surface tensions.

   • If this were to occur, the alveoli would sequentially empty their gases until large areas of deflated alveoli, hence nonfunctional lung units, would exist.

    – This situation is called *atelectasis* and exists in certain clinical situations where normal amounts of surfactant are *not* excreted. For example, the respiratory distress syndrome (RDS), or hyaline membrane disease, which has caused many deaths in premature infants, is attributed to an absence of surfactant.

    – If this situation occurs in adults, massive atelectasis occurs and a very high airway pressure is required to inflate and maintain the lungs. Toxic chemicals, aspiration of fluids, or near-drowning can cause diminished surfactant activity.

6.0 ARTERIAL BLOOD GASES
6.1 The importance of arterial blood gases

A thorough understanding of the terms and basic concepts of arterial blood gases (ABGs), the methods of obtaining and processing samples, and the methods of interpretation of ABGs is crucially important for the practicing therapist and technician. Arterial blood gases are often ordered in order to formulate a diagnosis and also to select appropriate therapy. Therefore the respiratory care practitioner must be well versed in blood gas interpretation in order to administer the therapy order by the physician in an intelligent manner.

1 Arterial blood gases are drawn and analyzed to determine if the patient is being well oxygenated and to determine the acid-base relationship of the blood. This relationship is determined by the ability of the lungs to eliminate CO_2 (up to 12,000 mEq/day) and by the kidneys, which excrete H^+ ion and N_3 ion and reabsorb[2] HCO_3^-.

2 Changes in the blood related to lung function are called *respiratory*. Those caused by renal action are called *metabolic*.

3 An arterial blood sample is used rather than venous because arterial blood is a better indicator of activity in all parts of the body, whereas a sample obtained from a vein would reflect information primarily about the extremity from which the sample was drawn. Arterial blood gives a better indication of how well the lungs are oxygenating the blood. Venous samples reflect the contributions of both the heart and lungs and cannot be used to isolate the failing organ.

4 In certain circumstances, whenever it is not possible to obtain an arterial sample, heat can be applied to an area such as the fingertip or earlobe and a capillary sample can be used. Heat causes capillaries near the surface to dilate, resulting in increased blood flow to the area, which is a mixture of venous and arterial

blood called *arterialized* blood. Samples of arterilized blood closely correspond to blood drawn from an artery. This concept is currently being used by various trancutaneous (skin) monitors to measure pH and oxygen pressure and does not require blood to be drawn.

7.0 BLOOD GAS PHYSIOLOGY

7.1 General terms relating to arterial blood gas interpretation and application

1 Absolute shunt. That part of the total physiologic shunt resulting from anatomic and capillary shunting (i.e., a true physiologic shunt).

2 Acid. A substance capable of giving up a hydrogen ion. Any substance with a pH of less than 7.0 (see *pH*, term no. 60).

3 Acid-base balance. The hydrogen ion concentration maintained at normal levels by the body's physiologic processes.

4 Acidemia. A condition where the blood is more acid than normal. The pH is below normal, which is usually 7.35 to 7.45.

5 Acidosis. An abnormal condition where the blood bicarbonate concentration is lower than normal, which is usually 22 to 26 mEq/L.

6 Acute. Rapid onset of situation; can also refer to severity.

7 Alkalemia. A condition where the blood is more alkaline than normal. The pH is above normal.

8 Alkali. A base substance (see *Base*, term no. 13).

9 Alkalosis. An abnormal condition where the blood bicarbonate concentration is above normal.

10 Alveolar-capillary membrane. The tissues that separate the air in the alveolus from the pulmonary blood in the surrounding capillaries.

11 Alveolar ventilation. The air that moves in and out of the alveoli and exchanges gases with the pulmonary blood.

12 Anatomic shunt. Blood that goes from the right side of the heart to the left side without passing through the pulmonary capillaries (i.e., unoxygenated blood).

13 Base. A substance capable of accepting a hydrogen ion; can neutralize an acid by taking up the acid's free hydrogen ions. Any substance with a pH greater than 7.0.

14 Base deficit. The number of milliequivalents per liter of bicarbonate below the normal base buffer level (22 to 26 mEq/L).

15 Base excess. The number of milliequivalents per liter of bicarbonate above the normal base buffer level (22 to 26 mEq/L).

16 Bicarbonate ion. The major blood base (HCO_3^-).

17 Blood gases. A general term identifying the gases dissolved in the blood. It relates to the measurement of the percent concentration and partial pressure of dissolved oxygen and CO_2 in the blood. A blood gas measurement usually includes pH as well.

18 BTPS. A measurement made at body temperature and pressure, saturated. This is 37° C at 760 mm Hg (torr) total pressure when PH_2O (water vapor pressure) is 47 mm Hg.

19 Buffer. A substance that can neutralize both acids and bases without noticeable change of the pH.

20 Carbon dioxide (CO_2). The waste product of the body's aerobic metabolism.

21 Carbon monoxide (CO). An extremely toxic substance that results from incomplete combustion. Carbon monoxide binds with hemoglobin (Hb) 200 times faster than oxygen, and asphyxia is caused by preventing Hb from combining with corresponding amounts of oxygen.

22 Carbonic acid (H_2CO_3). The primary acid in the blood formed from $H_2O + CO_2$.

23 Carboxyhemoglobin (HbCO). A compound resulting from the blood hemoglobin being bound with carbon monoxide.

24 Chronic. Problems or abnormalities of long standing; can also refer to reduced severity.

25 Clark electrode. The device used to measure oxygen tensions.

26 Dead space, alveolar. Alveolar air that does not exchange with blood (i.e., ventilation without blood flow).

27 Dead space, anatomic. That portion of the conducting airways not involved in gas exchange. Estimated at approximately 1 ml/lb body weight in the normal adult.

28 Dead space, mechanical. The addition of a device or tubing to the anatomic pathways, which results in the rebreathing of exhaled gases; deals primarily with rebreathed CO_2.

29 Dead space, physiologic. The sum of anatomic and alveolar dead spaces.

30 Dead space/tidal volume ratio (V_D/V_T). A measurement of that part of the tidal volume that does *not* come into contact with pulmonary blood.

31 Diffusion. The movement of gas molecules across a freely permeable membrane.

32 Electrolytes. Electrically charged particles (ions) in the blood responsible for electric and osmolar processes that take place; include bicarbonate (HCO_3^-), chloride (Cl^-), potassium (K^+), and sodium (Na^+).

33 Erythrocytosis (polycythemia). Refers to increased red blood cell count. Hypoxemia causes increased production of erythropoietin, a hormone that stimulates production of bone marrow. Erythrocytosis secondary to hypoxemia can be found in:
  a Normal fetal blood.
  b Exposure to high altitude.
  c Chronic pulmonary disease.
  d Chronic alveolar hypoventilation.

34 Exponential scale. The mathematic scale of the powers of base 10; the same as a logarithmic scale used to derive the Henderson-Hasselbalch equation.

35 External respiration. The exchange of gases between the alveoli and pulmonary capillaries.

36 FIo₂. The fraction of inspired oxygen, an alternate method of expressing oxygen percentage in the inspired air. Can be used to express the percentage of

any inspired gas by using the chemical symbol for the gas.

37 Hematocrit. The volume, in percent, of erythrocytes (red blood cells) in whole blood. Usually obtained by centrifuging whole blood and separating the blood solids from the plasma. Adult male normal is 40 to 54 volumes per 100 ml (45%), and adult female normal is 37 to 47 volumes per 100 ml (40%).

38 Hemoglobin (Hb). The red pigment responsible for carrying oxygen (see Module Four).

39 Hypercapnia. Above normal carbon dioxide in the blood; also hypercapnea.

40 Hyperkalemia. Above normal serum potassium.

41 Hypocapnia. Below normal carbon dioxide in the blood; also hypocarbia.

42 Hypokalemia. Below normal serum potassium.

43 Internal respiration. The exchange of gases between the blood and the body's tissues.

44 Interstitial edema. An accumulation of fluid *between tissue layers;* in pulmonary disease the fluid builds up between these layers and adversely affects the alveolar-capillary membrane.

45 Intrapleulra pressure. Normally subatmospheric pressure within the intrapleural space; also intrathoracic pressure.

46 Intrapulmonary pressure. Airway pressure; pressure within the lungs.

47 Ion. An element that has either a positive or negative net electric charge.

48 Kidney function. The performance of the kidney in either excreting acid (H^+ ions) or base (HCO_3^-).

49 Lactic acid. An acid produced by anaerobic (without oxygen) metabolism; an abnormal blood acid.

50 Lung function. The performance of the lungs in the elimination or retention of carbon dioxide.

51 Metabolism. The cellular process by which energy is produced and utilized; biochemistry of the life process.

52 Microcirculation. The capillary system; in the lung, the small vessels in which gas exchange takes place.

53 mm Hg. Millimeters of mercury, a unit of pressure equal to 1.36 cm H_2O

54 Oxygen affinity. The willingness of hemoglobin to accept or unwillingness to give up O_2 molecules.

55 Oxygen-carrying capacity. The capacity of the blood to carry oxygen; the total possible O_2 content of the blood, or 20.8 ml O_2/100 ml of blood.

56 Oxygen content. The sum of all oxygen in the blood; includes both oxygen bound to hemoglobin and dissolved oxygen, normally about 97.5%.

57 Oxygen dissociation curve. A graphic curve that shows the relationship between partial pressure of oxygen and percent saturation of hemoglobin with oxygen. A significance of this curve is the fact that the upper portion slopes very gradually, indicating that a relatively large drop in the oxygen tension results in only a small decrease in oxyhemoglobin (HbO_2) (Fig. 8-42).

58 Partial pressure. The pressure exerted by one gas in a mixture of gases.

59 Perfusion. The flow of blood throughout the body's tissues.

60 pH. A logarithmic scale used in expressing the hydrogen ion concentration (that is, how acid or alkaline the blood is in relation to normal).

61 Physiologic shunt. The percentage of cardiac output that does *not* exchange with the alveolar air; a small percentage is considered normal (1% to 5%).

62 Reduced hemoglobin. Hemoglobin with a depleted oxygen content but with enough oxygen still attached to maintain a partial pressure of approximatley 40 mm Hg.

63 Respiration. The exchange of gas molecules.

64 Respiratory failure. The "failure" or inability of the lungs to meet the metabolic needs of the body by providing oxygen and eliminating carbon dioxide.

65 Respiratory quotient (R.Q.). The ratio of carbon dioxide volume produced to the volume of oxygen consumed. For a 70 kg (150-pound) man, 200 ml of carbon dioxide is produced for every 250 ml of oxygen consumed for an R.Q. of 200/250 or 0.8.

66 Severinghaus electrode. A device used to measure carbon dioxide; can also be used to measure pH.

67 Shunt. Literally, a short circuit or a bypass of a normal route. In lung physiology an anatomic shunt is one in which there exists direct communication between an artery and a vein. A physiologic shunt is one where blood flows past alveoli with no ventilation.

68 Standard bicarbonate. The measurement of plasma bicarbonate referenced to a "normal" Pco_2 of 40 mm Hg.

69 Tension. The partial pressure of a gas.

70 Total physiologic shunt. The portion of cardiac output that does not exchange with alveolar air when one breathes room air or 21% oxygen.

71 True physiologic shunt. The portion of the cardiac output that does not exchange with alveolar air when one breathes 100% oxygen (see Absolute shunt, term no. 1).

72 Venous admixture. Shunting resulting from perfusion in excess of ventilation; uneven distribution of ventilation.

73 Ventilation. Movement of air into and out of the lungs; mechanical ventilation.

74 Ventilatory failure. The "failure" or inability of the respiratory system to eliminate carbon dioxide as fast as the body produces it.

75 Ventilatory insufficiency. Alveolar hypoventilation.

7.2 Symbols used in blood gas physiology

1 The following columnar material shows the use of *primary symbols* with examples:*

Symbols	Example
A, Alveolar	P_{AO_2}, Alveolar oxygen tension
C, Content in blood	Ca_{O_2}, Arterial oxygen content
D, Dead space	V_D, Dead space volume

---

*A dash above any symbol indicates a mean value; a dot above any symbol indicates a time limit, (e.g., $\dot{V}$, volume moved per unit of time or flow).

Symbols	Example
E, Expired	V_E, Expired volume of gas
F, Fraction of gas, concentration	FI_{O_2}, Fraction of inspired concentration of oxygen
I, Inspired	PI_{O_2}, Partial pressure of inspired oxygen
P, Pressure (blood or gas)	Pa_{O_2}, Arterial oxygen tension
Q, Blood volume	Qs, Volume of shunted blood
Q̇, Blood flow	$\dot{Q}a$, Arterial blood flow
S, Saturation	Sa_{O_2} Arterial oxygen saturation
a, Arterial	Pa_{CO_2}, Arterial carbon dioxide tension
c, Capillary	$\dot{Q}c$, Capillary blood flow
v, Venous	Qv, Venous blood volume
v̄, Mixed venous	$P\bar{v}_{O_2}$, Mixed venous oxygen tension
T, Tidal	V_T, Tidal volume
V, Volume of gas	V_A, Volume of alveolar gas
V̇, Gas volume per unit of time	$\dot{V}_{O_2}$, Oxygen consumption/minute

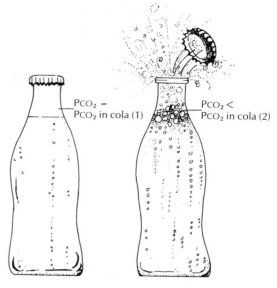

FIGURE 8-40 Demonstration by Henry's law. The dissolved CO_2 in cola is equal to the partial pressure of CO_2 in the space just under the cap. When the cap is lifted and the cola is exposed to the lower levels of atmospheric CO_2, the dissolved CO_2 comes out of solution and enters the atmosphere. This causes the cola to fizz.

The use of standard conditions permits an accurate comparison of multiple observations by the same operator or by different operators. The following abbreviations (commonly combined) refer to standard conditions: STP, standard temperature and pressure; D, dry gas; AT, ambient temperature; AP, ambient pressure; S, saturation.

  a STPD, Gas measurement at 0° C, 760 mm Hg (torr), dry

  b ATPS, Measurement made at ambient temperature and pressure, saturated with water vapor

  c BTPS, Body temperature (37° C), body pressure, saturated with water vapor

8.0 BASIC CONCEPTS OF ARTERIAL BLOOD GASES
8.1 Basic concepts relating to blood gases

 1 The study of blood gases is primarily related to understanding the exchange of oxygen and carbon dioxide between the inspired air and the body's tissues.

 2 In order to understand blood gases and their measurement, one must first understand the nature of gases in general and how they behave in liquids (i.e., blood).

  a The gases usually measured in blood are oxygen and carbon dioxide and are referred to by their partial pressures. The term "gas tension" is sometimes used instead of partial pressure.

  b Although not a "gas," the pH of blood is considered an integral part of blood gas measurement and does have an important relationship with CO_2 tension.

 3 Review the primary gas laws discussed in Unit 4.7:

  a Boyle's law (T = P × V)*

  b Charles' law $P = \dfrac{T}{V}$

  c Gay-Lussac's law $V = \dfrac{T}{P}$

  d Dalton's law ($P_{total} = P_1 + P_2 + P_3$, etc.)

  e Henry's law. When a liquid is exposed to a gas, the gas molecules will move into the liquid and exist in a dissolved state, providing the gas does not chemically combine with the liquid. The weight of gas dissolved in the liquid is proportional to the partial pressure of the gas.

  For example, the partial pressure of oxygen in a glass of water on a counter top will be exactly the same as the partial pressure of oxygen in the atmosphere.

  Further, the dissolved carbon dioxide in a cola (Fig. 8-40) is equal to the partial pressure of carbon dioxide in the half inch or so of free space under the unopened bottle cap *(1)*. This pressure causes a state of equilibrium to exist between the gas molecules in the liquid and the area above the liquid. When the cap is lifted the interfacing equalizing pressure is released, and the carbon dioxide comes out of solution as it moves into the room's atmosphere, which has relatively low CO_2. This movement causes the cola to fizz *(2)*. Eventually the cola will be "flat," because the carbon dioxide in the bottle reaches equilibrium with the carbon dioxide in the atmosphere.

  Similar gas movement occurs between the alveoli and the blood and between the tissues and the blood. This movement is not rapid enough to cause bubbles except when extreme pressure gradients exist such as is caused by a rapid ascent after a deep ocean dive, without allowing for time in decompression.

  f Graham's law. The speed with which a gas will diffuse through a liquid is directly proportional to its solubility coefficient and inversely proportional to the square root of its density. Remember the solubility coefficient is the amount of gas that can be dissolved by 1 ml of a given liquid at standard pressure

---
*T, temperature; P, pressure; V, volume.

and specified temperature. This is an important law to undestand because of the influence of the time factor involved in the exchange of gases across the alveolar-capillary membrane, which is primarily a fluid barrier.

  g The Fick principle. Similar to Graham's law in application (i.e., the rate of diffusion of a gas across a membrane or surface is proportional to the concentration gradient).

9.0 BASIC CONCEPTS OF PH
9.1 Basic concepts relating to pH

One of the most important concepts in studying blood gases is pH.

  1 The symbol "pH" is derived from the Scandinavian scientist S. P. L. Sörensen, who coined the term for puissance hydrogen (power of hydrogen).

  2 Hydrogen ion activity is a measure of dissociated hydrogen ions in solution. The free, and therefore unbuffered, hydrogen ion concentration depends on buffers that are available for use (i.e., the acids and bases).

  a The American biochemist L. J. Henderson developed an equation to express this buffer relationship:

$$(H^+) = K \frac{Acid}{Base}$$

  b This means that the hydrogen ion activity equals the physical solution constants of a given substance (K) times the acid (hydrogen ion donors), divided by the base (hydrogen ion recipients).

  c Since the hydrogen ion activity is between 0.0000001 mol/L* and 0.00000001 mol/L, it was decided to express this value logarithmically, or as exponents of the base 10:

$$10 = 10^1 \qquad 0.1 = 10^{-1}$$
$$100 = 10^2 \qquad 0.01 = 10^{-2}$$
$$1000 = 10^3 \qquad 0.001 = 10^{-3}$$
$$10,000,000 = 10^7 \qquad 0.0000001 = 10^{-7}$$

  • Therefore the normal hydrogen ion activity in the blood can be easily expressed as 10^{-7} to 10^{-8} mol/L.

  3 Also working on the concept of hydrogen ion activity, Danish biochemist and physician Karl Hasselbalch developed an expression for 10^{-7} mol/L as "the negative logarithm of the hydrogen ion activity" and pH could therefore be expressed as a positive number.

Hydrogen ion concentration in moles per liter	Fractional equivalent	Exponential notational equivalent	pH
0.0000001	$1/_{10,000,000}$	10^{-7}	7
0.00001	$1/_{100,000}$	10^{-5}	5
0.001	$1/_{1,000}$	10^{-3}	3
0.1	$1/_{10}$	10^{-1}	1

  a Note that pH corresponds to the number that appears as the minus power in the exponential form. pH equals "negative logarithm" times negative exponent

or a *positive* number. Note also that as hydrogen ion concentration *increases* (i.e., the blood becomes more acid), the pH *decreases*.

  b Henderson's original equation was applied directly, with the added concepts of Hasselbalch, to *blood* hydrogen ion activity as:

$$pH = pK + Log \frac{Base}{Acid}$$

or as what is now known as the Henderson-Hasselbalch equation.

  c Since the major blood base is the bicarbonate ion (HCO_3^-) and the major blood acid is carbonic acid (H_2CO_3), it is possible to work out a ratio by means of this equation. It is necessary, in addition, to know the pK (constant) of blood, which is 6.1. Plugging these values into the equation we get:

$$pH = pK + Log \frac{Base}{Acid}$$

  • $\dfrac{Base}{Acid} = \dfrac{HCO_3}{H_2CO_3} = \dfrac{25.4 \text{ mEq/L}}{1.27 \text{ mEq/L}} = \dfrac{20}{1}$

  • Logarithm of $\dfrac{20}{1} = 20 = 1.3$

  • Blood pK at BTPS = 6.1

  $pH = 6.1 + \log \dfrac{20}{1}$

  $ph = 6.1 + 1.3 = 7.4$

where BTPS is body temperature (37° C) atmospheric pressure, saturated with water vapor.

  4 By solving the Henderson-Hasselbalch equation, it is determined that the normal arterial blood pH is 7.4. Note that this is slightly more alkaline than pH 7.0, which is *neutral* (based on pure water).

  5 In homeostasis the pH of arterial blood is maintained within rather narrow limits; the normal phase of pH extends from *7.35 to 7.45*. Any value outside this range represents an acid-base imbalance.

  a A patient whose arterial blood displays a pH below 7.35 is said to be in *acidemia*. On the other hand, an arterial pH above 7.45 is said to represent *alkalemia*.

  • The literal definition of acidemia is "acid blood," and alkalemia means "basic blood or alkaline blood." These are relative terms, however, because they must be compared to what is normal for an individual as well as the textbook norm.

  – Technically in chemistry a pH reading below 7.0 must be reached before a solution can be called acid. In human physiology, acidemia is referred to as any pH reading "more acid than" 7.35. For example, chemically a pH of 7.05 is still in the alkaline range, although physiologically it would be considered extreme acidemia.

  • Acidemia is an important clinical consideration because of its interplay on cardiac function, bronchiole patency, and overall tissue perfusion. Continued survival is unlikely whenever a patient's arterial blood pH *drops below 6.8 or exceeds 8.0*.

---

*A mole is the formula weight of a substance expressed in grams.

10.0 PRODUCTION, TRANSPORTATION, AND ELIMINATION OF CARBON DIOXIDE

10.1 Transport of carbon dioxide

1 The partial pressure (tension) of CO_2 gas in physical solution within an arterial blood sample is reported as the "$Paco_2$."
   • This measurement provides a description of but one of the several ways that carbon dioxide is transported in the blood.
2 Carbon dioxide may be carried in the blood, *dissolved*, as *bicarbonate*, and in *combinations with proteins*.
3 Carbon dioxide is physically soluble in blood plasma. This combination results from a chemical reaction by which water and CO_2 combine to form carbonic acid. About 5% of the total carbon dioxide reacts in this manner.

$$CO_2 \text{ gas } + H_2O \rightarrow CO_2 \text{ solution (physical change)}$$
$$CO_2 \text{ solution } + H_2O \rightarrow H_2CO_3 \text{ (chemical change)}$$

4 H_2CO_3 is the formula for carbonic acid, a weak acid because of its tendency to form hydrogen ions as depicted by the following reaction:

$$H_2CO_3 \leftrightharpoons H^+ + HCO_3^-$$

The double arrows denote a reversible reaction showing that the reaction can go either way, depending on external conditions.
   a In the blood, carbonic acid (H_2CO_3) breaks down into hydrogen ions (H^+) and bicarbonate ions (HCO_3^-).
   b The free (dissociated) hydrogen ions (H^+) from the carbonic acid are responsible for determining blood pH.
5 Most of the total carbon dioxide in the blood (95%) is carried by the *erythrocyte* (red cell) in the following manner:
   a *Dissolved in the erythrocyte water:* a very small fraction.
   b *Combined with hemoglobin.* Known as reduced hemoglobin, the carbon dioxide rides on red blood cells, which have released their oxygen to the tissues. This protein is called "carbaminohemoglobin" or "carbino-Hb" and comprises approximately 10% of total blood carbon dioxide.

c This *protein is further changed chemically* into carbonic acid as a result of a chemical reaction helped along by the enzyme catalyst *carbonic anhydrase*.

10.2 Physiologic balance of carbon dioxide

1 The body's metabolic rate is balanced against the effectiveness of the lungs to remove carbon dioxide and the kidneys to retain or excrete bicarbonate.
   a The physical ability of the body to move air in and out of the lungs and its conducting passages is but one measure of ventilation. Physiologically the effectiveness of the lung to eliminate carbon dioxide is determined by a specific variable known as *alveolar* or *effective ventilation*.
   b Effective ventilation is only that portion of the inspired gas volume, natural or mechanical, that actually participates in gas exchange with the pulmonary blood.
2 Gas exchange between the blood and the alveoli occurs because of the pressure gradient differences (Fig. 8-41). Carbon dioxide continues to leave (diffuse from) the mixed venous blood that has returned from the tissue until the CO_2 tension in the blood equals the CO_2 tension in the alveoli. Oxygen leaves the alveoli and goes to the pulmonary blood in the same manner.
3 Three components must be present at the alveolar level for effective gas exchange and subsequent tissue oxygenation:
   a A fresh volume of gas must be available in the alveoli.
   b A pressure gradient must exist between the alveoli and the capillary blood.
   c Blood must circulate through the pulmonary capillaries that interface with alveoli.
      • If these conditions are not met in sufficient quantity, tissues will not receive adequate supplies of oxygen, nor will they be able to eliminate carbon dioxide, a by-product of cellular metabolism.
4 Although the lung is considered a single unit where ventilation and perfusion are perfectly matched, this is not actually the case. The lung has many functioning alveolar units that have different ventilation/perfusion ($\dot{V}A/\dot{Q}$) characteristics. Fortunately these units are reg-

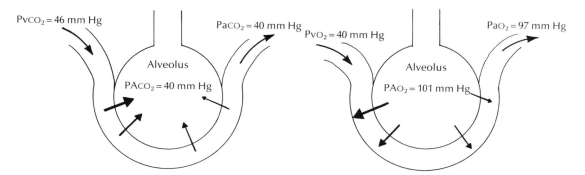

FIGURE 8-41 Pressure gradient differences between blood and alveoli cause gas exchange to occur.

ulated to the degree that some are overventilated in relation to their perfusion, whereas others are underventilated compared to their perfusion (i.e., homeostasis is maintained by an *average* of ventilation-to-perfusion relationships of all lung units). This relationship is normally maintained at a $\dot{V}A/\dot{Q}$ ratio of 1.

5 In sick patients, situations develop where there occurs wasted ventilation and/or wasted blood flow relative to the normal lung process.

a *Wasted ventilation* or *dead space* is identified as the sum of anatomic and alveolar dead space and is frequently referred to as "physiologic dead space."

• *Anatomic dead space.* The amount of air contained in the conducting airways that does not undergo gas exchange. It is a fairly constant figure and is related directly to body size. Anatomic dead space is equal to approximately *1 ml* for each pound of body weight in the adult.

• *Alveolar dead space.* This space occurs whenever air is entering and leaving the alveoli that are *not* being perfused by pulmonary blood. This type of dead space is difficult to measure, because it is subject to change constantly.

b Wasted blood flow (shunt) refers to circumstances that cause the pulmonary blood to bypass the ventilated lung altogether. This ultimately results in a mixing of unoxygenated blood with oxygenated blood from normally functioning lung units. This venous admixture decreases the percentage of oxygen available to the tissues. A similar situation occurs whenever the blood flow perfusing an alveolus exceeds the gas-exchanging potential of the alveolus. This abnormal ventilation-perfusion relationship results in venous admixture or physiologic shunt units.

• Wasted ventilation and perfusion are not desirable and result in hypoxic conditions and/or excessive CO_2 levels.

6 A measurement of CO_2 tension is the *best single indication* of whether alveolar ventilation is effective. In diffusion defects most patients will have an arterial CO_2 tension ($PaCO_2$) of 40 torr (mm Hg), because carbon dioxide is 21 times more soluble in water than oxygen, and carbon dioxide *is not* usually affected by the increased alveolar-capillary (a-c) distance that many pulmonary diseases cause.

a To estimate alveolar ventilation ($\dot{V}A$) measure the total amount of air exhaled in a minute ($\dot{V}E$) minus the estimated dead space ventilation (VD):

$$\dot{V}A = \dot{V}E - VD$$

• Note that 1 pound of body weight equals approximately 1 ml of anatomic dead space. Tracheostomy tubes and endotracheal tubes will reduce the anatomic dead space up to 50%, because they bypass the anatomic structures of the upper airway.

b It is frequently necessary, especially with mechanical ventilation, to calculate a ratio of dead space to total volume (VD/VT).

c The VD/VT ratio measures that portion of the tidal volume that is physiologic dead space or wasted ventilation because it did not participate in gas exchange with the blood. In normal young adults physiologic dead space is less than 30% of the tidal volume. This value increases with age.

• A formula for determining the VD/VT ratio is:

$$\frac{VD}{VT} = \frac{PaCO_2 - P\bar{E}CO_2}{PaCO_2}$$

where $PaCO_2$ is the arterial tension of carbon dioxide and $P\bar{E}CO_2$ is the mean expired CO_2 tension. A normal VD/VT is 0.2 to 0.4.

10.3 Carbon dioxide production

Carbon dioxide is normally produced at a rate equal to that eliminated by the alveoli (i.e., a state of homeostasis exists with the body eliminating the waste products of metabolism).

An increase in metabolic demands will cause an equal increase in ventilation to eliminate the increased amounts of carbon dioxide being produced.

1 To determine CO_2 production the following formula may be used:

$$\dot{V}CO_2 = \frac{\dot{V}A \times PACO_2}{Factor}$$

where $\dot{V}CO_2$ is the CO_2 production, $\dot{V}A$ is the alveolar ventilation, $PACO_2$ is the alveolar CO_2 tension, and there is a physiologic conversion factor.

a The physiologic conversion factor (0.863) equals a conversion of gas volume at BTPS* to gas volume at STPD* and correction for alveolar water vapor pressure.

EXAMPLE:
$$\dot{V}A = 5 \text{ L/min} - 150 \text{ VD}$$
$$\dot{V}A = 4.85 \text{ L/min}$$
$$PACO_2 = 40 \text{ mm Hg}$$
$$\dot{V}CO_2 = \frac{4.85 \times 40 \text{ mm Hg}}{0.863}$$
$$\dot{V}CO_2 = 224 \text{ ml/min}$$

11.0 TRANSPORTATION AND UTILIZATION OF OXYGEN
11.1 Transport of oxygen

1 Oxygen is required to support aerobic metabolism. Without an adequate supply of oxygen, energy cannot be generated by the cells, and death will occur. At rest or in a basal state, the individual requires about *250 ml* of oxygen per minute. During exercise this may increase to greater than 5 L O_2/min, or 20 times the basal needs. This is an important clinical consideration be-

*See Unit 7.2 *(1)*.

cause increased rates and depth of breathing cause increased O_2 consumption.

2 Most of the body's oxygen is present in loose chemical combination with *hemoglobin* (Hb). Hemoglobin is a pigmented protein with a molecular weight of 62,500 atomic mass units!

   a Each of these giant molecules has four iron-containing heme groups, and it is at these four sites that oxygen is bound (carried). The normal adult has 12 to 15 g Hb/100 ml blood, or expressed as grams percent (g %).

   b Oxyhemoglobin is defined as hemoglobin to which oxygen is bound and is symbolized as HbO_2.

3 As noted in Unit 10.1, carbon dioxide also combines with hemoglobin but at different sites, the amino group. Therefore hemoglobin carries oxygen and carbon dioxide simultaneously.

4 Carbon monoxide (CO) will also bind with hemoglobin and at the same heme sites as oxygen. The presence of carbon monoxide in breathing air is very hazardous, because hemoglobin has a much greater affinity for carbon monoxide than for oxygen (200 times), and carboxyhemoglobin (HbCO) is much less reversible than oxygen binding on the same site. Therefore the formation of carboxyhemoglobin severely limits the O_2 carrying capacity of hemoglobin.

5 It should be noted that O_2 molecules attached to hemoglobin are not dissolved oxygen and do not exert a partial pressure (tension).

6 The *partial pressure of oxygen* measured in the blood is that portion dissolved in the plasma, and this results from whatever is left over after all the hemoglobin sites have been filled.

7 For each 760 mm Hg of pressure a 0.023 ml of oxygen dissolves in each milliliter of blood. This is referred to in physiology as "volume percent" (vol %) or a certain number of milliliters of gas per 100 ml of plasma. Therefore for every 760 mm Hg of pressure there is a vol % of 2.3 of dissolved oxygen or 0.003 vol % for each millimeter of mercury.

   a *Oxygen capacity* is the amount of oxygen in milliliters that can be maximally bound to hemoglobin. Each gram of normal hemoglobin can bind with 1.34 ml of oxygen.

   b *Oxygen saturation* is defined as the ratio of hemoglobin O_2 content to O_2 capacity expressed as a percentage.

    • Oxygen capacity can be calculated by knowing the number of grams of hemoglobin per 100 ml of blood. Therefore an adult normally has 15 g Hb/ 100 ml blood; thus

$$(15 \text{ g Hb}/100 \text{ ml blood}) (1.34 \text{ ml } O_2/\text{g Hb}) =$$
$$20.0 \text{ ml } O_2/100 \text{ ml blood}$$

    • Oxygen saturation varies directly with O_2 tension (P_{O_2}), but the relation is nonlinear. If O_2 saturation is plotted on a graph ordinate and the P_{O_2} on the abscissa, the *oxyhemoglobin dissociation curve* results. The curve is sigmoid or S shaped (Fig 8-42).

    – The shape of this curve is very important. The relatively flat portion above 70 mm Hg P_{O_2} makes sure that most of the hemoglobin will be oxygenated even though there may be wide swings in alveolar (and arterial) oxygen tensions.

    – The steep portion of the curve between 10 and 50 mm Hg P_{O_2} ensures that large amounts of oxygen

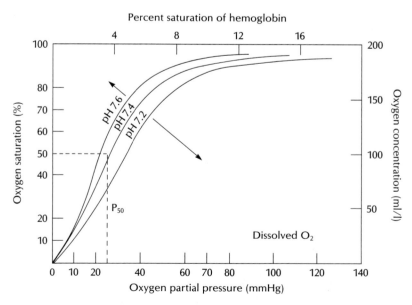

FIGURE 8-42 Oxyhemoglobin dissociation curve. (Modified from Current Reviews in Respiratory Therapy, lesson 14, vol 9, 1987.)

will be unloaded in the capillaries throughout the body.

- In other words, the shape of the curve means that the hemoglobin holds on to oxygen over a wide range at the upper end of the curve and readily lets go of the oxygen at the lower tension areas.

8 The concept of P_{50} is defined as the O_2 tension at which the O_2 saturation is 50%. If someone refers to a *higher* P_{50}, this means that the affinity of hemoglobin for oxygen is decreased, or it takes a higher O_2 pressure to load on the same amount of oxygen. As a result, hemoglobin will accept oxygen less readily and give up oxygen more readily to tissues.

  a A P_{50} *lower* than normal means the affinity of hemoglobin for oxygen is increased, or the same amount of oxygen can be loaded on the hemoglobin at a lower pressure. Therefore hemoglobin will accept oxygen more readily at the alveoli but release oxygen less readily at the tissues.

  b The normal P_{50} is 27 mm Hg (torr).

9 The entire oxyhemoglobin dissociation curve can be *shifted* left or right, thereby lowering or raising the P_{50}.

  a A "left shift" of the curve may be caused by:
  - Alkalemia ($\downarrow$ H^+)
  - Hypothermia ($\downarrow$ temperature)
  - Hypocapnia ($\downarrow$ CO_2)
  - Reduced 2,3-diphosphoglycerate (DPG): an enzyme that speeds the dissociation of oxygen from hemoglobin)

  b A "right shift" of the curve may be caused by:
  - Acidemia ($\uparrow$ H^+)
  - Hyperthermia ($\uparrow$ temperature)
  - Hypercapnia ($\uparrow$ CO_2)
  - Increased DPG

11.2 Oxygen uptake/shunts

1 Oxygen uptake is the difference between the amount of oxygen in the venous blood arriving at the lung and the amount leaving the lung in the systemic arterial blood.

2 As previously explained, the concept of ventilation and perfusion is defined by the ventilation/perfusion ($\dot{V}A/\dot{Q}$) ratio, which is simply the degree to which venous blood picks up oxygen from the alveolus.

  a This ratio will vary in the lung from place to place as a result of the effects of gravity on perfusion.

  b $\dot{V}/\dot{Q}$ abnormalities or inequality introduces the concept of *shunting*. A shunt is that portion of the blood that *does not exchange* with alveolar air.

3 There are basically three types of physiologic ventilatory shunts:

  a *Anatomic shunting*. A very small portion of blood ($\simeq$ 2%) goes directly into the left side of the heart without oxygenation. This is blood that comes from the bronchial, pleural, and thebesian veins. Specifically, any blood that leaves the right side of the heart and goes to the left side of the heart without going through the pulmonary capillaries is anatomic shunting.

  b *Capillary shunting*. Whenever blood flows past an alveolus that is unventilated, the blood will not exchange gases. Anatomic and capillary shunting added together constitute *true shunting*. True shunting (also called "absolute shunting") is *not* corrected by increasing the inspired oxygen concentration. Even with 100% oxygen, the patient's Pa_{O_2} will not respond when there is true or absolute shunting because of venous admixing. It is interesting to note that 100% oxygen actually increases the shunt.

  c *Perfusion in excess of ventilation*. Blood that passes a poorly ventilated alveolus, or blood in which there is an alveolar-capillary restriction to diffusion, will leave with a lower than normal Pa_{O_2}. This is called *venous admixture* or *shunt effect*. It is technically a ventilation perfusion inequality and is extremely variable.

12.0 ACID-BASE RELATIONSHIPS IN THE BLOOD
12.1 Control of acid-base balance

1 As was discussed in Unit 10.1, carbon dioxide's transport greatly influences the overall acid-base status of the blood and the body in general.

  a Because carbon dioxide is an acid producer, an increase or decrease in the arterial P_{CO_2} will result in a similar change in the arterial pH and vice versa.

  b The lungs can dispense with more than 12,000 mEq of carbonic acid as carbon dioxide per day compared with the kidneys, which excrete only 100 mEq of acid per day. This means that the lungs are the body's primary means of controlling CO_2 levels.

2 From an earlier discussion of the Henderson-Hasselbalch equation, it was noted that for every measure of acid, there are 20 measures of base. As long as the ratio remains the same, the pH will remain at 7.4 or normal. This bicarbonate proportion is provided by the kidneys, which retain or release acid and base through the urine.

  a It is critically important that the body maintain its pH balance within a very narrow range. It is doubtful that many people will survive a pH below 6.8 or above 8.0.

  b The pH can be affected by sickness, disease, emotional upsets (hyperventilation), food, and drink. The body is well equipped to deal with the constant chemical shifting necessary to maintain pH control.

3 If the blood pH should rise and become more alkaline, then a state of *alkalosis* is said to exist. If the pH falls and the blood is less alkaline, a state of *acidosis* is said to exist. These changes cause undesirable cardiac arrhythmias as well as vascular and airway changes.

4 There are two forms of acidosis and alkalosis: *respiratory* and *metabolic*.

  a If, as a result of respiratory disease, the lungs are not able to ventilate and "blow off" excessive carbon dioxide, then carbonic acid will accumulate and the pH will fall, causing a *respiratory acidosis*.

b If, on the other hand, some disturbance causes excessive hyperventilation and the lungs eliminate excessive amounts of carbon dioxide, then there would be a drop in carbonic acid (hydrogen ions) causing a rise in pH and *respiratory alkalosis*.

5 Simply stated, the causes of respiratory acidosis are conditions such as hypoventilation that lead to decreased elimination of carbon dioxide from the lungs. Similarly, the causes of respiratory alkalosis are conditions such as hyperventilation that lead to increased elimination of carbon dioxide by the lungs.

a Hypoventilation is primarily caused by conditions that prevent adequate ventilation. These include:
- Chest trauma
- Drug overdose
- Airway obstructions
- Chronic and acute pulmonary obstructive disease
- Neuromuscular defects
- Impaired diffusion and gas exchange
- Restrictive defects

b The *clinical signs of hypoventilation with CO_2 retention* are:
- Pinpoint pupils
- Lethargy, confusion, hallucination, coma
- Full bounding pulses with peripheral vasodilation
- Papilledema, headaches, insomnia, or reversal of sleep patterns

c The treatment for uncompensated respiratory acidosis is to remove the cause of, or compensate for, hypoventilation. This includes*:
- Establish satisfactory tidal volume (10 to 15 ml/kg in the adult).
- Reduce Pa_{CO_2} about 10 mm Hg/hr by mechanical ventilation.
- Give low percentage oxygen (1 to 3 L/min).
- Give sodium bicarbonate.
- Give potassium chloride if needed.

d Hyperventilation is primarily caused by conditions such as:
- Hypoxia
- Pulmonary emboli
- Emotional disturbances
- Pregnancy
- Mechanical ventilation

e The *clinical signs of hyperventilation* are:
- Dizziness
- Tingling or numbness of extremities
- Muscular spasms of hands and feet and possibly tetany

f The treatment for severe uncompensated respiratory alkalosis (hyperventilation)*:
- Give barbiturates, morphine, or tranquilizers.
- If the patient is connected to a mechanical ventilator, add 6-inch sections of mechanical dead space at 15-minute intervals until a Pa_{CO_2} of 35 to 45

torr is reached. O_2-CO_2 mixtures are not recommended.
- Give low percentage oxygen if hypoxia is present.

6 There are several different types of acids that are *not* associated with lung function and are usually controlled by the kidneys, which retain or excrete appropriate volumes of acids or base to maintain a normal blood pH. Acid-base disturbances caused by these acids are said to be *metabolic* and usually occur from chronic diseases over long periods of time.

a *Lactic acid*. This is produced whenever insufficient oxygen is available for normal aerobic metabolism to take place and the tissues are forced to shift to anaerobic metabolism. For example, this can occur with physical exertion beyond the body's ability to supply oxygen to itself. Recovery is achieved by reducing tissue or muscle action to reduce O_2 consumption. As the tissue resumes normal aerobic metabolism, the lactic acid will be metabolized and carbon dioxide will be produced as usual.

b *Keto acids*. This form of acid results from metabolism that occurs in the absence of insulin action. Glucose (sugar), necessary for normal metabolism, is controlled by the presence of insulin. Therefore a diabetic who is entering a "ketoacidosis" or metabolic acidosis because of insulin lack requires insulin to return metabolism to normal. It is rare, if ever necessary, to intervene with respiratory means in treating uncomplicated ketoacidosis.

c *Exogenous acids*. Since most food and drink are acidic, the action of the kidney is responsible for excreting these acids. When there is renal disease or failure, these acids accumulate, causing an exogenous or renal acidosis.

7 A summary of the more common causes of nonrespiratory metabolic acidosis follows:
a Diabetic ketoacidosis
b Poisonings
- Salicylate
- Ethylene glycol
- Methyl alcohol
- Paraldehyde

c Lactic acidosis
d Renal failure

8 The *clinical signs of metabolic acidosis* include:
a Kussmaul respiration
b Simple hyperventilation
c Nausea/vomiting
d Hypotension/cardiac arrhthmias
e Lethargy and coma

9 Another type of acid-base disorder is *metabolic alkalosis*. This occurs as a result of prolonged vomiting, which depletes the body of its stomach contents (hydrochloric acid), lowering its hydrogen ion level. Eating or drinking a strong alkali will accomplish the same effect.

10 A summary of the more common causes of nonrespiratory metabolic alkalosis follows:

---

*All treatment is delivered under medical orders by a physician.

a Excessive intake of milk

b Loss of the body's fixed acid by vomiting or naso-gastric suction

c Excessive loss of potassium (use of diuretics)
  • The clinical signs of metabolic alkalosis include muscular weakness and tetany.

11 To help regulate the acid-base balance the blood contains a system of *buffers* or alkaline reserves that will neutralize abnormal acids. These blood bases include sodium, calcium, potassium, and magnesium bound as bicarbonate salts. In this discussion the sodium bicarbonate buffer will be the primary system.

  a The bicarbonate ion concentration is expressed in milliequivalents per liter with a normal range of about 22 to 26 mEq/L.

  b Because bicarbonate ions readily associate with hydrogen ions, the bicarbonate ion can be considered a strong base. Therefore a high bicarbonate ion concentration is the same thing as a *base excess* and will thus tend to raise the pH (metabolic alkalosis).

  c A subnormal bicarbonate ion concentration (base deficit) tends to result in a surplus of hydrogen ions and a reduced pH (metabolic acidosis).

  d Whenever the bicarbonate level moves outside the normal range of 22 to 26 mEq/L, this means that there is some metabolic component to the disturbance in the blood gases.

12 Contrary to the quickness with which the lungs respond to a respiratory disturbance, the kidneys (metabolic component) are very slow to respond and usually take hours to days to adjust.

  a For example, if a primary respiratory acidosis develops, the kidneys will normally *compensate* by holding onto alkaline buffers to balance the increased acidemia. However, this compensation may not begin for several hours and may not be complete for up to 24 to 36 hours after the initial change.

  b As a result of this time lag, *acute* respiratory acidosis and respiratory alkalosis are uncompensated because of the length of time it takes for the kidneys to hold onto or speed excretion of bicarbonate (alkaline buffers). Long-term (chronic) respiratory acidosis and alkalosis are usually *well compensated*.

13 *Compensation* means that the source of the disturbance has *not* been eliminated. The body is simply trying to maintain the pH at a normal level. For example, a patient with chronic lung disease may have a Pco_2 of 60 mm Hg and a bicarbonate level of 34 mEq/L, which are certainly not normal. But this patient's pH of 7.38 is well within the normal range. Since the Pco_2 is unlikely to change, the kidneys will continue to compensate by retaining bicarbonate.

14 *Correction* means that the source of disturbance has been eliminated. If, for example, the patient cited in **13** could by some miracle "blow off" the excess carbon dioxide and return to a $Paco_2$ of 40 mm Hg, then the bicarbonate level would also fall back to around 24 mEq/L to maintain the pH at or near 7.4.

• Correction can also occur by respiratory means. The diabetic in severe ketoacidemia will have a characteristic form of hyperventilation called "Kussmaul respiration." This is the body's attempt by respiratory means to "blow off" the excessive metabolic acid.

13.0 ACID-BASE DISTURBANCES
13.1 Interpretation of acid-base disturbances

1 The first step in treating any problem is to *recognize the cause of the problem.*

2 A laboratory arterial blood gas report usually contains the following values:

  a Oxygen saturation %

  b Arterial O_2 tension (Pao_2) mm Hg

  c Arterial CO_2 tension ($Paco_2$) mm Hg

  d pH

  e Bicarbonate mEq/L

  f Hemoglobin (Hb)/hematocrit (hct)

  g Clinical status: fraction of inspired concentration of oxygen (FIo_2), respiratory rate, etc.

3 Each value provides a different look at a component of the blood sample, which must be considered separately and then together in reaching a conclusion about the patient's ventilatory status. A list of normal values for arterial and venous blood is presented in Table 8-7.

4 The following sequence should be followed in analyzing a blood gas report.

  a *Check the pH,* which indicates if the blood is too acid or too alkaline:
    • pH <7.35, acidemia
    • pH >7.45, alkalemia
      – The process causing acidemia is acidosis. The process causing alkalemia is alkalosis. Please note that both processes may be occurring simultaneously. If so, the pH will identify the *stronger process* (i.e., <7.35 if acidosis is stronger; >7.45 if alkalosis is stronger).

  b *Check the $Paco_2$,* which indicates how well the lungs are functioning. Remember $Paco_2$ refers to pressure or tension exerted by dissolved CO_2 gas in the blood and therefore is *influenced only by the lungs.*
    • Hypoventilation is a state caused whenever there is too much dissolved carbon dioxide in the blood (i.e., the lungs are not providing enough ventilation).

TABLE 8-7 Normal blood gas values

Value	Arterial blood	Mixed venous blood
pH	7.40 (7.35-7.45)	7.36 (7.31-7.41)
Pao_2	80-100 mm Hg	35-40 mm Hg
O_2 Saturation	95% or greater	70%-75%
$Paco_2$	35-45 mm Hg	41-51 mm Hg
HCO_3^-	22-26 mEq/L	22-26 mEq/L
Base excess	−2 to +2	−2 to +2

Note that only Pao_2, O_2 saturation, and $Paco_2$ are actual measurements of gases. The other values are indicators of metabolic involvement.

- Hyperventilation is a state caused whenever there is not enough dissolved carbon dioxide in the blood and the lungs are providing excessive ventilation.
- Carbon dioxide should be considered an acid because when it combines with water, it forms carbonic acid (H_2CO_3), which dissociates into a hydrogen ion (H^+) and bicarbonate (HCO_3^-). H^+ is buffered by plasma protein, whereas carbon dioxide must be eliminated by the kidneys as acid in urine and by the lung as CO_2 gas.

c Consider respiratory abnormalities:

Value	Condition	Cause
↑ Paco₂	Respiratory acidosis	↓ Ventilation
↓ Paco₂	Respiratory alkalosis	↑ Ventilation

d *Check bicarbonate* (HCO_3^-) and base excess (BE), which indicate whether or not the primary condition is metabolic or respiratory.
- HCO_3^- and BE are influenced only by metabolic processes that may be the result of anything other than respiratory disturbances that affects a patient's pH.
- Whenever a metabolic process causes an accumulation of acids in the body, or loss of bicarbonate occurs, HCO_3^- values will drop below normal range and the BE will become negative.
- Whenever a metabolic process causes a loss of acid, such as in vomiting, or accumulation of excessive HCO_3^-, bicarbonate values will rise and BE will be elevated from normal.

  NOTE: Base excess refers to HCO_3^- and also to plasma proteins and hemoglobin, which are bases in the blood.

e Consider metabolic abnormalities:

Value	Condition	Cause
↑ HCO₃⁻ or BE	Metabolic alkalosis	Acid ↓ or HCO₃⁻ ↑
↓ HCO₃⁻ or BE	Metabolic acidosis	Acid ↑ or HCO₃⁻ ↓

5 The body attempts to balance pH by two major mechanisms:

a Compensation. pH is normalized by altering the component not primarily affected. EXAMPLE: ↑ Paco₂, then HCO_3^- is retained.

b Correction. pH is normalized by altering the component primarily responsible. Example: ↑ Paco₂, then Pco₂ is ↓.

6 The body always strives to maintain a *balance between HCO_3^- and Pco₂ of 20:1.* At this ratio, pH is normal.

7 Paco₂ is inversely related to the pH and minute volume. Therefore an increase or decrease in Paco₂ of 10 torr from 40 torr will result in an increase or decrease of pH by 0.08 units.

EXAMPLE: Paco₂ increased by 20 torr (Paco₂ of 60 mm Hg),

$$pH = 2 \times .08 = 0.16$$

where 0.16 is subtracted from 7.40 because an increase in Paco₂ decreases pH to render a new pH of 7.24

8 In Fig. 8-43 the measurements of acid (Paco₂) and base

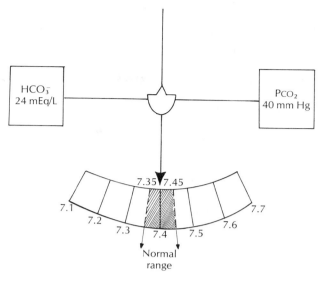

FIGURE 8-43 Measurements of acid (Pco₂) and base (HCO₃⁻) are balanced to a normal pH of 7.4.

TABLE 8-8 Blood gas states

Name of state	pH	Paco₂	HCO₃⁻
Respiratory acidosis			
Uncompensated (acute)	↓	↑	N
Partially compensated (subacute)	↓	↑	↑
Compensated (chronic)	N	↑	↑
Respiratory alkalosis			
Uncompensated (acute)	↑	↓	N
Partially compensated (subacute)	↑	↓	↓
Compensated (chronic)	N	↓	↓
Metabolic acidosis			
Uncompensated (acute)	↓	N	↓
Partially compensated (subacute)	↓	↓	↓
Compensated (chronic)	N	↓	↓
Metabolic alkalosis			
Uncompensated (acute)	↑	N	↑
Partially compensated (subacute)	↑	↑	↑
Compensated (chronic)	N	↑	↑

Arrows, Elevation or depression; N, normal.

(HCO_3^-) are balanced to a normal pH of 7.4. Remember, for a pH of 7.4, the base component would actually be *twenty* times "heavier" than the acid component.

9 For studying the states of acidemia and alkalemia, one needs the measurements of pH, Paco₂, and bicarbonate. Table 8-8 shows the relationship of the three values in the four areas of acid-base disturbance, and the following examples illustrate these concepts:

a pH, 7.45; Paco₂, 26; HCO₃⁻, 19
- The high pH is consistent with alkalemia.
- The subnormal Paco₂ indicates a respiratory alkalemia.
- The subnormal HCO_3^- reveals a metabolic acidemia.
  - Interpretation: partially compensated respiratory alkalosis.

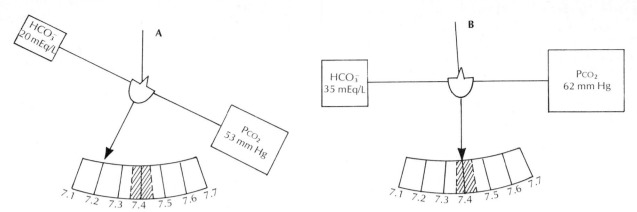

FIGURE 8-44 Respiratory acidosis. **A,** pH = 7.2; PCO_2 = 53 mm Hg; HCO_3^- = 20 mEq/L. Possible causes: respiratory failure, airway obstruction, central nervous system depression. Symptoms: Sluggishness, personality changes, central nervous system depression, somnolence. Treatments: restore the bicarbonate deficit, reverse central nervous system depression, mechanical ventilation; treat cause of respiratory failure. **B,** pH = 7.38; PCO_2 = 62 mm Hg; HCO_3^- = 35 mEq/L: compensated respiratory acidosis. Evidence: increased bicarbonate (kidney retention) has caused the pH to return to within normal range even though the PCO_2 is elevated.

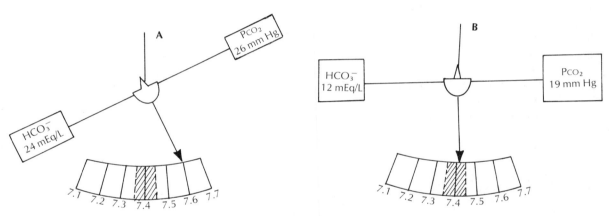

FIGURE 8-45 Respiratory alkalosis. **A,** pH = 7.6; PCO_2 = 26 mm Hg; HCO_3^- = 24 mEq/L. Possible causes: hyperventilation secondary to infection, central nervous system stimulation, cirrhosis, congestive heart failure, anxiety, excessive mechanical ventilation. Symptoms: any that reflect the possible causes; specifically, tingling of the extremities, dizziness, and possibly tetany. Treatments: eliminate cause for hyperventilation; do not administer mechanical dead space or oxygen–carbon dioxide mixtures in an attempt to increased PCO_2. **B,** pH = 7.42; PCO_2 = 19 mm Hg; HCO_3^- = 12 mEq/L: compensated respiratory alkalosis. Evidence: decreased bicarbonate (kidney excretion) has caused the pH to return to within normal range even though the pH is very low.

b pH, 7.48; $Paco_2$, 55; HCO_3^-, 38
- ↑ pH indicates alkalemia.
- ↑ $Paco_2$ indicates respiratory acidemia.
- ↑ HCO_3^- indicates metabolic alkalemia.
  - Interpretation: partially compensated metabolic alkalosis.

c pH, 7.13; $Paco_2$, 82; HCO_3^-, 24
- ↓ pH indicates acidemia.
- ↑ $Paco_2$ indicates respiratory acidemia.
- HCO_3^- shows a normal bicarbonate.
  - Interpretation: uncompensated respiratory acidosis.

10 Figs. 8-44 through 8-47 also illustrate the various acid-base states.

11 It may be helpful to memorize the following rules of thumb, which make it easier to determine whether or not a state is primarily respiratory:

a During acute changes HCO_3^- will increase 1 mEq/L for each 10 mm Hg increase in $Paco_2$ above 40 mm Hg (normal).

b During chronic changes HCO_3^- will increase 4 mEq/L for each 10 mm Hg increase in $Paco_2$ above 40 mm Hg.

c During acute changes HCO_3^- will decrease 2 mEq/L for each 10 mm Hg decrease in $Paco_2$ below 40 mm Hg.

12 The following two examples illustrate the use of the three rules to understanding bicarbonate:

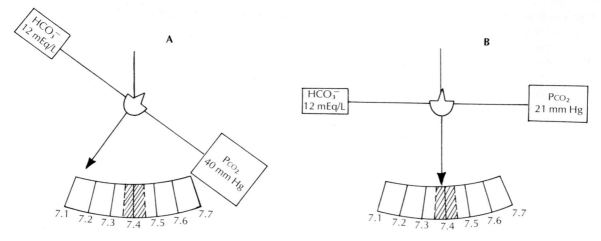

FIGURE 8-46 Metabolic acidosis. **A,** pH = 7.1; PCO_2 = 40 mm Hg; HCO_3^- = 12 mEq/L. Possible causes: kidney disease (uremic acidosis); abnormal production of metabolic acids, e.g., diabetic ketoacidosis; shock, causing lactic acidosis; loss of base (diarrhea, dysentery). Symptoms: extreme swings in pH may cause cardiac arrhythmias. Kussmaul respirations, possible lethargy and coma. Treatments: eliminate causative factor, depending on etiology; administer bicarbonate to restore base deficit; in extreme cases dialysis may be necessary. **B,** pH = 7.38; PCO_2 = 21 mm Hg; HCO_3^- = 12 mEq/L; compensated metabolic acidosis. Evidence: the lungs have "blown off" carbon dioxide to below normal levels but, in doing so, have caused the pH to return to within normal range.

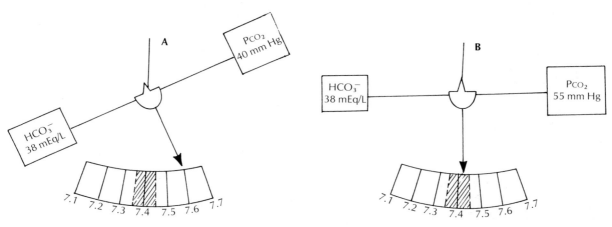

FIGURE 8-47 A, Metabolic alkalosis: pH = 7.6; PCO_2 = mm Hg; HCO_3^-. Possible causes: loss of hydrogen ions (acid) through vomiting, excessive intake of milk (milk alkali syndrome), potassium depletion (Diuretics, steroid therapy). Symptoms: muscular weakness, tetany, hypokalemia. Treatments: restore electrolyte balance; possible use of potassium chloride or ammonium chloride to raise blood acid levels; drugs to quicken bicarbonate elimination—acetazolamide (Diamox). **B,** pH = 7.43; PCO_2 = 55; HCO_3^- = 38: compensated metabolic alkalosis. Evidence: as a result of hypoventilation, carbon dioxide has accumulated in the blood to an above normal level, but the increased blood acid has caused the pH to return to within normal range.

a An otherwise healthy 22-year-old man suffers acute airway obstruction from a foreign body. ABGs on admission show:

pH	= 7.13
$Paco_2$	= 90 mm Hg
HCO_3^- (calculated)	= 28.2 mEq/L

It would seem that a bicarbonate of 28.2 mEq/L represents a metabolic alkalosis. Rule *a* in no. 11 shows, however, that at a $Paco_2$ of 90 mm Hg, the bicarbonate (HCO_3^-) should be in the range of 27 to 29 mEq/L if the increase is acute. Since 90 mm Hg less 40 mm Hg represents a

change of 5 units, subtracting this 5 mEq/L increase from the reported 28.2 mEq/L reveals a perfectly normal corrected value of 23.2 mEq/L. Since there is *no* metabolic component, the patient's normal state will be improved by restoring normal ventilation.

b A 60-year-old man with chronic obstructive pulmonary disease, chronic CO_2 retention, and an acute myocardial infarction is admitted to the critical care unit. ABGs on admission show:

pH	= 7.15
$Paco_2$	= 70 mm Hg
HCO_3^- (calculated)	= 23 mEq/L

These gases seem at first glance to reveal respiratory acidosis, but note that this patient has *chronic* lung disease and CO_2 retention. Rule *b* in no. 11 shows that the predicted HCO_3^- should be in the range of 33 to 44 mEq/L with a chronic $Paco_2$ of 70 mm Hg. Therefore the calculated HCO_3^- of 23 mEq/L is much less than it should be. This patient actually has a severe metabolic acidosis, possibly caused by cardiogenic shock brought on by the myocardial infarction, in addition to his chronic CO_2 retention.

- As demonstrated, the knowledge of what the HCO_3^- should be must be compared with what is actually found so that respiratory and metabolic components can be separated.

13 In the event of severe metabolic acidosis, the physician will sometimes give sodium bicarbonate or other "buffers" for pH correction.

14.0 OXYGEN TRANSPORT, CELLULAR DIFFUSION, AND METHODS OF ASSESSING CLINICAL EFFECTIVENESS OF OXYGEN THERAPY

14.1 Evaluation of arterial oxygen tension $Paco_2$

1 Checking $Paco_2$ and O_2 saturation indicates how well the arterial blood is being oxygenated. It does not necessarily reflect tissue oxygenation.

2 $Paco_2$ should be compared with the fraction of inspired oxygen (FIo_2) to determine degree of effective diffusion.

a Evaluation of a normal Pao_2 is based on the preexisting knowledge of the alveolar Pao_2, which will vary based on the FIo_2 and the alveolar Pao_2.

b The "textbook normal" for $Paco_2$ with an FIo_2 of 0.21 is 95 to 100 mm Hg and is based on a theoretical normal alveolar Po_2 of 100.

c Normal values for Po_2 should be based on altitude, age, and FIo_2.

$$\text{Altitude correction} = \frac{\text{Normal } Pao_2, \text{ at 760 torr} \times \text{Actual barometric pressure } (P_B)}{760}$$

$$\text{Age correction} = 90 - (0.3 \times \text{Age})$$

A normal Pao_2 should relate to FIo_2

3 Oxygen saturation (S) can be calculated by the formula:

$$O_2S \% = \frac{\text{Content}}{\text{Capacity}}$$

4 Oxygen content can be calculated thus:

O_2 content = Amount of oxygen carried (vol %)

= HbO_2 + Plasma

EXAMPLE: Content = 10 ml

$$S = \frac{10}{21} = 48\%$$

5 Oxygen tension does not directly relate to ventilation and is not used as a primary indicator of ventilation. It is interesting, however, to note that there is a reciprocal relationship between $PAco_2$ and Pao_2 (Table 8-9).

TABLE 8-9 Arterial blood gases: reciprocal relationship between alveolar Pco_2 and Po_2

$PAco_2$		PAo_2^*
20		120
40	Normal	100
60		75
80		50
100		25
120		0

*$P = 150 - (Pco_2 \times 1.25)$.

6 In healthy patients there is a difference (or gradient) between the alveolar Po_2 and the arterial Po_2 (A-a gradient).

a When O_2 concentrations above room air are inspired, it is necessary to calculate alveolar Po_2 so that any variation from normal given arterial Po_2 can be measured.

b Alveolar Po_2 may be calculated from the following formula:

$$[(P_B - 47) \times FIo_2] - Paco_2 \times 1.25$$

where

P_B = Barometric pressure,

47 = Vapor pressure of water at 37° C (in all pulmonary gas),

FIo_2 = Fraction of inspired oxygen,

$Paco_2$ = Arterial carbon dioxide tension (assumed to be equal to alveolar CO_2 levels), and

1.25 = Correction factor that is necessary when alveolar O_2 pressures are calculated while the patient is breathing room air. This is left out when working with levels of oxygen greater than 21%.

7 The *A-a gradient* can be used to evaluate the efficiency of lung function. If the lung were working as a perfect organ for gas exchange, there would be no difference between calculated alveolar (A) oxygen tension and measured arterial (a) O_2 tension. Obviously, A-a gradients *do* exist; thus increasing A-a gradients for oxygen signify deterioration in lung function.

8 Causes of increased A-a gradient in oxygen are:

a *Diffusion block* (alveolar-capillary block). Theoretically it is possible that there can be some substance that lies between the alveolus and the capillary inhibiting oxygen diffusion. This, however, is of little importance as a cause of acute hypoxemia.

b *Absolute shunt.* Any situation where blood passing through the lungs never comes in contact with an alveolus is said to be "shunted" past the diffusing surface. Venous admixture is created when the non-oxygenated blood mixes with blood that has been oxygenated. The amount of $\dot{V}/\dot{Q}$ shunt can be estimated by use of the following formula:

A-aO_2 gradient = 140 - (Po_2 torr)

Remember to subtract 5% from this value, which is a normal physiologic shunt.

EXAMPLE: A-aO_2 gradient = 140 s (62 + 40) = 38 mm

Hg = $\frac{38}{140}$ × 100 = 27% − 5% = 22% shunt

  c *Relative shunt* (decreased $\dot{V}/\dot{Q}$,* "shunt effect"). This occurs when alveoli have inadequate ventilation in relationship to the blood flow that passes them.

9 Diffusion block and relative shunts are corrected entirely when the patients are allowed to inspire 100% oxygen. In the case of an absolute shunt, however, increasing the inspired O_2 tension causes little improvement. (These disturbances are covered in more detail later in this module.)

10 On the surface one might assume that any decrease in arterial oxygenation would reflect changes in an absolute or relative shunt and accurately show deterioration. However, changes in *cardiac output,* by the nature of their effect on oxygen content in mixed venous blood, also ultimately affect PaO_2.

  a Increases in cardiac output tend to lessen the hypoxemia (and A-a gradient) that exists with any given amount of right-to-left shunt.

  b Decreases in cardiac output tend to accentuate the hypoxemia that occurs with any given amount of relative or absolute shunt.

  c Therefore procedures designed to improve arterial PO_2 (mechanical positive-pressure ventilation, positive end-expiratory pressure) may actually lower arterial PO_2 by causing a reduction in cardiac output.

14.2 Hypoxia

The clinical diagnosis of hypoxemia by presence of cyanosis is notoriously unreliable. Cyanosis is noted regularly only when hypoxemia is very severe, and many cases of clinical cyanosis result from impaired blood flow rather than low PaO_2. Arterial blood gas analysis is essential for accurate diagnosis.

Most modern blood gas laboratories measure PaO_2 directly by an oxygen (Clark) electrode system. Also, some type of oximetric or manometric measurement may provide a *direct* estimate of saturated arterial oxygen (of SaO_2). It is desirable to measure both PaO_2 and SaO_2 routinely as this provides an in-laboratory check on the validity of each determination.

Some laboratories report a SaO_2 calculated from the PaO_2 with a standard oxygen dissociation curve. This practice should *not* be used. The oxygen dissociation curve is not fixed; not only does it vary among individuals, but it may change with time in the same subject.

For example, although the hemoglobin is normally 50% saturated at PaO_2 of 27 mm Hg, this same degree of saturation may occur at 35 mm Hg or higher in a chronically hypoxemic individual, making it easier to unload oxygen in the peripheral tissues. In such cases calculated SaO_2 values are inaccurate and clinically misleading. A reduction in SaO_2 may occur for several reasons, and the differentia-

tion of the mechanism is important in differential diagnosis.

1 The following types of hypoxia are among the most well-known definitions, although definitions will vary somewhat from text to text. Clinically hypoxia is evident with the signs and symptoms of restlessness, headache, tachycardia, diaphoresis (excessive perspiration), and possibly cyanosis.

  a *Hypoxemic hypoxia.* An O_2 deficit in the tissues resulting from an O_2 tension may be caused by any of the following: high altitude, chronic obstructive pulmonary disease (COPD), pulmonary edema, suffocation, drug overdose, pneumonitis, pneumothorax, atelectasis, anatomic or intrapulmonary shunting, drowning, tracheal suctioning, pulmonary fibrosis.

  b *Stagnant hypoxia.* An O_2 deficit in tissue resulting from inadequate perfusion, which may be local, regional, or systemic. This disturbance in perfusion (blood flow) may be caused by shock, elevated intrapleural pressure (secondary to positive pressure ventilation or tension pneumothorax), polycythemia, disseminated intravascular coagulation (from sepsis of the blood), sickle cell anemia, and cardiac arrest.

  c *Anemia hypoxia.* An O_2 deficit in tissue resulting from decreased availability of hemoglobin and caused by chronic anemia, excessive blood loss, hemodilution, carbon monoxide poisoning and methemoglobinemia (methemoglobin in the blood as a result of toxic drug reaction or hemolytic processes).

  d *Histotoxic hypoxia.* An O_2 deficit in tissue resulting from the inability of the cells to use oxygen. This rarely seen disorder is caused by cyanide poisoning, nicotine poisoning, and profound electrolyte imbalances.

2 The mechanisms of hypoxia can be determined by relatively simple procedures available in most institutions and are summarized in Table 8-10.

  a *Decreased inspired oxygen tension.* This occurs with high altitude, rebreathing expired air, and excessive rates of external combustion of oxygen. Rebreathing is associated with a high Paco$_2$ and may be considered a form of hypoventilation.

  • The diagnosis of altitude hypoxemia presents no diagnostic problem as long as the practitioner is aware of the expected fall in PaO_2 with increasing altitude.

  • There are relatively little data concerning normal limits of PaO_2 at various elevations, particularly in older individuals. Table 8-11 offers a rough guideline.

  • Values at the lower ends of the normal range are unusual in young adults. Lower normal values for young children and older individuals reflect a higher degree of physiologic shunting at these ages.

  • With altitude hypoxemia, supplemental oxygen tends to raise PaO_2 by the same amount as the O_2 tension is increased in the inspired gas.

---

*Gas volume per unit of time per volume flow of blood per unit of time.

TABLE 8-10 Mechanisms of hypoxemia

			Arterial O_2 tension			
			Air breathing		28% O_2 breathing	100% O_2 breathing
Mechanism	Common causes	Arterial CO_2 tension	Rest	Exercise		
1 Decreased inspired O_2 tension	Altitude	Decreased	Decrease predictable from altitude	No significant change	Increases approx. 55 mm Hg	Increases to within 250 mm of barometric pressure >400 mm Hg
2 Alveolar hypoventilation	Depressed respiratory center Obesity syndrome Neuromuscular diseases Severe obstructive lung diseases	Increased	Decrease predictable from increase in Pa_{CO_2})	Variable (depends on effect on Pa_{CO_2})	Increases approx. 50 mm Hg minus the increase in Pa_{CO_2}	>400 mm Hg
3 Diffusion limitation (alveolar-capillary block)	An uncommon cause for hypoxemia	Normal or decreased	Little decrease, except terminally	Marked decrease	Increases >50 mm Hg	>400 mm Hg
4 Physiologic shunting	All types of pulmonary diseases	Normal or decreased (unless also hypoventilating)	Variable amount of decrease	Usually decreases	Increases <50 mm Hg	>400 mm Hg
5 Anatomic or anatomic-like shunts						
a Anatomic	Congenital heart disease Pulmonary atrioventricular fistula	Normal or decreased	Variable amount of decrease	Usually decreases	Increases <50 mm Hg	<400 mm Hg (<200 mm Hg if Pa_{O_2} is <55 mm Hg on room air) <400 mm Hg

TABLE 8-11 Range of normal Pa_{O_2}

	Mm Hg	
Altitude	Ages 10 to 60 yr	Under age 10; over age 60 yr
Sea level	84-110	>70
2000 feet	78-104	>67
4000 feet	73-98	>64
6000 feet	66-92	>61
8000 feet	60-86	>58

b *Alveolar hypoventilation.* Alveolar hypoventilation with hypercapnia must result in a decrease in Pa_{O_2}. For ordinary clinical purposes, the fall in Pa_{O_2} resulting from hypoventilation may be estimated to be equal to the rise in Pa_{CO_2}.

• When the respiratory exchange ratio (CO_2 production/O_2 consumption) is less than 1, as it is in most individuals, the fall in Pa_{O_2} will actually be slightly greater.

• Expected changes in Pa_{O_2} accompanying various levels of hypercapnia from alveolar hypoventilation are indicated in Table 8-10, in which a normal respiratory exchange ratio (respiratory quotient) of 0.8

and an environmental O_2 tension of 160 mm Hg are assumed.

• This reduction in Pa_{O_2} is caused by a right shift of the O_2 dissociation curve caused by elevated Pa_{CO_2}. This action is known as the *Bohr* effect (se Fig. 8-42).

• Greater reductions of Pa_{O_2} than shown in Table 8-10 indicate that there is an additional cause for the hypoxemia, most often an accompanying physiologic shunt.

• If ventilation is not further depressed, supplemental oxygen would be expected to increase Pa_{O_2} by the same amount as inspired O_2 tension is increased. Thus it is easy to increase the Pa_{O_2} in a pure hypoventilation problem.

c *Diffusion impairment.* Localized impairment of alveolar gas exchange may lead to a pattern of physiologic shunting. An overall problem with gas diffusion, however, leads to a different pattern of hypoxemia. This has been described as alveolar-capillary block.

• This type of impairment is rarely encountered in its pure form. More often some degree of alveolar-capillary block will complicate the more fundamental problem of physiologic shunting, but this is difficult to diagnose.

d *Ventilation/perfusion abnormalities (physiologic shunting).* Ventilation/perfusion abnormalities and physiologic shunting are the most common mechanism for hypoxemia. They simply indicate that some of the pulmonary blood does not become oxygenated even though it passes air-containing alveoli.

- Most commonly this results from a local underventilation problem. If some perfused alveoli do not receive their fair share of ventilation (a low ventilation/perfusion ratio), the blood perfusing them will be inadequately oxygenated, creating a shuntlike effect.

- Physiologic shunts tend to produce some CO_2 retention as well as hypoxemia, but since this can be readily compensated by an increase in overall ventilation, CO_2 retention is usually associated with alveolar hypoventilation.

- Compensation for hypoxemia cannot occur by increasing ventilation, since blood leaving normally ventilated alveoli is already almost fully saturated with oxygen.

e *Anatomic and anatomic-like shunts.* Abnormal vascular communications sometimes allow blood to totally bypass air-exchanging portions of the lung. Such communications may exist within the heart (congenital heart diseases), with reversed flow through a patent ductus arteriosus, or with intrapulmonary vascular shunts.

- Since the respiratory system is normal, hyperventilation can occur in response to blood gas changes, and Pa_{CO_2} is maintained at normal or even low levels.

- This type of hypoxia is very resistant to correction by supplemental oxygen. A pure anatomic shunt that leads to a Pa_{O_2} value near 50 mm Hg during air breathing will not allow the Pa_{O_2} to rise above 100 mm Hg even during inhalation of pure oxygen.

- Certain pulmonary disorders may lead to anatomic-like shunting even though no abnormal vascular channels are evident. With obstructive atelectasis, for example, blood moving through the airless lung behaves as if it were going through an anatomic shunt.

- Similar effects may be noted with acute pulmonary emboli, severe emphysema, bronchiectasis, or extensive parenchymal infiltrates.

3 Minor degrees of hypoxemia produce few obvious physiologic changes. Slight hyperventilation, minor impairment of intellectual performance, and subtle visual changes may be noted, but most clinically significant effects are not seen until the *Pa_{O_2} falls below 44 mm Hg*. The following may then be noted:

a Pulmonary hypertension, made worse by an coexisting respiratory acidosis. This is an important mechanism in the development of cor pulmonale.

b Increase in cardiac output, representing a further strain on cardiac function.

c Worsening effects on myocardial function, especially when there is associated coronary artery disease.

d Impaired renal function with a tendency to retain sodium.

e Altered central nervous system (CNS) function, usually characterized by headache, lethargy, or somnolence. With severe acute hypoxia, convulsions and permanent brain damage may result.

f A tendency for anaerobic metabolism with resultant lactic acidosis. This may lead to a severe reduction in pH in patients with coexisting respiratory acidosis.

4 *Cyanosis* is a bluish discoloration of the skin, nail beds, or mucous membranes and is usually the result of *excessive hemoglobin unsaturation*. Reduced hemoglobin is purple, whereas oxyhemoglobin is bright red. Cyanosis usually occurs when superficial capillaries contain more than 5 g of reduced Hb/100 ml of blood.

a However, the presence or absence of cyanosis is determined by the *subjective* impression of the observer and may be influenced by the thickness or pigmentation of the skin, the state of the superficial capillary bed, and even the ambient light source.

b Therefore cyanosis is not a sensitive indicator of oxygen supply to tissues. Many things associated with erythrocytosis may mimic cyanosis. On the other hand, severe hypoxemia in the presence of anemia will not produce cyanosis.

5 The following list shows situations in which discoloration suggestive of cyanosis may occur:

a Arterial hypoxemia
- Low inspired O_2 tension
- Alveolar hypoventilation
- Ventilation/perfusion abnormalities
- Physiologic shunting secondary to lung disease
- Anatomic right-to-left shunting
- Diffusion impairment (rare)

b Circulatory abnormality
- Low cardiac output
- Local reduction of blood flow
- Increased venous pressure
- Other causes of venous engorgement

c Abnormal blood or skin pigments
- Argyria
- Methemoglobinemia or sulfhemoglobinemia
- Exogenous pigments

d Erythrocytosis (polycythemia)

6 Arterial oxygen should always be measured whenever generalized cyanosis is observed. Because severe hypoxemia may exist before cyanosis is recognized clinically, the absence of this physical finding should never be taken as an indication of adequate arterial oxygenation.

7 Some relatively rare conditions may produce superficial discoloration that mimics cyanosis.

a Argyria resulting from silver ingestion may lead to a bluish-gray discoloration of the skin. Unlike true cyanosis, the discoloration of argyria does not blanch with pressure delivered to the skin.

   b Methemoglobin, which cannot combine reversibly with oxygen, is dark in color and produces the appearance of cyanosis. Methemoglobinemia should be suspected if the O_2 capacity of the blood is low in the presence of a normal total hemoglobin or if oximetric measurements indicate unsaturation in spite of a normal O_2 tension. It is confirmed by spectroscopic analysis of the blood.

8 Erythrocytosis (polycythemia) is the production of excess red blood cells in response to chronic severe O_2 deficiency. Any situation characterized by chronic hypoxemia may be associated with secondary erythrocytosis.

9 In patients with chronic respiratory disorders, there is often an associated increase in plasma volume, minimizing the increase in hematocrit. In these patients measurements of hemoglobin or hematocrit do not reflect accurately the actual increase in red cell mass.

15.0 PHYSIOLOGIC INFLUENCES ON BLOOD GASES
15.1 Physiologic determination of blood gases

The regulation of breathing is made possible by the constant analysis of the chemical state of blood.

1 This analysis is carried out in the brain by the *central chemoreceptor* and in the body by the *peripheral chemoreceptors.*

   a The central chemoreceptor is thought to be located somewhere on the ventrolateral surfaces of the medulla near the exit of the ninth and tenth cranial nerves.

   b Experiments on this area in laboratory animals show that a local application of hydrogen ions, carbon dioxide, acetylcholine, or nicotine rapidly produces increased breathing.

   c The medullary respiratory center is stimulated by hydrogen ions that diffuse into the cerebrospinal fluid (CSF) from the blood.

     • That is, the carbon dioxide of the blood diffuses across the blood-brain barrier to the CSF where it reacts with water to form bicarbonate (HCO_3^-) and hydrogen ion (H^+). The H^+ therefore is available to stimulate the respiratory center.

   d These receptors respond slowly to H^+ and HCO_3^- but rapidly to un-ionized dissolved carbon dioxide. This means that sudden increases in CO_2 levels rapidly elevate the H^+ concentration, which causes the medullary center to increase ventilation. The opposite occurs if CO_2 levels drop rapidly.

2 The peripheral chemoreceptors are small pieces of nervous tissue located in the angle of the bifurcation of the common carotid arteries and at the top of the aortic arch (Fig. 8-48)

   a These peripheral chemoreceptors primarily respond to a decrease in arterial blood Po_2, not to decreased O_2 content.

     • Even though decreased Pao_2 stimulates pulmonary

ventilation, the threshold for the stimulation is high and somewhat unpredictable.

     • Pao_2 must fall to the 50 to 60 mm Hg range, and the oxyhemoglobin saturation must fall to about 80% before significant hyperpnea occurs.

   b It should be noted that the normal operation of the peripheral chemoreceptors is blocked by giving a patient 100% oxygen to breathe.

   c The peripheral chemoreceptors are also sensitive to low arterial blood pH and to changes in the blood temperature and blood pressure; they also respond to changes to $Paco_2$. However, these responses are clearly secondary to the sensitivity of the receptors to hypoxia.

16.0 DRAWING AN ARTERIAL BLOOD GAS SAMPLE
16.1 Sampling technique for arterial blood gases

Each hospital has its own set of standards for drawing arterial blood samples. In some hospitals, respiratory care personnel are not allowed to draw gases, and this is the responsibility of the laboratory, physicians, or nursing staff.

Most hospitals, however, are allowing respiratory care personnel to draw at least arterial blood at the radial and brachial sites. Femoral puncture usually is performed only by physicians.

The technique is relatively simple but involves special skill, care, and caution.*

1 The patient (even one who appears comatose) should first have the procedure explained, since it does involve some pain and the patient should know what is coming. Care should be taken to prevent hyperventilation caused by anxiety or pain, since it will affect the results.

2 Equipment should be at the bedside and ready for use without wasting time fumbling around for proper equipment. Since one hand is on the patient at all times, supplies must be kept within easy reach. Necessary equipment includes

   a Alcohol or disinfectant swabs

   b Sterile 3 to 5 ml *glass* syringes

   c A selection of 1½-inch needles (20, 21, 22, 23 gauge)

   d Sodium heparin (1/1000)

   e Sterile gauze pads (4 × 4 inches)

   f Rubber cap or stopper to seal the needle

   g A container of ice

3 The most frequently used site is the radial artery although the physician may have left instructions or specific site preferences. If the radial site is used, the *Allen test* or modified Allen test described here should be done. The radial artery to the hand is usually joined by the collateral ulnar artery. However, not all individuals have sufficient blood flow through this second artery, and in the event of irreparable damage to the radial artery, the individual would have no blood flow to

---

*See Procedure 8-1 at the end of this module for a summary of drawing an arterial blood sample.

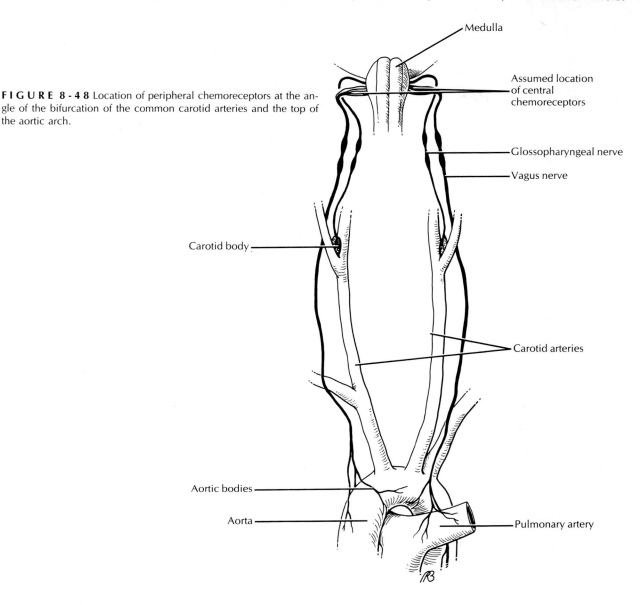

FIGURE 8-48 Location of peripheral chemoreceptors at the angle of the bifurcation of the common carotid arteries and the top of the aortic arch.

the hand. To perform a modified Allen test:

a Begin by compressing the patient's wrist so there is no blood flow past the radial or ulnar arteries (stop the pulses).

b Have the patient make a tight fist until the hand blanches, or in the unconscious patient, raise the hand above the chest so that the blood will drain by gravity.

c Carefully release the pressure on the ulnar artery while holding pressure on the radial artery.

d Look to see if the hand "pinks up" or if the color returns in 10 to 15 seconds.

e If it does not, ulnar circulation may be assumed to be inadequate. Do *not* draw a radial blood gas sample. Notify the physician.

4 The brachial artery is the second most likely site to be chosen and requires no special technique except that it is more difficult to palpate compared to the radial artery.

5 The femoral site is usually reserved for physicians primarily because it is very close to the femoral vein and nerve. Inadequate technique and uncertainty about the puncture site increase the possibility of drawing a mixed venous sample. Further, hemostasis is much more difficult in the large arteries, and hematomas may develop.

6 Before drawing the blood, the site should be *thoroughly* cleaned. A good technique is to use two or three swabs, one after the other.

NOTE: Obviously the practitioner's hands should be clean and gloved per Universal Precautions.

7 Once a site is chosen, a small amount of lidocaine (Xylocaine) may be injected under the skin in the area to be punctured. However, the practice is controversial, and many hospitals forbid respiratory care personnel from *injecting* medications.

a Its detractors say that the Xylocaine injection is just as painful, the procedure is time-consuming since

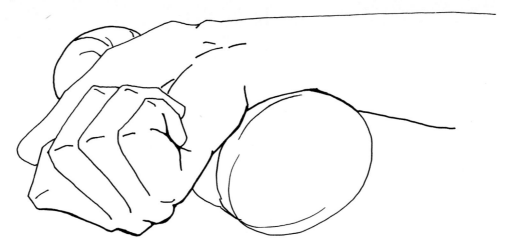

FIGURE 8-49 Proper positioning of patient's arm for a radial site puncture.

the Xylocaine takes several minutes to work, and a skilled technician can draw a blood sample with one stick and with little, if any, pain.

b The supporters of the Xylocaine procedures say that the use of anesthetic reduces hyperventilation, gives more time to work, permits multiple attempts without discomfort, and helps stabilize the tissue around the artery to prevent movement.

8 Careful palpation is necessary to fix the position of the artery. Correct positioning of the arm will aid the process.

9 For use of the brachial site, the practitioner should fully extend the arm, support the elbow with a towel pad, and extend the wrist moderately by placing a rolled towel or cloth under, using the free hand, if necessary, to push down the patient's hand (Fig. 8-49). Next, the practitioner cleans the site and checks again for the artery's position.

10 A glass syringe or newer plastic models provided with a commercially available sampling kit should be used so that once heparinized, it will fill with blood pumped by arterial pressure. Thus "pulling back" or aspirating the blood sample will *not* be necessary.

a Although heparin lubricates the plunger of the syringe, its primary use is to prevent clotting of blood in the needle and of the sample that is drawn.

b The practitioner draws about 0.5 ml of 1:1000 strength heparin into the syringe, using sterile technique; rotates the plunger and slides it in and out of the barrel; and after wetting the syringe, ejects the heparin, making sure there are no air bubbles in the syringe.

NOTE: Prepackaged sterile ABG kits can be purchased that contain preheparinized syringes.

11 The sample is drawn as follows:

a Hold the syringe firmly at its base, and stabilize the area to be punctured with your free hand. Use your free fingers to locate the best "pressure" spot.

b Hold the syringe at a 30- to 45-degree angle with the needle bevel pointing *up* and open toward the direction of the patient's heart, entering the skin in one smooth motion (Fig. 8-50). Advance the needle; when the artery is punctured, blood will flow into the syringe without help.

c When the flow starts, hold the syringe very still until 2 to 3 ml have entered the barrel.

d With your free hand, place a sterile (4 × 4 inch) pad on the puncture site, and withdraw the needle. *Firm pressure should be applied to the puncture for no less than 5 minutes* and up to *15 minutes* if the patient is receiving anticoagulant therapy. Some procedures call for wrapping the site with an elastic bandage after 5 minutes and after all signs of bleeding have stopped.

e While holding the site, hand the sample of blood to an assistant to prepare for icing and transport.

NOTE: Many clinicians, with practice, perform a very efficient "juggling act" and handle the whole procedure without any help.

12 After drawing, the assistant carefully eliminates any small air bubbles that may be in the syringe. Air bubbles in the blood will affect the gas values, because gaseous exchange will continue as long as the air-blood interface exists and the blood stays relatively warm.

13 When the bubbles are gone, the syringe is held horizontally while the needle is inserted in a rubber stopper or cap. This prevents air from accidentally entering by way of the needle. Some hospitals' procedures call for the needle to be removed and a syringe cap to be placed on the end of the syringe. Either way, the object is to keep air from the blood sample. The syringe is now ready to be placed in a container filled with ice. The ice slows the oxygen metabolism and will keep the sample "fresh" for up to 30 minutes. Before putting it into the ice, the practitioner rolls the syringe, while keeping it horizontal, back and forth between his or her

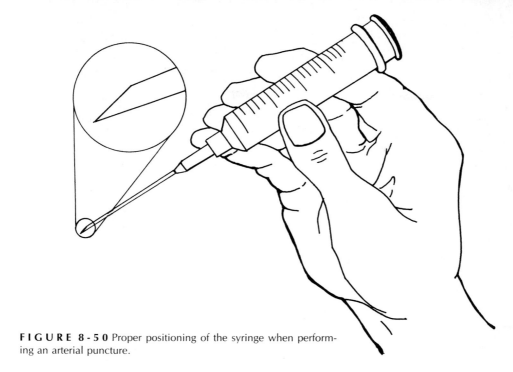

F I G U R E   8 - 5 0 Proper positioning of the syringe when performing an arterial puncture.

hands. This will ensure mixture of the heparin with the blood and will prevent clotting.

NOTE: Many hospitals prefer to use prepackaged and disposable kits for drawing ABG samples.

14 Necessary paperwork includes:

a Noting the patient's name and room number.

b Charting the exact time of collection. This verifies the time period between collection and processing of the sample.

c Noting the patient's most recent temperature. Remember the effect of temperature on the O_2 dissociation curve. If the patient had a high fever, the gas results, which are processed under standard conditions, may vary. The change in arterial PO_2 is about 6% for each centigrade degree temperature change. Although this problem may not significantly change the Pao_2, for the patient who is on the borderline between aggressive and conservative care, even a minute change in accuracy is important.

d Fraction of inspired concentration of oxygen FIo_2. It is *critically* important to note whether or not the patient is getting any supplemental oxygen, not only how much but in what manner delivered. Patients on mechanical ventilators should have all of the following reported at the time the blood is drawn:

• Tidal volume

• Dead space (if any)

• Rate

• FIo_2

• Positive end-expiratory pressure (PEEP) or continuous positive airway pressure (CPAP)—if any

• Intermittent mandatory ventilation (IMV) rate (if in use)

17.0 ARTERIAL BLOOD SAMPLE
17.1 Drawing an arterial blood sample for analysis

Procedure 8-1 presented at the end of this module may be used as an overview guide for drawing an arterial blood sample.

18.0 ANALYSIS OF ARTERIAL BLOOD GAS SAMPLES
18.1 Analysis of arterial blood samples

Once the gas has been delivered to the laboratory, it should be processed as soon as possible.

In today's hospitals the pH, $Paco_2$, and Pao_2 are measured directly by special electrodes contained in a device made for that specific purpose.

1 pH can be measured by the use of a special electrode, or it can be calculated from a known $Paco_2$ and bicarbonate. It can also be calculated from the total CO_2 content by use of the Henderson-Hasselbalch equation.

a The practitioner will most likely use the pH electrode method. The electrode is constructed of two half cells, which develop an electrical potential when connected together (Fig. 8-51).

• One side is the reference electrode *(1)*, which maintains a constant potential and is bathed in a known electrolytic solution, usually potassium chloride (KCl) *(2)*.

• The other side is the glass electrode, which develops an electrical potential that is proportional to the amount of hydrogen ion present *(3)*. Surrounding it is the test solution to be measured *(4)*.

b Between the two electrodes is a liquid junction potential *(5)*; the electrical is read on a meter calibrated in pH.

• This is a very simplified description of the pH mea-

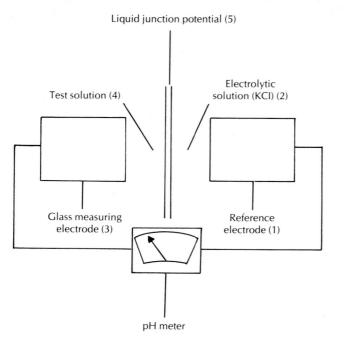

FIGURE 8-51 pH electrode.

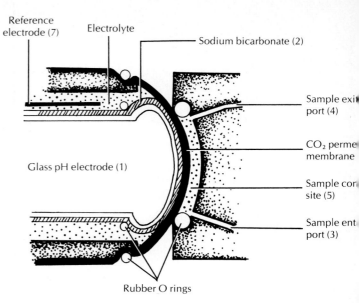

FIGURE 8-52 Severinghaus electrode used to measure PCO_2.

suring device, and the actual commercial type will not physically resemble it.

2 The $PaCO_2$ electrode was developed by *Severinghaus* and also operates on the principle of electric potential between electrodes (Fig. 8-52).

  a It consists of a glass pH electrode *(1)* with a tip that is in contact with a cellophane, Teflon, or some other semipermeable membrane, which is buffered with sodium bicarbonate *(2)*.

  b The arterial blood sample enters *(3)* and leaves *(4)* the sample area. In between *(5)*, the blood sample is in contact with a membrane *(6)* that is permeable to carbon dioxide but not to liquids or solids.

  c The carbon dioxide diffuses into the bicarbonate solution, and the change in pH is registered between the glass electrode *(1)* and the reference electrode *(7)* as an electric potential.

  d The electric potential is registered by either a needle meter or digital readout on a meter.

  e The Severinghaus electrode (CO_2) is reliable and usually accurate but needs preventive maintenance and gentle care. It should be calibrated with at least two known concentrations of carbon dioxide several times per day or more, if it is in heavy use.

3 The *Clark* or O_2 electrode is constructed from a platinum cathode (negative pole) and a silver anode (positive pole) (Fig. 8-53).

  a The cathode *(1)* is a thin platinum wire sealed in an insulating glass rod *(2)*. The anode *(3)* is a silver wire surrounded in an electrolyte bath *(4)*, which cuts down the effect of carbon dioxide on the electrode.

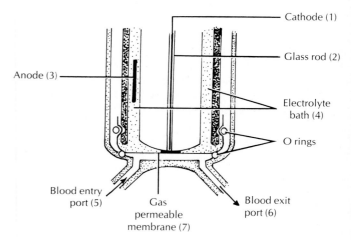

FIGURE 8-53 Clark electrode used to measure PCO_2.

  b The blood enters at *5* and leaves at *6*. The gas permeable polypropylene membrane *(7)* admits gas but not liquid or solids.

    • When a polarizing voltage is applied between the cathode and anode, electrons from the cathode combine with O_2 molecules, which are broken down.

      – The molecular breakdown causes a change in ionic current that is proportional to the surface area of the platinum, the electrolyte's diffusion characteristics, and the number of oxygen molecules around the electrode.

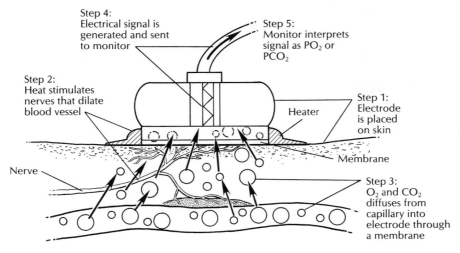

Step 4:
Electrical signal is generated and sent to monitor

Step 5:
Monitor interprets signal as PO_2 or PCO_2

Step 2:
Heat stimulates nerves that dilate blood vessel

Step 1:
Electrode is placed on skin

Heater

Membrane

Nerve

Step 3:
O_2 and CO_2 diffuses from capillary into electrode through a membrane

FIGURE 8-54 Transcutaneous monitor.

– Since there are no O_2 molecules around the cathode, a diffusion gradient is created between the sample and the cathode. The breakdown causes a small electrical current to be produced.

c The higher the tension of oxygen, the larger the gradient, and therefore the more current is produced. The current produced is amplified and displayed on a meter or digital readout.

d Oxygen electrodes are also fragile and require great care. As with the CO_2 electrode, the O_2 electrode should be calibrated against two known test references at least several times a day.

19.0 NONINVASIVE OXYGENATION MONITORING (TRANSCUTANEOUS) DEVICES

19.1 Noninvasive oxygenation monitoring

In the last few years a means of determining oxygenation in newborns, infants, and adults without having to draw blood has been developed.

A device called a *transcutaneous (tc)* O_2 monitor is able to detect Po_2 values directly through the skin.

1 Basically, a *tc monitor* is nothing more than a small Clark-type electrode recording instrument (Fig. 8-54).

  a The electrode is usually a gold cathode surrounded by a silver anode and a calibrated precision thermistor (heating element) and is about the size of a quarter. The electrode is connected by a cord to a power box similar to an O_2 analyzer.

  b Before application onto the skin, the electrode is calibrated to room Po_2 and equilibrated with humidified air.

2 The application site, preferably one without hair, is cleaned with alcohol and then covered with a special sensor gel. It is very important that there be an airtight seal between the electrode membrane and the skin. Typical sites are shown in Fig. 8-55.

3 The purpose of the thermistor is to maintain a constant 44° C temperature at the electrode site.* This improves local O_2 transport to the area by capillary dilation. The oxygen at this point is chemically reduced at the cathode, and a current is produced (Clark electrode method) proportional to the amount of diffusing oxygen.

4 The tiny current produced is amplified and then calibrated to display the O_2 tension in mm Hg (torr).

5 It is important to move the electrode sensor at least every 4 hours, since there is a slight tendency for it to cause skin burns. The thermistor is usually adjustable.

6 Occasional arterial blood samples still need to be drawn at 6- to 12-hour intervals to ensure reasonable correlation between Pao_2 and $tcPo_2$.

7 Under optimum conditions—i.e., good cardiac output, good perfusion, and no abnormal shunting—correlation between Pao_2 and $tcpo_2$ has been shown to be 3 to 5 mm Hg.

8 Companies manufacturing transcutaneous monitors include Critikon, Radiometer, and Novametrix.†

20.0 PATHOLOGY

Pathology is a science involved with the study of the nature and cause of disease and conditions caused by the disease. It is important for respiratory care personnel to recognize the clinical signs and symptoms of disease and any changes in normal laboratory values in order to participate in discussions and in the decision-making process.

---

*Temperature will vary depending on the model whether used for adults or infants.

†Critikon, 1410 N. Westshore Blvd., Tampa, FL 33607. Radiometer America, Inc., 811 Sharon Dr, Westlake, OH 44145. Novametrix Medical Systems, Inc., Wallingford, CT 06492.

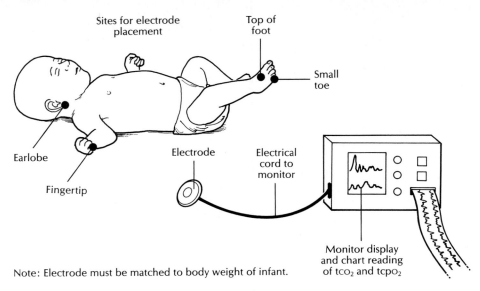

Sites for electrode placement

Top of foot

Small toe

Earlobe

Fingertip

Electrode

Electrical cord to monitor

Monitor display and chart reading of tco$_2$ and tcpo$_2$

Note: Electrode must be matched to body weight of infant.

FIGURE 8-55 Typical application sites for transcutaneous monitor.

20.1 Nature of pathology

1 The following units present various diseases by:
  a Identifying the *clinical diagnosis*
  b Pointing out primary *pathologic features*
  c Discussing the *causes* of the disease
  d Listing the *symptoms*
  e Describing *physical findings*
  f Discussing the *effects* of the disease as measured by pulmonary function studies
  g Suggesting *treatment* techniques
    NOTE: The suggested treatment techniques include many procedures that should be administered only by physicians. These techniques are mentioned so that the technician and therapist, aware of what is occurring at the bedside, will possibly be of more assistance to the physician.

2 The pathophysiology of various medical conditions caused by disease or trauma is discussed along with suggested treatment modalities.

3 For detailed presentation of all cardiopulmonary diseases the reader is encouraged to refer to pathology texts or supplemental materials available from manufacturers, the American Lung Association, professional journals, and hospital libraries.

4 A disease, as opposed to the general term "health," is:
  a Caused by a single factor (etiology)
  b Accompanied by certain structural changes (pathology)
  c Causing abnormal functions (physiology)
  d Reflecting a regular grouping of symptoms and clinical findings (syndrome)
    • Disease may be defined by *any one* or *all* of these four characteristics. However, their identification

and subsequent treatment will not always follow textbook norms. For this reason respiratory care personnel must be able to observe and *assess* a patient based on a *total* picture, rather than reach a foregone conclusion based on textbook facts alone.

5 Before studying each single pulmonary disease, it is appropriate to make some considerations and to focus attention on some common problems of pulmonary physiopathology.
  a Pulmonary diseases are developing into a major health problem. The incidence of pulmonary disorders appears to be high, since pulmonary changes are observed in 50% of autopsies in men over the age of 65 years.
  b Airway obstruction, in particular, is the keynote to a developing and steadily increasing pattern of pulmonary pathology.
  c It is not surprising that the American Lung Association and the American Thoracic Society, whose prime interest is combating respiratory diseases, are attempting to arouse professional and public interest in research that may lead to early recognition of chronic obstructive disease and its effective treatment.
  d According to the National Disease and Therapeutic Index, the diagnosis of obstructive lung disease during the first visit of a patient to a physician has greatly increased since 1960. Some of this increase may result from a greater awareness on the part of the physician that the condition may exist. It has been stated that the present knowledge of chronic obstructive lung disease is equivalent to the knowledge of tuberculosis about 70 years ago.

21.0 GLOSSARY

21.1 Terms related to pathology*

1 Diagnosis. (1) Identification of a disease or condition by a scientific evaluation of physical signs, symptoms, history, labortory tests, and procedures. (2) The name of a disease or condition. Kinds of diagnoses are clinical diagnosis, differential diagnosis, laboratory diagnosis, nursing diagnosis, and physical diagnosis.

2 Etiology. (1) The study of all factors that may be involved in the development of a disease, including susceptibility of the patient, the nature of the disease agent, and the way in which the patient's body is invaded by the agent. (2) The cause of a disease.

3 Gross specimen. Taking a large or coarse sample with no attention to preserving minutiae.

4 Microscopic specimen. A specimen whose detail can be examined only by microscope.

5 Morbidity. (1) An illness or an abnormal condition of quality. (2) (in statistics) (a): The rate at which an illness or abnormality occurs, calculated by dividing the entire number of people in a group by the number in that group who are affected with the illness or abnormality. (b): The rate at which an illness occurs in a particular area or population.

6 Moribund. Dying.

7 Mortality (1) The condition of being subject to death. (2) The death rate, which reflects the number of deaths per unit of population in any specific region, age group, disease, or other classification, usually expressed as deaths per 1000, 10,000, or 100,000.

8 Pathology. (1) The study of the characteristics, causes, and effects of disease, as observed in the structure and function of the body. (2) *Cellular pathology,* the study of cellular changes in disease. (3) *Clinical pathology,* the study of disease by the use of laboratory tests and methods.

9 Prodrome. (1) An early sign of a developing condition or disease. (2) The earliest phase of a developing condition or disease.

10 Prognosis. A prediction of the probable outcome of a disease based on the condition of the person and the usual course of the disease as observed in similar situations.

11 Syndrome. A complex of signs and symptoms resulting from a common cause or appearing, in combination, to present a clinical picture of a disease or inherited abnormality.

22.0 THE EFFECT OF PULMONARY DISEASE ON SOCIETY

22.1 General comments regarding pulmonary disease

1 It is interesting that emphysema and chronic bronchitis were relatively rare in England until soft coal was introduced as a fuel into the British economy.

2 US service personnel stationed in the Tokyo-Yokohama region of Japan suffered from chronic disease states characterized by dyspnea and wheezing. A change in environment resulted in immediate cessation of the symptoms, which were probably related to the high pollutant concentration and meterologic conditions existing in that area.

3 People exposed to air pollutants, however, do not *all* develop bronchitis and emphysema. A variety of host factors influence the development of the disease status. Heredity probably plays a subtle role by altering the resistance of the tracheobronchial tree to exogenous agents. Pertussis in childhood; viral bronchitis, especially in early age; and heavy smoking, paralyzing and ultimately destroying the cleansing action of the mucosal cilia, all appear to make the lung more susceptible to the action of pollutants.

4 The disease status and its treatment in pulmonary conditions may be complicated by many body changes secondary to the original damage. In tuberculosis, for example, the problem is largely bacteriologic. In this case it is a matter of eradicating, by the proper choice and application of drugs, a single type of organism, the tubercle bacillus. On the other hand, emphysema is often seriously complicated by bronchitis and pneumonia, which can be caused by almost any bacterium and fungus, all with different and varying drug sensitivity. This problem is compounded because the disease organism in a patient frequently varies or gets more complicated, even during treatment. In addition to the problem of infection, these patients are prone to bronchial spasm or asthma, which challenges the skill of the best physicians and technicians.

5 Heart failure (cor pulmonale), sputum accumulation, and lack of oxygen are frequent complications and are rarely easily resolved. For example, a tracheotomy may be the only way to handle airway and ventilatory complications. However, the measure in itself adds further therapeutic and precautionary measures. When the lungs no longer can eliminate carbon dioxide adequately, the patient is said to be in respiratory failure. This is a dangerous state—just as serious as impending coma in diabetes, kidney failure, or cardiac failure. This situation requires expert medical assistance to prevent respiratory paralysis, coma, and death.

6 Gastrointestinal bleeding in pulmonary patients is usually related to peptic ulceration and/or bleeding from the intestines. The exact causes of this disorder are not known, only that it occurs. The point is that it takes special training and people to handle these problems at any level. Critical care divisions for patients with respiratory failure have been established in many hospitals. Often the care of the patient is delegated to a team, just as for the patient scheduled for open-heart surgery. Physicians, nurses, an anesthesiologist, respiratory therapists and technicians, a pulmonary physio-

---

*Many of the definitions for these terms were taken from Mosby's medical, nursing, & allied health dictionary, ed 3, St Louis, 1990, The CV Mosby Co.

therapist, a blood gas technician, and trained aides may be found at the bedside of only one patient with respiratory failure.

7 The following units, which present various types of pulmonary diseases and recommended treatment, should be read and studied carefully and related to patients seen in the clinical situation.

23.0 PULMONARY DISEASES AND THEIR RECOMMENDED TREATMENTS

23.1 The common cold

The common cold is a highly communicable infection of the upper respiratory tract caused by *viruses* so small they cannot be seen under the ordinary microscope.

Other names include head cold (rhinitis), sore throat (pharyngitis), sinus (sinusitis), and chest cold (tracheobronchitis).

A cold usually starts as benign but, untreated, can spread to the lower respiratory tract where it causes more serious complications.

1 Colds are caused by any one of a large number of viruses. People who are fatigued or malnourished are more susceptible to the cold virus than healthy, rested individuals.

2 The method of spreading a cold is by the inhalation of droplets expelled by talking, coughing, or sneezing by an infected person. Colds are thought to be communicable only during the first 2 or 3 days of symptoms.

3 *Pathologically* the cold causes swelling of the mucosal lining, the nasal passages, and pharynx. Initially, copious (large) amounts of thin clear mucus are secreted. Subsequently the mucus becomes thick, tenacious, and pus filled, as indicated by yellow streaks. The infection may extend to involve the sinuses, the lower respiratory tract, and the middle ear (Fig. 8-56).

4 The *incubation period* for a cold is 1 to 3 days after contact with the virus.

5 *Initial symptoms* include a sore throat, followed by a feeling of fatigue (malaise) and "stopped-up nose." After a few days, nasal drainage begins, and the general symptoms subside.

6 Regardless of treatment, a cold may linger for from 10 days to 3 weeks.

7 The *complications* of a cold may be more serious than the cold itself, especially in pulmonary patients. Pneumonia, tracheobronchitis, earache, sinusitis, and laryngitis are all symptoms usually seen as complications. In pulmonary patients a cold can cause an exacerbation of underlying pulmonary disease, resulting in an increased airway resistance, hypoxemia, increased levels of dyspnea and shortness of breath, and even respiratory failure. Pulmonary patients must be protected against exposure to the cold virus.

8 The cold virus is always present, although it seems to reach epidemic levels most frequently during the fall and winter seasons. Older people have fewer colds, but the complications can be more serious. On the average, city dwellers have two or three colds a year.

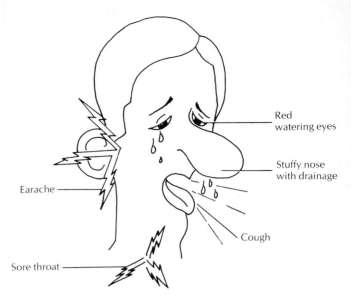

Red watering eyes

Stuffy nose with drainage

Earache

Cough

Sore throat

FIGURE 8-56 Typical cold symptoms.

9 *Laboratory tests* usually show common resident bacteria in the secretions from the nose or throat, but no viruses. This is because they cannot be seen with an ordinary microscope. Usually the white blood cell count is normal, although it may be slightly elevated if a fever is present.

10 Control and treatment of the cold usually is directed at isolating the patient to prevent its spread and relieving the symptoms.
  a Treatment includes:
   • A day or two of rest at onset
   • Isolation for 2 days or until symptoms subside
   • Aspirin to relieve muscle soreness and malaise
   • Nasal decongestants
   • A light diet with adequate fluid intake
   • When necessary for protection, wearing a protective mask to prevent the spread of droplets
  b The prevention of a cold is the best treatment
   • Avoid large gatherings during the cold season.
   • Avoid fatigue.
   • Eat a balanced diet supplemented with adequate vitamin intake.
   • Maintain cool, well-ventilated rooms for work and living.

23.2 Influenza

1 Influenza ("flu") is an infectious epidemic disease caused by the specific virus named *Influenzavirus*. It comes from a medieval Italian word meaning "influence," and it was believed that flu epidemics resulted from the influence of the stars.

2 The influenza virus has a special affinity for the respiratory tract.

3 There are four *known* types of influenza viruses: types A, B, C, and D. These types have been divided into groups that have caused epidemics known to be attributed to them since 1917.

a Types A_1, A_2 (Asian), B_2, and C are the most common causes of epidemics. The Hong Kong and England viruses are variations of the type A virus.

b The type D virus is probably a parainfluenza type, having fewer of the characteristics than the others.

4 *Legionnaires' disease* was suspected of being a new strain of virus but was proved to be a newly discovered gram-negative bacterium called *Legionella pneumophila*.

5 Like the cold, influenza is spread through the air by droplets from an infected person.

6 The *incubation* period is from 18 to 36 hours. After this period the patient becomes acutely ill with a fever. The patient will become physically exhausted and possibly psychologically depressed for some days. Like the cold, the secondary complications from bacterial infection may be worse than the virus itself, especially in patients with underlying pulmonary disease.

7 *Pathologically* the influenza virus attacks the epithelial lining of the respiratory tract, causing an exudate and detached cells. These cells may group up and/or slough off, causing inflammation of the respiratory tract all the way to the respiratory bronchioles. In the alveoli, blood may be present, and the alveolar membrane may be thickened by a hyaline membrane containing eosinophilic white cells that line the alveoli. This thickening of the alveolar membrane will decrease the effectiveness of the membrane to diffuse gases with the surrounding capillary bed, resulting in possible hypoxemia and later CO_2 retention. In patients who are predisposed to lung disease, this can cause death unless the condition is reversed.

8 Influenza usually occurs during the fall and winter seasons. Each epidemic usually lasts between 4 to 6 weeks. If a *pandemic* were to occur, as high as 20% to 40% of the population could become infected.

9 The symptoms of influenza are sudden, with chills, malaise, headache, muscle ache, fever of 38° to 40° C (101° to 104° F), and cough. The cough is usually nonproductive, and the patient has a sore throat and red eyes with a watery discharge. The face is usually red and flushed and hot to the touch. The lungs may be clear to slightly abnormal with auscultation. In pulmonary patients there may be rapid onset of dyspnea, malaise, depressed or elevated respiratory frequency, and stupor as ventilation becomes ineffective.

10 A chest radiograph would reveal normal markings or a poorly defined patchy pneumonitis, unless pneumonia has developed.

11 White blood cell count is normal initially, although it may become elevated from secondary bacterial infection. In pulmonary patients, arterial blood gases may reflect decreased arterial oxygen content initially and subsequently elevated CO_2 levels.

12 Like the common cold, influenza is difficult to avoid. Common-sense practices during an epidemic are probably the best methods for limiting the severity of the disease. Vaccines have been developed that are fairly effective and should be used by people with the greatest risk of developing a fatal disease. These include patients with respiratory, cardiac, and diabetic disease and those over 55 years of age.

13 There is no specific treatment for influenza. Bed rest, fluids, aspirin, and a balanced diet seem to work best for most people. Patients with underlying disease should be observed very closely for changes in respiratory rate or depth, fever, loss of appetite, and an increase or decrease in secretions. Elevated levels of dyspnea or any of the previously mentioned symptoms should be reported to the physician. Room humidity, tracheobronchial toilet, ventilation, and oxygenation must be observed and maintained especially in the pulmonary patient.

23.3 Bronchitis

1 Bronchitis is a general term describing an inflammation of the membrane that lines the airways. There are two types: *acute* and *chronic*. Both cause a productive cough of nonspecific origin, occurring primarily during the winter months. In Great Britain, the general term *bronchitis* is changed to chronic bronchitis and is used to describe a disease process that begins with simple bronchitis (inflammation of the bronchial tree), with hypersecretion of bronchial mucus manifested as a chronic cough producing mucoid sputum. This condition worsens, and recurrent episodes produce purulent sputum. Purulent sputum production becomes continuous, resulting in a chronic condition. This condition can cause impaired ventilation because of partial airway obstruction, which is diagnosed as emphysema in the United States. Emphysema is not diagnosed in England as a disease entity because of the confusion that exists between the diagnosis of emphysema versus chronic bronchitis.

2 In 1959 the Ciba Symposium attempted to standardize terminology. *Chronic bronchitis* was defined as a nonspecific cough, with sputum production present most days for at least 3 months during each of 2 successive years.

3 The primary differences between acute and chronic bronchitis is the *rapidity* of its onset.

4 The onset of *acute bronchitis* is very rapid and may follow the exposure of the airway to biologic agents, chemical or physical irritants, and allergy.

5 The most common infectious causes of acute episodes are viruses.

6 Clinically, acute bronchitis is preceded by a stuffy nose, mucus production, and a sore throat. Cough is always present, although it will vary in severity. Initially the cough will be dry, with progressing productivity. The patient may have a substernal burning discomfort, and dyspnea may or may not be present, depending on the severity of bronchospasm and mucus production.

7 On auscultation, rhonchi and/or wheezing and rales may be heard, especially during increased volume of

secretions. The chest radiograph will appear normal.

8 The treatment for acute bronchitis is:

  a Bed rest.

  b Controlled environment (i.e., warm temperature and high humidity).

  c Cough depressants and expectorants.

  d Respiratory therapy, which may include a room humidifier, administration of heated high humidity via enclosure or mask (with or without supplemental oxygen), and topical drugs delivered with intermittent positive pressure breathing (IPPB) or by aerosol.

23.4 Chronic bronchitis

1 Chronic bronchitis is a nonspecific chronic cough, with sputum production most days of the year for at least 3 months of the year and for at least 2 successive years.

2 The primary cause of chronic bronchitis is prolonged irritation of the bronchial mucosa with recurrent acute infections.

3 Air pollution, smoking, and long-term dust inhalation cause the mucous glands and cells to overproduce and the delicate ciliated membranes to thicken. These changes make the bronchial tubes more susceptible to infection. Organisms (most commonly isolated from the secretions) in chronic bronchitis are:

  a *Haemophilus influenzae* bacillus

  b *Streptococcus pneumoniae*

  c Klebsiella pneumoniae

  d Staphylococcus aureus

  e Streptococcus pyogenes

4 The main *pathologic* feature of chronic bronchitis is inflammation of the airways leading to:

  a Hypertrophy of the bronchial mucous glands and, to a lesser degree, an increase in the number of goblet cells in the respiratory mucosa. There are secretion of increased amounts of mucus with altered flow properties and associated chronic inflammatory cell infiltration and edema of the bronchial mucosa.

  b Narrowing of air tubes characterized by airway obstruction (increased airway resistance) resulting from the hypertrophy of the mucus-secreting glands, along with the excessive mucus production.

  c Some loss of cilia and multicellular thickening of the epithelium occurs as columnar cells change to squamous metaplasia. Also, there is a general destruction of ciliary action and slowing of phagocytic activity in smokers, and increased secretions leave the patient a perfect host for bacterial or viral infections.

  d Diffuse inflammatory changes in the thickened walls of the bronchi and cylindrical dilation of the bronchi are frequently seen. Diverticula (pockets), caused by openings of enlarged mucous glands and other irregularities that trap mucus and other bronchial secretions, may form.

  e Vascular changes, including development of pulmonary hypertension with increased vascular resistance

leading to right ventricular hypertrophy or cor pulmonale because of hypoxemia.

  f Chronic cough in the presence of increased bronchial secretions, which appear to affect the minute bronchioles to the point of total destruction from sharply elevated airway pressures and overdistended walls.

  g Bronchospasm. Bronchodilator administration may result in marked improvement in pulmonary mechanics.

5 Specific symptoms of chronic bronchitis include:

  a A productive cough that is usually loose and rattling. The cough is usually worse in the morning and evening than during the middle of the day. It also is worse on damp days or during cold weather.

  b Sputum varies in character from white (mucoid) to gray or yellow (mucopurulent) and may contain blood streaks at the end of a coughing episode. The amount of sputum raised may exceed an ounce per day.

  c Fever is present only during times of acute episodes.

  d Nutrition is usually well maintained, although the patient may be fatigued by excessive coughing.

  e Shortness of breath usually is not prevalent unless the patient is in congestive heart failure.

6 Radiographic studies usually are not significantly different from normal. Abnormalities such as hyperinflation or distorted and extended bronchi are present only if the more peripheral bronchioles are involved. The caliber of the bronchi is slightly narrowed, and a depressed diaphragm, which is caused by air trapping, may be seen.

7 Pulmonary function studies are usually normal unless small airways are specifically evaluated by a special test. The measurement of *closing volume* is one test that is occasionally used to determine the early presence of chronic bronchitis in the small airways.

8 The main pathophysiologic effect of chronic bronchitis is a ventilation-perfusion imbalance with an *increased* alveolar-arterial oxygen tension gradient (PA-ao_2) difference as one of the earliest signs.

9 Note that it may be difficult to differentiate between patients who have chronic bronchitis with emphysema and those without emphysema. Here many physicians use the more general term *chronic obstructive pulmonary disease* (COPD) to identify these patients.

  a COPD is a general term used to describe diseases or conditions resulting in chronic obstruction to air flow in the lungs. Most frequently this term relates to chronic bronchitis, asthma, and emphysema, although bronchiectasis and cystic fibrosis are sometimes included in this category.

  b Chronic bronchitis frequently leads to emphysema, and often the two disease states occur together, although the extent of each varies pathophysiologically from patient to patient. Increased airway resistance resulting from bronchospasm reduces the distribution of gas throughout lung units, causing a mismatch of ventilation-perfusion and decreased blood oxygen levels. The work of breathing is increased so that more oxygen goes to the muscles of breathing, with less available to other tissues. As hypoxemia and CO_2 levels increase, the patient may go into respiratory failure ($Paco_2 < 50$ mm Hg and $Paco_2 > 30$ mm Hg) and cor pulmonale while breathing room air.

10 Patients with chronic bronchitis and emphysema can be categorized as type A (those with *predominant emphysema*). The type A patient is characterized by:
   a Severe shortness of breath
   b Asthenic build with evidence of recent weight loss
   c Little cough or sputum production
   d Slight abnormality of blood gases
   e Radiologic evidence of hyperinflation, narrow mediastinum, and flat diaphragm
   f Increased thoracic gas volume
   g Reduction in CO uptake
   h Oxygen desaturation with exercise
   • Because of the tendency of these patients to hyperventilate, they maintain good color and in fact may be pink; hence they are called *pink puffers*.

11 COPD patients with *predominant bronchitis* are categorized as *type B* patients. These patients have a productive cough but are not as dyspneic or as prone to chest infection as the "pink puffer." Radiologic examination reveals chronic parenchymal infection rather than generalized emphysema. These patients show marked changes in arterial blood gases, and tend to develop cor pulmonale and respiratory failure more readily than the "pink puffer." Because of the cardiac involvement and secondary polycythemia, these patients are usually cyanotic, and since they tend to have stocky builds and a plethoric appearance, they are called "blue bloaters."
   • On *auscultation* the "blue bloater" usually has widespread wheezes and crepitations (crackling sounds) that may be heard during exhalation.

12 A summary of type A and B patients is presented in Tables 8-12 to 8-14.

13 Treatment of the patient with chronic bronchitis will vary depending on the degree of pathologic and physiologic involvement. General measures include:
   a Removal of sources of bronchial irritation—smoke, dust, pollen, radical changes in temperature and humidity.
   b Treatment of respiratory tract infections—preventive care: no exposure to persons with infection; vaccines to prevent influenza, use of antibiotics to treat secondary to bacterial infections as they occur.
   c Treatment of dyspnea—bronchodilators to control airway spasm, heated high humidity via room air or oxygen therapy, bronchial drainage combined with chest physiotherapy, exercise to promote an effective cough.
   d Prevention of respiratory failure. Education of patient and family to recognize signs of failure; following patient on a routine outpatient or in-hospital basis, monitoring pulmonary function and arterial blood gases, comparing results to baseline studies.

TABLE 8-13 Effect of emphysema and bronchitis on laboratory values

Laboratory value	Emphysema (type A)	Bronchitis (type B)
Arterial oxygen pressure	Early: N; later: −	−
Arterial CO_2 pressure	Early: N; later: +	+
pH	Early: N; later: −	−
Hemoglobin	N	+

N, normal; −, decreased; +, elevated.

TABLE 8-14 Comparison of diagnostic criteria for emphysema and bronchitis

	Emphysema (type A)	—Bronchitis (type B)
Clinical features	Dyspnea, cor pulmonale unusual, "pink puffing," progressive dyspnea	Cough, sputum (sometimes purulent), cyanosis, plethoric appearance, polycythemia, fluid retention, cor pulmonatel, "blue-bloated," progresses to respiratory failure
Radiology	Hyperinflated thorax, attenuated peripheral vessels	Normal or congested lung fields, evidence of previous infection, severe bronchitis
Pathology	Widespread emphysema	May have some centrilobular emphysema
Physiology	Airway obstruction, TLC may be high, elastic recoil low, CO diffusing capacity low, $Paco_2$ normal, Pao_2 often > 65 mm Hg	Airway obstruction, TLC may be normal, Elastic recoil usually normal, DLCO may be normal, $Paco_2$ raised, Pao_2 often < 65 mm Hg

TLC, Total lung capacity; CO, carbon monoxide; DLCO, diffusing capacity of lung for carbon monoxide.

TABLE 8-12 Effect of emphysema and bronchitis on pulmonary function results

Pulmonary function test	Emphysema (type A)	Bronchitis (type B)
Vital capacity (VC)	− or +	− −
Residual volume (RV)	++ or +++	N or +
Total lung capacity (TLC)	+ or ++	− or N
Single-breath nitrogen (SBN_2)	++++	+ or ++
Maximum voluntary ventilation (MVV)	− − −	− −
Airways resistance (R_{aw})	N or +	++ or +++
Static compliance (C_{st})	+++	N or −
Dynamic compliance (C_{dyn})	− − −	− −
Diffusing capacity for carbon monoxide (DLCO)	− −	N or −

−, Decreased, +, elevated; N, normal.

e Respiratory therapy modalities. Those most frequently used include:
  • Heated humidifier or nebulizer using a face tent or aerosol mask (with or without supplemental oxygen)
  • Mechanical or manual percussion and vibration
  • Incentive breathing devices
  • Bronchodilators delivered with intermittent positive breathing (IPPB) or aerosol units
  • Mechanical ventilator via cuffed endotracheal tube or tracheostomy tube, if patient is in ventilatory failure

23.5 Acute infectious bronchiolitis

1 This is an acute inflammation of the bronchioles usually caused by a viral infection.
2 This disease may occur in adults as well as children, although it is most *frequently* seen in children. It is especially dangerous in children under 2 years of age because of the relatively small size of their airways.
3 The onset of symptoms is preceded by cough and dyspnea. During the early stages the symptoms closely resemble those of an asthmatic attack.
4 The child will be apprehensive, restless, and cyanotic, and respirations will be shallow and labored with a grunt heard on exhalation.
5 On auscultation, the chest is hyperresonant to percussion, with scattered rhonchi and wheezes in both lung fields.
6 The degree of airway obstruction may be mild to severe and can led to ventilatory failure if untreated.
7 *Treatment* of this type patient includes administration of high-humidity therapy, with or without supplemental oxygen, depending on Pao_2, followed by bronchodilators and antibiotics to prevent secondary infection. Chest physical therapy, including postural drainage, percussion, and vibration, may be of benefit. More details involving the recognition and treatment of this disease are presented in Module Twenty-six, Neonatal and Pediatric Respiratory Care.

23.6 Bronchiectasis

1 Bronchiectasis is a disease of the air passages (bronchi) that become dilated as the result of inflammation and ulceration.
2 The term "bronchiectasis" is derived from the Greek "bronchos" meaning windpipe and "ektasis" meaning extension of airways.
3 Bronchiectasis is usually accompanied by a chronic discharge of thick purulent sputum that has a prominent foul odor. Patients with bronchiectasis usually are very sensitive about this odor and may have varying degrees of emotional problems concerning it.
4 The condition develops when the bronchial walls are weakened by chronic infections involving the bronchial mucosa, submucosa, and muscular covering.
5 The chronic infectious state causes by bronchiectasis will spread from segment to segment throughout the lungs if not controlled. This will cause successive infection of conducting airways and the lung parenchyma.
6 There is no single specific cause of bronchiectasis. It is a disease based on abnormal anatomy that may be present at birth or that may develop in early childhood.
  a *Kartagener's syndrome* is an example of bronchiectasis caused by a congenital defect associated with dextrocardia and sinusitis.
  b It is generally accepted that bronchiectasis develops after childhood diseases or other causes of airway obstruction or atelectasis. The assumption is that the high intrathoracic pressures required to overcome the resistance of an atelectatic lung pulls on the walls of surrounding bronchi, causing them to dilate. The degree of dilation depends on the size of the affected bronchi, with the small airways being more distorted than the larger ones. Distortion and stress on small airways cause edema and airway plugging, which usually results in secondary infection and destruction of the bronchial walls. As normal tissue is destroyed, it is replaced by fibrous tissue and fixed distorted bronchi. This process is self-destructive in that fibrous tissue causes further distortion, more infection and so on, until segments and even lobes may be affected.
7 Conditions associated with causing bronchiectasis include:
  a Cystic fibrosis
  b Bronchiolitis, measles, whooping cough, influenza complicated by pneumonia
  c Airway obstruction caused by tumor or aspiration of foreign objects
  d Pulmonary tuberculosis
  NOTE: Contrary to popular thought, bronchiectasis is *not* caused by chronic bronchitis but by a bronchial obstruction accompanied by infection.
8 *Pathologically* bronchiectasis can be classified (Fig. 8-57) thus:
  a Saccular—cystic *(1)*
  b Cylindrical *(2)*
  c Fusiform—varicose *(3)*
    • This identification is based on the distorted *configuration* (shape) of the bronchi as caused by the disease process, which destroys bronchial walls, causes mucosa to become inflamed and die, stops ciliary action, and blocks airways with secretions and cellular debris. The various shapes of affected bronchi that follow are usually revealed by the use of an opaque fluid instilled into the lung to make x-ray films of the small airways much more visible (bronchography).
9 The saccular type *(1)* is the classic advanced form characterized by irregular dilation and narrowing of the airways. The bronchi dilate progressively toward the periphery of the lung and end in "blind sacs," which collect pooled secretions and serve as a source for continuous infection. Microscopic examination shows:

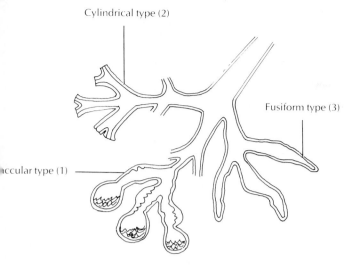

Cylindrical type (2)

Fusiform type (3)

accular type (1)

FIGURE 8-57 Bronchi affected by bronchiectasis. Three types are shown: saccular *(1)*, cylindrical *(2)*, and fusiform *(3)*.

TABLE 8-15 Effect of bronchiectasis on pulmonary function parameters

Test	Results
Vital capacity (VC)	−
Forced expiratory volume, one second (FEV_1)	−
Total lung capacity (TLC)	+ or −
Residual volume (RV)	+ or −
Maximum voluntary ventilation (MVV)	−
Single-breath nitrogen test (SBN_2)	++ or +
Airway resistance (R_{dw})	N or +
Static compliance (C_{st})	N or −
Partial pressure of oxygen in arterial blood (PaO_1)	−
Partial pressure of carbon dioxide in arterial blood ($PaCO_2$) (advanced stages)	+

−, Decreased; +, increased; N, normal.

a Destruction of walls of dilated bronchi

b Loss of cartilage, elastic tissue, and muscle

• Clinically, *clubbing* of the fingers is very common. This is related to hypertrophy of bronchial arteries combined with tissue hypoxemia. The saccular type is the most severe form of bronchiectasis and has the *worst* prognosis. "Dry" bronchiectasis is a true form of saccular bronchiectasis but without cough or expectoration.

10 Cylindrical (tubular) type bronchietasis *(2)* is characterized by the absence of normal bronchial tapering; it is usually a manifestation of severe chronic bronchitis rather than true bronchial wall destruction. Thus this type may be *reversed* as the obstructed condition is treated. In cylindrical bronchiectasis the bronchial walls are generally regular, with the bronchi ending squarely and abruptly. Mucous plugging and edema of the bronchial walls prevent the smaller branches from filling with the radiopaque medium, resulting in the cylindrical shape of the airways on the x-ray films.

11 In varicose (fusiform) bronchiectasis *(3)*, a radiograph will show irregularity produced by constrictions and dilations that deform the bronchial walls, giving it an appearance of varicose veins.

12 *Clinically,* the symptoms often date back to early childhood. Cough is usually present year-round but is especially aggravated by a cold or influenza.

a The sputum raised is usually purulent and copious, amounting to as much as 200 ml/day in severe cases. In some cases there is little or no sputum production; this is called "dry bronchiectasis." There is a close correlation between location of the disease and sputum production. For example, dependent bronchi produce more sputum than those in the upper lobes.

b *Hemoptysis* is common, with blood streaks or even large amounts of blood appearing in the sputum.

• Collected sputum, when left standing, settles out into three separate layers:

– Upper; watery, frothy

– Middle; turbid, mucopurulent

– Lower; opaque, purulent layer with small dirty-white and yellow masses (Dittrich's plugs)

c Occasionally brown or black specks or fibrouslike materials will be raised from lung tissues that have been destroyed.

d The patient in the more advanced stages may have clubbing of the fingers or may appear healthy except for expectoration of sputum and occasional dyspnea.

e Auscultation will reveal rales and rhonchi in the affected areas.

13 Pulmonary function studies will vary greatly among patients. For example, patients with little bronchial involvement will have normal pulmonary values as determined by routine spirometry and analysis of arterial blood gases. Patients with severe disease will exhibit changes including decreased vital capacities (VC), decreased forced expiratory volume in 1 second (FEV_1), decreased maximum voluntary ventilation (MVV), an increased functional residual capacity (FRC), and abnormal arterial blood gases (ABGs). Effects of bronchiectasis on pulmonary function are shown in Table 8-15.

14 The *prognosis* of severe untreated bronchiectasis is poor. Most patients die between 30 to 45 years after onset of symptoms. Death usually is by pneumonia, emphysema, right-sided heart failure, or other cardiopulmonary complications. Today, advances in medical treatment of these patients, especially antibiotic therapy and surgery, have resulted in normal life expectancy for many victims.

15 The *treatment* of bronchiectasis is directed primarily at measures to improve drainage of secretions, to control infection to prevent spreading, and to manage hypoxia and CO_2 levels. Respiratory care personnel play a major role in the treatment of these patients by:

a Hydration of the airways, using heated humidifiers and nebulizers.

b Administration of bronchodilators to control airway spasm.

c Implementation of chest physical therapy, including postural drainage, with clapping, vibration, and breathing control to produce an effective cough.

- In severe cases supplemental oxygen and/or mechanical ventilation may be required. If intermittent positive pressure is used, extreme care must be taken not to cause barotrauma resulting from rupture of blebs. In most cases incentive breathing techniques are adequate for hyperinflation of the lungs and promoting an effective cough.

23.7 Pneumonia

1 Pneumonia is an acute infection that causes inflammation of the lung. The inflammation then results in tissue swelling, which may lead to a filling of the air spaces with fluid. This congestion of the lung is called *consolidation.*

2 It can be caused by many bacterial agents: viruses and *Mycoplasma, Rickettsia,* and *Fungi* species. It can affect the lung as a primary disease or as a secondary disease. Pneumonia that strikes as a secondary insult to influenza has a very high mortality rate, especially in the elderly.

3 The major forms of pneumonia are bacterial, viral, secondary bacterial, and combined viral and bacterial pneumonia, which are discussed briefly in *4* through *7.* Other forms of pneumonia, many highly fatal, may be caused by the *Fungi* and *Rickettsia* spp., plague, and the aspiration of food, liquids, or other foreign substances into the lung.

4 Bacterial pneumonia. Most commonly caused by *pneumococci* bacterium, of which more than 80 strains have been identified. Other organisms frequently causing pneumonia are the *Streptococcus, Staphylococcus, Klebsiella,* and *Haemophilus influenzae* spp.

a Once bacteria have caused inflammation in the alveoli, the lungs respond by producing an exudate (fluid) that flows from the capillaries into the alveoli as a means of defense.

b The second stage of the lung's defense is the production of leukocytes. As the infection continues the infected alveoli are soon filled with bacterial debris, pus, and some red blood cells. As the alveoli fill, air is unable to flow or diffuse, and consolidation occurs. Hypoxia is usually evident.

c Consolidation can involve small, scattered areas of the lung (patchy consolidation) or can involve one large section or an entire lobe at one time. In the worst cases one entire side of the lung or more can be involved.

d As the infection runs its course, the leukocytes continue to clean up the cellular and bacterial debris as the bacteria count drops rapidly. The lung may be cleared in 2 to 3 weeks.

e Initial symptoms may be chills, chest pains, and a productive cough. Fever may exceed 40° C (104° F). Chest sounds heard by auscultation may reveal diffuse rales and distant breath sounds. Percussion shows a dull sound above areas of consolidation.

f Laboratory findings are as follows:

- Sputum cultures usually reveal the bacteria responsible for the infection.
- Blood cultures sometimes reveal the infective bacteria in the bloodstream (bacteremia).
- Radiology studies are very helpful in the bacterial pneumonias. Chest films reveal shadows of patchy or solid consolidation in the affected areas.
- Pulmonary function tests usually reveal a restrictive-type disease pattern with reduced compliance.

5 Viral pneumonia. Although up to 50% of all pneumonias are caused by viruses, many of which are not identified, no one form of viral pneumonia can be recognized by the clinical signs and symptoms it produces.

a First symptoms resemble an influenza infection with aches and muscle soreness, fever, headache, and dry cough. Shortness of breath increases, and cough becomes worse, producing scant amounts of bloody sputum. Breath sounds are usually good, and there is little evidence of consolidation.

b If the disease worsens, the most noticeable symptom is shortness of breath and extreme air hunger. Hypoxia is usually evident.

c Laboratory findings are as follows.

- There is usually a rise in viral antibodies and an elevated white blood cell count.
- In uncomplicated cases bacteria are rarely found.
- Diffuse shadows may show on x-ray films, but consolidation is not usually seen.
- Pulmonary function tests reveal a restrictive-type disease pattern.

6 Secondary bacterial pneumonia. Frequently the viral pneumonia will improve and symptoms subside only to suddenly worsen 2 to 3 weeks later.

a Symptoms are shaking chills, chest pains, and productive cough. Examination shows localized lung involvement and consolidation.

b Laboratory findings show bacterial infection from sputum and from blood samples (most often pneumococci and sometimes staphylococci).

7 Combined viral and bacterial pneumonia. This serious combination usually begins as an influenzal viral pneumonia, with bacterial infection following after several days. Symptoms and laboratory findings are similar to other forms, but the bacterial infection is most often caused by staphylococci.

8 Treatment of pneumonia depends on the cause. Widespectrum antibiotics are effective against the bacterial pneumonias and some of the rickettsial diseases. On the other hand, there is no effective treatment for viral pneumonia, only supportive therapy.

- Supportive therapy includes proper diet, relief from pain, bed rest, oxygen to relieve shortness of breath and hypoxia, and humidity to aid in the removal of secretions and to improve the cleansing mechanism of the cough.

NOTE: Because of the disturbances in ventilation (shunts), supplemental oxygen does not always reduce the hypoxemia.

23.8 Tuberculosis*

Tuberculosis (TB) is the disease caused by *Mycobacterium tuberculosis* and primarily involves the lungs, although it may also involve any other part of the body.

An infectious disease, it is spread primarily by airborne droplets produced by talking, eating, coughing, and sneezing. Although the introduction of chemotherapy has reduced mortality from tuberculosis, the number of cases has not declined as rapidly.† For example, in 1932 the new case rate was 76.7 per 100,000 population. In 1974, after chemotherapy the new case rate was still 14.2 per 100,000.

In the same period the mortality rate decreased from approximately 202 per 100,000 in 1900 to a low of 1.8 per 100,000 in 1974.

Nevertheless respiratory care personnel must be aware that patients with tuberculosis are still a source of cross-infection, and all precautions should be taken for protection against infection when treating them.

23.9 Fungal infections

1 The most common infection caused by fungus is *histoplasmosis,* which is caused by the *Histoplasma capsulatum.* The lungs are most often involved, and the disease may resemble tuberculosis.

   a The disease was not identified as a fungal involvement until 1934, and a diagnostic skin test, developed in 1945, revealed that this disease is widespread, although rarely fatal.

   b Although chronic infection with histoplasmosis is considered endemic in the Mississippi and Ohio River Valleys, it is found worldwide.

   c *H. capsulatum* is found on the droppings of birds and bats and whenever conditions of humidity, temperature, and fertility are ideal (such as in chicken coops, belfries, or bat-infested caves). *H. capsulatum* produces countless spores.

   • These spores are inhaled into the lung where phagocytes carry them to adjacent pulmonary lymph ducts. Here an allergic-type reaction occurs that becomes inflammatory and causes tubercle formation, caseation, scarring, calcification, and possibly cavity formation. At this stage only laboratory tests can differentiate between histoplasmosis and tuberculosis.

   d Fortunately the disease is not frequently serious, and an acute pulmonary infection carries an excellent prognosis and uneventful recovery. The chronic, generalized infections are more serious in the very

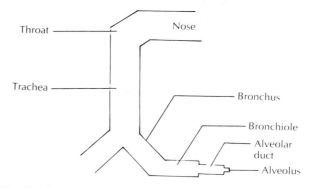

FIGURE 8-58 Air passages. (From American Lung Association: Breathing . . . what you need to know, New York, 1975, The Association, p 10.)

young and the elderly, and the cavitary form is usually terminal.

2 Symptoms of pulmonary infection include fever, malaise, and periods of weight loss. The generalized form demonstrates fever, rapid loss of weight, anemia, and liver and spleen enlargement.

3 Laboratory findings are as follows:

   a Sputum cultures in chronic histoplasmosis usually reveal the presence of *H. capsulatum;* the organism can also be detected from lymph node biopsy.

   b Special skin tests similar to the tuberculin test will reveal those individuals who are or have been previously infected.

   c Chest radiographs shows multiple, poorly defined shadows and enlargement of the lymph nodes during the acute phase. The chronic, cavitating disease shows calcification, scarring, and cavities indistinguishable from tuberculosis.

4 Although cases may take weeks or months to clear, most acute primary cases require no treatment. The chronic or persistent cases require hospitalization for long periods, and a drug, amphotericin B, has been found to be very effective in speeding recovery. Surgical resection of cavities may be necessary.

5 Other lung diseases caused by fungi and less common than histoplasmosis are:

   a Blastomycosis

   b Cryptococcosis

   c Actinomycosis

   d Nocardiosis

23.10 Bronchial asthma

1 Bronchial asthma is one of a series of diseases or conditions known as *chronic obstructive pulmonary disease* (COPD). These include asthma, chronic bronchitis, and emphysema, although cystic fibrosis and bronchiectasis are sometimes included because of small airway involvement.

   a Bronchial spasmodic asthma is characterized by intermittent episodes of bronchospasm, with increased responsiveness of the bronchioles and upper airway passages to various stimuli, causing sudden general-

---

*American Lung Association: Diagnostic standards and classification of tuberculosis and other mycobacterial diseases, New York, 1974, The Association.

†Weg JG: Pulmonary medicine.

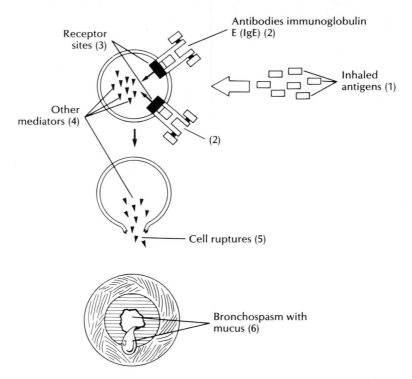

FIGURE 8-59 Symptoms of asthma are caused by the substances released by mast cells located in airway tissue.

ized narrowing of the airways and characteristic wheezing. Fig. 8-58, a schematic drawing of the air passages, provides perspective to involved disease areas. The figure illustrates only relative positions of parts of the tube system, not their relative sizes.

b Asthma comes from the Greek, meaning *panting*. This term vividly describes the clinical picture of the asthma patient.

c The medical axiom "all that wheezes is not asthma" means that a diagnosis of asthma should not be automatically assumed. Many diseases or conditions cause wheezes, such as bronchitis, tumors, or foreign objects in the airway.

d Asthma is a common respiratory disease that may begin at any age. In approximately 50% of the reported cases it begins before age 10 years. In one third of the cases it may be hereditary, with other family members having had asthma.

e Asthma seems to be more common among boys than girls, although later in life it seems to be more prevalent among women than men.

2 Although the one common characteristic is the hypersensitivity of the airways and resultant spasm, asthma can be categorized as *extrinsic* (atopic) or *intrinsic* (nonatopic).

a Patients with extrinsic asthma have some history of allergies, resulting in a hypersensitivity situation of an *antigen-antibody* type reaction. These patients usually have a family history of hypersensitivity and a personal history of *infantile eczema, dermatitis,*

hives, or *hay fever.* Extrinsic asthma results from the exposure (sensitization) of an atopic individual to an *allergen,* usually proteins such as pollen, molds, spores, animal dander, feathers, dust, lint, insecticides, certain foods (milk, seafood, nuts, chocolate), and even drugs such as aspirin.

b Intrinsic asthma cannot be linked to exogenous allergens. This type of asthma is frequently associated with respiratory tract infection and occurs most commonly in patients who contract asthma in later life.

3 In allergic patients the symptoms of asthma are caused by pharmacologically active substances that are released by mast cells located in the connective tissue (smooth muscle) of the airways (Fig. 8-59) or fixed to the basophils in the peripheral blood network. Individuals with extrinsic asthma respond to inhaled antigens *(1)* by producing antibodies, immunoglobulin E (IgE) *(2),* which become attached to the receptor sites located on mast cells in the respiratory tract *(3).* An *antigen* is any foreign substance tht stimulates the formation of an *antibody.* A specific antigen such as pollen does *not* produce a unique clinical picture; rather the clinical response will depend on the target (shock) organ. In one patient the same antigen may cause a runny nose; in another, asthma. Antibodies are proteins (immunoglobulin) that are formed in reaction to the antigen. When a reaction occurs between the antigen and antibody in the respiratory tract, the mast cell releases histamine and other mediators (4), which ruptures the cell *(5)* and causes bronchospasm, edema, and hypersecretion (6) in the affected air passages.

- Allergic reactions are not limited to causing respiratory impairment and may in fact cause hives, tearing of the eyes, or more severe anaphylactic reactions resulting in circulatory shock. Reactions have been classified by Coombs and Gell as type I, II, III, or IV.

4 In nonallergic asthmatic patients the increased hypersensitivity to stimuli such as infection, exertion, drugs, climatic changes, and emotional stress causes a *vagal* nerve reflex. This reflex, through cholinergic stimulation, also causes bronchospasm, edema, and hypersecretion of mucus.

5 Pathologic changes in asthma include:

a Hypertrophy of bronchial and bronchiole smooth muscle that contracts during an attack, causing bronchoconstriction.

b Hypertrophy of the submucosal mucous glands with an increase in the size and number of mucous goblet cells.

c Detachment of the epithelial lining of the bronchi and bronchioles, leaving the basement membrane exposed, resulting in its becoming inflamed and thickened with associated bronchial wall edema.

d Excessive submucosal infiltration by eosinophils.

e In *status asthmaticus,* thick tenacious plugs (Curschmann's spirals) blocking the small airways, which, on examination, contain portions of the epithelial lining (there is sloughing of ciliated cells).

f Hyperinflated lung parenchyma with areas of atelectasis (especially in status asthmaticus caused by the thick tenacious intraluminal plugs).

6 Asthma may be produced by an immunologic reaction.

7 *Clinical symptoms* usually include wheezing and dyspnea to varying degrees. Attacks may be insidious or sudden, with mild to severe involvement, depending on the circumstances. During an attack the patient will feel tightness in the chest and complain of dyspnea. He or she will usually assume an upright position and use accessory muscles for both inhalation and exhalation. A cough usually is not productive during the initial stage of the attack. Later it will be productive, with thick, stringy mucoid secretions that are difficult to raise. An attack may last from a few minutes to hours or days. An attack that does not respond to treatment is said to be *refractory* or that the patient is in *status asthmaticus.* Status asthmaticus is dangerous and should be treated aggressively in the hospital.

8 Radiographic examination of the chest during an attack reveals evidence of hyperinflation of lung volumes with hyperlucency of the lung fields.

9 *Auscultation* of the chest will reveal musical sounds or wheezes. Lung sounds are heard mostly during exhalation, although in severe attacks they will be present during both phases of ventilation.

10 *Paradoxical pulse* (marked fall in systolic and pulse pressure during inspiration) may be present because of the variation of systolic blood pressure during breathing. The increased work of breathing during an attack may cause the systolic blood pressure to be 10 mm Hg higher during exhalation than during inspiration, indicating severe airway obstruction. Changes in this sign can be used as an indicator of the progress of the attack and benefits of treatment.

11 Another useful test is to assess forced expiratory volumes by auscultation over the trachea. With the stethoscope bell placed above the suprasternal notch, the patient is asked to inhale deeply and exhale as quickly and completely as possible. Normally, expiration *should not continue beyond 1 to 2 seconds.* If expiratory gas flow exceeds 6 seconds, there is significant airway obstruction. This test is also useful in evaluating the patient's response to bronchodilator therapy.

12 Pulmonary function studies of the asthmatic patient will render grossly different results on the same person. Patients with spasmodic asthma are tested during one of the five pathophysiologic states:

a *Complete remission.* Patient completely without symptoms, and pulmonary function values are normal.

b *Partial remission.* Patient is clinically free of all symptoms between attacks, although there may be a continued slight increase in pulmonary resistance to air flow as well as a nonuniform distribution of inspired gas and a slight decrease in lung compliance.

c *Moderate bronchospasm.* In mild cases airway obstruction is limited to peripheral airways of 2 mm inner diamter or less. Because small airways account for such a small fraction of the total resistance to air flow, ventilatory function may still be relatively normal. Lung compliance will fall as respiratory rates are increased, showing the effects of air trapping by the small airways. As the attack worsens the larger airways become spasmodic and maximum breathing capacity (MBC), forced expiratory volume in 1 second (FEV_1), maximum expiratory flow rate (MEFR), and peak expiratory flow rate (PEFR) are affected.

d *Severe bronchopasm.* In severe cases large and small airways become spasmodic. The patient hyperventilates, characterized by hypocapnia ($Pa_{CO_2} < 40$ mm Hg) and dehydration resulting from water loss. As the condition worsens the Pa_{CO_2} begins to rise and Pa_{O_2} decreases because of the extreme shunting situation of mismatched ventilation-perfusion ratios. In severe bronchospasm, pulmonary function values as discussed in *c* are greatly altered. For example, PEFR becomes less than 100 L/min, with 400 to 600 L/min being normal. A PEFR less than 60 L/min is generally associated with high mortality.

e *Status asthmaticus.* A potentially *life-threatening* situation that requires hospital admission and close monitoring of ventilatory function. These patients may or may not be responsive to bronchodilator drugs. They have a severe reduction in their vital capacities and PEFRs, indicating gross air trapping. *Pulsus paradoxus* (paradoxical pulse) is usually

TABLE 8-16 General changes in pulmonary function parameters as caused by spasmodic asthma

Function tested	During attack	Symptomatic with frequent attacks	Asymptomatic with rare attacks
Vital capacity	$--$	$-$ or N	N
Residual volume	$++++$		N
Total lung capacity	$+++$	$++$	N
Single-breath nitrogen	$++++$	$+$	$+$
Maximum voluntary ventilation	$----$	$++$	N
		$-$ or N	
Airway resistance	$++++$	$+$ or N	N
Static compliance	$+$	N	N
Dynamic compliance	Yes$+++$	Yes$++$	$+$
Arterial oxygen tension		N	N
Arterial CO_2 tension	Late	N	N

$-$, Decreased; N, normal; $+$, elevated.

present and will correlate well with changes in the FEV_1. Spirometry tests discussed in *c* will be grossly altered, and the pattern of blood gases generally will reflect hypoxemia ($Pao_2 < 60$ mm Hg) with elevated CO_2 tensions > 45 mm Hg. The severity of these changes will depend on the severity and length of the attack.

13 General changes in pulmonary function tests caused by spasmodic asthma are presented in Table 8-16.

14 The following material summarizes principles and facts related to spasmodic asthma:

	Extrinsic (atopic/allergic) asthma	*Intrinsic (nonatopic/idiopathic/ infective)*
a	Family history usually positive	Family history usually negative
b	Attacks related to specific antigens (pollens, foods, drugs, dusts, danders)	Attacks related to infections, exercise, etc.
c	Skin test results usually positive	Skin test results usually negative
d	History of eczema in childhood	No history of eczema in childhood
e	Favorable response to hyposensitization	Unfavorable response to hyposensitization
f	IgE associated	IgE not associated
g	Attacks acute but usually self-limiting; prognosis favorable; conditions often outgrown but may become chronic; death rare	Attacks more fulminant and severe; prognosis poorer; condition may become chronic; death may occur
h	Usually during childhood	Usually in adults after age 30 years
i	No aspirin sensitivity	Aspirin sensitivity frequent
j	Sputum: many eosinophils, Charcot-Leyden crystals,* and Curschmann's spirals†	Sputum: few eosinophils
k	Blood eosinophils	May or may not have blood eosinophils
l	Expiratory wheeze, rhonchi scattered	Expiratory wheeze, rhonchi
m	"Allergic shiner" may be present; dark circles under the eyes	Nasal polyps in some cases

*Degenerative crystalloids of eosinophils.
†Tiny whorls arising as casts within the smaller airway; may be several centimeters in length.

15 The most common clinical signs of asthma are:
 a Respiratory distress
 b Apprehension
 c Flushing, cyanosis
 d Cough
 e Flaring of nares
 f Use of accessory muscles
 g Tachycardia
 h Perspiration
 i Hyperresonance of chest on auscultation
 j Distant breath sounds
 k Rhonchi
 l Eosinophilia (sputum)
 m Prolonged expiratory time
 n Hyperinflation of chest
 o Scant and viscid sputum, usually mucoid (white), perhaps purulent (yellow, gray, green)

16 *Treatment of asthma.* Patient education is an important component of the recognition and treatment of asthma. Patients must be able to recognize the signs and symptoms of an impending attack and begin self-care before it becomes a full-blown emergency. However, patients and their families must also recognize and realize the limitations of self-care and understand the importance of seeking medical assistance when it is indicated.

 a Precaution plays an important role in the treatment of asthma. A patient history and environmental profile may allow the physician to remove the unsuspecting asthmatic individual from irritants that can trigger an attack. A comprehensive care plan should be developed that covers all aspects of the patient's pathophysiologic status and life-style. This includes periodic assessment of airway obstruction and emphasis on mental health and relaxation.

 b An exercise program should be developed that will promote physical fitness but will not trigger an attack. Special breathing control methods such as relaxation exercises, diaphragmatic breathing, and *pursed-lip* breathing should be taught (Fig. 8-60). Pursed-lip breathing allows the patient to exhale against a partially closed proximal airway *(1)*. This mechanical maneuver creates a subtle back pressure that internally splints the small airways *(2)* open against increasing positive intrathoracic pressure of exhalation *(3)*. This splinting action allows more time for gas to be exhaled by reducing early airway closure. Many patients with COPD whistle or even unconsciously perform this maneuver.

 c Medications should be prescribed to prevent and control episodes of asthma. These may include bronchodilators, decongestants, steroids, iodides, antibiotics for secondary infections, and cromolyn sodium. Cromolyn sodium is a drug that has the unique property of blocking the release of histamine and slow-reacting substance of anaphylaxis from sensitized mast cells, preventing an attack. It, however, has no effect whatsoever once the attack is under way.

 d The specific treatment for a patient will depend on

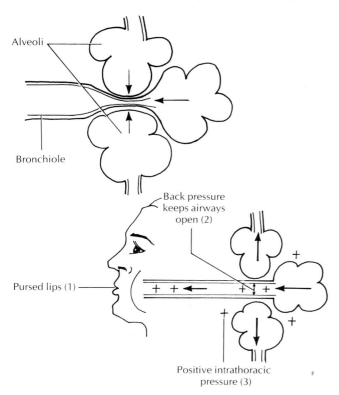

Alveoli

Bronchiole

Back pressure keeps airways open (2)

Pursed lips (1)

Positive intrathoracic pressure (3)

FIGURE 8-60 Pursed lip breathing.

whether the patient is in a mild, moderate, severe, or status attack.

Mild attacks usually can be self-treated at home by bronchodilation therapy. The drug may be administered with a metered dose inhaler; a gas-powered nebulizer, with or without intermittent positive pressure breathing (IPPB) and supplemental oxygen; or taken orally. Patients caring for themselves must be alerted against *abuse* of their medications through overdose, mixing of drugs, and contamination problems.

Patients having *moderate attacks* probably should seek medical advice. It is important that physicians be advised for any treatments that have been used in the past and any reactions to drugs. Patients seen on an outpatient basis will be given a thorough workup, including a history and physical examination. Auscultation of the chest will reveal musical sounds, especially during exhalation. A laboratory workup, including a complete blood count (CBC), urinalysis, sputum examination, and a chest radiograph may prove helpful.

- Typical sputum in an attack is white, thick, and viscous and stays stuck to the bottom of the container when it is inverted.
- Copious thin sputum suggests some other diagnosis.
- Purulent sputum suggests an infection.

- Sputum with small brown plugs suggests complicating allergic aspergillosis.
- Curschmann's spirals and bronchial casts suggest status asthmaticus.

Treatment may include bronchodilator therapy using hand-held nebulizer, breathing control (pursed lips), and IPPB.

NOTE: IPPB probably is *not* indicated if a patient can move adequate ventilation without assistance. Chest physical therapy combined with pulmonary drainage may assist in clearing the airways.

Treatment of *severe asthma* or *status asthmaticus* should be carried out in a step-by-step fashion, proceeding from the basic to more advanced techniques.

- Previous drug therapy should be noted.
- Adequate hydration should be maintained.
- Arterial blood gases (ABGs) should be monitored and oxygen given as needed by face mask or nasal cannula, if needed.
- Ventilatory support is a clinical decision that cannot be instituted from isolated ABG values.
- Theophylline and other drugs should be administered as indicated to achieve bronchial dilation.
- Chest physical therapy, including bronchial drainage, percussion, and vibration, may assist in removal of tenacious secretions.

e The patient must be carefully monitored at all times, as sudden movement of secretions from peripheral to major airways could cause major airway obstruction, atelectasis, pneumothorax, and other gas-flow, pressure-related incidents.

f The importance of developing *rapport* and *trust* between the clinician and patient cannot be overemphasized. In many cases such a relationship will allow the clinician to "talk a patient out of an attack," especially if it is tension or anxiety related.

g Atropine is being effectively used for bronchodilation in asthma. Its action as a parasympathetic blocker combined with its effect on reduction of secretions has made it of potential value as a bronchodilator in patients who are allergic to dust and other environmental contaminants.

23.11 Pulmonary emphysema

1 Pulmonary emphysema is another one of those diseases that is identified as being chronic obstructive pulmonary disease (COPD). It falls into the category of obstructive diseases, not because conductive airways are directly narrowed by disease, but because airways close prematurely on expiration. Premature closure is a result of destruction of normal supporting pulmonary tissue, which exerts an outward radial force that helps to maintain patency of the airways. Although it has been described in clinical, radiologic, and physiologic terms, it is best defined *morphologically*. Emphysema is a word from the Greek meaning "puffed out."

Emphysema is an enlargement of air spaces distal to

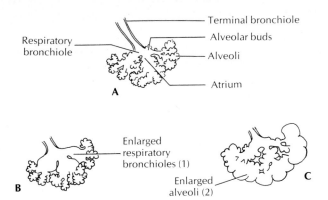

FIGURE 8-61 Classification of emphysema. **A,** Acinus of lungs affected by different types of emphysema. **B,** Centrilobar emphysema. **C,** Panlobular emphysema.

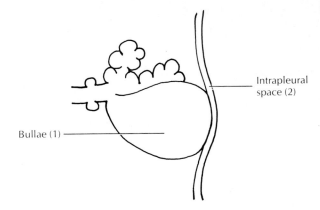

FIGURE 8-62 Acinus of lung affected by bullous emphysema.

the terminal nonrespiratory bronchiole, with subsequent destruction of alveolar walls.

The lung has approximately 35,000 terminal bronchioles, and their total internal cross section is at least 40 times as great as that of the lobar bronchi. The structure of the terminal bronchioles is primarily smooth muscle that is easily obstructed by secretions, by thickening of the walls because of edema, by inward collapse resulting from the loss of elasticity of the surrounding parenchyma, and by inspissation of exudate.

The terminal bronchiole is purely a conducting airway and does not have alveoli in its walls, as have the respiratory bronchioles.

The portion of the lung distal to the terminal bronchioles is called the *acinus.* The acinus is considered by many to be the anatomic unit of the lung. The acinus is the area of the lung primarily affected by emphysema.

2 Emphysema is classified according to which portion of the acinus is involved (Fig. 8-61, *A*).

a *Centrilobular emphysema* involves primarily the respiratory bronchioles, which become enlarged, with large areas of tissue destroyed adjacent to normal lung tissue (see Fig. 8-61, *B, 1*). This type of emphysema occurs primarily in the upper portion of the lung in males and is closely associated with bronchitis and smoking.

b *Panlobular emphysema* involves the acinus almost uniformly, with enlarged alveoli that have expanded to include the alveolar ducts. Septa separating alveoli disappear, and holes appear in the alveolar walls as they become nonfunctioning thin strands of tissue surrounded by capillaries (see Fig. 8-61, *C, 2*). Panlobular emphysema can occur anywhere in the lung but usually involves the lower regions. it is equally common in men and women and is not associated with bronchitis. It is related to a familial alpha₁-antitrypsin deficiency. Panlobular emphysema is often found in older people who do not have chronic bron-

chitis or clinical impairment of lung function. The term "senile emphysema" was formerly used to describe this condition. This term subsequently has fallen into disuse, because it is difficult for physiologists to determine where the normal aging of the lung ends and COPD begins.

c *Bullous emphysema (Fig. 8-62) describes a condition where there are isolated emphysematous changes with the development of bullae (1)* in the apparent absence of underlying generalized emphysema. A bulla is an air space that is larger than 1 cm when it is inflated. A smaller, more superficial air space is referred to as a *bleb.* The clinical significance of blebs and bullae is that their walls are usually thinner and less supported than normal alveoli, and they are more prone to rupture when exposed to elevated, internal gas pressures. If rupture of these structures occurs, gas will leak into the intrapleural space *(2)* and cause a *tension pneumothorax.*

At autopsy the lungs appear large, pale, and relatively bloodless, with many superficial blebs on the parenchymal surfaces. When the chest is opened the lungs do not collapse from the force of the atmosphere, indicating extensive air trapping. On histologic examination, numerous alveoli are seen to be distended and disrupted, with a decrease in the number and size of pulmonary capillaries. Chronic bronchitis is frequently found, and in severe emphysema the walls of the alveoli are incomplete and easily collapsed.

3 *Etiology.* The etiology (cause) of the emphysema cannot be linked to any known *single* source. Smoking and heredity are considered as strong factors, although the most immediate and frequent cause seems to be recurring or chronic inflammation of the bronchioles with functional obstruction of the air passages, primarily during exhalation. Obstructed air passages lead to distal air trapping and pooling of secretions, which cause infection and further edema and obstruction. Some air continues to enter lobules even when the primary air passages are blocked by collateral ventilation via Kohn's pores. This process results in a constant and

continuously increased stretching of the tissue connecting with the central bronchiole, until the alveolar walls and surrounding capillaries are destroyed. This process results in permanent destruction of tissue, which is not regenerated even though the obstructing process may be relieved. The destruction of alveolar septa and capillaries results in an inadequate blood supply to lung tissue itself, and eventually cellular hypoxemia and acidosis occur.

The boxed material includes general questions concerning respiratory symptoms, which can be used to obtain a history of a patient suspected of having emphysema.

4 *Clinical signs*. Emphysema begins insidiously, with the victim not able to pinpoint its onset. Repeated colds, increased sputum, and increasing dyspnea all seem to be common symptoms. Dyspnea is the chief and only essential symptom. It is noticed only on exertion initially and is usually attributed to age, body weight, smoking, or a lack of exercise. Dyspnea can be relieved at first by rest, until right-sided heart failure begins.

a There is some clubbing of the fingertips, and the chest is usually deep and almost spherical shaped, like a barrel—"barrel-chested." The patient appears to always be in a state of maximum inspiration despite forced efforts of exhalation.

b Accessory muscles are used for both inhalation and exhalation, and the patient usually assumes sitting or lying positions that are most conducive to fixing the accessory muscles for breathing (orthopnea).

c Emphysema patients will also use various conscious or unconscious airway maneuvers such as pursed-lip breathing or whistling to help stabilize the airways against early collapse during exhalation.

d Breath sounds are reduced in intensity and may be difficult to hear because of the increased distance of the chest from the lung tissue and the absence of conductive lung tissue itself.

5 A thorough patient history and physical workup are extremely useful in identifying patients with COPD. Simple questions may be indicative of the degree of COPD involvement.

A summary of physical signs generally found in COPD follows*:

Early: Examination may be negative or show only slight prolongation of forced expiration (which can be timed while auscultating over the trachea—normally 3 seconds or less); slight dimunition of breath sounds at the apices or bases; or scattered rhonchi or wheezes, especially on expiration, often best heard over the hili anteriorly. The rhonchi often clear after cough.

*American Lung Association: Chronic obstructive lung disease, ed 5, New York, 1977, The Association, p 64.

Respiratory symptoms questionnaire

Do you usually cough or have to clear your throat in the morning or when you get up?

Do you usually cough for as many as 3 months each year?

Do you usually bring up any mucus, sputum, or phlegm from your chest during the day?

Do you usually bring up any mucus, sputum, or phlegm for as many as 3 months each year?

Do you have to stop for breath when walking at your own pace on level ground?

Do you get short of breath when walking with other people of your own age on level ground?

Do you ever wheeze?

From American Lung Association: Chronic obstructive pulmonary disease, ed 5, New York, 1977, The Association, p 49.

Moderate: The above signs are usually present and more pronounced, often with decreased rib expansion; use of the accessory muscles of respiration; retraction of the supraclavicular fossae in inspiration; generalized hyperresonance; decreased area of cardiac dullness; diminished heart sounds at base; and increased anteroposterior distance of the chest.

Advanced: Examination usually shows the above findings to a greater degree, and often shows evidence of weight loss; depression of the liver; hyperpnea and tachycardia with mild exertion; low and relatively immobile diaphragm; contraction of abdominal muscles on inspiration; and inaudible heart sounds except in the xiphoid area; cyanosis.

Cor pulmonale: There is increased intensity and splitting of pulmonic second sound, right-sided diastolic gallop, left parasternal heave (right ventricular overactivity), and early systolic pulmonary ejection click with or without systolic ejection murmur.

With failure: distended neck veins, functional tricuspid insufficiency, V waves, hepatojuglar reflux, hepatomegaly, and peripheral edema.

6 Chest radiographs of patients with emphysema will reveal varied changes, including:

a Depressed and flattened diaphragms

b Narrowed mediastinum

c Reduced vascular markings

d Increased depth of space between the heart and sternum on lateral view

e Increased anteroposterior diameter of the chest

f Increased radiolucency of the lung fields

7 Because of the frequently occurring coexistence of bronchitis with emphysema, it has been difficult to clinically separate the two. Over the past two decades a great deal of effort has been devoted toward describing the pathophysiologic differences that do occur. These are summarized in Table 8-17.

8 *Pulmonary function tests.* Specific effects of emphysema on various pulmonary function tests are shown in Table 8-18.

9 Comparison of lung volumes to ventilatory impairment is presented in Table 8-19.

10 Pulmonary function values can be useful in predicting the degree of ventilatory impairment as shown in Table 8-20.

In severe stages the forced expiratory volume per second (FEV_1) can be used as an indication of survival. For example, patients with an $FEV_1 < 750$ ml usually die in less than 5 years.

11 Laboratory test values are varied as x-ray results, although generally:

a Red cell count increases (polycythemia) to compensate for lowered O_2 tension.

b White cell count is normal except during episodes of acute infection.

c With respiratory failure, actual blood gases reveal decreased Pao_2, indicating hypoxemia; increased $Paco_2$, signifying inadequate alveolar ventilation; elevated or decreased pH, depending on bicarbonate (HCO_3^-) levels; and elevated or decreased HCO_3^-, depending on the length of the failure. An analysis

TABLE 8-17 Pathophysiologic differences in chronic obstructive pulmonary disease

	Disease process		
Criteria	Emphysema	Bronchitis	Chronic asthma
Loss of tractional support	+		
Alveolar destruction	+		
Bronchial atrophy	+	Late minimal	
Bronchial obliteration	++	+	
Airway inflammation, edema		+	+
Airway mucus plugs		+	+
Airway muscle spasm	None	Small	+

+, Elevated.

TABLE 8-18 Pulmonary function tests

Description	Term used	Symbol	Comments
The maximum volume of air exhaled from the point of maximum inspiration	Vital capacity	VC	Slow vital capacity may be normal or reduced in COPD patients
Vital capacity performed with a maximally forced expiratory effort	Forced vital capacity	FVC	Forced vital capacity is often reduced in COPD because of air trapping
Volume of air exhaled in the specified time during the performance of forced vital capacity	Forced expiratory volume (qualified by subscript indicating the time interval in sec)	FEV_1 (usually FEV_1)	A valuable clue to the severity of the expiratory airway obstruction
FEV_1 expressed as a percentage of the forced vital capacity	Ratio of timed forced expiratory volume to forced vital capacity	$FEV_1/FVC\%$ (usually $FEV_1/FVC\%$)	Another way of expressing the presence or absence of airway obstruction
Mean forced expiratory flow between 200 and 1200 ml of the FVC	Forced expiratory flow	FEF 200-1200	Formerly called "maximum expiratory flow rate" (MEFR); an indicator of large airway obstruction
Mean forced expiratory flow during the middle half of the FVC	Forced midexpiratory flow	FEF 25%-75%	Formerly called "maximum midexpiratory flow rate"; slowed in small airway obstruction
Mean forced expiratory flow during the terminal portion of the FVC	Forced end-expiratory flow	FEF 75%-85%	Slowed in obstruction of smallest airways
Volume of air expired in a specified period during repetitive maximal effort	Maximal voluntary ventilation	MVV	Formerly called "maximum breathing capacity"; an important factor in exercise tolerance.

From American Lung Association: Chronic obstructive pulmonary disease, ed 5, New York, 1977, The Association, p 42.

of hematocrit (hct) levels usually reveals bleeding or erythrocythemia, both of which would interfere with normal pulmonary perfusion and gas transfer. Excessively high hematocrits (>60%) have been attributed to increased incidences of pulmonary *thromboembolism*.

The laboratory values in Table 8-21 are frequently used to assess the degree of diffusion-perfusion involvement in COPD patients.

12 In summary, the differential features of emphysema, chronic bronchitis, and asthma can be useful in identifying the disease entity (Table 8-22).

13 *Treatment of emphysema*. The treatment of emphysema is as varied as the symptoms of the disease process itself. Many things still are not understood about the disease process, although it is known that once lung damage has occurred, new tissue will *not* be generated, nor can it be repaired by medical science. For this reason therapeutic measures are directed at *relieving* the symptoms and taking measures to *slow progression* of the disease. A treatment plan should be designed based on addressing the presenting manifestations (i.e., bronchospasm, dyspnea, allergy, hypercapnia, hypoxemia, and psychologic disturbances).

The establishment of good therapist-patient rapport is extremely important to gain the patient's trust and maximum cooperation.

Other areas included in a treatment plan might include:

a Diet. Elevated fluid intake, combined with high-caloric foods and small feedings might prevent weight loss. The patient should not be overweight and probably should try to stabilize at a weight slightly less than the ideal weight.

b Climate and altitude. Climate changes usually are not beneficial unless related to a more temperate climate during the winter months. This will help prevent the bronchospasm associated with inhaling cold air. Altitudes above 4000 feet may not be well tolerated by patients with reduced Pao_2 at sea level. Even air travel may require supplemental oxygen, since most cabins are not pressurized until 6000 feet of altitude is reached.

c Clean air. Patients with emphysema should avoid any exposure to respiratory irritants. Cigarette smoking *must* be stopped, since it is a primary cause of lung deterioration. It is likely that lung deterioration will be slowed if a patient quits smoking. Other irritants such as dusts, fumes, and extreme temperature changes in inhaled air must be avoided to prevent bronchospasm and related problems.

Patients with emphysema should avoid persons with respiratory infections. A special effort during influenza outbreaks or other epidemics must be made to avoid crowds.

TABLE 8-19 Relationship of lung volumes to type of ventilatory impairment

Interpretation	FVC	FEV$_1$	FEV$_1$ FEC%	RV	TLC
Normal	Normal	Normal	Normal	Normal	Normal
Airway obstruction	Normal or low	Low	Low	High	High
Lung restriction	Low	Normal or low	Normal or high	Normal or low	Low
Obstruction and restriction	Low	Low	Low	Variable	Variable

From American Lung Association: Chronic obstructive pulmonary disease, ed 5, New York, 1977, The Association, p 45.
FVC, Forced vital capacity; FEV$_1$, forced expiratory volume per second; RV, residual volume; TLC, total lung capacity.

TABLE 8-20 Suggested categories of ventilatory impairment as percentage of predicted mean values

	VC, FVC, FEV$_1$, MVV	FEF$_{200-1200}$, FEF$_{25\%-75\%}$ FEF$_{75\%-85\%}$
Normal	>80	>75%
Mild	65-80	60-75
Moderate	50-64	45-59
Severe	35-49	30-44
Very severe	<35	<30

From the American Lung Association: Chronic obstructive pulmonary disease, ed 5, New York, 1977, The Association, p 45.
VC, Vital capacity; FVC, Forced vital capacity; FEV$_1$, forced expiratory volume per second; MVV, maximum voluntary ventilation; FEF, forced expiratory flow.

T A B L E 8 - 2 1 Blood gases and acid-base balance: terminology and values

Term	Definition	Remarks	Normal range (mean)
Arterial O_2 saturation (SaO_2)	Ratio of oxygen content and capacity	Influenced by the S-shaped O_2 hemoglobin dissociation curve, with its steep slope between 10 and 50 mm Hg PO_2 and flat portion between 70 and 100 mm Hg PO_2	93%-98% (97%) rises to about 100% if breathing 100% O_2
Arterial O_2 tension (PaO_2)	Partial pressure of oxygen	In equilibrium wth alveolar oxygen tension breathing 100% O_2	80-104 mm Hg (95%), 600 mm Hg
Arterial pH	Expression (negative logarithm) of the hydrogen concentration	Determined by the ratio of concentrations of bicarbonate ion and CO_2 (as dissolved CO_2, H_2CO_3, carbamino compounds) usually 20:1	7.38-7.44 (7.41)
Arterial CO_2 tension (PaCO_2)	Partial pressure of carbon dioxide	Regulated by volume and alveolar ventilation; CO_2 retention (hypercapnia) usually means hypoventilation	36-42 mm Hg (39)
Total CO_2 content or concentration of plasma (venous)	Carbon dioxide obtainable from bicarbonate dissolved CO_2, carbamino compounds, and H_2CO_3	Reflects both metabolic and respiratory disturbances; result is not a clear indicator of either	26-30 mEq/L (28) 58-67 vol % (64)
CO_2 combining power of plasma or serum "alklali reserve" (venous)	Total carbon dioxide content of plasma or serum when equilibrated at a PCO_2 of 40 mm Hg	May be expressed as plasma bicarbonate by subtracting dissolved CO_2 (1.2 mEq/L); reflects metabolic disturbances more reliably than respiratory disturbances	26-30 mEq/L (28) 58-67 vol % (64)
Serum or plasma bicarbonate (venous)	Bicarbonate ion concentration (PCO_2); total CO_2 content minus H_2CO_3 and dissolved CO_2	Most important plasma buffer; level regulated by kidney; compensatory increase when CO_2 retention occurs, but abnormal levels primarily reflect metabolic disturbances	25-28 mEq/L (26.5)
Standard bicarbonate of plasma (arterial or capillary)	Bicarbonate ion concentration measured at PCO_2 of 40 mm Hg in plasma of fully oxygenated blood	A term used by P. Astrup & Associates for bicarbonate concentration corrected to reflect HCO_3 concentration independent of respiratory changes (i.e., of changes in arterial PO_2 and PCO_2)	22-26 mEq/L (24)
Base excess concentration (arterial or capillary)	Expression of base excess in mEq/L over the normal value (which is zero for blood with a pH of 7.4 and PCO_2 of 40 mm Hg)	Astrup terminology; negative value indicates a base deficit of acid excess; independent of hemoglobin concentration; positive or negative values outside the normal range are more helpful in guiding therapy of metabolic rather than respiratory disturbances	−2.4 to +2.3 mEq/L (0)
Respiratory acidosis	Excess of CO_2 resulting from inadequate alveolar ventilation	Degree of compensation depends on the change in level of bicarbonate ion; this rises in attempts to maintain 20:1 ratio necessary for pH in normal range	Uncompensated pH 6.8-7.37 Compensated pH 7.438-7.41
Respiratory alkalosis	Deficit of CO_2 resulting from alveolar hyperventilation	Does not have the life-threatening potential for respiratory acidosis; kidney responds by excreting bicarbonate	Uncompensated pH 7.45-7.7 Compensated 7.41-744

T A B L E 8 - 2 1 Blood gases and acid-base balance: terminology and values—cont'd

Term	Definition	Remarks	Normal range (mean)
Metabolic acidosis	Bicarbonate deficit usually due to excess organic acid production, excess loss of base, or acid retention	Lung attempts to compensate by hyperventilation with removal of carbon dioxide; example: diabetic acidosis	Uncompensated pH 6.8-7.37 Compensated pH 7.38-7.41
Metabolic alkalosis	Bicarbonate excess usually due to excess loss of acids, excess intake of alkaline salts, or potassium deficit	Retention of carbon dioxide by alveolar hypoventilation may improve acid-base balance; example: prolonged vomiting	Uncompensated pH 7.45-7.8 Compensated pH 7.41-7.44

From the American Lung Association: Chronic obstructive pulmonary disease, ed 5, New York, 1977, The Association, p 56.

T A B L E 8 - 2 2 Differential features of chronic obstructive pulmonary disease

Feature	Emphysema	Chronic bronchitis	Asthma
Family history	Occasional (alpha; antitrypsin deficiency)	Occasional (cystic fibrosis)	Frequent
Atopy	Absent	Absent	Frequent
Frequent			
Smoking history	Usual	Usual	Infrequent
Sputum character	Absent or mucoid	Predominantly neutrophilic	Predominantly eosinophilic
Chest x-ray	Useful if bullae, hyperinflation, or loss of peripheral vascular markings is present	Often normal; occasional hyperinflation	Often normal; hyperinflation during acute attack
Spirometry	Obstructive pattern unimproved with bronchodilator	Obstructive pattern improved with bronchodilator	Obstructive pattern usually shows good response to bronchodilator

From American Lung Association: Chronic obstructive pulmonary disease, ed 5, New York, 1977, The Association.

14 *Medications.* Patients with emphysema may be given steroids to reduce bronchial inflammation, antibiotics to treat secondary infections, expectorants to thin secretions, bronchodilators to reverse airway spasm, oxygen to reduce hypoxemia, and mechanical devices to provide adequate alveolar ventilation. In addition, chest physical therapy combined with breathing exercises will help promote and maintain muscle tonus and bronchial clearance.

15 Respiratory therapy plays a major role in the continuous care of the emphysema patient. Specific techniques (modalities) will vary according to the manifestation being treated. For example, breathing exercises combined with high humidity and postural drainage may be used to help the patient clear secretions and maintain a patent airway. In the most severe cases involving respiratory failure, intubation or tracheotomy and prolonged support with a ventilator may be appropriate. The techniques used in emphysema patient care include:

a Incentive devices and breathing exercises to promote an effective cough, develop muscle tonus, and maintain exercise tolerance.

b Good hydration combined with postural drainage, percussion, and vibration to promote drainage and removal of secretions.

c Oxygen therapy to reduce hypoxemia, especially during exercise periods.

d Intubation and mechanical ventilation for ventilatory failure.

e Suction to remove secretions in the unconscious or uncooperative patient.

f Patient education to develop self-care programs and positive self image.

16 Emphysema patients must be closely monitored both in the hospital and at home because of the rapidity with which acute pulmonary episodes can occur. A patient's family, as well as respiratory care personnel, can be successfully used in this capacity.

23.12 Restrictive lung disease

1 Restrictive lung disease identifies a pattern of diseases, injuries, or situations that prevent or limit (restrict) the degree to which alveolar units can be expended in various parts of the lung. This situation leads to a nonuniform ratio of ventilation to perfusion in these areas and general hypoxemia, which result from the mixing of unoxygenated and oxygenated blood as the blood passes through the lung.

2 Causes of restrictive lung disease include:

a Decreased lung expansion because of *diffuse pulmonary fibrosis, pleural effusion, pneumothorax,* and *fibrothorax.*

b Limited thoracic expansion resulting from kyphoscoliosis, multiple rib fractures (flail chest), thoracic surgery, spinal arthritis, or neurologic depression.

c Decreased diaphragmatic movement caused by *abdominal surgery, ascites, peritonitis, pregnancy,* and *severe obesity.*

d Other restrictions such as tight clothing, strapping of the chest, and heavy weights on the chest or abdomen.

23.13 Fibrosis

1 Fibrosis is a term describing the formation and presence of an excessive amount of connective-type tissue in a part of an organ or other body structure.

2 Fibrotic tissue is thick scarlike tissue that develops as a natural process of tissue repair after inflammation or destruction of tissue.

3 Pulmonary fibrosis usually occurs after pneumonitis; pulmonary abscess; tuberculosis; or prolonged exposure to dust, fumes, or other irritants, including high concentrations of oxygen (>60%-80%) for longer than 24 hours at a time.

4 Pulmonary fibrosis may be diffused (spread throughout) or localized in specific areas.

5 Diffuse conditions involving both lungs usually are the result of a massive pulmonary infection or long-term exposure to pulmonary irritants such as inhalation of dust and fumes, certain collagen diseases, pulmonary infections, irradiation, chronic aspiration, oxygen toxicity, and exposure to certain drugs and toxins.

6 Regardless of the etiology, the characteristics of the disease are similar and include:

a Dyspnea

b Cyanosis

c Diffuse, mottled shadowing of lung fields on x-ray films

d Pulmonary hypertension and cor pulmonale

e A reduction in lung volumes without significant changes in airway resistance from normal

7 As the chest or lung unit becomes stiffer, *lung compliance* is greatly reduced. This probably accounts for the decreased lung volumes and increased breathing frequency experienced by most of these patients.

8 Because of nonuniform changes throughout the lung, an uneven ratio of ventilation to perfusion occurs, resulting in physiologic shunt units.

9 Depending on the degree of thickening of the alveolar membrane, diffusion of oxygen may be impaired, leading to generalized hypoxemia and dyspnea. Carbon dioxide diffusion is not usually affected, because its elimination is compensated for by the normal lung units and elevated breathing frequency.

10 Pulmonary function values differ for patients with restrictive lung diseases from various causes. The following material reflects *general* lung changes caused by restrictive diseases:

Test	*Results*
Vital capacity	↓
Residual volume	↓
Total lung capacity	↓
Single-breath nitrogen	↑
Airways resistance	Normal or ↓
Static compliance	↓
Diffusing capacity for carbon monoxide	↓
Arterial oxygen tension at rest	Normal or ↓
Arterial oxygen tension at exercise	↓
Arterial CO_2 tension	↓

11 Lung dysfunction resulting from inhalation of dust. Disorders and diseases caused by inhalation of dusts are called *pneumoconiosis*. As with most irritants, the degree of lung disorder is directly related to the degree of exposure. This is usually determined as a dose-time relationship. Changes in either variable can greatly influence the degree of lung dysfunction and permanent damage.

The diseases discussed in the following units are caused by patients' exposure to dust in their environment. Each disease is discussed in terms of cause, clinical signs, and basic treatment.

23.14 Asbestosis

1 Asbestos. A material commonly used in cement products, insulation, air filter, brake lining, car undercoating, and other commercial products. Some of these products undergo almost constant wear, which releases the by-products of asbestos into the atmosphere. Clinical asbestosis, however, is usually seen in patients with a prolonged and more intensified exposure to asbestos and who work in locations that manufacture materials containing asbestos.

2 According to recent research, the greatest danger from exposure to asbestos is cancer of the lung. Other pulmonary complications include pleural and/or pulmonary fibrosis and pleural effusion.

3 The initial pathologic responses from asbestos are irritation and inflammation of the distal airways and alveolar walls, causing fibrosis.

4 Fibrosis in asbetosis does not have a set cause in its development and varies greatly in the degree of complications.

5 In mild forms, alveolar septa are thickened; in more severe cases, the alveolar spaces are almost indistinguishable from the surrounding fibrotic tissue. The term "honeycombing of the lung" is sometimes used because of the appearance of the lung on the x-ray film.

6 The radiograph usually is not conclusive in identifying early development of asbestosis. The earliest evidence is the increased prominence of finer lung markings referred to as the "ground-glass appearance." By this time the radiograph is of assistance in making a diagnosis, and the patient probably already has fibrotic changes in the terminal lung units.

7 Clinically patients with asbestosis have increasing complaints of dyspnea (especially on exertion), cyanosis, basal pulmonary rales on auscultation, digital clubbing, and sometimes deformity of the chest itself.

8 The treatment of asbestosis includes removing the patient from the irritant, prohibiting smoking, relieving dyspnea with oxygen therapy, and reducing and controlling inflammation with cortisone.

23.15 Silicosis

1 Silicosis is the pneumoconiosis caused by inhalation of dust containing crystalline-free silica (SiO_2). The cause

of silicosis has been recognized as early as Roman times when it was known that miners and workers with stone had a high prevalence of lung disease. Current sources of exposure include dust from mining, tunneling, sandblasting, stonecutting, pottery making, and tile manufacturing.

2 The *factors* determining development of silicosis are:

  a Percentage of free silica dust inhaled

  b Concentration of dust inhaled

  c Size of dust particles (0.01-3 μg are deposited in alveoli)

  d The admixture of other dusts

  e Length of exposure

  f Individual differences in susceptibility (generally it takes at least 5 years of exposure in atmospheres of 5 million particles per cubic foot of dust with at least 50% silica to produce clinical symptoms)

3 Pathogenesis and pathology. Dust carried by inhaled air is deposited along the respiratory tract and in the alveoli (see Fig. 8-7).

  a Dust particles, which are deposited in the alveoli, are engulfed by phagocytes and transported by *lymph* to the pulmonary lymph nodes. Small particles tend to be deposited primarily in the lower half of the upper lobes and the upper half of the lower and middle lobes of the lungs.

  b The cause of fibrosis is suspected to be the death of macrophages and the release of dust and cellular debris in the lung areas.

  c The characteristic pathologic findings in silicosis are *silicotic nodules,* which are whorled and densely compacted fibrotic lesions scattered throughout the areas of the lung exposed to dust.

4 The three phases of lung change are:

  a Formation of nodules of collagen (fibrous connective tissue) along lymphatics and hilar lymph nodes.

  b X-ray identification of multiple discrete nodules from 2 to 5 mm in diameter throughout the lungs.

  c Formations of massive conglomerate fibrosis, which are scars formed in the upper and central portions of the lungs on both sides. These scars replace normal lung tissue, causing decreased perfusion and overdistension of lung tissue.

5 Clinical symptoms. Silicosis is a chronic disease that emerges over a period of 15 or more years.

  a A medical history can be useful, but its usefulness may be distorted by the fact that a worker is not constantly and uniformly exposed to dust for a long period of time.

  b The primary symptom is progressive dyspnea, with or without a cough. A productive cough is usually linked with cigarette smoking.

  c Other signs include *restricted chest expansion* with *scattered fine* crepitations or wheezes and related *prolonged expiration* similar to asthma.

6 Radiographic findings are marked reticular and nodular densities throughout both lungs. As the disease progresses, the upper lobes show less volume, with el-

evation of the hili and emphysematous changes in the lower lobes.

7 Laboratory findings, especially pulmonary function tests, are not conclusive in diagnosing silicosis. The test results are similar to those in other types of restrictive diseases resulting in a lower diffusing capacity, decreased pulmonary compliance, and reduced lung volume measurements.

8 Pulmonary tuberculosis is a possible complication of silicosis, because the cellular toxicity of silica tends to stimulate multiplication of the tubercle bacilli.

9 The treatment of silicosis should focus on *preventing* measures (i.e., preventing the problem from occurring). Once the clinical symptoms of conglomerate silicosis appear, the prognosis is not good. Oxygen therapy is required to relieve dyspnea (which is progressive even though the exposure to dust is removed). Because of the frequency of emphysema and heart failure, patients with silicosis must be closely observed for respiratory failure requiring mechanical ventilation. These patients, when ventilated, must be closely observed for a spontaneous or tension pneumothorax that may occur when the silicosis is accompanied by subpleural blebs.

23.16 Other pneumoconioses

1 Other diseases from the inhalation of minerals, metals, or organic dusts produce conditions in the lung identical or similar to silicosis.

2 Treatment, especially in the latter stages, is limited to supportive measures, since the fibrotic damage is irreversible. Most government and public agencies are attempting to limit this form of disease through education and prevention.

3 Other fibrosis-causing and/or pneumoconioses are:

  a "Black lung." Coal worker's silicosis.

  b Berylliosis. A fibrosis from inhaling the dust of the metal beryllium used in the alloy and metal industry.

  c Byssinosis. "Brown lung"—cotton worker's disease from the inhalation of cotton dust, leading to chronic bronchial irritation and emphysema.

  d Bagassosis. A disease whose reactions resemble berylliosis. Caused by exposure to dust from stored sugar cane or sugar cane fibers. Believed to be a reaction from molds in the dust.

  e Farmer's lung. Thought to be the result of moldy hay and silage and similar to bagassosis. However, recent research has not identified a specific fungus.

  f Coccidioidomycosis. By definition not a true pneumoconiosis. An infectious fungal disease caused by the inhalation of spores of the bacterium *Coccidioides immitis,* which is carried on wind-borne dust particles. Symptoms are similar to those of the common cold or influenza. Most frequently encountered in hot, dry regions of the United States that have been exposed to farm animals.

  NOTE: Silo-filler's disease should not be confused with the pneumoconioses. It is actually a chemical pneumonitis from breathing the nitrous gases generated by compacted grains in silos.

23.17 Cystic fibrosis

1 *Cystic fibrosis* (CF) of the pancreas *(mucoviscidosis)* is a *hereditary* disease occurring in approximately one out of every 1500 to 2500 births. Although it is considered to be a childhood disease, earlier medical treatment and improved techniques have extended the life expectancy of these patients to the young adult years. It is much more common among whites than blacks and essentially nonexistent in Asians.

2 Because it is a recessive hereditary disease, if one parent has CF, the child will have no clinical signs of the disease. If *both* parents have CF or are carriers, their offspring will have a 25% chance of having CF, a 50% chance of being carriers, and a 25% chance of having no trace of the disease.

3 Pathophysiologically, the CF patient has two distinct characteristics:

   a A high *concentration of sweat* electrolytes. A sweat test result of over 60 mEq/L is diagnostic of CF.

   b *Abnormal mucous secretion and elimination.* The abnormal viscid nature of pulmonary secretions results in blockage of small bronchi and bronchioles and resultant secondary infection. *Pseudomonas aeruginosa* and *Staphylococcus aureus* are frequently cultured from the pulmonary secretions of these patients. Stools are bulky and fatty because of poorly digested fat, reflecting the problems with the pancreas. Intestinal obstructions are common.

4 The major pathologic features of the lung of these patients are bronchitis, bronchiectasis, and bronchiolitis. Atelectasis, abscess formation, and pneumonia are frequently caused by airway plugging.

   a CF also involves the pancreas in many of these patients, causing pancreatic insufficiency, increased fibrous stoma, and mild dilation of the acini, with cysts in the acini and ducts. Normal tissue is replaced with fibrous and adipose tissue involving areas that may cause diabetes.

   b The small intestine also becomes involved in a small percentage of the newborns born with CF. The secretion of mucous glands in the intestinal walls may cause intestinal blockage with perforation, meconium peritonitis, or volvulus.

   c The tissue changes occurring in the liver are similar to those in the pancreas. The end results may include focal lesions and biliary cirrhosis that can be clinically associated with hypertension.

5 *Radiologic examination* of the chest shows areas of atelectasis, fibrosis, pneumonia, and bronchiectasis. Air trapping, as evidenced by diffuse hyperinflation, and flattened diaphragms are common. Lung markings are increased, with irregular but prominent densities.

6 Laboratory tests will reveal abnormal stools and a positive sweat test result.

7 *Pulmonary function tests* show a reduced vital capacity, elevated peak flow rates, increased airway resistance, decreased maximum voluntary ventilation, and a reduced dynamic compliance. These patients, because of lung involvement, have an ineffective cough caused by *collapse* of the large airways and the small airways during a cough maneuver.

8 Treatment of these patients should focus on removal of secretions, control of infection, preventive care, and treatment of any pancreatic insufficiency.

High-humidity therapy with aerosol generators that produce small particles is important to ensure maximum humidification of the airway and liquefaction of secretions. Ultrasonic nebulizers of pneumatic devices may be used with the addition of stabilizing agents to the reservoir solutions. Propylene glycol (10%) in distilled water is effective to produce a stable particle. Propylene glycol (5%) or 0.25% normal saline solution can be used with ultrasonic nebulizers to provide a stable particle. In addition, aerosols with antibiotics or bronchodilators can be given before or during airway clearance maneuvers. Postural drainage with clapping and/or vibration is necessary to help mobilize and remove secretions from all lung segments. Breathing exercises, especially controlled coughing techniques, are necessary and should be combined with chest physical therapy routines. Dry air and respiratory irritants should be avoided by the CF patient. Therefore room humidifiers and filtered air may be necessary. Intermittent positive pressure breathing (IPPB) should be avoided because it overdistends patent airways and underinflates obstructed ones. This increases air trapping and can lead to barotrauma and tension pneumothorax, which are frequent occurrences in these patients. Oxygen therapy may be useful to relieve episodes of severe dyspnea and in patients with advancing hypoxemia. Lung lavage and/or mechanical ventilation may be necessary to remove secretions and provide adequate alveolar ventilation in the more severe cases.

23.18 Pulmonary disease and heart disease

1 In the healthy state the lung's vascular bed is large enough so that the relatively weak *right* side of the heart can function easily against the low pulmonary vascular resistance. Even after major lung resection involving up to one half of the volume of both lungs, there are still sufficient vascular networks to maintain circulation without causing back pressure on the right side of the heart.

2 However, in conditions such as emphysema, fibrosis, and hypertension from any cause, the effect is to reduce the vascular bed to the point that increased pressure in the pulmonary artery (leaving the right side of the heart) may cause hypertrophy (overdevelopment) of the *right* side of the heart and eventually heart failure.

3 This right-sided failure of the heart from increased pulmonary vascular pressure is called *cor pulmonale,* which is characterized by edema (swelling) of the ankles and feet (gravity dependent) and of the liver.

4 Heart disease can also cause lung disease.

 a The normal low pressure of the lung's vast network of capillaries keeps the blood fluids (plasma) from seeping over into the air spaces (alveoli).

 b Whenever the *left* side of the heart fails to compensate for high blood pressure as a result of mitral stenosis, hypertension because of anteriosclerotic heart disease, or acute hypervolemia from too rapid infusion of fluid into the veins, the blood "backs up into the lungs."

 c This backing up of fluid causes increased capillary pressure and vascular congestion, which produce the symptoms of shortness of breath on exertion, breathlessness in bed (or whenever the person lies down), and the need to sit up to breathe more comfortably.

 d If this congestion and increased vascular pressure cannot be compensated by the lungs, the plasma fluid may actually leave the capillaries and go to the area of lower pressure, the alveoli.

 e This movement of fluid into the air spaces is known as *pulmonary edema*. When the plasma pours into the alveoli faster than the cough or lymphatics can clear it, airway obstruction occurs and death may soon follow.

5 Treatment for pulmonary edema from cardiac causes is best effected by improving cardiac function, reducing excess fluid volume (diuretics), and maintaining adequate oxygenation.

 NOTE: The use of intermittent positive pressure breathing (IPPB) to control plasma frothing in the airways and airway obstruction is controversial. At one time 70% ethyl alcohol was advocated as a means of lowering the surface tension of the plasma bubbles, but use of this technique has not found widespread favor.

23.19 Acquired immune deficiency syndrome

Although AIDS is addressed briefly elsewhere in this text, it is appropriate to discuss this newly discovered disease, which has infected approximately 40,000 according to the Center for Disease Control, since its recognition in 1980. This disease attacks and destroys the immune system of the body, leaving its victims hopelessly exposed to death by microorganisms that ordinarily would be harmless to most healthy individuals.

The etiology of AIDS has not been identified although its victims are primarily homosexuals and/or drug users. More recent cases also include intravenous drug users and the sex partners and offspring of infected victims. These occurrences have led researchers to believe that AIDS is caused by a blood-borne virus, named the *human T-cell lymphotrophic virus type III* (HTLV-III) by a group from the National Cancer Institute. Subsequently the International Committee on Taxonomy of Viruses named it the *human immunodeficiency virus* (HIV). This rationale was based on the fact that the HIV contains RNA and uses a special enzyme to ingrain its genetic code into the host cells' DNA.

Regardless of its etiology, the mortality rates are high, with 58% and more being reported.

In 1986 a conference was held by the U.S. Public Health Service to assess the AIDS problem and to predict future expansion. It was announced that from 1986 to 1991 there will be 235,000 new cases with more than 54,000 deaths in 1991 and 1.5 million infected.

The initial diagnosis of AIDS is very difficult, because there are no specific identifying clinical symptoms or laboratory tests.

1 Individuals with AIDS usually have symptoms such as:

 a Fatigue

 b Fever

 c Loss of appetite and weight

 d Enlarged generalized lymph nodes

 e Cough and related dyspnea

 f Cancerous lesions in the late stages

 g Pneumonia and other pulmonary conditions such as pneumocystosis

2 Because of respiratory complications with AIDS, especially in its advanced stages, respiratory care personnel frequently are involved in its treatment.

 Uncertainty as to the etiology of AIDS has caused widespread concern among health care personnel at all levels who must treat these patients.

 To date, literature has not reported any cases of AIDS resulting from such contact with patients.

 General infection control measures against infection from exposure to patients with AIDS include the following:

 a Skin or other contact with blood or other body fluids, including sputum, should be avoided.

 • Personnel should wear gloves and masks and should avoid injury from sharp instruments used on AIDS patients.

 b Patients should be isolated in a private room.

 c Personnel should use the same isolation procedure as is implemented for patients with hepatitis B and with pulmonary disease such as tuberculosis.

 d Gowns, gloves, and masks should be worn into the room, with appropriate disposal accommodations for these articles, before technicians leave a designated clean zone.

 e Ventilators, stethoscopes, and other instruments ideally should be dedicated for exclusive use and remain in the room.

 • If this is not possible, instruments should be decontaminated with an appropriate chemical agent, covered, and/or bugged, removing them from the room.

 • These instruments should then be thoroughly cleaned and decontaminated, preferably by ethylene oxide or steam, before use on other patients.

 NOTE: Life-threatening pulmonary edema is best treated with intubation and mechanical ventilation until the cause of the edema can be brought under control.

For more details on the HIV and other potential occupational infections see Module 9.

24.0 ADULT RESPIRATORY DISTRESS SYNDROME
24.1 Historical description

1 The adult respiratory distress syndrome (ARDS) is a common cause of acute respiratory failure. This unit will cover a review of definition, diagnosis, pathophysiology, pathology, and treatment of ARDS. An exhaustive review of mechanisms of lung injury will also be included since this may soon be important in pharmacologic therapy. Prognosis and epidemiology will be covered in another unit.

2 The adult respiratory distress syndrome has been called many different names over the decades, but all reflect the acute lung injury that results from a variety of insults (see list).

3 These insults can either directly or indirectly involve the lungs. All the processes lead to a clinical picture of respiratory distress, diffuse pulmonary infiltrates on chest x-ray film, decreased pulmonary compliance, and impaired oxygen transport.

4 The adult respiratory distress syndrome can be defined as a diffuse lung injury resulting in noncardiogenic (nonhydrostatic) pulmonary edema and acute respiratory failure. It can affect patients of all age groups and is particularly tragic since healthy young people are often afflicted.

5 Strict criteria have been developed to diagnose this syndrome (see list).

6 Since ARDS is a syndrome resulting from a variety of unrelated insults, it is important to adhere to strict criteria and eliminate patients with underlying chronic lung disease and lung disease resulting from left-sided heart failure.

Synonyms for adult respiratory distress syndrome
1 Acute respiratory distress in adults
2 Adult hyaline membrane disease
3 Bronchopulmonary dysplasia
4 Congestive atelectasis
5 DaNang lung
6 Hemorrhagic atelectasis
7 Hemorrhagic lung syndrome
8 Noncardiogenic pulmonary edema
9 Oxygen toxicity
10 Postperfusion lung
11 Posttransfusion lung
12 Posttraumatic atelectasis
13 Posttraumatic pulmonary insufficiency
14 Progressive respiratory distress
15 Pulmonary contusion
16 Pulmonary microembolism
17 Pump lung
18 Respiratory insufficiency syndrome
19 Respiratory lung
20 Shock lung
21 Stiff-lung syndrome
22 Transplant lung
23 Traumatic wet lung
24 Wet lung
25 White-lung syndrome

Criteria for diagnosing adult respiratory distress syndrome*
1 Clinical setting
   a Catastrophic event
   b Pulmonary
   c Nonpulmonary
2 Exclusions
   a Chronic pulmonary disease
   b Left-sided heart abnormalities
3 Respiratory distress (judged clinically)
   a Tachypnea > 20 BPM, usually greater
   b Labored breathing
4 Diffuse pulmonary infiltrates on x-ray film
   a Interstitial (initially)
   b Alveolar (later)
5 Physiologic
   a $Pao_2 < 50$ mm Hg with $F_Io_2 > 0.6$
   b Overall compliance < 50 ml/cm H_2O, usually 20 to 30 ml/cm H_2O
   c Increased shunt fraction ($\dot{Q}S/\dot{Q}T$) and deadspace ventilation (VD/VT)
6 Pathologic
   a Heavy lungs, usually > 1000 gm
   b Congestive atelectasis
   c Hyaline membranes
   d Fibrosis
7 Pulmonary collapse was known to occur even on the battlefields of World War I. With the advent of blood banking in World War II, patients with massive blood loss became salvageable, and renal failure emerged as the major cause of late death in these patients.
8 Burford and Burbank (1945) described a traumatic wet lung that appeared after a penetrating injury to the chest.
9 Mallory (1950) described pulmonary lesions in each necropsy case that he reviewed from World War II.
10 In 1950 Jenkins et al. described congestive atelectasis, which is the syndrome known as "shock lung."
11 Interestingly there were no reports documenting awareness of respiratory failure after trauma or shock during the Korean War in the early 1950s.
12 The Vietnam War in the 1960s brought a redescription of "shock lung." This was in part due to rapid helicopter evacuation, vigorous field resuscitation, and improved diagnostic methods.
13 In 1967 Ashbaugh, Bigelow, and Petty were the first to describe this syndrome after civilian trauma. Because of the similarities to infant respiratory distress syndrome, they coined the term "adult respiratory distress syndrome," ARDS.
14 Originally it was thought that lack of surfactant played an etiologic role, but later the defect in surfactant was found to be a result of the acute lung injury.
15 They were also the first group to describe the beneficial effects of positive end-expiratory pressure (PEEP) in the treatment of this syndrome.

---

*From Petty TC: Adult respiratory distress syndrome: definition and historial perspective, Clin Chest Med 3:3, 1982.

16 The adult respiratory distress syndrome is a common disorder and is associated with high mortality. It is estimated that ARDS develops in 150,000 patients each year.

17 More than 75% of patients requiring greater than 50% inspired oxygen concentration to maintain adequate oxygenation will die.

24.2 Clinical stages of adult respiratory distress syndrome

1 A variety of clinical conditions can give rise to the adult respiratory distress syndrome.

2 Sepsis, aspiration, near drowning, drug overdose, pancreatitis, inhalation of smoke and other inhaled gases, shock, trauma, consumptive coagulopathy, and high inspired oxygen fractions are among the causes.

3 No matter what the cause, four stages characterize the clinical course: (1) injury, (2) apparent stability, (3) respiratory insufficiency, and (4) terminal stage.

4 During initial injury there are usually no evident clinical signs, and the chest roentgenogram may be clear.

5 This phase may last as long as 6 hours. Hyperventilation and abnormalities of the chest roentgenogram and physical examination occur during the phase of apparent stability.

6 Approximately 12 to 24 hours after the injury the chest roentgenogram exhibits fine reticular infiltrates representing perivascular fluid accumulation and interstitial edema.

7 A diffuse, five-lobed alveolar and interstitial infiltrate is present during the phase of respiratory insufficiency that occurs during the next 12 to 24 hours.

8 Tachypnea and crackles are noted on physical examination.

9 There is a severe reduction in arterial oxygen tension, even when high concentrations of inspired oxygen are given.

10 The terminal stage is characterized by persistent, severe hypoxemia despite administration of 100% oxygen and CO_2 retention.

11 A number of investigators have tried to find the key to detecting early ARDS.

12 Weigelt et al. (1981) prospectively studied 73 patients with ARDS to identify those factors that would predict the onset of ARDS. They found that serial determinations of arterial oxygen tensions were the best indicator.

24.3 Physiology of adult respiratory distress syndrome

1 A maldistribution of ventilation, intrapulmonary shunting, is the major cause of hypoxemia in ARDS.

2 Shunting results when the alveolus is perfused and not ventilated.

3 Many alveoli are ventilated but not perfused, which results in increased physiologic dead space.

4 There is an increase in physiologic dead space and right-to-left shunting in ARDS.

5 In severe ARDS these abnormalities may exceed 50%. There are changes in lung compliance resulting from fluid accumulation in the interstitium and alveoli, and

resultant collapse of the terminal air spaces.

6 These factors produce the maldistribution of ventilation and right-to-left shunting. An increase in pulmonary vascular resistance may result from hypoxia, vasoconstriction, increased interstitial fluid pressure, or intravascular clotting.

7 Nonuniform increases in pulmonary vascular resistance can potentiate the ventilation-perfusion abnormalities. The pulmonary hypertension that is produced is an unfavorable prognostic sign.

8 The functional residual capacity is decreased in ARDS secondary to the microatelectasis and edema.

9 There is also a decrease in lung compliance or a stiffening of the lung.

10 All of these changes result in a widening of the alveolar-arterial oxygen tension gradient and produce profound hypoxemia that is resistant to high concentrations of inspired oxygen.

11 In the late stages there is no longer a sufficient number of functional respiratory units to maintain adequate ventilation, and CO_2 retention occurs.

12 Hypoxemia results in a decreased oxygen delivery to the tissues and their cellular mitochondria.

13 This produces a reduction in oxidative metabolism and results in the production of lactate.

24.4 Mechanisms of lung injury

1 The mechanism of the acute lung injury in ARDS is unknown. A large number of potential mediators have been shown to be able to produce or sustain the intense inflammatory response that is characteristic of the adult respiratory distress syndrome.

2 These mediators include arachidonic acid and its metabolites (prostaglandins, leukotrienes, thromboxane A_2), serotonin, histamine, β-endorphin, fibrin and fibrin degradation products, complement, superoxides, polymorphonuclear leukocytes, platelets, free fatty acids, bradykinins, proteolytic enzymes, and lysosomes.

3 ARDS is marked by increased lung vascular permeability, which leads to the noncardiogenic pulmonary edema.

4 The purpose of this unit is to review the experimental current understanding of the roles of many biochemical and cellular factors in the pathogenesis of ARDS and lung inflammation.

5 The inflammatory process in the lung in ARDS is accompanied by many cellular and biochemical processes, some of which probably initate the syndrome, others of which may perpetuate the syndrome, and some of which may be inactive by-products of inflammation.

6 An understanding of pathogenesis will come only when we can separate the various implicated mechanisms into *initiators*, *perpetrators*, or *bystanders*. Since sepsis and septic shock are the most common causes of ARDS, this unit will also review new possibilities that hold promise for the treatment of septic shock and ARDS when the pharmacologic agent is added as an adjunct to current accepted methods of therapy.

TABLE 8-23 Research models

Investigation	Model	Drug	Action
Snapper et al. (1983)	Sheep	Meclofenamate/ibuprofen	↓ Airway resistance/decrease in dynamic pulmonary compliance as result of endotoxin
Kopolovic (1984)	Porcine bacteremia	Ibuprofen	↑ Oxygenation ↓ Extravascular lung water ↓ Pulmonary hypertension
Adams and Traber	Endotoxin-treated sheep	Ibuprofen	↓ Chronotropic response/pulmonary hypertension
Bone et al. (1981)	Endotoxemia in canine	Ibuprofen	↑ Mean arterial pressure/cardiac output ↓ Pulmonary hypertension ↓ Metabolic acidosis ↑ Survival
Wise et al. (1980)	Streptococcal sepsis in neonatal rat	Ibuprofen	↑ Survival

24.5 Prostaglandins and the role of cyclooxygenase inhibitors, thromboxane synthetase inhibitors, and corticosteroids

1 Prostaglandins (PGs) are a group of carbon 20, unsaturated hydroxy fatty acids containing a cyclopentane ring. They are synthesized in most mammalian nucleated cells by a synthetase system associated with the microsomal fraction of cells.

2 PGs have been isolated from many tissues including the lung tissues of all species examined.

3 These PGs, however, are not stored in the tissues but are synthesized de novo and released in response to a variety of stimuli, including mechanical manipulation.

4 The lung has also been identified as a site of significant metabolism of the parent PGs, thus preventing the biologically active PGs released from other organs from reaching the arterial circulation.

5 Certain PGs and PG-like substances have been reported to exert physiologic and pharmacologic effects on pulmonary function.

6 PGF_2 is a potent bronchoconstrictor, whereas PGs of the E type are bronchodilators both in vivo *and* in vitro.

7 The enzyme 9-keto-PG reductase, which converts PGE to PGF, has been demonstrated to be present in a variety of tissues, including lung. This has led to some speculation that an increased activity of 9-keto-PG reductase in human lung could lead to bronchoconstriction.

8 PGs not only affect airway constriction but might participate in inflammatory responses by altering vascular permeability, modulating the release of other mediators, and affecting the function of cells such as polymorphonuclear leukocytes.

9 Because there are small-airway abnormalities as well as findings of tissue inflammation in ARDS, and since PGs can cause constriction of smooth muscle and can modulate certain features of the inflammatory reaction, it is of considerable importance that the specific role of PGs in ARDS be better delineated.

10 *Prostacyclin (PGI$_2$)* is a potent vasodilator and is thought to be responsible for the systemic hypotension in endotoxin shock.

11 *Thromboxane A$_2$* is a potent vasoconstrictor that is said to be responsible for the pulmonary artery hypertension in endotoxin shock.

12 Their stable end products, 6-keto-PGF$_{1\alpha}$ and thromboxane B$_2$, can be measured to assess their role in producing the hemodynamic events. Studies have shown favorable effects of PG inhibition on survival and hemodynamic events.

13 Based on the hypothesis that cyclooxygenase products of arachidonic acid metabolism increase septicemia-induced pulmonary hypertension and resistance to air flow, treatment with cyclooxygenase inhibitors has been used in various models of acute lung injury. Examples of these are presented in Table 8-23.

Cyclooxygenase inhibitors effectively reduce pulmonary hypertension and airway resistance in experimental animals with septic shock of acute lung injury. They may reduce the accumulation of extravascular lung water, although its effect is likely due to the diminished hydrostatic force that favors the movement of fluid across the microvascular bed.

14 In resting polymorphonuclear leukocytes, platelets, and macrophages, arachidonic acid is not free but, rather, covalently bound to complex lipids, usually associated with biologic membranes. When activated, these cells mobilize arachidonic acid through four or more pathway-catalyzed phospholipases; the rate-limiting step in initiating the arachidonic acid cascade is deacetylation of cellular phospholipids.

15 Corticosteroids inhibit the action of these phospholipases, perhaps by stimulating polymorphonuclear leukocytes to synthesize a protein (lipomodulin) that inhibits the activity of phospholipase. In addition, corticosteroids may act directly on the microvascular endothelium to "stabilize membranes."

16 Twenty years have elapsed since corticosteroids were first presented as being efficacious in treatment of septic shock. A testament to the continuing dilemma is the volume of discussion generated by the study by Sprung et al. (1984).

17 Perhaps the most impelling evidence in favor of corticosteroids derives from Shumer's prospective, randomized study of steroid administration in patients with

septic shock in 1976. These data include the methyl-prednisolone succinate (30 mg/kg) or dexamethasone (3 mg/kg) given once or twice reduced the mortality rate from 38.4% to 10.5%.

18 Sibbald et al. (1981) reported that corticosteroid treatment of patients with ARDS reduced the microvascular permeability injury as detected by accumulation of iodinated albumin in bronchoalveolar secretions.

19 Conversely, the prospective study of steroid administration by Sprung et al. (1984) suggests that steroid treatment may reduce multiorgan system injury but does not increase overall survival rate. Bone et al. wrote that corticosteroids do not help in treatment of septic shock. They also contend that corticosteroids increase the mortality rate of ARDS. Therefore corticosteroids should not be used for septic shock or ARDS.

20 Prostaglandins of the E series may have antiinflammatory properties. PGE_1 and PGE_2 decrease lymphokine production, depress lymphocyte mitogen response, and induce T-lymphocyte suppressor activity. They also diminish macrophage toxic oxygen radical production and plasminogen activator secretion, while perhaps enhancing Fc receptor expression.

21 PGE_1 is a potent inhibitor of platelet aggregation, either by augmenting cyclic adenosine monophosphate levels or by antagonizing the aggregatory effects of thromboxane.

22 Exogenous administration of PGE_1 can suppress immune complex–induced vasculitis in rats and immune complex–induced glomerulonephritis in mice.

23 Administration of PGE_1 to patients with ARDS is reported to reduce pulmonary artery pressures and increase arterial oxgyen content and cardiac output.

24 Most impressively, administration of PGE_1 to surgical patients with ARDS is reported to improve survival rates. These data are currently being expanded in a multicenter blinded trial of PGE_1 therapy for patients with ARDS that develops after trauma or sepsis or postoperatively.

25 As already stated, PGE_1 administration appears to result in diminished pulmonary hypertension in patients with ARDS. The effect of such therapy on airway resistance or microvascular permeability is not described.

26 Leukotrienes C, D, and E (LTC, LTD, LTE) have been shown to comprise slow-reacting substance of anaphylaxis (SRS-A). LTCs have been shown to be potent bronchoconstrictors in in vitro experiments.

27 Leukotrienes are released in significant amounts from lung and vascular tissue after immunologic activation. They are not preformed mediators, and there is thus no site of storage.

28 They are acidic, sulfur-containing molecules of approximately 500 molecular weight that are resistant to proteolytic enzymes such as trypsin, chromotrypsin, pepsin, and activated papain; peptidase and phospholipases A, B, C, and D; and neuraminidase.

29 They are inactivated by limpet and human eosinophil arylsulfatase.

30 SRS-A has been known to be released from sensitized human lung after antigen challenge.

31 SRS-A causes constriction of human bronchial smooth muscle in vitro, increases vascular permeability, and decreases pulmonary compliance independent of cholinergic mechanisms when injected intravenously into guinea pigs. Thus it appears that SRS-A may be a mediator in the vascular permeability component of the inflammatory reaction. Its role in ARDS is unclear.

24.6 Polymorphonuclear leukocytes

1 Polymorphonuclear leukocytes (granulocytes) are the most important cellular component of the acute inflammatory response.

2 Granulocytes accumulate in the lung interstitium early in the development of ARDS, but the mechanisms by which granulocytes remain there are related to both complement and leukotrienes.

3 Granulocyte adherence may be a key property in the capability of granulocytes to move out of the vascular space. Moreover suppression of granulocyte adherence could be an important mechanism of antiinflammatory agents.

4 Increased granulocyte adherence may be an early phenomenon in the development of ARDS, and the suppression of adherence may alter the manifestations of ARDS.

5 One recent study suggests that granulocyte entrapment in the lung after microembolization contributes to extravascular lung water.

6 As an effector of acute lung injury, the neutrophil is well equipped both to produce substances directly toxic to tissue in the microenvironment, and to amplify an inflammatory response.

7 Neutrophil azurophilic granules contain lysosomal enzymes, neutral proteases, and reactive oxygen species.

8 The latter two of these are found in increased quantities in the lavage fluid of patients with ARDS.

9 Oxidant tissue damage may be direct by lipid peroxidation or indirect by sulfhydryl oxidation of key enzyme systems and damage of nucleic acids.

10 Neutrophils further elaborate factors that contribute to injury, primarily by amplifying the inflammatory response, such as platelet activating factor, cyclooxygenase and lipoxygenase metabolites of arachidonic acid, and chemotactic factors including kallikrein, C5a, and plasminogen activator.

24.7 Alveolar macrophages in the inflammatory reaction

1 Alveolar macrophages are strategically located on the terminal airways and interstitial spaces of the lungs, an ideal position from which to orchestrate inflammatory responses.

2 The phagocytic function of macrophages was first described by Metchnikoff more than 70 years ago. Within the last decade immunologists and biochemists have recognized a vast constitutive and inducible secretory capacity for macrophages.

3 These secretory abilities confer to macrophages the potential to initiate and modulate an inflammatory response.

4 In addition to lysozyme, which accounts for the bulk of the enzymatic contents of secretory granules, macrophages produce abundant proteases, acting as neutral pH (elastase and collagenase), and acid hydrolases, which may be important as the pH in an inflammatory microenvironment falls.

5 Once activated, macrophages produce toxic oxygen radicals. These products may degrade components of vessel walls and perivascular tissues and may yield chemotactic products for mononuclear phagocytes and polymorphonuclear leukocytes.

6 Whereas the secretion of lysozyme is constitutive, secretion of neutral proteases and toxic oxygen species is inducible.

7 When macrophages are activated by stimuli such as endotoxins, a subsequent membrane perturbation (as with a phagocytic load or phorbol myristate acetate) will result in an increase in enzyme secretion and in production of reactive oxygen species.

8 Macrophages produce a number of bioactive lipids, including PGE_2, thromboxane A_2, lipoxygenase products, and platelet-activating factor.

9 These lipid mediators have direct cardiopulmonary activity (vasoconstriction or vasodilation, bronchoconstriction), may increase microvascular permeability to large molecular weight solutes, and are chemotactic for other inflammatory mediators.

10 Further, macrophages produce proteins that recruit neutrophils into the microenvironment, which in turn activate lymphocytes, and proteins that stimulate and inhibit the growth of fibroblasts.

24.8 Complement

1 Activation of the classical and alternate complement pathways may play an important, if not primary, role in many disease processes.

2 The complement activation sequence produces molecular complexes (C5b-9). These complexes cause membrane damage with cellular lysis or products such as anaphylatoxins (C5a and C3a), which have nonlytic cellular effects.

3 For instance, activation of either the classical or alternate complement pathway has been found to generate a factor that causes release of certain mediators from human leukocytes. In addition, there is simultaneous generation of chemotactic activity. Anti-C3 or anti-C5 inhibits the formation of this factor, and anti-C5 inhibits activity of this factor even after it is formed.

4 In addition, theophylline inhibits the subsequent release of some mediators, indicating that the reaction is through a membrane receptor cyclic adenosine monophosphate mechanism rather than cytolysis.

5 This releasing factor is throught to be C5a and/or C3a (an anaphylatoxin).

6 It is important to note that some mediators can also be released by antigen-IgE complex on the leukocytes and that this process is complement independent. Thus mediator release and perhaps several other related membrane processes can be complement dependent or complement independent.

7 There is now evidence that complement is involved in acute pulmonary disease.

8 The increased vascular permeability in the lung during *Pseudomonas* bacteremia is associated with complement.

9 Human pulmonary dysfunction during hemodialysis has been shown to be due to activation of complement by the cellophane dialysis tubing.

10 The findings of pulmonary leukostasis and interstitial edema were reproduced in experimental animals by activation of complement.

11 The important action of complement in direct cytolytic cellular damage as well as complement-induced release of mediators such as histamine and vasoactive amines, and the recent implication of complement in the pathogenesis of acute pulmonary dysfunction, make it necessary to examine complement activation and complement component levels during the development of ARDS.

12 One recent study by Webster et al. (1982) in an experimental model found the activation of complement in the intravascular compartment did not cause lung injury. Neutrophils were sequestered, but no vascular injury was observed.

13 These findings suggest that other factors are needed in addition to neutrophils and complement to produce lung injury.

14 Jose et al. (1981) found that C5a, polymorphonuclear leukocytes, and PGE_2 were necessary to increase permeability in a systemic capillary bed.

24.9 Platelets in the injury reaction

1 The recognition of a variety of substances that stimulate platelet aggregation and secretion of platelet contents has led to the implication that they, in addition to their hemostatic function, may also play a role in inflammatory reactions.

2 Platelets are known to accumulate in blood vessels adjacent to tissue damage and inflammation.

3 In experimental studies, platelet and leukocyte microthrombi have been demonstrated in the lung, while at the same time leukopenia and thrombocytopenia were demonstrated in peripheral blood.

4 The platelet may participate in alteration of vascular permeability and is reportedly involved in stimulating a neutrophil chemotactic activity through cleavage of C5.

5 Intrapulmonary sequestration of platelets in ARDS is commonly observed, although the contribution of platelets to pulmonary injury is not clearly established.

6 The best evidence suggests that platelets are recruited and activated in the lung by macrophage- and neutro-

phil-derived platelet activating factor (acetyl glyceryl ether phosphocholine).

7 These platelets then release vasoactive cyclooxygenase products, probably thromboxane A_2, that contribute to the increased pulmonary vascular tone airways resistance characteristic of bacteremia and endotoxemia.

8 The time lapse relationship between the appearance of metabolic products of thromboxane synthesis in the blood and lymphatic fluid and the amelioration of the pulmonary hypertension and bronchospasm with thromboxane synthetase inhibitors or cyclooxygenase inhibitors supports the role of these vasoactive mediators, possibly platelet derived, in the response of ARDS.

24.10 Antioxidant agents and therapeutic agents

1 Natural defense mechanisms against toxic oxygen radicals include antioxidant enzymes superoxide dismutase, catalase, glutathione reductase, and nonspecific free radical scavengers such as vitamins E and C.

2 It is postulated that toxic oxygen species produced by cells in the lung cause injury when these antioxidant defenses are overwhelmed.

3 For instance, tolerance to hyperoxia can be induced by preexposure to sublethal levels of atmospheric oxygen, by preexposure to hypoxia, and by prior injection of small doses of endotoxin. Each of these therapies increases the antioxidant enzyme contents (superoxide dismutase and catalase) of the lung and decreases the accumulation of pulmonary edema.

4 It should therefore be possible to reduce the pulmonary oxygen radical–induced toxicity by increasing the concentration of antioxidant agents.

5 Protection against hyperoxia can be afforded to cells in short-term tissue culture by the addition of antioxidant enzymes to the bathing medium.

6 The difficulty in administration of antioxidant enzymes to a host, however, is that in order to be effective, these enzymes must be incorporated intracellularly at the site of injury.

7 Free enzymes rapidly degrade peripherally and therefore are often of little use.

8 Entrapment of antioxidant enzymes in liposomes is theoretically an efficient method for delivery of these proteins to target organs in vivo.

9 Consistent with the hypothesis that oxygen radicals affect tissue injury through peroxidation of lipids, which are major components of biologic membranes, oxygen radical injury is characterized by an increase in microvascular permeability to large molecular weight substances.

10 Treatment with antioxidant agents generally affords protection against the accumulation of extravascular lung water and is without effect on the pulmonary hypertension of increased airways resistance of acute lung injury.

24.11 Heavy metal chelators as treatment modalities

1 It has long been recognized that iron, by virtue of the role as a redox agent, can alter the oxygen metabolites derived from leukocytes.

2 There is increasing evidence that the Haber-Weiss reaction ($O2^- + H_2O_2 \rightarrow O_2 + OH + OH^-$) is catalyzed in the presence of iron.

3 Repine et al. (1981) and Nathan et al. (1980) have shown that the production of OH' by neutrophils is essential for microbicidal activity.

4 Liposomes incubated with FD^{+3} undergo lipid peroxidation, a reaction that can be inhibited by apolactoferrin. These data suggest a role for iron in leukocyte-dependent tissue injury.

5 Heavy metal chelators are believed to be efficacious by virtue of their capacity to reduce the toxic oxygen species in the microenvironment.

6 As one might predict from this role, chelators are primarily effective in reducing the microvascular permeability injury associated with leukocyte activation in animal models of injury, and they have little or no activity with respect to the pulmonary hypertension or increased airways resistance of acute lung injury.

24.12 Oxygen radical scavengers as treatment modalities

1 To overcome the difficulties of delivering large antioxidant enzymes to target organs, some investigators have employed chemical scavengers such as mannitol and ethanol to protect against oxidant injury.

2 These compounds, however, have relatively low reactivity with the hydroxyl radical so that the use of effective concentrations of these agents is precluded by toxicity.

3 Dimethylsulfoxide is many times more potent than mannitol or ethanol and is a relatively specific scavenger of the hydroxyl radical. It protects against hydroxyl radical injury or *Staphylococcus aureus* and against complement-induced acute lung injury in rats.

4 As discussed, oxygen radical scavengers act primarily to protect the pulmonary system against an increase in microvascular permeability and are without any recognized effects on the pulmonary hypertensive or bronchoconstrictive response to sepsis.

24.13 Niacin

1 Nicotinamide adenine dinucleotide (NAD) is a critical compound in cellular metabolism, serving as a coenzyme for multiple essential synthetic pathways.

2 In higher organisms, de novo synthesis of NAD involves the conversion of quinolinic acid to nicotinic acid mononucleotide (NAMN), a reaction catalyzed by a phosphoribosyl transferase. This enzyme is rapidly inactivated by hyperoxic exposure.

3 An alternative pathway to NAD synthesis utilizes the substrate niacin, which is converted to NAMN by a separate transferase enzyme. Niacin, then, may serve to reduce oxygen toxicity by acting as a substrate for an alternative pathway for NAD synthesis.

4 Niacin addition to the bathing solution of alveolar macrophages reduces oxygen toxicity as determined by phagocytic function.

5 The protection afforded by niacin is only partial, an observation that the authors attribute to free radical damage to membrane lipids, DNA, and other enzymes.

6 The efficacy of niacin in protecting against any of the pathophysiologic manifestations of acute lung injury is unknown, since its use has been reported only in macrophages maintained in short-term tissue culture.

24.14 Surfactant replacement in treatment of neonatal respiratory distress syndrome

1 Phospholipids of alveolar surfactant are secreted by granular pneumocytes (type II alveolar lining cells) and serve to reduce the surface tension in the terminal airways so that the alveoli may remain in the expanded state.

2 It is now recognized that neonatal respiratory distress syndrome (RDS) results from quantitative or qualitative deficiency of surfactant.

3 Further, hyperoxia is known to impair synthesis of surfactant proteins and phospholipids. Once this deficit in surface-active compounds was recognized, investigators began attempts to replace these compounds with natural or synthetic surfactants.

4 Exogenous surfactant replacement in premature lambs can improve initial lung function, even when administered after many hours of ventilatory support.

5 Human infants with RDS treated with tracheal instillation of human surfactant isolated from amniotic fluid show dramatic increases in arterial oxygentation, decreases in lavage elastase levels, and an increase in alpha$_1$-protease inhibitor when compared to values of control infants.

6 These results are promising; however, the role for surfactant replacement in adults with respiratory distress has yet to be established.

7 Surfactant replacement in animal models of acute lung injury has been effective in reducing the increased pulmonary resistance to air flow by maintaining the alveoli in the expanded state. Surfactant replacement therapy does not affect pulmonary hypertension or microvasular permeability.

8 Although there are no specific therapies for septic shock or acute lung injury that have proven efficacy in multicenter trials in humans, a growing understanding of mechanisms of tissue injury has suggested interventions that may prevent or treat this injury.

9 These therapies range from immunization against the glycopolysaccharide core of endotoxin, to cyclooxygenase inhibitors, to specific oxygen radical scavengers. Some of these therapies have been tested in man with promising preliminary results. Each of these treatments is effective in ameliorating at least one of the pathophysiologic manifestations of acute lung injury, although the long-term effect of any of these agents is unknown.

10 Interaction between several factors and mediators is likely necessary for the development of acute lung injury. It is hoped that with additional knowledge regarding mechanisms of injury, gained through basic science and clinical research, we can apply definitive therapy that may salvage people who now die with sepsis and acute lung injury.

Since sepsis is the most frequent cause of ARDS, a brief review of developing treatment modalities for sepsis follows.

24.15 Immunization against *Escherichia coli* endotoxin for septic shock

1 More than 10 years ago Zinner and McCabe (1976) and McCabe, Kreger, and Johns (1972) reported that patients with high humoral antibodies against the common core glycolipid of gram-negative bacteria had fewer episodes of septic shock and that fewer died.

2 Because most gram-negative bacteria and rough mutants of *E. coli* have similar core lipopolysaccharide components, cross-specific immunity may develop for the purpose of protecting against cardiopulmonary alternations of gram-negative bacteremia.

3 Sheep actively immunized with the core glycoprotein fraction of *E. coli* were protected against the pulmonary hypertension, decrease in cardiac output, and decrease in Pao$_2$ that they exhibited in response to *Serratia marcescens* endotoxin before immunization. Passive immunization in this model also afforded a lesser but significant protection.

4 Pollack et al. (1984) have demonstrated a good correlation between survival in patients with *Pseudomonas aeruginosa* bacteremia and high levels of antibodies (both IgG and IgM) to the *E. coli* endotoxin core.

5 Ziegler et al. (1982) have described improved survival in patients with gram-negative septicemia treated with human antiserum to the J5 mutant of *E. coli* endotoxin core. Although this therapeutic approach is encouraging, confirmation of these results in a multicenter, blinded trial is needed.

6 Since immunization protects against the development of the systemic response to bacteremia, it could therefore be considered effective in preventing all pathophysiologic manifestations of acute lung injury that occur in the setting of sepsis.

24.16 Endorphins in endotoxin shock

1 Endorphins are natural opiates that act as neurotransmitters or hormones within the central and autonomic nervous systems.

2 Injections of endorphins into animal and human subjects cause hypotension, tachycardia, and diminished cardiac output, which simulate the hemodynamic changes in endotoxin shock.

3 Previous work by Holaday and Faden (1978) and others supports the hypothesis that endorphins are involved in the pathophysiology of endotoxin shock.

4 Previous work of Bone et al. (1985) with canine endotoxin shock has shown an associated fivefold increase in β-endorphins.

5 Specific blockade of the opiate receptors with naloxone resulted in improved blood pressure and cardiac index in dogs with endotoxin-induced shock.

6 Since plasma β-endorphins are elevated in endotoxin shock and hypotension is blocked by specific opiate antagonists, it was concluded that endorphins were causally related to the hypotension of endotoxin shock.

7 Acidosis is still present after naloxone treatment of endotoxin shock. Thus the systemic perfusion defect produced by endotoxin was not alleviated despite marked improvement of hemodynamics.

24.17 Pathophysiology of adult respiratory distress syndrome

1 The alveolar-capillary membrane is the primary site of injury in the adult respiratory distress syndrome.

2 In many experimental models of ARDS there are swelling and retraction of the capillary endothelial cells. This results in a larger intracellular gap that leads to increased alveolar permeability and interstitial edema.

3 Increased interstitial fluid produces stiffer, noncompliant lungs.

4 As the process continues, alveolar edema results and alveolar collapse occurs.

5 There is microatelectasis, and eventually alveolar disruption and hemorrhagic edema result.

6 In the normal state the intracellular junctions of the alveolar epithelium are tight, and the membrane has low permeability to lipid-insoluble substances other than water.

7 The normal loose junctions separating capillary endothelial cells allow small molecules (less than 10,000 molecular weight) to pass.

8 In the adult respiratory distress syndrome the first leak occurs through the capillary endothelium.

9 Surfactant, a phospholipoprotein produced by the type II pneumocyte, has decreased activity in ARDS. Its normal function is to reduce alveolar surface tension. In its absence the alveolar surface tension is high, and alveoli tend to collapse.

10 The terminal bronchiole may also be a site of increased permeability. Histamine has been shown to produce leakage of proteins and fluid from the bronchiolar venous plexus at the terminal bronchiole level before the development of alveolar edema.

11 A similar leakage has also been described in endotoxin shock.

12 It has been suggested that fluid movement across the terminal bronchioles may be important in pulmonary edema.

24.18 Pathologic changes in adult respiratory distress syndrome

1 Despite the diverse causes of ARDS, the pathologic changes are uniform and nonspecific.

2 Both acute and chronic states are described.

3 The lungs may appear grossly normal during the first few hours after the initial insult.

4 The *acute stage* reveals interstitial and alveolar edema that is secondary to the damage to the epithelial and endothelial cell layers. The alveolar spaces are inhomogenously filled with a proteinaceous and often a hemorrhagic fluid. White blood cells, macrophages, cell fragments, amorphous material, protein, fibrin strands, and remnants of surfactant are also present, along with an occasional hyaline membrane. Whereas light microscopy reveals little interstitial change, electron microscopy shows widening of the interstitial space with fluid accumulation, blood cells, and occasional fibrin strands. Endothelial cells appear to have better preservation than the epithelial cells, which may indicate a greater reparative capacity of the endothelial cells. When antecedent disseminated intervascular coagulation is present, there may be free intravascular fibrin.

5 The *chronic stage* is marked by a proliferative tissue reaction, with epithelial transformation, distinct alveolar septal thickening by cell proliferation, and infiltration with a variety of interstitial cells. These changes may occur within a few days of the initial insult. There is an increase in the number of cuboidal cells resembling type II pneumocytes that line the alveolus during the reparative process. Evans et al. (1973) have shown that these cells are able to transform into type I cells in approximately 48 hours. The protein-rich fluid in the alveolar space may become organized and create a pattern of intraalveolar fibrosis. This can lead to an additional reduction in the gas-exchanging surface area.

24.19 Treatment of adult respiratory distress syndrome

1 There is no specific therapy for ARDS.

2 The treatment is directed toward maintaining adequate tissue oxygenation of vital organs, particularly the brain and heart, through respiratory and circulatory support. If possible, treatment of the underlying cause of lung damage should also be instituted.

3 Once the alveolar-capillary membrane is damaged, the clinical problem is essentially the same regardless of the inciting event.

4 This supportive therapy should continue until the integrity of the alveolar-capillary membrane is reestablished.

5 The critical factors in treatment include (1) optimal distension of alveoli to increase functional residual capacity, (2) careful attention to fluid balance and maintenance of adequate tissue perfusion, and (3) control of the primary problem.

6 One of the major objectives of therapy is to obtain optimal distension of alveoli and reverse alveolar collapse.

7 Positive end-expiratory pressure (PEEP) is used to increase the functional residual capacity and correct the progressive atelectasis.

8 The use of PEEP creates a distending pressure that is sufficient to overcome the elastic forces in the alveolar walls and to maintain the functional residual capacity. The use of PEEP allows maintenance of adequate oxygenation, with a decrease in required oxygen concentration. This helps to minimize the potential toxic effects of high oxygen tension to the lung and yet maintain adequate arterial oxygenation.

9 A number of excellent reviews deal with the use of PEEP.

10 PEEP has been an integral part of the treatment of ARDS for almost 15 years.

11 PEEP allows the airway and alveolar pressures to remain increased at the end of expiration, at levels greater than atmospheric pressure. This produces a continuous positive distending pressure across the walls of the airways and alveoli and maintains the patency of many closed or atelectatic gas-exchanging units.

12 The result is improved ventilation of alveoli that were previously sites of shunting or low ventilation in relation to perfusion. This recruitment increases the Pao_2.

13 The use of PEEP may also stabilize fluid-filled alveoli and allow the fluid to occupy a relatively flattened and thinned layer on the alveolar wall that would permit gas exchange.

14 There is no evidence that the use of PEEP decreases extravascular lung water. In fact, with high lung volumes there may be an increase in extravascular lung water.

15 Improved compliance results from the increase in functional residual capacity produced by the use of PEEP.

16 This results from a shift of the end-expiration point to a steeper portion of the pressure-volume curve of the lung and chest wall.

17 It is important to note that there is no linear relationship between improved compliance and increased PEEP.

18 With a high PEEP, alveoli may become overdistended and may be underperfused as a result of high intraalveolar pressure and a reduction in cardiac output.

19 Other beneficial effects that may be attributed to the use of PEEP include conservation of alveolar surfactant and a reduction in alveolar surface tension.

20 It has been shown that ventilation with high tidal volumes can cause surfactant to aggregate, and thus its effectiveness in lowering alveolar surface tension is diminished. There are also several reports, primarily in the surgical literature, that suggest that early use of PEEP may prevent the development of ARDS.

21 The selection of the optimal level of PEEP has been a controversial issue.

22 Most agree that PEEP should be increased in small increments, and the cardiac output requirements of the patient should be monitored during these changes. If the cardiac output falls, it should be supported with volume infusions and inotropic drugs.

23 The goal of PEEP is to allow a reduction in the FIo_2 to 50% or less.

24 Suter et al. (1975) have defined "optimal PEEP" as the level of PEEP that produces maximal pulmonary compliance.

25 Gallagher, Civetta, and Kirby (1978) defined "best PEEP" as the level of PEEP that reduces the intrapulmonary shunt fraction to less than 15% of the cardiac output. Which, if either, of these levels is the ideal is still a matter of debate.

26 At present the level of PEEP should be guided by the ability to reduce the inspired oxygen concentration and maintain adequate tissue oxygen delivery.

27 The use of PEEP has a variety of hemodynamic effects including impaired venous return, increased pulmonary vascular resistance, reduced left ventricular afterload, and altered right and left ventricular geometry and compliance.

28 Most patients with ARDS require ventilatory assistance. If the arterial oxygen tension is less than 60 mm Hg on room air in a patient with previously normal lungs, the patient is a candidate for supplemental oxygen.

29 Ventilatory assistance becomes necessary if the arterial oxygen tension does not reach adequate levels despite administration of high oxygen concentrations.

30 Volume-cycled ventilators are preferred, and the suggested tidal volume is between 10 and 13 ml/kg.

31 If the patient requires the use of PEEP, the tidal volume may need to be reduced to avoid pulmonary barotrauma.

32 PEEP can be used to maintain adequate arterial oxygen tension when inspired oxygen concentrations are above 50%.

33 Oxygen toxicity usually occurs after 2 to 3 days of an FIo_2 that exceeds 60%.

34 With an inspired oxygen concentration of 40% or less, there have been no reports of oxygen toxicity.

35 It is well documented that a number of potential complications are associated with assisted ventilations, and it is important to carefully monitor the patient.

36 Sepsis is one of the most frequent causes of the adult respiratory distress syndrome, and its early recognition is important in order that effective treatment may be instituted. Proper bacterial cultures and immunologic techniques should guide the choice of appropriate antibiotics when infection is present.

37 It is also vitally important to maintain proper fluid balance. This helps to ensure adequate perfusion and oxygen delivery to vital organs such as the brain, heart, and kidneys.

38 This is guided by the physical examination, hemodynamic information, and laboratory data.

39 The use of the flow-directed, balloon-tipped pulmonary artery catheter has greatly aided this evaluation by allowing ready access to pulmonary capillary wedge pressure, mixed venous oxygen tension, and thermodilution cardiac output determinations.

40 A mixed venous oxygen tension below 30 mm Hg is an indicator of severe tissue hypoxia. Unfortunately the mixed venous oxgyen tension is not as reliable a prog-

nosticator in the presence of sepsis.

41 Correction and proper treatment of the underlying disorder are also a necessity in the proper care of these seriously ill patients. This therapy must be individualized, since a variety of causes are attributed to this syndrome.

42 It is important to remember that more than one cause may be present in a single patient.

43 Adequate ventilatory support in an intensive care unit is required to allow the lung to recover. Proper nursing care with strict attention to detail is invaluable.

44 The list herein summarizes the goals of treatment of ARDS.

Treatment goals for adult respiratory distress syndrome

1 Good nursing care
2 Prevention and control of infection
3 Adequate fluid balance with maintenance of tissue perfusion
4 Bronchodilators if signs of increased airway resistance are present
5 Ventilatory assistance if indicated
  a Use volume-cycled ventilators
  b Use tidal volumes of 10 to 13 ml/kg (to maintain optimum compliance)
  c Keep inspired oxygen concentration as low as possible, consistent with adequate arterial oxygenation (Pao_2 >60 mm Hg) and mixed venous oxygenation (PvO_2 >30 mm Hg)
  d Keep inflation pressure as low as possible
  e Provide adequate humidification
  f Use PEEP of an inspired oxygen concentration >50% is required

24.20 Complications of adult respiratory distress syndrome

1 With improvements in treatment and supportive therapy, patients now survive longer. Unfortunately multiorgan failure and other complications develop in some of these patients.

2 The following list contains a number of complications that are prone to occur in these seriously ill patients.

3 Among the pulmonary complications is pulmonary embolic disease, which is difficult to diagnose in these patients without a pulmonary angiogram.

Complications associated with the adult respiratory distress syndrome*

1 Pulmonary
  a Pulmonary emboli
  b Pulmonary barotrauma
  c Pulmonary fibrosis
  d Pulmonary complications of ventilatory and monitoring procedures
    1. Mechanical ventilation
      a Right main stem intubation
      b Alveolar hypoventilation

---

*Pingleton S: Complications of acute respiratory failure. In Bone RC, ed: The Medical Clinics of North America, 1983, WB Saunders Co.

2 Balloon catheterization
  a Pulmonary infarction
  b Pulmonary hemorrhage
2 Gastrointestinal
  a Gastrointestinal hemorrhage
  b Ileus
  c Gastric distension
  d Pneumoperitoneum
3 Renal
  a Renal failure
  b Fluid retention
4 Cardiac
  a Arrhythmia
  b Hypotension
  c Low cardiac output
5 Infection
  a Sepsis
  b Nosocomial pneumonia
6 Hematologic
  a Anemia
  b Thrombocytopenia
  c Disseminated intravascular coagulation
7 Other
  a Hepatic
  b Endocrine
  c Neurologic
  d Psychiatric

4 Pingleton et al. (1981) have shown that the use of prophylactic low-dose heparin decreased the incidence of documented pulmonary emboli in a respiratory intensive care unit from eight cases to one case per year. Low-dose heparin was found to be safe and should be routinely used unless there is a specific contraindication, such as bleeding diathesis of lesion, head injury, malignant hypertension, or severe liver disease.

5 Pulmonary barotrauma includes pneumothorax, pneumomediastinum, and subcutaneous emphysema. The predisposing factors for the development of pulmonary barotrauma include the use of volume ventilators, high inflation pressures in the presence of decreased compliance, high levels of PEEP, high tidal volumes, a complication of intravascular catheter placement, necrotizing pneumonias, and bronchoscopy during mechanical ventilation.

6 The gastrointestinal complications include gastrointestinal hemorrhage, ileus, gastric distension, and pneumoperitoneum.

7 Gastrointestinal hemorrhage has an impact on survival, and current recommendations include prophylaxis with sulcafate. Antacids used for prophylaxis were shown in 1988 to increase nosocomial colonization and subsequent pneumonia.

8 Cardiovascular complications include arrhythmias, hypotension, and decreased cardiac output.

9 Almost all patients have flow-directed, balloon-tipped pulmonary artery catheters that allow determination of pulmonary capillary wedge pressure, cardiac output, and mixed venous oxygen tension.

10 Unfortunately such catheterization may also be arrhythmogenic, especially when coupled with acidosis, alkalosis, or hypoxemia.

11 Other complications include renal failure, which is associated with a 60% mortality in ARDS.

12 Nosocomial infections are important causes of late morbidity and death. It is also important to maintain the nutritional status of the patient and to prevent the development of protein calorie starvation.

13 An aggressive approach toward these potential complications is vital for patient management. Strict attention to detail, the use of prophylactic measures, and keen anticipation are the cornerstones of good management. When a complication develops, prompt recognition and treatment are essential.

PROCEDURE 8-1

Draw an arterial blood sample for gas analysis

No.	Steps in performing the procedure
	The practitioner will draw an arterial blood gas sample from an adult patient in the clinical facility as ordered per institutional policy.
1	Verify physician order.
2	Collect necessary apparatus.*
	2.1 Alcohol or disinfectant swabs
	2.2 Sterile 3 to 5 ml glass syringe
	2.3 Assortment of needles (20 to 23 gauge)
	2.4 $\frac{1}{1000}$ sodium heparin
	2.5 Sterile gauze pads
	2.6 Seal for needle
	2.7 Container of ice
3	Wash hands.
4	Heparinize the syringe and needle.
5	Introduce yourself.
6	Identify and greet patient.
7	Discuss procedure with patient.
8	Assemble apparatus for accessibility.
9	Position patient and carry out Allen test (if radial stick).
10	Prepare site with alcohol or disinfectant swab.
11	Palpate artery to be punctured.
12	Gently insert the needle, with bevel up, into the tissue. When artery is punctured, the syringe plunger will rise.
13	If unsuccessful, withdraw needle and try again.
14	Allow 1 to 2 ml blood to flow into syringe.
15	Remove needle from tissue and eject air bubbles from blood sample.
16	An assistant will apply pressure to the puncture site with clean gauze pad.
17	Cover needle and mix sample by rolling between hands.
18	Label the sample according to hospital's procedure. Place in an ice container.
19	Fill out required paperwork.
20	Transport sample immediately to laboratory.

*Many hospital prefer to use prepackaged commercial ABG kits.

BIBLIOGRAPHY

Adams F et al: Lung phospholipid of human fetuses and infants with and without hyaline membrane disease, J Pediatr 77:833, 1970.

Adams T Jr and Traker DC: The effects of prostaglandin synthetase inhibitor, ibuprofen, on the cardiopulmonary response to endotoxin in sheep, Circ Shock 9:481, 1982.

American Lung Association: Diagnostic standards and classification of tuberculosis and other mycobacterial disease, New York, 1974, The Association.

American Lung Association: The tuberculin skin test (suppl to Diagnostic standards and classification of tuberculosis and other mycobacterial diseases), New York, 1974, The Association.

Anderson RR, Holliday RL, and Driedger AA: Documentation of pulmonary capillary permeability in the adult respiratory distress syndrome accompanying human sepsis, Am Rev Respir Dis 119:869, 1979.

Anggard E: The isolation and determination of prostaglandins in lungs of sheep, guinea pig, monkey and man, Biochem Pharmacol 14:1507, 1965.

Anthony CP and Thibodeau GA: Textbook of anatomy and physiology, ed 12, St Louis, 1987, The CV Mosby Co.

Anthony CP and Thibodeau GA: Structure and function of the body, ed 8, St Louis, 1988, The CV Mosby Co.

Appel P and Shoemaker W: Hemodynamic and oxygen transport effects of prostaglandin E_1 in patients with adult respiratory distress syndrome, Crit Care Med 12:528-529, 1984.

Arand DL, McGintz DJ, and Littner MR: Respiratory patterns associated with hemoglobin desaturation during sleep in chronic obstructive pulmonary disease, Chest 80:183, 1981.

Arnoux B, Duval D, and Benveniste J: Release of platelet activating factor (PAF-acether) from alveolar macrophages by the calcium ionophore A23187 and phagocytosis, Eur J Clin Invest 10:437, 1980.

Ashbaugh DG et al: Acute respiratory distress in adults, Lancet 2:319, 1967.

Askin FB and Katzenstein AA: Pneumocystis infection masquerading as diffuse alveolar damage: a potential source of diagnostic error, Chest 79:420, 1981.

Ayres SM: Mechanisms and consequences of pulmonary edema: cardiac lung, shock lung and principles of ventilatory therapy in adult respiratory distress syndrome, Am Heart J 103:97, 1982.

Bachafen M and Weibel ER: Structural alterations of lung parenchyma in the adult respiratory distress syndrome, Clin Chest Med 3:35, 1982.

Bartlett RH: Pulmonary pathophysiology in surgical patients, Surg Clin North Am 60:1323, 1980.

Bitterman P, Rennard S, and Hunninghake G: Human alveolar macrophage growth factor for fibroblasts, J Clin Invest 70:806, 1981.

Blaisdell FW: Controversy in shock research. Con: the role of steroids in septic shock, Circ Shock 8:673, 1981.

Bone RC: Treatment of adult respiratory distress syndrome with diuretics, dialysis and positive end expiratory pressure, Crit Care Med 6:136, 1978.

Bone RC, Francis PB, and Pierce AK: Intravascular coagulation associated with the adult respiratory distress syndrome, Am J Med 61:585,1976.

Bone RC, Francis PB, and Pierce AK: Pulmonary barotrauma complicating positive end expiratory pressure, Am Rev Respir Dis 1135:921, 1976.

Bonnet F, Richard C, Glaser P et al: Changes in hepatic flow induced by continuous positive pressure ventilation in critically ill patients, Crit Care Med 10:703, 1982.

Bowers RE, Brigham KL, and Owens PJ: Salicylate pulmonary edema: the mechanism in sheep and review of the clinical literature, Am Rev Respir Dis 115:261, 1977.

Bowers RE, Ellis EF, Brigham KL et al: Effects of prostaglandin cyclic endoperoxides on the lung circulation of unanesthetized sheep, J Clin Invest 63:131, 1979.

Brigham K: Pulmonary edema—cardiac and noncardiac, Am J Surg 138:361, 1979.

Brigham KL: Mechanisms of lung injury, Clin Chest Med 3:9, 1982.

Brigham K et al: Prostaglandins and lung injury, Chest 83:70S, 1983.

Brigham KL et al: Increased vascular permeability caused by pseudomonas bacteremia, J Clin Invest 54:792, 1974.

Brocklehurst WE: Slow-reacting substance and related compounds, Prog Allergy 6:539, 1962.

Brocklehurst WE: The release of histamine and formation of a slow-reacting substance (SRS-A) during anaphylactic shock, J Physiol 151:416, 1960.

Brooks SM and Paynton-Brooks N: The human body: structure and function in health and disease, ed 2, St Louis, 1980, The CV Mosby Co.

Bruck-Kan R: Introduction to human anatomy, New York, 1979, Harper & Row Publishers Inc.

Burford TH and Burbank B: Traumatic wet lung: observation on certain physiological fundamentals in thoracic trauma, J Thorac Cardiovasc Surg 14:415, 1945.

Burton GG, Gee GN, and Hodgkin JE, editors: Respiratory care: a guide to clinical practice, Philadelphia, 1977, JB Lippincott Co.

Burton WN, Vender J, and Shapiro BA: Adult respiratory distress syndrome after placidyl abuse, Crit Care Med 8:4, 1980.

Bywaters EGL: Ischemic muscle necrosis: a type of injury seen in air raid casualties following burial beneath debris, JAMA 124:1103, 1944.

Camussi G et al: Release of platelet activating factor (PAF) and histamine. II. The cellular origin of human PAF: monocytes, polymorphonuclear neutrophils and basophils, Immunology 42:191, 1981.

Casciari RJ et al: Effects of breathing retraining in patients with chronic obstructive pulmonary disease, Chest 79:393, 1981.

Cassan SM: PEEP and barotrauma, West J Med 131:47, 1979.

Chand N: FPL 55712—an antagonist of slow reacting substance of anaphylaxis (SRS-A): a review, Agents Actions 9:133, 1979.

Christensen EE et al: Initial roentgenographic manifestations of pulmonary *Mycobacterium tuberculosis, M. kansasii,* and *M. intracellularis* infections, Chest 80:132, 1981.

Christensson P, Arborelius M, and Lilja B: Salbutamol inhalation in chronic asthma bronchiole: dose aerosol vs jet nebulizer, Chest 79:416, 1981.

Clowes GHA: Pulmonary abnormalities in sepsis, Surg Clin North Am 54:993, 1974.

Clowes GHA et al: Septic lung and shock lung in man, Ann Surg 181:681, 1975.

Cobin HS et al: Structure function correlations in cardiovascular and pulmonary diseases: Ebstein's anomaly in the elderly, Chest 80:212, 1981.

Cockcroft DW and Horne SL: Localization of emphysema within the lung: an hypothesis based upon ventilation/perfusion relationships, Chest 82:483, 1982.

Craddock PR et al: Complement and leukocyte-mediated pulmonary dysfunction in hemodialysis, N Engl J Med 296:769, 1977.

Cuthbert MF: Prostaglandins and respiratory smooth muscle. In Cuthbert MF, editor: The prostaglandins, Philadelphia, 1973, JB Lippincott, pp 253-285.

Dan MR and Walker BK: Noncardiogenic pulmonary edema associated with hydrochlorothiazide therapy, Chest 79:482, 1981.

Dantzker DR: Gas exchange in the adult respiratory distress syndrome, Clin Chest Med 3:57, 1982.

Dantzker DR et al: Ventilation-perfusion disturbances in the adult respiratory distress syndrome, Am Rev Respir Dis 120:1039, 1979.

Dechert R et al: Use of PEEP in acute respiratory distress syndrome in dogs, Crit Care Med 9:10, 1981.

Dee P, Teja K, and Korzeniowski O: Miliary tuberculosis resulting in adult respiratory distress syndrome: a surviving case, Am J Roentgenol 134:569, 1980.

Demling RH, Staub NC, and Edmisnels LH Jr: Effect of end-expiratory airway pressure on accumulation of extravascular lung water, J Appl Physiol 38:907, 1975.

Demling RH et al: The effect of prostacyclin infusion on endotoxin-induced lung injury, Surgery 89:257, 1981.

Demling R et al: Methylprednisolone prevention of increased lung vascular permeability following endotoxemia in sheep, J Clin Invest 67:1103, 1981.

Demling RH et al: Pulmonary injury and prostaglandin production during endotoxemia in conscious sheep, Am J Physiol 240:H348, 1981.

Divertie MB: The adult respiratory distress syndrome, Mayo Clin Proc 57:371, 1982.

Editorial. Neutrophils and adult respiratory distress syndrome, Lancet 2:790, 1984.

Egan E et al: Natural and artificial lung surfactant replacement therapy in premature lambs, J Appl Physiol 55:865, 1983.

Elias J et al: Human alveolar macrophage inhibition of lung fibroblast growth, Am Rev Respir Dis 131:94, 1985.

Ellman H and Dembin H: Lack of adverse hemodynamic effects of PEEP in patients with acute respiratory failure, Crit Care Med 10:706, 1982.

Esbenshade AM et al: Respiratory failure after endotoxin infusion in sheep: lung mechanics and fluid balance, J Appl Physiol 53:967, 1982.

Evans MJ et al: Renewal of alveolar epithelium in the rat following exposure to NO_2, Am J Pathol 70:175, 1973.

Faden AI and Holaday JW: Experimental endotoxin shock: the pathophysiologic function of endorphins and treatment with opiate antagonists, J Infect Dis 142:229, 1980.

Fantone J and Ward P: Role of oxygen-derived free radicals and metabolites in leukocyte dependent reactions, Am J Pathol 197:397, 1982.

Fenster LF, Wheelis RF, and Ryan JA Jr: Acute respiratory distress syndrome after peritoneovenous shunt, Am Rev Respir Dis 125:244, 1982.

Fisher A, Durandy A, and Griscelli C: Role of prostaglandin E_2 in the induction of nonspecific T-lymphocyte suppressor activity, J Immunol 126:1452, 1981.

Fletcher JR and Ramwell PW: Prostaglandins in shock: to give or to block, Adv Shock Res 3:57, 1980.

Fletcher JR, Ramwell PW, and Harris RH: Thromboxane, prostacyclin and hemodynamic events in primate endotoxin shock, Adv Shock Res 3:145, 1980.

Ford-Hutchison A et al: Leukotriene B, a potent chemotactic and aggregating substance released from polymorphonuclear leukocytes, Nature 286:264, 1980.

Fox R: Prevention of granulocyte-mediated oxidant lung injury in rats by a hydroxyl radical scavenger, dimethylthiourea, J Clin Invest 74:1456, 1984.

Frank L: Protection from O_2 toxicity by preexposure to hypoxia: lung antioxidant enzyme role, J Appl Physiol 53:475, 1982.

Frank L: Endotoxin reverses the decreased tolerance of rats to >95% FIO_2 after pre-exposure to los O_2, J Appl Physiol 51:577, 1981.

Frank L and Massaro D: Oxygen toxicity, Am J Med 69:117, 1980.

Gallagher TJ, Civetta JM, and Kirby RR: Terminology update: optimal PEEP, Crit Care Med 6:323, 1978.

Girotti M et al: Effects of immunization on cardiopulmonary alterations of gram-negative endotoxemia, J Appl Physiol 56:582, 1984.

Glenney CU, Teres D, Sweet S et al: The effect of renal and respiratory failure on surgical ICU mortality, Crit Care Med 7:134, 1979.

Gong H: Positive pressure ventilation in the adult respiratory distress syndrome, Clin Chest Med 3:69, 1982.

Goodwin RA and Des Prez RM: Apical localization of pulmonary tuberculosis, chronic pulmonary histoplasmosis, and progressive massive fibrosis of the lung, Chest 83:801, 1983.

Gordon D, Bray M, and Morley J: Control of lymphokine secretion by prostaglandins, Nature 262:401, 1976.

Gossling HR and Donohue TA: The fat embolism syndrome, JAMA 241:2740, 1979.

Greisman S, Dubuy J, and Woodard C: Experimental gram-negative bacterial sepsis: prevention of mortality not prevented by antibiotics alone, Infect Immunol 25:538, 1979.

Gross N and Smith D: Impaired surfactant phospholipid metabolism in hyperoxic mouse lungs, J Appl Physiol 51:1198, 1981.

Guenter CA and Welch MH, editors: Pulmonary medicine, Philadelphia, 1977, JB Lippincott Co.

Gutteridge J: Inhibition of lipid peroxidation by the iron binding protein lactoferrin, Biochem J 199:259, 1981.

Hammerschmidt D: Leukocytes and lung injury, Chest 83:16S, 1983.

Hammerschmidt DE et al: Association of complement activation and elevated plasma C5a with adult respiratory distress syndrome, Lancet 2:947, 1980.

Harlan J et al: Selective blockade of thromboxane A_2 synthesis during experimental *E. coli* bacteremia in the goat, Chest 83:75S, 1983.

Hayes MF Jr, Rosenbaum RW, and Zibelman M: Adult respiratory distress syndrome in association with acute pancreatitis, Am J Surg 127:314, 1974.

Heffner J et al: Platelet induced pulmonary hypertension and edema, Chest 83:78S, 1983.

Heflin AC Jr and Brigham KL: Prevention by granulocyte depletion of increased vascular permeability of sheep lung following endotoxemia, J Clin Invest 68:1253, 1981.

Hegyi T and Hiatt IM: The effect of continuous positive airway pressure on the course of respiratory distress syndrome: the benefits of early initiation, Crit Care Med 9:38, 1981.

Henson PM and Cochrane CG: The effect of complement depletion on experimental tissue injury, Ann NY Acad Sci 256:426, 1975.

Hill RN, Spragg R, Wedel, MK, et al: Adult respiratory distress syndrome associated with colchicine intoxication, Ann Intern Med 83:523, 1975.

Hinman L et al: Elastase and lysozyme activities in human alveolar macrophages, Am Rev Respir Dis 121:263, 1980.

Hinshaw L, Beller-Todd B, and Archer L: Review update. Current management of the septic shock patients: experimental basis for treatment, Circ Shock 9:543, 1982.

Hinshaw L et al: Survival of primates in LD_{100} septic shock following steroid/antibiotic therapy, J Surg Res 28:151, 1980.

Holaday JW and Faden AI: Naloxone reversal of endotoxin hypotension suggests role of endorphins in shock, Nature 275:450, 1978.

Holbrook PR, Taylor G, Pollack MM et al: Adult respiratory distress syndrome in children, Pediatr Clin North Am 27:677, 1980.

Hosea S, Brown E, Hammer C et al: Role of complement activation in a model of adult respiratory distress syndrome, J Clin invest 66:375, 1980.

Hudson LD: Causes of the adult respiratory distress syndrome—clinical recognition, Clin Chest Med 3:195, 1982.

Hunninghake G: Release of interleukin I by alveolar macrophages of patients with active pulmonary sarcoidosis, Am Rev Respir Dis 129:569,1984.

Hunninghake G, Gallin J, and Fauci A: Immunologic reactivity of the lung, Am Rev Respir Dis 117:15, 1978.

Hurewitz A and Bergofsky EH: Treatment of adult respiratory distress syndrome, Pract Cardiol 6:79, 1980.

Hyers TM: Pathogenesis of adult respiratory distress syndrome: current concepts, Semin Respir Med 2:104, 1981.

Ikegami M, Jacobs H, and Jobe A: Surfactant function in respiratory distress syndrome, J Pediatr 102:443, 1983.

Jacob HS: Role of complement and granulocytes in septic shock, Acta Chir Scand Suppl 499:97, 1980.

Jacobs ER et al: Ibuprofen in canine endotoxin shock, J Clin Invest 70:536, 1982.

Janssen HF and Lutherer LO: Ventriculocisternal administration of naloxone protects against severe hypotension during endotoxin shock, Brain Res 194:608, 1980.

Jenkins MT et al: Congestive atelectasis: a complication of the intravenous infusion of fluids, Ann Surg 132:327, 1950.

Jenkinson SG: Pulmonary oxygen toxicity, Clin Chest Med 3:109, 1982.

Jobe A et al: Saturated phosphotidylcholine secretion and the effect of natural surfactant on premature and term lambs ventilated for 2 days, Exp Lung Res 4:259, 1983.

Johnson A and Malik AB: Effect of granulocytopenia on extravascular lung water content after microembolization. Am Rev Respir Dis 122:561, 1980.

Johnson TH, Altman AR, and McCaffree RD: Radiologic considerations in the adult respiratory distress syndrome treated with positive end expiratory pressure (PEEP), Clin Chest Med 3:89, 1982.

Jose PJ, Forrest MJ, and Williams TJ: Human C5a des Arg increases vascular permeability, J Immunol 127:2376, 1981.

Kadowitz PJ, Joiner PD, and Hyman AL: Physiological and pharmacological roles of prostaglandins, Am Rev Pharmacol 15:285, 1975.

Kahn F et al.: Results of gastric neutralization with hourly antacids and cimetidine in 320 intubated patients with respiratory failure, Chest 79:409, 1981.

Kapit W and Elson LM: The anatomy coloring book, New York, 1977, Harper & Row Publishers Inc.

Kaplan RL, Sahn IA, and Petty TL: Incidence and outcome of the respiratory distress syndrome in gram negative sepsis, Arch Intern Med 139:867, 1979.

Kinsman RA et al: Symptoms and experiences in chronic bronchitis and emphysema, Chest 83:755, 1983.

Kopolovic R et al: Effects of ibuprofen on a porcine model of acute respiratory failure, J Surg Res 36:300, 1984.

Kuckelt W et al: Effect of PEEP on gas exchange, pulmonary mechanics, and hemodynamics in adult respiratory distress syndrome (ARDS), Intensive Care Med 7:177, 1981.

Kunkel S et al: Modulation of inflammatory reactions by prostaglandins, Oxford, 1982, Oxford University Press, pp 633-640.

Lamy M et al.: Pathologic features and mechanisms of hypoxemia in adult respiratory distress syndrome, Am Rev Respir Dis 114:267, 1976.

Lee C et al: Elastolytic activity in pulmonary lavage fluid from patients with adult respiratory distress syndrome, N Engl J Med 304:192, 1981.

Lemaire I, Tseng R, and Lemaire S: Systemic administration of β-endorphin: potent hypotensive effect involving a sereotonergic pathway, Proc Natl Acad Sci U S A 75:6240, 1978.

Leslie CA and Levine L: Evidence for the presence of a prostaglandin E_2-9-keto reductase in rat organs, Biochem Biophys Res Commun 52:717, 1973.

Levine E, Senior R, and Butler J: The elastase activity of alveolar macrophages: measurements using synthetic substrate and elastin, Am Rev Respir Dis 113:25, 1976.

Mallory TB: The general pathology of traumatic shock, Surgery 27:629, 1950.

Marks MB: Nebulization of cromolyn sodium in the treatment of childhood asthma, Respir Care 28:1282, 1983.

Martin L; respiratory failure, Med Clin North Am 61:1369, 1977.

Martin T et al: Leukotriene B₄ production by the human alveolar macrophages: A potential mechanism for amplifying inflammation in the lung, Am Rev Respir Dis 129:106, 1984.

Marx JL: The leukotrienes in allergy and inflammation, Science 215:1380, 1982.

Masson RG, Ruggieri J, and Siddiqui MM: Amniotic fluid embolism: definitive diagnosis in a survivor, Am Rev Respir Dis 120:187, 1979.

Matte AA: Studies on actions of prostaglandins in the lung, Acta Physiol Scand 441:1, 1976.

Maulding TS: The case for routine supervision of tuberculosis treatment with the medication monitor (editorial), Chest 79:377, 1981.

McCabe W, Kreger M, and Johns M: Type specific and cross-reaction antibodies in gram-negative bacteremia, N Engl J Med 287:262, 1972.

McCord J: Oxygen radicals and lung injury, Chest 83:35S, 1983.

McPherson SP and Spearman CB: Respiratory therapy equipment, ed 3, St Louis, 1985, The CV Mosby Co.

Merritt T et al: Reduction of lung injury by human surfactant treatment in respiratory distress syndrome, Chest 83:27S, 1983.

Metzger Z, Hoffeld J, and Oppenheim J: Regulation by PGE₂ of the production of oxygen intermediates by LPS-activated macrophages, J Immunol 127:1109, 1981.

Modell JH, Graves SA, and Ketover A: Clinical course of 91 consecutive near drowning victims, Chest 70:231, 1976.

Morgan WKC: Pulmonary disability—can't work? won't work? Respir Care 28:471, 1983.

Murphy TL et al: Rise of platelet serotonin in the canine pulmonary response to endotoxin, J Appl Physiol 50:178, 1981.

Murray H and Cohn Z: Macrophage oxygen-dependent antimicrobial activity. I. Susceptibility of *Toxoplasma gondii* to oxygen intermediates, J Exp Med 150:938, 1979.

Murray JF: Mechanisms of acute respiratory failure, Am Rev Respir Dis 115:1071, 1971.

Murray JF: Pathophysiology of acute respiratory failure, Respir Care 28:531, 1983.

Nathan C, Murray H, and Cohn Z: The macrophage as an effector cell, N Engl J Med 303:622, 1980.

Nicholson D: Corticosteroids in the treatment of septic shock and the adult respiratory distress syndrome, Med Clin North Am 67:717, 1983.

O'Flaherty J: Lipid mediators of acute allergic and inflammatory reactions. In Lynn W, editor: Inflammatory cells and lung disease, Boca Raton, Fla, 1983, CRC Press Inc.

Ogletree M and Brigham K: The effect of cyclooxygenase inhibitors on pulmonary vascular responses to endotoxin in unanesthetized sheep, Prostaglandin Leukotriene Med 8:489, 1982.

Ogletree M et al: Increased flux of 5-HETE in sheep lung lymph during pulmonary leukostasis after endotoxin, Fed Proc 40:767, 1981.

Orange RP, Stechschulte DJ, and Austen KF: Cellular mechanisms involved in the release of slow-reacting substance of anaphylaxis, Fed Proc 28:1710, 1969.

Packham NA, Nishizawa EE, and Mustard JF: Response of platelets to tissue injury, Biochem Pharmacol 171:84, 1968.

Parker J et al: Prevention of free radical mediated vascular permeability increases in lung using superoxide dismutase, Chest 83:52S, 1983.

Pearl R and Raffin T: Niacin reduces oxygen toxicity in mouse alveolar macrophages, Pharmacology 27:219, 1983.

Petty T and Ashbaugh DG: The adult respiratory distress syndrome, Chest 60:233, 1971.

Petty TL: Adult respiratory distress syndrome: definition and historical perspective, Clin Chest Med 3:3, 1982.

Pingleton SK: Complications associated with the adult respiratory distress syndrome, Clin Chest Med 13:143, 1982.

Pingleton SK et al: The efficacy of low dose heparin in the prevention of pulmonary emboli in a respiratory intensive care unit, Chest 79:647,1981.

Pollack M et al: Enhanced survival in *Pseudomonas aeruginosa* septicemia associated with high levels of circulating antibody to *Escherichia coli* endotoxin core, J Clin Invest 72:1874, 1984.

Pontoppidan H, Geffin B, and Lowenstein E: Acute respiratory failure in the adult, N Engl J Med 287:690, 743, 799, 1972.

Ramwell RW and Shaw JE: Biological significance of the prostaglandins, Recent Prog Horm Res 26:139, 1970.

Repine J, Fox R, and Berger E: Hydrogen peroxide kills *Staphylococcus aureus* by reacting with staphylococcal iron to form hydroxyl radical, J Biol Chem 256:7094, 1981.

Reynolds DG et al: Blockage of opiate receptors with naloxone improves survival and cardiac performance of canine endotoxic shock, Circ Shock 7:38, 1980.

Reynolds HY: Lung inflammation: role of endogenous chemotactic factors in attracting polymorphonuclear granulocytes, Am Rev Respir Dis 1327:S16, 1983.

Rinaldo JE and Rogers RM: Adult respiratory distress syndrome—changing concepts of lung injury and repair, N Engl J Med 306:900, 1982.

Risberg B and Heideman M: The cascade systems in post-traumatic pulmonary insufficiency, Acta Chir Scand Suppl 499:107, 1980.

Rister M and Baehner R: The alteration of superoxide dismutase, catalase, glutathione peroxidase, and NAD(P)H cytochrome c reductase in guinea pig polymorphonuclear leukocytes and alveolar macrophages during hyperoxia, J Clin Invest 58:1174, 1976.

Rossman MD, Daniele RP, and Dauber JH: Nodular endobronchial sarcoidosis: a study comparing blood and lung lymphocytes, Chest 79:427, 1981.

Sandhaus R et al: Elastolytic proteinases of the human macrophage, Chest 83:60S, 1983.

Schmidt GB et al: Continuous positive airway pressure in the prophylaxis of the adult respiratory distress syndrome, Surg Gynecol Obstet 143:613, 1976.

Schneider R, Zapol W, and Carvalho A: Platelet consumption and sequestration in severe acute respiratory failure, Am Rev Respir Dis 122:445, 1980.

Schnells G et al: Electron-microscopic investigation of lung biopsies in patients with post-traumatic respiratory insufficiency, Acta Chir Scand Suppl 499:9, 1980.

Schumer W: Controversy in shock research. Pro: the role of steroids in septic shock, Circ Shock 8:667, 1981.

Schumer W: Steroids in the treatment of clinical septic shock, Ann Surg 184:333, 1976.

Shoemaker WC et al: Pathogenesis of respiratory failure (ARDS) after hemorrhage and trauma, Crit Care Med 8:504, 1980.

Short B, Miller M, and Fletcher J: Improved survival in the suckling rat model of group B streptococcal sepsis after treatment with non-steroidal antiinflammatory drugs, Pediatrics 70:343, 1982.

Sibbald WJ, Anderson RR, and Holliday RL: Pathogenesis of pulmonary edema associated with the adult respiratory distress syndrome, Can Med Assoc J 120:445, 1979.

Sibbald W et al: Alveolo-capillary permeability in human septic ARDS, Chest 79:133, 1981.

Simmons DH: Therapy of ARDS: positive end-expiratory pressure, West J Med 130:229, 1979.

Slonim NB and Hamilton LH: Respiratory physiology, ed 4, St Louis, 1981, The CV Mosby Co.

Snapper J et al: Effects of cyclooxygenase inhibitors on the alterations in lung mechanics caused by endotoxemia in the unanesthetized sheep, J Clin Invest 72:63, 1983.

Spearman CB, Sheldon RL, and Egan DF: Egan's fundamentals of respiratory therapy, ed 4, St Louis, 1982, The CV Mosby Co.

Sprung C et al: The effects of high dose corticosteroids in patients with septic shock: a prospective controlled study, N Engl J Med 311:1137, 1984.

Staub NC: Pulmonary edema. Physiol Rev 54:678, 1974.

Stein M and Thomas DP: Role of platelets in the acute pulmonary responses to endotoxin, J Appl Physiol 23:47, 1967.

Stothert JC Jr et al: Randomized prospective evaluation of cimetidine and antacid control of gastric pH in the critically ill, Ann Surg 192:169, 1980.

Suter PM, Fairly HB, and Isenberg MD: Optimum end-expiratory airway pressure in patients with acute pulmonary failure, N Engl J Med 292:284-289, 1975.

Suttorp M AND Simon L: Lung cell oxidant injury: enhancement of PMN leukocyte mediated cytotoxicity in lung cells exposed to sustained in vitro hyperoxia, J Clin Invest 70:342-350, 1982.

Tacker WA: Recent developments in the treatment of sudden death syndrome, Respir Care 27:682, 1982.

Traker DL, Adair TH, and Adams T Jr: Hemodynamic consequences endotoxemia in sheep, Circ Shock 8:551, 1981.

Turrens J, Crapo J, and Freeman S: Protection against oxygen toxicity by intravenous injection of liposome-entrapped catalase and superoxide dismutase, J Clin Invest 73:87, 1984.

Vaage J: The role of platelets in post-traumatic pulmonary insufficiency, Acta Chir Scand Suppl 499:141, 1980.

Valdes ME et al: Continuous positive airway pressure in prophylaxis in adult respiratory distress syndrome in trauma patients, Surg Forum 29:187, 1978.

Van Dorp DA: Aspects of the biosynthesis of prostaglandins. Prog Biochem Pharmacol 3:71, 1967.

Waldker JR, Smith MJH, and Ford-Hutchinson AW: Prostaglandins and leukotaxis, J Pharm Pharmacol 28:745, 1976.

Ward P et al: Evidence for role of hydroxyl radical in complement and neutrophil-dependent tissue injury, J Clin Invest 72:789, 1983.

Wasserman SI, Goetzl EJ, and Austen KF: Inactivation of slow-reacting substance of anaphylaxis by human eosinophil arylsulfatase, J Immunol 114:645, 1975.

Webb PJ et al: Do prostacyclin and thromboxane play a role in endotoxic shock? Br J Surg 68:720, 1981.

Webster RO et al: Absence of inflammatory lung injury in rabbits challenged intravascularly with complement-derived chemotactic factors, Am Rev Respir Dis 125:335, 1982.

Weigelt JA, Mitchel RA, and Snyder WH III: Early positive end-expiratory pressure in the adult respiratory distress syndrome, Arch Surg 114:497, 1979.

Weigelt JA, Snyder WH, and Mitchell RA: Early identification of patients prone to develop adult respiratory distress syndrome, Am J Surg 142:687, 1981.

Weiso JW, Drazen JM, and Coles N: Bronchoconstrictor effects of leukotriene C in humans, Science 216:196, 1982.

Weksler BB and Coupal E: Platelet-dependent generation of chemotactic activity in serum, J Exp Med 137:1419, 1973.

Wentzell B and Epand R: Stimulation of the release of prostaglandins from polymorphonuclear leukocytes by the calcium ionophore A 23187, FEBS Lett 86:355, 1978.

Whitcomb ME: The normal lung and its diseases, St Louis, 1982, The CV Mosby Co.

White MK, Shepro D, and Hechtman B: Pulmonary function and platelet-lung interaction, J Appl Physiol 34:697, 1973.

Wise W et al: Ibuprofen improves survival from endotoxic shock in the rat, J Pharmacol Exp Ther 215:160, 1980.

Wise WC, Cook JA, and Halushka PV: Implications for thromboxane A_2 in the pathogenesis of endotoxic shock, Adv Shock Res 6:83, 1981.

Witek TJ and Schachter EN: Air pollution and respiratory health, Respir Care 28:442, 1983.

Witek TJ, Schachter EN, and Leaderer BP: Indoor air pollution and respiratory health, Respir Care 29:147, 1984.

Wolter N et al: Production of cyclooxygenase products by alveolar macrophages in pulmonary sarcoidosis, Chest 83:79S, 1983.

Zapol WM and Snider MT: Pulmonary hypertension in severe acute respiratory failure, N Engl J Med 296:476, 1977.

Ziegler E et al: Treatment of gram-negative bacteremia and shock with human antiserum to a mutant *Escherichia coli*, N Engl J Med 307:1225, 1982.

Ziment I: Expectorants in chronic bronchitis, Respir Care 27:1398, 1982.

Zimmerman GA, Morris AH, and Gengiz M: Cardiovascular alterations in the adult respiratory distress syndrome, Am J Med 73:25, 1982.

Zinner S and McCabe W: Effects of IgM antibody in patients with bacteremia due to gram-negative bacilli, J Infect Dis 133:37, 1976.

Microbiology and decontamination

9.25 Discuss the risk of acquiring other infections of workers with AIDS.

9.26 Point out considerations for handling and decontaminating items and waste exposed to AIDS.

9.27 Appraise the risk of acquiring AIDS from workers sharing the same environment with an AIDS carrier.

9.28 Identify other issues besides cross-infection that must be considered when making decisions about employment of persons with AIDS.

1.0 TERMINOLOGY AND PRINCIPLES

1.1 Definitions

1 Aerobic. To live in an atmosphere containing oxygen.

2 Anaerobic. To live in an atmosphere without oxygen. In the discussion of anaerobic bacteria, the term "facultative" means that the bacteria prefer environments without oxygen (O_2) but will grow in an O_2 atmosphere.

3 Antiseptic. A substance that opposes sepsis, putrefaction, or decay; one that prevents or arrests the growth or action of microorganisms either by inhibiting their activity or by destroying them.

4 Asepsis. The state or condition of *complete absence* of all bacteria, an ideal state. Functionally, it refers to the state of being as free from bacteria or microorganisms as is possible.

5 Autoclave. A device for sterilizing medical supplies and equipment by steam under pressure.

6 Autotrophic. Refers to organisms that derive their energy from the oxidation of inorganic materials.

7 Bacilli. Bacteria that appear under the microscope as rods. The word comes from the Latin "bacillum," meaning little staff or rod.

8 Bacteremia. The presence of bacteria in the blood; does not imply growth of bacteria.

9 Bacteria. Microscopic, unicellular plants containing no chlorophyll, which reproduce by binary fission.

10 Bacteriophage. A bacterial virus. The virus or phage particle attacks a susceptible bacteria cell in the following three phases:

  a An absorption of a part of the surface of the bacteria cell occurs.

  b The entrance of at least a portion of the phage particle into the cell follows with a replication of the viral substance.

  c The continued reproduction of the viral substance eventually causes a swelling and then bursting (lysis) of the bacterial cell.

11 Binary fission. A simple means of cellular reproduction; the division (splitting) of true bacteria cells into two equal, identical cells.

12 Biologic transmission of infection. The mode of disease transmission from host to host by an animal or insect, in which the causative agent (such as a protozoan) undergoes a cycle of development in the animal's or insect's body, e.g., malarial development in the mosquito.

13 Capsule. The gelatinous outer wall found around some bacteria, which serves as an effective barrier against adverse environmental conditions.

14 Carrier. An individual who internally or externally carries the causative agent of a disease without developing any symptoms or showing ill effects of the disease.

15 Cidal. Refers to actual killing power or action of a substance.

16 Cocci. The bacteria appearing under the microscope as circles, dots, or spheres. "Coccus" comes from the Latin corruption of the Greek "kokkos" meaning seed.

17 Commensalism. A symbiotic association between two organisms without causing harm to either; in fact, one host may benefit from the relationship, e.g., the relationship of the shark and remora fish.

18 Communicable disease. A disease that may be transmitted directly or indirectly from one individual to another.

19 Contagious disease. Communicable disease with reference to the organism that causes the disease.

20 Culture. The growth or production of microorganisms on or in a nutrient substance (medium).

21 Culture media. The nutritive substances that are used to grow microorganisms in the laboratory. The media may be:

  a Liquid—usually a nutrient "broth" or body fluid.

  b Solid—usually contains agar (a gel derived from a species of seaweed) and the same nutrients as the liquid medium.

22 Disinfectant. A chemical agent that destroys disease germs or other harmful microorganisms or inactivates them. Most commonly refers to chemicals that kill the growing forms (vegetative forms) but not necessarily the resistant spore forms of bacteria. Disinfectant usually describes substances that are applied to inanimate objects.

23 Ecology. The relationship of organisms to their environment.

24 Ehrlich, Paul (1854-1915). The "Father of Chemotherapy," noted for his development of an arsenic treatment for syphilis.

25 Endemic disease. A disease that is in constant presence in a region or class of individuals but of relatively slow incidence, e.g., histoplasmosis is endemic to the Mississippi Valley area of the United States (in contrast to the suddenly flaring epidemic disease that affects large numbers of people within a short period of time).

26 Epidemic disease. A disease that suddenly flares, affecting large numbers of people in a short period of time, e.g., plaque, influenza, typhoid (in contrast to the endemic disease that is constantly present in a given region or location).

27 Etiology. The total body of knowledge regarding the cause of a disease, dealing with such factors as the source, mode of transmission, and pathway by which the pathogens enter the body.

28 Flora, resident. The bacteria that reside below the surface of the skin, in the pore openings, and among the

cracks, crevices, and folds of the skin. They cannot be removed by ordinary washing.

29 Flora, transient. The bacteria on the surface of the skin, which can be easily removed by normal washing.

30 Fungicide. Anything that destroys fungi (yeasts and molds); applied especially to chemical agents that kill both pathogenic and nonpathogenic fungi other than bacteria; commonly used for substances applied to both living tissue and inanimate objects.

31 Germicide. Anything that destroys bacteria; applied especially to chemical agents that kill disease "germs," but not necessarily spores.

32 Gram-negative organism: An organism that appears *red* as a result of treatment with Gram's staining technique.

33 Gram-positive organism. An organism that appears *blue* as a result of treatment with Gram's staining technique.

34 Halophilic. A propensity for high salt concentration.

35 Heterotrophic. Refers to organisms that obtain their energy from the breakdown of organic material.

36 Host. An animal or human that has a pathogen present on or within the body, whether or not the pathogen produces symptoms.

37 Hypertonic. A condition or situation in which the solute concentration (osmotic pressure) is higher than normal body fluid.

38 Hypotonic. A condition or situation in which the solute concentration (osmotic pressure) is lower than normal body fluid.

39 Incubation. A procedure in which microorganisms are grown under carefully controlled temperature and humidity conditions.

40 Incubation period. The period between the beginning of an infection and the appearance of symptoms.

41 Infectious disease. Any disease caused by the growth of pathogenic microorganisms in the body; may or may not be contagious.

42 Killing time. The time required to kill microorganisms under specified conditions of temperature, concentration, size of the organism, specimen, and nature of the killing agent.

43 Koch, Robert (1870). First to demonstrate that bacteria actually cause disease (bacteria life forms were recognized in 1675).

44 Leeuwenhoek, Anton (1675). First to develop a microscope (although much different from that with which we are familiar) and first to see and therefore understand bacteria.

45 Lister, Joseph (1827-1912). Recognized as the "father of aseptic surgery" because of his efforts to reduce surgical infections through the use of carbolic acid sprays.

46 Microorganisms. Bacteria, spiral organisms, algae, rickettsial bacteria, viruses, molds, yeasts, and protozoa are all microscopic organisms.

47 Parasitism. The state or condition in which an organism lives within, on, or at the expense of another organism, called the host, e.g., fleas, mistletoe, etc.
NOTE: A "good" parasite does not kill its host.

48 Pasteur, Louis (1822-1895). The chemist and bacteriologist recognized for his discovery of the anthrax vaccine, rabies vaccine, etc.

49 Pathogen. Any disease-producing microorganism or material; *any* organism may be pathogenic under the correct circumstances.

50 Petri dish. A flat dish containing a growth medium with agar on which bacteria are grown (cultured) for laboratory purposes.

51 pH. The symbol used in expressing hydrogen ion concentration; the measure of alkalinity and acidity. All life can exist within only a narrow range. A pH of 7.0 is neutral, with numbers below 7.0 called acid and numbers above 7.0 called alkaline.

52 Phagocyte. A cell capable of ingesting bacteria or other foreign particles.

53 Phenol coefficient. A number indicating the disinfection value of a substance. It represents the quotient obtained by dividing the number representing the dilution of a disinfectant that kills an organism in a fixed time by the number representing the degree of dilution of phenol that kills the organism in the same time.

54 Plate count. A method of determining the number of living bacteria in a sample; based on the growth of colonies of bacteria on a nutrient in a Petri dish.

55 Rickettsias. Very small gram-negative organisms appearing within cells as either short bacilli or cocci; the causative agent for Rocky Mountain spotted fever.

56 Sanitizer. An agent that reduces the bacteria count to "safe levels" as judged by public health requirements for food-handling equipment, eating and drinking utensils, etc.

57 Spirochetes. Slender, flexuous, or corkscrew-shaped organisms that are highly motile. The causative agent of syphilis.

58 Spores. Structures formed by bacteria, which permit survival under adverse environmental conditions through the formation of a thick, heavy coating that serves as a protective shield. This coating is resistant to staining by dyes, heat, cold, and many chemical agents. The structures are capable of developing into a new bacterial cell. The reproductive cells of true molds are also called spores.

59 Staining. Procedure in which microscopic specimens are subjected to special chemicals that give color to them so that they can be more easily seen under the microscope.

60 Stasis. Refers to inhibition or prevention of growth; does not necessarily kill organisms.

61 Sterilize. Any process, physical or chemical, that will destroy *all* forms of life, including bacteria, mold, spores, and viruses.

62 Surveillance. To identify baseline information about the frequency and type of endemic nosocomial infection to permit rapid identification of deviations from that baseline.

63 Symbiosis. Mutual beneficial relationship between two hosts.

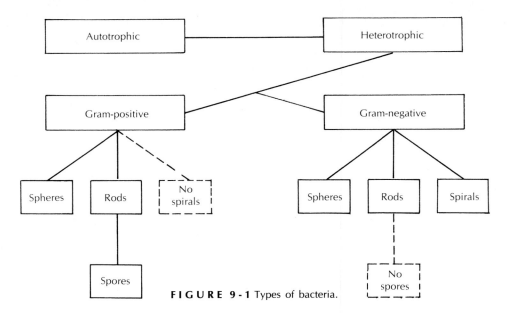

FIGURE 9-1 Types of bacteria.

64 Synergism. Cooperative effort by two or more harmless species to produce something that each alone is incapable of doing.

65 Toxins. Metabolic products secreted by bacteria in their growth.

66 Viricide. Anything that destroys or inactivates viruses.

67 Virulence. Refers to an organism's disease-producing power.

1.2 Principles of basic microbiology

1 Microbiology is one branch of the greater science of biology that includes studies of the nature of all living matter.

2 Microbiology is a practical subject concerned with microscopic organisms: their form, structure, mode of life, and effect on human beings.

3 Most people are already somewhat aware of microbiology because they are taught from early childhood to wash their hands before eating. They did this to kill "germs"—microorganisms that exist everywhere.

4 The one particular group of microorganisms or microbes that is of interest to respiratory care personnel is *bacteria*.

  a However, not all bacteria are pathogenic. Many are harmless and some are very helpful to humans.

    • Strains of bacteria normally live in the digestive tract and help produce vitamin K necessary to control bleeding. Other normally present bacteria produce folic acid, a vitamin that prevents anemia.

  b The major classifications of microorganisms are algae, protozoa, yeasts, molds, bacteria, rickettsias, and viruses.

5 The nature of bacteria can be illustrated by Fig. 9-1, which shows two distinct divisions of bacteria, grampositive and gram-negative. The basis for identifying bacteria as gram-positive or gram-negative will be presented later.

6 Note that there are three basic types of bacteria shapes (Fig. 9-2):

  a *Bacilli* (bacillus). Rod shaped organisms *(A)*.

  b *Cocci* (coccus). Round or ball-shaped organisms *(b)*.

  c *Spirals* (spirochetes). Comma-shaped or spiral-shaped organisms *(C)*.

7 In more detail, Fig. 9-2 also shows the different forms of each of the three major divisions:

  a Two rods that are connected together are called a *diplobacillus (4)*.

  b Four rods together in a chain are called a *streptobacillus (5)*.

  c A single sphere is a *coccus (6)*.

  d Two (paired) cocci form a *diplococcus (7)*.

  e A chain of cocci is referred to as a *streptococcus (8)*.

  f A cluster of cocci (like grapes) is called a *staphylococcus (9)*.

  g A curved rod with less than one spiral turn is a *vibrio (10)*.

  h A rigid spiral with one or more turns is a *spirillum (11)*.

  i A flexible curved rod with several complete spiral turns is a *spirochete (12)*.

8 The bacterial structure is illustrated by the schematic of the hypothetical rod-shaped cell in Fig. 9-3.

  a The slime layer (capsule, gelatinous coat) *(1)* is probably on all bacteria to some degree. The extent of this slime layer apparently has some effect on the virulence of selected bacteria. It is thought to serve a protective role, either by conserving fluid within the cell or by providing a shield against the host's attacking defenses.

  b The cell wall *(2)* is best described as the cell's outer skin. This outer shell is a rather tough and yet flexible structure lying just inside the slime layer. A number of vital functions are handled by the cell wall of this unicellular organism, which has no

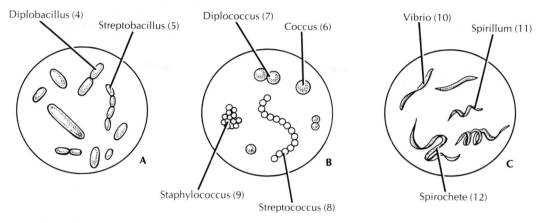

FIGURE 9-2 Basic bacterial forms. **A,** Bacilli (rod-shaped). **B,** Cocci (round-shaped). **C,** Spirals.

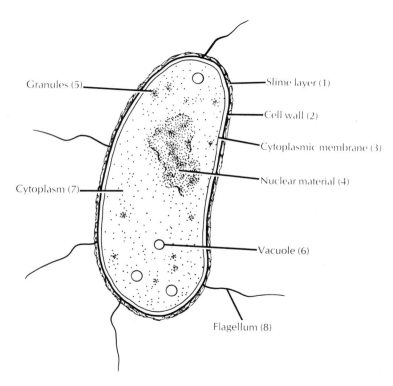

FIGURE 9-3 Rod-shaped bacterial cell structures.

mouth parts or any well-defined structures for handling food digestion and excretion of metabolic wastes.

c The cytoplasmic membrane is best described as the cell's inner skin *(3)*. It is semipermeable; hence, selective in character. This is because it only passes certain substances in and out of the cell like a filter.

d Whether or not bacteria actually have well-defined nuclei *(4)* is controversial. However, it is probably safe to guess that bacteria have *some* kind of DNA-containing nucleus or regulatory body to govern reproduction and metabolism.

e Granules *(5)* are scattered throughout the cell's "body." It is suggested that they are either:
  • Accumulations of waste material not yet eliminated through the cell wall.
  • Reserves of food to be used in times of need.
  • Both of these.

f The vacuole *(6)* is a clear space in the protoplasm or cytoplasm of a cell. It may represent the space left behind by a particle of digested food.

g As with most living things, much of the internal substance of bacteria is *water*. The cell's cytoplasm *(7)* is its water content or life substance.

h Bacteria move about with the aid of flagella *(sing. flagellum—8),* meaning "little whips." The configuration illustrated is hypothetical. Actually there may be only one, two at the one end, twelve around the middle, or any other combination that nature can provide. Some bacteria have been "clocked" moving at 100 µ per second, or equal to approximately 100 miles per hour!

9 Bacteria receive nutrition in solution by *osmosis.* Food passes through the cell wall and cytoplasmic membrane, which are both semipermeable. Waste products pass out by the same process.

10 Bacteria produce different types of waste products.
   a Some give off various gases.
   b Some produce enzymes, some of which are necessary to the life functions of their host.
   c Some produce toxins that are poisonous to the host.

11 Bacteria are classified as one of the following:
   a *Psychrophilic* (cold-liking)—living and growing between 0° and 25° C.
   b *Mesophilic* (middle-liking)—living and growing between 20° and 45° C (37° C is normal for humans).
      • Some bacteria that are mesophilic may not grow at temperatures above 45° C but, by spore formation, will survive temperatures above 200° C.
   c *Thermophilic* (heat-liking)—living and growing between 45° and 70° C.

Bacterial *growth factors,* which are also referred to as incubation, consist of:
   a Water. Nutrients dissolve in surrounding liquid and, in this form, pass through the cell wall.
   b Osmotic pressure. Because of the difference in osmotic pressure inside and outside the cell, nutrient-carrying pressure inside and outside the cell, nutrient-carrying liquid outside the cell (with its higher pressure) is "pulled" into the cell's lower interior pressure. Materials are drawn out of the cell by a reversal of this pressure difference.
   c Nutrients. Cells need exactly the same raw materials for metabolism and growth as humans. These include carbon, hydrogen, oxygen, phosphorus, potassium, iodine, nitrogen, sulfur, calcium, iron, and magnesium.
   d Surface tension. If surface tension of a medium is low, materials in solution that are responsible for lowering the surface tension will tend to be concentrated at the cell's surface. If this material is slightly toxic, such as soap or alcohol, it may inhibit or prevent the cell's growth.
   e Oxygen needs. Microorganisms are mostly either aerobes or anaerobes; faculative bacteria can function with or without oxygen.
   f pH. All living organisms function in a narrow range of pH acid and base ratio.

12 *Reproduction.* The process necessary for continuation of a species is carried out by bacteria in the following manner:

a Cells grow to maximum size and split along the short axis (at right angles to the organism) to form new cells. This process is called *binary fission* and continues for as long as suitable conditions for growth continue.

b The rate of cell division is rapid: every 20 to 30 minutes when all conditions are ideal.

c Spore formation is a higher form of reproduction. Offspring lie dormant and have protective walls that are more resistant to physical or chemical changes than the original organism.

13 Differences in bacteria groups are characterized by the Gram method of staining.
   a This method was first described by a Danish bacteriologist named Gram in 1884. This process involves the following steps:
      • A heat-fixed smear on a glass slide is stained with crystal violet, preferably a solution buffered to a slightly alkaline pH.
      • The specimen is then washed in water and treated with a dilute solution of iodine. This is followed by a decolorizing rinse of alcohol or alcohol-acetone mixture.
      • Some kinds of bacteria are not decolorized and remain purple (the color of the crystal violet) and these are called *gram-positive.*
      • Others lose all their color, and since they are difficult to see, they are usually stained with a mild dye that is easily distinguished from the violet, usually safranine, a red dye. These are called *gram-negative.*
      • It is not the color of the cells that is important; rather the reaction to the stain is related to *deep-seated differences* between the organisms.
      • Gram-positive organisms are inhibited by certain dyes, penicillin, halogens, etc.; may form spores; and have a cell wall different from gram-negative organisms.
      • The gram-positive character is associated with certain yeasts and molds, as well as certain bacteria. All other organisms are gram-negative.
   b The gram-negative rods group (the largest) can be divided into the following four groups:
      • The highly *oxidative rods.* These are important for their ability to fix nitrogen in the soil; very few pathogens.
      • The *fermentative rods.* These are important in water analysis and enteric disease; several pathogens.
      • The *"fastidious" rods* (require special growth media); most are pathogenic.
      • The *others;* as with any groups there are loners that do not fit in anywhere else; few pathogens.
   c There are no known pathogenic gram-negative cocci.

14 Bacteria are also characterized by the *acid-fast test.* Acid-fast bacteria, especially *Mycobacterium tuberculosis,* are not readily decolorized by acids after staining.

15 *Viruses* are considered the simplest form of life. Their chief characteristics are as follow.
   a Viruses are smaller than bacteria and cannot be seen with an ordinary light microscope.

b They are able to pass through filters that trap bacteria.

c They are grown only *on living tissue* and cannot grow on culture media.

d They are not true cells and live as parasites on living cells or even on bacteria, which they use to help replicate their genetic material for reproduction and to produce food.

e Usually they are classified by the type of disease they cause, e.g., polio, cold, smallpox, influenza, mumps, measles, or yellow fever.

f Once a virus has attached itself to a cell, it "plugs in" to that cell's life functions and begins to manufacture basic viral components out of the host's cellular material until the cell bursts, releasing millions of duplicate viruses, which then invade other cells.

g It has also been shown that a virus can force a cell to manufacture new cells if it needs more raw material; hence the discovery that viruses *may* be responsible for at least some forms of cancer.

h Viruses also produce toxins and, because of their small sizes, are regarded as antigens by the host, which then produces antibodies in defense, except in the HIV.

2.0 DECONTAMINATION AND SURVEILLANCE PROGRAM

2.1 The problem of nosocomial infections caused by contaminated equipment

1 Nosocomial infections are those infections acquired by a patient while in the hospital.

2 In 1970, Drs. J.P. Sanford and A.K. Pierce, in a report for the Centers for Disease Control, presented the following summary.

a Respiratory infections represent an important facet of the broad problem of nosocomial infections. From 0.5% to 5.0% of all patients admitted to general hospitals developed hospital-acquired pneumonias.

b These pneumonias are caused by pathologic agents, including both gram-positive cocci (especially staphylococci) and aerobic gram-negative bacilli.

- It appears that the gram-negative bacilli are taking on a greater role in the evolution of nosocomial respiratory infections.
- One of the causes of gram-negative bacillary pneumonia in the moderately ill to the moribund patient is the autoinfection produced by aspiration of oropharyngeal secretions.

c However, *respiratory care equipment,* especially those items that utilize nebulization, constitutes the major potential source of nosocomial gram-negative bacillary pneumonias.

- Elimination of the potential danger of contaminated respiratory therapy equipment requires ongoing decontamination and surveillance programs.

3 Thus far, respiratory care equipment has been named as a definite causative agent in the spread of the

pseudomonas, flavobacterium, herellea, alcaligenes, and *achromobacter species*.

4 The initial source of contamination may be any one of the following:

a Contaminated medications (water, normal saline).

b Contaminated water reservoirs.

c Contaminated nebulizer jets and Venturi tubes.

- Contaminated nebulizers are especially hazardous in spreading infections. Aerosols deposited beyond the level of ciliated bronchial epithelium cause colonization of the area, which subsequently spreads to other areas of the lung.

5 Current research indicates devices that deliver only humidity (vapor), even if heated, are much less likely to cause nosocomial infection, because of the lack of physical particles on which bacteria can travel.

a The "cascade" *humidifier* has been named as relatively safe with regard to being a bacteria producer.

b However, the spinning disk and ultrasonic *nebulizers* have been specifically named as chief sources of bacteria production in the hospital environment.

6 Nosocomial infections are determined by the occurrence of several common factors.

a Infections occur in the hospital environment where antibiotic-resistant bacteria are in the majority.

b Infections develop in those patients with anatomic and/or physiologic weaknesses in their ability to fight bacteria.

c The incriminated bacteria have in common the following characteristics:

- All can acquire *resistance* to antibiotics.
- All are *omnipresent* in their distribution.
- Most can survive wide temperature ranges, especially those consistent with human life.

7 The bacteria commonly responsible for nosocomial infections are the staphylococci, the *klebsiella-enterobacter* species, *pseudomonas aeruginosa, serratia marcescens,* the *herellea* and *mima* species, and the *flavobacterium* species.

a Many of these are *secondary invaders,* which means that they will take advantage of an individual's lowered resistance and cause an infection. For example, *Serratia* species is not normally pathogenic, but it is *opportunistic* and will multiply rapidly when the host is weakened by a primary problem such as chronic obstructive pulmonary disease (COPD) or extensive burns.

2.2 The problem of contamination resulting from hospital personnel as carriers

1 Since the discovery of "Thyphoid Mary," it has been known that certain individuals can harbor (carry) pathogens without themselves being affected.

2 Today Typhoid Mary's counterpart works in our hospitals.

3 Studies have shown that from 30% to 50% of hospital personnel are colonized with *staphylococcus aureus* in their nasal passages.

4 A further question arises: if a pathologic strain is identified in an individual, did the employee acquire the organism in the hospital?

5 *Staphylococcus aureus* is not the only pathogen carried by hospital personnel. Studies have shown an increasing incidence of gram-negative nosocomial infections in hospitals.

  a These include carriers of *pseudomonas aeruginosa* (found in up to 16% of hospital employees) and *proteus* species (in up to 33%).

  b It should be noted that actual transmission of these gram-negative flora from personnel to patients is not *known* to be significant, but it is at least important to realize that we need to guard our patients from ourselves, as well as from our equipment.

2.3 Decontamination and surveillance programs in the respiratory care department

1 Although it is not general practice, routine culturing of hospital personnel can uncover individuals who, for whatever reason, are harboring pathogenic organisms.

2 One recommended control is improving the health and hygiene of hospital personnel through the use of the employee-health clinic. Health clinics can be used for:

  a Preemployment examination.

  b Routine purified protein derivative (PPD) (TB skin tests).

  c Chest radiographs.

  d Immunizations (influenza shots).

  e Reporting and treatment of acute infections.

3 Respiratory care personnel must be especially careful to maintain their health and level of hygiene because of constant exposure to infections.

  • A person with lowered resistance and/or poor hygiene can easily become sick or a carrier who could accidentally transmit pathogenic organisms to his or her patients.

4 Departments of respiratory care should be constantly on guard through programs of decontamination and surveillance.

  a *Decontamination* means that equipment used in delivering therapy should be thoroughly cleaned, rinsed, and then exposed to a sterilizing agent to minimize pathogen transfer or growth.

  b *Surveillance* means that material and equipment used to deliver therapy are inspected and checked by microbiologic means to discover the existence of pathogenic organisms on items presumed "clean" and ready for use.

5 Strangely, one of the chief areas of contamination, hence concern, is not the surfaces of the equipment itself, but any water left standing *in* the equipment. This water serves as a *growth medium* for bacteria.

  a Recovery rooms, critical care areas, patient rooms, emergency rooms, etc., contain containers of water functioning as humidifiers, nebulizers, bottles of "distilled water" for rinsing and washing, and bottles of water for diluting medications and other uses.

  b Many groups of bacteria, especially *pseudomonas* and *flavobacteria* spp., survive and thrive in such a warm, moist, and shielded environment.

  c Companies manufacture prepackaged sterile water for respiratory care. It is true that this water is sterile when the container has not been opened. However, this sterility *ends* once the seal to the nebulizer has been broken and the unit is left hanging from a wall outlet in a patient care area for longer than 8 to 12 hours. The technician who changes humdifier or nebulizer units must wash his or her hands between changes to reduce the chances of contaminating a unit as it is being changed.

6 The respiratory care department can help control the spread of nosocomial infections by:

  a Proper *decontamination* of equipment.

  b Proper *storage* of clean equipment to prevent recontamination.

  c Insisting that employees protect themselves against infection by maintaining their health.

  d Not permitting employees to work if they are sick.

  e Enforcing hospital policy regarding isolation procedures and hand washing techniques.

  f Insisting that all employees wash their hands between patients and when handling equipment or medications.

  g Developing and implementing an effective surveillance program for respiratory care equipment.

  h Implementing an effective follow-up program that investigates any positive surveillance results.

3.0 PATHOGENS
3.1 Various types of pathogens

This unit outlines most of the pathogenic bacteria known to infect humans and discusses hepatitis B and HIV. These bacteria are listed by shape and Gram's stain reaction. This outline does include conditions caused by molds, yeasts, rickettsias, or other viruses. The words in italics refer to the bacterium genus; the common name or disease that it causes is in parenthesis.

1 Gram-positive pathogens (cocci):

  a *Staphylococcus aureus* (staph). Lives on the skin, the mouth, and on nasal and other mucous membranes. Responsible for the following diseases and conditions: pimples (boils), carbuncles, abscesses, wound infections, respiratory infections (pneumonia), septicemia (septic condition of the blood), and food poisoning.

  b *Streptococcus pneumoniae* (diploccus or pneumococcus). Responsible for up to 80% of human lobar pneumonia. Eighty serologic strains or types have been identified.

  c *Streptococcus pyogenes* (strep). Beta-hemolytic streptococci are responsible for "strep throat," fever, puerpueral fever, tonsillitis, acute glomerulonephritis, and mastitis.

2 Gram-negative pathogens (cocci):

  a *Neisseria gonorrhoeae* (gonorrhea).

b *Neisseria meningitidis.* Responsible for meningococcal meningitis.

3 Gram-positive pathogens (rods);

a *Corynebacterium diphtheriae* (diptheria).

b *Corynebacterium minutissimum.* Responsible for erythrasma, a chronic skin infection.

c *Mycobacterium leprae* (leprosy). This bacterium cannot be grown in the laboratory.

d *Mycobacterium tuberculosis.* The causative agent of tuberculosis (Tests gram + and/or −).

4 Gram-positive pathogens (spore-forming rods):

a *Bacillus anthracis* (anthrax).

b *Clostridium botulinum* (botulism). Food poisoning.

c *Clostridium novyi.* Gas gangrene.

d *Clostridium welchii* or *C. perfringens.* Gas gangrene.

e *Clostridium tetani* (tetanus).

5 Gram-negative pathogens (enteric disease rods):

a *Actinomyces israelii* (lump jaw). An infection of the deep tissues and mucous membranes, particularly around the head and neck.

b *Bordetella pertussis* (whooping cough).

c *Brucella abortus* (brucellosis).

d *Escherichia coli.* Part of the normal intestinal flora of humans and other animals. Pathogenic species cause urinary tract infections and epidemic diarrheal diseases.

e *Haemophilus aegyptius.* Causes contagious conjunctivitis or "pinkeye."

f *Haemophilus influenzae.* Once thought to be a type of "flu," now known to cause a highly fatal form of meningitis, especially in infants.

g *Klebsiella pneumoniae.* Causative agent of Friedländer's pneumonia and other respiratory infections; a dangerous *secondary* invader.

h *Pasteurella multocida.* The causative agent of hemorrhagic septicemias.

i *Yersinia pestis* (plague, black death).

j *Pasteurella tularensis* (tularemia, rabbit fever).

k *Proteus vulgaris.* Causes cystitis and is often found as a *secondary* invading agent.

l *Pseudomonas aeruginosa.* An aggressive *secondary* invader (opportunist), forming blue-green pus. *Pseudomonas* is a water-loving bacterium that is implicated in many respiratory infections.

m *Salmonella enteritidis.* The causative agent of gastroenteritis in humans.

n *Salmonella typhi* (typhoid).

o *Serratia marcescens.* A water-loving bacterium seen in many respiratory and burn patients as a *secondary* invader. Noted for its blood-red pigment, it was once thought harmless and was used by microbiology students to demonstrate transmission among themselves.

6 Gram-negative pathogens (spirals):

a *Borrelia vincentii.* Associates with the *Fusobacterium fusiforme* to cause Vincent's angina or trench mouth.

b *Leptospira icterohaemorrhagiae.* Causative agent of Weil's disease (infectious jaundice).

c *Treponema pallidum* (syphilis).

d *Vibrio cholerae* (Asiatic cholera). Not generally found in the United States.

4.0 IDENTIFYING PATHOGENS
4.1 Methods of culturing microorganisms

Once a specimen to be cultured is delivered to the laboratory, some of it is specially prepared so that the suspected microorganisms will be more visible.

1 After the sample has been properly prepared, it will be stained by various dyes and rinsed by a solvent.

a A contrasting stain is added to detect any organisms that did not "pick up" the first stain. (See the previous discussion on Gram staining.)

b A *second* staining test that is important when dealing with respiratory infections is the *acid-fast stain.*

2 The acid-fast tests uses special stains and an acid-alcohol solvent. If the cells show red after the acid solvent rinse, they are called acid-fast because of the inability of the solvent to remove the red stain.

a If the cells are blue, the acid rinse did remove the red dye and the cells are therefore nonacid-fast.

b This test diagnoses the presence of acid-fast bacteria in a specimen, which usually means the presence of the *tuberculosis* bacterium.

3 After specimens are prepared, they are examined under the microscope for the type and number and to provide a means of early diagnosis.

a To know more about the bacteria, it is necessary to grow large numbers of them in a special medium, which may be liquid or solid.

b A nutrient liquid (broth) may be used that contains all the necessary elements for cellular growth. The bacteria are introduced into this previously sterile container, and then it is placed into an environment ideal for cellular growth.

c The most common method of obtaining cultures is to add *agar* (a complex polysaccharide made from seaweed, which resembles thick gelatin in appearance) to the broth and place these in a Petri dish, Fig. 9-4. The Petri dish shown is a common one, but many other styles and types are also used, depending on the type of bacteria grown and growth medium used.

• With the Petri dish filled with the proper nutrient "soil," the "seeds" (bacteria) are "planted" (inoculated) by using a sterilized wire with a small loop at the end (Fig. 9-5).

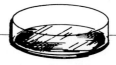

F I G U R E   9 - 4 Petri dish used for culturing bacteria.

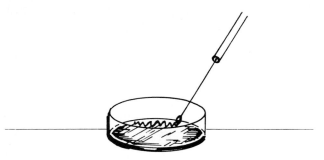

FIGURE 9-5 Inoculation of nutrient media with bacteria.

  • The loop is placed in the specimen to be cultured and is then carefully streaked along the surface of the nutrient agar medium.
4 Different types of bacteria require different media and different conditions in which to grow. For example, some require cultures containing blood (the hemophilic bacteria), others need special nutrients because of high metabolic demands (the fastidious bacteria), and some may require growing conditions without oxygen (the anaerobic bacteria).
  a Once the inoculated medium shows sufficient growth, the pathologist or microbiologist can identify the types of bacteria and their frequency and perform many types of analyses on them.

Obviously, this is a simplified description of culturing bacteria. Most laboratory treatments are much more complex. Growing the viruses, fungi, and other microorganisms requires much more difficult procedures.

If possible the reader should visit a laboratory to observe the procedures discussed in this module.

5.0 TRANSMISSION OF DISEASE
5.1 Accidental transmission

1 The spread of most microbial diseases is through the four F's. (See Module Five for definitions.)
  a Fingers
  b Flies
  c Fomites
  d Food
2 Transmission of microorganisms may be *direct* or *indirect*.

"Direct" means sufficient contact with the infected person; actual body contact is not necessary. Microorganisms certainly may be spread by touch, but just as effectively by a sneeze or cough.
  a Sneezing, coughing, talking, and even yawning spray countless microbe-laden particles of moisture into the air.
  b An uncovered sneeze can throw droplets of moisture as far away as 10 feet. A similar situation occurs as exhaled particles are sprayed from the exhalation valve of a ventilator or intermittent positive pressure breathing (IPPB) machine.

  c Sneezed or coughed particles float about for hours in the air, long after the unthoughtful person who spreads infection has gone.
  d The microorganisms, even after the droplet of moisture has evaporated, settle on dust particles, hair, clothing, and other inanimate articles where they can still cause infection.

"Indirect" means that the microorganism has been passed to a person through handling articles that have been touched or used by an infected person or by an intermediate host, such as food, water, clothing, money, dust, other animals, insects, and other carriers. The *stethoscope* can be a major source of microorganism transmission unless it is properly cleaned after each use.
  e Microorganisms usually enter or leave the body by way of the nose, throat, mouth, gastrointestinal (GI) tract, urinary tract, the eyes, and any break in the skin.
  f Fortunately, most of us live in relative harmony with pathogens that inhabit our bodies.
  g However, it is important to realize that the microorganisms that are presently harmless to us may *seriously* infect and eventually *kill* someone else who has a *lowered resistance*.
3 The accidental transmission of microorganisms is the cause of most nosocomial infections.

The most dangerous nosocomial infections, i.e., *Pseudomonas, Serratia, Klebsiella,* and *Staphylococcus* spp., are usually spread by *negligence* of procedure, *ignorance* of their presence, and *apathy* toward the spread of infection.
4 It is necessary to understand that *people* are almost always responsible for nosocomial infections.
  a *Staphylococcus. Escherichia coli, Klebsiella,* and *Enterobacter* spp. are carried by *people*.
  b Pseudomonas, Serratia, and the *Herellea* spp. are grown in water as a result of *people* who did not properly clean and maintain the equipment.
5 Since humidification is one of the chief causes of pathogen spread, it is helpful to review the known facts about respiratory therapy equipment and the growth of microorganisms. More specific details on the operation of humidifiers and nebulizers are presented in Modules Eleven and Twelve.
6 Humidification systems may be one of several types of humidifiers and nebulizers.
  a By strict definition, a *humidifier* is a device that saturates the gas with *water vapor* by directing a gas flow through water, causing a bubbling action or by blowing the gas over the surface of the water.
  b In either case humidification is achieved by water molecules moving from an area of high water vapor pressure to a decreased pressure area.
  c Water vapor is another form of gas and, therefore, water particles are not visible.
  d Although it was once believed that water molecules could not carry bacteria, more recent research has

shown that it *may* be possible for bacteria and viruses to be carried on molecules. Whether bacteria can be carried on molecules or not, humidifiers should receive the same care in cleaning as other types of equipment.

e *Nebulizers* are frequently referred to as humidifiers. They produce increased humidity by passive evaporative methods and by producing water droplets as a *mist* (aerosol).

f Most nebulizers used in respiratory therapy are pneumatically powered and in some way pull in room air, which is used to transport the mist or aerosol.

g This room air (laden with bacteria) is drawn into the nebulizer and deposited on the water or medication solution and on the internal parts of the nebulizer. When the solution is heated, the risk for contamination is rapidly increased (unless the temperature is extreme and would then be too hot for safe usage).

h *Spinning disk* or *ultrasonic nebulizers* also utilize room air to transport the aerosol to the patient. Most brands use filters for entrained air. These, in most instances, filter out gross contaminants, such as dust or dirt, but are not effective against microorganisms.

7 An important concept to remember is that even though a piece of equipment has been decontaminated, it can very easily be *recontaminated* by careless handling, a cough, a sneeze, or improper storage.

8 The question of bacteria-laden air or oxygen being delivered through the piping system has been raised but not documented.

9 Small-volume medication nebulizers (4 to 6 ml) generally have not been found to be a cause of nosocomial infections unless they are not cleaned every day or unless they are passed from patient to patient without decontamination between patients.

5.2 Isolation procedures

A review of isolation procedures (see Module Five) is appropriate because of the importance of preventing cross-infection.

1 Isolation procedures and the use of the gown, mask, gloves, and head gear as protective devices are designed to break the chain of direct and indirect contact by *isolating* the practitioner's body surfaces from the patient's.

2 The other common isolation measures are:
  a Special rooms.
  b Special hand washing and other techniques.
  c Special material handling.

3 The easiest and most often used method is *hand washing*.
  a Contaminated material is removed by soap, simple friction, and running water.
  b Special bacteriostatic soaps may be used to aid the process.
  c Hands should be washed before and after every patient and equipment contact.

4 Special rooms usually require the following:
  a A *closed* door to stop the spread of particles from leaving the room.
  b Special ventilation to filter bacteria out of the hospital air-circulation system.
  c Special built-in air systems over, under, or around the patient's bed (currently being researched for use with large-percentage burn patients).

5 The following refer to the use of caps, gowns, masks, and gloves.
  a All are used to impose a clean barrier between the practitioner and the patient, sometimes for the practitioner's and sometimes for the patient's protection (protective isolation).
  b Caps cover the hair, which can carry great numbers of bacteria on loose hairs, dust settled on the hair, and skin normally shed from the scalp (dandruff).
  c Excessively long hair should be trimmed to a length that is easy to cover.
  d Beards, mustaches, and other facial hair are just as bacteria-infested as the scalp hair. In fact, beards and mustaches may be heavily colonized because of residual food and drink particles left around the mouth.
  e The gown is used to put a clean covering over the practitioner's street clothes, which are usually bacteria covered. Yes, germs *do* get on white jackets! Clinic or laboratory jackets should be washed every night to prevent "today's germs from growing into tomorrow's nosocomial epidemic."
  f The primary purpose of masks is to cover the mouth. Regardless of what one would like to think, the human mouth is a dirty place, teeming with bacteria.
  g Masks fairly effectively filter the air that leaves and enters via the mouth and nose.
    NOTE: Masks are *not* to be worn below the nose, and they should be changed as soon as they become damp. This period depends on the type of mask material being used, with cloth being the least efficient.
  h The Center for Disease Control in Atlanta has advocated masking the patient instead of the staff since the individual with the disease is the one who needs the protection the most.
  i Gloves are useful for the following reasons.
    • They make it esthetically easier to deal with blood, mucus, vomit, pus, and fecal material.
    • They protect the minute nicks, cuts, and scrapes on the practitioner's hands from infection from these sources.
    • They protect the patient's susceptible surfaces and orifices from invasion by the caretaker's bacteria.

Special material handling is discussed in Unit 8.1 of this module.

Procedures at the end of Module Five may be used for sterile gowning and gloving practice.

6.0 THE BODY'S NATURAL DEFENSE SYSTEMS
6.1 Mode of entry and defensive mechanisms

1 The skin is the body's first line of defense. It is important that hospital personnel protect their skin against breaks or cuts, especially if they are exposed to contaminated wounds or other sources of contact infection.

2 Most infecting bacteria enter the human body through the *respiratory* or *digestive* tract.

  a Examples of diseases that are caused by respiratory entry are tuberculosis, smallpox, and almost all viral diseases, as well as certain types of pneumonias and certain fungal growths such as histoplasmosis.

  b Examples of diseases that can be caused by entry through the digestive system are typhoid, cholera, dysentery, and various types of food poisoning.

3 On the other hand, venereal diseases such as gonorrhea, syphilis, and herpes infections (oral or venereal herpes) are spread almost exclusively by sexual and oral contact.

4 Some diseases (e.g., malaria, rickettsiosis, plague) require direct blood transmission via mosquitoes, ticks, fleas, or other vectors.

5 Regardless of the mode of entry, the body has several means to repel and fight the invading organisms.

  a The *macrophages* are neutrophilic leukocytes capable of phagocytosis. These cells seek out and "eat" (ingest) foreign microorganisms and other particles that find their way into the lungs, blood, and body tissues. This defense process, as evidenced by pus formation (the collection of dead white blood cells), is effective against only a small range of bacteria, primarily the staphylococci.

  b The body's ability to successfully fight off numerous diseases or rapidly overcome them must be the result of some form of *immuity*.

6 *Immunity refers to what happens when a foreign substance (bacteria) enters the body. Simplified, this process is as follows.*

  a The bacteria enter the bloodstream.

  b The body has special cells or structures that are alerted to produce *antibodies*. The invading substance is called an *antigen*.

  c The body can synthesize different kinds of antibodies to deal with different kinds of antigens.

  d For most antigens, the body maintains a "file" of successful antibodies that can be quickly synthesized whenever that particular antigen reinvades the body.

    • For example, mumps usually are contracted only once, because the body has developed "anti-mumps" antibodies that will not allow the mumps virus to survive a second time. These antibodies are present in the patient's blood for his or her lifetime.

    • On the other hand, other diseases, such as the common cold, may infect a person time and time again, because there are either thousands of *different* types of cold viruses or the human body cannot manufacture a successful "anticold" antibody.

7 Immunity may be acquired by:

  a Antibodies transmitted prenatally, passed to the baby from the mother via breast milk, or already present in the baby's genetic make-up (natural immunity).

  b Inoculation with either dead tissue organisms (*vaccine*) or by injection of a *serum* taken from another person or animal already immune to that particular disease (acquired immunity).

8 Immunity, as well as its science, immunology, is the subject of much study and speculation regarding the body's ability to protect itself. It has been demonstrated that immunity to certain diseases can be affected by the following:

  a Genetics. The tendency to acquire a disease or successfully fight diseases seems to be determined by hereditary factors.

  b Sex. Some diseases are more prevalent in one sex than the other.

  c Race. Different races have different abilities to fight diseases and are sometimes more prone to develop certain diseases than others. For example, sickle-cell anemia is much more prevalent among blacks than whites.

  d Age. Newborn infants, children, and old people do *not* have the same ability to produce antibodies as young adults and middle-aged people.

  e Physical state. Chronically sick people are described as having "lowered resistance." What this means is that sick people whose vitamin intake and nutrition are poor and who do not get proper rest, simply do not have the reserve energy and raw materials to fight infections *in addition to* what is needed to produce heat, metabolize food, and maintain life.

    In addition, there are many other environmental factors that affect resistance and immunity.

    NOTE: The acquired immunodeficiency syndrome (AIDS) is a medical concern that has prompted major investigative efforts. With this condition the body's cells lose their ability to develop an immunity to disease. This leaves the body prey to infections and tumors that are lethal in a majority of cases. Details concerning AIDS are presented in Unit 9.3 of this module and in Module Eight, "Human Respiratory Anatomy, Physiology, Pathology, and Applied Physics."

9 Tissues with specialized functions also help protect the body against infection.

  a Cilia. These structures (see Module Eight), located in the large airways and trachea, constantly "sweep" bacteria and other particles out of the lungs and down from the nose to be coughed out or swallowed. The cilia are easily injured by irritating agents (e.g., smoking) and by a lack of humidity.

  b Mucous membranes. A layer of mucus literally traps the bacteria and particles in the lungs, nose, mouth, and throat where either the macrophages can engulf them or the cilia can sweep them out.

  c The stomach. The stomach acid will readily kill *most*

pathogens that are swallowed, provided there is sufficient time. A large meal with a large quantity of liquid will dilute the acid and "push" the food through too quickly for the bacteria to be harmed. Also, the *enteric pathogens* (e.g., dysentery, diarrhea, cholera) can pass through the stomach with little or no harm.

d The skin. This envelop of tissue is, for the most part, impervious to water, oil, dirt, and microorganisms as long as it is not broken. Naturally, an opening in the skin allows passage to any organism.

e Many microorganisms, pathologic and nonpathologic, make their homes on and in the skin. They reside in the cracks, pores, hair follicles, and folds.

f Washing and scrubbing help to keep microbe numbers within reasonable limits, but keep in mind that any antiseptic advertising the ability to *kill* germs would probably be too powerful to use on human skin. Most antiseptics simply *arrest* or *inhibit* bacteria growth rather than kill the bacteria.

7.0 DECONTAMINATION
7.1 Methods and techniques

1 The principal factors that influence the ability to kill bacteria and other microorganisms are:

a The *strength* of the killing agent, e.g., concentration of the agent means that an organism that will survive 105° C may quickly die when the strength (intensity) is pushed to 110° C. Also, an organism that thrives in a 0.1% solution of disinfectant may simply stop growing in a 1% solution and quickly die in a 2% solution.

b The *time* that the agent has to act, e.g., 15 minutes in glutaraldehyde may kill growing microorganisms but not spores. Spores may take hours to kill.

c The *temperature* of the environment in which the killing takes place; i.e., the higher the temperature of the environment surrounding the organism, the faster the killing. It is calculated that the rate of microbe death doubles with every 10° C rise in temperature.

d The *type* of microorganism being killed, e.g., that which kills one microbe may only arrest the growth of another. In addition, some microbes develop spores or capsules for protection against adverse environmental conditions.

e The environment *around* the area to be decontaminated, e.g., a tightly wrapped or poorly immersed piece of equipment may not allow the killing properties of some agents to reach all areas to be sterilized. Also, an environment that uses heat may enhance the killing effects of a certain agent, e.g., ethylene oxide.

f The *number* of microbes to be killed.

2 A method for testing the killing power of some compounds and agents is called the *phenol coefficient (P.C.) test,* which was developed in 1903 by Rideal and Walker.

a The P.C. is a number that measures the killing power of an agent relative to the killing power of phenol under a set of controlled conditions.

b Phenol is assigned the number *1,* and other chemicals or agents are assigned numbers relative to the *1,* depending on the amount of their dilution.

For example, when used to kill a test culture of *Salmonella typhi,* Lysol has a P.C. of 5. This means that Lysol can be diluted 500 times whereas phenol can only be diluted 100 times to be effective; or Lysol is five times more effective than phenol under the same conditions:

$$P.C. = \frac{X}{100}$$

$$P.C. = \frac{500 \text{ (Lysol)}}{100 \text{ (phenol)}}$$

$$P.C. = 5$$

c The phenol coefficient test was originally designed to be used in comparing phenol with other phenol-type compounds such as Lysol, hexylresorcinol, tincture of iodine, and mebromin (Mercurochrome). It has little if any use in comparing phenol with nonphenol compounds.

3 Microorganisms may be killed by any of the following:* (Table 9-1 comparing the use and effectiveness of decontamination agents and techniques evaluates the list in no. *4.*)

a Liquid chemicals: iodines, phenols, mercurials, alcohols, chlorine and bromine compounds, quaternay ammonium compounds, formaldehydes, and glutaraldehydes.

b Radiation: radiographs, gamma rays, certain wave lengths of light (ultraviolet), electron beam (cathode), radiation, accelerated particles (protons, neutrons, and electrons), and atomic fission fragments.

c Desiccation (drying). Once an organism that is over 90% water dries out, osmotic pressure causes structural damage to the cell wall and death to the organism. As previously explained, some bacteria can prevent this structural damage (and therefore death) by developing into *dormant spores.*

d Pressure. Pressure by itself does not harm many bacteria, e.g., some have been known to survive over 12 atmospheres for hours without harm. However, pressure and heat (autoclaving) is very effective. *Autoclaving* consists of *moist* heat (steam) at 120° C under a pressure of 15 psi for varying lengths of time, depending on the size, shape, and material to be sterilized.

e Osmotic pressure. A *hypotonic* solution around the organism causes the organism (or cell) to swell (plasmoptysis). As the pressures outside and inside the organism seek equality through the cellular membrane, the organism usually bursts. A *hypertonic* so-

---

*This listing does not take into account the antibiotic drugs or preparations. For more details on individual compounds, refer to alternate texts.

TABLE 9-1 A comparison of decontamination techniques and agents

	Usefulness as			Range of effectiveness against	
	Disinfectant	Antiseptic	TBC	Bacteria	Spores
CHEMICALS					
Iodine	Fair	Very good	Good to very good	Good	None
Phenols	Good	Poor	Good	Good	Poor
Mercurials	None	Poor	None	Fair	None
Alcohols	Good	Good	Very good	Good	None
Chlorine	Good	Fair	Fair	Fair to good	Fair
Quaternary ammonium compounds	Good	Good	None	Poor to good	None
Formaldehydes	Good	None	Very good	Good	Good
Glutaraldehydes	Good	None	Good	Good	Good
Formalin (aqueous)	Fair	None	Good		Fair
GASES/STEAM/PASTEURIZATION					
Ethylene oxide	Sterilization	—	—	—	—
Beta propriolactone		None	Good	Very good	Very good
Steam	Sterilization	—	—	—	—
Pasteurization	Good	None	Good	Good	Fair

All agents must be used in appropriate strength and for designated exposure time and according to other conditions in order to be effective as designated.

lution around the organism causes the cell to lose water and shrink. This loss of water causes plasmolysis (cellular shrinking). This principle is used in the sugar or salt "drying" of meat or fish. The hypertonic concentration of the sugar or salt "curing" stops the growth of damaging bacteria.

f Ultrasonic vibrations: those sound waves above 20,000 cycles per second. Ultrasonic sound waves literally vibrate the organism until it shatters. Their effectiveness depends on the "construction" of the microbe.

g Pasteurization: kills vegetative cells of yeasts, molds, bacteria, and tuberculosis organisms, but not spores. It consists of heating material in somewhat less than boiling (55° to 60° C) water for 20 to 30 minutes. Pasteurization can be used with detergents to lower surface tension characteristics of microbes and to enhance killing power.

h Dry heat: not particularly effective. However, organisms are killed at temperatures maintained above 160° C for relatively long periods.

i Acid/alkali extremes: can kill bacteria, e.g., using an acid (as in the stomach) when the pH is lower than 4.5. Bacteria are also killed by alkali (as in lye) when the pH is greater than 9.0.

j Poison gases (such as ethylene oxide): very popular for sterilizing equipment, especially pieces that cannot get wet. Note that oxygen can also be toxic under the right circumstances.

4 The following outline lists the most common decontamination methods used in respiratory therapy (see also Table 9-1). Each method is described first in terms of its good points, then in terms of its less desirable points.

a Radiation. Disposable items like endotracheal tubes or cardiac catheters are packaged first, then irradiated with gamma particles. This system is not practical for routine hospital sterilization.

b Steam. Autoclave (120° C at 15 psi):
• Kills all pathogens
• Quick procedure.
• Leaves no toxic residue.
• Simple quality control; equipment can be wrapped before procedure.
• Inexpensive to operate; however:
   – Cannot use on all equipment.
   – Expensive to purchase and install.
   – Can be dangerous.

c Pasteurization (immersion in 60° C water for 30 minutes):
• Kills vegetative pathogens, not spores.
• Inexpensive to operate.
• Fairly easy to use.
• No corrosion; however:
   – Sterilization not guaranteed; material must be dried and handled after procedure.
   – Expensive to purchase and install.
   – Burn and scald hazard.
   – Careful loading necessary.
   – Cannot do larger pieces of equipment.
   – Limited to articles that can be wetted.

d Activated glutaraldehyde (Cidex, Sonocide):
• Inexpensive procedure.
• Easy to use.
• Quick procedure (15 minutes).
• Minimum corrosion.
• Kills all pathogens (spores require longer exposure); however:
   – Sterilization not guaranteed; material must be rinsed, dried, and handled after procedure.
   – Irritating to skin, eyes, respiratory tract; allergy risk.

– Cannot do larger pieces of equipment.
– Limited to articles that can be wetted.
– Expensive to use, must be changed at frequent intervals.

e Ethylene oxide (toxic gas):
• Kills all pathogens.
• Can use with all equipment.
• Simple quality control; equipment is wrapped before procedure.
• Long shelf life, depending on wrapping.
• Minimum corrosion; however:
– Expensive equipment required.
– High installation cost.Careful training necessary.
– Leaves residue.Toxic.
– Requires time-consuming aeration after procedure (24 hours to 7 days).
– Gas is fire and thus explosion hazard.

8.0 A RESPIRATORY CARE DECONTAMINATION PROGRAM

8.1 Organizing a program

The basic program includes *gathering* equipment, *washing* it, and then *storing* it.

Since space problems plague most respiratory therapy departments, assessing exact space needs to operate the program is a prerequisite in designing a decontamination program.

1 One partial solution to having to clean large amounts of equipment is to use *disposable* equipment, a solution that has acquired tremendous popularity because of personnel shortages and equipment problems.

a Generally, disposable equipment provides certain assets. It ensures quality control for a relatively low expense, when compared with a traditional cleaning and decontamination service. It makes efficient use of respiratory therapy personnel time, i.e., time is spent delivering therapy not processing equipment, and it provides prepackaged, easy-to-use systems.

b It should be noted that disposable equipment is rarely sterile when packaged, although *some* are sterilized after packaging by gas. Sterile items are more expensive and are labeled as sterile on the package. Most disposable respiratory care supplies are not sterile, but considered *clean,* e.g., cannulas, airways, IPPB circuits, etc. The primary disadvantages of disposable equipment are its requirements of a great deal of storage space and maintenance of large inventories because of potential problems such as shortages and strikes. It also means a regular monthly outflow of cash from department revenues. Finally, disposable nebulizers and other devices do not generally work as efficiently as do their permanent counterparts.

2 Most departments use a combination of both disposable and permanent equipment.

3 Permanent equipment is usually much more expensive initially but is eventually used "free" if regularly maintained in good working order. The only expense is the cost of decontamination which, as noted, will vary considerably depending on the method used and minor routine maintenance necessary.

a The relative "savings" of reusing permanent equipment may be absorbed by the expense of decontamination equipment, sinks, dryers, dirty areas, clean areas, packaging areas, and paying someone to do the work.

b Further disadvantages of permanent equipment and supplies are noted in the remainder of this unit.

4 The following outlines a hypothetical department decontamination program. Obviously, it may or may not be identical to the reader's hospital's plan, but it contains the *minimum* requirements for an effective program.

a "Dirty" shall refer to all contaminated equipment and supplies. "Clean" shall refer to all equipment and supplies that have undergone decontamination and are ready for packaging.

b Dirty supplies should *never* be carried in the open down the halls or from room to room.

c A dirty piece of equipment should be carried to the department inside a plastic bag (as is used in housekeeping) or covered with a clean sheet if it is a ventilator. Personnel should always use the service elevator (if there is one) and then go directly to the department's cleaning area (Fig. 9-6).

d In the process of changing smaller pieces of equipment such as nebulizers or humidifiers, the dirty ones should be carried in a large plastic bag that *will not leak*. Otherwise, the contaminated water from the dirty nebulizers will drip their "bacterial soup."

e Dirty and clean equipment should not ride on the same cart. If it is absolutely necessary that they do, the dirty bags of equipment should be carried on one side of the cart and clean supplies on the other side.

f The dirty water from nebulizers should *not* be poured down the patient's sink. It should be disposed of in the toilet or bedpan hopper.

g Dirty equipment goes *directly* to the dirty receiving area. The dirty area should be separate from the clean area, unless it can be closed, and should not have an opening communicating with the clean area. It is strongly recommended that the dirty room have its own ventilation system with a filtered exhaust fan that does not communicate with the rest of the hospital.

h All incoming dirty equipment should be *completely* disassembled to discover (1) hidden areas for contaminated material to lodge and (2) flaws, defects, and needed repairs and to allow *total* drying after washing.

i Once the pieces are disassembled and checked, they should be scrubbed in a detergent solution to loosen dried material, blood, or secretions. A long-handled brush will be necessary for tubing, and various small brushes will be required for small orifices and jets.

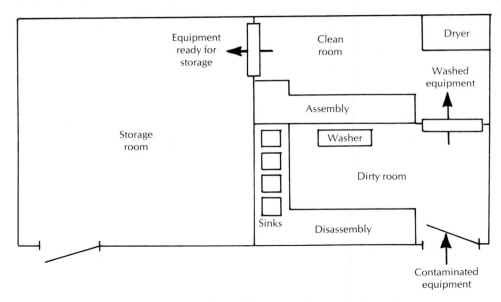

FIGURE 9-6 Hypothetical department decontamination setup.

j Following rinsing in hot water, the material is ready for the sterilizing procedure. This will differ from hospital to hospital but may utilize the autoclave, the pasteurizer, ethylene oxide, or activated glutaraldehyde.

k After the sterilizing cycle, the material should go directly to the clean area. Although it is probably better if two crews of people work on equipment—one "dirty" and one "clean"—this system is not always feasible. Therefore great care *must* be taken to wash the hands, change aprons, and even wipe the bottoms of the shoes to prevent spread of contamination from the dirty room into the clean room.

l Carts and transporting equipment should be carefully wiped down with a disinfectant solution or spray before going back into storage. Some hospitals have special cart cleaning areas.

m After clean equipment is received in the clean room, it should be dried if it has come out of a liquid rinse following liquid sterilization. Drying must be *complete*. Where there is water, bacteria can grow. Following autoclaving and gassing, the material is generally ready for packaging. Wrapping must be secure and firmly taped. If gas was used, it will be necessary to aerate the equipment to "flush" the toxic ethylene oxide. This is usually done in warmed, forced air cabinets that speed the process. Although aeration can be passive by placing the equipment on a counter, this defeats the sterilization.

n Dried pieces are now ready to be reassembled. Reassembly requires a clean assembly area, a clean assembly table, and clean hands to put it together. A useful accessory would be a plastic shield over the table similar to those seen in cafeterias and over salad bars. This device would prevent thoughtless

people from sneezing and coughing on the clean equipment as they assemble it. A forced "clean-air" duct could also be used over the clean table.

5 The assembled equipment may now be packaged. A popular method is placing it into "clean" food storage bags and sealed with a taping machine or a metallic twist.

6 All packaged equipment and supplies must be dated so that the shelf life can be monitored. Shelf life refers to the length of time an article will remain sterile once it has been sterilized and packaged. Shelf life varies according to sterilization method and wrapping method. The following applies to the shelf life of gas-sterilized items.

Wrapping material	Storage (shelf) life
Cloth wrap	15-30 days
Paper wrap	30-60 days
Plastic wrap (sealed with tape)	90-100 days
Plastic wrap (heat sealed)	1 year

7 Monitoring the length of time that materials have been in storage is important, and those pieces that have outlived their shelf life should be routinely rerun through the decontamination process.

8 Items that cannot be immersed, gassed, or autoclaved must be treated differently (see no. *9* in Unit 8.2).

a Most of these items should be wiped down with a strong disinfectant, although it is doubtful that nosocomial infections can be picked up from the surfaces of dry equipment.

b Nebulizers that use electric motors can be run daily for a short time with a solution of 0.25% acetic acid in the reservoir to *reduce* contamination. Acetic acid does *not* sterilize an item, although it is effective in controlling the growth of certain gram-negative organisms, especially *Pseudomonas* species.

c Chemical disinfectants and sterilizing agents must not be left in material to be used. For example, a nebulizer jet that was not carefully rinsed may still contain glutaraldehyde, which would be nebulized into the lungs of a patient. This must *not* happen.

d For the most part, compounds containing quaternary ammonias, phenols (popular in many sprays), and hexachlorophenes are not recommended for use with respiratory therapy equipment, because they may leave residues that can be harmful if they come into contact with inhaled gases or tissue.

8.2 Contamination and prevention

The following suggestions, which deal more with prevention than with decontamination, should be addressed at this time.

1 Equipment in the patient breathing circuit should be changed *at least* every 24 hours. Many hospitals change circuits every 8 to 12 hours. In-line bacteria filters on incoming and outgoing gas lines may be used although recent evidence does not indicate that they significantly reduce infection rates.

2 Nebulizers, humidifiers, and ultrasonic equipment should be rotated (changed) every 24 hours. Condensed water that collects in the tubing of these devices must *never* be drained back into their reservoirs. It should be disposed of in an appropriate disposal unit.

3 Sinks are for *hand washing only,* not for the disposal of contaminated materials.

4 Water to refill reservoir should be *sterile*. The popular "deionized" water for respiratory therapy grows bacteria with ease.

All water used in respiratory therapy must be sterile, especially medication water.

5 Small-dose vials or unit doses are preferable to multiple dose bottles, which are *easily* contaminated (this includes *all* respiratory therapy medications).

6 Medications should be stored in a refrigerator, dated, and discarded 24 hours after opening.

7 Standby equipment at the bedside should be left dry until ready to use, and articles such as manual resuscitators, aerosol T pieces, and ventilator adapters must be kept wrapped and protected against contamination.

8 Although not required in many hospitals, personnel assigned to specialty areas (e.g., critical care, intensive care nursery, recovery room, burn unit) should be allowed to wear scrub clothes. The wearing of street clothes in these areas is inconsistent with hospital aseptic technique. "Scrubs" should be donned whenever entering these areas and removed whenever leaving them unless for very short periods.

"Scrubs" are *not* to be worn in the cafeteria, library, or anywhere else in the hospital, even with a laboratory jacket. They are certainly not to be worn home. It is a very *unprofessional* person who leaves the hospital with "scrubs" on and stethoscope draped around his or her neck.

9 Equipment such as ventilators and ultrasonic nebulizers require special care.

The following precautions should be taken with ventilators.

a After an item such as the Bennett PR series or Bird Mark series ventilator has been received in the dirty area, all disposable accessories should be discarded.

b Nondisposable accessories should be disassembled and processed as previously discussed.

c The ventilator cabinet, cascade heating elements, electric cords, high pressure hose, and stand should be sprayed with a disinfectant spray or foam, allowed to stand, and then wiped dry.

d The wheels should be sprayed with a disinfectant and then wiped dry with paper toweling.

e The ventilator cabinets should be gassed at least once a month.

f The nebulizer line and main flow outlet bacterial filters should be autoclaved or gassed at least once a month, preferably between patients. Care should be taken to see that these filters do not get clogged from trying to stretch their lifetime.

- With larger ventilators like the Bennett MA series or Bourns BEAR series, one follows the same wipedown described in *a* through *f*.
- In addition, the larger ventilators have cool-air intake filters that clean the air used to dissipate the heat generated by compressor motors and other electrical devices. These filters must be removed at least once a week and sent through the decontamination cycle. If not, the lint and dirt that collects will block air flow to the unit, as well as provide a place where bacteria can grow.
- The Bennett MA-1 ventilator has other in-line filters that should be cleaned according to the manufacturer's schedule.*

The following precautions should be taken with ultrasonic nebulizers.

a Ultrasonic nebulizers have stands, housings, and wheels that should be sprayed with a disinfectant spray or foam and then wiped down.

b The transducer disk should not be sprayed, since the spray may prevent the ultrasonic nebulizer from working properly.

c Air intake filters can be decontaminated after each patient or at least every 24 hours, depending on how the nebulizer is used.

d Transducer units from ultrasonic nebulizers should never be *immersed* in sterilization solutions. It is possible to pour the solution *into* the transducer, let it sit for 15 minutes, pour it out, and rinse the transducer carefully with clean, warm water.

e Another method of decontaminating ultrasonic nebulizers is to run 2% acetic acid in them for 10 to 15

---

*The reader is encouraged to refer to the Bennett MA-1 operating manual for details on cleaning the fresh-air intake filter and silencer and the oxygen filter.

minutes once a day, although this will not sterilize the unit.

    f Items like the Wright respirometer can be cleaned by gently wiping the inside with a cotton applicator dipped in 70% alchol.

- To wipe off the respirometer's external surface, a paper towel that has been sprayed with disinfectant may be used.
- Respirometers may be dried by running an oxygen flow through them as needed. Note manufacturer's instructions regarding high flows that can damage the jeweled movements.
- Respirometers should be gassed between patients.

8.3 Decontaminating a Puritan-Bennett all purpose nebulizer

Procedure 9-1 describes the steps in decontaminating a Puritan-Bennett all-purpose nebulizer.

9.0 EVALUATING THE EFFECTIVENESS OF DECONTAMINATION TECHNIQUES

1 Disassembling
2 Washing
3 Rinsing
4 Placing into a sterilization solution
5 Rinsing
6 Drying
7 Assembling
8 Packaging

9.1 Organizing a surveillance program for equipment decontamination

1 A surveillance program for a hospital decontamination program should have the following objectives:

    a To determine the kind and frequency of nosocomial infections.

    b To establish a baseline of infections so that deviations can be detected.

    c To gather information so that studies can be done.

    d To determine where control measures are needed.

    e To establish policies relating to surveillance and decontamination procedures.

    f To protect the patient and community from infections arising from the hospital.

    g To meet guidelines of regulatory agencies.

    h To update the knowledge on nosocomial infections for the hospital staff.

2 Officially, the hospital-wide surveillance program should have at minimum: a *nurse* in charge of infection control and a *physician-epidemiologist* (full or part-time).

The job description of these two individuals will vary from hospital to hospital. Since it is beyond the scope of this module to present detailed job descriptions, it is sufficient to note that both of these individuals work together to:

    a Monitor hospital infections.

    b Determine their cause.

    c Develop and implement a plan to control and eliminate nosocomial infection.

    d Work with all service areas on a hospital-wide surveillance program.

3 A third staff need for the surveillance program is an infections control person. Although most respiratory therapy departments have no full-time person, certainly someone should be assigned this task on a part-time basis.

One of the primary functions of this person will be to collect cultures, at random, of various pieces of equipment. Typically, this function will include:

    a Cultures of equipment in the dryer or on the assembly table, especially nebulizer jets, reservoirs, tubing, and any other small part.

    b Cultures of equipment in storage, including any part of the device, and especially those concealed areas that by reputation hide microorganisms, e.g., cracks, jets, etc.

    c Cultures of equipment in use should include the nebulizer/humidifier reservoirs, the jets or nebulizing parts, and the tubing.

4 How thoroughly a department or individual area needs to be cultured depends on the deviation from baseline; for instance:

    a Areas with high levels of contamination may require numerous specific cultures to discover the contaminating agent or person.

    b It may be necessary to take personnel cultures if it is suspected that someone in the department is a carrier. This culture will be done by the infections control person.

5 Another primary function of the infections control person will be to observe decontamination, assembly, and packaging procedures to discover careless or negligent handling.

6 Respiratory care personnel are rarely responsible for doing their own plate streaking or culture inoculation.

However, the surveillance team member from respiratory care may use a small cardboard or paper wand that is sterile and suspended above an ampule of nutrient material. The culturing procedure is as follows.

    a The wand is carefully withdrawn from its sterile tube.

    b The sterile end (usually wrapped with cotton or similar material) is introduced into the area to be cultured and a brief swabbing action will pick up any bacteria.

    c The contaminated end of the wand is then reintroduced into its holder and pushed against the ampule, which is broken, releasing the nutrient to surround the tip of the wand.

    d The wand should be numbered and a form, labeled with the date, place, time, and piece of equipment cultured, should be filled out.

7 Other, more sophisticated culturing methods may be used, for example:

    a Filter samples of water; the filter will then be removed and cultured.

b Pour a nutrient broth through tubing, filter the broth, and then culture the filter.

c Culture the air or oxygen that has passed through a humidifier or nebulizer, and deposit the aerosol onto an agar plate. Devices like the Anderson Air Sampler can be used to pull in room air for culturing.

8 Reports of cultures grown should be filed with the epidemiologist's office and with the department head.

9 In addition to checking decontamination procedures, culturing equipment, and analyzing results, the individual responsible for the surveillance should also do the following:

a Keep abreast of hospital infections, and evaluate respiratory care's part (if any) in them.

b Make reports on patients' infections to all respiratory care personnel so that special procedures can be put into effect if needed.

c Make routine checks of patient charts to discover infection trends.

d Visit the laboratory often to be recognized and to establish good relations.

e Maintain close contact with the nurse clinician or epidemiologist in charge of the surveillance program.

f Use charts, graphs, and other visual aids to improve departmental knowledge of infection status and results of decontamination surveillance.

9.2 Hepatitis B virus

1 The hepatitis B virus (HBV) consists of an outer shell of hepatitis B surface antigen (HB$_s$Ag) surrounding a nucleocapsule containing the hepatitis B core antigen (HB$_c$Ag). Infected patients also carry two other spherical and tubular noninfectious viral particles in the blood.

2 An infected patient will have HB$_c$Ag present in hepatocyte nuclei and HB$_s$Ag in serum samples.

3 HBV is a very contagious infection that is transmitted primarily by exposure of personnel to infected blood, skin puncture, body secretions, sexual contact, and from mother to newborn.

4 Its prevalence is 3% to 5% in the general population and 15% to 22% in hospital personnel who work with blood.

5 After exposure, its symptoms usually occur after 4 to 6 weeks. They may be so minimal that they are attributed to the flu or so involved as to cause nausea and jaundice with elevated liver enzymes and possible permanent hepatic damage.

6 If the infection is controlled, Hb$_s$Ag will disappear from the serum and will be replaced first by anti-HB$_c$ and eventually by anti-HBs.

7 Precautions to prevent infection include isolation barriers, avoidance of accidental puncture wounds or cuts, and immunization.

8 An exposed person's immunity level can be elevated by inoculation with hepatitis B immune globulin.

9 Two vaccines are currently available in the United States.

a Heptavax B; derived from the plasma of HBV carriers.

b Recombivax; HB developed from HB$_s$Ag produced in bread yeast.

10 After vaccination, the individual is protected against reinfection for a period up to five years.

9.3 Etiology of human immunodeficiency virus (HIV)

1 Statistics regarding the historical growth and the impact of the acquired immunodeficiency syndrome were presented in Module Eight.

2 AIDS is caused by the human T-lymphotropic virus type III now referred to as the human immunodeficiency virus (HIV). HIV is a retrovirus that contains single strand ribonucleic acid (SSRNA) and the reverse transcriptase enzyme. These viruses are so named because of their ability to carry out reverse (retro) transcription from RNA to deoxyribonucleic acid (DNA). When attacking a cell the retrovirus carries out a series of events that confuses the normal defense mechanisms of the cells, allowing the virus to survive and reproduce.

A simplified explanation of the retrovirus and how it affects cellular transformation is presented in Fig. 9-7 through 9-10.

3 In Fig. 9.7, the retrovirus, which measures only one ten-thousandth of a millimeter, has an outer protective shell with spiney nubs that enable it to attach itself to a host cell (1).

4 The inner core of the shell contains the retrovirus (2) with reverse transcriptase (3).

5 This reverse transcriptase is the genetic information needed by the virus to permit its own replication.

6 This genetic information constitutes the primary structure of a virus because it must gain access to a host cell to replicate.

7 Once the virus has gained access to the body, the cells literally reach out and attempt to engulf the cell as they would other foreign organisms (1) (Fig. 9-8).

8 Helper T cells are summoned by the host to identify and combat the virus.

9 Once the helper T cells arrive, they are confused by the virus and do not establish the defense mechaisms that ordinarily result in the mustering of killer T cells to fight the infection. (Fig. 9-9).

10 Instead, the killer T cells are not summoned and therefore do not sacrifice the host cell by chemically penetrating it.

11 Had this occurred, the host cell would have died along with the virus.

12 The virus unchecked eats the host cell and helper T cells, replicates, and moves to new cells throughout the body, (Fig. 9-10).

13 Of equal concern, the AIDS virus has now confused the body's immune system, making it vulnerable to other opportunistic infections, as listed in 9-4.

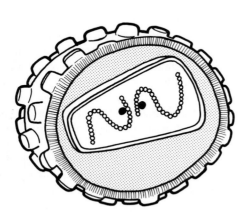

FIGURE 9-7 Structure of HIV-1 virus.

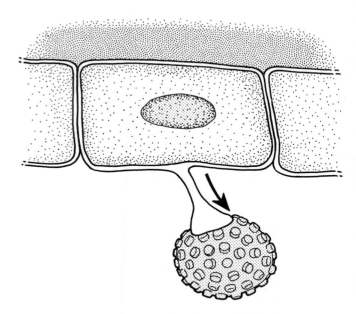

FIGURE 9-8 Body cells grasp HIV-1 virus.

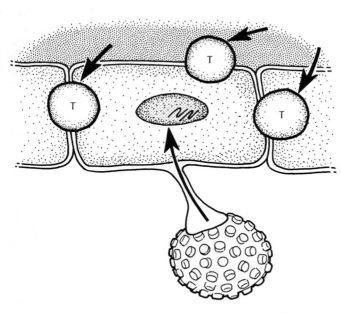

FIGURE 9-9 Helper T cells arrive but are confused by virus.

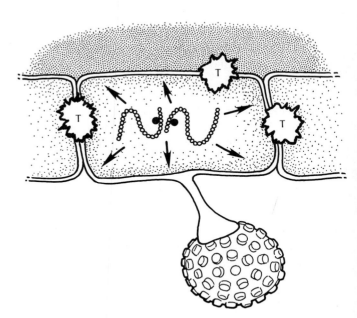

FIGURE 9-10 AIDS virus eats host cell annd helper T cells replicate and spread to other cells.

9.4 Infectious complications

1 The most commonly diagnosed infectious complication of AIDS is Pneumocystis carinii pneumonia.

2 It occurs in greater than 60% of AIDS patients and results in 30% mortality.

3 Symptoms include:
   a Dyspnea
   b Malaise
   c Fever
   d Nonproductive cough
   e Chest pain
   f Chills

4 Physical examination may reveal:
   a Fever
   b Tachycardia
   c Normal breath sounds

5 Chest roentgenogram reveals:
   a Diffuse bilateral interstitial infiltrates
   b Enlarged hilar and mediastinal lymph nodes

6 Pulmonary function tests show:
   a Decreased diffusing capacity for CO
   b Gallium scintigraphy reveals diffuse intake in lung parenchyma

7 Arterial blood gases show low PaO_2 with increased A–a gradient.

8 Laboratory tests show:
   P. carinii organism with Gomori methenamine-silver or Giemsa staining of lung tissue or secretions.

9 Other organisms may be encountered alone or in combination include:
   a *Mycobacterium avium*-intracellular
   b *Cytomegalovirus*
   c Cryptococus neoformans
   d Herpes simplex
   e Toxoplasma gondii

10 After airway and ventilation is assured, the initial treatment of choice is trimethoprim-sulfamethoxazole (TMP-SMX) administered intravenously in a dose of 20 mg/kg TMP and 100 mg/kg of SMX daily, divided into four doses for 14 to 21 days.

11 Secondary treatment may include administration of pentamidine isethionate intramusularly or intravenously. The usual adult dosage is 4 mg/kg/day.

9.5 Noninfectious complications

1 Noninfectious complications include:
   a Kaposi's sarcoma
   b Nonspecific pneumonitis
   c Lymphocytic interstitial pneumonitis
   d Adult respiratory distress syndrome (ARDS).

2 It is important to note that AIDS patients usually test positive for multiple organisms, leading to multiorgan failure.

9.6 Antibody tests for HIV-1 (AIDS)

The following information was extracted from a booklet distributed by the Arizona Department of Health Services titled *Information and Guidelines Regarding HTLV-III Infections*.

1 The only tests currently licensed for detecting antibodies to HIV-1 in blood and blood products are the enzyme-linked immunosorbant assays (ELISA), also known as enzyme immunoassay (EIA), using disrupted whole virus antigen.

2 The currently licensed ELISA tests are both highly sensitive and specific. A variety of other ELISA tests (some using cloned antigen), a fluorescent antibody test, and other procedures are being developed and tested and may be licensed in the future.

3 In addition, the Western blot test, which is an immuno-electroprecipitin test using disturbed whole virus antigen, is available through many laboratories.

4 The Western blot test is a reference laboratory procedure and must be performed carefully with appropriate standards. It is a useful additional test to help assess the significance of a positive ELISA test.

9.7 Definition of a positive ELISA

Because several ELISA test kits to detect antibodies to HIV-1 have been licensed and each has unique characteristics and slightly different methods of determining a positive test, no single definition of a positive antibody test is possible. In determining whether reactive results represent a positive test, some general principles apply:

1 To be positive, the reactive test must be reproducible and yield approximately the same degree of reactivity when repeated several times independently or with different specimens from the same person.

2 The more highly reactive the test, the greater the probability that the test is truly positive. Test results that cluster near the test cut-off value are likely to be nonspecific reactions or "false positives."

3 Specimens that have a reactive ELISA test and that are also reactive by a second type of test, such as Western blot or fluorescent antibody, should be considered true positives.

4 A strongly reactive repeated ELISA test that is nonreactive using a second type of test or a repeated weakly reactive ELISA test that is reactive using a second type of test probably is positive, but this represents an equivocal result and additional testing is warranted.

5 A weakly reactive repeated ELISA test that is nonreactive using a second type of test usually denotes a nonspecific or falsely reactive test reaction. Additional follow-up for testing often is warranted to ensure the correctness of the finding.

9.8 Public health service blood screening recommendations

1 The Food and Drug Administration (FDA) has issued guidelines for implementing HIV-I antibody testing of all donated blood and plasma. Although these guideline are voluntary, pending the establishment of regulations requiring testing, virtually all blood and plasma collected in Arizona and the nation since April 1985 has been screened.

2 An important aspect of HIV-I antibody screening is public education about who should not donate blood;

no person who has a risk factor for HIV-I infection or AIDS should donate blood or plasma.

3 After prospective donors have read appropriate information materials, completed the medical history and screening, and have been accepted to donate blood or plasma, the donated unit should be tested for HIV-I antibody using one of the licensed tests.

4 All reactive units should be tested several times as outlined by the test kit manufacturer. Positive units are destroyed and the donor's name added to the donor deferral register.

5 Each blood and plasma center has its own guidelines for additional testing and donor notification. The degree of ELISA test reactivity, as well as additional tests such as the Western blot, may provide guidance about the significance of the test results and the probability of HIV-I infection in the donor.

6 Future refinement in the test systems may eliminate most nonspecific test results.

9.9 General principles (See Bibliography for documents distributed by the Center for Disease Control in Atlanta, Ga.)

1 People with HIV-I antibody are likely to be infected with the virus persistently and may transmit it to others.

2 Since a diagnosis of AIDS or of infection with HIV-I may create considerable anxiety and stress, it is important that each person understand the implications of the antibody test before being tested and be given the opportunity to decline being tested.

  a The HIV-I antibody test is used to detect the presence of antibody to HIV-I, which denotes that the person is or has been infected with HIV-I. Used alone, the HIV-I antibody test is not a test to diagnose acquired immunodeficiency syndrome (AIDS).

  b The HIV-I antibody test is an extremely important procedure for protecting the nation's blood supply, and is a valuable test to assist research efforts into AIDS and HIV-I–related problems. The test has other selective clinical and public health applications, and has been added as a criterion in the application of the recently revised case definition of AIDS.

  c At the present time, the HIV-I antibody test has limited utility for purposes other than stated above. The HIV-I test should not be used for generalized screening or as a condition for employment, evidence of insurability, admission to hospitals, or admission to schools.

  d HIV-I antibody test should only be performed with the individual's consent. That consent should include specific reference to the test, and should not be part of blanket consent procedures.

  e Because of the serious potential for social and psychologic harm to the individual resulting from the HIV-I antibody test results, great care must be taken

to inform the public and health care professionals about limitations in current understanding of the test results and of the entire disease process related to HIV-I infection, including AIDS.

  f Information gathered from the testing or counseling of individuals must be kept strictly confidential.

3 Physicians and other health personnel must recognize the need to maintain confidentiality about reactive test results.

4 Disclosure of this information for purposes other than medical or public health could lead to serious and unwarranted consequences for an individual with a reactive blood test (such as discrimination in employment).

5 Screening procedures should be designed with safeguards to protect against unauthorized disclosure. Donors should be given a clear explanation of how information about the results of the test will be handled.

6 Facilities should develop contingency plans in the event that disclosure is sought through legal process.

9.10 Medical evaluation

1 If a patient with a reactive test for HIV-I is referred to a physician, the patient should be questioned about possible exposures to the virus or possible risk factors for AIDS, such as sexual orientation, history of intravenous drug use, hemophilia, history of transfusion of blood or blood products, and sexual contact with members of AIDS risk groups.

2 A second ELISA test should be obtained on a follow-up serum if it has not already been done and, if reactive, a Western blot or another antibody test should be considered for additional confirmation.

3 This is particularly important if the patient has no identified risk factors or exposures to the virus.

4 The patient should be examined for signs for AIDS or related conditions with focus on general systemic problems, including unexplained weight loss, fever, diarrhea, dyspnea, dysphagia, lymphadenopathy, and oral thrush.

5 The examination should include abdominal palpation, genital, rectal, skin, and fundoscopic examinations, and special attention to skin or mucous membrane lesions suggestive of Kaposi's sarcoma.

6 Laboratory studies should include a complete blood count including platelets, differential, VDRL, and sedimentation rate.

7 Enumeration of the T-lymphocyte subset is an expensive test, and should be used selectively to demonstrate decreased lymphadenopathy and oral thrush immune function.

8 Anergy to multiple skin tests with common antigens, such as Streptococcus, Candida, mumps, Trichopyton, diphtheria, or tetanus is another indicator of depressed cellular immunity.

9 Testing for antibodies to HIV-1 in the individual's sexual partners may also be useful in establishing whether the test results represent true infection.

9.11 Follow-up recommendations for individuals with positive test results

1 Individuals with positive test results should be advised to establish a relationship with a physician who can, by reason of training and experience, continue to evaluate the patient for signs and symptoms of AIDS or related conditions. It is also recommended that these individuals be advised of the following:

2 The early clinical manifestations of HIV-I infection, AIDS, and AIDS-related conditions, and advised to seek immediate medical attention if any signs or symptoms occur.

3 Currently, the prognosis for a person infected with HIV-I is uncertain. However, studies being conducted among seropositive persons with HIV-1–related risk factors indicate that most will remain infected and must be considered infectious.

4 Seek medical evaluation and follow-up as recommended by their physicians.

5 Although they may be asymptomatic, there is a risk of infecting others through sexual intercourse and by sharing hypodermic needles. It is remotely possible, but not proven, that HIV-I may be transmitted through saliva by intimate kissing. The risk of transmission through oral-genital contact is unknown. The efficacy of condoms in preventing infection with HIV-I is not definitely proved, but the consistent use of them may reduce transmission and should be promoted strongly among all persons at risk for HIV-I infection. In vitro efficacy of condoms as a resistant barrier to passage of the virus has been established.

6 Their blood, plasma, breast milk, sperm, body organs, or other tissues must not be donated, and the exchange of blood, semen, saliva, urine, and feces should be avoided.

7 Toothbrushes, razors, and other implements that could become contaminated with blood should not be shared.

8 Children born since 1978 to women with a positive HIV-I test should be clinically and serologically evaluated.

9 If they are women and they are HIV-I antibody positive, they have a high risk of transmitting HIV-1 to their offspring, and the offspring may develop AIDS or another HIV-I–related condition. Until further evidence is available, these women should be advised to avoid pregnancy.

10 Women who are sexual partners of men with positive test results are at increased risk of acquiring HIV-I infection. These women should be advised to postpone pregnancy. (Refer to the following section on perinatal transmission for further recommendations.)

11 Inform their sexual contact(s) and/or needle-sharing partner(s), and recommend that they receive medical evaluation, including a test for HIV-I antibody.

12 In the absence of intimate sexual or needle-sharing contact, household contacts need not be referred for testing.

13 After accidents resulting in bleeding, contaminated surfaces should be cleaned with household bleach freshly diluted 1:10 in water.

14 Devices that have punctured the skin, such as hypodermic acupuncture needles, must be steam sterilized by autoclave before reuse, or safely discarded. Whenever possible, disposable needles and equipment should be used and disposed of promptly.

15 When seeking medical, dental, or eye care, they should inform those responsible for their care of the positive HIV-I results so appropriate evaluation and precautions can be undertaken.

16 Most persons with positive HIV-I test results need not consider a change in employment or pursuit of education. If an individual is employed in medical, dental, or other health care occupations, the precautions successfully used to limit the spread of hepatitis B should be taken. (The primary action to be taken is to use gloves and extreme caution during any invasive procedures.)

17 If they have donated organs, tissue, semen, breast milk, or blood (dating back to 1977), they should inform the collecting agency.

9.12 Recommendations for preventing HIV-I transmission in the workplace

1 The information and recommendations that follow have been developed with particular emphasis on health care workers and others in related occupations who might be exposed to blood from persons infected with HIV-I.

2 Because of public concern about the purported risk of transmission of HIV-I by persons providing personal services and those who prepare and serve food and beverages, recommendations for workers in these industries are included in this chapter. These recommendations address workplaces in general where there is no known risk of transmission of HIV-I.

3 Because AIDS is a bloodborne, sexually transmitted disease that is not spread by casual contact, the Center for Disease Control (CDC) and the Department of Health Services do not recommend routine HIV-I antibody screening for the groups addressed. Nor should workers known to be infected with HIV-I be restricted from work unless they have another infection or illness that would warrant such a restriction.

4 The following summary of recommendations contains instructions to prevent transmission of all bloodborne infectious diseases to people exposed in the course of their duties to blood from persons who may be infected with HIV-I. Health care workers should take all possible precautions to prevent needlestick injury.

5 The recommendations, based on well-documented modes of HIV-I transmission, are patterned on the hepatitis B model of transmission, a virus that is hardier and more infectious than HIV-I. Practices that will prevent transmission of hepatitis B virus (HBV) will also prevent transmission of HIV-I.

6 Persons at increased risk of acquiring infection with HIV-I include homosexual and bisexual men, intravenous drug abusers, persons transfused with contaminated blood or blood products, heterosexual contacts of persons with HIV-I infection, and children born to infected mothers. HIV-I is transmitted through sexual contact, parenteral exposure to infected blood or blood components, and perinatal transmission from mother to neonate. The kind of nonsexual, person-to-person contact that generally occurs among workers and clients or consumers in the workplace does not pose a risk for transmission of HIV-I.

9.13 Comparison with hepatitis B virus

1 The epidemiology of HIV-I infection is similar to that of HBV, and much that has been learned over the last 15 years related to the risk of acquiring hepatitis B in the workplace can be applied to understanding the risk of HIV-I transmission in health care and other occupational settings. Current evidence indicates that, despite epidemiologic similarities of HBV and HIV-I transmission, the risk for HBV transmission in health care settings far exceeds the risk for HIV-I transmission. The risk of acquiring HBV infection after a needle stick from an HBV carrier ranges from 6% to 30%, far in excess of the risk of HIV-I infection after a needlestick involving a source patient infected with HIV-I, which is less than 1%.

2 Routine screening of all patients or health care workers for evidence of HBV infection has never been recommended. Control of HBV transmission in the health care setting has emphasized the implementation of recommendations for the appropriate handling of food, other body fluids, and items soiled with blood or other body fluids.

9.14 Risks of health care workers acquiring HIV-I in the workplace

1 Using the HBV model, the highest risk for transmission of HIV-I in the workplace would involve parenteral exposure to a needle or other sharp instrument contaminated with blood of an infected patient.

2 The risk of acquiring the infection has been evaluated in several studies and has been determined to be extremely low.

3 In spite of the extremely low risk of transmission of HIV-I infection, even when needlestick injuries occur, more emphasis must be given to precautions to prevent needlestick injuries in workers caring for any patient, since such injuries continue to occur even during the care of patients who are known to be infected with HIV-I.

9.15 Precautions to prevent acquisition of HIV-I infection by health care workers in the workplace

1 These precautions represent prudent practices that apply to preventing transmission of HIV-I and other bloodborne infections and should be used routinely.

2 Items such as needles, scalpel blades, and other sharp instruments should be considered potentially infective

and handled with extraordinary care to prevent accidental injuries.

3 Disposable syringes and needles, scalpel blades, and other sharp items should be placed in puncture-resistant containers located as close as practically possible to the area in which they are used.

4 To prevent needlestick injuries, needles should not be recapped, purposefully bent, broken, removed from disposable syringes, or otherwise manipulated by hand.

5 When the possibility of exposure to blood or other body fluids exists, routinely recommended precautions should be followed. The anticipated exposure may require gloves alone, as in handling items soiled with blood or equipment contaminated with blood or other body fluids, or may also require gowns, masks, and eye-coverings when procedures are performed that involve more extensive contact with blood or potentially infective body fluids, as in some dental or endoscopic procedures or postmortem examinations. Hands should be washed thoroughly and immediately if they accidentally become contaminated with blood.

6 To minimize the need for emergency mouth-to-mouth resuscitation, mouthpieces, resuscitation bags or other ventilation devices should be strategically located and available for use in areas in which the need for resuscitation is predictable.

7 Pregnant health care workers are not known to be at greater risk of contracting HIV-I infections than health care workers who are not pregnant; however, if a worker develops HIV-I infection during pregnancy, the infant is at increased risk of infection resulting from perinatal transmission.
Because of this risk, pregnant health care workers should be especially familiar with precautions for preventing HIV-I transmission.

9.16 Precautions for health care workers during home care of persons infected with HIV-I

1 Persons with AIDS can be safely cared for in home environments. Studies of family members of patients infected with the virus have found no evidence of HIV-I transmission to adults who were not at risk for parenteral transmission.

2 Health care workers providing home care face the same risk of infection as workers in hospitals or other health care settings, especially if there are needlesticks or other parenteral or mucous membrane exposures to blood or other body fluids. Thus, infection control measures similar to those used in hospitals are appropriate.

9.17 Precautions for providers of prehospital emergency health care

1 The risk of transmission of infection, including HIV-I infection, from infected persons to providers of prehospital emergency care should be no higher than that for health care workers providing emergency care in the hospital if the same appropriate precautions are taken to prevent exposure to blood or other body fluids.

9.18 Management of parenteral and mucous membrane exposures of health care workers

1 If a health care worker has a parenteral (e.g., needle stick or cut) or mucous membrane (e.g., splash to the eye or mouth) exposure to blood or other body fluids, the source patient should be assessed clinically and epidemiologically to determine the likelihood of HIV-I infection.

2 If the assessment suggests that infection may exist, the patient should be informed of the incident and requested to consent to serologic testing for evidence of HIV-I infection.

3 If the source patient has AIDS or other evidence of HIV-I infection, declines testing, or has a positive test, the worker should be evaluated clinically and serologically for evidence of HIV-I infection as soon as possible after the exposure.

4 If seronegative, the worker should be retested after six weeks and on a periodic basis thereafter (e.g., three, six and 12 months after exposure) to determine if transmission has occurred.

5 During this follow-up period, especially the first six to 12 weeks when most infected persons are expected to seroconvert, exposed health care workers should receive counseling about the risk of infection and follow U.S. Public Health Service (PHS) recommendations for preventing transmission of AIDS.

6 If the source patient is seronegative and has no other evidence of HIV-I infection, no further follow-up of the health worker is necessary.

7 If the source patient cannot be identified, decisions regarding appropriate follow-up should be individualized based on the type of exposure and the likelihood that the source patient was infected.

9.19 Serologic testing of patients

1 Routine serologic testing of all patients for antibody to HIV-I is not recommended to prevent transmission of HIV-I infection in the workplace. Results of such testing are unlikely to further reduce the risk of transmission, which, even with documented needle sticks, is already extremely low.

2 The risk of infection could be reduced by emphasizing and consistently implementing routinely recommended infection control precautions (e.g., not recapping needles).

9.20 Risk of transmission from health care workers to patients

1 Although there is no evidence that health care workers infected with HIV-I have transmitted infection to patients, a risk of transmission of virus infection from workers to patients would exist in situations in which there is both (1) a high degree of trauma to the patient that would provide a portal of entry for the virus (e.g., during invasive procedures), and (2) access of blood or serous fluid from the infected worker to the open tissue of a patient, as could occur if the worker sustains a needlestick or scalpel injury during an invasive procedure.

2 Health care workers known to be infected with HIV-I need not be restricted from work unless they have evidence of other infection or illness for which any health care worker should be restricted. Additional recommendations for workers who perform invasive procedures are outlined below.

9.21 Precautions to prevent transmission

1 These precautions apply to all health care workers, regardless of whether they perform invasive procedures.

  a All health care workers should wear gloves for direct contact with mucous membranes or nonintact skin of all patients. Gloves should be changed between all patient contacts.

  b Health care workers who have exudative lesions or weeping dermatitis should refrain from all direct patient care and from handling patient care equipment until the condition resolves.

2 In addition, special emphasis should be placed on the following precautions for heatlh care workers performing invasive procedures (operative, obstetric, or dental procedures).

  a Extraordinary care must be taken to prevent accidental injuries to hands caused by needles, scalpel blades, and other sharp instruments during invasive procedures.

  b Health care workers who perform or assist in invasive procedures should be educated regarding the epidemiology, modes of transmission and prevention of HIV-I infection, and in the need for routine use of appropriate barrier precautions.

  c If a glove tear, needle stick, or other instrument injury occurs during any invasive procedure, the glove should be changed as promptly as safety permits and the needle or instrument replaced.

9.22 Management of parenteral and mucous membrane exposure of patients

1 If an incident occurs in which blood from a health care worker in an institutional setting contaminates tissue or mucous membranes of a patient, the patient should be informed of the incident and an evaluation conducted according to institutional policies for management of such an incident.

2 When such an incident occurs in a noninstitutional setting, the patient should be informed and the need for further action should be determined on a case-by-case basis by the practitioner in consultation with other individuals or agencies as deemed appropriate.

9.23 Serologic testing of health care workers

1 Routine serologic testing of health care workers who do not perform invasive procedures (including providers of home and prehospital emergency care) is not recommended to prevent transmission of HIV-I infection.

2 The risk of transmission is extremely low and can be further minimized when routinely recommended infection control precautions are followed.

3 Health care workers who perform invasive procedures and who have reason to believe that they may have been infected with HIV-I should be encouraged to participate in periodic serologic testing so that, if positive, they can be assessed as outlined below and follow other existing recommendations for persons infected with HIV-I.

9.24 Management of health care workers with HIV-I infection who perform or assist in invasive procedures

1 Health care workers with HIV-I infection who perform or assist in invasive procedures should be counseled individually so that the modes of transmission of HIV-I and the need for barrier and other infection control precautions can be reemphasized.

2 The health care worker's personal physician, in consultation with the institution's personnel health care, infection control committee, or medical director, as deemed appropriate, should assess the infected health care worker on an individual basis and determine whether the infected worker can adequately and safely perform or assist in invasive procedures.

3 If the assessment indicates that the infected worker cannot adequately and safely perform or assist in an invasive procedure, or if appropriate precautions cannot be taken to prevent transmission, then the worker should be restricted from such procedures.

4 If health care workers infected with HIV-I have evidence of other infection or illness for which any health care worker would routinely be restricted from performing such procedures in accordance with established institutional policies, they should also be restricted.

5 For health care workers who perform or assist in invasive procedures in locations not covered by institutional policies, this case-by-case assessment should be made by the worker's personal physician in consultation with the local health department or other individuals or agencies deemed applicable to the individual case.

9.25 Risk of occupational acquisition of other infections diseases by health care workers infected with HIV-I

1 Health care workers who are known to be infected with HIV-I and who have defective immune systems are at increased risk of acquiring or experiencing serious complications of other infectious diseases.

2 Of particular concern is the risk of severe infection after exposure to patients with infectious diseases that are easily transmitted if appropriate precautions are not taken (e.g., tuberculosis).

3 Workers should be counseled about this potential risk and should continue to observe recommended infection control procedures to minimize their risk of exposure to other infectious agents.

4 A determination about whether a health care worker can adequately and safely perform patient care duties should be made on an individual basis by the worker's personal physician(s) in conjunction with the personnel health service or medical director of the facility.

5 Recommendations of the Immunization Practices Advisory Committee and institutional policies concerning requirements for vaccinating health care workers with live-virus vaccines should also be considered.

9.26 Sterilization, disinfection, housekeeping, and waste disposal

1 Sterilization and disinfection procedures currently recommended for use in health care dental facilities are adequate to sterilize or disinfect instruments, devices, or other items contaminated with the blood or other body fluids from individuals infected with HIV-I.

2 Instruments or other nondisposable items that enter normally sterile tissue or the vascular system through which blood flows should be sterilized before reuse.

3 Surgical instruments used on all patients should be decontaminated after use rather than rinsed with water.

4 Decontamination can be accomplished by machine or by hand cleaning by trained personnel wearing appropriate protective attire and using appropriate chemical germicides.

5 Instruments or other nondisposable items that touch intact mucous membranes should receive high-level disinfection.

6 Several liquid chemical germicides commonly used in laboratories and health care facilities have been shown to kill HIV-I at concentrations much lower than are used in practice.

7 When decontaminating instruments or medical devices, chemical germicides that are registered with and approved by the U.S. Environmental Protection Agency (EPA) as "sterilants" can be used for either sterilization or for high-level disinfection, depending on contact time; germicides that are approved for use as "hospital disinfectants" and are mycobactericidal when used at appropriate dilutions can also be used for high-level disinfection of devices and instruments.

8 Germicides that are mycobacterial are preferred because mycobacteria are one of the most resistant groups of microorganisms; therefore, germicides that are effective against mycobacteria are also effective against other bacterial and viral pathogens. Instruments or devices to be sterilized or disinfected should be thoroughly cleaned before exposure to chemical germicide and the manufacturer's instruction for use should be followed.

9 Laundry and dishwashing cycles commonly used in hospitals are adequate to decontaminate linens, dishes, glassware, and utensils.

10 Housekeeping procedures commonly used in hospitals are adequate when cleaning environmental surfaces; surfaces exposed to blood and body fluids should be cleaned with a detergent followed by decontamination using an EPA-approved hospital disinfectant that is mycobactericidal. Individuals who clean up such spills should wear disposable gloves.

11 In addition to hospital disinfectants, a freshly prepared solution of household bleach is an inexpensive and very effective disinfectant.

12 Dilution ratios of household bleach ranging from 1:10 to 1:100 are effective, depending on the amount of organic material present on the surface to be cleaned and disinfected.

13 Sharp items should be considered potentially infective and should be handled and disposed of with extraordinary care to prevent accidental injuries.

14 Other potentially infective waste should be contained and transported in clearly identified impervious plastic bags.

15 Recommended practices for disposal of infective waste are adequate for disposal of waste contaminated by HIV-I. Blood and other body fluids may be carefully poured down a drain connected to a sanitary sewer.

9.27 Other workers sharing the same work environment

1 No known risk of transmission to co-workers, clients, or consumers exists from HIV-I–infected workers in other settings (e.g., offices, schools, factories, construction sites).

2 This infection is spread by sexual contact with infected persons, injection of contaminated blood or blood products, and by parenteral transmission.

3 Workers known to be infected with the virus should not be restricted from work solely on the basis of this finding. Moreover, they should not be restricted from using telephones, office equipment, toilets, showers, and water fountains. Equipment contaminated with blood or other body fluids of any worker, regardless of HIV-I infection status, should be cleaned with soap and water or a detergent.

4 A disinfectant solution or a fresh solution of household bleach should be used to wipe the area after cleaning.

9.28 Other issues in the workplace

1 These recommendations do not address all the potential issues that may have to be considered when making specific employment decisions for persons with HIV-I infection.

2 The diagnosis of this infection may evoke unwarranted fear and suspicion in some co-workers.

3 Other issues that may be considered include the need for confidentiality; applicable federal state or local laws governing occupational safety and health; civil rights of employees; workers' compensation laws; provisions of collective bargaining agreements; confidentiality of medical records; informed consent; employee and patient privacy rights; and employee right-to-know statutes. The reader is encouraged to seek additional information regarding AIDS and other infectious diseases from employers and state and federal agencies.

PROCEDURE 9-1

Decontamination procedure for nebulizer unit

No.	Steps in performing the procedure
	The practitioner will disassemble, wash, rinse, place into sterilization solution, rinse, dry, assemble, and package a Puritan-Bennett* all-purpose nebulizer according to the following procedure.
1	Don apron and gloves (where available).
2	Disassemble nebulizer completely:
	2.1 Make certain the screw-in jet assembly is taken apart.
	2.2 Remove siphon tube from jet assembly, and disconnect and disassemble intake filter.
	2.3 Check all pieces for wear and needed repair.
3	Place all items in a warm, detergent solution and allow to soak for a short time.
4	Scrub all surfaces, using a small brush, especially the small orifices.
5	Rinse all pieces after scrubbing in clean, warm water.
6	Remove all pieces from rinse, shaking all excess water free.
7	Immerse all pieces individually to guarantee *complete* submersion of all pieces into the sterilizing solution (e.g., Cidex, Sonocide).
8	Remove all pieces from the sterilizing solution after 15 minutes, shaking excess solution free.
9	Rinse all pieces in clean, warm water.
10	Make certain all *traces* of sterilizing solution are rinsed from the equipment, especially the siphon tube, filter, and jet.
11	Place all pieces in a heated dryer after shaking excess water free.
12	Optional step: Blow all excess moisture free with a compressed air gun from a *filtered* source, especially the siphon tube and jet assembly.
13	Reassemble all pieces after they are *completely* dry.
	13.1 Replace the jet assembly and wire cleaner.
	13.2 Replace the wire carefully to avoid bending.
	13.3 Test the push-button jet cleaner before completing assembly.
	13.4 Replace the gasket, and snap gasket retainer ring into proper position.
	13.5 Replace the siphon tube firmly, and attach the intake filter, taking care not to tear the filter fabric.
	13.6 Screw on the reservoir jar.
	13.7 Replace the "pop-off" valve *firmly.*
	13.8 Replace the metal plug for the immersion heater port *firmly.*
	13.9 Turn the oxygen diluter to the 100% position.
14	Place the reassembled nebulizer in a clean storage bag; label it with your name, shift, and the date.

*Another brand nebulizer may be substituted if Puritan-Bennett is unavailable.

BIBLIOGRAPHY

ACIP: Update on hepatitis B prevention, MMWR 36:343, 1987.

Bageant RA et al: In-use testing of four glutaraldehyde disinfectants in the cidematic washer, Respir Care 26:1255, 1981.

Berry AJ, Isaaison IJ, Knae MA et al: A multicenter study of the prevalence of hepatitis B viral serologic markers in anesthesia personnel, Anesthesia 63:738, 1984.

Boucher RMG: Stability of glutaraldehyde disinfectants during storage and use in hospitals, Respir Care 23:1063, 1978.

Bruck-Kan R: Introduction to human anatomy, New York, 1979, Harper & Row, Publishers, Inc.

Burton GG, Gee GN, and Hodgkin JE, editors: Respiratory care; a guide to clinical practice, Philadelphia, 1977, JB Lippincott Co.

Center for disease control: Recommendations for prevention of HIV transmission in health-care settings, MMWR 36 (Serial No. 2 S):3S, 1987.

Curran JW et al: The epidemiology of AIDS: current status and future prospects, Science 229:1352, 1985.

Darin J: Respiratory therapy equipment and the development of nosocomial respiratory tract infections, Curr Rev Respir Ther 4 (lesson 11)83-86, 1982.

Dominquez B, Englender S, and Coldwell G: AIDS acquired immunodeficiency syndrome—Information and guidelines regarding HTLV-III infections, Arizona Department of Health Services, 1986.

George WL and Finegold SM: Today's practice of cardiopulmonary medicine: bacterial infections of the lung, Chest 81:502, 1982.

Hazalens RE, Cole J, and Berdischewsky M: Tuberculin skin test conversion from exposure to contaminated pulmonary function testing apparatus, Respir Care 26:53, 1981.

Leach ED: A new synergized glutaraldehyde-phenate sterilizing solution and concentrated disinfectant, Infect Control 2:26, 1981.

Lukomsky GI, Ovchinnikov AA, and Bilal A: Complications of bronchoscopy: comparison of rigid bronchoscopy under general anesthesia and flexible fiberoptic bronchoscopy under topical anesthesia, Chest 79:316, 1981.

Murray JF et al: Pulmonary complications of the acquired immunodeficiency syndrome, N Engl J Med 310:1682, 1984.

Stenson W, Aranda C, and Bevelaqua FA: Transbronchial biopsy culture in pulmonary tuberculosis, Chest 83:883, 1983.

Stover DE et al: Spectrum of pulmonary diseases associated with the acquired immune deficiency syndrome, Am J Med 78:429, 1985.

Straffran K: Microbiology of pneumonia. II. Disinfectants, antiseptics and sterilization, Curr Rev Respir Ther 2 (lesson 1)3, 1979.

Wallace J et al: Bronchoscopy and transbronchial biopsy in evaluation of patients with suspected active tuberculosis, Am J Med 70:1189, 1981.

Witek TJ et al: The acquired immune deficiency syndrome (AIDS): current status and implications for respiratory care practitioners, Respir Care 29:35, 1984.

Medical gas therapy

LEARNING OBJECTIVES

On completion of this module the reader will be able to:

1.1 Explain terms related to assembly and operation of a nasal cannula unit.

1.2 Discuss the purpose and special factors related to the placement and operation of a nasal cannula.

1.3 Show appreciation for the need to economize in the use of oxygen without jeopardizing quality of care by explaining the theory of operation and utilization of the Oxymizer™ cannula.

1.4 Describe possible hazards and complications related to nasal cannula therapy.

2.1 Check correct operation of a nasal cannula.

3.1 Explain terms related to assembly and operation of a nasal catheter.

3.2 Discuss the purpose and special operational factors related to the placement and operation of a nasal catheter.

3.3 Administer oxygen via nasal catheter.

3.4 Describe possible hazards and complications related to nasal catheter therapy.

4.1 Check correct operation of a nasal catheter system.

5.1 Explain terms related to assembly and operation of a Venturi mask.

5.2 Discuss the purpose and special factors related to the placement and operation of a Venturi (jet) mask.

5.3 Administer oxygen through a Venturi (jet) mask.

5.4 Describe possible hazards and complications related to Venturi (jet) mask therapy.

6.1 Check correct operation of Venturi (jet) mask.

7.1 Explain terms related to assembly and operation of a simple and partial rebreathing oxygen mask.

7.2 Discuss purpose and special operational factors related to the placement and operation of the simple and rebreathing oxygen mask.

7.3 Administer oxygen using a simple and/or rebreathing oxygen mask.

7.4 Describe possible hazards and complications related to simple oxygen mask therapy and the rebreathing oxygen mask.

8.1 Check correct operation of simple and rebreathing oxygen mask.

9.1 Explain terms related to the assembly and operation of a nonrebreathing oxygen mask.

9.2 Discuss the purpose and special factors related to placement and operation of nonrebreathing oxygen masks.

9.3 Administer oxygen via nonrebreathing oxygen mask.

9.4 Describe possible hazards and complications related to oxygen therapy using a nonrebreathing oxygen mask.

10.1 Check correct operation of a nonrebreathing oxygen mask.

10.2 State the approximate FIO_2 for various types of oxygen therapy equipment at given liters per minute.

11.1 Identify various indications for oxygen therapy.

11.2 Identify contraindications for oxygen therapy.

11.3 Explain the concept of oxygen free radicals and how it relates to lung injury from oxygen therapy.

11.4 List four antioxidants and explain how each may protect the cell against free radicals.

12.1 Explain the theoretic basis for and the methods of providing CPAP, EPAP, and PEEP.

13.1 Discuss the theory of operation for the transtracheal oxygen catheter.

13.2 Point out the advantages of using transtracheal oxygen as compared with other methods.

13.3 Discuss possible complications from transtracheal oxygen.

The appliances presented in the following module begin the study of a number of devices used to administer medical gas therapy. Any form of medical gas therapy ultimately requires a physician's written order. Under certain circumstances, a situation may require the clinician to initially act on an *oral order*, or *treatment protocol* established by standing orders or department policy. If standing orders are used, they must be established in writing and signed by the medical authority.

1.0 NASAL CANNULA UNIT

1.1 Terminology/facts

1 Anterior aperture. Nares (nostrils).

2 Dehydration. State of lack of fluid (moisture); dryness.

3 FIo_2. Fraction of oxygen gas to be inspired by patient expressed as a decimal equivalent of 100%, e.g., 0.5 = 50% oxygen.

4 Humidifier. A device that provides humidity (H_2O vapor) to gas administered to a patient (therapy gas), usually by passing oxygen (gas) through a reservoir of H_2O.

5 Internal nares. The nose is separated internally into right and left chambers (vestibules) by the nasal septum.

6 Low-flow oxygen delivery. Room air is mixed with the gas flow of the apparatus to fully meet the patient's inspiratory demands.

7 Mucous membrane. Capillary enriched lining covering structures of the nasal passages.

1.2 Purpose of nasal cannula (See also McPherson, in the index under "Cannula, nasal."*)

1 The nasal cannula is a simple nontraumatic means of providing low to moderate concentrations of oxygen to a patient.

2 The maximum comfortable gas flow is 1 to 6 L/min. Flows greater than this will irritate the mucosa and cause patient discomfort.

---

*McPherson SP and Spearman CB: Respiratory therapy equipment, ed 4, St Louis, 1990, The CV Mosby Co.

3 Contrary to popular belief, the FIo_2 is inconsistent (21% to 90%), depending on the patient's respiratory frequency and tidal volume.

4 The components and function of nasal cannula assembly are as follows (Fig. 10-1).

a Nasal cannula (prongs) *(1)*. Provides connection of oxygen source to patient via one nasal tip placed in each nostril *(2)*.

b Restraining band *(3)*. Adjustable strap that fits around patient's head to hold cannula in position. Its adjustment is critical to comfort of patient and effectiveness of therapy. If the band is too loose, the tips may fall out of the nares; if it is too tight, the tips will press against the surface of the nares, causing irritation.

c Delivery tube. Small bore delivery tube *(4)*, normally 3 or 5 feet in length, connecting nasal cannula to humidifier outlet (Fig. 10-2).

d Humidifier *(1)*. Screws onto flowmeter outlet *(2)* and provides humidity to source gas, which is extremely dry as it comes from wall outlet or cylinder. If a jet-type humidifier is used, care must be taken to prevent water deposits in the delivery tube from being blown into the patient's nose. Although tradition has dictated its use, studies do not show a need for humidifying oxygen at 4 L/min or less.

e Flowmeter. Provides controlled delivery of gas (L/min) from wall station outlet.

f Cylinder regulator. If a wall outlet is not used, the pressure regulator attaches to a cylinder outlet to provide controlled gas flow (liters per minute) to humidifier unit (not shown).

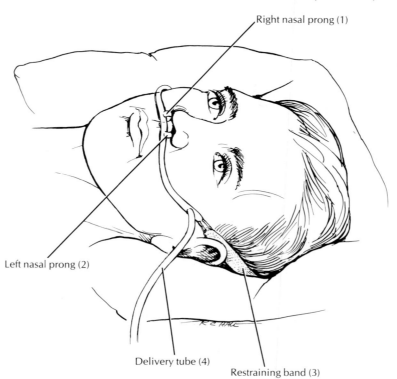

Right nasal prong (1)

Left nasal prong (2)

Delivery tube (4)

Restraining band (3)

FIGURE 10-1 Nasal cannula.

1.3 Economizing cannula

1 A modified version of the standard nasal cannula (described above) was developed for the purpose of providing required blood oxygen saturation levels at reduced flowrates.

2 The operating principle is based on the fact that at the end of each inspiration, fresh gas fills a patient's anatomic deadspace but does not participate in gas exchange. During the initial phase of exhalation this still-fresh gas is exhaled and captured by the reservoir of the economizing cannula and used as a portion of the next inspiration.

3 This principle is the same as that applied by rescuers in exhaled air resuscitation.

4 With standard cannulas, if oxygen is being administered, the patient wastes oxygen-enriched gas with each exhalation.

5 The reservoir cannula and cannula pendant developed by Oxymizer capture the first portion of a patient's exhalation and use it to provide an 18-ml bolus of oxygen-enriched gas with each subsequent inhalation. (Fig. 10-3, *A* and *B*).

6 The components and function of the reservoir nasal cannula are shown in Figure 10-4.

7 The Oxymizer pendant functions in a similar manner but is more desirable to some patients because the cannula is not as visible. The Oxymizer concept results in reported oxygen utilization savings of 25% while maintaining desired blood oxygen saturation levels.

It also enables patients on portable systems to go longer between refills from the main oxygen supply.

NOTE: The general steps in operating a nasal cannula are presented in Procedure 10-1 at the end of this module. The procedure may be used as a guide for administering nasal cannula therapy or as a checklist for evaluating someone else's performance. Before using this procedure compare it with the hospital procedure for any variances in technique. When using a nasal cannula,

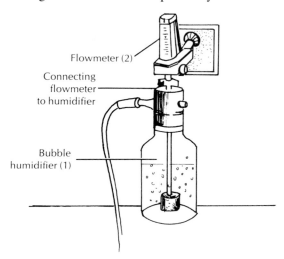

Flowmeter (2)

Connecting
flowmeter
to humidifier

Bubble
humidifier (1)

F I G U R E   1 0 - 2 Nasal cannula tubing connected to humidifier.

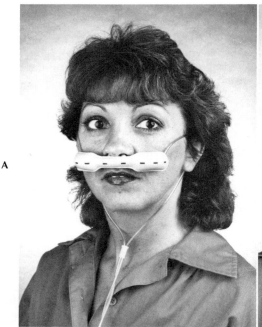

A

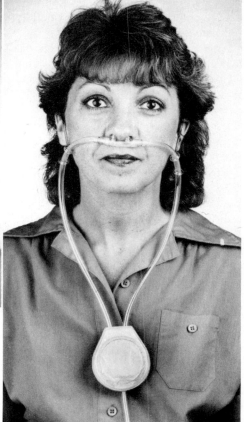

B

F I G U R E   1 0 - 3 A, Reservoir nasal cannula unit **B,** Reservoir pendant nasal cannula unit. (Courtesy Chad Therapeutics, Inc, Chatsworth, Calif.)

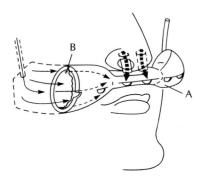
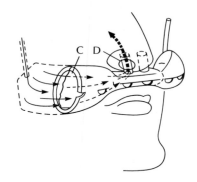

WHILE PATIENT IS EXHALING, oxygen is accumulating in the reservoir (A) formed by the inflated diaphragm (B) and the back wall of the Oxymizer.

WHEN PATIENT INHALES, the diaphragm (C) collapses, and the oxygen-enriched air from the reservoir is released to the patient (D).

FIGURE 10-4 Component parts of the Oxymizer™ nasal cannula showing operation during exhalation and inspiration. (Courtesy Chad Therapeutics, Inc, Chatsworth, Calif.)

position the tips comfortably and accurately inside the nares and adjust the oxygen flow to prescribed levels.

1.4 Possible hazards/complications of nasal cannula therapy

A nasal cannula is one of the least complicated and safest devices for oxygen therapy. However, the following potential hazards and complications should be carefully checked for and prevented.

1 Fire. Always enforce the "no smoking" rule for patients and anyone else in the area when oxygen is being administered. Although oxygen alone will not explode, it will support combustion and cause flammable substances such as nasal cannula to burn rapidly.

2 Nasal trauma. Tissue damage may result from pressure of nasal tips resting on the mucosa of internal nares or a nasal cannula that has been left in place too long without a change (8 to 12 hours).

3 Dehydration. Excessive gas flow (greater than 8 L/min) or poorly humidified gas can result in drying of the mucosal surface of airway passages. Dehydration can result in a nosebleed, substernal pain, earache, laryngitis, and bronchospasm.

4 Over-oxygenation. A low-flow oxygen system provides very inconsistent FIo_2 (21% to 90%) depending on:
  a Patient's respiratory frequency (rate)
  b Patient's tidal volume (depth of breathing)
  c Placement of cannula
  d Liter flow of oxygen
  CAUTION: When using a low-flow oxygen delivery system, such as a nasal cannula, a reduced liters per minute flow rate does *not* ensure a low FIo_2. This must be considered in patients with whom an exact FIo_2 is required. This includes patients with chronic

pulmonary disease with elevated carbon dioxide (CO_2) levels and a diminished hypoxic drive to breathe; excessive FIo_2 can cause these patients to stop breathing, resulting in death from asphyxia.

5 Under-oxygeneration. An improperly positioned cannula or too low a flow of oxygen to meet the patient's inspiratory demands may result in inadequate FIo_2 and under-oxygenation (hypoxia). It is important to note that studies have shown little difference in the tracheal oxygen levels of patients with nasal cannulas who breathe through their mouths as compared with those who breathe through their noses.

2.0 OPERATION OF NASAL CANNULA UNIT
2.1 Equipment check

1 Patients receiving oxygen therapy should be routinely checked according to the severity of their condition. For example, a patient with chronic obstructive pulmonary disease with elevated arterial carbon dioxide tension ($PaCO_2$) should be watched constantly because the oxygen could depress the hypoxic drive, causing the patient to quit breathing. A less acute patient may require rounds once each shift.

2 The following are comments regarding check rounds for patient receiving nasal cannula therapy.
  a Check the patient and the equipment. Check rounds should be patient *and* equipment oriented.
  b Speak to the patient; note any strange or radically changed behavior patterns from previous rounds.
  c Question the patient as to his or her comfort and note any oxygen-related discomforts (e.g., substernal discomfort or drying of the nose, mouth, or throat).
  d Build rapport with the patient and staff by being

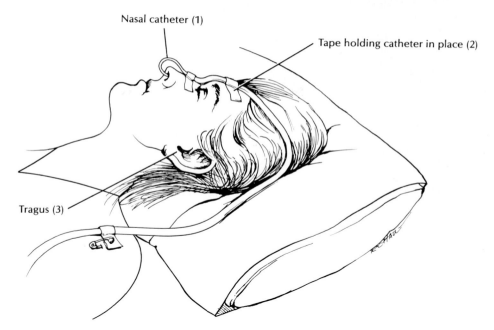

F I G U R E 1 0 - 5 Proper stabilization of nasal catheter by taping to nose and forehead.

alert, professional, and helpful. Procedure 10-2 may be used as a guide for conducting patient rounds.

3.0 NASAL OXYGEN CATHETER UNIT
3.1 Terms related to assembly/operation

1 Nasal oxygen catheter. A tube that is placed into the nasopharynx (Fig. 10-5, *1*) for delivery of low to moderate flows of oxygen. The oxygen concentrations are very similar to those obtained by the nasal cannula, although patient discomfort is usually greater because of catheter position and external taping (Fig. 10-5, *2*). This mode of therapy is still preferred by some physicians, although it is rapidly being replaced by the nasal cannula.

2 Tragus. The cartilaginous, tonguelike fleshy projection just below the external opening of the ear (Fig. 10-5, *3*); this is used as a landmark for determining the insertion distance of a catheter.

3 Uvula. A fleshy mass hanging from the soft palate area above the base of the tongue (Figs. 10-6 and 10-7). It can be seen with the use of a flashlight and tongue depressor; it is a landmark used to determine the resting position of a properly placed oropharyngeal nasal catheter.

4 Nasopharynx. The area of the pharynx that lies above the soft palate.

5 Oropharynx. The area of the pharynx lying behind the mouth and tongue and above the upper edge of the epiglottis.

6 Components and function of a nasal oxygen catheter assembly. (See McPherson, in the index under "Catheter, nasal."*) The *basic components and function* of a nasal oxygen catheter are presented here.

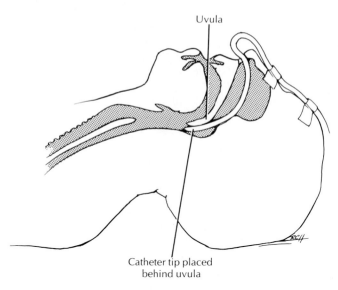

F I G U R E 1 0 - 6 Placement of nasal catheter in nasopharynx.

a An oxygen catheter (sizes 10, 12, 14 French for adults) is inserted into the most open nostril for delivery of moderate flows of oxygen (6 to 8 L/min) (Fig. 10-5, *1*).

b A connecting tube (of small bore tubing) connects the catheter to the humidifier outlet. The oxygen tubing should be of adequate length to allow patient motion (6 to 9 feet) (Fig. 10-8). One must be careful to monitor *the actual gas flow* through the catheter as

*McPherson SP and Spearman CB: Respiratory therapy equipment, ed 4, St Louis, 1990, The CV Mosby Co.

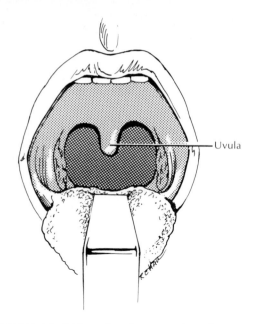

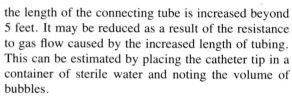

FIGURE 10-7 View of uvula as seen through open mouth.

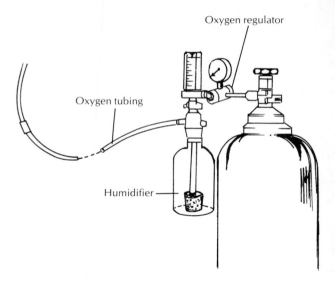

FIGURE 10-8 Nasal catheter connected to humidifier via small bore oxygen tubing.

the length of the connecting tube is increased beyond 5 feet. It may be reduced as a result of the resistance to gas flow caused by the increased length of tubing. This can be estimated by placing the catheter tip in a container of sterile water and noting the volume of bubbles.

c A film of water-soluble lubricant is placed on the catheter to reduce friction trauma during insertion and to facilitate removal.

d A tongue depressor is used to depress the base of the tongue so that the position of the catheter tip can be seen after insertion.

e A flashlight is used to check the catheter position in the oropharynx before taping it in place.

f An oxygen flowmeter can be used to deliver gas flow (liters per minute).

g An oxygen regulator valve with a flowmeter is required if a cylinder is used (Fig. 10-8).

h A humdifier (bubble-type) is required to humidify or add moisture to inhaled oxygen, if the liter flow is greater than 4 L/min.

i Sterile distilled water is used to fill the humidifier reservoir.

j Adhesive tape (¾ inch) is used to tape the catheter in position (Fig. 10-5, 2).

k A NO SMOKING sign should be posted over the flowmeter and/or entrance to the room to warn patients and visitors against smoking in the room.

l All cigarettes and other smoking items should be removed from the patient's room. (Disoriented patients or those with an uncontrollable smoking habit are burned every year from attempting to smoke while using nasal oxygen.)

3.2 Purpose and placement of nasal catheter

1 The purpose of a nasal catheter is to provide low to moderate oxygen flows in situations in which a nasal cannula will not work, e.g., as a result of facial trauma.

2 Once the catheter is placed, the nasal and oral passages serve as an oxygen reservoir.

3 The usual oxygen flow rate is 4 to 8 L/min, resulting in a FIo_2 of 25% to 50%.

CAUTION: A nasal catheter functions as a low-flow oxygen delivery system, which does *not* provide constant oxygen concentrations. The actual FIo_2 will depend on initial L/min flow and the patient's respiratory frequency and tidal volume. It will vary as much as 25% to 90% as the patient's tidal volume and breathing frequency change.

4 The distance that the catheter is inserted into the nose is determined by placing the catheter along the face from the tip of the patient's nose to the tragus of the ear, and also by viewing the catheter tip just behind the uvula.

5 Before placement, a catheter should be lubricated using a water-soluble lubricant. Petroleum lubricants should not be used because they can be hazardous, resulting in possible aspiration of droplets into the lungs and causing lipid pneumonia. However, water-soluble lubricants are absorbed by the mucosa and may cause the catheter to adhere to the mucosa. It is recommended that a low flow of oxygen be administered through the catheter during insertion to prevent possible blockage of the tip by the lubricant or secretions. For this reason, nasal catheters must be checked every 8 hours and alternated between nostrils to minimize possible dam-

age resulting from tissue reaction and adhesions. If a catheter becomes impacted, it must be carefully removed using warm soaks or surgery. Forceful removal will cause trauma to the mucosa and severe bleeding.

6 The catheter must be securely taped in place over the nose and across the forehead to prevent accidental removal or uncontrolled insertion (see Fig. 10-5).

3.3 Administration of oxygen therapy via nasal catheter

1 Procedure 10-3, which is included at the end of this module, may be used as a procedure for inserting a nasal catheter.

2 If the patient violently objects or if bleeding occurs during insertion of the catheter, stop the procedure and request from the physician another mode of therapy, such as the nasal cannula or Venturimask.

3.4 Possible hazards and complications related to use of nasal catheter therapy

1 Nasal catheter oxygen therapy is a simple technique, although it does present more potential hazards and complications than does a nasal cannula.

2 The following are some of the most frequent complications and hazards experienced as a result of using nasal catheter oxygen therapy.

a Fire hazard. Neither the patient nor visitors should be allowed to smoke when oxygen is in use. A patient who smokes with a catheter in place may become frightened if the cigarette flames and the sparks drop onto the bedding, possibly causing a fire.

b Trauma to nasal passages during insertion.

c A catheter that is inserted too deeply into the distal area of the pharynx may press on the epiglottis, causing the patient to swallow oxygen into the stomach. This is uncomfortable and may result in gastric distention and possible rupture of the stomach.

d A catheter that is not carefully monitored and managed may cause inflammation and swelling of the internal nares and nasopharynx resulting in irritation from gas flow, movement of the catheter against the mucosa, or adhesions from accumulation of secretions.

e Accidental connection to suction equipment by inexperienced personnel. Fortunately, this type of situation does not occur very frequently because of the green color coding for nasal catheters. However, as a safeguard, oxygen should never be connected to a catheter that is in place unless it is green and properly located.

4.0 OPERATION OF A NASAL CATHETER UNIT
4.1 Equipment check

1 As with all therapy, check rounds should be patient *and* equipment oriented.

2 Speak to the patient and note any strange or radically changed behavior patterns.

3 Question the patient as to comfort and note any oxygen-related problems (e.g., substernal discomfort or drying of the mucosa).

4 Check the position of the catheter and note any irritations of the mucosa, stomach distension, or patient's swallowing gas.

5 Change the catheter to the opposite side of the nose if irritation is noted or if 8 hours have passed since its insertion into the nostril.

6 Build rapport with the patient and staff by being alert, professional, and helpful.

7 Procedure 10-4, which is included at the end of this module, may be used as a procedure for conducting check rounds.

5.0 VENTURI-TYPE MASK
5.1 Terms and facts related to assembly and operation of a Venturi (air entrainment) mask

The injection of oxygen through a Venturi to draw in (entrain) room air into a face mask is a technique that is used by many different manufacturers. Although the principle is similar, the masks have different names, such as Mix-O-Mask, jet mask, or Venturi mask. All related to the same type of device that uses room air to dilute and hence control the concentration of oxygen being delivered to the patient. The major clinical advantage to all these devices is that a predetermined oxygen percentage can be delivered to the patient, regardless of a wide deviation of changes in the patient's respiratory rate and minute ventilation. However, one must be careful not to assume that all masks are equally accurate under all conditions. Recent studies have shown that Venturi-type devices can be in error as much as $\pm 8\%$ or even greater from the indicated FI_{O_2}.

This is an important consideration especially if the expected delivered FI_{O_2} is not the actual tracheal FI_{O_2}, which directly affects the arterial oxygen pressure (PA_{O_2}) used to calculate the alveolar-arterial gradient.

In this situation the calculated alveolar to arterial gradient would be greater than it actually is and may cause the physician to initiate tracheal intubation and other unneeded therapy to treat what was believed to be a patient in severe respiratory failure.

1 Venturi. The Venturi effect is a physical phenomenon describing the ability of moving fluid (gas) in a tube (Fig. 10-9, *1*) to create a decreased pressure gradient (zone) *(4)* relative to surrounding fluid *(2)* (gas) when it is ejected *(5)* into the opening of a downstream, funnel-shaped tube with an entrance angle of not greater than 15 degrees *(3)*. Higher surrounding pressure *(2)* will cause gas to move toward the decreased pressure gradient (entrained) *(4)* until the pressure is equalized. In a constant output situation (i.e., mask), this gradient will *not* equalize, and mixing of room air *(2)* with driving gas *(1)* will continue in a specific proportion.

2 Back pressure. A build-up of pressure from some distal point in a system to the proximal (origin) source, usually caused by a restriction at a downstream point.

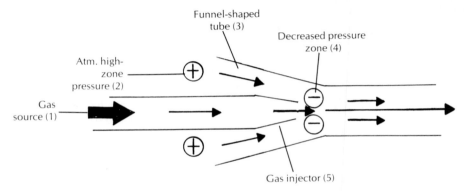

FIGURE 10-9 Air entrainment via the Venturi effect.

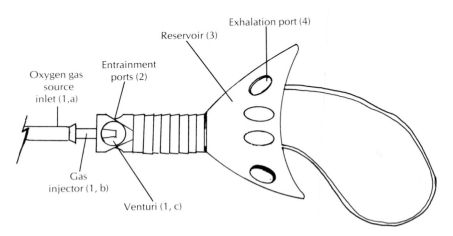

FIGURE 10-10 Parts of Venturi mask.

3 Mix-O-Mask,* Accur-Ox Mask,† Multi-Vent Mask,‡ Ventimask§. Brand names for different types of entrainment mask systems.

4 Components and functions of the Venturi-type mask are as follows (Fig. 10-10).

a Injector *(1b)*. Attaches to oxygen connecting tube *(1a)* and compresses gas for accelerated injection into opening (throat) of the Venturi *(1c)*. Changing of the injector orifice (opening) will alter FIo_2.

b Venturi *(1c)*. Receives compressed gas from injector and produces decreased pressure gradient along lateral walls, causing room air to flow into the opening toward the decreased pressure zone.

c Entrainment ports *(2)*. Openings that allow room air (surrounding gas) to be pushed into the Venturi as a result of existing pressure gradient, causing a mixing of environmental gas with source gas in the Venturi.

d Reservoir *(3)*. Cone-shaped structure that receives gas from Venturi.

e Exhalation ports *(4)*. Permit the patient to freely exhale to atmosphere with minimum back-pressure created on the Venturi. Occlusion or alteration of these ports would cause increased back-pressure during exhalation and result in a *Venturi stall* (i.e., pressure equalized so that room air is not entrained as efficiently). Any decrease in entrainment of room air will cause a rise in the oxygen concentration breathed by the patient.

f Restraining strap (Fig. 10-11, *1*). Used to position and hold the mask in place.

g Oxygen connecting tube *(2)*. Connects Venturi mask oxygen inlet to gas source. Relationship between liters per minute flow and mask determines FIo_2. Oxygen flow to mask should match indicated recommended flow labeled on the mask *(3)*.

NOTE: Flows greater than those indicated on the mask will be compensated for by the size of the inlet orifice. Flows *less* than those indicated on the mask will result in decreased entrainment of air and an elevated and *inaccurate* FIo_2 (Table 10-1).

---

*Mix-O-Mask, OEM Medical (a unit of Whittaker Corp.), 8741 Landmark Rd., Richmond, VA 23260.

†Accur-Ox Mask, Inspiron Respiratory Div., C.R. Bard, Inc., 8600 Archibald Ave., Rancho Cercamonga, CA 91730.

‡Multi-Vent Mask Hudson, 27711 Diaz Rd., Temecula, CA, 92390-0066.

§Ventimask, Vickers Medical Products Corp., P.O. Box 101, U.S. Hwy 22, Whitehouse Station, NJ 08889.

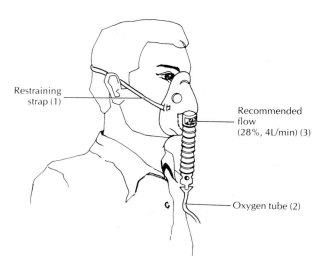

FIGURE 10-11 Proper placement of Venturi mask.

TABLE 10-1 Typical oxygen: air entrainment ratios

	Oxygen- (L/min)		Air—O_2 mixing ratio		Total flow
24% Venturi mask	4	=	25 : 1	=	97 L/min
28% Venturi mask	4	=	10 : 1	=	44 L/min
35% Venturi mask	8	=	5 : 1	=	48 L/min
40% Venturi mask	8	=	3 : 1	=	32 L/min

NOTE: These numbers do not apply to all Venturi type masks.

5.2 Purpose of and factors related to placement and operation of the Venturi mask

1 The purpose of a Venturi mask or any oxygen/air-type mixing mask is to provide a *specific* FIo_2 to the patient without having to use a premixed gas source.

2 To operate effectively, the Venturi mask must be placed so that the face cone (mask) is positioned directly in front of the patient's nose and mouth with restraining straps comfortably positioned around the lower portion of the head above the ear (see Fig. 10-11, *1*).

3 The connecting tube should be attached directly to an oxygen source *without* a humdifier. If a humidifer is used, it must be of the vapor type—not an aerosol-producing device. Water droplets will occlude the injector (oxygen inlet) to the mask and alter entrainment characteristics. If humidity is required, a humidity adaptor collar should be used. However, studies have shown that these adaptors alter specific FIo_2 by as much as 8% in some masks.

5.3 Administration of oxygen via Venturi mask

1 Procedure 10-5, which is included at the end of this module, may be used as a guide for administering a Venturi mask or a similar type of mask.

2 With supervision, assemble components and administer oxygen to patients using prescribed oxygen percentages and according to Procedure 10-5. Remember to monitor the FIo_2 in patients by drawing the sample from the hypopharynx. Tracheal oxygen levels are the closest indicators of Pao_2 levels.

5.4 Possible hazards and complications related to air/oxygen mask therapy

1 Venturi-type masks are simple to use and relatively safe as long as fire regulations are observed and as long as one realizes that this type of mask is not precise under all conditions.

2 Inaccurate FIo_2. Studies have shown that FIo_2 may vary from that indicated on the mask. Patients who retain CO_2 or who otherwise may require accurate FIo_2 should be closely observed initially regardless of stated FIo_2 controls. Humidity collars can alter FIo_2 by as much as 8% from stated levels. If in doubt, arterial oxygen tension (Pao_2) should be tested and compared with tracheal FIo_2. A dyspneic patient may require peak inspiration flow rates greater than 90 L/min. If these flow rates are not delivered by the mask, room air will be entrained and cause a duressed FIo_2. A rule of thumb for estimating a patient's inspiratory peak flow rate is 4 to 6 times the measured minute ventilation, ($V_M \times$ 4-6).

3 Dehydration. Air/oxygen mixing masks provide high flows of gas to the patient of 84 L/min or greater. This gas is usually not properly humidified and can result in dehydration of airways, causing a drying of secretions and impairment of ciliary function after the humidity of gas in contact with mucosa decreases to 72% relative humidity.

6.0 OPERATION OF VENTURI-TYPE MASK
6.1 Equipment/patient check rounds

1 Patient and equipment check rounds should be conducted on a Venturi mask the same as for other oxygen therapy devices. The key is to evaluate the patient first and then the equipment.

2 Procedure 10-6, which is included at the end of this module, may be used to conduct check rounds for patients receiving oxygen/air mask therapy.

7.0 SIMPLE AND PARTIAL REBREATHING-TYPE OXYGEN MASKS
7.1 Terms and facts related to assembly and operation

1 Oxygen masks were one of the earliest methods of providing high concentrations of oxygen to the patient. The key to using an oxygen mask is to use a gas flow that is adequate to meet the minute ventilatory demands of the patient. One must remember that with most masks, room air is pulled into the mask whenever the gas flow is too low for the patient's inspiratory demands.

2 Oronasal mask. A mask that covers both the mouth and nose of the patient.

3 There are two major types of oronasal masks.

a A *partial rebreathing* system in which part of the exhaled gas is rebreathed during subsequent inhalation.

This rebreathed gas does *not* normally include higher levels of CO_2.

b A *nonrebreathing* system in which exhaled gas is *not* rebreathed in any amount. This is usually accomplished by placement of a one-way (check) valve between the face mask and the reservoir bag to prevent exhaled gas from re-entering the bag during exhalation.

4 Other classifications* further divide masks into:

a High-flow systems. Masks that supply all the patient's inspired gases at a given FIo_2.

b Low-flow systems. Masks that do *not* meet the patient's inspiratory flow needs; room air is entrained to make up the difference.

5 Besides the one-way valve described earlier, nonrebreathing masks usually also incorporate an exhalation valve on the exhalation ports of the mask that are opened to the atmosphere by exhaled gas flow. During inhalation, these one-way valves reseat to prevent air entrainment, which would dilute the FIo_2.

6 An entrainment valve is a one-way valve that opens in response to a preset pressure gradient to allow atmospheric air to enter (entrain) into a mask. This valve allows patients to pull in room air whenever the gas flow into the mask is not sufficient to meet the inspiratory demands; it is also sometimes called a safety valve.

7 The so-called simple mask (Fig. 10-12) is a variation of the face cone mask. Oxygen is provided through an inlet connection *(1)*, and exhalation occurs through open ports in the face piece *(2)*. It has no valves and depends on the gas flow from the flowmeter to wash out any accumulating CO_2 and provide an elevated FIo_2. At flows of 10 L/min, an FIo_2 of approximately 55% can be delivered to the patient.

8 An *oronasal partial rebreathing face mask* includes the following parts.

---

*First described by Shapiro Barry A, et al: Clinical application of respiratory care, Chicago, 1975, Year Book Medical Publishers, Inc, p. 135.

a Face piece. Portion of mask that covers patient's mouth and nose; normally contains ports for venting of exhaled gases (Fig. 10-13, *1*).

b Reservoir bag *(2)*. A collection chamber for containment of gases used to meet patient's inspiratory demands.

• In a partial rebreathing mask, both inhaled and exhaled gases are mixed in the reservoir. The exhaled gas to the bag is made up of the last one third of the previously inspired gas that filled the anatomic reservoir of the mouth, nose, and upper trachea (anatomic dead space), where the oxygen was not used, plus the incoming oxygen from the connecting tubing. The last two thirds of the previously inspired gas is that which underwent internal respiration, contains higher levels of CO_2, and is vented to the room through the exhalation ports (Fig. 10-13, *1*). If the reservoir bag collapses *completely* during the patient's inspiration, a deficit will be created between the patient's tidal volume (V_T) and volume available from the bag and liters per minute flowing into the mask.

• Any deficit volume will be satisfied by room air that enters the system via the exhalation ports. When this occurs, the FIo_2 will be decreased and the patient's breathing effort may be increased.

c Connecting tube *(3)*. Oxygen tube that connects the mask to the humidifier unit. The tubing should be of sufficient length to permit patient movement without accidental removal of the mask. Care must be taken

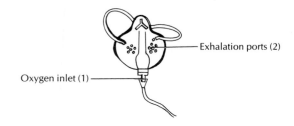

FIGURE 10-12 Simple oxygen mask.

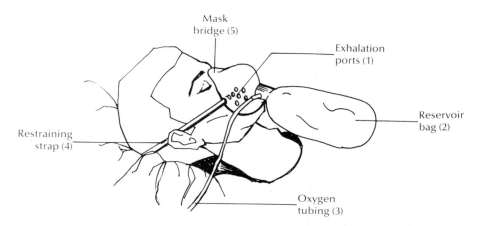

FIGURE 10-13 Parts of partial rebreathing oronasal oxygen mask.

not to kink or occlude this tube as the mask is being placed on the patient.

d Restraining strap *(4)*. Holds the mask in position on the patient's face. Note that the upper portion of the bridge of the mask should rest on the superior aspect of the nasal bone and against the patient's forehead *(5)*. An improperly fitted mask can result in dilution of the FIo_2 with room air and cause irritation of the patient's eyes. If the leak is around the bridge of the mask, oxygen will flow into the patient's eyes.

e Humidifier unit. A bubble-type humidifier may be used with sterile distilled water.

f If a piping system is used, a flowmeter with appropriate wall outlet adapter provides oxygen from the wall outlet to the humidifier.

g Pressure regulator, if a cylinder is used to provide oxygen. In this situation, the humdifier is attached to the flowmeter for delivery of humidified gas to the patient.

7.2 Purpose of and factors related to operation of oronasal oxygen masks—partial rebreathing type

1 The oronasal oxygen mask (with reservoir bag) is used to provide oxygen therapy to patients requiring moderate to high FIo_2. Table 10-2 shows approximate FIo_2 at a given liters per minute flow based on a normal inspiratory flow rate of 30 L/min. For example, at 8 L/min the patient would receive a FIo_2 of approximately 0.45 or 45%.

NOTE: As with any low-flow delivery system, the FIo_2 will vary as tidal volume (V_T), peak inspiratory flow rate (PIF), and breathing frequency (f) change from that which was present when the mask was initiated.

2 When a patient is using the mask, the liters per minute gas flow into the mask must be adequate to keep the reservoir bag *partially inflated* during the patient's inspiratory efforts. A deflated bag will result in decreased FIo_2 because room air will be entrained through the expiratory ports of the mask.

3 When the practitioner is placing the mask on the patient, the face piece must be adjusted for the patient's maximum comfort and delivery of FIo_2. As previously stated, care must be taken to position the bridge of the mask against the patient's forehead to prevent the escape of the gas around the mask into the patient's eyes, which can cause drying and irritation.

TABLE 10-2 A comparison of FIo_2 at various oxygen flow rates

Flow rate (L/min)	Approximate FIo_2
6	0.35
7	0.40
8	0.45
9	0.50
10	0.60

7.3 Oxygen administration via simple and partial rebreathing oxygen masks

1 Procedure 10-7, which is included at the end of this module, may be used for administration of mask oxygen therapy.

2 When administering oxygen therapy the physician's order for FIo_2, duration of therapy, and monitoring should be followed.

7.4 Possible hazards and complications related to oxygen therapy via partial rebreathing oxygen mask and simple oxygen mask

1 It is important that respiratory care personnel be aware of each of these hazards and complications and check for their presence in the clinical setting.

2 Hyperoxygenation of a patient with chronic obstructive pulmonary disease and CO_2 retention. An elevated FIo_2 can depress the patient's respiratory drive as a result of hypoxia and result in apnea and death.

3 Aspiration. *Any* covering of the face may hide the fact that a patient is vomiting. This is potentially dangerous because the mask can trap vomitus and/or blood, with the result of possible aspiration by the patient. Aspiration of stomach contents, especially acid, is extremely toxic to the airway and can cause chemical burns and potentially lethal pneumonitis.

4 Oxygen toxicity. Oxygen percentages greater than a FIo_2 of 0.60 for periods longer than 72 hours can result in lung changes such as consolidation, shunting of blood flow, bronchospasm, and other adverse responses leading to increased levels of hypoxia and CO_2 retention. X-ray films reveal white patchy areas consistent with the adult respiratory distress syndrome (ARDS).

5 Dehydration. High oxygen flows (8 to 10 L/min) can result in dehydration of airway mucosa and subsequent thickening of secretions.

6 Eye irritation. Improperly positioned masks can result in gas escaping around the edges and into the patient's eyes.

8.0 OPERATION OF SIMPLE OR PARTIAL REBREATHING OXYGEN MASKS
8.1 Equipment/patient check rounds

1 Patients receiving O_2 therapy via a face mask must be observed regularly (see Hazards).

2 The humidifier must be serviced and water levels maintained for continuous humidification.

3 Oxygen liter flow must be maintained at prescribed levels.

4 The patient's safety from fire must be assured by removal of smoking implements and posting of NO SMOKING signs.

5 The patient must be observed for the following.

a Mental awareness. Ask the patient questions.

b General skin color, warmth, turgor. These can be checked as vital signs are taken.

c General comfort. Adjust as necessary, position the

beds, fluff the pillow, check for adequate humidity.

d Face care. The face must be checked for pressure ridges resulting from mask placement.

e Respiratory rate and depth. Rate may decrease in a patient receiving oxygen therapy; check to make sure the resevoir bag does not collapse during inspiration.

f Effectiveness of therapy to relieve hypoxic condition (clinical signs combined with arterial blood gas analysis).

NOTE: An accurate determination of effective therapy can only be confirmed by assessment of partial pressure of oxygen in the arterial blood (Pao_2).

6 Procedure 10-8, which is included at the end of this module, may be used to conduct patient and equipment rounds.

9.0 NONREBREATHING ORONASAL OXYGEN MASK
9.1 Terms and facts

1 Disposable. Any item that is used and discarded. Disposable units are used to reduce expense and problems involved with service and decontamination of permanent items. Disposables generally do not perform as well as permanent items.

2 One-way valve. A valve that allows gas to flow only in a predetermined direction. Used to prevent exhaled gases from flowing back into the reservoir bag.

3 Nonrebreathing. Ideally, patients breathe only that which comes from the reservoir bag with no mixing of inspiratory and expiratory gases.

4 Nonrebreathing oxygen masks provide higher FIo_2 than partial rebreathing masks at the same liters per minute flow.

5 Most nonrebreathing oxygen masks function as a low-flow delivery system because of small reservoirs (600 to 800 ml) and liter flows (8 to 10 L/min). They do not always completely meet the constantly changing peak inspiratory flow rates and tidal volume demands of the patient.

6 Ideally, a nonrebreathing oxygen mask should function as a *high* percentage oxygen system and should do so as long as the patient's tidal volume and flow demands are met. In this situation, a leak-free mask system should deliver a FIo_2 of approximately 1.0.

7 An approximation of FIo_2 delivered by a nonrebreathing *permanent* vs. *disposable* oxygen mask system is compared with a partial rebreathing type oxygen mask in Table 10-3.

8 Components and functions of nonrebreathing oronasal oxygen masks (Fig. 10-14) are as follows.

a One-way valves *(1* and *2)* are positioned to cause gas to flow in one direction only.

b Inhalation valve *(2)* isolates reservoir bag from mask to prevent backflow of exhaled gas into bag.

c Exhalation valve(s) *(1)* (most nonrebreathing-type oxygen masks will have one or two valves) is opened by the patient's expiratory gas flow, allowing the exhaled gases to exit. These valves reseat during inspiration to prevent inflow of room air.

d Inspiratory relief valve is a spring-loaded valve *(4)* that opens to allow passage of room air if oxygen flow is interrupted or inadequate to meet inspiratory flow demands of the patient; sometimes called an entrainment valve *(3)*.

e Reservoir bag *(5)* (600 to 800 ml) serves as a reservoir for inlet gas only. A one-way valve prevents backflow of exhaled gases into the bag.

TABLE 10-3 A comparison of FIo_2 using permanent vs. disposable oxygen masks

Administrative device	FIo_2	Approximate L/min (V)
Permanent O_2-type mask	90%-100%	Reservoir distended
Disposable O_2-type mask	95% ± 5%	Reservoir distended
Partial rebreathing-type mask	60%	Reservoir distended

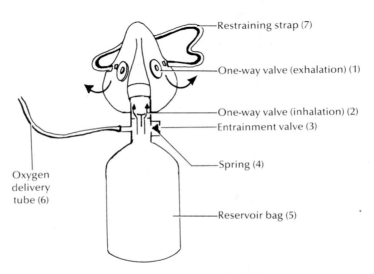

Restraining strap (7)

One-way valve (exhalation) (1)

One-way valve (inhalation) (2)

Entrainment valve (3)

Spring (4)

Oxygen delivery tube (6)

Reservoir bag (5)

FIGURE 10-14 Parts of nonrebreathing oronasal oxygen mask.

f Delivery tube *(6)* connects the mask to the humidifier.

g Humidifier may be bubble type or jet.

h Strap *(7)* is used to secure the mask on the face. A leak-free fitting must be ensured if a FIO_2 of 1.0 is desired.

9.2 Factors related to placement/operation of a nonbreathing oxygen mask

1 Select a *proper size* mask to fit the face of the patient.

2 In preparation for positioning the mask adjust an adequate gas flow (the reservoir bag will be inflated [distended]).

a Place the mask over the patient's chin.

b Expand the sides of the mask and position the mask along the patient's cheek.

c Place the bridge of the mask last, making sure that the tip of the mask rests snugly, but comfortably, over the bridge of the patient's nose and against the forehead.

d Tighten the restraining strap to maintain mask position and to prevent leaks.

e Check the mask for leaks by feeling for gas escape and noting the movement of the reservoir bag. In a tight system, the bag will respond to the patient's slightest inspiratory efforts.

CAUTION: Do not use excessive gas flows into the mask. Once the reservoir is inflated, use only enough gas to keep it *partially inflated* during the patient's inhalation. Avoid excessive flows that can cause the inhalation and exhalation valves to remain open, resulting in a decreased FIO_2.

3 Observe the patient for any signs of nausea, and if possible place the patient in a modified Fowler's position to decrease the risk of aspiration should vomiting occur.

4 Provide facial care as required to prevent pressure ridges from face mask and reddening of skin from gas contact.

9.3 Administering oxygen therapy via oronasal nonrebreathing oxygen mask

1 By tradition nonrebreathing masks are assumed to be capable of delivering an oxygen percentage of 95% or more. Clinically, this is usually not the case, especially with disposable masks that deliver 50% to 70% oxygen.

2 Nonrebreathing masks function as low-flow systems in most instances, and the FIO_2 will vary in response to changes in the patient's breathing.

3 Nonrebreathing masks can be used to administer other gas mixtures, such as helium/oxygen and carbon dioxide/oxygen, provided an airtight system is maintained.

4 Procedure 10-9, which is included at the end of this module, may be used for administering mask oxygen therapy.

5 When using a face mask remember that a leak-proof system is necessary to deliver FIO_2 90% or greater.

9.4 Potential hazards and complications related to nonrebreathing oxygen mask therapy

1 Fire. (See previous comments regarding fire safety.)

2 Aspiration. Masks hide the fact that a patient has vomited. For this reason, masks have the potential to trap regurgitated stomach contents and other body fluids, such as aspirated blood. To minimize this possibility, the patient should be placed in a Fowler's position if possible or on one side; the patient must be observed closely.

3 Excessive flow rates. Gas flows greater than 30 L/min may cause the epiglottis to open in the unconscious patient, allowing gas to enter the stomach. This situation can cause vomiting or possible rupture of the stomach.

4 Oxgen toxicity. Oxygen toxicity has been shown to have a dose and time relationship. At FIO_2 of 0.4 few to no lung changes were noted in patients requiring therapy for 48 to 72 hours.

10.0 OPERATION OF NONREBREATHING OXYGEN MASKS

10.1 Equipment/patient rounds

1 One of the most important functions of respiratory care personnel is to monitor the patient and routinely check this equipment for proper operation.

2 Patients receiving oxygen therapy via a face mask must be observed regularly (see Hazards).

3 The humidifier must be serviced and water levels must be maintained for continuous humidification.

4 The liter flow must be maintained at prescribed levels or at levels necessary to maintain bag inflation.

5 The patient's safety from fire should be ensured by removal of smoking implements and posting of signs.

6 The patient must be observed for the following.

a Mental awareness

b General skin color, warmth, turgor

c General comfort; adjust mask as necessary

d Face care; face must be checked for pressure ridges resulting from mask placement

e Respiratory rate and depth

f Effectiveness of therapy to relieve hypoxic condition (clinical signs combined with arterial blood gas analysis)

NOTE: An accurate determination of effective therapy can be confirmed only by assessment of partial pressure of oxygen in the arterial blood (Pao_2). Clinically, a rule of thumb is to administer a FIO_2 that will achieve a Pao_2 of not less than 50 mm Hg and still not exceed 0.6.

7 Procedure 10-10, which is included at the end of this module, may be used for conducting patient and equipment rounds.

10.2 Summary of performance characteristics for various types of oxygen therapy devices

1 In respiratory care, equipment and techniques are prescribed to provide an enriched FIO_2 and high humidity therapy.

2 Table 10-4 presents a summary of the FIo_2 that can be obtained by various techniques at various liters per minute gas flow. The relative humidity provided by the aerosol and/or humidity devices will vary between 40% and 90% and will depend on various conditions that will be discussed in more detail in Modules Eleven and Twelve. Table 10-5 compares Venturi ratio with gas flow rates. The box below contains a formula for calculating total gas flows and/or the liters per minute of oxygen needed to produce a given FIo_2.

3 One way of solving for the proper oxygen to air ratio to provide a desired FIo_2 at any given rate is to use the "Magic Box" approach as explained below.

- *Step one:* Draw a box and enter the *desired* percentage of oxygen in the center.
- *Step two:* Draw a dotted line *horizontally* through the center of the box continuing beyond the right side of the box. The area *above the line* (the top of the box) will represent oxygen, and the area *below the line* (the bottom of the box) will represent air.
- *Step three:* Enter *100* at the upper left corner of the box.
- *Step four:* Enter *20 or 20.93* (room air) at the bottom left corner of the box.
- *Step five:* Enter the equation *Part O_2 = Desired O_2 − Room Air* at the upper right corner of the box. (Results should be entered above the dotted line.)
- *Step six:* Enter the equation *Part air = 100 − desired O_2* in the bottom right corner. (Results should be entered below the dotted line.)
- *Step seven:* Reduce the fraction created by the number above and below the line. Report it as a ratio of 1:_____

TABLE 10-4 Approximate oxygen concentration delivered through various devices*

Administration device	Flow rate (L/min)	Approximate FIo_2
Nasal cannula	1	0.24
	2	0.28
	3	0.31
	4	0.34
	5	0.37
	6	0.40
Venturi mask (24%)	4	0.24
(28%)	4	0.28
(35%)	8	0.35
(40%)	8	0.40
Simple mask	6	0.35
	7	0.40
	8	0.45
	9	0.50
	10	0.55
Partial rebreathing mask	6	0.35
	7	0.40
	8	0.45
	9	0.50
	10	0.60
Permanent nonrebreathing mask	Sufficient flow to maintain distended reservoir and effective mask seal	1.0
Disposable nonrebreathing mask		0.95% ± 5%
Face tent (40%)	15	0.30-0.40
(70%)	15	0.45-0.55
(100%)	15	0.45-0.55
Aerosol/tracheal mask		
(40%)	15	0.35-0.40
(70%)	15	0.45-0.60
(100%)	15	0.45-0.60
T-tube reservoir (40%)	15	0.40
(70%)	15	0.60-0.70
(100%)	15	0.70-1.0

*Based on normal inspiratory flowrates of 30 L/min. FIo_2 will also vary, depending on patient's inspiratory flow, tidal volume, and breathing rate.

| 100 | (O₂ | Part O_2 = Desired O_2 − Room Air = _____ |
	% Desired	
	O₂ Percent	Part Air = 100 − Desired O_2 Part Air = _____
20	(AIR)	

TABLE 10-5 Venturi ratios and gas flows

FIo_2	O_2 flow rate	Air entrainment ratio	Total gas flow (L/min)
0.24	4	25:1	97
0.28	4	10:1	44
0.35	8	5:1	48
0.40	8	3:1	32
0.70	10	0.6:1	16
1.0	10	0:1	10

Formula for computing total flows or oxygen entrainment

$$\text{Liter flow} = \dot{V}\, \frac{(FIo_2 - .2)}{.8}$$

Total flow (air + o₂) q 15 liters per minute
Desired FIo_2 = 60%
Amount of oxygen required is 8 liters per minute.

EXAMPLE:
$$\frac{15(.60 - .2)}{.8}$$
$$\frac{15(.4)}{.8}$$
$$\frac{6}{.8} = 7.5 \text{ (rounded off) approximately 8 liters oxygen.}$$

EXAMPLE: A physician prescribes a FIo_2 of 0.30 (30%) to be delivered to the patient. Calculate the air to oxygen ratio for any given liter per minute flow rate, following the steps listed above.

100	Part $O_2 = 30 - 20 = 10$
	30
20	Part air $= 100 - 30 = 70$

O_2 to air ratio $= {}^{10}\!/_{70} = 1:7.$

For any given flow rate situation, seven times as much air as oxygen would be used.

11.0 INDICATIONS AND CONTRAINDICATIONS FOR OXYGEN THERAPY

11.1 Indications for oxygen therapy

1 As previously stated, hypoxia not only wrecks the machine, it stops the machinery.

2 The primary indication for oxygen therapy is to prevent or relieve hypoxemia.

3 Current medical evidence indicates that mild hypoxemia, as indicated by an arterial blood partial pressure of 60 torr or greater, is not dangerous in the otherwise normal patient.

4 The administration of oxygen to these patients probably is not clinically beneficial and cannot be justified financially.

5 In many medical centers the measurement of venous blood for oxygen tension is used as a guide to the adequacy of tissue oxygenation. This technique is useful, and when compared with arterial samples it presents a clearer picture of the effectiveness of oxygen therapy. A mixed venous oxygen tension ($P\bar{v}o_2$) of less than 30 torr is considered abnormal and indicates a need for oxygen therapy and/or changes in the therapy procedures.

6 The causes of hypoxemia and the mathematics for calculating hypoxemia were discussed in detail in Module Eight. In review, the causes of hypoxemia are hypoventilation, right-to-left shunts, diffusion impairments, and ventilation-perfusion mismatch. It was pointed out in Module Eight that *normal* Pao_2 values vary according to a person's age, anatomic position, and altitude above sea level. Clinically the concept of predicted (expected) normal Pao_2 is very important. A misinterpretation of what a normal Pao_2 should be for a patient can lead to the administration of *unnecessary* therapy that may even harm the patient. It was also learned in Module Eight that one way of assessing a patient's need for oxygen therapy was to determine the alveolar-arterial oxygen gradient (A-ao_2). A normal A-ao_2 in hypoxemia usually indicates that the hypoxia is caused by hypoventilation and that oxygen therapy alone will *not* help. An otherwise widening gradient usually indicates hypoxemia caused by oxygen deficit where oxygen therapy may be of assistance unless it is caused by a large shunt. (If these concepts are not clear please review Module Eight before proceeding.)

7 To review, in *hypoventilation,* oxygen therapy is of little benefit unless ventilation is restored to physiologic levels. *Do not* make the mistake of assuming that oxygen therapy will substitute for inadequate breathing frequency and/or tidal volume.
   - In these situations, low concentrations of oxygen ($FIo_2 = 0.30$) may be of benefit to supplement other problems that develop with mechanical ventilation. It is estimated that increasing the FIo_2 by as little as 4% to 7% will double the oxygen available to the tissues.

8 In *right-to-left shunts,* oxygen therapy is of little value because of the mixing of oxygenated blood with unoxygenated blood. Some increase in the dissolved oxygen levels in the plasma may occur, although probably not enough to supply the body's needs.
   - In such cases, the application of continuous positive airway pressure (CPAP) or positive end expiratory pressure (PEEP) may be of assistance by reducing the shunt, thus decreasing the magnitude of arterial venous mixing.

9 *Diffusion impairments* are caused by diseases or conditions that widen the distance between the alveolar membrane and the pulmonary capillaries. Pulmonary edema, hyaline membrane, and interstitial fibrosis pneumonia all cause a widening of the diffusion distance for oxygen into the capillary blood. Moderate-to-high concentrations of oxygen in these patients may be useful in relieving the hypoxemia.

10 In patients with a *ventilation-perfusion mismatch,* such as occurs in chronic obstructive pulmonary disease, oxygen therapy is usually very effective in raising the arterial blood oxygen level. In such cases, care must be taken not to reduce the hypoxia levels to the point that apnea is induced. One should also be aware that the administration of O_2 will cause an increase in the arterial carbon dioxide tension ($Paco_2$). In these patients a FIo_2 of 0.24 to 0.35 is usually sufficient to control hypoxemia and not depress respirations.

11 The conditions included in Table 10-6 usually result in hypoxemia that can be improved through the use of supplemental oxygen (indications). In each condition it is assumed that the patient is able to maintain an adequate minute ventilation or that one is provided through mechanical support in conjunction with supplemental oxygen. The oxygen dosage and administering oxygen therapy techniques will vary from hospital to hospital.

In addition to the medical conditions in Table 10-6, recent studies have clearly pointed out that hypoxic episodes are more common in patients with diseases that predispose them to hypoxemia when they are asleep than when they are awake. These patients should be carefully observed to prevent acute hypoxemia or they should be given nocturnal oxygen therapy. This therapy usually involves the use of a nasal cannula at 2 to 4 L/min. Patients who receive nocturnal oxygen

TABLE 10-6 Conditions resulting in hypoxemia that can be improved by supplemental oxygen administration*

Medical condition	FIo$_2$
Acute cerebral vascular accident	0.60-1.0
Acute cor pulmonale	0.60-1.0
Anaphylactic shock	1.0
Acute sepsis	0.50-1.0
Asphyxia neonatorium	0.60-1.0
Asphyxia	1.0
Asthma	0.40-0.60
Bullar polio	0.60
Bronchiolitis	0.40-0.60
Burn shock	0.60-1.0
Bronchial obstruction	0.80-1.0
Congestive heart failure	0.40-0.60
Carbon monoxide poisoning	0.90-1.0
Chronic cor pulmonale	0.60-1.0
Cesarean delivery	0.25-4.0
Eclampsia	1.0
Electroshock	1.0
Fetal bradycardia	0.40-1.0
Gas poisoning (other than monoxide)	0.60-1.0
Hemorrhagic shock	0.60-1.0
Laryngotracheobronchitis	0.60-1.0
Myocardial infarction	0.60-1.0
Neurosurgery	0.40-0.60
Pulmonry emphysema	0.40-1.0
Pulmonary embolism	1.0
Pulmonary edema	0.60-1.0
Pneumonia	0.40-1.0
Premature infants	0.21-0.40
Postoperative surgery	0.30-0.40
Postoperative atelectasis	0.40
Tetanus	0.60-1.0
Traumatic shock	0.60-1.0

*Refer to Table 10-4 for therapy modes for these conditions.

therapy overall have a marked decrease in the number of sleep apneas, and an increase in the level of ventilation monitoring is required. An ear oximeter may be used in place of invasive techniques.

12 In many cases the physician will prescribe the use of continuous positive airway pressure (CPAP) or positive end expiratory pressure (PEEP) before increasing the FIo$_2$ above 0.60. It has been proved that concentrations of oxygen above 60% after approximately 72 hours will cause a decrease in lung volumes and diffusing capacity and produce chest pain, cough, anorexia, weakness, and a pneumonia-like exudate.

11.2 Contraindications for oxygen therapy

The contraindications for oxygen therapy are primarily a concern over too much oxygen, causing oxygen toxicity. In the premature infant, too much oxygen may cause retrolental fibroplasia and/or oxygen toxicity. Too little oxygen, on the other hand, will cause cellular hypoxia.

1 The classic description of oxygen toxicity pathology in animals was made in 1897 by Dr. J. Lorrain Smith. Subsequently, oxygen toxicity has sometimes been called the Lorrain Smith effect. It was known as long ago as 1775 that oxygen could both give and take life.

2 The clinical symptoms of oxygen toxicity are listed below. It is important to realize that the changes inherent with oxygen toxicity cause decreases in ventilation, diffusion defects, increased shunting as a result of atelectasis, and an interstitial exudate that causes the lungs to have a white-out appearance on chest films because of consolidation. These symptoms are commonly referred to as adult respiratory distress syndrome (ARDS).

  a Early symptoms
- Retrosternal discomfort and/or tracheobronchitic pain
- Restlessness
- Cough
- Lethargy
- Vomiting
- Dyspnea

  b Late signs
- Respiratory insufficiency
- Cyanosis
- Frothy or bloody sputum
- Asphyxia

3 Healthy individuals will begin to develop symptoms after 4 to 12 hours of breathing 100% oxygen at 1 atmosphere. Unfortunately, the symptoms are more subtle in patients with lung disease because it is felt that the presence of pulmonary diseases and hypoxia may actually help protect the patients against a rapid onset of symptoms. All patients have an increasing level of hypoxia with dyspnea, even though the oxygen percentage may be increased. Oxygen toxicity is a trap that may cause the unaware clinician to continue to increase inspired FIo$_2$ in an attempt to treat the obvious increased hypoxia; hence a vicious cycle develops.

4 Experience has shown that the following conditions and drugs may increase a patient's susceptibility to oxygen toxicity
  a Viral and bacterial infection
  b Extremes in humidity
  c Hypercapnia
  d Acidosis
  e Hyperthermia
  f Corticosteroids
  g Catecholamines
  h Hyperthyroidism
  i Pulmonary edema

5 The factors listed above cause the patient to develop the symptoms of oxygen toxicity at lower levels of FIo$_2$ and in a shorter time than would occur in a patient without the factors but receiving the same dose of oxygen for the same time.

6 To minimize the risk of hyperoxygenation or hypooxygenation, the practitioner must be aware of the patient's needs and efficacy of the therapy to meet these needs. Methods of measuring oxygen saturation and utilization in the body include arterial blood gases, Module Eight, Unit 16.0, and oximetry Module Sixteen, Unit 14.0.

11.3 Mechanisms of oxygen injury in the lung

1 Contraindications for oxygen administration were described above.

2 The mechanisms for cellular injury caused by oxygen is caused by the metabolic process itself and by phagocytosis as the cell attempts to fight infection.

3 Once oxygen arrives at the cell, the molecule is metabolized to create adenosine triphosphate (ATP).

4 In the presence of the enzyme cytochrome oxidase, the oxygen molecule is reduced to form two molecules of water.

5 This process results in the formation of a superoxide anion (O_2), the hydroxyl radical ($OH-$), and hydrogen peroxide (H_2O_2). These active products, called free radicals, are believed to be the cause of tissue damage linked with oxygen toxicity.

6 The inhalation of normal atmospheric oxygen concentrations results in the release of relatively low concentrations of radicals near the mitochondria of the cell, compared with the greatly elevated levels released as increased oxygen concentrations are given.

7 Free radicals react with polyunsaturated fatty acids, which are sidechains of membrane lipids, causing the formation of lipid peroxides.

8 These peroxides inhibit the active catalic actions of many enzymes and decompose further to form agents, which can result in protein sulfhydryl oxidation and cause holes in cell membranes.

9 As holes occur, the cells leak fluids into extracellular spaces.

10 When inflammation occurs in the cells, additional free radicals are released as phagocytosis occurs.

11.4 Protecting against free radicals

1 Research has shown that the molecule glutathione, an intracellular tripeptide, may protect intracellular enzymes and neutralize oxygen free radicals.

2 Chemicals that protect the cell against free radicals include:

  a Cytochrome oxidase. Reduces oxygen with the production of large numbers of free radicals.

  b Superoxide dismutases. Eliminates the superoxide anion.

  c Peroxidase. Eliminates hydrogen peroxides and lipid peroxides.

  d Glutathione peroxidase. Reduces hydrogen peroxide and lipid peroxides.

  e Vitamin E. A nonspecific free oxygen scavenger. It donates a free atom and stops lipid peroxidation.

3 Vitamin E acts as an antioxidant defense and, along with other agents, protects the cell against free radicals at 1 atmosphere. This is not true, however, at elevated oxygen concentration levels.

12.0 ELEVATED AIRWAY BASELINE PROCEDURES— CPAP/PEEP

12.1 Physiology

1 In Module Eight the lung and its various compartments, known as volumes and capacities, were presented.

2 It was emphasized that respiration is *not* a simple process of moving air into the lung during inspiration and out during exhalation.

3 Instead, respiration involves a combination of events whereby air flows into the airways during inspiration, with the various lung units filling at different rates (slow- and fast-filling units).

4 During exhalation, air flows out of the lung in a similar manner. Different units (portions) of the lung empty their volumes at different times during the expiratory process until the airways close off, causing gas flow to cease from a particular lung unit (closing volume).

5 An important consideration is that not all of the air leaves the various lung units during exhalation. A certain volume remains as a *residual* force to stabilize alveoli against collapse and as reservoir for gas exchange to constantly occur between the alveoli and the pulmonary capillaries.

6 This remaining volume of gas is called the *residual volume* (RV), which when combined with the expiratory reserve volume forms the *functional residual capacity* (FRC). At the level of the residual volume, gas flow becomes negligible and gas movement is primarily by diffusion.

7 It is from the functional residual capacity that the alveoli acquire the gas used for exchange with the pulmonary capillaries. It follows therefore that increasing or decreasing the volume and oxygen percentage of gas in this compartment can greatly influence the ability of alveoli to achieve effective diffusion with the adjacent pulmonary capillaries.

8 Research and clinical experience have shown that manipulation of the patient's expiratory reserve volume (ERV) is the best method of changing the size of the functional residual capacity.

9 This volume can be mechanically altered by creating variations of continuous positive pressure breathing (CPPB) on the airway in the form of positive end expiratory pressure (PEEP) or continuous positive airway pressure (CPAP). These can be life-saving procedures for patients who have a reduced Pao_2 because of a decreased functional residual capacity and/or atelectasis. Conditions that cause a decreased FRC include:

  a Patient positioning

  b Obesity

  c Abdominal pain

  d Anesthesia

  e Acute pulmonary disease

  f Thoracic or abdominal surgery

10 Historically CPPB was used by Poulton and his associates and by Barack primarily to prevent or treat pulmonary edema by reducing the return of venous blood to the right side of the heart. The pulmonary application of this procedure was not appreciated until the mid-1960s when Asbaugh and his associates used a positive end expiratory pressure (PEEP) *with mechanical venti-*

lation to treat hypoxemia associated with ARDS. In 1969 Gregory and his associates used expiratory positive pressure to treat hypoxia in the *spontaneous non-ventilated infant* and called it continuous positive airway pressure (CPAP).

11 For the first decade of its use, PEEP meant the delivery of an elevated airway baseline pressure provided at the end of exhalation when used *in conjunction with a ventilator*. CPAP was the term describing elevated airway baseline pressure when it was used with a spontaneously breathing patient without a ventilator.

12 Currently these definitions have changed so that the distinguishing difference between PEEP and CPAP is the manner in which the elevated airway pressure is provided rather than whether or not it is being used with a ventilator.

13 A *CPAP system* uses a high pressure reservoir that delivers a constant flow of gas that exceeds the patient's inspiratory peak flow demands. With this system a continuous positive airway pressure is maintained during both inspiration and exhalation.

14 In comparison, a *PEEP system* uses an open-ended reservoir that allows gas to flow in response to the pressure gradient created as the patient inhales. To accomplish this gradient the patient must first drop the airway pressure from a positive end expiratory level to below ambient baseline to open the one-way valve and generate the flow necessary for the subsequent inspiration.

15 For this reason a PEEP system requires more work by the patient to operate it than does a CPAP system. Physiologically this may or may not be beneficial, although studies have shown that the work of lowering the airway pressure in a PEEP system may augment venous return and increase cardiac stroke volume in patients with a compromised circulation. CPAP, on the other hand, may be hemodynamically more beneficial in some patients than PEEP because it reduces left ventricular afterload and results in a more effective ejection of blood from the left side of the heart.

16 CPAP may also be more effective than an equal pressure of PEEP in increasing Pao_2. The mechanism for this increased effectiveness is not clear, although it has been suggested that the benefits of PEEP may be counteracted because patients on PEEP have a tendency to force exhalation by actively contracting their expiratory muscles.

17 PEEP and CPAP may be created in a breathing circuit by inserting a *flow or threshold* resistor valve. Most modern PEEP and CPAP systems use a threshold resistor valve instead of a flow resistor to generate the desired elevated airway pressure.

18 This valve is inserted at the distal end of the expiratory side of a breathing circuit. During exhalation the pressure in the breathing circuit falls until it reaches an opposing level preset on the threshold resistor valve. When this occurs the threshold resistor closes to prevent any further drop in the system pressure, causing a positive end expiratory pressure to be maintained. With this type of valve a constant elevated airway pressure may be provided independent of expiratory flow rates and without increasing the work of breathing.

19 Additional information on resistor valves will be presented in Module Twenty-Three on mechanical ventilation.

20 The use of CPAP with a face mask is an example of how CPAP may be used in an alert and spontaneously breathing adult without ventilatory support to improve the Pao_2/FIo_2 ratio.

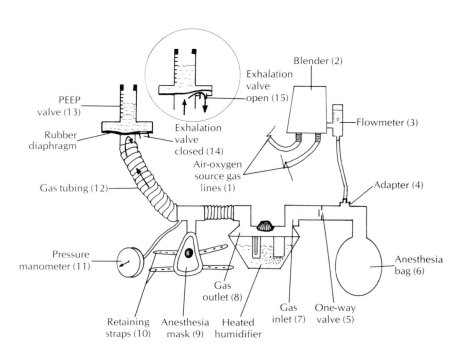

FIGURE 10-15 Components of typical face mask—CPAP system.

21 An example of a typical face mask CPAP system is presented in Fig. 10-15.*

a In this example an air/oxygen blender *(2)* is connected to source gases *(1)* that are administered via a flowmeter capable of delivering 70 to 90 L/min *(3)* through an adapter *(4)* to a 5 L anesthesia bag *(6)*.

b The flow rate is adjusted to keep the anesthesia bag *fully* distended, forcing gas to flow past a one-way valve *(5)* to the inlet side of a heated humidifier *(7)*.

c Humidified gas leaves the humdifier via the outlet *(8)* and is breathed by the patient, who is attached to an anesthesia type mask *(9)*.

d This mask is held in place by a four-prong retaining strap *(10)*.

e During inspiration, gas is inhaled by the patient at a preset positive pressure level as determined by the distention (fullness) of the anesthesia bag and height of the water column in the PEEP valve *(13)*.

f Exhalation is permitted only to the point that the positive airway pressure force created by the patient during exhalation is able to overcome the weight of the water holding the exhalation valve closed *(14)*.

g At this point the rubber diaphragm is lifted and exhalation occurs *(15)*.

h When the airway pressure generated by exhalation no longer exceeds the downward resistance caused by the weight of the water pushing down on the valve, the valve will close, causing the breathing circuit to equalize with the patient force generated by distension of the anesthesia bag.

22 An advantage to the CPAP system is that the constantly pressurized breathing circuit makes it easy for the patient to generate a pressure gradient and acquire inspiratory gases. A combination of work vs. breathing adjustments can be set by regulating the flowmeter and observing airway pressure on the manometer *(11)*.

---

*In this example the water column PEEP valve is modified after the device produced by JH Emerson Co, Cambridge, Massachusetts. The CPAP system is modified after the design used by Michael Banner, RRT and Robert Smith, RRT et al, while they were at Jackson Memorial Hospital in Miami, Florida. A similar system is published in Current Reviews in Respiratory Therapy, vol. 1, lessons 1 and 2, 1978.

23 A face mask PEEP system (Fig. 10-16) is easier to assemble than the CPAP system described above. (The equipment and design of this system are modified from previous designs. (See the footnote.)

a In a PEEP mask system an oxygen flow is delivered from a flowmeter *(1)* through a mechanical nebulizer *(2)* with an adjustable FIo_2 capability.

b The humidified gas with a preset FIo_2 (40%, 50%, etc.) flows to a one-way *(3)* that is held closed.

c The opposing force that is holding the valve closed is established by the height of the water column pressing down to close the PEEP valve *(6)* on the expiratory side of the breathing circuit.

d To inspire fresh gas the patient must first generate enough subambient force within the breathing circuit to overcome the opposing pressure caused by PEEP level plus the mechanical opening resistance of the one-way valve.

e The sensation is similar to that of trying to drink a viscous liquid through a straw.

f In this example the work of drinking (sucking on the straw) is determined by the viscosity of the fluid plus the internal diameter and length of the straw.

g In a PEEP system the work of overcoming the opposition of the closed one-way valve is directly related to the height of the water column and the inertia of the valve to open. Some clinicians claim that the work of breathing characteristic of a PEEP system is hemodynamically advantageous. This claim is based on the fact that while the patient is generating a subambient circuit pressure his or her intrapleural pressure decreases and causes an increase in venous return to the right side of the heart.

h The purpose of the reservoir tube *(4)* is to store gas at a fixed FIo_2. This is necessary because as the FIo_2 is increased by closing the nebulizer diluter valve the flow rate probably will not meet the inspiratory peak flow demands of the patient.

i When this occurs the patient will pull gas at the preset FIo_2 from the reservoir.

j As the FIo_2 is enriched, the reservoir tube will need to be lengthened. A rule of thumb is to keep the vol-

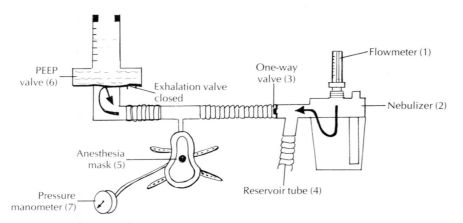

FIGURE 10-16 Components of typical face mask—PEEP system.

ume of the reservoir tube at approximately one and a half times the patient's tidal volume.

k If a decrease in FIo$_2$ is noted at the patient's airway, the reservoir volume should be increased until the desired FIo$_2$ is achieved.

13.0 TRANSTRACHEAL OXYGEN SYSTEM (FIG. 10-17)

13.1 Theory of operation

1 Dr. H. J. Heimlich presented the physiologic and economic benefits from administering oxygen through a transtracheal catheter in Annals of Otology, Rhinology and Laryngology.

2 This system as originally described, but later modified by others, allows the administration of a continuous low flow of oxygen via a connecting tube *(1)* directly to the lower trachea through a no. 16 intravenous catheter or specially designed catheter. This catheter is placed using a needle inserted directly into the cervical trachea of the lower anterior neck *(2)*.

13.2 Advantages of transtracheal oxygen

The advantages to such a system are:

1 Safety, comfort, and convenience. The small opening in the lower anterior neck can be performed under local anesthesia, and is safe, comfortable, and convenient because the catheter does not interfere with shaving, washing, kissing, and other activities that would be hindered by a cannula or other devices attached to the face.

2 Cosmetic acceptability. The small catheter inserted in the lower neck and secured by a lariat around the neck is barely noticed, even when it is not hidden by clothing.

3 Greater mobility. The use of lower oxygen flowrates (1 to 3 LPM) is more economic and enables the patient to use lighter and more compact portable oxygen sources that provide extended time between refills.

4 Greater efficacy. The administration of oxygen directly to the lower trachea eliminates wasted gas caused by anatomic dead-space, as is common with other devices. It reduces the work of breathing and frequently allows patients who are refractory to nasal cannula oxygen or facial oxygen devices commonly used in a hospital to be treated at home.

5 Reversibility. Once the small catheter has been removed, the trachea will close on its own without treatment.

13.3 Complications

1 Morbidity with transtracheal oxygen appears to be minor and acceptable.

2 Most patients tolerate transtracheal oxygen and will prefer it over the oxygen devices.
Possible complications include:
a Accidental removal of the catheter.
b Irritation and infection of the insertion site and trachea.
c Inspired secretions.

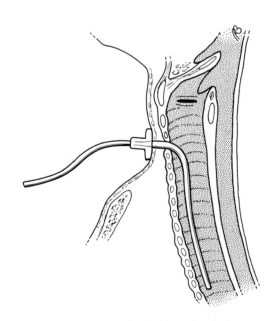

F I G U R E 1 0 - 1 7 Transtracheal catheter inserted transtracheally.

PROCEDURE 10-1

Initiation of oxygen therapy through nasal cannula

No.	Steps in performing the procedure
1	The practitioner will implement this procedure when initiating oxygen therapy via nasal cannula in a clinical area supplied with a wall mounted quick-connect oxygen outlet. Assemble equipment **1.1** Flowmeter **1.2** Humidifier **1.3** Sterile water **1.4** Connecting tube **1.5** Cannula
2	Verify physician order on patient's chart.
3	Wash hands.
4	Introduce yourself to patient and verify patient's identity by wrist band.
5	Explain the procedure as appropriate to the patient's condition and familiarity with the procedure. Stress the fire hazards involved in oxygen administration.
6	Fill humidifier jar to appropriate line with sterile distilled water.
7	Attach humidifier to flowmeter.
8	Connect flowmeter to oxygen source and check operation of flowmeter, humidifier pressure relief valve, and humidifier.
9	Open cannula package and attach to humidifier with care to avoid contamination of cannula nasal tips.
10	Loosen strap of cannula and place cannula into patient's nares. (Care should be taken to avoid pressure on the patient's skin, and the patient is made as comfortable as possible.)
11	Turn on oxygen flowmeter to prescribed liter flow. (Optional: where an accepted procedure, record flow rate on label and attach to flowmeter.)
12	Affix NO SMOKING sign to patient's door and reemphasize the fire hazard to the patient.
13	Observe patient for any unfavorable signs or symptoms. Special observation should be used when patient has a known history of chronic obstructive lung disease.
14	Reassure patient.
15	Wash hands.
16	Record procedure on patient's chart and on additional forms as necessary.

PROCEDURE 10-2

Operational check—nasal cannula

No.	Steps in performing the procedure
	The practitioner will visit each patient and check operation of nasal cannula according to the following steps.
1	Verify physician order.
2	Review patient's progress notes.
3	Review respiratory therapy notes.
4	Wash hands.
5	Introduce yourself to patient.
6	Identify patient by wrist band.
7	Verify correct liter flow from flowmeter.
8	Remove connecting tube.
9	Occlude delivery tube and note operation of safety relief valve on humidifier.
10	Reconnect delivery tube.
11	If needed, turn flowmeter "off."
12	Empty water from humidifier reservoir.
13	Rinse reservoir jar and refill with sterile distilled water.
14	Where applicable, replace humidifier according to departmental quality assurance program (maximum q 9 to 12 hours).
15	Adjust flowmeter to "on" and set prescribed liter flow.
16	Note operation of flowmeter.
17	Check placement of nasal cannula for the following. **17.1** Band comfort **17.2** Position of cannula tips
18	Note and report any tissue reaction to nasal cannula or oxygen flow.
19	Question patient as to comfort.
20	Wash hands.
21	According to hospital or department policy, record check round activity in patient's chart, noting any special directions or circumstances related to patient's progress and care. Replace cannula if occluded or according to department replacement schedule (q 8 to 12 hours).

PROCEDURE 10-3

Initiation of therapy through nasal catheter

No.	Steps in performing the procedure
1	The practitioner will set up, insert, and maintain oxygen therapy through a nasal catheter on order of attending physician. Great care should be taken to avoid undue pain and possible hemorrhage during insertion.
	Collect necessary equipment
	1.1 Flowmeter
	1.2 Humidifier
	1.3 Oxygen connecting tube
	1.4 Nasal catheter
	1.5 Water soluble lubricant
	1.6 Sterile glove
	1.7 Flashlight
	1.8 Tongue depressor
2	Assemble apparatus (except catheter) and fill humidifier with sterile distilled water.
3	Verify physician order.
4	Wash hands.
5	Identify patient, then introduce yourself.
6	Discuss the purpose and steps of procedure with the patient. Measure proper insertion length on patient. Place catheter to one side in a sterile manner.
7	Plug flowmeter to oxygen source.
8	Check pressure relief valve on the humidifer.
9	Place the nasal catheter into the nasopharynx in a sterile, nontraumatic manner.
10	Turn on oxygen flow.
11	Instruct the patient to refrain from adjusting the catheter and to call for assistance if discomfort occurs.
12	Observe patient for any unfavorable signs or symptoms. Special observation should be used when a patient has a history of chronic obstructive lung disease.
13	Reassure patient.
14	Wash hands.
15	Hang NO SMOKING sign on the door.
16	Chart the procedure in the patient's chart.
17	Change the catheter every 8 hours to the opposite nostril.

PROCEDURE 10-4

Operational check—nasal oxygen catheter

No.	Steps in performing the procedure
	The practitioner will visit each patient and check operation of nasal oxygen catheter according to the following steps.
1	Verify physician order.
2	Review patient's progress notes.
3	Review respiratory therapy notes.
4	Wash hands.
5	Introduce yourself to patient.
6	Identify patient by wrist band.
7	Verify correct liter flow from flowmeter.
8	Remove connecting tube.
9	Occlude delivery tube and note operation of safety relief valve on humidifier.
10	Reconnect delivery tube.
11	If needed, turn flowmeter "off."
12	Empty water from humidifier reservoir.
13	Rinse reservoir jar and refill with sterile distilled water.
14	Where applicable, replace humidifier according to departmental quality assurance program (maximum q 9 to 12 hours).
15	Adjust flowmeter to "on" and set prescribed liter flow.
16	Note operation of flowmeter.
17	Check placement of nasal catheter for the following.
	17.1 General comfort and taping
	17.2 Position of catheter
18	Change catheter and insert it in alternate nostril if it is occluded or if it has been in place for 8 hours.
19	Note and report any tissue reaction to nasal catheter or oxygen flow.
20	Question patient as to comfort.
21	Wash hands.
22	According to hospital or departmental policy, record check round activity in patient's chart, noting any special directions or circumstances related to patient's progress and care.

PROCEDURE 10-5

Initiation of oxygen therapy through Venturi mask

No.	Steps in performing the procedure
1	The practitioner will implement this procedure when initiating oxygen therapy via Venturi mask in a clinical area supplied with a wall mounted quick-connect oxygen outlet. Assemble equipment **1.1** Flowmeter with nipple **1.2** Connecting tube **1.3** Venturi mask (with appropriate percentage Venturi) NOTE: Humidification of the humiditity or aerosol collar is optional.
2	Verify physician order on patient's chart.
3	Wash hands.
4	Introduce yourself and verify patient's identification by wrist band.
5	Explain the procedure as appropriate to patient's condition and familiarity with the procedure.
6	Attach one end of connecting tube to Venturi mask jet and the other end to nipple of flowmeter.
7	Turn on oxygen to proper liter flow, double-check O_2 percentage marked on mask; listen for the "hiss" of the Venturi jet entraining room air.
8	Place mask over patient's mouth and nose; adjust strap for snug fit.
9	Observe patient for unfavorable reaction to therapy.
10	Instruct patient to terminate smoking in room.
11	Inform other patients to terminate smoking.
12	Hang a NO SMOKING sign on patient's door.
13	Reassure patient.
14	Wash hands.
15	Chart procedure in chart and fill out necessary forms.

PROCEDURE 10-6

Operational check—Venturi mask

No.	Steps in performing the procedure
	The practitioner will visit each patient and check operation of Venturi mask according to the following steps.
1	Verify physician orders.
2	Review patient's progress notes.
3	Review respiratory therapy notes.
4	Wash hands.
5	Introduce yourself to patient.
6	Identify patient by wrist band.
7	Verify correct liter flow from flowmeter to mask according to chart and verify mask percentage specifications.
8	Check placement of Venturi mask for the following. **8.1** Band comfort **8.2** Position
9	Note and report any tissue reaction or pressure ridges resulting from mask or band placement.
10	Question patient as to comfort.
11	Wash hands.
12	According to hospital or departmental policy, record check round activity in patient's chart, noting any special directions or circumstances related to patient's progress and care.
13	Verbally report any circumstances needing attention to appropriate superior.

PROCEDURE 10-7

Initiation of oxygen therapy through simple and/or partial rebreathing oxygen mask

No.	Steps in performing the procedure
1	The practitioner will set up oxygen therapy via either a simple or partial rebreathing oxygen mask in a clinical area supplied with a wall-mounted quick-connect oxygen outlet. Assemble equipment **1.1** Flowmeter **1.2** Humidifier **1.3** Sterile water **1.4** Oxygen mask
2	Verify physician order on patient's chart.
3	Wash hands.
4	Introduce yourself, then verify the patient's identity by wrist band.
5	Explain the procedure as appropriate to the patient's condition and familiarity with the procedure. Stress the fire hazards.
6	Fill humidifier jar to appropriate line with sterile distilled water.
7	Attach humidifier to flowmeter.
8	Connect flowmeter to oxygen source and check operation of flowmeter, humidifier pressure relief valve, and humidifier.
9	Attach oxygen mask tubing to humidifier.
10	Place mask on patient's mouth and nose. NOTE: If using the partial rebreathing mask, cover your thumb or index finger with a clean tissue and occlude the reservoir bag opening, allowing the oxygen flow to fill the bag before placing it on the patient.
11	Check oxygen flow. Adjust to ordered liter flow if simple mask or adjust to prevent bag deflation if partial rebreathing mask.
12	Instruct patient to terminate smoking in room.
13	Instruct other patients to terminate smoking in room.
14	Observe patient for any unfavorable reaction from therapy.
15	Hang NO SMOKING sign on patient's door.
16	Reassure patient.
17	Wash hands.
18	Chart procedure in chart and fill out necessary forms.

PROCEDURE 10-8

Operational check—simple and partial rebreathing oxygen mask

No.	Steps in performing the procedure
	The practitioner will visit each patient and check operation of simple oxygen mask according to the following steps.
1	Verify physician order.
2	Review patient's progress notes.
3	Review respiratory therapy notes.
4	Wash hands.
5	Introduce yourself to patient.
6	Identify patient by wrist band.
7	Verify correct liter from flowmeter.
8	Remove connecting tube.
9	Occlude delivery tube and note operation of safety relief valve on humidifier.
10	Reconnect delivery tube.
11	If needed, turn flowmeter "off."
12	Empty water from humidifier reservoir.
13	Rinse reservoir jar and refill with sterile distilled water.
14	Where applicable, replace humidifier according to departmental quality assurance program (maximum q 9 to 12 hours).
15	Adjust flowmeter to "on" and set prescribed liter flow.
16	Note operation of flowmeter.
17	Check placement of simple oxygen mask for the following. **17.1** Strap position and patient comfort **17.2** Mask position Check placement of partial rebreathing mask for the following. **17.3** Mask and strap position and patient comfort. **17.4** Oxygen flow and whether bag remains inflated during inspiration.
18	Note and report any pressure ridges at facial pressure point.
19	Question patient as to comfort.
20	Wash hands.
21	Replace mask if needed according to department replacement schedule.
22	According to hospital or departmental policy, record check round activity in patient's chart, noting any special directions or circumstances related to patient's progress and care.
23	Verbally report any circumstances needing attention to appropriate supervisor.

PROCEDURE 10-9

Setting up a nonrebreathing oxygen mask

No.	Steps in performing the procedure
	The practitioner will set up a nonrebreathing oxygen mask on the appropriate order of a physician. The flow of oxygen must be adjusted to allow reservoir bag to remain partially inflated during inspiration and follow-up arterial blood gas analysis should be suggested. Prolonged use of high concentrations of oxygen should be suspected in the development of oxygen toxicity.
1	Collect necessary equipment.
	1.1 Flowmeter
	1.2 Humidifier
	1.3 Oxygen connecting tubing
	1.4 Nonrebreathing oxygen mask
2	Verify physician's order.
3	Identify patient and introduce yourself.
4	Wash hands.
5	Assemble apparatus and fill the humidifier with sterile distilled water.
6	Discuss purpose of procedure with patient.
7	Plug flowmeter/humidifier into oxygen source.
8	Check pressure relief valve on humidifier.
9	Place mask over patient's nose and mouth in most comfortable position possible after allowing the oxygen flow to fill the reservoir bag.
10	Check the humidifier operation and adjust flow appropriately to keep bag inflated.
11	Readjust mask as needed and instruct patient and others to terminate smoking in the room.
12	Wash hands.
13	Hang NO SMOKING sign in the room.
14	Chart the procedure in the patient's chart and fill out necessary forms.

PROCEDURE 10-10

Operational check—nonrebreathing oronasal oxygen face mask

No.	Steps in performing the procedure
	The practitioner will visit each patient and check operation of nonrebreathing oronasal oxygen face mask, according to the following steps.
1	Verify physician order.
2	Review patient's progress notes.
3	Review respiratory therapy notes.
4	Wash hands.
5	Introdce yourself to patient.
6	Identify patient by wrist band.
7	Verify correct liter flow from flowmeter.
8	Remove connecting tube.
9	Occlude delivery tube and note operation of safety relief valve on humidifier.
10	Reconnect delivery tube.
11	If needed, turn flowmeter "off."
12	Empty water from humidifier reservoir.
13	Rinse reservoir jar and refill with sterile distilled water.
14	Where applicable, replace humidifier according to departmental quality assurance program (maximum q 9 to 12 hours).
15	Adjust flowmeter to "on" and set prescribed liter flow.
16	Note operation of flowmeter.
17	Check placement of mask for the following.
	17.1 Band comfort
	17.2 Position
	17.3 Leaks
	17.4 Deflation of bag during inspiration; adjust oxygen flow accordingly
18	Note and report any tissue reaction to mask pressure on oxygen flow.
19	Provide facial care according to departmental policy.
20	Question patient as to comfort.
21	Wash hands.
22	Replace mask as needed or according to departmental replacement schedule.
23	According to hospital or department policy, record check round activity in patient's chart, noting any special directions or circumstances related to patient's progress and care.
24	Verbally report any circumstances needing attention to appropriate supervisor.

BIBLIOGRAPHY

Anthonisen NR: Hypoxemia and O_2 therapy, Am Rev Respir Dis 126:729, 1982.

Ashbaugh DG, Bigelow DB, Petty TL et al: Acute respiratory distress in adults, Lancet 2:319, 1967.

Banner NR and Govan JR: Long term transtracheal oxygen delivery through microcatheter in patients with hypoxaemia due to chronic obstructive airways disease, Br Med Jrnl 293:111, 1986.

Barack AL, Martin J, and Eckman M: Positive pressure respiration and its application to the treatment of acute pulmonary edema and respiratory obstruction, Proc Soc Clin Invest 16-664, 1937.

Block ER: Oxygen therapy. In Fishman AP, editor. Update: pulmonary diseases and disorders, New York, 1982, McGraw-Hill.

Christopher KL et al: The safety, efficacy and efficiency of a new transtracheal procedure and catheter, Am Rev of Resp Dis 133(4):A209, 1986.

Christopher KL et al: Transtracheal oxygen therapy for refractory hypoxemia, JAMA 256:494, 1986.

Christopher KL et al: Transtracheal oxygen therapy (submitted).

Covelli HD, Weled BJ, and Beekman JF: Efficacy of continuous positive airway pressure administered by face mask, Chest 81:147, 1982.

Demeri RR: Oxygen delivery systems for use in acute respiratory failure, Respir Care 28:533, 1983.

Dorinsky PM and Whitcomb ME: The effect of PEEP on cardiac output, Chest 84:210, 1983.

Ellman H and Dembin H: Lack of adverse hemodynamic effects of PEEP in patients with acute respiratory failure, Crit Care Med 10:706, 1982.

Findley LJ, Whelan DM, and Moser KM: Long-term oxygen therapy in COPD, Chest 4:671, 1983.

Fisher AB and Forman HJ: Oxygen utilization and toxicity in the lungs. In Fishman AP et al (editors). The respiratory system: circulation and nonrespiratory functions, Bethesda, 1984, American Physiological Society.

Frank L and Massaro D: The lung and oxygen toxicity, Arch Internal Med 139:347, 1979.

George RB: Intermittent CPAP to prevent atelectasis in postoperative patients, Respir Care 28:71, 1983.

Gregory GA, Kitterman JA, Phibbs RH et al: Treatment of idiopathic respiratory distress syndrome with continuous positive airway pressure, N Engl J Med 284:1333, 1971.

Heimlich HJ: Respiratory rehabilitation with transtracheal oxygen system, Ann Otol Rhinol Laryngol 91:643, 1982.

Henry WC, West GA, and Wilson RS: A comparison of the oxygen cost of breathing between a continuous-flow CPAP system and a demand-flow CPAP system, Respir Care 28:1273, 1983.

Jenkinson SG: Pulmonary oxygen toxicity. In Bone RC, editor. Clinics of chest medicine, Philadelphia, 1982, WB Saunders.

Kacmarek RM et al: Technical aspects of positive end expiratory pressure (PEEP). Part I, Physics of PEEP devices, Respir Care 27:1478, 1982.

Kacmarek RM et al: Technical aspects of positive end expiratory pressure (PEEP). Part II, PEEP with positive pressure ventilation, Respir Care 27:1490, 1982.

Kacmarek RM et al: Technical aspects of positive end expiratory pressure (PEEP). Part III, PEEP with spontaneous ventilation, Respir Care 27:1505, 1982.

Kirillof LH et al: Nasal cannula and transtracheal delivery of oxygen (abstract), Chest 86:313, 1984.

Mathewson HS: Carbon dioxide: therapeutic for what? Respir Care 27:1272, 1982.

McDonald GJ: Long-term oxygen therapy delivery systems, Respir Care 28:899, 1983.

McNicholas WT et al: Beneficial effect of oxygen in primary alveolar hypoventilation with central sleep apnea, Am Rev Respir Dis 125:773, 1982.

Op't Holt TB et al: Comparison of changes in airway pressure during continuous positive airway pressure (CPAP) between demand valve and continuous flow devices, Respir Care 27:1200, 1982.

Poulton EP and Oxon DM: Left-sided heart failure with pulmonary oedema: its treatment with the "Pulmonary Plus Pressure Machine," Lancet 231:981, 1936.

Saul GM, Feelez TW, and Mihm FG: Effect of graded administration of PEEP on lung water in noncardiogenic pulmonary edema, Crit Care Med 10:667, 1982.

Shapiro BA, Cane RD, and Harrison RA: Positive end-expiratory pressure in acute lung injury, Chest 83:558, 1983.

Spofford BT and Christopher KL: Tight control of oxygenation, Chest 89(suppl):486S, 1986.

Tyler DC: Positive end expiratory pressure: a review, Crit Care Med 11:300, 1983.

Humidity therapy

On completion of this module the reader will be able to:

1.1 Explain terminology related to understanding physical and physiologic concepts of humidification.

2.1 Interpret facts relative to application of physical and physiologic concepts of humidity.

2.2 Discuss concepts relative to understanding how humidity is generated and depleted and its effects on patients with and without pulmonary disease.

2.3 Explain clinical indications for humidity deficit.

2.4 Point out situations requiring humidification.

2.5 Identify contraindications for addition of humidity.

3.1 Explain the theory of operation for a surface humidifier.

3.2 Describe how a Wick humidifier adds moisture to unhumidified gas.

3.3 Discuss how a bubble humidifier adds moisture to unhumidified gas.

3.4 Compare the principle of operation of a Cascade humidifier to the bubble humidifier.

3.5 Point out the primary difference between the Bennett Cascade II Servo humidifier and the earlier model.

3.6 Describe the Win-Liz (jet) humidifier.

3.7 Describe the spinning disk humidifier.

3.8 Discuss clinical applications of the hygroscopic condenser humidifier and explain its theory of operation.

4.1 Assemble and operate various types of humidifiers in conjunction with various modes of medical gas therapy.

5.1 Conduct patient and equipment check rounds.

6.1 Appraise effectiveness of various humidifiers to prevent humidity deficit in various clinical situations.

7.1 Measure relative and absolute humidity using various types of electrical and mechanical hygrometers.

7.2 Describe the principles of operation for the gravimetric hygrometer.

8.1 Perform service and maintenance on various types of humidifiers.

Humidity is a broad term describing water vapor and particles contained in an environment. For this reason certain terms and concepts presented in this module may also be applied to the module on aerosol therapy.

1.0 PHYSICAL AND PHYSIOLOGIC CONCEPTS OF HUMIDIFICATION

1.1 Terminology

The following terms and definitions will be useful in understanding the language and concepts related to the production of humidity and deposition of aerosol in the tracheobronchial tree.

1 Absolute humidity. Total mass of water vapor or particles present in a unit volume of gas expressed as grams per cubic meter or as a partial pressure, e.g., 47 mm Hg.

2 Ambient. Surrounding on all sides; encompassing. Used to denote the surrounding pressures and temperatures.

3 Atom. Smallest part of an element that has all the properties of that element.

4 Body humidity. The relative humidity of a gas corrected to what the gas could carry at body temperature (37° C) (see Table 11-1).

5 Boiling point. Temperature/pressure at which vapor pressure of a liquid equals atmospheric pressure. The boiling point decreases as one ascends above sea level. For example, boiling water at Denver, Colorado (5000 feet elevation) is barely warm to the touch because the atmospheric pressure is approximately 623 mm Hg as compared to 760 mm Hg at sea level. This means that less heat is required to cause the H_2O molecules to escape to the atmosphere.

6 Brownian movement. Random erratic movement of particles caused by buffeting of molecules of the gas carrying the aerosolized particles.

7 Calorie. Amount of heat needed to raise the temperature of 1 g of water 1° C.

8 Coalescence. To unite. Aerosol particles strike each

TABLE 11-1 H_2O vapor pressure, content, and saturation

Temperature (° C)	Vapor pressure (mm Hg)	H_2O content (mg/L)	% Saturation warmed to body temperature (Body humidity)
0	4.58	4.85	11
5	6.54	6.80	15
10 (50° F)	9.10	9.30	21
20	17.54	17.30	39
25	23.76	23.04	52
30	31.82	30.35	69
35	42.18	39.60	90
37 (98.6° F)	47.07	43.80	100

other as they move in an air stream and grow larger through coalescence.

9 Compound. Combination of two or more elements whose bond requires that they must be separated chemically.

10 Density. Number of droplets (particles) per gas volume. A mist that is heavy like a fog is said to be a dense mist. In this environment particles themselves become a source for vaporizing humidity to surrounding gas molecules.

11 Dewpoint. Temperature at which condensation of water vapor in the air takes place.

12 Diffusion. Movement of a gas from an area in *high* concentration to an area of *lower* concentration across a fully permeable membrane. (See McPherson in the index under "Diffusion."*)

13 Dwell time. The elapsed time in which a substance remains at a location. When a patient inhales an aerosol, it is important to increase the time in which the particles remain in contact with the airways (dwell time).

14 Dynamic equilibrium. A condition of stabilization that is reached when as many molecules re-enter a liquid as leave it (no evaporation loss).

15 Element. Contains only one kind of atom.

16 Evaporation. The transition of a substance from a liquid to the gaseous state that occurs at the surface of the liquid. Energy used to accomplish this process is taken from the remaining portion of the fluid, which grows progressively cooler as molecules are evaporated, or is provided by an external heat source. For example, the constant bubbling of a fish tank or a bubble humidifier will cause the water to cool unless the temperature is maintained with a heater.

17 Fluid. A term that applies to either a liquid or gas medium. In science, fluid is used when the same physical laws apply.

18 Gram (g). Basic unit of mass of the metric system. Equivalent to 15.432 grains or 1 milliliter (ml). One ounce equals 28.35 g.

19 Humidity. General term relating to the amount of H_2O particles or vapor present in the air.

20 Hygrometer. Device used to measure humidity. Principles usually incorporate change in weight of water-seeking materials (hydroscopic) as moisture is absorbed or the change in temperature of a thermometer that is exposed to evaporating water or a change in the resistance of an electrical wire to a current as the wire becomes exposed to humidity.

21 Laminar flow. Fluid flow situation describing straight line movement of fluid through a passageway (Fig. 11-1). Most desirable in terms of volume moved per unit of time at a given pressure gradient. (See McPherson in the index under "Reynolds' number."*)

22 Latent heat of vaporization. Number of calories required to change 1 ml of a liquid to a vapor without actually heating the liquid; for water this is equal to 540 calories. The expense of calories causes a cooling effect whenever evaporation occurs; the sensation that is felt when alcohol is placed on the skin.

23 Mechanical nebulizer. A gas-powered (air or oxygen) device that produces aerosol through Venturi action with selective baffling to control the particle size.

24 Milliliter (ml). A metric unit of volume; 1000th of a liter.

25 Mixture. Two or more solutions. Can be separated by physical means with each component retaining its original properties.

26 Molecule. Smallest unit of a substance that still possesses the distinctive properties of the substance formed from two or more atoms.

27 Relative humidity (RH). Ratio between H_2O vapor actually present in a volume of gas at a given temperature to that which the gas would be capable of holding if it were 100% saturated. Usually expressed as a percentage of 100% saturation, e.g., 79% relative humidity. (See McPherson in the index under "Humidity, relative."*)

$$\% \text{ RH} = \frac{\text{Actual water vapor}}{\text{Potential water vapor}} \times 100$$

The maximum amount of water that air can carry as a vapor at a given temperature (100% relative humidity) can be determined by Table 11-1.

28 Saturation deficit. Amount of water vapor necessary in addition to that already present per unit volume of air to produce saturation at existing temperature and pressure.

29 Settle. To drop from suspension. Aerosol particles have a tendency to drop out of the carrier gas as they move further away from the nebulizer, with larger particles settling first.

30 Stability. Ability to retain original mass (size). Aerosol particles that float in the carrier gas stream or remain in suspension in the airway are said to be stable.

31 Super-heated mist. Mist warmed above body temperature but less than approximately 52° C (125° F). Super-

*McPherson SP and Spearman CB: Respiratory therapy equipment, ed 4, St. Louis, 1990, The CV Mosby Co.

*McPherson SP and Spearman CB: Respiratory therapy equipment, ed 4, St. Louis, 1990, The CV Mosby Co.

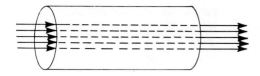

FIGURE 11-1 Laminar flow. Straight line movement of fluid through a passageway.

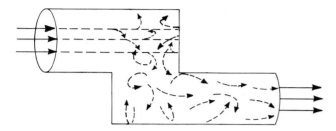

FIGURE 11-2 Turbulent flow. Nonstraight line flow resulting in eddy formations.

heated mist will cause water to be added to the airway.

32 Surface tension. Attraction of molecules at the surface of a fluid causing them to stick together. Attraction is greatest along walls of the container and directly below molecules at fluid surface. This attraction causes fluids to be pulled downward, tending to make the surface smaller. For example, if you look directly across the surface of a glass of water, you will notice the surface has a tendency to bend upward. A needle will float on the surface of a glass filled with water as a result of the surface tension.

33 Tepid mist. Mist warmed to a body temperature of 37° C (98.6° F).

34 Terminal settling velocity. Speed (movement) at which the influence of gravity overpowers forward suspended movement of an aerosol particle, causing it to drop from suspension (see Settle).

35 Turbulent flow. Fluid flow situation describing a nonstraight line flow resulting in eddy formations (Fig. 11-2). Turbulent flow results in a decreased volume of gas moved per unit of time per pressure gradient.

36 Ultrasonic nebulizer. Aerosol produced by mechanical vibration of an electronically powered transducer sending sound waves upward through a liquid reservoir. Sound energy causes fluid particles to be torn away from the surface of the liquid. Speed of *vibration* (frequency) determines droplet size, which is stable within a specified range.

37 Vapor. A substance in the gaseous state as distinguished from the liquid or solid state.

38 Vapor pressure. Molecular pressure exerted by a fluid in all directions. The difference between the vapor pressure and another interface causes a gradient to occur that results in a molecular movement from the area of higher pressure.

39 Vaporization. A process that causes the molecules of a liquid to escape to the surrounding environment (evap-

oration). This occurs whenever vapor pressure in the surrounding environment is less than that of the exposed liquid. (See McPherson in the index under "Matter, state of."*)

40 Viscid. Having a glutinous consistency; thick, sticky. Secretions that are dried on the surface from exposure to poorly humidified gas will become viscid and difficult to expectorate.

2.0 HUMIDITY/HUMIDIFICATION
2.1 Facts and principles

The following facts and principles will be useful in applying gas flow physics and humidity to clinical situations.

1 In medical gas therapy, *two humidity deficits* are created. The *first* is created as the gas is delivered from its source: either the cylinder or patient station outlet. The *second* is created as the gas is inhaled and raised to 100% relative humidity at 37° C. Humidifiers correct the first deficit by saturating the gas at the humidifier to 100% relative humidity at approximately 50° F. However, this gas, when compared to a body temperature of 98.6° F or 37° C, is only 50% saturated, resulting in the body's having to correct the secondary humidity deficit.

2 Bernoulli's theorem. Describes fluid flow in a horizontal tube with varying constrictions. In this situation lateral wall pressure is least where the forward velocity of the fluid is the greatest. (See McPherson in the index under "Gas flow."*)

3 Venturi principle. Application of Bernoulli's theorem to gas entrainment or nebulizer devices. (See Module Ten, Unit 5.1.)

4 Kinetic gas theory. A theory describing the attraction and movements of molecules in a fluid (gas or liquid). The theory states that:

a Gases are comprised of molecules.

b Molecules move rapidly in all directions at different speeds (Brownian movement).

c The average distance between molecules is large compared to the size of the molecules. This space allows room for the molecules to be compressed, a characteristic of a gas.

d Movement of the molecules is increased with temperature, resulting in an increased gas pressure.

5 Reynold's number. A numerical value assigned to describe the flow point at which laminar gas flow becomes turbulent in a tube system. Reynold's formula is derived to the base 2000. When the *value exceeds 2000*, flow will become turbulent and resistance to flow will geometrically increase according to the increase in flow.

6 Humidity (water in vapor form) replaces a volume of air, in part. The amount of volume replaced depends on temperature. For example:

a At 25° C, the water vapor pressure is 23 mm Hg,

---

*McPherson SP and Spearman CB: Respiratory therapy equipment, ed 4, St. Louis, 1990, The CV Mosby Co.

and the water vapor is 3.44% or 0.023 ml/L.

b At 37° C, the water vapor pressure is 47 mm Hg, and the water vapor is 6.2%, or 0.44 ml/L.

c At 85° C, the water vapor pressure is 468.7 mm Hg, and the water vapor is 61.7% or 0.0367 ml/L.

d At 100° C, the water vapor pressure is 760 mm Hg, and the water vapor is 100%, or 0.574 ml/L.

7 When the *temperature* of a gas *drops,* the *water vapor content rises* above the saturation point. For example, in a heated aerosol being delivered through a large bore tubing, excess water forms microcloud particles around condensation nuclei in the air. As the dewpoint continues to fall to 37° C, 0.044 ml/L of water (100% relative humidity) is reached. This is the saturation point of the gas volume at 37° C, i.e., all that the air will hold as humidity. Any water vapor that is present above 0.044 ml/L condenses out on condensation nuclei, of particles already formed, causing a doubling in particle size every 20° C drop in temperature. Water also condenses out in the tubing. With a temperature drop from 100° to 37° C, the humidity rainout would be 0.530 ml/L. This causes a snowball effect in which the rapidly growing particles in the lighter and less viscous air "rain out," causing water to collect on tubing walls. This results in progressively less humidity being delivered to the patient as more water vapor condenses and collects in the delivery tubing.

8 Humidity is water in the vapor state that cannot be seen with the unaided eye. Because it is a vapor, positive pressure will cause condensation to occur with subsequent rainout of water, much the same as one "wrings water from a sponge." In many humidifiers, humidity is converted to particulate matter by the pressure generated by the source gas that is flowing through the unit. For example, if a gas flow of 6 lpm is to be delivered through a $\frac{3}{16}''$ inside diameter (I.D.) tubing 3 feet long, a pressure head of approximately 21 psi must be generated to cause the gas flow to the patient. This causes a compression "rain out" of approximately 50% of the water vapor that originally left the humidifier, resulting in a relative humidity of the inspired gas at the patient of 12% to 13%. This causes a humidity deficit that must be satisfied by the patient.

9 A humidity deficit is also caused by the difference in temperature between the gas that receives water vapor at the humidifier at approximately 27° C (80° F) and the same gas that is inhaled and warmed by the patient to 37° C (98.6° F). A rough approximation of this deficit can be obtained by comparing the humidity content of air 100% saturated at 20° C (68° F) and the same volume of air 100% saturated at 37° C (Table 11-1). The deficit is 43.80 mg/L at 37° C − 17.30 mg/L at 20° C or a 26.5 mg/L difference. This deficit must be corrected by the body as the air is inhaled. The heating of the air and the adding of humidity by the body *causes work and dehydration of the airway* in the already compromised pulmonary patient.

10 Humidity naturally comprises part of an air volume unless it is dehumidified. Humidity does not *add* water to the lungs. Unless it is supersaturated by heating, humidity prevents the lungs from *evaporating* water, at an expense of 603 g calories/ml of water evaporated by the airway. Rarely in the natural state does an individual breathe 100% humidified air. Heating air removes 1 calorie/L. When heat liberation is blocked through the lungs, increased capillary perfusion to the skin must be produced to get rid of the extra heat. Breathing accounts for one third of body heat loss. This is very apparent in the animal that pants to cool itself. If heat is added to the body from condensation of water that is inhaled from heated air humidifiers, 603 calories/ml of water condensed is added to body heat. This excess must be eliminated if a normal body temperature is to be maintained.

11 Air has weight. Dry air is heavier than humidified air at the same temperature. Cold air is heavier than hot air.

a At 22° C, dry air weighs 1.2929 g/L; humidified air is 1.2837 g/L.

b At 37° C, dry air weighs 1.1389 g/L; humidified air is 1.1123 g/L.

c At 87° C, dry air weighs 0.6453 g/L; humidified air is 0.5638 g/L.

d At 100° C, dry air weights 0.4989 g/L; humidified air is 0.3925 g/L.

12 A given volume of air will support, or temporarily hold in suspension, aerosol particles in proportion to its weight. Humidified air at body temperature is two times the weight of air at 85° C and four times as heavy as air at 100° C. This means that for a given size aerosol particles moving at the same velocity will settle out faster in heated air than in cool air.

2.2 Application of concepts of humidity/humidification

1 Humidity is a general term that describes water or vapor present in the atmosphere.

2 As a vapor, humidity is *not* visible *unless its dewpoint is reached,* causing it to condense and appear as dew, fog, mist, or clouds.

3 The water vapor present in a volume of air is measured as relative humidity and absolute humidity.

4 The amount of moisture (humidity) that air can hold is dependent on its pressure and temperature.

5 Clinically, gas delivered to a patient containing less than 1.18 g of water per cubic foot (43.90 mg/L) at 37° C (98.6° F) will create a humidity deficit as it is inhaled. (See Unit 2.1, No. 9.)

6 A gas that is 100% saturated at temperature/pressure will not hold more moisture unless the *temperature is increased* and/or *pressure decreased.* Beyond the point of 100% saturation, a molecule of water vapor will be deposited as condensate from the air for every water molecule that is evaporated into the air, causing a state of dynamic equilibrium to be reached. In closed con-

tainers the water in the container does not evaporate because the air in the space above the water is 100% saturated and a state of dynamic equilibrium exists.

7 Humidity is derived from any open source of water, such as:

a Lakes, rivers, oceans

b Plants, animals, humans

c Food, wood, materials

8 Air acquires humidity through the process of vaporization. In this process, water molecules move from an area of *high to low* vapor pressure until equilibrium is achieved.

9 Equilibrium of water vapor pressure is achieved when as many molecules re-enter a liquid as leave it (dynamic equilibrium).

10 Dynamic equilibrium occurs when water vapor pressure (gas) surrounding a liquid is 100% saturated. As previously explained, this occurs when a liquid is stored in a closed container.

11 Vaporization (evaporation) expends heat energy causing temperature of the fluid to decrease. If no actual heat is used, the energy comes from *within the fluid itself,* and is known as the *latent heat of vaporization.*

12 Condensation releases energy, causing the temperature of the surrounding area to increase. This phenomenon is seen in nature as the outside temperature rises just before a large snow storm because of the condensation of water vapor to form snow crystals. Clinically this occurs in croupettes or other closed chambers in which condensation exceeds vaporization.

13 Pulmonary airways adhere to the principles of vaporization and condensation.

14 Therefore tissues and secretions in the pulmonary airways also adhere to the principles of vaporization and condensation.

15 Dewpoint temperature is the temperature at which gas becomes saturated with water vapor, causing it to condense and "rain out" as a particulate water, e.g., fog.

16 Clinically, dewpoint is reached in gas delivery tubes and in patient's airways, causing condensate to be deposited. In delivery tubes this is undesirable as water may be aspirated into the airways or cause an obstruction to gas flow through the tube. In the airways, this may be desirable as a means of adding water to lubricate dried secretions.

17 The cilia are *hair-like projections* extending from epithelial cells of upper airways that constantly move secretions at a rate of approximately 2 cm/min toward the surface by wavelike motions. Studies have shown that the ciliary action is impaired when relative humidity falls below 70%, and ceases if humidity falls below 30%.

18 The *purpose for controlled humidity* in man includes:

a The control of body temperature through evaporation of perspiration

b The source of moisture to mucosal lining of airways to support ciliary function

c The source of moisture to help keep the mucous blanket fluid and mobile

d The source of moisture for secretions to prevent dryness and incrustation

e A means of preventing a humidity deficit in inspired gases, especially from oxygen therapy sources

19 Anatomic structures of the body serve to warm and humidify inhaled gases so that gas in the bronchiolar region is constantly maintained at 98.6° F and 100% relative humidity (RH). The *approximate* humidity added by each region is presented below.

a Vascular structure of nose/pharynx   75% RH

b Structure below larynx   25% RH

c Carina region   100% RH

2.3 Clinical indications of humidity deficit

The signs of humidity deficit should be quickly recognized by alert respiratory care personnel. These signs include:

1 Reduced ciliary action and reduced tracheobronchial toilet (cleaning). In this situation, the patient usually has a dry, hacking, *nonproductive cough,* although the presence of secretions is suspected.

2 Inspissated secretions, resulting in elevated airflow resistance, increased level of infection, and atelectasis. When this occurs the patient usually has increased bronchial sounds, labored breathing, and low-grade temperature.

3 Earache. This may be caused by pressure on the eardrum. The patient complains that swallowing does not clear the pressure. This is because a swollen eustachian tube does not permit an equalization of pressure to occur.

4 Substernal pain. Inflammation of airway tissue from contact with dry gas. Patient complains that it burns whenever a deep breath is taken.

5 Sore throat. Exposure of laryngopharyngeal region to dry gas. Patient complains of pain and a feeling of obstruction whenever he attempts to swallow.

6 Dryness of skin. The patient's skin appears dry and wrinkled and the sclera of the eye appears to have lost its turgor (not full).

7 Unstable control of body fluids. In a normal environment a healthy person loses 250 to 300 ml of water daily to humidify inspired air. A pulmonary patient loses 1000 to 2000 ml of fluid, which can result in a fluid imbalance with possible electrolyte complications if it is not recognized and resolved through fluid intake or humidification of inhaled gases.

2.4 Situations requiring humidification

The following conditions require the addition of humidity to the inspired air. This humidity may be provided in the form of water vapor or as particulate droplets (aerosol).

1 Administration of medical gases from a cylinder or pipeline.

2 An environmental relative humidity of less than 40% in a patient *without* lung disease.

3 An environmental relative humidity of less than 70% in a patient *with* lung disease.

4 A patient with known secretions or a condition that causes an increase in the production of secretions.

5 Any situation in which a patient's normal anatomic routes for humidification are bypassed, such as a tracheal tube.

2.5 Contraindications for addition of humidity

The administration of humidity, like oxygen, should be controlled. One must not assume that all patients require humidity or fall in the trap of illogically thinking that "if a little bit is good, a lot must be better." The following conditions do *not* require the addition of humidity.

1 Situations in which the environment is already at 100% relative humidity at a fixed temperature.

2 Situations in which the patient's body temperature may increase beyond desired levels.

3 Situations in which equipment may be damaged to the point that it can be ineffective and dangerous to the patient.

4 Situations in which secretions may swell and block the patient's airway.

5 Situations in which humidity will add excessive water to the patient's system causing an undesirable fluid and electrolyte imbalance.

6 Situations in which humidity may saturate a surgical dressing, causing a site for infection or delayed healing.

7 These are only some of the contraindications for the use of humidity. Respiratory care personnel should be aware that others do exist and request advice whenever a questionable situation arises.

3.0 PRINCIPLES OF OPERATION OF HUMIDIFIERS
3.1 Surface humidifiers (blow-by, pass-over)

1 Humidifiers are devices that add water to the air in the form of a water vapor. There are many brands of humidifiers. The following materials do not represent any particular brand and are presented to provide *operational concepts* that can be applied to the wide variety of humidifiers encountered in the hospital.

2 Surface (pass-over) humidifiers refer to devices that add water vapor to the gases as they come into contact with (pass over) the surface of the water (liquid-air interface). These types of devices are used in small tents; they are sometimes used in rooms.

3 The humidifiers shown in Figs. 11-3 and 11-4 are examples of surface or pressure-type humidifiers.

4 As shown in Figs. 11-3 and 11-4 unhumidified gas enters through an inlet *(1)* and is exposed to open liquid.

5 Humidification results from water molecules moving from liquid to gas at the gas-liquid interface (evaporation) *(2)*. The humidified gas leaves the humidifiers at the outlet *(3)*.

6 Examples of devices using pass-over humidifiers include:

  a Isolettes

  b Incubators

  c "Hot pot" or Emerson ventilator

7 The *effectiveness* of a surface-type humidifier is determined by the:

  a Volume and temperature of liquid reservoir

  b Length of time the gas is exposed to the water (flow rate)

  c Humidity deficit of the gas being exposed

  d Temperature/pressure of the gas being exposed

8 The limitation of the surface (pass-over) humidifier is that it is generally ineffective in situations in which gas flows rapidly over the reservoir surface.

9 The chief hazard of the pass-over humidifier is that the reservoir serves as a potential source of infection from *Pseudomonas* and other water-bred microbes, and its

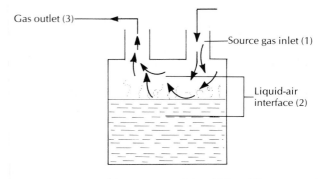

FIGURE 11-3 Surface (pass-over) humidifier. Water vapor is added to gas as it passes over water surface.

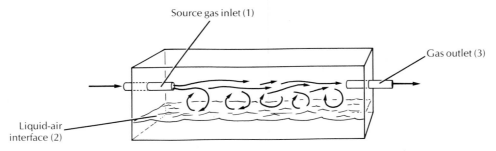

FIGURE 11-4 Water molecules move from liquid to gas (evaporate) at the gas-liquid interface.

general ineffectiveness causes a humidity deficit to occur in the patient.

3.2 Wick humidifier

1 The wick humidifier was initially developed for vaporization of anesthesia gases. Currently it is also used to humidify gases for mechanical ventilator breathing circuits (Fig. 11-5).

2 In this type system, *unhumidified* gas enters through an inlet *(1)* and is exposed to a cloth or sponge (wick), which is partially submerged in a reservoir of liquid (water) *(2)*.

3 *Capillary action* causes water to fill the pores of the wick *(3)* until it is saturated.

4 Gas, when exposed to the wick, picks up humidity by evaporating water molecules from the wick into the gas *(4)*. The humidified gas leaves the humidifier through an outlet to the patient *(5)*.

5 Examples of manufacturers who are producing wick humidifiers for use with ventilators include Bird, Travenol, and Respiratory Care, Inc.

6 Effectiveness of the wick humidifier is determined by the temperature of the water bath, temperature and pressure of the exposed gas, and the humidity deficit of the exposed gas.

7 Limitations of the wick humidifier will vary from model to model. However, it is moderately effective, provided the wick surface is large enough to provide adequate exposure for the volume of gas to be humidified and the exposed gas is in contact with the wick long enough for humidification to occur. Heating the water seems to increase the effectiveness of the wick. The amount of resistance to gas flow is a consideration whenever the system is used.

8 Potential hazards of this type of humidifier are that it serves as a potential breeding environment for *Pseudomonas* and other types of water-bred microbes, and it may not be effective as a humidifier under certain conditions involving large tidal volumes or rapid respiratory rates.

3.3 Diffusion (bubble) humidifier

1 The diffusion or bubble-type humidifier is the most popular type of humidifier. These devices are used primarily with oxygen therapy masks, catheters, and cannulae in an attempt to raise the humidity content of the dry oxygen to acceptable levels. These humidifiers may be heated or unheated. Unheated bubble humidifiers are *not* effective in preventing a humidity deficit because of the difference between 100% saturation of the gas at the humidifier as compared to 30% to 40% relative humidity when the gas is warmed by the body to 37° C (98.6° F) (Fig. 11-6).

NOTE: When environmental humidity is adequate, the use of humidifiers with oxygen therapy equipment probably is not necessary whenever gas flow rates are provided at 4 L/min or less.

2 In the following example of a bubble humidifier, the unhumidified inlet gas is forced down a diffuser tube from a regulated gas source *(1)* to be released as bubbles from a diffuser *(2)* under the surface of a volume of water.

3 Bubbles of gas are exposed to a liquid-air interface on all sides as they float to the surface.

4 During ascent to the surface, the bubbles acquire humidity from the surrounding water by vaporization *(3)*.

5 When the bubbles "pop" *(4)* at the surface, they release water vapor into the gas-filled area above the water's surface, causing it to be humidified.

6 *Simultaneously,* vaporization is constantly occurring at the surface as water molecules are more actively attracted to the gas molecules with decreased water vapor pressure.

7 The humidified gas is carried by the constantly flowing gas to the patient *(5)*.

8 To prevent a build up of excessive pressure in the humidifier reservoir, a relief valve *(6)* is preset by either spring tension or by the weight of the valve to open and release excess pressure to the atmosphere.

9 *Effectiveness of a bubble humidifier* is determined by:

a Number and size of bubbles released from the humidifier diffuser head. Large bubbles generally are *not* as effective as small bubbles because the total gas surface exposed by a few large bubbles is not as great as the area exposed by many small bubbles.

b Time of exposure to reservoir water, both as bubbles and as a gas above the liquid.

c Temperature of the reservoir water. This is impor-

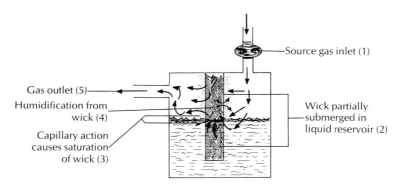

FIGURE 11-5 Wick humidifier.

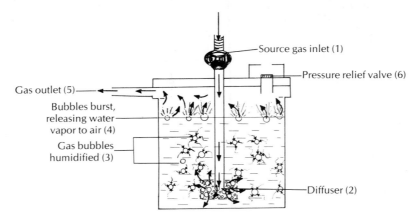

FIGURE 11-6 Bubble-type humidifier.

tant, since vaporization (the source of humidification) constantly cools the water of the reservoir.

d Length and temperature of the delivery tube. If the gas is warmed in the tube by the room as it travels to the patient, the relative humidity will decrease and condensation will occur in the tube. As this gas is inhaled, it is again warmed to body temperature and the relative humidity is still further decreased.

NOTE: Unless the reservoir and delivery tube are heated and maintained at a physiologic temperature, the cooling process that occurs as a result of vaporization and of gas being cooled as it travels to the patient will result in a relative humidity of only 20% to 30% at a body temperature of 37° C (98.6° F). This deficit will cause drying of secretions and other undesirable circumstances related to administration of relatively dry gas.

10 Calculations of required humidity to saturate a given liters per minute flow of gas at 37° C (98.6° F) are as follows:

a Reference to Table 11-1 shows that 43.8 g of water are required to saturate 1 cubic meter of air at 37° C (98.6° F).

b Given:

$$1 \text{ milliliter (ml)} = 1 \text{ gram (g)}$$
$$1 \text{ liter (L)} = 1000 \text{ milliliters (ml)}$$

Factor to determine number of grams necessary to saturate 1 L of gas at 98.6° F = 1000th of 44 g or 0.044 g.

EXAMPLE: A patient is receiving a nasal cannula at
- 6 L/min oxygen flow from a bubble humidifier
- 6 L/min gas × 60 = 360 L/hr of gas to patient
- 360 × 0.044 g = 15.8 H_2O needed per hour to saturate oxygen with humidity at 98.6° F at 6 L/min.

ADDITIONAL CONSIDERATION: A patient breathing at a rate of 12/min allows 5 seconds for each complete cycle of inspiration and exhalation.
- Assuming a desired inspiration to expiration breathing ratio (I:E) of 1:2, 1.6 seconds is al-

lowed for inspiration; 3.4 seconds is allowed for exhalation. This means that two thirds of the time, moisture content originally calculated did not allow for exhalation—two thirds of the breathing cycle. To correct the original requirement of 15.8 g/hr to saturate 360 L of gas (6 L/min × 60 min), the original 15.8 g/hr of water calculated only for the inspiratory phase must be doubled.
- This increases the total moisture requirement for 6 L/min gas flow for 1 hour to 47.4 g or 2 × 15.8 = 31.6. To accomplish this, the gas flow through the humidifier must be increased to 18 L/min or 1080 L/hr.
- *This is impossible* because the maximum output for most bubble humidifiers is 13 L/min or 780 L/hr. Therefore, if 1 L of gas fully saturated at 98.6° F contains 0.0443 g of H_2O/min, 780 L would only contain 34.4 g in 1 hour.

11 In this example, the bubble humidifier *would not be adequate* to meet the required 18 L/min flow rate resulting in 47.4 g H_2O/hr required to saturate the patient's 6 L/min of oxygen flow. This situation results in a relative humidity *deficit* of 13 g H_2O/hr or 27% at 98.6° F.

12 To further complicate the problem, most bubblers deliver gas at approximately 12° to 20° F below room temperature or 50° F. If this gas were warmed to 98.6° F, reference to Table 11-1 would show that air at 50° F or reservoir temperature can only carry 9.3 g H_2O/cubic meter compared to body temperature of 98.6° F and 43.8 g, the maximum body humidity for a bubbler operating without a heater, is reduced to 21.2%.

13 Clinically, this situation results in having the patient supply the energy and moisture necessary to make the differences for humidity of inhaled gases to bring them to 98.6° F at 100% relative humidity (body).

14 Limitations. Bubble humidifiers *generally are ineffective* as humidifiers unless modifications are made to compensate for humidity deficit, such as adjusting the fluid intake of the patient, heating the humidifier and

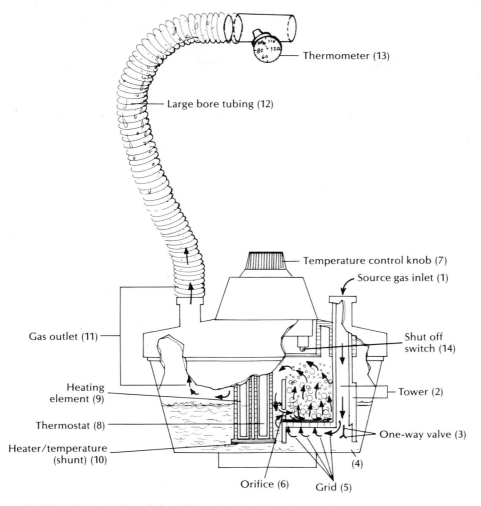

Thermometer (13)

Large bore tubing (12)

Temperature control knob (7)

Source gas inlet (1)

Gas outlet (11)

Shut off switch (14)

Heating element (9)

Tower (2)

Thermostat (8)

One-way valve (3)

Heater/temperature (shunt) (10)

(4)

Orifice (6)

Grid (5)

FIGURE 11-7 Cascade humidifier. (Modified from drawing by Puritan-Bennett Corp.)

delivery tube, or complementing oxygen therapy with periodic heated mist therapy.

15 Hazards. The primary hazard is ineffective humidity at body temperature, resulting in dehydration of the airways and secretions. Although it may not be a hazard, the use of humidifiers whenever they are not indicated is an economic consideration.

3.4 Cascade humidifier

1 The Cascade-type humidifier is based on the cascading principle—the water falls or pours across a surface. In this example, a film of water pours across the surface of a grid that is exposed to the gas to be humidified. Vaporization occurs and the air picks up moisture.

2 Dry gas enters the humidifier inlet from a gas source (Fig. 11-7, *1*).

3 As pressure is built up in the tower *(2)*, water is displaced downward past a one-way valve *(3)* to evacuate the tower *(4)*.

4 The gas then flows upward through a grid that is covered with a film of water that has entered the grid *(5)* by cascading through an orifice *(6)*.

5 The water that spreads across the grid surface has been heated by exposure to a heating element *(9)*. The water temperature is controlled by a control knob *(7)* that is linked to a thermostat housed in a water-tight shield (thermal well) *(8)* and a heating element *(9)*.

6 The heater and switch are interconnected by a metal plate (shunt) *(10)* that keeps the *temperature of the heater controlled* even if the reservoir were to run dry.

7 Humidified gas leaves the humidifier through the outlet port *(11)*.

8 As the gas travels to the patient *(12)*, it will cool to room temperature, causing condensation to occur along the walls of the tube and to pool in bends because of gravity.

9 As condensation occurs, the humidity content will *decrease,* although 100% relative humidity will be maintained at each temperature point as the gas cools.

10 If 100% body humidity is desired, the gas leaving the humidifier must be heated until the temperature of the gas at the distal end of the delivery tube (at the patient's proximal airway) is approximately 98° F.

11 To accomplish this, a thermometer *(13)* must be placed

in the delivery tube at the patient's proximal airway and the temperature of the humidifier adjusted via a control switch until the desired temperature is reached at the end of the delivery tube.

12 Other components of the Bennett Cascade Humidifier include a shut-off switch *(14)* that stops the heater whenever the jaw is removed exposing the thermal wells.

13 A one-way valve *(3)* prevents heated vapors from flowing *backward* whenever gas is not flowing through the unit.

14 A color-coded and numbered control switch *(7)* allows one to estimate output temperatures based on a color-coded and numerical system.

15 Cascade-type or large volume heated humidifiers are manufactured by several companies, although the most popular brand is manufactured by the Puritan-Bennett Corporation.

16 Effectiveness. The Cascade-type humidifier can provide approximately 100% relative humidity at body temperature, if the heater is properly controlled so that gas temperature is about 90° + F at the patient's proximal airway.

CAUTION: The patient must be closely observed when temperatures in this range are used to assure that airway tissue is not harmed as a result of constant exposure to heated gas.

17 Limitations. The Cascade-type humidifier must be operated as a heated unit if it is to provide high levels of humidity. Approximately 20 minutes warm-up time must be allowed before operational temperatures are reached. When used as a heated unit, the delivery tube must be positioned and checked to prevent large accumulations of condensate, which could restrict gas flow and/or be accidentally carried into the patient's airway. When used as part of an assisted ventilation circuit, the Cascade-type humidifier will usually present a small resistance to inhalation as a result of the valve action in the tower.

18 Hazards. As with most electrical devices, possible danger from electrical shock and burns are the greatest potential hazards. With the Puritan-Bennett unit, strict isolation of electrical parts from contact with liquid has reduced this potential considerably.

19 Airway burn resulting from excessive heating of inhaled gases must be carefully guarded against by prescription and careful monitoring of inhaled gas temperatures.

20 In addition, the operator may be burned when changing any heated humidifier. Thermal wells can reach 120° F and the bare heating rod can produce severe burns if touched.

3.5 Bennett Cascade II Servo Controlled Heated Humidifiers

The Bennett Cascade II Servo Controlled Heated Humidifier incorporates a servo mechanism that *automatically adjusts* the heating elements to maintain a *preselected* temperature for the gas at the patient's proximal airway. Although an unlikely occurrence, a potential problem with this type of system is excessive heating that may occur if the thermometer at the patient's airway malfunctions or becomes disconnected from the breathing tube.

3.6 Win-Liz (jet humidifier)

1 The Win-Liz humidifier is a device that adds water vapor by using aerosol particles as an evaporation source (Fig. 11-8).

2 This type of device is used primarily for oxygen therapy devices such as masks, tents, chambers, and T pieces. Some departments use the Win-Liz in ventilation circuits.

3 In Fig. 11-8, a flow of dry gas is directed from a controlled source *(1)* through a "down tube" *(2)* connected to a jet assembly floating just below the surface of the water *(3)*.

4 Gas leaves the jet *(4)* with great forward velocity and causes water particles to be formed as it breaks through the surface of the water *(5)*.

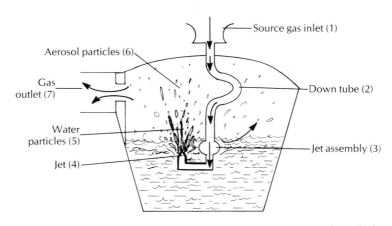

F I G U R E 1 1 - 8 Win-Liz humidifier. This humidifier generates aerosol particles, which serve as an evaporation source.

5 These particles are baffled (blocked) from leaving the humidifier chamber but serve as a massive source for vaporization to occur *(6)*.

6 Humidified gas leaves the humidifier at the outlet *(7)*.

7 As the water level drops, the "down tube," which is flexible *(2)*, is extended so that the jet is always in the proper position.

Notably, the Win-Liz unit has been replaced in many hospitals by Cascade and/or other equally efficient humidifiers. It is presented here primarily because it represents a theoretic approach to humidity production.

3.7 Spinning disk humidifier

1 The spinning disk humidifier is used primarily in large volume devices for humidification of rooms, tents, and chambers. An earlier model was used by Airshields in its ventilator circuit (Fig. 11-9).

2 A spinning disk with vanes *(1)* is powered by an electric motor *(2)*. The spinning disk causes water to be pulled upward *(3)* from a reservoir as a result of cylonic action.

3 The centrifugal force of the spinning disk throws water against a baffle *(4)* on the sides of the reservoir, which breaks it into small particles that are dispersed into the environment by gas flow through the gas outlet *(5)*.

4 Once the particles are dispersed in the room, the suspeneded particles serve as a water source for vaporization to occur as they interface with drier gas molecules in the room.

5 Effectiveness. This type of humidifier usually is *not* effective unless a small area is to be treated. Droplets leaving the humidifier are usually large and raise relative humidity primarily in the area immediately above and around the outlet. The total increase in relative humidity usually is not sufficient to effectively influence relative humidity in a room.

6 Limitations. The unit must be used in a small confined space if it is to be effective in changing relative humidity of surrounding environment. "Rain out" from large droplets can wet the sheets and patient.

7 Hazards. The unit may *not* be effective as a humidifier and cause a false sense of security, leading one to believe that the patient is receiving humidified air. The unit's reservoir serves as a potential breeding chamber for *Pseudomonas* and other types of gram-negative infections. Water droplet dispersion into the environment is a definite source of spreading any contamination present in the reservoir.

3.8 Artificial nose (Fig. 11-10, A and 11-10, B)

1 Hygroscopic condenser humidifier (HCH), the artificial nose, and the heat and moisture exchanger (HME) are all terms describing a device that utilizes a patient's exhaled gas to warm and humidify each subsequent inspiration.

2 This device has been used in Europe for many years but is only now beginning to have increased use in the United States.

3 The HCH is positioned in the patient breathing circuit as close as possible to the patient connection (Fig. 11-10, A).

4 The HCH utilizes the physical principle that exhaled gas is approximately 90% to 95% saturated with water vapor at approximately 1 to 2° C lower than body temperature.

5 As this gas is exhaled through the HCH core, it comes into contact with hygroscopic (water-seeking) material contained in the chamber, its dewpoint is reached, and water condenses onto the surface of the hygroscopic materials and is absorbed (Fig. 11-10, B).

6 With the next inspiration, unhumidified gas passes through the HCH core where it is exposed to the water vapor-enriched hygroscopic materials.

7 These materials, because of the lower existing water content in the inhaled gas, vaporize (release) water vapor to the gas at a prewarmed temperature.

8 These gases are then provided with additional humidity and heat by the body as they are delivered to the patient's lungs.

9 To be effective, these units should have a heat and moisture output of at least 21 to 24 mgH$_2$O/L.

Advantages of the HCH:

1 Inhaled gas can be humidified from 70% to 90% of body humidity.

2 The device is small, is not position sensitive, and does not contain free water that can be spilled.

3 The device does not require a special heat source or water replacement.

Disadvantages

1 Performance of the HCH is indirectly related to the inhaled volume and breathing frequency. As the volume and breathing frequency increase, the ability of the HCH to provide adequately humidified gas at body temperature is decreased.

2 Patients may experience increased resistance to gas flow as tidal volume and flowrates are increased.

3 The unit, if it is not properly secured, may place stress on the patient's airway. HCH production depends on the state of the patient's systemic hydration and body temperature.

4 It may not provide adequate humidification for ventilator patients after 48 to 72 hours.

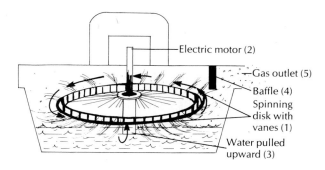

Electric motor (2)
Gas outlet (5)
Baffle (4)
Spinning disk with vanes (1)
Water pulled upward (3)

FIGURE 11-9 Spinning disk humidifier.

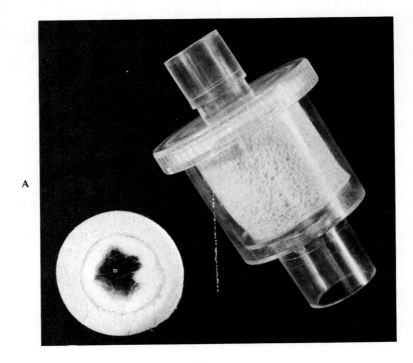

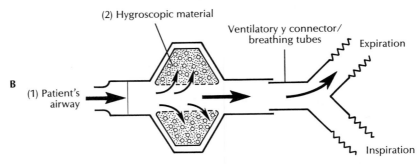

F I G U R E 1 1 - 1 0 A, The Servo Humidifier 150 by Siemens-Elema Ventilation Systems. (Courtesy of Siemens Corp, Union, NJ) **B,** Schematic of hygroscopic condenser humidifier during exhalation.

5 The HCH also should not be used for patients who require humidity therapy.

4.0 OPERATION OF VARIOUS TYPES OF HUMIDIFIERS
4.1 Operation of humidifiers

The following are basic considerations that must be observed when operating any type of humidifier.

1 The humidity output (mg) ml/min must be adequate to prevent airway *complications* such as those described in Unit 4.1 as a result of humidity deficit.

2 The gas flow must be adequate through the unit to allow adjustment of desired liters per minute output to accommodate the patient's minute ventilation.

3 In order for it to operate, the humidifier must be connected to a *proper power* source (compressed air, oxygen, or electricity).

4 All parts must be properly assembled (air-tight) and in good working order.

5 A safety relief valve must be present and operating to prevent an undesirable pressure buildup in the humidifier reservoir container.

6 If a heating unit is used, the control switch must be operative and accurate as measured by a thermometer.

7 When activated, the humidifier must function as designed (i.e., a bubble humidifier should bubble).

8 If a heating device is used, it must be properly grounded and insulated to prevent possible electrical shock to the patient and operator.

9 In all cases, proper reservoir levels must be maintained.

10 Units must be routinely serviced to ensure continued proper operation.

11 Units must be replaced or cleaned at least q 12h or according to a hospital's quality assurance program.

12 Examples of typical procedures for operation of a bubble humidifier with mask oxygen, a Cascade humidifier, and a spinning disk humidifier are included at the end of this module as Procedures 11-1 to 11-3.

5.0 OPERATIONAL CHECKS OF HUMIDIFIERS
5.1 Operational checks

1 Patients receiving humidity therapy must be routinely

assessed for response to therapy and for proper operation of the equipment.

2 During operational checks of equipment, the operator must also consider radical changes in the patient's attitude, level of comfort, restlessness, skin color and condition, body temperature, and mental awareness.

3 A humidifier reservoir must be changed according to a set schedule—water must not be added to already existing water. If the complete humidifier unit is not changed, the reservoir jar must be emptied and rinsed and the humidifier cap assembly rinsed and dried before adding clean distilled water and reconnecting the patient.

NOTE: In prefilled disposable systems, the humidifier is frequently used until the water is depleted to minimal operational limits.

4 Procedures 11-4 to 11-6, at the end of this module, may be used as examples of how to conduct operational checks of various types of humidifiers.

6.0 CLINICAL EVALUATION OF EFFECTIVENESS OF HUMIDIFIERS

6.1 Clinical assessment of effectiveness of humidity therapy

1 The purpose of humidification is to prevent dehydration of airway tissue and secretions leading to accumulation of immobile mucous pooling, infection, increased airway resistance, decreased ventilation of lung areas distal to mucous plug formation (atelectasis), and pneumonia.

2 To facilitate bronchial toilet, inflammatory exudates and secretions must be *thin* enough or free enough in the bronchial airways to be *evacuated* or readily *reabsorbed*. Ventilation must be maintained effectively enough either to mobilize the material or to aid in reabsorption by pulmonary lymphatics.

3 A humidifier is clinically effective if:
a A patient's secretions are thin and easy to evacuate
b The patient does not complain of dryness resulting from gas therapy.
c Lung segments are free of atelectasis
   NOTE: This may require *deep breathing,* as well as intense humidification.
   CAUTION: If the humidifier is effective, the patient may loosen large amounts of secretions that were immobile, causing transient hypoxia. If so, judgment concerning continuation of humidity therapy should be exercised. In most cases humidity therapy should be continued and the patient assisted in evacuation of secretions by cough instructions, postural drainage, and/or airway suction.

7.0 MEASURING HUMIDITY USING HYGROMETERS

7.1 Measurement of humidity (optional)

1 The actual measurement of clinical humidity is a relatively new science. To accomplish this, an instrument known as a *hygrometer* is used.

2 Hygrometers may be used to measure absolute and relative humidity.

3 One method of measuring absolute humidity is to force a known volume of air through tubes with phosphorus pentoxide or calcium chloride. These hygroscopic materials absorb any moisture in the air, causing their weight to increase. Humidity can be determined by measuring the *increase* in weight of the tubes. Tubes are arranged so that no weight gain in the last tubes indicates that all water vapor has been captured by previous tubes.

4 Relative humidity can be measured by:
a A hygrometer, which uses some hygroscopic material that responds by altering its length to humidity changes (cotton string, human hair, etc.)
b Humidity transducers, which change electrical characteristics when they absorb water. An integral substance serves as a resistor or capacitor and changes in capacitance as a result of water loss or gain, which is detected by an electronic circuit and recorded on a meter.
c Regnault's hygrometer. This is a silver tube cooled by the evaporation of liquid ether that reaches the dew-point of surrounding air. Water droplets form on the tube as the temperature of ether is measured. The temperature at which droplets form indicates the pressure of humidity and the absolute humidity can be read from a table.
d The sling psychrometer. This is a form of hygrometer consisting of a pair of accurate thermometers, a *wet* bulb and a *dry* bulb (Fig. 11-11). This device must be moved through the air to obtain readings.

5 The operation of a wet/dry bulb thermometer (hygrometer) (Fig. 11-12) is as follows:
a One thermometer is covered with a wick or woven cloth, and draws water to it from an attached container.
b Evaporation occurs from around the bulb covered by the water-saturated wick.
c The rate of evaporation is governed by the dryness of the surrounding air.
d As evaporation occurs, heat is lost, causing the thermometer temperature to decrease.
e The lower temperature of the wet bulb thermometer is compared with the higher temperature of the dry bulb thermometer.
f The difference in temperatures, which is determined by tables and charts provided with each instrument, is used to translate temperature into relative humidity determinations.

6 Procedure 11-7, which is included at the end of this module, is an example of how to use a sling psychrometer for calculating relative humidity.

7.2 Gravimetric hygrometer

1 The gravimetric hygrometer is a device that measures humidity using a static sample by determining the weight, volume pressure, and temperatures of the sample.

2 Once these values have been measured on the sample,

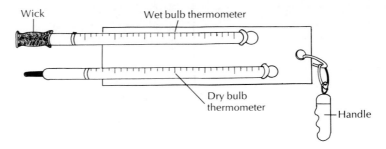

FIGURE 11-11 Sling psychrometer consisting of wet bulb and dry bulb thermometers. Must be moved through air to obtain reading.

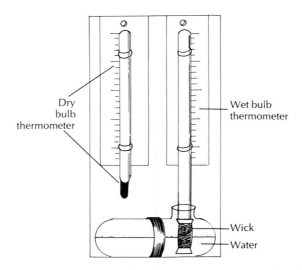

FIGURE 11-12 Operation of a web/dry bulb thermometer.

it is passed through a drying chamber and the weight of the absorbed water is determined.

3 Absolute humidity is then calculated by dividing the weight of the water by the volume of the gas sample.

8.0 SERVICE/MAINTENANCE OF HUMIDIFIERS
8.1 Service/maintenance of humidifiers

Since it is impossible in this module to adequately cover all brands of humidifiers, the Puritan-Bennett bubble-jet unit will be used as an example of general service and maintenance procedures that should be observed with most humidifiers of this type.

NOTE: Difficult repairs should *not* be attempted by respiratory care personnel and, as with all life support equipment, the unit should be given to a qualified biomedical technician for repair (Fig. 11-13).

Symptom	Action
1 Unit will not bubble with function lever on bubble setting *(1)*.	Check liter per minute gas flow. Remove and clean down tube *(2)*. Check diffuser for damage *(3)*. Clean or replace.
2 Relief valve sticks "closed" *(4)*.	Remove/check popett plunger assembly. Clean popett *(5)*, valve seat *(6)*, and valve cavity *(7)* in lid of humidifier.
3 Relief valve sticks "open" *(4)*.	Same as above.
4 Gas leaks around reservoir jar and lid *(8 and 9)*.	Check jar for tight seal and proper thread alignment. Remove/check top of jar edge for possible cracks or chips; replace if needed *(9)*. Remove gasket retainer *(10)* and check gasket *(11)* located inside lid for tears, improper position, missing.
5 Leak around small bore tubing adapter *(12)*.	Check for tight fit by rotating adapter in cavity. Remove adapter and check O ring *(13)* for tears, improper shape (flattened), missing. Replace if needed.
6 Leak around gas inlet connector *(14)*.	Loosen threaded connector and check for cross-threading. Reconnect and check for leak. If leak persists, return to factory for repair.

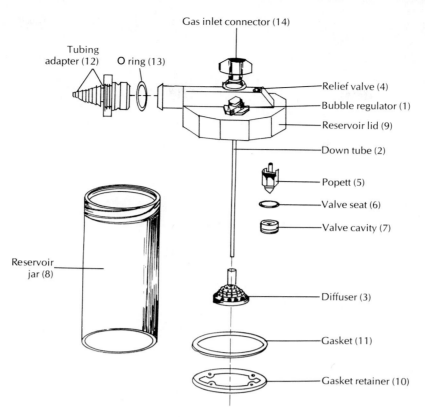

Gas inlet connector (14)

Tubing adapter (12)   O ring (13)

Relief valve (4)

Bubble regulator (1)

Reservoir lid (9)

Down tube (2)

Popett (5)

Valve seat (6)

Valve cavity (7)

Reservoir jar (8)

Diffuser (3)

Gasket (11)

Gasket retainer (10)

F I G U R E   1 1 - 1 3 Parts of Puritan-Bennett bubble-jet type humidifier. (Modified from drawing by Puritan-Bennett Corp.)

7 To reduce any possible hazard of cross-infecton, a humidifier should be cleaned and decontaminated, using chemical disinfectant, gas, or steam autoclaving after each use.

8 More detailed service and maintenance instructions can be acquired on each unit by contacting individual manufacturers.

9 A representative replacement parts inventory for most humidifiers should include:
  a Reservoir jar
  b Retaining ring (gasket in top of jar)
  c Relief valve assembly
  d Diffuser

PROCEDURE 11-1

Use of bubble humidifier for mask oxygen therapy

No.	Steps in performing the procedure
	The practitioner will connect and operate a bubble humidifier using the following steps for mask oxygen therapy.
1	Receive order notification.
2	Wash hands.
3	Select bubble unit from among other available types.
4	Check assembly of unit for gasket, relief valve, needed connectors.
5	Select appropriate flow control device—flowmeter or reducing valve.
6	Attach humidifier to flow control device.
7	Take equipment to patient area; verify physician order; scan chart. Note diagnosis.
8	Wash hands, introduce yourself to patient.
9	Check patient's identification.
10	Explain procedure to patient.
11	Attach flowmeter to oxygen source or reducing valve, if cylinder is ordered.
12	Remove/fill water reservoir with sterile distilled water; or, if unit is disposable, properly connect sterile water unit to flowmeter adapter.
13	Reattach reservoir jar to humidifier cap.
14	Position patient.
15	Adjust flowmeter to prescribed liter flow, check safety "pop-off" by pinching tubing; note proper audible signal, then release.
16	Place oxygen administration device on patient.
17	Observe patient's tolerance to therapy.
18	Ensure patient's comfort.
19	Place NO SMOKING sign on door.
20	Wash hands.
21	Chart therapy and complete department record forms.

PROCEDURE 11-2

Initiation of therapy by Cascade humidifier

No.	Steps in performing the procedure
	The practitioner will follow this procedure when connecting a Cascade humidifier to deliver heated humidity therapy in conjunction with a selected therapy appliance. The practitioner will be especially aware of electrical and heating hazards.
1	Receive order notification.
2	Wash hands.
3	Select, assemble, and check appropriate equipment.
	3.1 Cascade humidifier
	3.2 Flowmeter
	3.3 Adapter tubing from flowmeter to Cascade
	3.4 Sterile distilled water
4	Take equipment to patient area. Verify physician order. Scan chart. Note diagnosis.
5	Wash hands, introduce yourself.
6	Check patient information.
7	Explain procedure to patient.
8	Attach Cascade to appropriate gas source.
9	Remove reservoir jar.
10	Fill reservoir with sterile distilled water.
11	Reattach reservoir to humidifier cap.
12	Attach electrical cord to electrical source.
13	Adjust temperature control for desired level.
14	Attach appropriate tubing with device to measure temperature proximal to patient.
15	Position patient.
16	Allow equipment to warm up (time for warm-up is approximately 20 minutes).
17	Establish prescribed gas flow to Cascade inlet.
18	Observe patient's tolerance to therapy.
19	Note temperature at patient's proximal airway and adjust temperature control as needed.
20	Ensure patient's comfort.
21	Wash hands.
22	Chart therapy and complete department record forms.

PROCEDURE 11-3

Initiation of therapy by spinning disk humidifier

No.	Steps in performing the procedure
	The practitioner will follow this procedure when using a spinning disk humidifier for aerosol therapy. The practitioner will be particularly aware of danger of water with electrical equipment.
1	Receive order notification.
2	Wash hands.
3	Select, assemble, and check appropriate equipment for electrical function.
4	Take equipment to patient area. Verify physician order.
5	Wash hands, then introduce yourself.
6	Check patient's identification.
7	Explain procedure to patient.
8	Fill water reservoir with sterile distilled water.
9	Place spinning disk on reservoir tub.
10	Connect humidifier to electrical source.
11	Adjust directional port.
12	Position patient.
13	Turn on humidifier—note production of mist.
14	Observe patient's tolerance of therapy.
15	Ensure patient's comfort.
16	Wash hands.
17	Chart therapy and complete department record forms.

PROCEDURE 11-4

Operational check for a bubble humidifier

No.	Steps in performing the procedure
	The practitioner will assess the patient and check equipment according to the following steps.
1	Verify order for continuation of therapy.
2	Wash hands.
3	Greet patient.
4	Explain procedure.
5	Disconnect patient from humidifier by removing therapy appliance.
6	Turn off gas flow.
7	Remove humidifier reservoir, empty, rinse container, and refill with sterile distilled water, or replace unit at least every 12 hours, or according to department quality assurance program.
8	Remove humidifier cap assembly from flowmeter, rinse, and dry.
9	Reconnect humidifier cap to jar.
10	Readjust flow acccording to prescription and note proper bubble action of humidifier.
11	Pinch delivery tube and note visual/audible signs of pressure release.
12	Replace therapy appliance on patient's face to ensure maximum therapy/comfort.
	CAUTION: Steps 5-12 must be completed quickly (maximum 1 minute) because the patient's Pa_{O_2} will rapidly decrease once oxygen therapy is interrupted. In critical patients, a substitute oxygen source should be used to provide continuous oxygen therapy while humidifier is being changed or serviced.
13	Observe patient's tolerance to therapy.
14	Ensure patient's comfort.
15	Clear area of used oxygen equipment.
16	Wash hands.
17	Chart activity and complete department record forms.

PROCEDURE 11-5

Operational check for Cascade humidifier

No.	Steps in performing the procedure
	The practitioner will assess the patient and check equipment according to the following steps.
1	Verify order for continuation of therapy.
2	Wash hands.
3	Greet patient.
4	Explain procedure.
5	Disconnect patient from humidifier by removing therapy appliance.
6	Turn off gas flow.
7	Disconnect electrical cord.
8	Remove Cascade reservoir, rinse, and refill with sterile distilled water to proper level, or remove lid/reservoir assembly and replace with a clean unit every 12 hours, or according to department quality assurance program.
9	Fill reservoir to proper level with sterile distilled water.
10	Plug electrical cord into electrical outlet.
11	Adjust gas flow to humidifier inlet.
12	Empty connecting tube of any condensate.
13	Position therapy appliance on patient for maximum effectiveness/comfort.
14	Observe patient's tolerance to therapy.
15	Check gas temperature at patient's airway.
16	Clear area of used equipment.
17	Wash hands.
18	Chart therapy and complete department record forms.

PROCEDURE 11-6

Operation check for spinning disk humidifier

No.	Steps in performing the procedure
	The practitioner will assess the patient and check equipment according to the following steps.
1	Verify order for continuation of therapy.
2	Greet patient, explain procedure.
3	Wash hands.
4	Check equipment for electrical function.
5	Check patient's identification.
6	Disconnect humidifier from electrical source.
7	Empty, rinse, and clean water reservoir.
8	Replace with a clean unit every 12 hours or according to department quality assurance program.
9	Reassemble unit.
10	Adjust directional port.
11	Position patient.
12	Turn on humidifier; note production of mist.
13	Observe patient's tolerance to therapy.
14	Ensure patient's comfort.
15	Wash hands.
16	Chart therapy and complete department record forms.

PROCEDURE 11-7

Use of sling psychrometer to calculate relative humidity

No.	Steps in performing the procedure
	The practitioner will keep the psychrometer moving to prevent air from being saturated with water vapor near the bulb of the wet thermometer.
1	Check water reservoir for fullness.
2	Telescope and swivel psychrometer.
3	Moderately sling psychrometer.
4	Observe readings of both thermometers.
5	Use slide rule or calculator and tables to compute relative humidity.
6	Record date and complete department record forms.

BIBLIOGRAPHY

American National Standard for Humidifiers and Nebulizers for Medical Use ANSI 279: 9. Available from American National Standards Institute Inc, 1430 Broadway, New York, NY 10018.

Hay R and Miller WC: Efficacy of a new hygroscopic condenser humidifier, Crit Care Med 10:49, 1982.

Knudsen J, Lomholt N, and Wisborg K: Postoperative pulmonary complications using dry and humidified anaesthetic gases, Br J Anaesth 45:363, 1973.

McPherson SP and Spearman CB: Respiratory therapy equipment, ed 4, St. Louis, 1990, The CV Mosby Co.

Primiano FP Jr, Montague FW Jr, and Saidel GM: Measurement system for water vapor and temperature dynamics, J Appl Physiol 56:1679, 1984.

Shelly M, Bethune DW, and Latimer RD: A comparison of five heat and moisture exchanges, Anesthesia 41:527, 1986.

Aerosol therapy

LEARNING OBJECTIVES

On completion of this module the reader will be able to:

1.1 Define terminology relating to aerosols.

2.1 Explain facts and principles of aerosol production and deposition.

3.1 Describe factors influencing aerosol density.

3.2 Describe factors influencing particle size.

4.1 Explain the deposition of aerosol.

5.1 List criteria for classification of nebulizers.

5.2 Identify basic types of nebulizers.

6.1 Explain operation of mechanical nebulizers.

6.2 Explain operation of the orifice-type nebulizer.

6.3 Explain operation of the Babington nebulizer.

6.4 Describe history, operation, advantages, and safety components of the ultrasonic nebulizer.

7.1 Describe administration of aerosol via nebulizers.

7.2 Describe administration of ultrasonic nebulization.

8.1 Identify general complications from the use of aerosol.

8.2 Identify potential hazards from using ultrasonic nebulizers.

9.1 Describe ancillary equipment for administration of aerosol therapy.

10.1 Perform patient and equipment check rounds.

11.1 Carry out general care and maintenance of mechanical and ultrasonic nebulizers.

12.1 List pathologic conditions and situations requiring aerosol therapy.

13.1 Describe the expected clinical response to aerosol therapy.

1.0 TERMINOLOGY OF AEROSOLS

1.1 Terminology of aerosols

1 Aerosol. Liquid or solid particles that are produced by an aerosol generator and carried by a flowing gas stream to the patient.

2 Atelectasis. Localized nonexpansion of alveoli.

3 Atomizer. A device that produces an aerosol that *varies* in *particle size*.

4 Agglomerate. To group together in a mass.

5 Baffle. An obstruction that is placed in a gas pathway to cause turbulence or to serve as a surface for impaction of rapidly moving aerosol particles.

6 Coalesce. To unite; to grow together.

7 Condensation. Changing from a gas to a liquid. When this occurs, energy is released to the surrounding medium, causing the temperature to rise.

8 Density. Number of droplets (particles) per gas volume.

9 Diffusion. Movement of a gas from an area of *high* concentration to an area of *lower* concentration across a freely permeable membrane.

10 Dwell time. The elapsed time in which a substance remains at a location.

11 Gram. A metric unit of mass and weight; 1000th part of a kilogram (weight of 1 ml of water).

12 Hypertonic solution. One that has a higher salt content than the blood. Hypertonic solutions when inhaled may cause bronchial irritation and bronchospasm.

13 Hypotonic solution. One that has a lower salt content than the blood.

14 Inertia. Tendency of a mass once started in a direction to continue to move in that direction.

15 Mechanical nebulizer. A nebulizer powered by a gas source of air or oxygen (O_2). Nebulization occurs when gas at high velocity is passed through a stream of liquid, causing particles to be fractured away from the moving stream and forced against baffles.

16 Micro. A prefix used in naming a unit of measurement

that is one millionth the size of the unit to which it is joined. Example: microgram = one millionth of a gram.

17 Micron (μm). A measurement of length. One micron equals one thousandth of a millimeter or 1/25,000 inch. The unit of measurement describing the size of aerosol particles.

18 Nebulizer. A device that produces aerosol particles that are within a *specific size* range because of the arrangement of baffles and the size of the nebulizer jet.

19 Peristaltic movement of the bronchioles. Wavelike progression of alternate contraction and relaxation of the smooth muscle fibers moving foreign particles up the bronchioles toward the proximal airway.

20 Saturation deficit. Amount of water vapor necessary, in addition to that already present per unit volume, to produce saturation at existing temperature and pressure.

21 Settle. To drop from suspension.

22 Stability. Ability of aerosol particles to retain their original mass (size).

23 Superheated mist. Mist warmed above body temperature but less than 52° C (125° F).

24 Tepid mist. Mist warmed to body temperature of 37° C (98.6° F).

25 Terminal settling velocity. Point at which the influence of gravity overpowers forward suspended movement of an object, causing it to drop from suspension.

26 Ultrasonic nebulizer. An electrically powered transducer that produces aerosol sending sound waves upward through a liquid reservoir. Sound energy causes fluid particles to be torn away from the surface of the liquid. Speed of vibration (frequency) determines droplet size, which is stable within a specified range.

2.0 FACTS/PRINCIPLES OF AEROSOL PRODUCTION/DEPOSITION

2.1 Production and deposition of aerosols

1 An aerosol is any liquid or dry particulate matter suspended (floating) in the air.

2 In respiratory care aerosols are produced by mechanical and electrical devices called nebulizers.

3 Nebulizers produce aerosols in the form of particulate liquid viewed as a mist.

4 This mist may appear light or heavy (dense) in quantity.

5 The mist may quickly settle out of the air (rain out) or remain suspended for some time (stable).

6 Each aerosol particle is formed from the solution in the reservoir of the nebulizer and has a particular size and weight (mass) depending on the characteristics of the particular nebulizer.

7 If a mixture is used as a solution, the particle will contain a portion of liquid (solvent) and a portion of particulate (solute).

8 The size of an aerosol particle is described in terms of microns (1 micron = 1/25,000 of an inch) and is many times smaller than the period ending this sentence.

9 Size (mass), combined with the total number of particles produced in a given period of time by a nebulizer (density), *should* determine the amount of aerosolized solution presented to the patient for inhalation.

10 This is *not* true. however, because of the influence of other factors on an aerosol that cause it to alter its mass and density from the time it is produced in the nebulizer until it is deposited at the described location somewhere in the patient's airway.

11 In an aerosol what is seen being produced is definitely not what results at the deposition site.

12 Forces that interplay to change the mass and density of aerosols include:

a Vaporization. An aerosol is a microliquid source (humidifier) that will evaporate its liquid to the surrounding environment according to the difference in water vapor pressure of the particle and surrounding gas molecules. This will continue until each particle reaches a state of *dynamic equilibrium* with its environment. Given normal room temperature and pressure, the rate of vaporization is approximately 10% of the mist volume for every foot away from the nebulizer.

b Coalescence. Aerosol particles are in constant motion from the time they are produced until they are deposited. The microscopic particles are buffeted by *brownian* forces and constantly come into contact with other particles. These microscopic particles, which have not vaporized, grow larger (snowball effect) as they join (coalesce). The larger particles, which have not vaporized and grown smaller, coalesce and grow still larger. Condensation also results in the *rebirth* of aerosol particles, which were initially vaporized as the particles left the nebulizer. Rebirth occurs as *dew point temperature is reached,* causing condensation in the delivery tube. This process is similar to the way in which rain is formed from cloud formations and micronuclei in the upper atmosphere.

c Agglomeration. During the constant growth and evaporation process, particles of all sizes are buffeted by turbulence as they are carried by the moving flow of gas to the patient. *Turbulence* caused by excessive gas flow or bends or obstructions in the delivery tube and connecting equipment causes many of the moving particles to impact (hit) each other as well as the walls of the bent tubing and other obstructions. Particles that are in contact stick together, forming a larger mass.

d "Rain out." Particles that become too large will settle as they strike each other and the walls of the tube and other obstructions. As particles settle in a moving gas stream, they coalesce with the particles below them, causing spaces of unsaturated gas. These spaces are quickly filled with other particles that are influenced by the decreased water vapor pressure and grow smaller.

e Condensation. Tubing, or any container holding or transporting gas containing aerosol, is influenced by the *dew point* temperature. This effect is most noticeable in delivery tubes, which quickly develop pools of condensate from exposure to aerosolized gases. This is especially true when the aerosolized gas is heated. This occurs because the delivery tube is normally at room temperature. As the aerosolized gas comes into contact with the cooler surface of the delivery tube, condensation occurs. This is because the carrier gas contains 100% relative humidity, compared to reservoir temperature, as well as that of the particulate liquid. Pooled condensate increases the process of condensation because of the difference in temperature of the condensate mass and the carrier gas and the added influence of impaction and coalescence.

f Terminal settling velocity (gravity settlement). Factors that determine how long a particle will remain suspended (float) in an air mass depend on the *size* of the particle *(Archimedes' principle)* and the *speed* (velocity, flow rate) of the gas containing the aerosol. The further a particle moves away from the nebulizer, the greater is the tendency to settle. This is based on the fact that particles fall through space at a constant velocity so that with suspended particles the resistance of the air equals the weight of the molecules *(Archimedes' Principle)*. Whenever the particle diameter becomes smaller than the free space between the molecules (Bernoulli—kinetic gas theory), supportive resistance is absent and particles settle out. This factor can be directly related to increase in size and decrease in flow rate. Once inhaled, particles continue to be influenced by all the factors (items a–f) above and especially the influence of inertia and impaction caused by turbulent gas flow. If particles remain suspended long enough to reach the respiratory bronchioles, gas flow becomes a minor factor as very small particles (less than one micron) are suspended as floating agents. Movement in this region is primarily by diffusion and deposition of gravity settlement.

Brownian movement, molecular collision (kinetic gas theory), and even pulsation from the heart beat cause movement and deposition of these very small particles. This movement causes the particles in the lung to coalesce, agglomerate, and settle as they grow too heavy to remain suspended.

13 Air will support and temporarily hold particles in suspension in proportion to the volume of molecules displaced. At body temperature, humidified air is two times the weight of air at 85° C (heated humidifier temperatures) and four times heavier than air at 100° C.

14 Aerosolized water or liquids must be temporarily suspended in the air if it is to be delivered. Only suspended particles can be delivered. Water weighs more than air. Water also changes weight with temperature.
a At a standard, 4° C, 1 L of water weighs 1000 g.
b At 22° C, 1 L of water weighs 997 g.
c At 37° C, 1 L of water weighs 993 g.

d At 85° C, 1 L of water weighs 968 g.
e At 100° C, 1 L of water weighs 958 g.
Particulate water does not change weight with temperature fluctuation as readily as does air.

15 Air at body temperature can only temporarily hold in suspension a given weight and volume of water. The *minimum* effective particle number at 2- to 5-micron particle size is 100 particles/ml. The *maximum* particle-carrying capacity is 1000 particles/ml. This amounts to 1 million particles in 2 to 5 microns/L^3. Particle populations above this size coalesce to form large, heavy particles and "rain out" too rapidly to be carried sufficiently long enough to be transported.

16 Injecting particulate water into 100% humidified air at 100° C results in an aerosol volume of one fourth of that which can carry at 37° C. Injecting particulate water into 85° C 100% humidified air will result in an aerosol delivery of one half the volume as that of air at 37° C.

17 When particles are produced from a fluid, energy is expended. *Electrical charges* are placed on the particles, proportional to the energy expended to produce them. Particles stay suspended longer with larger charges. Naturally formed particles (water condensation around condensation nuclei to form cloud particles) have the least charge and rain out fastest. On the other hand, ultrasonically produced particles have an extreme charge and are unusually stable. Electrical repulsion of particles, one by the other, occurs in proportion to the charge on the particles. This principle is used in Germany as a means of depositing aerosol in the lungs.

18 Nebulizers are of many types. The primary purpose of a nebulizer is to produce particulate material to be delivered into the lungs. The *oldest* type of prototype nebulizer is the *handbulb-operated atomizer*. This device has been used with a number of medications. The particle size produced is dependent upon the speed and force of the hand squeeze. The dose received is dependent upon:
a The exhalation before the squeeze
b The inhalation with the squeeze
c The time of breath holding allowing for "rain out" following the squeeze
d The friction, resulting from flow rate, when squeezed
e The capillary tube and jet size
Because of a *lack* of baffles, most particles produced by the handbulb atomizer are above 10 microns on delivery into the mouth. This constitutes the most inefficient type of nebulizing.

19 The *ultrasonic nebulizer* puts out a very high-density, small particle spray. This is produced by a very high energy expenditure. This puts an extremely high electrical charge on the particles. The particles are very stable because of this charge and do not "rain out" easily. The charges cause electrical repulsion of the particles for each other. This *electrical repulsion* will cause particles to move down a tube in which there is no

flow. Air at body temperature will still carry only 0.1 ml particulate and 0.044 ml/L as humidity. This is the ma.:imum air-carrying capacity regardless of the volume of particles produced. The small, highly charged particles from an ultrasonic nebulizer seem to travel much deeper into the lungs than other nebulizer outputs.

20 Archimedes' principle. A body immersed in a fluid is buoyed up by a force equal to the weight (mass) of the fluid displaced. This is true whether it is a liquid or a gas, e.g., particles in a flowing gas stream are suspended in the stream as long as their weights are less than the weight of air molecules being displaced.

3.0 DENSITY OF AEROSOLS

3.1 Factors influencing aerosol density

The following factors can act separately or together to determine the *density* of an aerosol.

1 Mechanical. In a gas-powered nebulizer, *gas velocity* (L/min flow rate) determines output volume (mist density).

2 Electrical. In ultrasonic nebulizers, *amplitude* of the radio signal determines the degree that the transducer will "expand and contract," creating the strength of the signal that generates the mist.

3 Space into which aerosol is evacuated from nebulizer. The greater the space, the less dense is a given volume of aerosol.

4 Depth of jet below the surface of the liquid. In a Win-Liz floating island nebulizer, the aerosol is produced by forcing a jet of air through the liquid surface creating a mist. The greater the depth, the more dense will be the mist until performance capability of the jet is exceeded and no mist is produced.

5 Surface tension of fluid. In the Babington nebulizer, a thin film is exposed to a jet of gas that causes the film to be broken into aerosolized particles. As the surface tension of the film increases, aerosol production decreases.

3.2 Factors influencing particle size

The following factors determine the *mass* of the aerosol droplet. REMEMBER: Density × Mass × Flow rate = Volume of mist delivered to the patient.

1 Mechanical. In a gas-powered nebulizer, the *size of the jet orifice* determines the size of the particle. The larger the jet orifice, the greater the mass of the particle. The original size or mass of the particle is of primary concern, because the mass of a particle is proportional to the cube of its radius. This means that a particle having a radius twice as large as another will have eight times its mass.

EXAMPLE: A 1-micron particle = 1 × 1 × 1, giving a mass of 1.
A 2-micron particle = 2 × 2 × 2, or 8 times the mass of a 1-micron particle.

Particle size is an important consideration when one is attempting to determine treatment levels of medication where time exposure and particle size vary.

2 Electrical. In ultrasonic nebulizers the *frequency* of the radio signal is preset around 1.35 megacycles. Frequency of the signal when matched with the transducer determines the particle size. The higher the frequency, the smaller the particle produced.

3 Chemical. Because of external influences such as vaporization and condensation, chemical *composition* of the aerosol particle mass will determine size at the time of deposition. For example, if the particle content corresponds to 1% sodium chloride (NaCl) solution, or 2.5% propylene glycol solution, particles will be deposited at the original size. If 80% NaCl solution is used to generate particles in a humidified environment, particles will grow to three times their original mass. Bronchodilators have greater molecular weights than either NaCl or propylene glycol. Therefore, if a nebulized solution contains 0.25% pure bronchodilator, the solvent of the particle mass will be evaporated into the carrier gas, causing the mass of the particle to be approximately half that of when it leaves the nebulizer. This factor not only will alter deposit sites with the airway but also may cause an undesirable drug reaction because of the increasing strength of the medication being delivered. This occurs because of the evaporation of the solvent, leaving increasingly pure levels of solute (drug) in the nebulizer cup—*reconcentration effect*.

4 Environmental. The temperature of the carrier gas and tubing, combined with the relative humidity and density of the aerosol, will directly influence the effects of vaporization and condensation on the aerosol. These factors will cause the particles to decrease or grow in size, depending on the length of exposure and changing temperatures. Effects of vaporization and condensation must be minimized if the particle size is to remain stable from production to the site of desired deposition. Special insulated and/or heated delivery tubes provide a constant temperature between the nebulizer and the patient and greatly minimize the influence of vaporization and condensation. Any aerosolized particles that are introduced into a main gas flow must be at the same temperature and relative humidity as the main flow of gas; otherwise a change in the particle size will occur. Cool mist (less than body temperature) warms as it travels to the patient and tends to evaporate, causing deposition in the smaller airways. Heated mist cools on the way to the patient and grows larger, causing deposition in larger airways. If cool mist is introduced via a sidestream nebulizer into a warmed gas environment, the mist particles will grow larger and be deposited in the patient's mouth and larger airways.

5 Particle size and deposition can be controlled initially by placing *baffles* in the path of moving aerosol particles. This process was successfully demonstrated by Dautrebande as a selective filtration of microaerosols resulting in the output of particles of a specific size. Structural baffles may be designed or, they may be un-

intentional (such as bends in the delivery tubing or restrictions in the inner diameter of the tube caused by connectors or adapters). In his laboratory, Abramson demonstrated that the most effective baffle is a turn or angle in the delivery tube of *180 degrees.* Any change in the structural configuration of the gas conduit from a low resistance gasflow state will result in increased gas-flow turbulence, aerosol mixing, and "rain out." Anatomic and physiologic baffles have the same net effect on particle size and deposition as designed baffles. Turbinates of the nose, angles in the airways, and decreases in the inner diameter of the distal airway structures all serve as baffles influencing the size of particles and site of deposition. The effect of turns or angles on deposition of particles, at a flow rate of 15 L/min gas flow, is presented here:

Degree of bend or angle	% "Rain out" (aerosol deposited)
1 mm	1%
3 mm	10%
5 mm	20%
7 mm	33%

4.0 DEPOSITION OF AEROSOLS
4.1 Deposition of aerosol

To be of maximum efficiency with minimum side effects, aerosols should be administered with a primary deposition target site identified *(predetermined site).* Frequently, a "shotgun approach" is used for selecting nebulizers that produce an aerosol with a broad spectrum of particle sizes. This approach will cause particles to be deposited throughout the respiratory tract and may be functional if the delivery of water is the treatment objective. If drugs are used, the "shotgun approach" frequently results in the patient experiencing side effects before the desired therapeutic results are accomplished. Primary factors determing the *deposition site* of aerosols include:

1 Mass. Numerous studies have shown that mass of the aerosol particle is the most influential determinant of the deposit site. The following can serve as a general guide to the site of deposition for various sizes of particles:

Particle size in microns	Site of deposit
30 or larger	Nose, mouth, upper airway
29-10	Bronchioles
9-3	All of respiratory tract to alveolar ducts
2-0.5	Alveoli
Less than 0.5	Remain suspended, float in-and-out

Smaller droplets reach distal portions of the lung but carry less mass. Therefore, to gain the desired effect, longer periods of administration are required, resulting in systemic reaction caused by *deposition of larger particles in upper airways first.* To deliver functional dosages of medication to lung periphery without untoward effects, the practitioner should use a nebulizer that produces particles in the range of the 2-micron size:

Particle size (micron)	Percent deposit
5	96%
0.5	42%
0.2	21%
Less than 0.2	2.6% (majority float in-and-out)

NOTE: Because of the direct relationship factors that determine the size of the particle, deposit site will also be influenced.

2 Baffles (see Unit 3.2). Baffles, either designed or unplanned, cause particles to be deposited. *Inertial impaction is* the primary mechanism for deposition since particles according to their mass and speed hit surfaces because they cannot turn to follow gas flow around or across the obstruction. Deposition is proportional to the square root of the diameter of the particles. Four times more particles are removed when a particle size is doubled.

  a Particles of 8 to 10 microns are primarily deposited by inertial impaction.

  b Particles of 1 to 8 microns are deposited by sedimentation (gravity settlement)

  c Particles of less than 1 micron are deposited by Brownian motion or diffusion.

3 Temperature/humidity content (see Unit 3.2).

4 Chemical content (see Unit 3.2).

5 Distance traveled. A direct relationship exists between the distance an aerosol particle must travel and the site of deposit. As previously discussed, size will constantly vary. In addition, speed or linear velocity will decrease as distance traveled from the aerosol generator increases, causing the particle to reach its terminal settling velocity and be deposited.

6 Length of exposure. Time is probably the second most influential factor in determining where and how much aerosol will be deposited. The length of time that aerosol remains at the lung site is referred to as *dwell time.* Dwell time in the human lung is determined by:

  a Speed of inhalation (peak flow)

  b Length of breath hold

  c Speed of exhalation (peak flow)

7 The *peak flow rate* of healthy adults on inspiration is approximately 100-300 L/min. Exhalation is 400 to 600 L/min.

8 Ideal breathing pattern. The suggested ideal breathing pattern for maximum deposition of aerosol should be with the subject breathing through an open mouth at the rate of 5 breaths per minute, peak flow of approximately 300 ml/sec, maximum VT of 1350 ml, a breath hold of 5 seconds, and slow exhalation. Slow, deep breaths will primarily deposit large droplets of greater than 8 microns in the depths of the lungs. Rapid, shallow breathing will deposit large particles of greater than 8 microns in the upper airways.

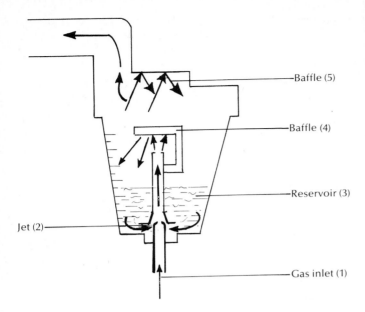

FIGURE 12-1 Small volume jet nebulizer.

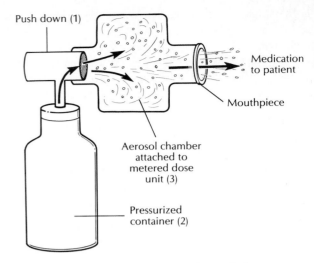

FIGURE 12-2 Metered dose nebulizer.

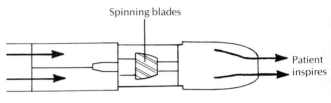

FIGURE 12-3 Spinhaler.

A study by Edward Palmes et al.* showed that fewer particles are exhaled compared to those inhaled during periods of breath-holding up to 30 sec. To gain maximum effective deposition in the alveoli of particles of 0.2 to 0.4 microns, the breath should be held for a maximum of 15 sec before exhalation.

9 Turbulence. Excessive turbulence during pressure breathing and inspiratory airflow will cause particles to be deposited early. To reduce turbulence, delivery tubes should be straight and have a large inner diameter.

5.0 CLASSIFICATION OF NEBULIZERS
5.1 Criteria for classification of nebulizers

Nebulizers are identified according to the following criteria:
1 Size of the reservoir. Small or large volume. A small volume nebulizer usually holds 6 ml of liquid; a large volume nebulizer holds 500 ml or more.
2 Power source. Gas-powered (pneumatic) or electrically powered.
3 Method of aerosol production. Mechanical (jet), ultrasonic, orifice wick, or spinning disk.
4 Placement in patient's breathing tube. Mainstream, sidestream, slipstream.

5.2 Basic types of nebulizers

1 Small volume nebulizer (Fig. 12-1). Reservoir capacity 3 to 6 ml maximum. Powered by O_2 or compressed air *(1)*, the jet entrains medication *(2)* from the reservoir *(3)*. The particles are baffled first at *(4)* and then again at *(5)* before being delivered to the patient.

*Palmes E et al: Deposition of aerosols in the human respiratory tract during breath holding, Institute of Environmental Medicine, 1966, New York University.

2 Large volume nebulizer. Reservoir capacity 250 ml to 1000 ml maximum.
3 Metered dose nebulizer (may or may not have aerosol chamber). A self-contained device powered by an inert gas (Fig. 12-2). Operation of the unit will provide a single dose of medication per maneuver. Total volume is normally 6 to 8 ml. Pushing down *(1)* on the pressurized container *(2)* causes the medication to spray out. If an aersol chamber is used the aerosol is suspended until a breath is taken *(3)* On exhalation the chamber captures exhaled particles to prevent waste.
4 Spinhaler (Fig. 12-3). Brand name for a small volume nebulizer that disperses dry powdered aerosol via the action of spinning impeller blades, which are activated by the patient's inspiratory airflow.
5 Micronebulizer (not shown). A device that administers microaerosolized particles of a specific size through a process of filtering out undesired sizes.
6 Mainstream nebulizer (Fig. 12-4). A device positioned so that a *major* portion of the gas being delivered to the patient passes through the nebulizer *(1)*. The nebulizer jet is powered *(2)* by an additional source of gas. The mainstream is usually a large volume device.
7 Sidestream nebulizer (Fig. 12-5). A nebulizer positioned so that nebulized gas enters the mainstream as a side accessory. The mainstream of gas does not pass through this device. Gas required to power the sidestream nebulizer is added to the volume of main gas flow.

8 Slipstream (Fig. 12-6). Brand name for a device manufactured by Puritan-Bennett Corporation. Incorporates characteristics of both sidestream and mainstream nebulizers in that only a portion of the main gas stream passes through side nebulizer. An additional gas source is required to power the unit and is added to the main gas stream.

6.0 OPERATION OF NEBULIZERS

There are many different brands of nebulizers manufactured for medical purposes. Rather than attempt to identify and explain the operation of each manufacturer's product, this instructional unit categorizes nebulizers according to principles of operation. These principles can be applied to understanding the operation and application of most mechanical and electrical nebulizers.

6.1 Mechanical nebulizers

1 The mechanical nebulizer is one that utilizes a high-pressure gas stream in conjunction with Bernoulli's

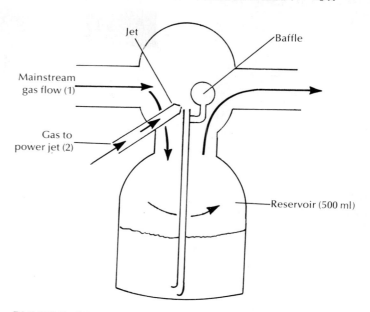

FIGURE 12-4 Mainstream nebulizer. Major portion of gas passes through nebulizer.

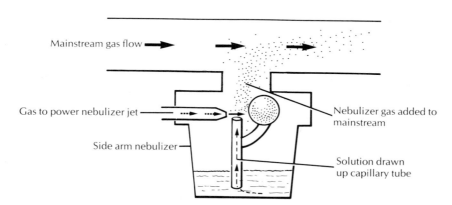

FIGURE 12-5 Sidestream nebulizer. Nebulized gas enters mainstream as side accessory.

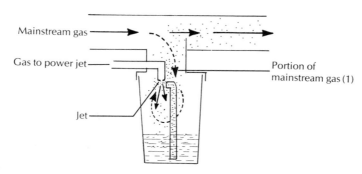

FIGURE 12-6 Slipstream nebulizer. Portion of main gas stream passes through side nebulizer. Unit is powered by additional gas source, which is added to main gas stream.

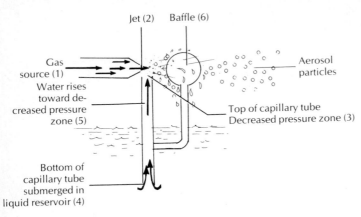

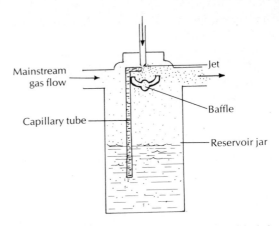

FIGURE 12-7 Mechanical nebulizer. Uses Bernoulli's theorem and Venturi's application to produce an aerosol.

FIGURE 12-8 Bird mechanical nebulizer. (Modified from a drawing courtesy Bird Products Corp, Palm Springs, Calif.)

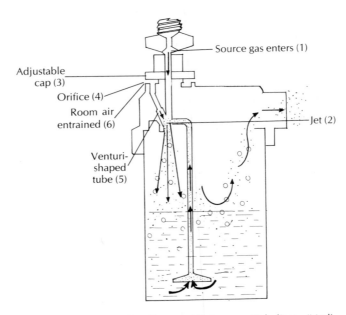

FIGURE 12-9 Puritan-Bennett All Purpose Nebulizer. (Modified from a drawing courtesy Puritan-Bennett Corp, Overland Park, Kan.)

theorem and Venturi's application to produce an aerosol (Fig. 12-7).

2 The power source of this unit is a high-velocity gas stream, which is created as gas is forced by a high pressure source (1) past a jet nozzle (2).

3 As gas leaves the jet nozzle, it passes over the top portion of a capillary tube (3) whose bottom is submerged in a liquid (4).

4 As the jet passes across the opening capillary tube, a decreased pressure gradient is created immediately above the tube—Bernoulli's theorem (3).

5 Atmospheric pressure acting downward on the surface of the liquid causes it to rise toward the decreased pressure zone (5).

6 As the liquid reaches the top of the capillary tube (3), it comes into contact with the high velocity gas leaving the jet nozzle (2).

7 The jet gas breaks the liquid into particles, which are blown toward a designed baffle (6).

8 Because of inertia, large particles cannot follow the gas flow around the baffle and strike the baffle and other surfaces such as the nebulizer lid, the wall, and liquid surfaces.

9 Baffled droplets return to the reservoir and smaller suspended particles are carried by the existing gas flow to the patient.

10 An application of this principle is the Bird 500 ml nebulizer as illustrated by Fig. 12-8.

11 Nebulizers use the Venturi principle to entrain room air to provide gas flow in addition to that powering the jet.

12 If supplemental room air is used, however, the humidity content (mist density) and fraction of inspired oxygen (FIo_2) of source gas used to power the jet will be diluted.

T A B L E 1 2 - 1 Correlation of FIo_2 to gas entrainment

Gas flow L/min	Unrestricted gas flow from nebulizer (L/min) based on Venturi setting including jet flow		
	40%	*70%*	*100%*
2	8	3.2	2
4	16	6.4	4
6	24	9.6	6
8	32	12.8	8
10	40	16.0	10
12	48	19.2	12

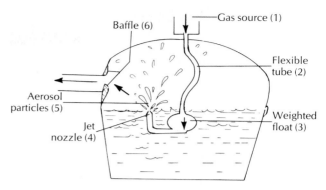

F I G U R E 1 2 - 1 0 Win-Liz unit. Primarily used as room humidifier. Aerosol it produces is used as source of vaporization.

13 The Puritan-Bennett All Purpose Nebulizer represents air entrainment in addition to the primary action of nebulization (Fig. 12-9).

   a In this unit, source gas enters the jet nozzle *(1)* from the flowmeter and leaves with greatly increased linear velocity *(2)*.

   b An adjustable cap *(3)* is positioned so that a series of variable-size orifices can be set *(4)*, allowing the operator to select an FIo_2 for the patient based on the amount of air mixing (entrainment).

   c Gas flow from the jet *(2)* causes a decreased pressure zone along the walls of the Venturi-shaped tube *(5)* and room air is entrained *(6)*.

   d The ratio of room air entrained is determined by the size of the adjustable orifice *(4)*. The relationship is presented in Table 12-1.

6.2 Orifice-type nebulizer (Win-Liz)

The Win-Liz unit is presented in Module Eleven. This nebulizer functions as a humidifier because the aerosol it produces is used as a source of vaporization for the gas that passes through the nebulizer chamber. Particulate liquid (aerosol) is not delivered directly to the patient (Fig. 12-10).

1 A high velocity gas jet *(1)* is connected via a flexible tube *(2)* to a float just below the surface *(3)* of the reservoir liquid with its jet nozzle pointing upward toward the surface of the liquid *(4)*.

2 Source gas leaves the jet with increased forward linear velocity forcing its way through the surface of the liquid.

3 At the surface, liquid particles (aerosol) are created by the jet gas as it breaks through the liquid surface *(5)*.

4 Aerosol density and initial particle size are determined by velocity of the jet gas and by the distance the jet is located below the surface of the liquid.

5 Baffling is used as a secondary means of controlling particle size *(6)*.

6.3 Babington nebulizer (hydrosphere)

This device utilizes the principle of a jet stream of gas being directed through a thin film of continually flowing liquid spread across a rounded surface. The gas penetrates the liquid surface causing aerosol particles to be formed (Fig. 12-11).

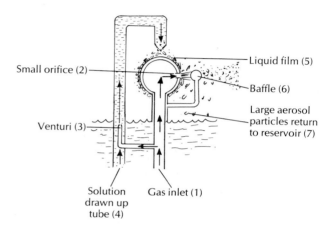

F I G U R E 1 2 - 1 1 Babington nebulizer (hydrosphere). Jet stream of gas passes through thin film of continually flowing liquid spread across rounded surface.

1 Source gas is supplied to the nebulizer through the inlet connection *(1)*.

2 Gas is compressed and its forward velocity is greatly increased as it exits from a very small orifice *(2)*.

3 Pressurized gas also operates a Venturi *(3)* that entrains solution to be nebulized *(4)*.

4 A continuous flow of this liquid spreads as a thin film over a hollow sphere *(5)*.

5 High velocity gas leaving the jet orifice in the dome of the sphere ruptures the surface of the liquid into aerosol particles *(2)*.

6 A baffle keeps particle size controlled *(6)*.

7 Unused liquid is returned to the reservoir for reuse *(7)*.

8 Particle size is determined by the thickness of the film velocity of fluid flow and configuration of the surface. Density is determined by the number of jet orifices located in the sphere.

6.4 Ultrasonic nebulizer

The ultrasonic nebulizer is an outgrowth of paint sprayers, which required uniform particle production. In the ultrasonic nebulizer, aerosol is produced by ultrasonic sound waves emitted from a vibrating transducer and directed upward through a reservoir of liquid. As the ultra-high frequency (1.35 megahertz [MHz]) sound waves break the liquid surface, particles are torn away, creating an aerosol mist.

1 The specific mechanism for mist formation is not clearly understood, although two theories are proposed:

 a The creation of energy reserves on the surface of the liquid in response to directed energy. This energy causes the liquid particles to tear away from the surface of the liquid in the reservoir.

 b Formation and bursting of resonance bubbles as they are created at the liquid surface by the escaping energy.

2 Historically, the Currie brothers discovered in 1880 that a crystal will emit an electrical charge.

3 It was further discovered that the molecules of a crystal will realign themselves in response to an electrical charge.

4 This realignment causes the crystal to grow either larger or smaller.

5 As an alternating charge is applied to a crystal, it will grow larger and smaller (vibrate) at the same rate (frequency) of the charge (Fig. 12-12). Crystal movement is exaggerated to show vibration.

6 A rapid rate will result in a vibration as the transducer rapidly increases and decreases its size.

7 If water is dropped on a rapidly vibrating crystal, the water will be broken into many tiny parts (droplets).

8 If the crystal is submerged under the surface of a liquid, the ultrasonic sound waves forced to the surface will be transferred up through the solution much the same as a rock thrown in a pool will cause ripples that extend outward from the point of impact.

9 One cannot hear ultrasonic energy as it is produced and released because of its ultra high frequency. Sounds greater than 20,000 cycles per second (hertz) are not usually detected by the human ear.

10 There are many brands of ultrasonic nebulizers, although all of them will operate on the same principle (Fig. 12-13).

 a Each type has an electrical module that generates sound waves like a radio transmitter.

 b The sound waves are controlled by frequency—how rapidly they occur *(1)*—and by amplitude—strength of the signal *(2)*.

 c A frequency somewhere between 1.35 to 3 MHz is set by the manufacturers in accordance with the Federal Communications Commission and should not be altered.

 d This frequency determines the particle size ranging from 1 to 10 microns, with an average size of 3 microns overall.

 e The consistent particle size combined with slight electrical charges that are present on the aerosol particle make the ultrasonic aerosol very stable compared with most mechanical nebulizers.

 f Amplitude of the unit *(2)* can be controlled by the operator the same as turning the volume control on a radio. Amplitude determines the volume of mist produced.

 g The wider the control is opened, the stronger is the signal *(2)* and the volume of mist produced (density).

 h The mist density is calculated by measuring the volume of a liquid that a nebulizer will aerosolize in 1 minute (output volume).

 i The output volume will vary depending on the brand of unit between maximums of 3 and 6 ml/min.

 j The electrical module (Fig. 12-14, *1*) should not be immersed in liquid or operated on a wet surface.

11 The transducer assembly *(2)* is comprised of a transducer *(3)* and couplant chamber with water *(4)*. The transducer assembly is connected to the electrical module with a shielded *coaxial cable* to prevent electrical leakage *(5)*. The transducer is matched (tuned) to receive the radio signal produced by the electrical module via the coaxial cable.

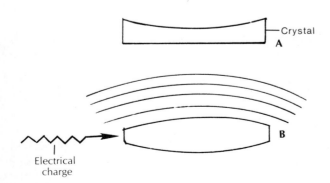

FIGURE 12-12 An alternating charge applied to crystal causes it to vibrate at same frequency as charge. **A,** Crystal before charge applied. **B,** Crystal after charge applied.

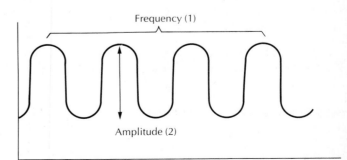

FIGURE 12-13 Sound waves generated by ultrasonic nebulizers.

a Once the unit is turned on, the electrical signal causes the transducer to pulsate at a preset frequency and according to the operator's selection of amplitude. The amplitude also controls mist density.

b Sound waves are generated and directed from the face of the transducer upward toward the surface of the liquid in the reservoir.

c If a flat transducer is used, the sound waves penetrate the surface in vertical lines causing aerosol production.

d If a focused transducer is used, the energy waves peak just below the surface. This causes all the energy to be focused at one point. This type of transducer produces more mist per unit of power than a flat one.

e Transducers may be constructed of very brittle ceramic material or more durable magnetostrictive or nickel sandwiched metals.

f Ceramic transducers used in nebulizers are fragile and are easily broken, even though they may be covered with a metal shield.

g Transducers should not be handled roughly or pressed upon during cleaning.

h Transducers generate heat when operating and should not be used unless they are covered by water.

i Rapid changes in the temperature of water in the cooling chamber must be avoided to prevent cracking the transducers.

j Transducers must not be exposed to salt, soap, or other strong chemicals.

k Transducers carry a small electrical charge for a short period of time even *after* they have been turned off and should *not* be handled unnecessarily.

l Factors causing damage to transducers include:
 • Cavitation—wear caused by holes, like cavities in a tooth

 • Working the transducer too hard (overdriven—mismatch of electrical module to transducer)
 • Overheating—a transducer must be submerged in water at all times during operation to prevent excessive heat build-up and damage to transducer.
 • Physical abuse—because of their fragile structure, transducers cannot be dropped, removed by unqualified persons, or otherwise abused.

12 The couplant chamber (Fig. 12-14, *4*) is so named because it couples (links) the transducer to the nebulizer chamber *(7)* via a separation membrane *(8)*.

a The couplant chamber contains water to cool the transducer during operation. As previously stated, the nebulizer must not be operated unless water is kept in this chamber at all times.

b When the nebulizer is turned on by a master switch *(9)* and the amplitude set by the output control *(6)*, a signal is carried to the transducer *(3)*, which vibrates, sending energy waves up through the water in the couplant chamber and across the reservoir-separation membrane *(8)* to aerosolize the solution in the nebulizer chamber *(7)*.

c A constant level of solution in the nebulizer chamber can be obtained by connecting a tube from the feeder attachment *(10)* to an intravenous (IV) type bottle *(11)*.

d Fluid flow into the nebulizer chamber should equal nebulizer output.

13 Once an aerosol is produced in the nebulizer chamber, it must be carried to the patient by means of a blower module *(12)*.

a To accomplish this, various arrangements are employed, depending on the brand of nebulizer and the therapy modality.

b Some ultrasonic nebulizers contain blowers that are connected to the nebulizer. Others use external

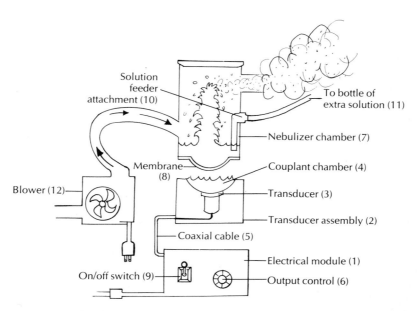

FIGURE 12-14 Components of ultrasonic nebulizer.

blowers (Fig. 12-15, *A*) or gas flow from ventilators *(B)* or flowmeters attached to a cylinder or wall outlet to evacuate the nebulizer cup *(C)*.

c If a flowmeter is used, a small bore tubing adapter must be used to modify the nebulizer inlet to receive the smaller tubing.

d Blowers deliver 20 to 30 L/min of air to the nebulizer cup.

e If a blower is not used, an adequate gas flow must be established to evacuate the volume of mist being produced.

f The L/min of gas required to evacuate a nebulizer must be set according to the volume output setting of the nebulizer.

g The minimum flow of gas necessary to evacuate a nebulizer can be estimated by multiplying the output volume of the nebulizer at any given setting by 2 or approximately 1 L/min gas flow for every 0.5 ml of aerosol produced. EXAMPLE: A nebulizer producing 3 ml/min of aerosol would require a minimum of 6 L/min gas flow to evacuate the nebulizer chamber.

h CAUTION: An ultrasonic nebulizer *must* be evacuated whenever it is operating to prevent heat buildup from condensation occurring in the nebulizer cup and the heat generated by the operating transducer.

i If heat buildup does occur, the nebulizer may stop operating until the transducer has cooled to a proper operating range.

j The practitioner must remember that mist density is dependent on amplitude settling and flow to carrier gas. The higher the gas flow in proportion to the volume of aerosol being produced, the lower the aerosol density.

14 The following are cited advantages of using ultrasonic nebulizers (USN) over mechanical nebulizers:

a Aerosol production is independent of airflow. In mechanical jet nebulizers, the output volume depends on L/min airflow going through the nebulizer. In a USN, production is dependent on total output range as determined by adjusting amplitude.

b USNs produce 100% relative humidity. Aerosol output volume is approximately 10 times greater than that required to saturate a volume of gas 100% at 37° C (98.6° F).

c Airflow used to evacuate the nebulizer can be filtered.

d Nebulizer parts are easily disconnected and can be decontaminated by any of several methods.

e Nebulizers can be operated using a constant water supply to the nebulizer.

f USNs are quiet. With the transducer being ultrasonic (above human hearing range), the only sound comes from the blower.

g USNs produce a dense, stable mist. Approximately 97% of mist produced is within effective range (1 to 5 microns) compared to approximately 55% for pneumatically powered jet nebulizers.

h USNs can add water to the airway. This can be a double-edged sword in that adding water will lubricate and moisten secretions, making it easier for them to be evacuated. However, swelling secretions may increase airway resistance and cause elevated levels of dyspnea resulting from hypoxia. In infants the ultrasonic mist can cause fluid overload and symptoms of drowning. CAUTION: Ultrasonic nebulizers must *not* be used unless the patient's airways are patent or methods (suctioning) have been provided to handle the increased volume in secretions.

It should be noted that ultrasonic nebulizers are not as widely used as they were 10 years ago and in some places are restricted to use for raising sputum samples.

15 Most ultrasonic nebulizers incorporate the following safety features:

a Fuses. Fuses are used to interrupt power to the electrical module and to the transducer if electrical line surges, shorts, or excessive heat buildup occurs. Most units will cease to operate whenever the transducer temperature approaches 77° C (170° F).

b Low-level cut-off switch. This is an open switch that will not complete the electrical circuit from the electrical module to the transducer until a safe water level is present in the couplant assembly. NOTE: This feature is not present in all units and should not be relied upon as an excuse to let the couplant chamber run dry.

7.0 CONSIDERATIONS WHEN ADMINISTERING AEROSOLS
7.1 Administration of aerosol via mechanical nebulizers

Patients receive aerosol therapy intermittently or on a long-term basis. *Intermittent* therapy is normally delivered via a small volume (4 to 6 ml) nebulizer and may be administered with an aerosol mask, directional flow device, or intermittent positive pressure breathing (IPPB) machine. *Long-term* aerosol therapy is usually provided using a large volume (500 ml) mechanical nebulizer, which may be heated, unheated, or ultrasonic. Whichever device is used, the following areas should be considered when administering aerosol.

1 Receipt of proper prescription. The physician's order should contain:

a Type of nebulizer—heated or unheated

b Length/frequency of treatment

c Medication dosage

d Any special related instructions such as special positions, airway care, supplemental O_2 or chest physical therapy

NOTE: Recent evaluation of various brands of nebulizers indicates that the ability to heat the reservoir is most significant in providing optimal humidity for the patient.

2 Patient instruction. Patients must be informed as to the purpose of the aerosol treatment, expected outcomes, proper procedures, and safety factors. They must be placed completely at ease so that respiratory rates and

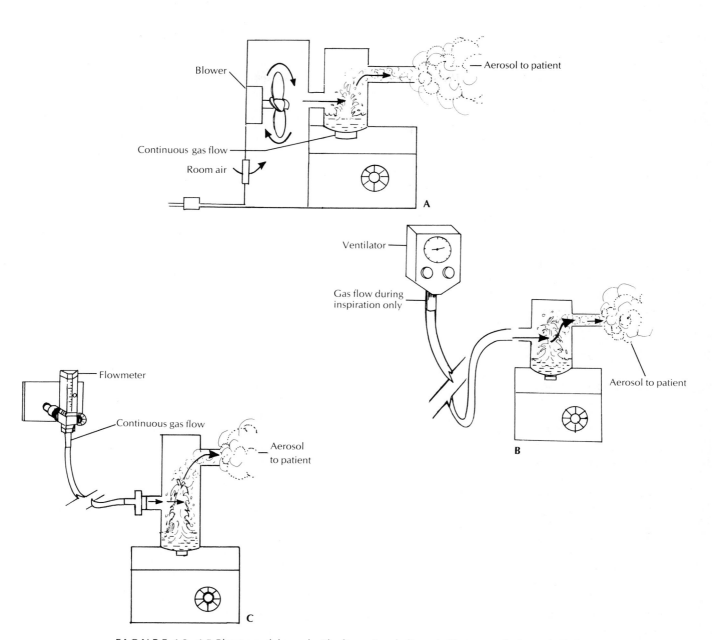

FIGURE 12-15 Blower module used with ultrasonic nebulizer. **A,** Blower attached to unit. **B,** Gas flow from ventilator acts as blower. **C,** Flowmeter utilized as blower.

volumes can be controlled. If patients have copious secretions, they must be instructed in deep breathing and coughing techniques. For maximum benefit, patients should be instructed to take slow, deep breaths at a rate of 5/min, with a pause for a minimum of 5 sec at the end of each breath. If patients are unable to raise and expectorate secretions, equipment and staff must be provided to assist in airway maintenance.

3 Equipment. The nebulizer type should be according to the physician's orders. It must be clean and in proper working order. If it is working properly, an aerosol mist will be seen at the nebulizer outlet port.

4 Patient positioning. It is important to predict at what level the aerosol will be deposited in the bronchial tree. To help accomplish this, the patient's position can be altered to provide maximum ventilation; hence, the flow of aerosol can be directed to specific lung areas.

For example, an upright position will result in maximum ventilation of the upper lobes. To obtain maximum aerosol delivery to the small airways, the mist should be inhaled through an open mouth with teeth and tongue out of the way. Delivery tubes should be free of obstructions to prevent baffling out of larger particles. A 90-degree bend in the tubing will remove up to 25% of mist volume.

5 Special therapy techniques. In addition to proper instructions and positioning, the patient may require additional assistance, such as deep breathing, coughing, or even suctioning. These procedures are necessary to achieve maximum delivery and deposition of aerosol to the bronchial tree.

6 Procedure 12-1 included at the end of this module can be used for administering a small volume nebulizer.

7.2 Administration of ultrasonic nebulization

1 As with any other treatment, USN must be administered according to a physician's orders.

2 The patient's history must be carefully reviewed to note any tendency of episodic hypoxia and dyspnea.

3 The USN must be clean, and sterile water, .9 or .45 NaCl, must be used in the nebulizer cup.

4 The output volume should be adjusted to obtain maximum desired results with minimum patient discomfort from coughing, hypoxia, dyspnea, or tightness of the chest caused by increased airway resistance.

5 The treatment must be explained to the patient. Also, the patient should understand that the unique stable characteristic of ultrasonic nebulization is that it causes secretions to be expectorated up to 1 hour following a treatment.

6 Proper technique should be used with the patient inhaling the mist through the mouth using slow, deep breaths with a pause at the end of each inhalation before exhalation.

7 If a tracheostomy is present, the patient should be instructed to take slow, deep breaths, with a pause to allow "rain out" at the end of each inhalation.

8 CAUTION: Patients receiving USN must be observed for acute changes in airflow characteristics, depth and rate of ventilation, and signs of hypoxia or atelectasis.

9 Procedure 12-2 can be used for administering ultrasonic nebulization.

8.0 POTENTIAL PROBLEMS/COMPLICATIONS OF AEROSOL THERAPY
8.1 General complications from the use of aerosol

Humidification by artificial means has not always been accepted without reservations by a number of authorities.

1 In 1955 Hoffman and Feinberg attributed an increase in incidence of *Pseudomonas* in newborns to high humidity in nurseries.

2 In 1958 McPherson found extensive bacterial contamination of humidifier units and of the carts used to transport the water for filling the humidifiers.

3 Studies have disclosed that significant quantities of bacteria may be disseminated by mist aerosols.

4 In 1960 Modell and others reported tracheal erosion, bronchopneumonia, and death in puppies exposed to an atmosphere of ultrasonically generated saline mist for long periods (72 hours).

5 In 1962 Herzog showed disorders in fluid and electrolyte balance that can occur from the use of high density mist on children.

6 In 1964 Johnson described alterations in lung mechanics and alveolar surface tension following the instillation of normal saline solution into the pulmonary tree of experimental animals.

7 In a follow-up study Huber and Finley confirmed that lavaging the pulmonary tree with saline solution results in marked changes in alveolar structure and loss of surface-active lung extracts.

8 In 1968 a group from Baltimore described atelectasis, interstitial edema, and bronchopneumonia in animals exposed to ultrasonic nebulization.

9 In 1979 problems encountered with the use of aerosol therapy were reported in the Proceedings of the Conference on The Scientific Basis Of In-Hospital Respiratory Therapy sponsored by the National Heart, Lung, and Blood Institute. These problems included:

a Difficulty in estimating or measuring dosages given to a patient by aerosol

b Difficulty in assuring deposition site

c Failure of nebulizers to provide a reproducible dose

d Infection of patients from contaminated nebulizers with primarily *Pseudomonas, Proteus, Alcaligenes, Herellea,* and *Flavobacterium* organisms.

It is important to point out that nebulizers with air entrainment devices cause room air to be drawn into the nebulizer. If this air is contaminated it will infect the solution being delivered to the patient.

In multiple patient rooms care must be taken not to spread infection from one patient to another. In these areas cross-contamination can be minimized by closing the air entrainment port on the nebulizer and powering it with compressed air or 100% O_2.

8.2 Potential hazards from using ultrasonic nebulizers

1 Electrical hazards. USN generate very high voltages and must be grounded to prevent possible shock to the operator or patient. Coaxial cables and other fittings must be routinely inspected to guard against electrical leakages that may interfere with patients who have pacemakers or other electronic devices. Ultrasonic units must be operated on a dry surface and the electrical module protected from submersion or high temperatures during the decontamination process. Only tap water should be used in the type of USN that has a couplant chamber. If distilled water is used, the unit may not operate because of the absence of electrolytes needed to complete the low water-level circuit.

2 Cross-infection. Ultrasonic aerosol presents the same potential source for cross-infection as any other nebulizer. Special attention must be given to the nebulizer cup and air module during cleaning operations. The couplant chamber should be cleaned but is not directly exposed to patient gas because of the separation membrane. Other USN brands have nebulizer cups that *do* come in direct contact with the patient's breathing circuit and therefore should be cleaned as carefully as any other piece of equipment in the patient's breathing circuit. CAUTION: An ultrasonic nebulizer must *not* be operated so that the liquid in the couplant chamber is aerosolized and delivered to the patient.

3 Overhydration of airways. Increased wheezing may occur following administration of ultrasonic aerosol.

  a A jet nebulizer at 40 L/min gas flow delivers 0.5 ml H_2O equal to 13 mg H_2O/L or 0.25 of 100% body humidity.

  b An ultrasonic nebulizer can deliver 4 g of H_2O or 400 mg H_2O/L, which exceeds 53 mg/L required to achieve 100% body humidity.

  c The USN is most effective in removing secretions if used in conjunction with a bronchodilator.

4 Atelectasis. Increased water in the airways increases airway resistance because of swelling of secretions and causes a shift in the opening and closing volumes of small airways. This may cause focal atelectasis if the treatment is not combined with bronchodilator, deep breathing/coughing, and other airway clearance maneuvers such as chest physical therapy.

5 Pathologic changes. In long-term exposure to ultrasonic aerosol (greater than 6 hours), changes resulting in exudate similar to pneumonia have developed.

6 Changes in drug dosage. The drug *reconcentration* effect as a result of evaporation of solvent in the nebulizer cup results in an increasingly stronger dosage being delivered as a treatment progresses. For example, a treatment that begins with normal saline may end with the patient receiving a hypertonic solution.

7 Elevated level of dyspnea. Increased airway resistance combined with inhalation of a dense ultrasonic mist may cause increased hypoxia. A low concentration of supplemental O_2 may be desirable if the patient experiences hypoxia during an aerosol treatment.

8 Changes in fluid electrolyte balances. In infants, especially premature infants, changes in fluid levels and chemistry similar to those seen in fresh and salt water drowning may occur.

9 Excessive cough. High density mist may prove irritating to many patients and result in uncontrolled coughing. This may be eliminated by reducing the volume of mist produced and/or changing the solution being nebulized.

9.0 APPLICATION OF AEROSOLS USING ANCILLARY PIECES OF EQUIPMENT

9.1 Ancillary equipment for administration of aerosol therapy

The following items may be used to deliver aerosol to the patient. The specific mode chosen should depend on desired volume of mist, FIO_2, and patient comfort.

1 Aerosol mask. An aerosol face mask (Fig. 12-16) resembles an oxygen mask with the exception that a large bore inlet adapter *(1)* is provided to attach corrugated tubing from the nebulizer outlet to the mask, and the exhalation ports are also large *(2)* to accommodate exhalation of aerosol without increased resistance resulting from condensate.

  a Either O_2, air, or a combination mixture may be used to power the unit.

  b Gas flow to the mask should be sufficient to prevent CO_2 accumulation or undesired entrainment of room air through the expiratory ports on the face mask. A rule of thumb to observe for selecting an adequate flow rate is to adjust gas flow rate until aerosol can be seen escaping from the expiratory ports during both inhalation and exhalation (Fig. 12-17).

  c Procedure 12-3 can be used for administering an aerosol mask.

2 Face tent. A less confining method of administering aerosol is via an open top mask called a face tent— sometimes called a face shield (Fig. 12-18).

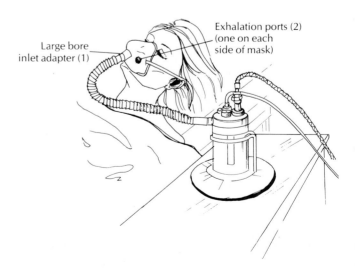

FIGURE 12-16 Continuous aerosol therapy assembly.

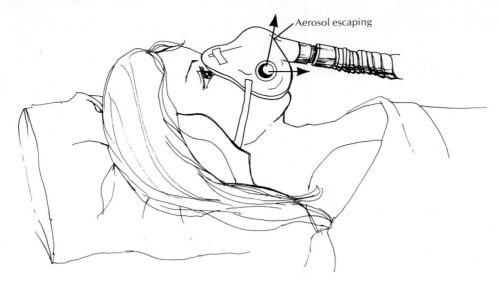

FIGURE 12-17 Aerosol mask. When gas flow is properly adjusted, aerosol can be seen escaping from expiratory ports during inhalation and exhalation.

Aerosol escaping

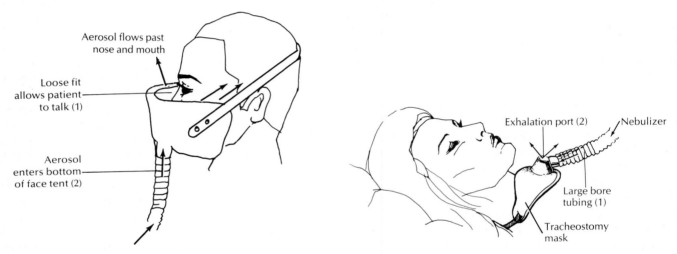

Aerosol flows past nose and mouth

Loose fit allows patient to talk (1)

Aerosol enters bottom of face tent (2)

FIGURE 12-18 Face tent.

Exhalation port (2)

Nebulizer

Large bore tubing (1)

Tracheostomy mask

FIGURE 12-19 Tracheostomy mask (collar).

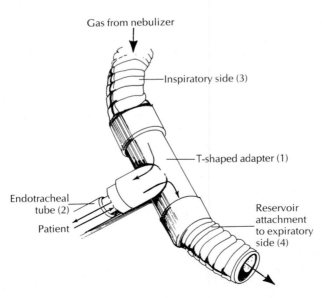

Gas from nebulizer

Inspiratory side (3)

T-shaped adapter (1)

Endotracheal tube (2)

Patient

Reservoir attachment to expiratory side (4)

FIGURE 12-20 Aerosol T (Brigg's) adapter for attachment to endotracheal or tracheostomy tube.

a The face tent allows the patient to talk more freely because it fits loosely about the face and is less confining than an aerosol mask *(1)*.

b A concentration of mist is maintained proximal to the nose and mouth at all times by aerosol entering the bottom of the tent from the nebulizer *(2)*. Ultrasonic mist delivered in this manner is very effective.

c If an elevated FIo_2 is desired, it should be noted that the face tent does *not* deliver as high an FIo_2 (50%) as the aerosol mask (60%) at O_2 flows of 15 L/min.

d Procedure 12-4 can be used for setting up and operating a face tent.

3 Tracheostomy mask (collar). A mask that fits over a patient's tracheostomy tube (Fig. 12-19).

a Aerosol and a controlled FIo_2 is maintained by a large bore tube connected to a nebulizer *(1)*. O_2 therapy for patients with tracheostomies is delivered with either a tracheostomy collar or an aerosol T piece (Fig. 12-20, *1*). In these cases, aerosol is delivered primarily to replace the moisturizing functions of the nose and pharynx, which are bypassed by the tracheostomy or endotracheal tube. O_2 may or may not be used, but when needed it is relatively easy to regulate FIo_2 since it can be controlled with a minimum of air dilution (review oxygen delivery in Module Ten).

b When operating the mask a gas flow is adjusted until a mist is viewed leaving the exhalation port during the patient's inhalation and exhalation (Fig. 12-19, *2*).

c Caution should be observed when using this mask to prevent accidental movement of the patient's tracheostomy tube or contamination of the stoma site.

d Procedure 12-5 can be used for assembly and application of a tracheostomy mask.

4 Aerosol T adapter. A T-shaped adapter (see Fig. 12-20, *1*) can be connected to a patient's tracheostomy tube or to an endotracheal tube *(2)* for administration of aerosol and a controlled FIo_2.

a To prevent CO_2 accumulation, a constant flow of gas from the nebulizer must be provided that meets the patient's peak inspiratory flow demands *(3)*.

b A practical way of determining this is to increase gas flow until an aerosol mist can be seen leaving the expiratory side of the T adapter during inhalation and exhalation.

c A higher FIo_2 (up to 1.0) can be achieved if a reservoir attachment is added to the expiratory side of the T *(4)*. This short piece of tubing helps prevent the patient from pulling in room air through the expiratory side, which would dilute the gas flow from the nebulizer with room air.

d T adapters are used in lieu of tracheostomy masks (collars) and as O_2 therapy attachments to endotracheal tubes. T adapters can be modified to provide continuous positive airway pressure (CPAP) in special circumstances where arterial oxygen tension (Pao_2) cannot be maintained using ambient pressure conditions.

e Procedure 12-6 can be used for assembly and application of a T adapter.

NOTE: In some situations where a high FIo_2 is required a single nebulizer may *not* be capable of providing a flow rate sufficient to meet the patient's inspiratory demands without pulling in room air. One solution is to operate two nebulizers in tandem (dual nebulizers). In this situation the peak flow available to the patient will be the total flow available from both nebulizers.

The final FIo_2 may be calculated using the following formula:

$$\text{Final } FIo_2 = \frac{\% FIo_2 \, (\dot{v} \text{ tot}) \text{ of A} + \% FIo_2 \, (\overline{v} \text{ tot}) \text{ of B}}{60} \times 100$$

5 Environmental chambers. Incubators, pediatric croup tents, hoods, and tents can be used primarily to provide an enriched FIo_2 and/or high humidity therapy. The operation and application of these and other environmental chambers are covered in detail in Module Fourteen.

10.0 PATIENT/EQUIPMENT CHECK ROUNDS
10.1 Patient/equipment check rounds

As with other therapy modalities, the patient's overall *mental* and *physical* condition should be assessed.

1 Any acute changes should be reported to the appropriate medical personnel.

2 Equipment checks should include the adequacy of aerosol output and the temperature control if heated aerosol is being administered.

3 Special care must be observed to ensure that the patient receiving an aerosol is tolerating the treatment well and that expected outcomes are being observed.

4 Caution must be practiced to prevent an uncontrollable accumulation of secretions in the airway or overhydration of the patient's airway, causing swelling and obstruction.

5 If medications are administered, vital signs must be routinely monitored.

6 Procedures 12-7, 12-8, and 12-9 can be used for conducting patient and equipment check rounds.

11.0 GENERAL CARE AND MAINTENANCE OF NEBULIZERS
11.1 General care/maintenance of nebulizers

All equipment should be cleaned and maintained per department policy and manufacturer's instructions. The following are general rules but will apply to most units.

1 Mechanical jet nebulizers (Fig. 12-21)

a Change frequently. Nebulizers are potential sources for water-bred microorganisms and should be changed at least every 12 to 24 hours according to the hospital's quality assurance program.

b Maintain fluid level in reservoir. A nebulizer will not function unless fluids are maintained above minimum levels in nebulizer jars. To refill a reservoir, the practitioner must empty the remaining fluid,

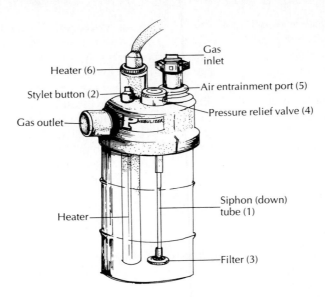

FIGURE 12-21 Care and maintenance of mechanical jet nebulizer. (Modified from a drawing courtesy Puritan-Bennett Corp, Overland Park, Kan.)

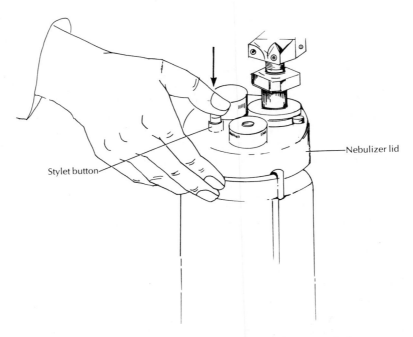

FIGURE 12-22 Depressing a button atop Puritan-Bennett All Purpose Nebulizer causes a built-in wire stylet to be inserted into jet orifice and thus remove any built-up deposits.

rinse the jar, and add fresh fluid. Topping off a nebulizer by adding fluid is dangerous in that it allows more time for microorganisms that are already present to grow in the reservoir.

c Keep jets and tubes clear. The two major components of any jet nebulizer are the jets and the tubes. After a period of operating, mineral deposits, solutes from medications, or sodium chloride (NaCl) collect and occlude the jet at the proximal end of the siphon (down) tube *(1)*.

In the Puritan-Bennett All-Purpose Nebulizer, a built-in wire stylet can be inserted into the jet orifice by depressing a button atop the nebulizer lid *(2)*. In other brands a stylet can be inserted and rotated to clear the orifice (Fig. 12-22). CAUTION: The stylet must be of the proper outside diameter to prevent damage to the orifice. An enlarged jet orifice will result in modified nebulizer performance and particle size. The siphon or liquid tube should be checked and cleared as necessary.

d Change filters frequently. Some nebulizers use a gross filter on the bottom of the siphon tube to prevent any large particles from entering and subsequently obstructing the jet *(3)*. These filters must be cleaned and/or changed each time the unit is decontaminated. An obstructed filter will result in a decreased flow of fluid to the jet and subsequent reduction in aerosol output.

e Check pressure relief valves. All nebulizer units should have pressure relief valves *(4)* that give a *visual* and *audible signal* when operating. These devices are calibrated to open to release gas whenever excessive pressure builds up in the nebulizer circuit. Many units are set to open whenever the circuit pressure exceeds 2 psi. Some manufacturers provide interchangeable relief valves set to vent at various pressures. If a nebulizer incorporates *air entrainment (5)*, the relief valve will *not* work on any setting except 100% because any pressure is vented back through the air entrainment port. Relief valves can be checked by running a low flow of gas (2-3 L/min) into the nebulizer and obstructing the nebulizer gas outlet. As the pressure builds, the relief valve should open. If a relief valve does not work, the practitioner should check for leaks around the jar and nebulizer lid as well as the relief valve. All units must be checked for leaks and operational relief valves each time they are cleaned and during patient/equipment check rounds.

f Check heaters. If heating devices such as elements *(6)* or cuffs are used, they must be checked for accuracy using a thermometer. Damaged wires and electrical leaks should be checked for whenever the nebulizer is cleaned. As a rule, heating devices should not be submerged in a liquid during the decontamination process. Specific service and decontamination instructions should be followed according to department policy and manufacturer's instructions.

g Follow manufacturer's instructions. Manufacturers are required to provide instructions on the care and operation of their devices. These instructions should be followed in addition to department procedure when servicing a unit.

2 Ultrasonic nebulizers

a Check for electrical leaks. Ultrasonic devices generate extremely high voltage and should be checked for frayed cords, loose fittings, and any electrical leaks by qualified service personnel.

b Disassemble and clean nebulizer cup. The nebulizer cup contains the medication (solution) the patient will be breathing. This chamber must be cleaned at least every 12 hours or according to department policy. Ideally, it should be changed between patients if the nebulizer is used for short-term treatments. When decontaminating the nebulizer cup, all fittings should be removed and scrubbed. Parts should then be sterilized using chemicals or other means. Steam should not be used unless the manufacturer states that steam autoclaving can be used.

c Blower. If present, the air filter should be cleaned or exchanged each time the unit is decontaminated and the blower cleaned according to manufacturer's recommendations. REMEMBER: The blower generates gas flow that evacuates the nebulizer chamber. For this reason, if it is not properly decontaminated, the blower can become a *major source for cross-infection*. For specifics on decontamination processes, see Module Nine. Service to the blower may include lubrication of bearings and other parts per manufacturer's instructions.

d Couplant chamber. Some brands have a couplant chamber that contains water to cool the transducer and to transmit sound waves to the nebulizer cup. The water in this chamber should not come into contact with the aerosol being delivered. Saline solution must *not* be used as a coolant. If distilled water is used, some units with water level devices may fail to operate because of a lack of electrolytes in the water. Addition of a small amount of tap water will remedy this problem. The couplant chamber should be washed whenever the unit is decontaminated with a detergent. Soap should not be used to clean the couplant chamber or the nebulizer cup because the fatty composition of soap hinders the ultrasonic activity even though the unit is operating. If this situation occurs, the addition of a small amount of alcohol in the nebulizer cup or couplant chamber should remedy the situation. Do *not* press on the transducer during cleaning or completely submerge the couplant chamber in a cleaning solution. The transducer should be exposed to harsh decontamination chemicals only per manufacturer's instructions.

e Electrical module. The electrical module must *not* be tampered with. For cleaning purposes the outside cabinet should be washed and wiped with a decontamination agent. If the unit has been operated in isolation, it should be gas autoclaved or otherwise decontaminated per the manufacturer's instructions.

12.0 INDICATIONS FOR AEROSOL THERAPY

12.1 Pathologic conditions and situations requiring aerosol therapy

The following pathologic conditions or situations usually require heated or cool mist therapy. Specifics regarding the treatment should be prescribed by the physician.

1 Laryngotracheobronchitis (croup)
2 Status asthmaticus
3 Tracheostomy
4 Refractory chronic bronchitis
5 Bronchiectasis
6 Cystic fibrosis
7 Bronchopneumonia
8 Acute pharyngitis/sinusitis
9 Prolonged ventilatory support
10 Glottic and subglottic edema
11 Other situations resulting in dehydration of the airway and tenacious secretions

13.0 EXPECTED CLINICAL RESPONSES TO AEROSOL THERAPY

13.1 Expected response to aerosol therapy

1 Laryngotracheobronchitis. Reduction of edema in laryngeal region with decreased airway resistance and croupy cough.

2 Status asthmaticus. Thinning of airway secretions with expectoration of ropy, stringy, thick bronchiolar secretions resulting in decreased airway resistance and increased ventilation.

3 Tracheostomy. Prevention of encrustation of secretions distal to the tube with improved general bronchial hydration.

4 Refractory chronic bronchitis. Thinning and expectoration of secretions resulting in decreased inflammation, edema, and cough.

5 Bronchiectasis. Expectoration of voluminous, purulent sputum resulting in decreased bronchial obstruction and bronchitis. Aerosol therapy usually is most effective if combined with postural drainage and other airway evacuation maneuvers.

6 Cystic fibrosis. Thinning of secretions with increased expectoration of thick tenacious secretions.

7 Bronchopneumonia. Expectoration of mucopurulent secretions with reduction in airway resistance and increased ventilation to involved lung areas.

8 Acute pharyngitis/sinusitis. Heated aerosol therapy should result in increased drainage of blocked sinuses with a reduced level of infection and subsequent clearing of inflammation.

9 Prolonged ventilatory support. Mechanical ventilation causes large volumes of dry source gas to be delivered to the patient unless moisture is added using a humidifier or a nebulizer. To be effective, the unit should provide gas at 100% relative humidity at 37° C (98.6° F). Inadequately humidified gas must be avoided because it will result in increased airway resistance resulting from edema of airway tissue and drying of airway secretions.

10 Glottic and subglottic edema. Swelling that may follow traumatic tracheal intubation and extubation is reduced with medication and aerosol.

11 Other situations possibly requiring aerosol therapy include airway burns or other forms of trauma, such as chemical exposure and smoke inhalation. William F. Miller, M.D. of Dallas, Texas, commented that the only way that water can be effectively added to the distal airway is to superheat (greater than 37° C [98.6° F], but less than 59° C [125° F]) and saturate inhaled gases with moisture that will cool, causing condensate to be deposited in the airways.

PROCEDURE 12-1

Initiation of small volume nebulizers for medication delivery

No.	Steps in performing the procedure
	The practitioner will implement the following procedure for either short-term aerosol bronchodilator or other medications given as a treatment.
1	Receive order notification.
2	Wash hands.
3	Select, assemble, and check the following:
	3.1 Small volume nebulizer
	3.2 Connecting tube
	3.3 Flowmeter or cylinder regulator
4	Check patient's chart for order and diagnosis.
5	Wash hands; introduce yourself to patient.
6	Check patient's identification.
7	Explain therapy.
8	Attach flowmeter to gas source; check flowmeter for operation.
9	Unscrew nebulizer reservoir.
10	Place medication in reservoir.
11	Screw on reservoir to nebulizer cap.
12	Attach tubing to flowmeter.
13	Attach tubing to nebulizer jet.
14	Attach equipment such as ancillary tubings and mouthpieces.
15	Give patient treatment instructions.
16	Set flowmeter to desired flow.
17	Position patient and equipment.
18	Administer aerosol; check patient's comfort and vital signs.
19	Observe patient's tolerance to therapy throughout treatment.
20	Instruct and encourage patient to breathe properly.
21	Discontinue therapy when medication is delivered.
22	Have patient cough and breathe deeply.
23	Reposition patient; check for comfort.
24	Wash hands.
25	Chart therapy.

PROCEDURE 12-2

Initiation of aerosol therapy through ultrasonic nebulizer

No.	Steps in performing the procedure
	The practitioner will use this procedure whenever an order for aerosol therapy by ultrasonic nebulization is received. The practitioner should be attentive to electrical hazards and therapy contraindications.
1	Receive order notification.
2	Wash hands.
3	Select, assemble, and check appropriate equipment, being attentive to electrical hazards.
4	Check patient's chart for order and diagnosis and possible contraindications to therapy.
5	Wash hands; introduce yourself to patient.
6	Check patient's identification.
7	Explain therapy.
8	Fill couplant compartment with water or electrolyte as needed (where applicable).
9	Check nebulizer chamber.
10	Place nebulizer chamber in couplant compartment.
11	Secure nebulizer chamber.
12	Attach tubing to blower or gas source.
13	Attach tubing to patient's accessories.
14	Add solution to nebulizer chamber.
15	Place lid on nebulizer chamber. (Omit if disposable unit is used.)
16	Connect electrical cord.
17	Select output.
18	Turn switch on.
19	Properly position patient.
20	Instruct patient on proper breathing techniques.
21	Evaluate effectiveness of treatment and adjust output if required.
22	Assist patient in proper coughing techniques.
23	Monitor patient's progress and level of comfort.
24	Discontinue treatment.
25	Reassure patient and have patient cough.
26	Wash hands.
27	Chart results.

PROCEDURE 12-3

Application of an aerosol mask

No.	Steps in performing the procedure
	The practitioner will administer aerosol and/or oxygen therapy using a heated or unheated nebulizer as prescription indicates.
1	Verify physician's orders.
2	Wash hands.
3	Collect equipment:
	3.1 Flowmeter or reducing valve
	3.2 Nebulizer
	3.3 Large bore connecting tube
	3.4 Aerosol mask
	3.5 Distilled water
4	Introduce yourself to patient.
5	Identify patient.
6	Explain procedure.
7	Wash hands.
8	Assemble equipment in aseptic manner.
9	Fill nebulizer jar with sterile water.
10	Connect flowmeter to gas source.
11	Adjust gas flow for desired FI_{O_2} as indicated.
12	Assess adequacy of aerosol production.
13	Activate and set temperature (if heated aerosol is prescribed).
14	Position patient.
15	Place aerosol mask over patient's mouth and nose.
16	Adjust retaining strap for comfort.
17	If heated aerosol is used, check mist temperature at aerosol mask.
18	Adjust temperature as required.
19	Instruct patient on self-care (coughing) when using the mask.
20	Provide for patient's safety (NO SMOKING sign).
21	Evaluate patient's tolerance of treatment.
22	Wash hands.
23	Chart procedure.

PROCEDURE 12-4

Application of a face tent

No.	Steps in performing the procedure
	The practitioner will administer aerosol and/or oxygen therapy using a heated or unheated nebulizer.
1	Verify physician's order.
2	Wash hands.
3	Collect equipment:
	3.1 Flowmeter or reducing valve
	3.2 Nebulizer
	3.3 Large bore connecting tube
	3.4 Face tent
	3.5 Distilled water
4	Introduce yourself to patient.
5	Identify patient.
6	Explain procedure.
7	Wash hands.
8	Assemble equipment in aseptic manner.
9	Fill nebulizer jar with sterile water.
10	Connect flowmeter to gas source.
11	Adjust gas flow for desired FI_{O_2} as indicated.
12	Assess adequacy of aerosol production.
13	Activate and set temperature (if heated aerosol is prescribed).
14	Position patient.
15	Place face tent in proper position in front of mouth and nose.
16	Adjust face tent for comfort.
17	If heated aerosol, check mist temperature at face tent.
18	Adjust temperature as required.
19	Instruct patient on self-care (coughing) when using face tent.
20	Provide for patient's safety (NO SMOKING sign).
21	Evaluate patient's tolerance of treatment.
22	Wash hands.
23	Chart procedure.

PROCEDURE 12-5

Application of a tracheostomy mask (collar)

No.	Steps in performing the procedure
	The practitioner will administer aerosol and/or oxygen therapy using a heated or unheated nebulizer and a tracheostomy mask.
1	Verify physician's order.
2	Wash hands.
3	Collect equipment:
	3.1 Flowmeter or reducing valve
	3.2 Nebulizer
	3.3 Large bore connecting tube
	3.4 Tracheostomy mask (collar)
	3.5 Distilled water
4	Introduce yourself to patient.
5	Identify patient.
6	Explain procedure.
7	Wash hands.
8	Assemble equipment in aseptic manner.
9	Fill nebulizer jar with sterile water.
10	Connect flowmeter to gas source.
11	Adjust gas flow for desired F_{IO_2} as indicated.
12	Assess adequacy of aerosol production.
13	Activate and set temperature (if heated aerosol is prescribed).
14	Position patient.
15	Place aerosol mask over tracheostomy site, taking care not to accidentally strike tracheostomy tube or contaminate the stoma.
16	Adjust retaining strap for comfort.
17	If heated aerosol, check mist temperature at mask (collar).
18	Adjust temperature as required.
19	Instruct patient on self-care, and explain how to call respiratory care or nurse for assistance (call button).
20	Provide for patient's safety and comfort (NO SMOKING sign).
21	Evaluate patient's tolerance of treatment.
22	Wash hands.
23	Chart procedure.

PROCEDURE 12-6

Application of T adapter

No.	Steps in performing the procedure
	The practitioner will administer aerosol and/or oxygen therapy using a heated or unheated nebulizer and a T adapter.
1	Verify physician's order.
2	Wash hands.
3	Collect equipment:
	3.1 Flowmeter or reducing valve
	3.2 Nebulizer
	3.3 Large bore connecting tube
	3.4 T adapter
	3.5 Distilled water
	3.6 Reservoir tube
4	Introduce yourself to patient.
5	Identify patient.
6	Explain procedure.
7	Wash hands.
8	Assemble equipment in aseptic manner.
9	Fill nebulizer jar with sterile distilled water.
10	Connect flowmeter to gas source.
11	Adjust gas flow for desired F_{IO_2} as indicated.
12	Assess adequacy of aerosol production.
13	Activate and set temperature (if heated aerosol is prescribed).
14	Position patient.
15	Connect aerosol T adapter to patient's tracheostomy tube, taking care not to accidentally displace tracheostomy tube or otherwise traumatize or contaminate the stoma site.
16	Position adapter so that minimum tension is placed on the tracheostomy tube.
17	If heated aerosol is used, check mist temperature at site of T.
18	Adjust temperature as required.
19	Instruct patient on self-care, and explain how to call respiratory care or the nurse for assistance (call button).
20	Provide for patient's safety (NO SMOKING sign).
21	Evaluate patient's tolerance of treatment.
22	Wash hands.
23	Chart procedure.

PROCEDURE 12-7

Assess patient and operation of an unheated nebulizer using an aerosol mask

No.	Steps in performing the procedure
	The practitioner will assess the patient and the operation of an unheated nebulizer and aerosol mask.
1	Verify continuation of physician's order.
2	Review patient's progress notes and other relevant data.
3	Wash hands.
4	Greet patient.
5	Question patient on treatment progress.
6	Assess patient's physical status/mental awareness.
7	Remove aerosol mask from patient's face.
8	Check for skin pressure ridges, red area, and other undesirable reactions.
9	Empty condensate from delivery hose into an appropriate container, *not* back into nebulizer reservoir.
10	Operate nebulizer and evaluate aerosol output; if inadequate, take corrective action:
	10.1 Check gas flow.
	10.2 Remove nebulizer jar and assure patency of filter on bottom end of siphon tube.
	10.3 Clear aerosol jets.
	10.4 Clear inlet orifice.
11	Wash reservoir jar and refill with sterile solution.
12	Adjust gas flow to 3 to 4 L/min and occlude nebulizer gas outlet to check for gas leaks and operation of pressure relief valve.
13	Adjust gas flow to prescribed liter flow.
14	Attach delivery hose.
15	Clean or change aerosol mask.
16	Place mask on patient's face and adjust head strap for comfort.
17	Observe adequacy of gas flow and nebulizer output.
18	Reassure patient and have patient cough as required.
19	Wash hands.
20	Remove any used equipment from room.
21	Chart procedure.

PROCEDURE 12-8

Assess patient and operation of unheated nebulizer using a tracheostomy mask (collar)

No.	Steps in performing the procedure
	The practitioner will assess the patient and the operation of an unheated nebulizer and a tracheostomy mask.
1	Verify continuation of physician's order.
2	Review patient's progress notes and other relevant data.
3	Wash hands.
4	Greet patient; introduce youself.
5	Question patient on treatment progress.
6	Assess patient's physical status/mental awareness.
7	Remove tracheostomy mask from patient's neck.
8	Check tracheostomy stoma for signs of infection, bleeding, encrustation of secretions, and other unusual conditions.
9	Check tracheostomy tube for patency and security.
10	Take appropriate action to correct abnormal situations according to department policy.
11	Empty condensate from delivery tube into appropriate container, *not* back into nebulizer reservoir.
12	Operate nebulizer and evaluate aerosol output; if inadequate, take corrective action:
	12.1 Check gas flow.
	12.2 Remove nebulizer jar and assure patency of filter on bottom end of fluid tube.
	12.3 Clear aerosol jets.
	12.4 Clear inlet orifice.
13	Wash reservoir jar and refill with sterile solution.
14	Adjust gas flow to 3 to 4 L/min and occlude nebulizer gas outlet to check for gas leaks and operation of pressure relief valve.
15	Adjust gas flow to prescribed L/min flow.
16	Attach delivery hose.
17	Clean or change tracheostomy mask.
18	Place mask over patient's tracheostomy tube, taking care not to strike tracheostomy tube, and adjust neck strap for comfort and mask position.
19	Observe adequacy of gas flow and nebulizer output.
20	Reassure patient and have patient cough as required. Suctioning, if needed, should be done *only* by preceptor.
21	Wash hands.
22	Remove any used equipment from room.
23	Chart procedure.

PROCEDURE 12-9

Assess patient and operation of an unheated nebulizer using T adapter

No.	Steps in performing the procedure
	The practitioner will assess the patient and the operation of an unheated nebulizer and a T adapter.
1	Verify continuation of physician's order.
2	Review patient's progress notes and other relevant data.
3	Wash hands.
4	Greet patient; introduce yourself.
5	Question patient on treatment progress.
6	Assess patient's physical status/mental awareness.
7	Disconnect T adapter from tracheostomy tube.
8	Check stoma site for signs of infection, bleeding, encrustation of secretions, and other unusual conditions.
9	Check tracheostomy tube for patency and security.
10	Take appropriate action to correct abnormal situation according to department policy.
11	Empty condensate from delivery tube into appropriate container, *not* back into nebulizer reservoir.
12	Operate nebulizer and evaluate aerosol output; if inadequate, take corrective action:
	12.1 Check gas flow.
	12.2 Remove nebulizer jar and assure patency of filter on bottom end of fluid tube.
	12.3 Clear aerosol jets.
	12.4 Clear inlet orifice.
13	Wash reservoir jar and refill with sterile solution.
14	Adjust gas flow to 3 to 4 L/min and occlude nebulizer gas outlet to check for gas leaks and operation of pressure relief valve.
15	Adjust gas flow to prescribed liter flow.
16	Attach delivery hose.
17	Clean or change T adapter.
18	Attach T adapter to patient's tracheostomy tube and adjust so that minimum stress is placed on tube.
19	Observe adequacy of gas flow and nebulizer output.
20	Reassure patient and have patient cough as required. Suctioning, if needed, should be done *only* by preceptor.
21	Wash hands.
22	Remove any used equipment from room.
23	Chart procedure.

BIBLIOGRAPHY

Burton GG, Gee GN and Hodgkin JE, editors: Respiratory care: a guide to clinical practice, Philadelphia, 1977, JB Lippincott Co.

Heebink DM: The treatment of sinusitis by aerosol therapy—nothing to sniff at? Respir Care 27:976, 1982.

Hill TV and Sorbello JG: Humidity outputs of large reservoir nebulizers, Respir Care 32:255, 1987.

Klein EF: Performance characteristics of conventional and prototype humidifiers and nebulizers, Chest 64:690, 1973.

Marks MB: Nebulization of cromolyn sodium in the treatment of childhood asthma, Respir Care 28:1282, 1983.

McFadden ER et al: Thermal mapping of the airways in humans, J Appl Physiol 58:564, 1985.

McPherson SP and Spearman CB: Respiratory therapy equipment, ed 4, St Louis, 1990, The CV Mosby Co.

Slonim NB and Hamilton LH: Respiratory physiology, ed 4, St. Louis, 1981, The CV Mosby Co.

Spearman CB, Sheldon RL and Egan DF: Egan's fundamentals of respiratory therapy, ed 5, St Louis, 1990, The CV Mosby Co.

Oxygen analyzers

1.0 MONITORING INSPIRED OXYGEN LEVELS (FIo_2)

1.1 The need for measuring (monitoring) FIo_2

1 Oxygen (O_2) is a drug and should be administered with the same precautions as any other medication.

  a The potential danger from inhalation of too much O_2 is a real concern to clinicians.

  b Of equal importance, however, is the potential harm from hypoxemia that can occur if O_2 therapy is withheld because of the fear of administering toxic levels.

  c This clinical dichotomy points out the need for accurately and closely measuring the percentage of O_2 that is being administered to a patient.

2 It is important to point out that one cannot rely on gas flow rate or sampling of inspired O_2 as accurate measurements of adequate or therapeutic O_2 levels.

  a Determination of reliable O_2 levels in the blood is best assessed by measuring the partial pressure of O_2 in an arterial blood sample.

  b Other techniques such as transcutaneous monitoring, ear oximetry, and venous blood sampling are outcome measurements and are discussed in a subsequent module.

c In O_2 therapy the patient's treatment must be under the control of the clinician from the point of accurately determining the percentage of gas being administered to measuring its effectiveness to achieve the desired therapeutic effects.

d This first step of determining the percent of O_2 being administered is crucial because many outcome evaluations are based on this initial FIO_2 measurement.

3 Determination of the fraction of inspired oxygen (FIO_2) in a given volume of inhaled gases can be accomplished by using oxygen analyzers to sample the inspired gases on a *periodic* or *continuous* basis.

4 The role of O_2 in sustaining life and causing death has been reported in the literature since the days of Lavoisier, Scheele, and Priestley.

5 There is a physiologic range below which hypoxemia will occur and above which O_2 toxicity and cellular destruction will take place. E.J. Campbell has shown that an arterial oxygen tension (PaO_2) of less than 20 mm Hg is inconsistent with cellular survival.

6 On the other end of the scale it has been shown that our bodies have antioxidant defenses against the toxic defects of O_2.

a Cellular metabolism that is the basis for life is totally dependent on an adequate supply of O_2.

b O_2, like so many other drugs, is a double-edged sword. For example, the oxygen free radicals produced as a by-product of the action of O_2 have been identified as the cause of aging and eventual cellular death.

c As metabolism occurs over time, waste by-products are accumulated in the cell until it can no longer function and dies. This is the so-called Clinker Theory of aging.

7 Therefore O_2 therapy should not be prescribed without a great deal of forethought. Generally, it should be used only when the advantages outweigh the disadvantages and no higher concentrations should be used than are necessary to achieve the desired effect.

8 The following list comprises the primary untoward effects of O_2 therapy with which the respiratory care practitioner must be familiar.

a Oxygen toxicity. Oxygen toxicity is caused in adults and children as a result of exposure to O_2 concentrations that cause the PaO_2 to exceed 50 mm Hg for extended periods of time (more than 48 to 72 hours) or by breathing O_2 concentrations greater than 60% ($FIO_2 = 0.60$) for more than 48 to 72 hours (see Modules Eight and Ten).

b Pulmonary exposure. Pulmonary exposure to high concentrations of O_2 causes:
- Hyaline membrane formation in the alveoli with alveolar thickening
- Interstitial edema and the development of interstitial fibrosis
- Alveolar cell hyperplasia

c Systemic toxicity (high arterial tensions or PaO_2 greater than 150 mm Hg). Systemic toxicity has been shown to cause gastrointestinal symptoms, convulsions, and *retrolental fibroplasia*. Retrolental fibroplasia describes a type of fibrotic tissue that forms behind the lens of the eye of premature infants, causing blindness. Retrolental fibroplasia can be prevented completely by not exposing premature infants to an FIO_2 in excess of 0.40.

d Elevated $PaCO_2$ and reduced PaO_2. A chronic pulmonary disease patient who has a chronically elevated arterial carbon dioxide tension ($PaCO_2$) and a chronically reduced PaO_2 may stop breathing when exposed to an FIO_2 greater than 0.30. This patient is often said to be breathing on *hypoxic drive*. This means that the stimulus to breathe no longer responds to elevations in CO_2. The patient breathes now because of reduced O_2 (hypoxic drive). When the body's need for O_2 is satisfied with a high percentage O_2 device, the body's O_2 need (hypoxia) is satisfied (temporarily) and the patient stops breathing.

9 Guidelines for the safe administration of O_2 are as follows:

a Do *not* use an FIO_2 above 0.30 with a chronic pulmonary disease patient without careful monitoring and arterial blood gases.

b Do *not* use an FIO_2 above 0.40 with a premature infant and newborn unless necessary to sustain life.

c Although there is no hard scientific evidence that breathing 100% O_2 for less than 24 hours causes any irreversible harm in adults, do *not* exceed an FIO_2 of 0.60 in routine situations.

d Always use the minimum concentration necessary to achieve the desired effect.

e Use alternate methods such as PEEP and CPAP to obtain the desired PaO_2 once the FIO_2 has reached 0.60.

10 Calculating the difference between a patient's FIO_2 and PaO_2 can be used as an index for determining whether a patient has a diffusion or ventilation-perfusion abnormality and as a clinical prognostic indicator for patients received O_2 therapy (see Module Eight, Unit 14.1).

2.0 OPERATING AND SERVICING THE PARAMAGNETIC OXYGEN ANALYZER

2.1 Principles of measurement of the paramagnetic analyzer

1 Linus Pauling, a physicist, discovered that O_2 and nitrous oxide are unique because of their strongly paramagnetic atomic configuration—*attracted* into a magnetic field. All other gases are diamagnetic—repelled from the magnetic field.

2 This magnetic attraction by O_2 causes the O_2 molecule to behave like a temporary magnet when it is placed in an electromagnetic field.

3 The density (number) of O_2 molecules attracted by a magnetic field is directly related to the number of available O_2 molecules in a given sample of gas.

4 Movement of O_2 will cause the magnetic field to be altered.

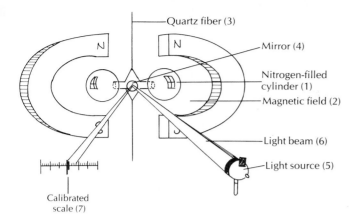

FIGURE 13-1 Beckman D-2 analyzer.

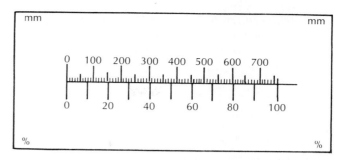

FIGURE 13-2 Calibrated scale for Beckman D-2 analyzer showing O_2 percentage and mm Hg.

5 The greater the density of O_2, the more the magnetic field is altered.

6 The paramagnetic oxygen analyzer allows one to visualize the degree to which the magnetic field is altered by the movement of a light beam on a calibrated scale.

7 The popularity of this type of analyzer has slowly diminished with the availability of electrochemical and polarographic analyzers. It is presented in this module because it is still widely used by many hospitals.

2.2 Principles of operation of the Beckman D-2 oxygen analyzer (Figs. 13-1 and 13-2)

1 A nitrogen-filled, dumbbell-shaped cylinder *(1)* is suspended between a magnetic field *(2)* by a quartz fiber *(3)*.

2 A mirror (galvanometer) *(4)* is located midpoint along the shaft of the dumbbell.

3 A battery-powered light source is generated by depressing a switch and activating the lamp *(5)*.

4 The light beam *(6)* strikes the mirror *(4)* and is reflected on a calibrated scale *(7)*.

5 The position of the light beam on the scale is determined by the angle of the mirror to the fixed light source.

6 Increases or decreases in the O_2 content in the gas sample from 20.9% will cause the dumbbell to be twisted in response to the molecular density.

7 As the mirror is twisted, the light beam strikes the scale calibrated to provide a reading of O_2 percentage and also in mm Hg (see Fig. 13-2).

8 A *blue* silica gel located in a tube at the rear of the analyzer removes moisture from the sample gas before its entrance into the testing chamber. Moisture in the testing chamber will alter gas density and cause inaccurate O_2 readings.

2.3 Potential problem areas with the Beckman D-2 analyzer

The Beckman D-2 analyzer is a simple unit to operate and is accurate provided it is not exposed to abuse and receives basic maintenance. The following are potential problem areas that should be avoided or recognized and corrected:

1 Battery failure. There will be no light beam.

2 Calibration. The unit must be adjusted for high and low O_2 concentrations to establish an accurate baseline for measurement.

3 Position. The unit is position-sensitive and must be set in a horizontal position so that the light beam will strike the scale correctly.

4 Fragile. The unit is easily broken if dropped or handled roughly.

5 Altitude. The unit must be corrected for altitude because of changes in tension of the quartz fiber. This is corrected by increasing the torque on the dumbbell fibers by rotating the dumbbell at less dense altitudes. A correction scale for altitude is provided with each unit. As the altitude increases from sea level, percentages shown by the analyzer *will be lower* than the actual concentration. Values shown on the conversion table should be added to correct the scale values shown by the analyzer.

2.4 Brands employing the paramagnetic principle

The analyzer made by Beckman Instruments is the only currently known brand incorporating the paramagnetic principle. This type of analyzer is accurate and specific to the measurement of O_2 with the *exception* of nitrous oxide, which is also attracted into a magnetic field.

2.5 Operation of the Beckman D-2 analyzer

1 Procedure 13.1 for operating the Beckman analyzer to measure FIO_2 on a patient receiving O_2 therapy is included at the end of this module.

2 The light, silica gel, and baseline FIO_2 of 20.9% should be checked before each use.

2.6 Preventive maintenance of the Beckman D-2 oxygen analyzer

1 Daily, check analyzer for accuracy, using a room air sample of 20.9% O_2.

2 Daily, check color of silica gel and note the following:
   a Blue indicates active (dry).
   b Pink to white indicates inactive (damp).

3 Remove and dry lamp crystals by exposing them to dry heat.

4 Check light image on scale. If there is no image, change the battery and/or lamp.

5 If light still does not appear on the scale, the test body is probably broken. Return the analyzer to the factory or vendor.

6 Test the analyzer for leaks. Close off sample tube inlet, squeeze bulb, and release. If the bulb reinflates, check for leak in the circuit.

7 Keep external cabinet clean and free of dust.

8 *Do not* submerge unit in chemical decontamination agents after using it in isolation. Also, do not steam autoclave or use ethylene oxide gas. Wipe the unit down completely with a disinfectant and allow to air.

3.0 OPERATING AND SERVICING THE THERMOCONDUCTIVE ANALYZER

3.1 Principles of measurement of the thermoconductive analyzer

1 O_2 conducts heat at a faster rate than any other known gas.

2 The rate of heat conduction from a surface (cooling) by a gas mixture is directly proportional to the concentration of O_2 in the mixture.

3 A cool wire has a lower resistance to current flow than a hot wire.

3.2 Principle of operation of the thermoconductive analyzer (Fig. 13-3)

1 The thermoconductive analyzer employs a *wheatstone bridge* circuit attached to a voltmeter.

2 A wheatstone bridge is comprised of a four-sided circuit system *(1-4)* connected to a switch *(6)* and a voltmeter *(7)*.

3 Two sides of the circuit *(1 and 2)* are exposed to the gas to be analyzed with the other two sides *(3 and 4)* exposed to a reference gas—normally room air.

4 Before analyzing a gas sample, the practitioner draws room air into the reference cell by squeezing a handbulb and uses a variable resistor (adjustment knob; *5*) to adjust the bridge and calibrate the needle *(7)* on the voltmeter to reflect 20.9% (or room air).

5 The sample gas is drawn into the analysis cell by equalizing a handbulb attached to the analyzer.

6 A switch *(6)* is depressed and the bridge circuit is activated.

7 If O_2 is present at greater than 20.9%, the wires exposed to the gas sample in the analysis cell *(1 and 2)* cool more rapidly than those exposed to room air in the reference cell *(3 and 4)*.

8 As the wires in the analysis cell cool, their resistance to current flow is reduced compared with those in the reference cell.

9 The difference in resistance unbalances the bridge circuit, which is reflected by the voltmeter *(7)* as O_2 percentage.

10 This type of analyzer usually incorporates a silica gel that should be *pink* (containing moisture) to equalize moisture at the reference and analysis elements. NOTE:

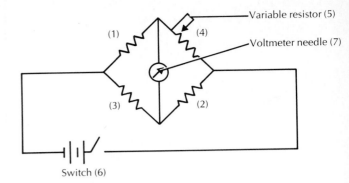

FIGURE 13-3 Thermoconductive analyzer employing a wheatstone bridge circuit attached to a voltmeter.

the Mira analyzer uses pink gel; other brands may use different colors of silica gel.

3.3 Potential problem areas of the thermoconductive analyzer

1 It is neither as stable nor as accurate as the electrochemical and paramagnetic analyzers. Like the paramagnetic analyzer it too is slowly being replaced by more accurate and fast-response electrochemical and polarographic units.

2 The silica must be changed frequently.

3 It may be affected by other gases.

4 It cannot be used in flammable gas atmospheres (surgery).

5 It responds differently to flowing versus static gas situations.

6 It should be used only on inspiration due to the influence of CO_2 molecules.

7 It should not be used with anesthesia gases.

3.4 Brands employing the thermoconductivity principle

1 Mira Corporation

2 OEM Medical, Inc.

3 Bourns Life Systems Division

3.5 Operation of the Mira analyzer

Procedure 13-2 at the end of this module can be used for operating the Mira analyzer or similar brand.

3.6 Preventive maintenance of a Mira oxygen analyzer

The following schedule should be followed to ensure peak performance of the unit and minimize "down time."

1 Calibrate for 21% and 100% O_2 percentages daily.

2 Replace the battery if the analyzer reads less than 95% on pure O_2 after a 20.9% adjustment on air.

3 Check pink silica gel daily and replace if it turns blue.

4 Check the analyzer for leaks in the handbulb, tubing, or caps on the silica gel container. Replace or repair worn parts.

5 After the unit is used in isolation, *do not* submerge it in chemical decontamination agents. Also, do not steam autoclave or use ethylene oxide gas. The practitioner

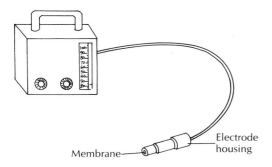

FIGURE 13-4 Polarographic analyzer.

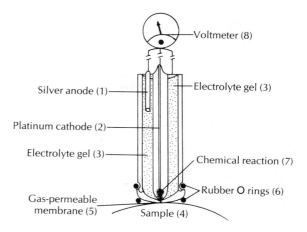

FIGURE 13-5 Components of polarographic electrode.

should wipe the unit down completely with a disinfectant and allow to air.

4.0 OPERATING AND SERVICING THE ELECTROCHEMICAL POLAROGRAPHIC ANALYZER

4.1 Principles of measurement of the electrochemical polarographic analyzer

1 O_2 molecules diffusing through a permeable membrane and exposed to an electrolyte solution will produce an electric current caused by a chemical reaction.
2 The amount of current generated is dependent on the density of the O_2 molecules exposed to the electrolyte solution.
3 A voltmeter measures the difference in current between the two sides of the membrane and displays it as partial pressure and O_2 percentage.

4.2 Principle of operation of the polarographic analyzer
(Figs. 13-4 and 13-5)

1 The heart of a polarographic analyzer is an electrode, originally described by Clark to measure O_2 concentration in the blood.
2 The electrode contains a silver anode *(1)* and a platinum cathode *(2)*, which are attached to a control box that houses a voltmeter *(8)*.
3 The silver anode and platinum cathode are connected through an electrolyte gel *(3)*.
4 The anode and cathode are separted from the sample *(4)* by a gas-permeable membrane *(5)*, which is held on by rubber O rings *(6)*.
5 A low-voltage current (0.8 V) is passed between the cathode *(2)* and anode *(1)*. This voltage causes an oxidation-reduction (redox) chemical reaction to occur *(7)* with O_2 diffusing in through the membrane toward a decreased pressure gradient caused by the redox reaction.
6 Chemically, this redox equation is initiated as O_2 enters the cell to produce:

$$O_2 + 2 H_2O + 4e^- \underline{\quad\quad} > 4 OH^-$$

These hydroxyl ions are attracted to the silver anode

where a reaction occurs generating four electrons to produce:

$$4 OH^- + 4 Ag \underline{\quad\quad} > 2 Ag_2 + 2 H_2O + 4e^-$$

7 Additional current is generated proportional to the partial pressure of O_2 in the sample *(4)*.
8 Current flow is reflected on a previously balanced voltmeter so that the greater the O_2 present, the greater the current flow will be.
9 The amount of current generated is measured by the voltmeter *(8)* and presented on a scale as partial pressure and O_2 percentage.

4.3 Potential problem areas with the polarographic analyzer

The following is a list of the complications most frequently experienced when using the polarographic analyzer. Although this device is highly accurate, the older models need frequent service and careful use to maintain their accuracy.

1 The electrolyte solution dries up and must be replaced.
2 O rings that secure the membrane become flattened and leak fluid.
3 The membrane becomes contaminated (dirty) or torn and must be cleaned or replaced.
4 Blood samples usually read 4% lower than gas samples.
5 The unit is mostly glass and is fragile; damage easily occurs to the electrode body because of accidental impact.
6 If the analyzer is placed in line for continuous measurement of oxygen in a ventilator circuit, readings must be corrected for:
   a Peak inspiratory pressure. A higher FIo_2 is reported during inspiration than during exhalation.
   b PEEP. Levels greater than 13 cm H_2O would cause the FIo_2 to read higher than actual volume.
   c Humidity. Condensate on the membrane will cause the analyzer to read a lower FIo_2 than is actually be-

ing delivered. Procedures for correcting the above situations should be obtained from the manufacturers of each respective analyzer.

4.4 Brands employing the polarographic electrochemical principle

1 Instrumentation Laboratory, Inc.
2 Critikon, Division of McNeil Laboratories
3 International Biophysics Corporation (IBC)
4 Beckman Instruments
5 Ohio Medical Products
6 Cavitron KDC Cardiopulmonary Group
7 IMI, Division of Becton, Dickinson and Company

4.5 Operation of the polarographic analyzer

1 Operation rarely involves more than occasional calibration and turning the unit on. If the electrode is being used in a tubing system, a special adapter may be required.
2 Procedure 13-3 can be used to set up and operate a Critikon or other polarographic oxygen analyzer.
3 No preventive maintenance is required on a Critikon analyzer other than periodically changing the O_2 sensor whenever the O_2 level drifts rapidly downscale, when high calibration cannot be attained, or if obvious damage has occurred to the membrane.
4 Other brands, especially older designs, may require more detailed maintenance. Refer to the manufacturer's service manual for each unit.

5.0 OPERATING AND SERVICING THE ELECTROCHEMICAL GALVANIC ANALYZER

5.1 Principles of measurement of the electrochemical oxygen analyzer (galvanic cell)

1 The power source for this type of analyzer is a galvanic cell containing a gold cathode and a lead anode in a basic electrolyte paste of potassium hydroxide.
2 Diffusion of O_2 molecules through a permeable membrane into the electrolyte cell causes a redox reaction, producing a low-voltage current proportional to the partial pressure of the O_2.

$$O_2 + 2 H_2O + 4e^- \rightarrow 4 OH$$

where 4e stands for released electrons.

5.2 Principle of operation of the galvanic oxygen analyzer
(Figs. 13-6 and 13-7)

1 A cell encapsulated in an inert plastic container contains a gold cathode (positive) (1) and a lead anode (negative) (2) surrounded by a base electrolyte paste (potassium hydroxide) (3).
2 A permeable membrane allows O_2 molecules to enter the cell (4).
3 O_2 molecules coming in contact with the electrolyte paste cause a redox reaction that generates a low electrical current.
4 Electrons flow from the cathode to the anode.
5 The amount of current is proportional to the partial

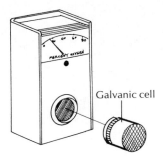

FIGURE 13-6 Galvanic cell oxygen analyzer.

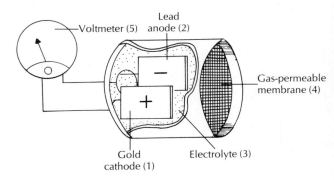

FIGURE 13-7 Components of galvanic cell.

pressure of the O_2 and is displayed on a voltmeter (5) as O_2 percentage.
6 The life of a cell is directly related to the length of time that it is exposed to O_2.
7 The average life is 3 to 9 months with normal use in O_2 atmospheres below 100%.

5.3 Potential problem areas with the galvanic analyzer

1 If the unit is to be used in an atmosphere of less than 40% O_2, it should be calibrated using 100% instead of 21% O_2.
2 Cells are expensive to replace and should be capped when not in use.
3 Use in O_2 enriched atmospheres of more than 40% will reduce cell life greatly.
4 Moisture accumulation on the surface of the membrane will decrease O_2 reading. Use in wet atmospheres may result in inaccurate readings.
5 Galvanic cells need to be pressure compensated with a special attachment when used in a ventilator circuit to prevent positive pressure from moving the membrane closer to the electrodes and decreasing their accuracy.
6 Electrochemical processes are increased because of increases in temperature. To compensate and prevent a reading that is too high, the temperature must be controlled and a compensating thermistor inserted to decrease current flow to the amp meter.

5.4 Brands employing the galvanic principle

1 Teledyne Analytical Instruments

2 BioMarine Industries, Inc. (BMI)

3 Hudson Photographic Industries, Inc.

5.5 Operation of a BMI Oxygen Analyzer

Procedure 13-4 may be used for operation of a BioMarine (BMI) Oxygen Analyzer or other galvanic analyzer to measure FI_{O_2} of a patient receiving various modes of therapy. The following may be useful when using this type of analyzer.

1 Operation rarely involves more than occasional calibration and placing the membrane in contact with the gas to be measured.

2 If the membrane is placed in a tubing system, a special adapter may be necessary. Care should be taken to avoid getting the membrane wet. It should never be left in a wet atmosphere for more time than it takes to get a reading.

3 The galvanic cell must be replaced whenever calibration is unstable or the unit delivers unstable readings. Refer to the manufacturer's directions.

5.6 Preventive maintenance of the galvanic analyzer

1 Since the unit has few moving parts and is not battery powered, little maintenance is required.

2 The screen protecting the membrane must be kept clear of moisture, dust, and other obstructions.

3 The meter should be checked daily and calibrated for 21% and 100% O_2.

4 The galvanic cell must be replaced whenever it becomes impossible to obtain a stable reading.

PROCEDURE 13-1

Operation of Beckman D-2 oxygen analyzer

No.	Steps in performing the procedure
	The practitioner will use a Beckman D-2 oxygen analyzer to measure FI_{O_2} on a patient receiving O_2 therapy through a Croupette (mist tent) and infant hood
1	Collect Beckman D-2 oxygen analyzer.
2	Check *blue* silica gel; change if not blue.
3	Check light beam (battery, bulb).
4	Replace battery or bulb as necessary.
5	Test all tubes and fittings for leaks.
6	Check accuracy of analyzer using room air (21%).
7	Check accuracy of analyzer when exposed to 100% O_2 by drawing a sample of O_2 from a reservoir containing pure O_2.
8	Use analyzer to measure FI_{O_2} of patient receiving various modes of O_2 therapy as listed above.
9	Wash hands.
10	Operate analyzer correctly by:
	10.2 Positioning analyzer in a horizontal position
	10.2 Inserting sampling tube near patient's proximal airway
	10.3 Squeezing and releasing sampling bulb at least five times to allow bulb to inflate completely between squeezes
	10.4 Depressing switch button on top of analyzer cabinet to activate the lamp
	10.5 Holding switch down until light beam stabilizes on scale
11	Flush O_2 from the analyzer system by squeezing handbulb six to eight times.
12	Recheck initial reading according to steps 10.1 to 10.5.
13	Compare reading to prescribed FI_{O_2}.
14	Wash hands.
15	Chart results.

PROCEDURE 13-2

Operation of a Mira* oxygen analyzer

No.	Steps in performing the procedure
	The practitioner will use a Mira oxygen analyzer to determine FI_{O_2} delivered to patients receiving O_2 therapy through a Croupette (mist tent) and infant hood.
1	Collect Mira analyzer.
2	Test and calibrate unit for correction operation by:
	2.1 Purging instrument of previous samples (squeezing bulbs four to six times)
	2.2 Depressing switch and checking meter for room air reading of 21% O_2
	2.3 Using adjustment screw to calibrate needle to 21%
	2.4 Placing sample tube in 100% O_2 source and adjusting needle as necessary to reflect 100% on meter:
	a. Remove nickel-plated cap in back of cabinet
	b. Turn exposed adjustment screw in clockwise direction to adjust needle to 100%
	2.5 If 100% setting cannot be maintained, replace battery.
	2.6 Recheck meter for 21% setting by sampling room air.
3	Check and replace silica gel as required:
	3.1 Pink color is normal.
	3.2 Blue indicates need for replacement.
	NOTE: Other brands may use different color silica gel.
4	Wash hands.
5	Use analyzer to test FI_{O_2} of patient receiving various modes of O_2 therapy as listed above.
6	Wash hands.
7	Chart results.

*Or similar brand.

PROCEDURE 13-3

Operation of a Critikon* oxygen analyzer

No.	Steps in performing the procedure
	The practitioner will operate the Critikon oxygen analyzer to measure FI_{O_2} on a patient receiving O_2 therapy through a Croupette (mist tent), T piece, mechanical ventilator, and infant hood therapy.
1	Collect Critikon analyzer and appropriate adapters.
2	Check accuracy in room air environment.
3	Check accuracy in 100% O_2 environment.
4	Change membrane cartridge if necessary.
5	Change batteries if necessary.
6	Clean silver anode if necessary.
7	Wash hands.
8	Use analyzer in upright position to measure FI_{O_2} of patient in the required modes. Allow to stabilize.
9	Accurately read the O_2 percentage on the dial.
10	Wash hands.
11	Chart results.

*Or similar brand.

PROCEDURE 13-4

Operation of a Biomarine* oxygen analyzer

No.	Steps in performing the procedure
	The practitioner will assemble parts of a Biomarine oxygen analyzer to measure FI_{O_2} of a patient receiving O_2 therapy through a Croupette (mist tent), T piece, mechanical ventilator,† and infant hood therapy.
1	Collect Biomarine analyzer with appropriate adapters.
2	Check accuracy in room air environment.
3	Check accuracy in 100% O_2 environment.
4	Wash hands.
5	Use analyzer in upright position to measure FI_{O_2} of patient in the required modes, making sure cell membrane is not obstructed by moisture or other objects. Allow to stabilize.
6	Accurately read the O_2 percentage on the dial.
7	Wash hands.
8	Change galvanic cell if required.
9	Chart results.

*Or similar brand.
†A pressure compensator should be available for this measurement.

BIBLIOGRAPHY

Bageant RA: Oxygen analyzers, Respir Care 21:410, 1976.

McPherson SP and Spearman CB: Respiratory therapy equipment, ed 4, St Louis, 1990, The CV Mosby Co.

Pauling L et al: An instrument for determining the partial pressure of oxygen in a gas, J Am Chem Soc 68:795, 1946.

Rau JL and Rau MY: Fundamental respiratory therapy equipment, Sarasota, Fla, 1977, Glenn Educational Medical Services, p 175.

Spearman CB, Sheldon RL, and Egan DF: Egan's fundamentals of respiratory therapy, ed 5, St Louis, 1990, The CV Mosby Co.

Wilson RS and Laver MB: Oxygen analysis: advances in methodology, Anesthesiology 37:112, 1972.

Environmental therapy

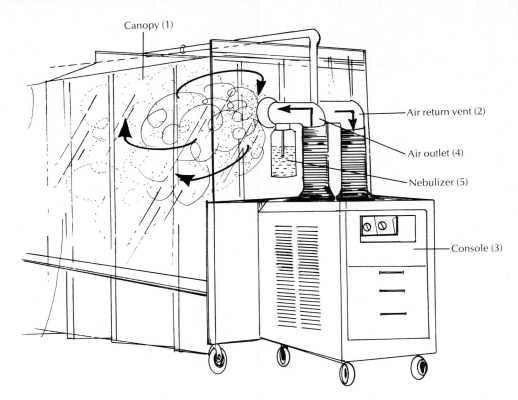

FIGURE 14-1 High humidity oxygen tent.

1.0 DEFINITION OF ENVIRONMENTAL CHAMBERS

1.1 Environmental chambers

Environmental chambers are transparent canopy-type enclosures that fit over a patient's head or body, such as a hood or tent, or rigid enclosures such as an Isolette or hyperbaric chamber.

2.0 THEORY OF ELECTRICALLY POWERED OXYGEN TENTS

2.1 Oxygen tents

1 Oxygen tents are rarely used today except as a means of cooling or warming and maintaining the relative humidity of the patient's environment. Even these therapies can be more efficiently administered in other ways that do not require isolating the patient in a canopy.

2 Oxygen tents provide poor oxygen (O_2) therapy, even with the best techniques. The available inspired O_2 averages 30% to 40%.

2.2 Temperature control

1 The temperature inside a tent canopy is controlled by various methods, depending on the manufacturer.

2 One of the following methods is typically used:
  a Mechanically forced air—air conditioners (Ohio 350)
  b Mechanically cooled circulated liquid—conduction (CAM tent)
  c Radiation-cooled forced air—(Ohio Pediatric Mist Tent)

2.3 High humidity oxygen tent

1 Most tents work on a principle similar to a room air conditioner with Freon 12 used as the cooling agent (Fig. 14-1).

2 Air within the canopy *(1)* is constantly removed from the canopy through a return vent *(2)*, circulated across cooling coils inside the tent console *(3)*, and recirculated into the canopy through an outlet *(4)*.

3 The circulating gas is cooled according to a preset temperature selected by the operator.

4 If high humidity is required, a nebulizer *(5)* can be activated to inject aerosol into the circulating gas.

2.4 Problem areas in tent therapy

1 Low levels of inspired oxygen (FIo_2)
2 Fire hazard
3 Isolation of the patient, hindering good nursing care
4 Failure by patient, family, and staff to comply with good operating procedure, e.g., leaving canopy open
5 Negative psychologic impact on patient and family

2.5 Typical oxygen tent operating procedure

1 Turn tent on and allow it to cool before placing canopy over patient.

2 Initially, flood canopy with 15 L/min of O_2 for 15 to 20 minutes or whenever the canopy is opened.

3 After 15 to 20 minutes, decrease the O_2 flow to 10 to 12 L/min for standard operation.

4 Set the temperature control at 20° to 22° C (68° to 72°

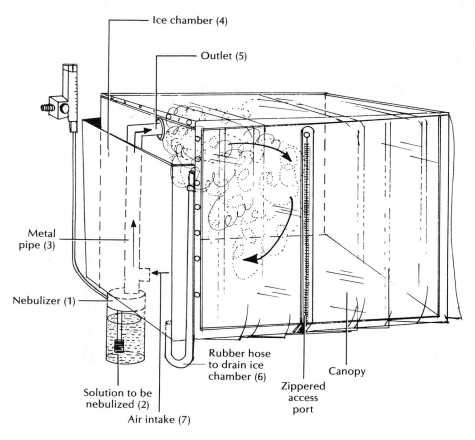

Ice chamber (4)

Outlet (5)

Metal pipe (3)

Nebulizer (1)

Solution to be nebulized (2)

Air intake (7)

Rubber hose to drain ice chamber (6)

Zippered access port

Canopy

FIGURE 14-2 Croupette.

F) or no more than 8.3° C (15° F) below room temperature.

5 Adjust humidity to desired output.

6 Tuck the canopy under the patient's mattress tightly.

7 Empty the condensate tray as required to prevent spillage and possible icing of coils.

8 Check FIo_2 at least every 4 hours.

9 Protect against fire hazards by removing all smoking devices, electrical devices, or anything else that could generate a spark from the room.

10 Post a NO SMOKING sign on the door and on the tent. Inform everyone involved, e.g., the patient, family, roommate, of the extreme fire hazard of an oxygen tent.

3.0 HIGH HUMIDITY OXYGEN TENTS FOR AEROSOL/OXYGEN THERAPY
3.1 Operation of a high humidity oxygen tent

Procedure 14-1 for operating a high humidity oxygen tent on an adult patient is included at the end of this module.

4.0 CHECK ROUNDS FOR PATIENTS IN OXYGEN TENTS
4.1 Procedure for check rounds

1 Procedure 14-2 for conducting check rounds on a patient receiving high humidity oxygen therapy is included at the end of this module.

2 Check rounds are conducted to evaluate the patient as well as the equipment.

3 During these rounds special care must be taken to assess the patient's response to therapy.

4 Mental awareness, changes in breathing and coughing patterns, expectoration of secretions, and general condition should be assessed. Any undesirable effects should be reported *at once*.

5.0 OPERATION OF CROUP TENTS (MIST TENTS)
5.1 Croupette

1 The pediatric croup tent (Croupette or similar brand) is a small version of the oxygen tent initially developed for the treatment of croup in children by using high humidity (Fig. 14-2).

2 As with the oxygen tent, there are many different brands and models. They all are used primarily to treat infants and toddlers who have croup, bronchiolitis, pneumonia, atelectasis, and other respiratory complications.

3 Older children are too big for Croupettes and should be placed in a larger type of mist chamber such as the Child Adult Mist (CAM) Tent manufactured by Mistogen, Inc. or the Ohio Pediatric Mist (OPM) tent manufactured by Ohio Medical Products, Inc.

4 Tent-type devices are better for active children who do not understand or who are not willing to cooperate by using a face tent or aerosol mask for aerosol therapy.

5.2 Clinical situations involving the croup tent

1 Mist tent therapy is used to prevent insensible water loss and subsequent dehydration of the patient's airways. This situation leads to bronchospasm, airway plugging, infection, and eventually, atelectasis.
2 The diseases most frequently treated with mist include:
 a Croup (laryngotracheobronchitis)
 b Bronchiolitis
 c Cystic fibrosis (CF)
 d Pneumonia
 e Epiglottitis

5.3 Operation of a Croupette

1 The conduction-cooled Croupette uses an O_2 source or compressed air to power a nebulizer *(1)* that produces an aerosol from the solution in the nebulizer jar *(2)*.
2 The aerosol passes through a metal pipe *(3)* leading to the tent that is cooled externally by ice in a chamber *(4)*.
3 The mist is cooled by heat transfer (conduction) as it flows through the pipe and leaves an outlet *(5)* into the canopy forming a tent closure.
4 The entrainment action of the nebulizer jet causes gas to leave the tent where it is replenished with aerosol and O_2 and recirculated to the patient.
5 This process results in the patient's receiving a constant level of aerosol that will eventually dampen the patient.
6 If the humidity level is high enough in the canopy, *evaporation will be minimized* and the patient will not be chilled.
7 Melted ice, which is used for cooling, is routinely drained from the chamber by an attached rubber hose.

5.4 Considerations when operating a Croupette

1 The reservoir container must be kept filled.
2 If ice is used, the level must be maintained and condensate drained.
3 If a nebulizer is used, the jets, liquid tube, and filter must be kept clean and changed frequently to prevent the growth of microorganisms.
4 The canopy must be securely tucked and access ports closed at all times to maintain an elevated FI_{O_2} (if prescribed) and adequate humidity levels.
5 The patient's temperature should be checked frequently to assess the chill factor.
6 The manufacturer's instruction should be followed for operating and cleaning the unit.
7 Occasionally, mist tents or Croupettes are ordered without O_2 and must be powered by compressed air from the wall or electric compressors. In this case the canopy must not be tucked under the mattress and gas flow must be adequate to prevent the accumulation of carbon dioxide (CO_2). Air-oxygen blenders may also be used.

6.0 CROUP TENT FOR AEROSOL/OXYGEN THERAPY
6.1 Operation of croup tents in the home

Croup tents are frequently used in the home to treat asthmatic patients or those with cystic fibrosis. The procedure for operating the tent in the home is the same as that outlined above.

7.0 CHECK ROUNDS FOR PATIENTS IN CROUP TENTS
7.1 Procedures for check rounds

Procedures 14-3 and 14-4 for operation of a croup tent and conducting check rounds on a patient receiving croup tent therapy are included at the end of this module.

8.0 OPERATION OF ADULT AEROSOL TENTS
8.1 Operation of larger size aerosol tents

1 Larger versions of the croup tent are available from several manufacturers for children too large to fit inside a regular Croupette.
2 The Child Adult Mist (CAM) Tent is one example developed primarily for the delivery of a high density mist therapy to an adult or pediatric patient (Fig. 14-3).

8.2 Gas flow through the CAM Tent

1 A high density jet nebulizer *(1)* delivers an aerosol mist into the tent canopy via large pipes *(2)*.
2 The circulation of gas within the canopy by the nebulizer flow causes gas to contact a metal plate with exposed coils *(3)*.
3 Chilled water is constantly circulated through the coils by inflow and outflow tubing *(4)* to a refrigeration unit contained within the tent housing *(5)*.
4 The coils serve as a heat exchanger causing the warm air in the canopy to be cooled by the chilled coils *(3)* through the process of convection.
5 This cooled air is recirculated through the tent, resulting in a controlled temperature within the canopy as determined by the refrigeration unit.

8.3 Considerations when using the CAM Tent

1 To be effective, the canopy must be *tightly* tucked under the mattress at all times.
2 A minimum of 10 L/min gas flow should be delivered to the nebulizer to prevent CO_2 accumulation inside the canopy.
3 Setting up an adult aerosol tent is similar to setting up an adult oxygen tent and a child's croup tent. The practitioner should follow manufacturer's instructions for specific details.
4 The procedure for checking the patient and equipment is similar to the rounds for the adult tent and child's croup tent.

9.0 INFANT OXYGEN HOOD
9.1 Function of the infant oxygen hood

1 This is a transparent plastic enclosure that comes in various sizes to deliver high concentrations of O_2 and aerosol to infants up to 18 pounds (Fig. 14-4).
2 The hood can be used with heated or cooled aerosol.

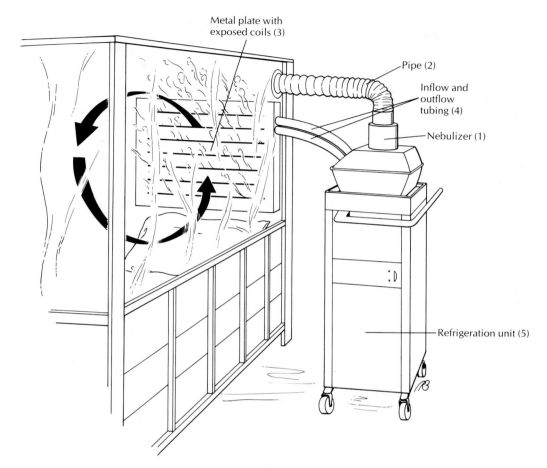

F I G U R E 1 4 - 3 Child Adult Mist (CAM) Tent.

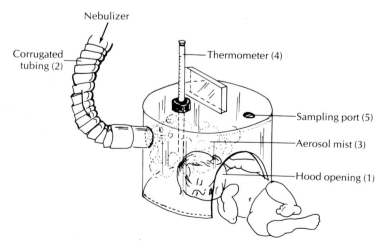

F I G U R E 1 4 - 4 Infant oxygen hood.

3 When using the hood, extreme care must be taken to closely monitor and control the FIO_2, temperature of the aerosol, and body water of the infant. More details on hood therapy are presented in Module Twenty-Six.

9.2 Principle of hood operation

1 A transparent enclosure is placed over the infant's head so that the body opening fits just proximal to the baby's chin or jaw *(1)*.

2 Heated or unheated aerosol is delivered to the hood via a corrugated tube *(2)* attached to an external nebulizer unit.

3 Aerosol leaving the tube fills the hood and provides the baby with a controlled FIO_2 and humidity *(3)*.

4 Temperature inside the hood can be constantly observed by a thermometer inserted through the lid *(4)*.

5 Infant hoods are frequently used inside incubators so that accurate O_2 percentages can be maintained while preventing insensible water loss.

6 The FIO_2 in the hood can be monitored via a sampling port *(5)* without removing the lid.

7 Easy access to the infant in the hood can be achieved by lifting and removing the lid by the handle.

8 Problems encountered when using hoods include:
 a High noise levels inside the hood caused by incoming gas.
 b Pooling of O_2 resulting in an uneven FIO_2 in all parts of the hood.
 c Reduced visibility even through the hood is transparent.
 d Dampened bedding under infant.
 e Inaccessibility of infant to good nursing care without loss of desired FIO_2.

10.0 INFANT OXYGEN HOOD FOR AEROSOL/OXYGEN THERAPY
10.1 Procedures for administering oxygen/aerosol therapy

Procedures 14-5 and 14-6 for operating an infant oxygen hood and for conducting patient check rounds are included at the end of this module.

11.0 CHECK ROUNDS FOR PATIENTS IN OXYGEN HOODS
11.1 Considerations when checking patients in oxygen hoods

When checking an infant in an oxygen hood one should observe the patient's overall appearance, degree of restlessness, body temperature, respiratory rate, and any signs of airway obstruction. In addition the hood should be inspected for cracks, noise level, temperature, and FIO_2.

12.0 INFANT INCUBATORS
12.1 Function of infant incubators

1 Newborns, and especially premature infants, require a closely regulated environment for O_2, temperature, humidity, and clean air (Figs. 14-5 and 14-6).

2 The incubator is an enclosure that provides this support until the baby's body and organ development are ma-

ture and functional enough to survive outside the chamber.

3 There are many types of incubators available with just as many features designed for the care of the infant. Thus general rules of good care are presented in the following units. For details on the operation of a specific incubator, the practitioner should read the manufacturer's instruction manual and hospital procedure manual.

12.2 Major incubator components and operational characteristics

The following components and functions will be present in most incubators. The model illustrated is the Isolette, manufactured by Air Shields, Inc.

1 Fig. 14-5 shows a transparent plastic hood with access ports that can be quickly opened and closed to provide care of the baby *(1)*.

2 Fig. 14-6 illustrates a main power unit, which electrically operates a blower *(2)* to circulate air throughout the unit *(3)*.

3 In Fig. 14-5 a heater and thermostat are manually set by the operator or "servoed" by the patient *(4)*. Servo-controlled units are operated by taping a temperature probe to the skin or inserting it into the rectum of the infant. The operator sets the desired infant temperature on the control panel and the incubator will automatically maintain the infant at this temperature by intermittently heating the unit to raise the infant's body temperature to the preset control temperature.
CAUTION: Servo units should be *fail-safe*. If the temperature probe accidentally becomes disconnected from the infant, the unit should *not* heat up in an attempt to raise the environment to that of the constantly cooling probe. The temperature should revert back to some safe level of 31° to 32° C (88° to 90° F) until a reconnection can be made.

4 An ice chamber cools the incubator if the temperature becomes too high (Figs. 14-5 and 14-6, *5*).

5 A passover-type humidifier (which can be heated or unheated) is usually located beneath the infant's mattress, inside the plastic hood (Fig. 14-6, *6*).

6 A clearly marked O_2 delivery system permits the maintenance of FIO_2 and clearly indicates an FIO_2 greater than 40%. In many models this is controlled by lifting a red flag-type lever that indicates an FIO_2 greater than 0.40 is being used.

7 Filters reduce cross-contamination from air being drawn into the blower from the room.

8 Alarms indicate excessive FIO_2, acute temperature changes, or power failure.

12.3 Differences between manually controlled incubators and servo-controlled units

1 The primary difference between manual and servo-controlled incubators is the *automatic* adjustment of the incubator's heating/cooling systems to maintain a preset level based on a desired infant temperature. A servo

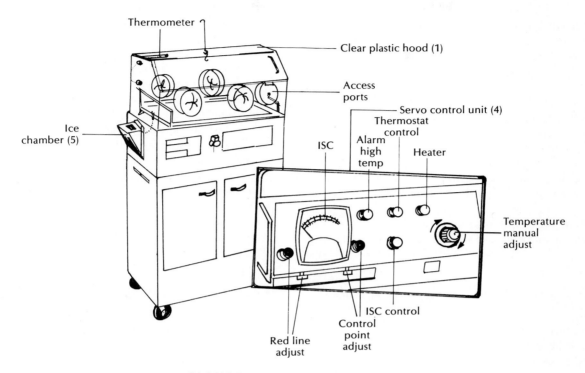

FIGURE 14-5 Front view of incubator.

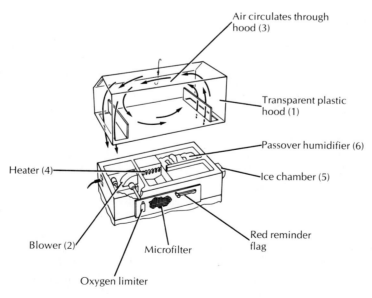

FIGURE 14-6 Back view of incubator.

unit is controlled by a temperature probe that monitors the infant's temperature and feeds this information to the heating and cooling unit of the incubator. The incubator automatically heats or cools to bring the infant's temperature to the preset range.

2 If the probe becomes detached from the infant, the incubator will continue to heat until air around the probe reaches the temperature that was preset for the infant. This situation can cause the incubator to overheat, causing harm to the infant.

12.4 Special precautions when using an incubator

1 O_2 is a drug and should not be administered to anyone without a physician's order.

2 CAUTION: In newborns weighing less than 5 pounds, O_2 concentrations greater than 40% will cause a scarring destruction in the eye known as retrolental fibroplasia. This condition may lead to permanent partial or complete blindness of the infant.

3 To help prevent this serious clinical incidence, the American Academy of Pediatrics passed the following guidelines, which should be followed whenever infants are receiving O_2 in an incubator-type chamber.

12.5 AAP guidelines for administering O_2 via incubators

1 Except in an emergency, O_2 should be prescribed only by medical order.

2 O_2 should *not* be administered routinely but only upon specific medical indication.

3 The O_2 concentration should be kept at the lowest possible level that will relieve the symptoms for which it is given, if possible, not over 40%.

4 O_2 therapy should be discontinued as soon as the indication for it has passed.

5 Ordinarily, the clinical indications for supplemental O_2 are general cyanosis and dyspnea. This method of diagnosis, however, is not as reliable as arterial blood gas analysis or percutaneous O_2 monitoring. The urgency of treating these symptoms must rest with the clinical judgment of the attending physician.

6 The O_2 concentration must be determined by means of an oxygen analyzer as often as necessary, but at least every 4 hours, to keep the FIo_2 properly stabilized.

7 An O_2 source that does not contain or deliver more than 40% O_2 will ensure against exceeding that concentration but may not be adequate where higher concentration is desired. If such a restricted source of O_2 is employed, additional O_2 should be available for those special instances where it is indicated.

8 There are no apparent contraindications to the use of supplemental O_2 in infants weighing more than 5 pounds other than the same precautions observed when administering O_2 to an adult patient.

12.6 Measuring FIo_2 in incubators

1 As an additional safety measure, the FIo_2 in incubators should be initially checked every 30 minutes and then hourly, using any type of reliable analyzer.

2 NOTE: When checking the FIo_2, the practitioner should place a sampling tube or sensor, and *not* the analyzer, inside the canopy.

12.7 Administering aerosols to an infant in an incubator

When administering aerosols to an infant in an incubator, the following facts should be considered:

1 Small particle sizes (1 to 5 microns) are desirable.

2 Newborns may have bronchospasm and may need bronchodilators administered with the aerosol.

3 Liquefying agents or detergents that are administered by aerosol are helpful in loosening thick secretions for subsequent suctioning.

4 Fine mists aid in the hydration of newborns.

5 Ultrasonic mists are so dense that they must be used with caution, and the premature infant must be weighed during the course of continuous administration to assess any positive water gain.

6 Only *sterile* distilled water should be used in incubators.

7 The humidifier and nebulizer should be changed at least every 12 hours to prevent growth of gram-negative microbes.

12.8 Operating an Air Shields 150 Model Isolette

1 Before putting it in service, ensure that the Isolette has been thoroughly cleaned, sterile linen is available, and the unit is within its service due date. This service date should be found at the back on the top of the microfilter assembly.

2 Fill the humidity chamber with sterile distilled water and add 20 ml of acetic acid. Check the water level each 8-hour shift and fill as required.

12.9 Manually controlling the Isolette

The following procedure applies when the Isolette is to be used on a *manual* thermostat control basis only:

1 Connect the power cord to an electrical outlet. One of two white lights will illuminate to indicate power is reaching the unit and the circulating system is operating.

2 Turn the thermostat knob to the thermostat control position. The white thermostat control light will remain on continuously.

3 Adjust the thermostat control knob to raise the incubator temperature to the desired limit. It will take up to 1 hour for the Isolette to warm up to 30° to 32° C (88° to 90° F).

4 If desired, the infant's skin temperature can be monitored. Insert the plug of the patient probe into the socket on the underside of the control panel and tape the tip of the patient probe to the infant's abdomen. Use an opaque, nonirritating tape and ensure that the entire tip is covered with tape.

12.10 Automatically operating the Isolette

The following procedure applies when the Isolette is to be operated on the *Infant Servo Control* (ISC) unit:

1 Connect the incubator to an electrical outlet. One of the two white lights will illuminate to indicate power to the unit and that the air circulating system is operating.

2 Turn the thermostat knob fully clockwise to the infant servo control position. The white infant servo control light will then remain on continuously.

3 Check the calibration of the temperature meter. To do this, remove the patient probe from the socket on the underside of the control panel and then press the red "line adjust" button. The needle on the meter should move up slowly and stop on the red line.

4 Check the temperature control point. This is done by pressing the "control point adjust" button and waiting for the needle on the meter to come to a stop. It should come to rest at a meter reading of 36° C (97° F).

5 Tape the tip of the patient probe to the infant using an opaque, nonirritating tape. The patient probe should be secured to the patient at the midline of the abdomen, halfway between the umbilicus and xiphoid. Caution should be taken to ensure that the entire tip is covered by tape.

6 If cooling is desired, fill the ice chamber with about 10 pounds of ice and 1 quart of water. Then turn the thermostat control knob counterclockwise. Wait until the desired temperature has been reached and then turn the thermostat control knob clockwise until the amber heater light comes on. This will maintain the temperature at plus or minus 1° F of the thermostatic control setting.

12.11 Care of incubator

The following general steps should be observed when using an incubator:

1 Damp-dust the canopy and other parts with a disinfectant solution daily.

2 Clean arm ports daily with a disinfectant solution.

3 Change plastic sleeves as needed.

4 Change baby to freshly cleaned Isolette every 3 days.

5 Fill humidity chamber with sterile distilled water and add 20 ml of acetic acid to restrict the growth of *Pseudomonas* and gram-negative organisms.

6 Add sterile distilled water as needed.

7 Clean humidifier at least every 12 hours.

8 *Do not* attach accessories that are *not* specifically designed for use with the Isolette.

13.0 PROVIDING A CONTROLLED ENVIRONMENT FOR OXYGEN, TEMPERATURE, AND HUMIDITY
13.1 Operation of the Ohio Servo-Controlled Heating Unit with a Model 190-A Incubator

1 The Ohio Servo incubator represents an example of how a heating device can be operated by a feedback signal from the temperature probe attached to the baby's skin.

2 As with similar units, placement of the probe is critical as is the calibration of the unit before leaving the infant on automated control.

3 It is critical that appropriate safeguards be established

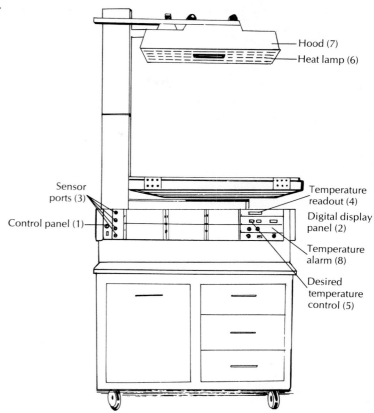

FIGURE 14-7 Open incubator.

to ensure that the infant is routinely monitored by unit personnel as well as by the alarm devices.

4 Procedure 14-7 for operation of an Ohio Servo Model Incubator (or similar brand) is included at the end of this module.

14.0 CHECK ROUNDS FOR PATIENTS IN INCUBATORS
14.1 Procedure for conducting check rounds

Procedure 14-8 for conducting check rounds on infants in incubators is also included at the end of this module.

15.0 OPEN INCUBATORS (INFRARED WARMERS)
15.1 Operation of an open-tube incubator system

1 Since 1975 many infant care units have changed to open incubators, which are heated by infrared energy lamps positioned in a hood above the baby (Fig. 14-7).

2 The heating lamp is servo-controlled by the baby's skin temperature as monitored by a temperature probe usually attached by tape to the baby's skin.

3 The major benefit to such a system is easy access to the baby for positioning, treatments, and attachment of supportive aids such as drains and ventilator tubing.

4 NOTE: There are many models of infrared warmers. For this reason, the type shown below will vary somewhat from manufacturer to manufacturer, although the principles of operation will be similar for any open incubator. One notable difference between the Healthdyne IW-10 Infant Warmer and the Puritan Infa-Care Unit

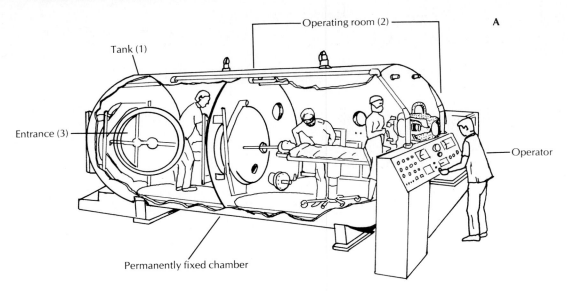

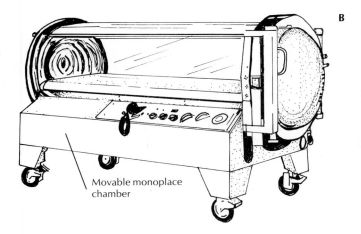

FIGURE 14-8 A, Fixed hyperbaric chamber. **B,** Monoplace chamber.

(see Fig. 14-7) is the addition of a phototherapy accessory light to the warmer to treat bilirubinemia.

15.2 Theory of operation for the Puritan Infa-Care Unit

1 A control panel provides power outlets, timers, alarms, and memory functions for the entire system *(1)*.
2 A master control switch, when depressed, will activate the panel *(2)* including all digital displays.
3 The temperature probe is plugged into one of the sensor ports located on top of the cabinet *(3)*.
4 The baby's skin temperature is monitored by a skin temperature probe and is shown by digital light presentation *(4)*.
5 The desired skin temperature is set by the temperature control *(5)* and a meter.
6 The heat lamp *(6)* housed in a hood *(7)* will automatically turn on and off to keep the baby's temperature at the preset level (normally 36.6° C [98° F]).
7 An alarm will sound if temperature probe exceeds 2.5° F of preset temperature *(8)*.
8 For details on operation, see the manufacturer's instruction manual that accompanies a particular model or the hospital procedure manual.

15.3 Key points when using an infant infrared warmer

1 Heating lamps must be positioned no closer than 12 inches from the Infa-Care unit.
2 The temperature sensor must be securely and properly taped in place. CAUTION: The temperature sensor controls the heating time of the lamp. If the sensor probe becomes disconnected, or is left out of the basket, the hood will keep heating to maximum temperature, possibly overheating the infant.

16.0 HYPERBARIC CHAMBERS
16.1 Application of a hyperbaric chamber

1 Hyperbaric refers to pressures above 1 atm. A hyperbaric chamber is capable of being operated at pressures greater than 1 atm (14.7 psi). Pressure vessels have been used for various applications since their introduction by Alexander the Great in 332 B.C. as diving chambers.
2 Today, hyperbaric chambers are constructed of rigid steel and concrete or special plastic. They may be large concrete and steel permanently fixed rooms or a single-person (monoplace) transparent movable chamber (Fig. 14-8, *A* and *B*).

3 Medical centers used permanent fixed chambers for medical treatment and as operating rooms.

4 Diseases treated by hyperbaric pressures include circulatory insufficiency, traumatic arterial injury, cerebrovascular accidents, myocardial infarction, peripheral vascular disease (ulcers), frostbite, burns, carbon monoxide poisoning, barbiturate poisoning, cyanide poisoning, gas gangrene, tetanus, respiratory insufficiency, pulmonary edema, and caisson disease (bends).

5 The chamber may be a single room or consist of several tanks with different pressure ratings connected together *(1)*.

6 Operating rooms are usually 16 to 19 feet in diameter *(2)* and 30 feet long, having various entrance and exit locks *(3)*.

7 Pressure levels will vary according to the chamber rating, although most large chambers are rated to 45 psi or 3 atm.

8 Atmospheres in the chambers will vary according to the "depth of the dive" (pressure referred). Most chambers will use a gas mixture of 80% nitrogen (N_2) and 20% O_2, although helium-oxygen mixtures may be used.

9 The atmosphere and pressure within the chamber are controlled by an operator who remains outside the chamber. It is important that this person be especially qualified as a chamber operator by the U.S. Navy or other qualified agencies.

10 Respiratory care personnel are frequently trained to operate the small monoplace chambers that are becoming more commonplace in community hospitals and even outpatient care facilities.

16.2 Hazards and special considerations

1 Hazards in hyperbaric chambers include an increased fire potential because of complete saturation of materials with chamber gas. A spontaneous pneumothorax may occur because of changes in lung pressure, and persons with occluded eustachian tubes may have their eardrums ruptured. Other considerations include central nervous system (CNS) toxicity and pulmonary toxicity.

2 Equipment used in hyperbaric chambers *must be modified* because of the increased density and resistance to gas flow through orifices above 1 atm absolute (ATA).

3 Persons must not submit themselves to a chamber "dive" until they have had a complete physical examination clearing them for hyperbaric work.

PROCEDURE 14-1

Operating a high humidity electric oxygen tent for delivery of aerosol/oxygen therapy

No.	Steps in performing the procedure
1	The practitioner will assemble and operate an electric humidity/oxygen tent to deliver prescribed therapy to patient. Collect necessary equipment:
	1.1 Tent console with nebulizer
	1.2 Disposable canopy
	1.3 Flowmeter with small bore tubing adapter
	1.4 Oxygen delivery tube
	1.5 Sterile distilled water
	1.6 Oxygen analyzer
2	Verify physician's order.
3	Review chart for relevant data.
4	Wash hands.
5	Greet patient; introduce yourself.
6	Verify patient identification.
7	Explain procedure/reassure patient.
8	Wheel equipment into room.
9	Assemble equipment and attach flowmeter to gas source.
10	Fill nebulizer reservoir with sterile distilled water.
11	Turn tent on and adjust temperature between 68° to 72° F or no greater than 15° below room temperature.
12	Adjust gas flow into nebulizer to flush or to 15 L/min and note aerosol density.
13	Adjust gas flow as necessary to produce adequate mist.
14	Position tent in appropriate location adjacent to bed.
15	Open canopy and place over patient, taking care not to contact patient's face.
16	Tuck canopy tightly under mattress on all sides.
17	Secure canopy across patient's abdominal region with a draw sheet or across the foot of bed, if tent is being used with child.
18	Check FIO_2 and readjust O_2 flow to between 10 and 12 L/min after 15 min on flush.
19	Remove all fire hazards from patient's room.
20	Position call bell where patient can summon help.
21	Post NO SMOKING signs.
22	Reassure patient.
23	Wash hands.
24	Chart procedure.

PROCEDURE 14-2

Operational check—high humidity electric oxygen tent

No.	Steps in performing the procedure
1	The practitioner will visit assigned patients, assess patients' progress, and check operation of electric humidity/oxygen tent. Collect necessary equipment: **1.1** Sterile distilled water **1.2** Fresh supplies **1.3** Oxygen analyzer
2	Verify continuation of therapy.
3	Review patient's progress notes.
4	Review relevant laboratory/therapy data.
5	Wash hands.
6	Greet patient; introduce yourself.
7	Verify patient's identification.
8	Observe patient's mental and physical status. Note any acute changes in respirations or behavior.
9	Verify L/min gas flow.
10	Insert oxygen analyzer sensor into canopy through slightly opened zipper or appropriate opening. Allow to stabilize. Note O_2 percentage and compare to physician's ordered FIo_2.
11	Assess aerosol output and correct if inadequate.
12	Check nebulizer and siphon tube.
13	Rinse nebulizer jar and refill with sterile distilled water.
14	Inspect canopy for damage. Replace if necessary or according to department quality control procedure.
15	Change nebulizer according to departmental quality control procedure.
16	Ensure that canopy is properly fitted to bed and draw sheet is in proper position.
17	Empty condensate tray or bottle into appropriate container. *Do not* pour into patient's sink.
18	Wash hands.
19	Chart rounds.

PROCEDURE 14-3

Operating an Air Shields Model D or Universal Croupette*

No.	Steps in performing the procedure
1	The practitioner will assemble and operate a Croupette to deliver prescribed aerosol/oxygen therapy to patient. Collect necessary equipment: **1.1** Croupette **1.2** Canopy **1.3** Ice **1.4** Sterile distilled water **1.5** Flowmeter **1.6** Connecting tubing **1.7** Draw sheet
2	Verify physician's order.
3	Wash hands.
4	Identify patient; introduce yourself to family.
5	Orient family to therapy.
6	Attach flowmeter to gas source.
7	Attach drain tubing to bottom of ice chamber.
8	Slip end of drain tube into retaining clip on ice chamber.
9	Assemble nebulizer jet and appropriate nozzles.
10	Fill water jar with sterile distilled water.
11	Check nebulizer for proper position in base assembly.
12	Attach water jar to base assembly of nebulizer.
13	Firmly secure unit to bed.
14	Attach canopy to canopy frame.
15	Attach small bore tubing to flowmeter and nebulizer inlet.
16	Set flow rate to 10 L/min minimum.†
17	Evaluate adequacy of aerosol output.
18	If inadequate, correct situation.
19	Place canopy over patient.
20	Securely tuck sides of canopy under mattress and use draw sheet to secure foot of canopy.
21	Place ice in ice chamber.
22	Remove all fire hazards from room.
23	Post NO SMOKING signs.
24	Reassure patient/family.
25	Wash hands.
26	Chart therapy.

*Or similar device.
†If compressed air is being used, do not tuck sides of canopy.

PROCEDURE 14-4

Operational check—croup tent

No.	Steps in performing the procedure
1	The practitioner will visit assigned patients, assess patients' progress, and check operation of a croup tent. Collect necessary equipment: **1.1** Sterile distilled water **1.2** Fresh supplies **1.3** Oxygen analyzer
2	Verify continuation of order for therapy.
3	Review patient's progress notes.
4	Review relevant laboratory/therapy data.
5	Wash hands.
6	Greet patient and/or family. Introduce yourself.
7	Verify patient identification.
8	Assess patient's mental and physical status. Note any acute changes in respirations or behavior.
9	Verify L/min gas flow.
10	Insert oxygen analyzer sensor into canopy through slightly opened zipper or appropriate opening. Allow to stabilize. Note O_2 percentage and compare to physician's ordered FI_{O_2}.
11	Assess aerosol output and correct if inadequate.
12	Check nebulizer filter and siphon tube.
13	Rinse nebulizer jar and add sterile distilled water.
14	Inspect canopy for damage, cleanliness, and fit. Replace if necessary or according to departmental quality control procedure.
15	Drain ice compartment.
16	Empty nebulizer and melted ice into appropriate container. *Do not* pour into patient's sink.
17	Change nebulizer according to departmental quality control procedure.
18	Add ice to ice compartment.
19	Wash hands.
20	Chart rounds.

PROCEDURE 14-5

Operating Olympic Oxyhood to administer elevated FI_{O_2} and aerosol to infant*

No.	Steps in performing the procedure
1	The practitioner will assemble and operate an Olympic Oxyhood to deliver prescribed therapy to patient. Select proper size hood: **1.1** Infant under 2½ pounds: small, 6-inch diameter **1.2** Infant 2½-8 pounds: medium, 8-inch diameter **1.3** Infant 8-18 pounds: large, 10-inch diameter
2	Collect other necessary equipment: **2.1** Nebulizer **2.2** Large bore tubing **2.3** Flowmeter **2.4** Sterile distilled water **2.5** Oxygen analyzer **2.6** Heater†
3	Verify physician's order.
4	Review chart for relevant data.
5	Wash hands.
6	Identify patient/introduce yourself to family.
7	Orient family to therapy.
8	Ready equipment for operation.
9	Adjust nebulizer to prescribed FI_{O_2}.
10	Adjust gas flow to produce desired aerosol density.
11	Place hood over infant's head with space provided between infant's neck and hood's opening.
12	Check infant's position in hood.
13	Check FI_{O_2} with analyzer and correct to prescription, as necessary.
14	Wash hands.
15	Chart procedure.

*Or similar brand.
†Hoods are not routinely heated; check orders.

PROCEDURE 14-6

Operational check—oxygen hood

No.	Steps in performing the procedure
1	The practitioner will visit assigned patients, assess their progress, and check operation of an infant hood. Collect necessary equipment: **1.1** Sterile distilled water **1.2** Fresh supplies **1.3** Oxygen analyzer
2	Verify continuation of order for therapy.
3	Review patient's progress notes.
4	Review relevant laboratory/therapy data.
5	Wash hands.
6	Greet patient and/or family. Introduce yourself.
7	Verify patient identification.
8	Assess patient's physical status. Note any acute changes in respirations or airway patency since prior report.
9	Verify FIO_2. Insert oxygen analyzer sensor into hood and close lid. Allow to stabilize. Note O_2 percentage and compare to physician's ordered FIO_2.
10	Adjust gas flow or mixture as required.
11	Assess nebulizer aerosol output and correct as needed.
12	Check all connections and lid for tightness and seal.
13	Check temperature inside hood and adjust as necessary. NOTE: Hoods are not routinely heated; check orders.
14	Empty condensate from delivery tube into an appropriate container, *not* back into nebulizer jar or patient's sink.
15	Change nebulizer, tubing, and hood according to departmental quality control procedure.
16	Check placement of hood and change as necessary.
17	Recheck FIO_2.
18	Wash hands.
19	Chart rounds.

PROCEDURE 14-7

Operating an Ohio Servo-Controlled Heating Unit in conjunction with 190-A Incubator*

No.	Steps in performing the procedure
1	The practitioner will use servo control to automatically regulate an infant's temperature at a preset level. Special care will be taken to properly attach the temperature probe to the infant's skin. Collect necessary equipment: **1.1** Ohio 190-A Incubator with servo heat control **1.2** Temperature probe **1.3** Flowmeter **1.4** Nebulizer, if prescribed **1.5** Nonirritating tape **1.6** Connecting tubing **1.7** Oxygen analyzer
2	Verify physician's order.
3	Review chart for relevant data.
4	Wash hands, observing special nursery technique precautions.
5	Verify patient identification.
6	Prepare equipment.
7	Connect power cord.
8	Place selector to "start."
9	Set temperature control to "start."
10	Adjust flowmeter to correct L/min flow.
11	Preheat incubator until stable using thermometer inside hood.
12	Adjust black needle on temperature meter to 36° C (red mark).
13	Set control temperature to 36.4° C (97.6° F) (movable red needle) by adjusting knob on meter.
14	Plug probe into socket beneath temperature meter.
15	Place infant in incubator in appropriate position.
16	Attach temperature probe to infant's abdomen midway between umbilicus and xiphoid using nonirritating tape, being sure to cover tip of probe completely.
17	Read infant's temperature from meter.
18	Move selector control to "servo" position (automatic).
19	Measure FIO_2 in incubator and adjust O_2 L/min flow as needed.
20	Monitor q. 30 min for first hour.
21	Monitor q. 1h for next 4 hours.
22	Monitor q. 4h after FIO_2 stable.
23	Wash hands.
24	Chart therapy.

*Or similar brand.

PROCEDURE 14-8

Operational check—incubator

No.	Steps in performing the procedure
1	The practitioner will visit assigned patients, assess their progress, and check operation of a Servo incubator. Collect necessary equipment: **1.1** Sterile distilled water **1.2** Fresh supplies **1.3** Oxygen analyzer
2	Verify physician's order.
3	Review patient's progress notes.
4	Review relevant laboratory/therapy data.
5	Wash hands.
6	Check patient identification and position.
7	Assess patient's physical status. Note any acute changes in respirations or airway patency since prior report.
8	Verify L/min gas flow.
9	Insert oxygen analyzer sensor into access port. Allow to stabilize. Note O_2 percentage and compare to physician's ordered FIo_2.
10	Measure FIo_2 and adjust gas flow or mixture required.
11	Check all ports and access sleeves for seal and operation.
12	Check, and if necessary, change air filter.
13	Check patient's temperature and attach temperature probe.
14	Retape temperature probe, if necessary.
15	Check temperature inside incubator and adjust as needed.
16	Check operation of servo unit according to the manufacturer's check procedure.
17	Check and refill humidifier, if being used.
18	If nebulizer is being used, empty water from reservoir jar; rinse jar and refill with steile distilled water.
19	Evaluate aerosol output density and correct as needed.
20	Recheck FIo_2.
21	Wash hands.
22	Chart rounds.

BIBLIOGRAPHY

Beckham RW and Cominsky MS: Sound levels inside incubators and oxygen hoods used with nebulizers and humidifiers, Respir Care 27:33, 1982.

Burton GG, Gee GN, and Hodgkin JE, editors: Respiratory care: a guide to clinical practice, Philadelphia, 1977, JB Lippincott Co.

Engle WD et al: Effect of increased radiant warmer power output on state of hydration in the critically ill neonate, Crit Care Med 10:673, 1982.

Hyperbaric oxygen therapy: a committee report, revised, Bethesda, Md, 1986, Undersea and Hyperbaric Medical Society.

McPherson SP and Spearman CG: Respiratory therapy equipment, ed 4, St Louis, 1990, The CV Mosby Co.

Shilling CW, and Faiman MD: Physics of diving and physical effects on divers. In The physician's guide to diving medicine, New York, 1984, Plenum Press, pp 35-69.

Spearman CB, Sheldon RL, and Egan DF: Egan's fundamentals of respiratory therapy, ed 5, St Louis, 1990, The CV Mosby Co.

Pharmacology

On completion of this module the reader will be able to:

1.1 Demonstrate an understanding of the need for pharmacology by discussing drugs and procedures when questioned about various drugs, dosages, their actions, and routes of administration.

2.1 Use correct terminology and abbreviations when charting results of patient care involving the administration of drug therapy.

2.2 Define commonly used abbreviations in prescription orders.

3.1 Differentiate between various agencies and regulations involved in the manufacturing, distribution, and selling of drugs.

4.1 Compare the *United States Pharmacopeia* to the *National Formulary* as information resources on drugs.

4.2 Describe the current system for catagorizing and naming drugs.

4.3 Use the *United States Pharmacopeia,* the *National Formulary,* and the *Physicians' Desk Reference* to look up drugs used in respiratory care.

5.1 Identify factors influencing the effects of administering single and combined drugs.

6.1 Explain factors determining the metabolism of drugs within the body.

7.1 Discuss drug action theory as it relates to the combination of drugs with cellular sites, interaction with cellular enzymes, and action potential on changing cellular membrane structures.

7.2 Explain the drug receptor theory.

7.3 Discuss the role of enzymes within the cell.

8.1 List various routes for administering drugs.

8.2 Discuss factors determining routes of administration.

9.1 Explain general responsibility of the physician, nurse, and respiratory care personnel for the administration of drugs.

10.1 Relate principles to be observed by respiratory care personnel when administering drugs.

11.1 Describe guidelines for preparation of drugs for administration.

12.1 Explain general concepts and precautions to be observed when using a nebulizer to administer medications.

13.1 Identify components comprising a properly written medical order for a treatment involving respiratory drugs.

14.1 Use a needle and syringe to draw a prescribed amount of medication from a vial and ampule.

14.2 Use a unit dose vial to dispense a prescribed amount of medication into a container.

15.1 Discuss the need for accurately measuring drugs before administering them to patients.

15.2 Define terms used in preparing solutions and use formulae to solve problems related to drug calculation.

15.3 Discuss special dosage considerations for infants and children.

16.1 and **16.2** Describe theory of the pharmacologic and physiologic bases of drug action.

17.1 through **17.4** Discuss principles of medications that can cause respiratory depression.

18.1 Discuss the use of central nervous system depressants in respiratory care.

19.1 Discuss anesthetic drugs and their use.

20.1 Discuss principles of medications that can cause central nervous system stimulation.

21.1 and **21.2** Discuss the use of antibiotics and describe specific antibiotic agents.

22.1 Discuss drugs that affect metabolism (e.g., steroids).

23.1 Define histamine reaction and treatment.

24.1 and **24.2** Discuss action of the autonomic nervous system and describe classification of drugs affecting the autonomic nervous system.

25.1 Discuss cardiac-related drugs.

26.1 Discuss diuretic drugs.

27.1 Discuss xanthine-related drugs.

28.1 through **28.13** Discuss and describe the use of specific drugs in and/or in conjunction with respiratory therapy according to:

1 Generic name

2 Proprietary name

3 Action

4 Use

5 Dosage

6 Cautions

7 Side effects

29.1 Discuss drugs used in cardiopulmonary emergencies.

30.1 Demonstrate the importance of having a working knowledge of cardiorespiratory drugs by listing and discussing the application of aerosolized drugs covered in this module.

30.2 Define bronchospasm and compare the various drugs and their actions used to treat this condition.

30.3 Discuss the source of mucus and differentiate between the various drugs used to control airway secretions.

30.4 Describe the pathologic changes noted in severe asthma and compare actions of the various drugs used for Steps I, II, and III therapy.

1.0 IMPORTANCE OF PHARMACOLOGY IN RESPIRATORY CARE

1.1 Need for pharmacology

1 Pharmacology is the science of studying drugs; their origin, nature, properties, and effects on living things.

2 Drugs refer to any substance (including gases) that is applied or taken into the body to cure, relieve, prevent, and diagnose disease.

3 A thorough understanding of the clinical aspects of the drugs given to respiratory patients is one of the most important competencies a respiratory care practitioner must acquire to be safe and effective at the bedside.

4 *All substances* that are administered to a patient via the pulmonary route are potentially dangerous as a result of a drug action or as a source for infection. To minimize the risk of drug reactions, the clinician must know the indications, contraindications, average dosages, desired effects, untoward effects, and precautions for every drug used. In addition, a clinician must learn to use the *Physicians' Desk Reference* (PDR), the *United States Pharmaopeia* (USP), and the *National Formulary* (NF) as resources. A clinician is legally accountable for what is administered to a patient.

2.0 TERMINOLOGY AND ABBREVIATIONS

2.1 Glossary of useful terms*

1 Absorption. (1) The incorporation of matter by other matter through chemical, molecular, or physical action, as the dissolving of a gas in a liquid or the taking up of a liquid by a porous solid. (2) (in physiology) The passage of substances across and into tissues, as the passage of digested food molecules into intestinal cells or the passage of liquids into kidney tubules. Kinds of absorption in physiology are agglutinin absorption, cutaneous absorption, external absorption, interstitial absorption, intestinal absorption, parenteral absorption, and pathologic absorption. (3) (in radiology) The absorption of radiant energy by living or nonliving matter with which the radiation reacts.

2 Addiction. Compulsive, uncontrollable dependence on a substance, habit, or practice to such a degree that cessation causes severe emotional, mental, or physiologic reactions. (compare Habituation.*)

3 Adverse reaction. A response in opposition to a substance, treatment, or other stimulus, such as an antigen-antibody reaction in immunology, a hypersensitivity reaction in allergy, or an adverse reaction in pharmacology.

4 Affinity. A likeness or special relationship; an attraction.

5 Agonist. (1) A contracting muscle whose contraction is opposed by another muscle (an antagonist). (2) A drug or other substance having a specific cellular affinity that produces a predictable response.

6 Allergy. A hypersensitive reaction to intrinsically harmless antigens, most of which are environmental. Studies show that 1 of every 6 Americans has a severe allergy and that more than 20 million Americans have allergic reactions to airborne or inhaled allergens, such as cigarette smoke, house dust, and pollens. Allergic rhinitis, which is associated with airborne allergens, affects perdominantly young children and adolescents but occurs in all age groups. Allergies are classified according to Types 1, 11, 111, and IV hypersensitivity. Types I, II, and III involve different immunoglobulin antibodies and their interaction with different antigens. Type IV allergy is associated with contact dermatitis and with T-cells that react directly with the antigen and cause local inflammation. Allergies are divided into those that produce immediate or antibody-mediated reactions and those that produce delayed or cell-mediated reactions. Immediate allergic reactions involve Types I, II, and III hypersensitivity and antigen-antibody reactions that activate certain enzymes, creating an imbalance between these enzymes and their inhibitors. Immediate allergic reactions also release certain substances into the circulation, such as histamine, bradykinin, acetylcholine, gamma globulin G, and leukotaxine, Delayed allergic reactions are caused by antigens but do not seem to depend on antibodies. Depending on the type of hypersensitivity involved, some common symptoms of allergy are bronchial congestion, conjunctivitis, edema, fever, urticaria, and vomiting. Severe allergic reactions, such as anaphylaxis, can cause systemic shock and death. Symptoms of limited dura-

---

*Most of these definitions were taken from Mosby's medical, nursing, & allied health dictionary, St Louis, ed 3, 1990, The CV Mosby Co.

*See Mosby's medical, nursing, & allied health dictionary, ed 3, St Louis, 1990, The CV Mosby Co.

tion, such as those associated with hay fever, serum-sickness, bee stings, and urticaria, can be suppressed by glucocorticoids administered as supplements to primary therapy. The effect of such steroids may be considerably delayed. Severe allergic reactions, such as anaphylaxis and angioneurotic edema of the glottis, commonly require immediate therapy with epinephrine administered subcutaneously. When allergic reactions are life-threatening, steroids, such as dexamethasone sodium phosphate, may be administered intravenously. For milder diseases, such as serum sickness and hay fever, antihistamines are usually administered.

7 Ampule. A small, sterile glass or plastic container that usually contains a single dose of a solution to be administered parenterally.

8 Analeptic. See Central nervous system stimulant.*

9 Analgesic. (1) Relieving pain. (2) A drug that relieves pain.

10 Anaphylaxis. An exaggerated hypersensitivity reaction to a previously encountered antigen. The response, which is mediated by antibodies of the IgE class of immunoglobulins, causes the release of histamine, kinin, and substances that affect smooth muscle. The reaction may be a localized wheal and flare of generalized itching, hyperemia, angioedema, and, in severe cases, vascular collapse, bronchospasm, and shock. The severity of symptoms depends on the original sensitizing dose of the antigen, the amount and distribution of antibodies, and the route of entry and size of the dose of antigen producing anaphylaxis. Insect stings, contrast media containing iodine, aspirin, antitoxins prepared with animal serum, and allergens used in testing and desensitizing patients who are hypersensitive produce anaphylaxis in some individuals. Penicillin injection is the most common cause of anaphylactic shock. Kinds of anaphylaxis are aggregate anaphylaxis, antiserum anaphylaxis, cutaneous anaphylaxis, cytotoxic anaphylaxis, indirect anaphylaxis, and inverse anaphylaxis.

11 Anesthesia. The absence of normal sensation, especially sensitive to pain, as induced by an anesthetic substance or by hypnosis or as occurs with traumatic or pathophysiologic damage to nerve tissue. Anesthesia induced for medical or surgical purposes may be topical, local, regional, or general and is named for the anesthetic agent used, the method or procedure followed, the area or organ anesthetized, or the age or class of patient served.

12 Antagonist. (1) One who contends with or is opposed to another. (2) (in physiology) Any agent, such as a drug or muscle, that exerts an opposite action to that of another. Kinds of antagonists include associated antagonist, competitive antagonists, direct antagonist. (3) (in dentistry) A tooth in the upper jaw that articu-

lates during mastication or occlusion with a tooth in the lower jaw.

13 Antibiotics. (1) Of or pertaining to the ability to destroy or interfere with the development of a living organism. (2) An antimicrobial agent, derived from cultures of a microorganism or produced semisynthetically, used to treat infections. The penicillins, derived from species of the fungus *Penicillum* or manufactured semisynthetically, consist of a thiazolidine ring fused to a beta-lactam ring connected to side chains; these agents exert their action by inhibiting mucopeptide synthesis in bacterial cell walls during multiplication of the organisms. Pencillin G and V are widely used in treating many gram-positive coccal infections but are inactivated by the enzyme penicillinase produced by some strains of staphylococci cloxacillin, dicloxacillin, methicillin, nafcillin, and oxacillin are penicillinase-resistant penicillins. Broad-spectrum penicillins effective against gram-negative organisms are ampicillin, carbenicillin, and hetacillin. Hypersensitivity reactions, such as rash, fever, bronchospasm, vasculitis, and anaphylaxis are relatively common side effects of penicillin therapy. Aminoglycoside antibiotics, composed of amino sugars in glycoside linkage, interfere with the synthesis of bacterial proteins and are used primarily for the treatment of infections caused by gram-negative organisms. The aminoglycosides include gentamicin derived from *Micromonospora*, semisynthetic amikacin, kanamycin, neomycin, streptomycin, and tobramycin. These agents commonly cause nephrotoxic and ototoxic reactions as well as gastrointestinal disturbances. Macrolide antibiotics, consisting of a large lactone ring and deoxyamino sugar, interfere in protein synthesis of susceptible bacteria during multiplication without affecting nucleic acid synthesis. Oleandomycin, which is added to feed to improve the growth of poultry and swine, and broad-spectrum erythromycin, used to treat various gram-positive and gram-negative infections, are macrolides derived from species of *Streptomyces*. Erythromycin may cause mild allergic reactions and gastrointestinal discomfort, but nausea, vomiting, and diarrhea occur infrequently with the usual oral dose. Polypeptide antibiotics derived from species of *Streptomyces* or certain soil bacilli vary in their spectra, most of these agents are nephrotoxic and ototoxic. Bacitracin and vancomycin are polypeptides used to treat severe staphylococcal infections; capreomycin and vancomycin are antituberculosis agents; and gramicidin is included in ointments for topical infections. Antifungals, including amphotericin B and nystatin, apparently bind to sterols in fungus cell membranes and change their permeability; griseofulvin grossly distorts terminal hyphae of fungi. Amphotericin B is effective against many kinds of fungi; it may cause fever, vomiting, diarrhea, generalized pains, anemia, renal dysfunction, and other adverse effects when administered intravenously. Oral

---

*See Mosby's medical, nursing, & allied health dictionary, ed 3, St Louis, 1990, The CV Mosby Co.

griseofulvin is used to treat various fungal infections of the skin and nails and may cause hypersensitivity reactions, gastrointestinal disturbances, fatigue, and insomnia. Nystatin is applied locally for the treatment of oral and vaginal candidiasis; it is also used for vaginal candidiasis. The tetracyclines, including the prototype derived from *Streptomyces,* chlortetracycline, demeclocyline, doxycycline, minocycline, and oxytetracycline, are active against a wide range of gram-positive and gram-negative organisms and some rickettsiae. Antibiotics in this group are primarily bacteriostatic and are thought to exert their effect by inhibiting protein synthesis in the organisms. Tetracycline therapy may cause gastrointestinal irritation, photosensitivity, renal toxicity, and hepatic toxicity, and administration of a drug of this group during the last half of pregnancy, during infancy, or before the age of eight may result in permanent discoloration of the teeth.

The cephalosporins, derived from the soil fungus (*Cephalosporium* or produced semisynthetically, inhibit bacterial cell wall synthesis, resist the action of penicillinase, and are used in treating infections of the respiratory tract, urinary tract, middle ear, and, bones as well as septicemia caused by a wide range of gram-positive and gram-negative organisms. The group includes cefadroxil, cefamandole, cefazolin, cephalexin, cephaloglycin, cephaloridine, cephalothin, cephapirin, and cephradine. The cephalosporins are divided into three groups. The first group—the first-generation cephalosporins—includes cephalothin, cephapirin, cefadroxil, cefazolin, cephalexin, cefaclor, cephaloridine, and cephradine. The second generation includes cefamandole, cefoxitin, and cefuroxime. The third generation includes cefotaxime, moxalactam, and cefoperazone. New cephalosporins are rapidly being released. Treatment with a cephalosporin may cause nausea, vomiting, diarrhea, enterocolitis, or an allergic reaction, such as rash, angioedema, or exfoliative dermatitis; use of antibiotics in the group may cause an allergic reaction in patients who have shown hypersensitivity to a penicillin. Chloramphenicol, a broad-spectrum antibiotic initially derived from *Streptomyces venezuelae,* inhibits protein synthesis in bacteria by interfering with the transfer of activated amino acids from soluble RNA to ribosomes. Since the drug may cause life-threatening blood dyscrasias, its use is reserved for the treatment of acute typhoid fever, serious gram-negative infections (including *Hemophilus influenzae* meningitis), and rickettsial diseases.

14 Antibody. An immunoglobulin, essential to the immune system, produced by lymphoid tissue in response to bacteria, viruses, or other antigenic substances. An antibody is specific to an antigen. Each class of antibody is named for its action. Among the many antibodies are agglutinins, bacteriolysins, opsonins, and precipitin.

15 Antidote. A drug or other substance that opposes the action of a poison. An antidote may be mechanical, acting to coat the stomach and prevent absorption; or chemical, acting to make the toxin inert; or physiologic, acting to oppose the action of the poison, as a sedative given to a person who has ingested a large amount of a stimulant.

16 Antitoxin. A subgroup of antisera usually prepared from the serum of horses immunized against a particular toxin-producing organism, such as botulism antitoxin given therapeutically in botulism and tetanus and diphtheria antitoxin given prophylactically to prevent those infections.

17 Atonic. (1) Weak. (2) Lacking normal tone, such as in the case of a muscle that is flaccid. (3) Lacking vigor, such as an atonic ulcer, which heals slowly.

18 Atrophy. A wasting or diminution of size or physiologic activity of a part of the body owing to disease or other influences. A skeletal muscle may undergo atrophy because of lack of physical exercise or as a result of neurologic or musculoskeletal disease. Cells of the brain and central nervous system may atrophy in old age because of restricted blood flow to those areas.

19 Autonomic nervous system. The part of the nervous system that regulates involuntary vital function, including the activity of the cardiac muscle, the smooth muscle, and the glands. It has two divisions: the sympathetic nervous system accelerates heart rate, constricts blood vessels, and raises blood pressure; the parasympathetic nervous system slows heart rate, increases intestinal peristalsis and gland activity, and relaxes sphincters.

20 Bactericidal. Destructive to bacteria.

21 Bacteriostatic. Tending to restrain the development or the reproduction of bacteria. Compare bactericidal.

22 Barbiturate. A derivative of barbituric acid that acts as a sedative or hypnotic.

23 Beta activity. Used in electroencephalography to describe electrical activity with a frequency greater than 13 H_Z. Can be caused chemically by administration of barbiturates and benzodiazepine agents.

24 Beta receptor. Any one of the postulated adrenergic components of receptor tissues that responds to epinephrine and such blocking agents as propranolol. Activation of beta receptors causes various physiologic reactions, such as relaxation of the bronchial muscles, increased cardiac rate, and the force of cardiac contraction. Also called beta-adrenergic receptor.

25 Bradycardia. An abnormal circulatory condition in which the myocardium contracts steadily but at a rate of less than 60 contractions a minute. The heart normally slows during sleep, and, in some physically fit people, the pulse may be quite slow. Pathologic bradycardia may be symptomatic of a brain tumor, digitalis toxicity, or vagoteria. Cardiac output is decreased, causing faintness, dizziness, chest pain, and, eventually syncope and circulatory collapse. Treatment may include administration of atropine, implantation of a pacemaker, or reduction of digitalis dosage.

26 Bronchoactive. Any agent that causes dilation or restriction of the pulmonary bronchioles.

27 Bronchoconstriction. A narrowing or reduction in the
caliber of the airways of the bronchial tree. This action may be caused by disease (inflammation) or by a
reflex response to irritants such as smoke, dust, or
chemicals.

28 Bronchodilator. A substance, especially a drug, that
relaxes contractions of the smooth muscle of the bronchioles to improve ventilation to the lungs. Pharmacologic bronchodilators are prescribed to improve aeration in asthma, bronchiectasis, bronchitis, and emphysema. Commonly used bronchodilators include
corticosteroids, ephedrine, isoproterenol, theophylline, and various derivatives and combinations of
these drugs. The adverse effects vary, depending on
the particular class of the bronchodilating drug. In
general, bronchodilators are given with caution to
people with impaired cardiac function. Nervousness,
irritability, gastritis, or palpitations of the heart may
occur.

29 Capsule. (1) (Compare Tablet.*) A small, soluble
container, usually made of gelatin, used for enclosing
a dose of medication for swallowing. (2) A membranous shell surrounding certain microorganisms, such
as the pneumococcus bacterium. (3) A well-defined
anatomic structure that encloses an organ or part,
such as the capsule of the adrenal gland.

30 Cardiac arrest. A sudden cessation of cardiac output
and effective circulation, usually precipitated by ventricular fibrillation and, in some instances, by ventricular asystole. When cardiac arrest occurs, delivery of
oxygen and removal of carbon dioxide stop, tissue
cell metabolism becomes anaerobic, and metabolic
and respiratory acidosis ensue. Immediate initiation of
cardiopulmonary resuscitation is required to prevent
heart, lung, kidney, and brain damage.

31 Cardiac arrhythmias. An abnormal rate or rhythm of
atrial or ventricular myocardial contraction. The condition may be caused by a defect in the ability of the
sinoatrial node to maintain its pacemaker function, or
by a failure of the bundle of His, the bundle branches,
or the Purkinje network to conduct the contractile impulse. Increased metabolic demand, such as in exercise or fever, or altered metabolic function, such as
acidosis, alkalosis, hypokalemia, or hypocalcemia,
result in an arrhythmia if the capacity of the heart to
adjust to the particular stress is exceeded. Kinds of arrhythmia include bradycardia extrasystole, heart
block, premature atrial contraction, premature ventricular contraction, and tachycardia.

32 Cardiac decompensation. Failure of the heart to perform its function.

33 Cardiac depressant. A drug or other agent that retards

the action of the heart either in rate and/or force of
contraction.

34 Cardiac stimulant. A pharmacologic agent that increases the action of the heart. Cardiac glycosides,
such as digitalis, digitoxin, digoxin, delanoside, lanatoside, acetyldigitoxin, and ouabain, increase the
force of myocardial contractions and decrease the
heart rate and conduction velocity, allowing more
time for the ventricles to relax and become filled with
blood. These glycosides, which are composed of a steroid nucleus, a lactone ring, and a sugar, are used in
the treatment of congestive heart failure, atrial flutter
and fibrillation, paroxysmal atrial tachycardia, and
cardiogenic shock. Toxic signs and symptoms, resulting from an overdose or the cumulative effect of
slowly eliminated digitalis preparations, include anorexia, nausea, vomiting, diarrhea, abdominal pain,
headache, muscle weakness, confusion, drowsiness,
irritability, visual disturbances, bradycardia or tachycardia, ectopic heart beats, bigeminy, and a pulse deficit. Epinephrine, a potent vasopressor and cardiac
stimulant, is sometimes used to restore heart rhythm
in cardiac arrest but is not employed in treating heart
failure or cardiogenic shock. Isoproterenol hydrochloride, which is related to epinephrine, may be used in
treating heart block. Dobutamine hydrochloride and
dopamine are employed in the short-term treatment of
cardiac decompensation owing to depressed contractility.

35 Cardiotonic drugs. (1) Of or pertaining to a substance
that tends to increase the efficiency of contractions of
the heart muscle. (2) A pharmacologic agent that increases the force of myocardial contractions. Cardiac
glycosides, derived from certain plant alkaloids, exert
a tonic effect by altering the transport of electrolytes
across the myocardial membrane, causing an increased influx of sodium and calcium and an increased efflux of potassium. Digitalis, digitoxin, and
digoxin, widely used cardiac glycosides obtained
from leaves of a species of foxglove, increase the
force of myocardial contractions, extend the refractory period of the atrioventricular node, and, to a
lesser degree, affect the sinoatrial node and the
heart's conduction system. Other cardiac glycosides
are ouabain and strophanthin, obtained from species
of *Strophanthus;* scillaridin, derived from squill; and
bufotalin, obtained from the skin and saliva of a Eu-
ropean toad.

36 Cardiovascular system. The network of structures, including the heart and the blood vessels, that pump
and convey the blood throughout the body. The system includes thousands of miles of vessels, capillaries, and venules and is vital to maintaining homeostasis. Numerous control mechanisms of the system assure that the blood is delivered to the structures where
it is most needed and at the proper rate. The system
delivers nutrients and other essential materials to the
fluids surrounding the cells and removes waste prod-

---

*See Mosby's medical, nursing, & allied health dictionary, ed 3, St
Louis, 1990, The CV Mosby Co.

ucts, which are conveyed to excretory organs, such as the kidneys and the intestine. The cardiovascular system functions in close association with the respiratory system, transporting oxygen inhaled into the lungs and conveying carbon dioxide to the lungs for expiration. Sympathetic and parasympathetic impulses from the medulla and cardiac baroreceptors sensitive to changes in pressure control the function of the heart, which pumps the oxygenated blood carried by the arteries and receives deoxygenated blood from the veins. Cardiovascular diseases affect a large number of individuals throughout the world, and half a million Americans die each year from coronary diseases. A variety of factors, such as diet, exercise, and stress, affect the cardiovascular system.

37 Central nervous system (CNS). One of the two main divisions of the nervous system of the body, consisting of the brain and the spinal cord. The central nervous system processes information to and from the peripheral nervous system and is the main network of coordination and control for the entire body. The brain controls many functions and sensations, such as sleep, sexual activity, muscular movement, hunger, thirst, memory, and the emotions. The spinal cord extends various types of nerve fibers from the brain and acts as a switching and relay terminal for the peripheral nervous system. The 12 pairs of cranial nerves emerge directly from the brain. Sensory nerves and motor nerves of the peripheral system leave the spinal cord separately between the vertebrae but unite to form 31 pairs of spinal nerves containing sensory fibers and motor fibers. More than 10 billion neurons constitute but one tenth of the brain cells, the other cells consisting of neuroglia. The neurons and the neuroglia form the soft, jellylike substance of the brain, which is supported and protected by the skull. Flowing through various cavities of the CNS, such as the ventricles of the brain, the subarachnoid spaces of the brain and spinal cord, and the central canal of the spinal cord, is the cerebrospinal fluid. This fluid helps to protect surrounding structures and affects the rate of respiration through changes in its content of carbon dioxide. The brain and the spinal cord are composed of gray matter and white matter. The gray matter contains primarily nerve cells and associated processes; the white matter consists of bundles of predominantly unmyelinated nerve fibers. The central nervous system develops from the embryonic neural tube, which first appears as the neural folds in the third week of pregnancy. The cavity of the neural tube is retained after birth in the ventricles of the brain and in the central canal of the spinal cord. (Compare Peripheral nervous system.* See also Brain, Spinal cord.*)

---

*See Mosby's medical, nursing, & allied health dictionary, ed 3, St Louis, 1990, The CV Mosby Co.

38 Chemotherapy (unsealed radioactive). The oral or parenteral administration of a radioisotope, such as iodine-131 (^{131}I) for the treatment of hyperthyroidism or thyroid cancer, phosphorus-32 (^{32}P) for leukemia or polycythemia vera, or gold-198 (^{198}Au) for lung cancer or peritoneal ascites resulting from widely disseminated carcinoma.

METHOD: Before unsealed radioactive chemotherapy is administered, the patient receives an explanation of the procedure and of the need for isolation during the half-life of the radioisotope (8.1 days for ^{131}I, 14 days for ^{32}P, and 2.7 days for ^{198}AU). The room in which the patient is isolated adjoins a private bathroom and is equipped with convenient furniture, a freshly made bed placed next to the building's outer wall, a functioning phone and television set, adequate lighting, reading and hobby materials, and containers for contaminated linen, dressings, and excreta. Radioactive tags are posted on the door. The patient's chart and individual radioactive badges, which are kept at the door, are worn by each staff member entering the room to record the amount of radiation exposure; pregnant staff members are not assigned to the patient's care. Disposable dishes, utensils, and trays are used for the patient's preferred diet, which is ordered before the isolation period. Prior to receiving the radioisotope, the patient bathes or showers and is assisted in notifying family and friends that visits are not allowed in the initial 24 hours of therapy and are thereafter limited to 2 hours if the person remains 6 feet or more from the patient. During isolation, the patient, if able, performs daily self-care measures and the staff member caring for the patient limits the time spent in the room by planning the observations and procedures to be accomplished beforehand. Urine excreted by a patient treated with ^{131}I is collected directly or via an indwelling catheter, in a lead-lined container, which is sent to the laboratory for assay of the radioisotope. Feces, sputum, and vomitus are placed in the toilet and decontaminated with a dropperful of a saturated solution of potassium iodide before the bowel is flushed. If excreta are spilled on the skin, the area is rinsed in running water for 2 minutes and washed in soap and water for an additional 3 minutes. If the bed or another surface in the room is contaminated with excreta, the radiation control officer is notified and the area is monitored before being cleaned. Dressings and bed linen are handled with rubber or plastic gloves; contaminated linens are placed in a hamper and trash is placed in plastic bags; they are not removed from the room until monitored with a Geiger-Miller counter. The staff member limits exposure by repositioning the debilitated patient with a turn sheet, by bathing only the soiled body areas, and by preparing and cutting food on the diet tray before entering the room. The patient treated with ^{131}I is observed for evidence of neck tenderness, changes in exophthalmia, a transient productive cough, hypoparathyroidism, hypothyroidism, and hyperthyroidism. Similar procedures of care are followed for the patient treated with ^{32}P, but since the beta rays emitted by this radionuclide are absorbed by the patient's body, there is no danger of external exposure. If ^{33}P is administered intravenously or injected into the body cavity, no special precautions are needed for disposal of excreta, but dressings and linen contaminated by seepage from wounds are placed in lead-lined containers, as is the vomitus of the patient who is given the radionuclide orally. Special precautions are required in caring for the patient treated with radioactive gold, which emits gamma and beta rays. After purple liquid ^{198}Au is injected into the body cavity, the patient is turned with a sheet every 15 minutes for 2 hours to tissues contaminated by the purple seepage from wounds are burned immediately; linen in contact with wounds is placed in special containers. The patient injected with ^{198}Au is usually terminally ill, and, if death occurs, a tag is placed on the body to alert the mortician to the presence of the radionuclide.

NURSING ORDERS: The nurse wears a radiation badge when entering the patient's room and limits exposure by performing planned procedures efficiently. Routine the patient is ambulatory, but emotional support is provided in brief hourly visits at the door and via the intercommunication system. The nurse anticipates and fulfills the isolated patient's requests as promptly as possible, arranges diversional activities, and assures the patient that when a certain period of time has passed the patient will no longer be a source of radioactivity.

OUTCOME CRITERIA: Radioactive iodine usually counteracts hyperthyroidism and is frequently used in conjunction with surgery in the treatment of thyroid cancer. Radioactive phosphorus often controls polycythemia vera, but other agents are generally more effective in leukemia therapy. Radioactive gold is usually administered as a last resort in advanced lung cancer or peritoneal ascites resulting from malignant disease.

39 Cholinergic. (1) Of or pertaining to nerve fibers that elaborate acetylcholine at the myoneural junctions. (2) The tendency to transmit or to be stimulated or to stimulate by the elaboration of acetylcholine. (Compare Adrenergic.*)

40 Clinical pharmacology. The science of using drugs and other chemicals to treat patients, usually in the hospital setting.

41 Contraindication. A factor that prohibits the administration of a drug or the performance of a procedure in the care of a specific patient, such as pregnancy is a contraindication for the prescription of tetracycline, immunosuppression is a contraindication for vaccina-

tion, and complete placenta previa is a contraindication for vaginal delivery.

42 Demulcent. (1) Any of several oily substances used for soothing and reducing irritation of surfaces that have been abraded or irritated. (2) Soothing, such as a counterirritant or balm.

43 Depressant. (1) (of a drug) Tending to decrease the function or activity of a system of the body. (2) Such a drug, such as a cardiac depressant or a respiratory depressant.

44 Detergent. (1) A cleansing agent. (2) Cleansing.

45 Detoxification. To remove or reduce the poisonous properties of a chemical agent.

46 Disinfectant. A chemical or agent that rapidly kills microorganisms usually at relatively low concentrations.

47 Diuretic. (1) (of a drug or other substance) Tending to promote the formation and excretion of urine. (2) A drug that promotes the formation and excretion of urine. The more than 50 diuretic drugs available for prescription in the United States and Canada are classified by chemical structure into several basic pharmacologic groups: anthralinecs, ethacrynics, mercurials, steroids, sulfonamides, and thiazides. A diuretic medication may contain drugs from one or more of these groups. Diuretics are prescribed to reduce the volume of extracellular fluid in the treatment of many disorders, including hypertension, congestive heart failure, and edema. The particular drug to be prescribed is selected according to the action desired and the physical status of the patient. Hypersensitivity to sulfonamides prohibits use of this class of drug, and diabetes mellitus may be aggravated by thiazide medications; thus the presence of a particular condition may prohibit the use of a particular agent. Several adverse reactions are common to all diuretics, including hypovolemia and electrolyte imbalance.

48 Dose. The amount of a drug or other substance administered at one time.

49 Dose-response relationship. The amount (dose) of a drug that is required in order to attain a desired physical and/or physiologic response.

50 Double-blind study. An experiment designed to test the effect of a treatment or substance using groups of experimental and control subjects in which neither the subjects nor the investigators know which treatment or substance is being administered to which group. In a double-blind test of a new drug, the substance may be identified to the investigators only by a code. The purpose of a double-blind study is to eliminate the risk of prejudgment by the participants, which could distort results. A double-blind study may be augmented by a cross-over experiment in which experimental subjects unknowingly become control subjects, and vice versa, at some point in the study.

51 Drug. (1) Also called medicine. Any substance taken by mouth, injected into a muscle, the skin, a blood vessel, or a cavity of the body, or applied topically to

*See Mosby's medical, nursing, & allied health dictionary, ed 3, St Louis, 1990, The CV Mosby Co.

treat or prevent a disease or condition. (2) *Informal.* A narcotic substance.

52 Drug action. The means by which a drug exerts a desired effect. Drugs are usually classified by their actions, as a vasodilator, prescribed to decrease the blood pressure, acts by dilating the blood vessels.

53 Drug reaction. (See Adverse reaction.)

54 Edema. The abnormal accumulation of fluid in interstitial spaces of tissues, in the pericardial sac, intrapleural space, peritoneal cavity, or joint capsules. Edema may be caused by increased capillary fluid pressure, venous obstruction, such as in varicosities, thrombophlebitis, or pressure from casts, tight bandages, or garters, congestive heart failure, overloading with parenteral fluids, renal failure, hepatic cirrhosis, hyperaldosteronism, such as in Cushing's syndrome, corticosteroid therapy, and inflammatory reactions. Edema may also occur because of loss of serum protein in burns, draining wounds, fistulas, hemorrhage, nephrotic syndrome, or chronic diarrhea, in malnutrition, especially kwashiorkor, in allergic reactions, and in blockage of lymphatic vessels owing to malignant diseases, filariasis, or other disorders. Treatment of edema is directed to correction of the basic cause, but potassium-sparing diuretics may be administered to promote excretion of sodium and water and care is exercised in protecting edematous parts of the body from prolonged pressure, injury, and temperature extremes. When a limb is edematous because of venous stasis, elevating the extremity and applying an elastic stocking or sleeve facilitates venous return.

55 Efficacy (of a drug or treatment). The maximum ability of a drug or treatment to produce a result, regardless of dosage. Narcotics have a nearly identical efficacy but require various dosages to obtain the effect. (Compare Potency.)

56 Elixir. A clear liquid containing water, alcohol, sweeteners, and flavors, used primarily as a vehicle for the oral administration of a drug.

57 Embolism. An abnormal circulatory condition in which an embolus travels through the bloodstream and becomes lodged in a blood vessel. The symptoms vary with the degree of occlusion that the embolism causes, the character of the embolus, and the size, nature, and location of the occluded vessel. Kinds of embolism include air embolism and fat embolism.

58 Emetic. (1) Of or pertaining to a substance that causes vomiting. (2) An emetic agent. Apomorphine hydrochloride, acting through the central nervous system, induces vomiting 10 to 15 minutes after the parenteral administration. Syrup of ipecac is used in the emergency treatment of drug overdosage and in certain cases of poisoning, but it can be cardiotoxic if it is absorbed and not vomited.

59 Emulsion. (1) A system consisting of two immiscible liquids, one of which is dispersed in the other in the form of small droplets. (2) (in photography) A composition sensitive to actinic rays of light, consisting of one or more silver halides suspended in gelatin applied in a thin layer to film.

60 Enzyme. A protein produced by living cells that catalyzes chemical reactions in organic matter. Most enzymes are produced in minute quantities and catalyze reactions that take place within the cells. Digestive enzymes, however, are produced in relatively large quantities and act outside the cells in the lumen of the digestive tube.

61 Etiology. (1) The study of all factors that may be involved in the development of a disease, including the susceptibility of the patient, the nature of the disease agent, and the way in which the patient's body is invaded by the agent. (2) The cause of the disease (Compare Pathogenesis.*)

62 Excretion. The process of eliminating, shedding, or getting rid of substances by body organs or tissues, as part of a natural metabolic activity. Excretion usually begins at the cellular level where water, carbon dioxide, and other waste products of cellular life are emptied into the capillaries. The epidermis excretes dead skin cells by shedding them daily.

63 Expectorant. (1) Of or pertaining to a substance that promotes the ejection of mucus or other exudates from the lung, bronchi, and trachea. (2) An agent that promotes expectoration by reducing the viscosity of pulmonary secretions or by decreasing the force with which exudates adhere to the lower respiratory tract. Expectorant drugs include acetycysteine, guaifenesin, terpin hydrate, and tyloxapol.

64 FDA. Abbreviation for Food and Drug Administration.

65 Formula (of a drug). A simplified statement, generally using numerals and other symbols, expressing the constituents of a chemical compound, a method for preparing a substance, or a procedure for achieving a desired value or result.

66 FTC. Abbreviation for Federal Trade Commission.

67 Fungicide. A drug that kills fungi.

68 Ganglionic blocker. Any one of a group of drugs prescribed to produce controlled hypotension, as required in certain surgical procedures or in emergency management of hypertensive crisis. The drugs act by occupying receptor sites on sympathetic and parasympathetic nerve endings of autonomic ganglia, preventing response of these nerves to the action of acetylcholine liberated by the presynaptic nerve endings. Trimethaphan and mecamylamine are the most commonly prescribed ganglionic blocking agents. They are used with great caution in treating patients who are affected with coronary, cerebrovascular, or renal insufficiency or who have a history of severe allergy. Adverse reactions to the drugs include sudden marked

---

*See Mosby's medical, nursing, & allied health dictionary, ed 3, St Louis, 1990, The CV Mosby Co.

hypotension, paralytic ileus, urinary retention, constipation, visual disturbances, heartburn, and nausea.

69 Generic name. The official, established nonproprietary name assigned to a drug. A given drug is licensed under its generic name, and all manufacturers of the drug list it by its generic name. However, a drug is usually marketed under a trade name chosen by the manufacturer.

70 Grain. The smallest unit of mass in avoirdupois, troy, and apothecaries' weights, being the same in all and equal to 0.06479891 gram. The troy and apothecaries' ounces contain 480 grains; the avoirdupois ounce contains 437.5 grains.

71 Gram (g). A unit of mass in the metric system equal to 1/1000 of a kilogram, 15.432 grains, and 0.03 ounce avoirdupois.

72 Half-life of drug. The time that it takes for a drug to lose half its potency or be eliminated by natural or artificial means.

73 Hallucinogenic. A substance that causes excitation of the central nervous system, characterized by hallucination, mood change, anxiety, sensory distortion, delusion, depersonalization, increased pulse, temperature, and blood pressure, and dilation of the pupils. Psychic dependence may occur, and depressive or suicidal psychotic states may result from the ingestion of hallucinogenic substances. Some kinds of hallucinogens are lysergic acid diethylamide (LSD), mescaline, peyote, phencyclidine, psilocybin.

74 Hormone. A complex chemical substance produced in one part or organ of the body that initiates or regulates the activity of an organ or a group of cells in another part of the body. Hormones secreted by the endocrine glands are carried through the bloodstream to the target organ. Secretion of these hormones is regulated by other hormones, by neurotransmitters, and by a negative feedback system in which an excess of target organ activity signals a decreased need for the stimulating hormone. This principle is integral to oral contraceptive pills. A steady supply of estrogen and progesterone in the medication causes a reduction in the secretion of the pituitary hormones that ordinarily stimulate the ovary to develop the follicle, release the egg, and secrete the estrogen and progesterone. Other hormones are released by organs for local effect, most commonly in the digestive tract.

75 Hypersensitivity. An abnormal condition characterized by an excessive reaction to a particular stimulus.

76 Hypertension. A common, often asymptomatic disorder characterized by elevated blood pressure persistently exceeding 140/90 mm Hg. Essential hypertension, the most frequent kind, has no single identifiable cause, but the risk of the disorder is increased by obesity, a high sodium level in serum, hypercholesterolemia, and a family history of high blood pressure. Known causes of hypertension include adrenal disorders, such as aldosteronism, Cushing's syndrome, and pheochromocytoma, thyrotoxicosis, toxemia of pregnancy, and chronic glomerulonephritis. The incidence of hypertension is higher in men than in women and is twice as great in blacks as in whites. Persons with mild or moderate hypertension may be asymptomatic or may experience suboccipital headaches, especially on rising, tinnitus, lightheadedness, easy fatigability, and palpitations. With sustained hypertension arterial walls become thickened, inelastic, and resistant to blood flow and, as a result, the left ventricle becomes distended and hypertrophy may lead to congestive heart failure. High blood pressure associated with hypersecretion of catecholamines in pheochromocytoma is often accompanied by anxiety attacks, palpitation, profuse sweating, pallor, nausea, and in some cases, pulmonary edema. malignant hypertension, characterized by a diastolic pressure higher than 120 mm Hg, severe headaches, blurred vision, and confusion, may result in fatal uremia, myocardial infarction, congestive heart failure, or a cerebral vascular accident. Drugs used to treat hypertension include diuretics, such as furosemide and thiazide derivatives, vasodilators, such as hydralazine and prazosin; sympathetic nervous system (SNS) depressants, such as rauwolfia alkaloids; SNS inhibitors, such as guanethidine and methyldopa, and ganglionic blocking agents, such as clonidine and propranolol. Patients with high blood pressure are advised to follow a low-sodium, low-saturated fat diet, to reduce calories and countrol obesity, to exercise, to avoid stress, and to take adequate rest.

77 Hypoglycemia. A less-than-normal amount of glucose in the blood, usually caused by administration of too much insulin, excessive secretion of insulin to the islet cells of the pancreas, or by dietary deficiency. The condition may result in weakness, headache, hunger, visual disturbances, ataxia, anxiety, personality changes, and if untreated, delirium, coma, and death. The treatment is the administration of glucose in orange juice by mouth if the person is conscious or in an intravenous glucose solution if the person is unconscious. (Compare diabetic coma.*).

78 Idiosyncrasy. (1) A physical or behavioral characteristic or manner that is unique to an individual or to a group. (2) An individual's unique hypersensitivity to a particular drug, food, or other substance.

79 Immune. (1) (in civil law) Exemption from a duty or an obligation generally required by law, such as an exemption from taxation, exemption from penalty for wrongdoing, or protection against liability. (2) The quality of being insusceptible to or unaffected by a particular disease or condition.

80 Indication. A reason to prescribe a medication or perform a treatment, such as a bacterial infection may be an indication for the prescription of a specific antibi-

---

*See Mosby's medical, nursing, & allied health dictionary, ed 3, St Louis, 1990, The CV Mosby Co.

otic or an appendicitis is an indication for appendectomy.

81 Infusion. (1) (Compare Injection, Instillation,* Insufflation.*) (a) The introduction of a substance, such as a fluid, electrolyte, nutrient, or drug, directly into a vein or interstitially by means of gravity flow. Sterile techniques are maintained, the equipment is periodically checked for mechanical difficulties, and the patient is observed for swelling at the site of infection and for cardiac or respiratory difficulties. (b) The substance introduced into the body by infusion. (2) The steeping of a substance, as an herb, in order to extract its medicinal properties. (3) The extract obtained by the steeping process.

82 Inhalant. Any medication or other agent that is adminsitered by inhalation.

83 Inhibition. (1) The act or state of inhibiting or of being inhibited, restrained; prevented; held back. (2) (in psychology) The unconscious restraint of a behavioral process, usually resulting from the social or cultural forces of the environment; the condition inducing such restraint. (3) (in psychoanalysis) The process in which the superego prevents the conscious expression of an unconscious instinctual drive, thought, or urge. (4) (in physiology) Restraining, checking, or arresting the action of an organ or cell or the reduction of a physiologic activity by an antagonistic stimulation. (5) (in chemistry) The stopping or slowing down of the rate of a chemical reaction.

84 Injection. (1) (Compare Infusion, Instillation,* Insufflation.*) (a) The act of forcing a liquid into the body by means of a syringe. Injections are designated according to the anatomic site involved; the most common are intra-arterial, intradermal, intramuscular, intravenous, and subcutaneous. Parenteral infections are usually given for therapeutic reasons, although they may be used diagnostically. Sterile technique is maintained. (b) The substance injected. (2) Redness and swelling observed in the physical examination of a part of the body, caused by dilation of the blood vessels secondary to an inflammatory or infectious process.

85 Intoxication. (1) The state of being poisoned by a drug or other toxic substance. (2) The state of being inebriated owing to an excessive consumption of alcohol. (3) A state of mental or emotional hyperexcitability, usually euphoric.

86 Intractable. Having no relief, such as a symptom or a disease that remains unrelieved by the therapeutic measures employed.

87 Intravenous. Of or pertaining to the inside of a vein, as of a thrombus or an infection, infusion, or catheter.

88 In vitro. (of a biologic reaction) Occurring in a laboratory apparatus. (Compare In vivo.)

89 In vivo. (of a biologic reaction) Occurring in a living organism. (Compare In vitro.)

90 Isotonic. (of a solution) Having the same concentration of solute as another solution, hence exerting the same amount of osmotic pressure as that solution, as an isotonic saline solution that contains an amount of salt equal to that found in the intracellular and extracellular fluid. Also called isosmotic.

91 Kilogram. A unit for the measurement of mass in the metric system. One kilogram is equal to 1000 g or to 2.2046 pounds avoirdupois.

92 Label (in radiology and immunology). (1) A substance with a special affinity for an organ, tissue, cell, or microorganism in which it may become deposited and fixed. (2) The process of depositing and fixing a substance in an organ, tissue, cell, or microorganism.

93 Lethargic. (1) The state or quality of being indifferent, apathetic, or sluggish. (2) Stupor or coma resulting from disease or hypnosis. Kinds of lethargy include hysteric lethargy, induced lethargy, lucid lethargy.

94 Liquid. A state of matter, intermediate between solid and gas, in which the substance flows freely with little application of force and assumes the shape of the vessel in which it is contained. (Compare Fluid.*)

95 Lotion. A liquid preparation applied externally to protect the skin or to treat a dermatologic disorder.

96 Maintenance therapy. The minimum dose of a drug that is required to provide continuous desired effects.

97 Mediator. A chemical or agent that causes a change. (see Mediate.*)

98 Metabolism. The aggregate of all chemical processes that take place in living organisms, resulting in growth, generation of energy, elimination of wastes, and other bodily functions as they relate to the distribution of nutrients in the blood after digestion. Metabolism takes place in two steps; anabolism, the constructive phase, in which smaller molecules (such as amino acids) are converted to larger molecules (such as proteins); and catabolism, the destructive phase, in which larger molecules (such as glycogen) are converted to smaller molecules (such as pyruvic acid). Exercise, elevated body temperature, hormonal activity, and digestion can increase the matabolic rate, which is the rate determined when a person is at complete rest, physically and mentally. The metabolic rate is customarily expressed (in calories) as the heat liberated in the course of metabolism.

99 Mucolytic. Capable of dissolving mucus.

100 Mucus. Of or pertaining to mucus or the secretion of mucus.

101 Narcotic. (in pharmacology) (1) Of or pertaining to a substance that produces insensibility or stupor. (2) A narcotic drug. Narcotic analgesics, derived from

---

*See Mosby's medical, nursing, & allied health dictionary, ed 3, St Louis, 1990, The CV Mosby Co.

opium or produced synthetically, alter perception of pain; induce euphoria, mood changes, mental clouding, and deep sleep; depress respiration and the cough reflex; constrict the pupils; and cause smooth muscle spasm, decreased peristalsis, emesis, and nausea. Repeated use of narcotics may result in physical and psychologic dependence. Among the narcotic drugs administered clinically for relief of pain or butorphanol tartrate, hydromorphone hydrochloride, morphine sulfate, pentazocine lactate, and meperidine hydrochloride. These drugs act by binding to opiate receptors in the central nervous system; narcotic antagonists, as naloxone hydrochloride, which is used in treating narcotic overdosage, apparently displace opiates from receptor sites.

102 *National Formulary (NF).* A publication containing the official standards for the preparation of various pharmaceuticals not listed in the *United States Pharmacopeia.* It is revised every 5 years.

103 Nausea. A sensation often leading to the urge to vomit. Common causes are sea and other motion sicknesses, early pregnancy, intense pain, emotional stress, gall bladder disease, food poisoning, and various enteroviruses.

104 Nerve impulse. A self-propagating wave of electrical negativity that travels along the surface of a neuron's cytoplasmic membrane.

105 Nerve synapse. (1) The region surrounding the point of contact between two neurons or between a neuron and an effector organ, across which nerve impulses are transmitted through the action of neurotransmitter, such as acetylcholine or norepinephrine. When an impulse reaches the terminal point of one neuron, it causes the release of the neurotransmitter, which diffuses across the gap between the two cells to bind with receptors in the other neuron, muscle, or gland, triggering electrical changes that either inhibit or continue the transmission of the impulse. Synapses are polarized so that nerve impulses travel in only one direction; they are also subject to fatigue, oxygen deficiency, anesthetics, and other chemical agents. (2) To form a synapse or connection between neurons. (3) (in genetics) To form a synaptic fusion between homologous chromosomes during meiosis. Kinds of synapses include axoaxonic synapse, axodendritic synapse, axodendrosomatic synapse, axosomatic synapse, dendrodentritic synapse. (Compare Ephapse.*)

106 Neuroleptic. (1) Of or pertaining to neurolepsis. (2) A drug that causes neurolepsis, as the butyrophenone derivative, droperidol.

107 Neuromuscular. Of or pertaining to the nerves and the muscles.

108 Neuromuscular blocker. A chemical substance that interferes locally with the transmission or reception of impulses from motor nerves to skeletal muscles. Nondepolarizing agents, such as metocurine, pancuronium, and tubocurarine, competitively block the transmitter action of acetylcholine at the postjunctional membrane. Depolarizing blocking agents, such as succinylcholine chloride, compete with acetylcholine for cholinergic receptors of the motor end plate. Neuromuscular blocking agents are used to induce muscle relaxation in anesthesia, endotracheal intubation, and electroshock therapy and as adjuncts in the treatment of tetanus, encephalitis, and poliobronchospasm, hyperthermia, hypotension, or respiratory paralysis and are used with caution, especially in patients with myasthenia gravis, renal, hepatic, or pulmonary impairment, and in elderly and debilitated individuals.

109 Neuron. The basic nerve cell of the nervous system, containing a nucleus within a cell body and extending one or more processes. Neurons are classified according to the direction in which they conduct impulses and according to the number of processes they extend. Sensory neurons transmit nerve impulses to the spinal cord and the brain. Motor neurons transmit nerve impulses from the brain and the spinal cord to the muscles and the glandular tissue. Multipolar neurons, the bipolar neurons, and the unipolar neurons are classified according to the number of processes they extend to the different kinds of neurons. Multipolar neurons have one axon and several dendrites, as do most of the neurons in the brain and the spinal cord. Bipolar neurons, which are less numerous than the other types, have only one axon and one dendrite. Unipolar bodies fuse dendrites and axons in a single fiber that stretches for a short distance from the cell body before separating again into the two processes. All neurons have at least one axon and one or more dendrites and have a slightly gray color when clustered, as in the brain and the spinal cord. As the carriers of nerve impulses, neurons function according to electrochemical processes involving positively charged sodium and potassium ions and the changing electrical potential of the extracellular and the intracellular fluid of the neuron.

110 Nostrum. A drug that makes dishonest claims for its effectiveness.

111 Ointment. A semisolid, externally applied preparation, usually containing a drug. Various ointments are used as local analgesic, anesthetic, anti-infective, astringent, depigmenting, irritant, and keratolytic agents. Also called salve, unction, unguent.

112 Opiate. (1) A narcotic drug that contains opium, derivatives of opium, or any of several semisynthetic or synthetic drugs with opium-like activity. (2) *Informal.* Any soporific or narcotic drug. (3) Of or pertaining to a substance that causes sleep or relief or pain. Also called opioid.

113 Oxidation. (in chemistry) (1) Any process in which the oxygen content of a compound is increased. (2)

---

*See Mosby's medical, nursing, & allied health dictionary, ed 3, St Louis, 1990, The CV Mosby Co.

Any reaction in which the positive valence of a compound or a radical is increased owing to a loss of electrons.

114 Parasympathomimetic. (1) Of, or pertaining to a substance producing effects similar to those caused by stimulation of a parasympathetic nerve. (2) An agent whose effects mimic those resulting from stimulation of parasympathetic nerves, especially the effects produced by acetylcholine. The parasympathomimetic drugs include bethanechol chloride, neostigmine bromide, neostigmine methylsulfate, and pyridostigmine bromide, variously used to treat myasthenia gravis, acute postoperative and postpartum nonobstructional urinary retention, and to reverse or antagonize the action of nondepolarizing muscle relaxants. Also called cholinergic.

115 Parenteral. Not in or through the digestive system.

116 Paroxysm. (1) A marked, usually episodic increase in symptoms. (2) A convulsion, fit, seizure, or spasm.

117 Pertussis. An acute, highly contagious respiratory disease characterized by paroxysmal coughing that ends in a loud whooping inspiration. It occurs primarily in infants and in children less than 4 years of age who have not been immunized. The causative organism, *Bordetella pertussis,* is a small, nonmotile, gram-negative coccobacillus. A similar organism, *B. parapertussis,* causes a less severe form of the disease called parapertussis. Also called whooping cough. OBSERVATIONS: Transmission occurs directly by contact or by inhalation of infectious particles, usually spread by coughing and sneezing, and indirectly through freshly contaminated articles. Diagnosis consists of positive identification of the organism in nasopharyngeal secretions. The initial stages of the disease are difficult to distinguish from bronchitis or influenza. A fluorescent antibody staining technique specific for the *B. pertussis* is an accurate means of early diagnosis. The incubation period averages 7 to 14 days, followed by 6 to 8 weeks of illness divided into three distinct stages: catarrhal, paroxysmal, and convalescent. Onset of the catarrhal stage is gradual, usually beginning with coryza, sneezing, a dry cough, a slight fever, listlessness, irritability, and anorexia. The cough becomes paroxysmal after 10 to 14 days and occurs as a series of short rapid bursts during expiration followed by the characteristic whoop, a hurried, deep inhalation that has a high-pitched crowing sound. There is usually no fever, and the respiratory rate between paroxysms is normal. During the paroxysm there is marked facial bulge, the tongue may protrude, and the facial expression usually indicates severe anxiety and distress. Large amounts of a viscid mucus may be expelled during or following paroxysms, which occur from four to five times a day in mild cases to as many as 40 to 50 times a day in severe cases. Vomiting frequently occurs after the paroxysms because of gagging or choking on the mucus. In infants, choking may be more common than the characteristic whoop. This stage lasts from 4 to 6 weeks, with the attacks being most frequent and severe during the first 1 to 2 weeks, then gradually declining and disappearing. During the convalescent stage, a simple persistent cough is usual. For a period of up to 2 years following the initial attack, paroxysmal coughing may accompany respiratory infections. INTERVENTION: Routine treatment consists of bed rest, a good diet, and adequate amounts of fluid. Erythromycin or another antibacterial may be prescribed to reduce contagiousness or to control secondary infection. Hospitalization may be necessary for infants and children with severe or prolonged paroxysms and for those with dehydration or other complications. Oxygen may be needed to relieve dyspnea and cyanosis; intravenous therapy may be necessary when prolonged vomiting interferes with adequate nutrition. Intubation is rarely necessary but may be lifesaving in infants if the thick mucus cannot be easily suctioned from the air passages. Pertussis immune globulin is available, but its efficacy has not been established and its use is not recommended. Active immunization is recommended with pertussis vaccine, usually in combination with diphtheria and tetanus toxoids in a series of three injections. One attack of the disease usually confers immunity, although some second, usually mild episodes have occurred. NURSING CONSIDERATIONS: Severe paroxysms in an infant may require oxygen, suction, and intubation. The child needs to be kept calm and protected from respiratory irritants like dirt, smoke, or dust. Overstimulation, noise, or excitement may precipitate paroxysms. A good diet and adequate fluids are encouraged through frequent, small feedings. Common complications of the disease include bronchopneumonia; atelectasis; bronchiectasis; emphysema; otitis media, convulsions, hemorrhage, including subarachnoid, subconjunctival, and epistaxis; weight loss; dehydration; hernia; prolapsed rectum; and asphyxia, especially in infants.

118 Pharmacology. The study of the preparation, properties, uses, and actions of drugs.

119 Pharmacopeia. (1) A compendium containing descriptions, recipes, strengths, standards of purity, and dosage forms for selected drugs. (2) The available stock of drugs in a pharmacy. (3) The total of all authorized drugs available within the jurisdiction of a given geographic or political area.

120 Phenol. (1) A highly poisonous, caustic, crystalline chemical derived from coal tar or plant tar or manufactured synthetically. It has a distinctive, pungent odor and, in solution, is a powerful disinfectant, commonly called carbolic acid. (2) Any of a large number and variety of chemical products closely related in structure to the alcohols and containing a hydroxyl group attached to a benzene ring. The phenols are components in dyes, plastics, disinfectants, and in antimicrobials and other drugs, including salicylic acid.

121 *Physicians' Desk Reference (PDR).* A compendium compiled annually, containing information about drugs, primarily prescription drugs and products used in diagnostic procedures, supplied by their manufacturers.

122 Pill. Mixtures of a drug with some cohesive material that have been molded into a globular, oval, or flattened body convenient for swallowing.

123 Placebo. An inactive substance, such as saline, distilled water, or sugar, or a less than effective dose of a harmless substance, such as a water-soluble vitamin, prescribed as if it were an effective dose of a needed medication. Placebos are used in experimental drug studies to compare the effects of the placebo with those of the experimental drug. They are also prescribed for patients who cannot be given the medication they request or who, in the judgment of the health care provider, do not need that medication. Placebo therapy is effective in some cases, and side effects often occur as they would from the actual medication. The benefit to the patient of a placebo should clearly outweigh the ethical, moral, and legal problems posed by its administration.

124 Poison. Any substance that impairs health or destroys life when ingested, inhaled, or absorbed by the body in relatively small amounts. Some toxicologists suggest that, depending on dosages, all substances are poisons. Many experts state that it is impossible to categorize any chemical as either safe or toxic and that the real concern is the risk or hazard associated with the use of any substance, as the high risk that may be associated with a life-saving drug that would not be acceptable as a food additive. Clinically, all poisons are divided into those that respond to specific treatments or antidotes and those for which there is no specific treatment. Research continues to develop effective antitoxins for poisons, but there are relatively few effective antidotes and the treatment of poisoned individuals is based mainly on eliminating the toxic agent from the body before it can be absorbed. Maintaining respiration and circulation is the most important aspect of such treatment. Some substances that may be poisonous are the saps of certain plants, bacterial toxins, animal venoms, corrosives, heavy-metal compounds, certain gases, various volatile and nonvolatile substances, industrial chemicals, and numerous drugs. The toxic effects of poisons may be reversible or irreversible. The capacity of body tissue to recover from poison determines the reversibility of the effect. Poisons that injure the central nervous system (CNS) create irreversible effects because CNS neurons of the brain cannot regenerate. Toxic effects of chemicals may be divided into local effects and systemic effects. Local effects, such as those caused by the ingestion of caustic substances and the inhalation of irritants, involve the site of the first contact between the biologic system and the toxicant. Systemic effects depend on the absorption and the distribution of the toxicant. Systemic toxicity most often affects the CNS but may also affect the circulatory system, the blood and hematopoietic system, the skin, and the visceral organs, as the liver, kidney, and lung. The muscles and the bones are less often affected by system toxicity. The precise incidence of poisoning in the United States is not known, but about 150,000 cases are voluntarily reported to the National Clearinghouse for Poison Control Centers each year. Authorities, however, estimate that the real incidence is at least 10 times the number of reported cases. The total number of poisoning cases increases each year, but the incidence of poisoning in children under 5 years of age has significantly decreased, probably because of safer packaging of household drugs and products. About 60% of all poisoning involves children 1 to 2 years old and the ingestion of chemicals other than drugs. Approximately 75% of the cases of poisoning in individuals over 15 years of age are drug-related. About 4000 persons die each year in the United States from poisoning by toxic liquid and solid substances. Another 7000 persons are bitten by poisonous snakes, such as the pit viper and coral snake. Such bites may cause severe pain and swelling, numbness, respiratory distress, paralysis, impaired coagulation, coma, and death. Snake bites may be treated with antivenin, tetanus toxoid, and broad-spectrum antibiotics. Antihistamines and topic antipyretics are commonly used to treat toxic skin reactions from poisonous plants, as poison ivy, poison sumac, and poison oak. The saps or juices of such plants may cause severe reactions through skin contact or through ingestion. Authorities stress the importance of prompt treatment of acute poisoning from toxic chemicals and liquid. Some common treatments in such cases involve emesis and gastric lavage. Most toxic effects of drugs occur shortly after administration, but carcinogenic effects of chemicals may take 15 to 45 years to develop fully. chemical carcinogenesis is a complex process involving the conversion of secondary carcinogens into primary carcinogens and the possible development of tumors through reactions of the toxicant with deoxyribonucleic acid.

125 Potency. (in embryology) the range of developmental possibilities of which an embryonic cell or part is capable, regardless of whether the stimulus for growth or differentiation is natural, artificial, or experimental.

126 Potentiation. A synergistic action in which the effect of two drugs given simultaneously is greater than the effect of the drugs given separately.

127 Prescription. An order for medication, therapy, or a therapeutic device given by a properly authorized person to a person properly authorized to dispense or perform the order. A prescription is usually in written form and includes the name and address of the patient, the data, the Rx symbol (superscription), the medication prescribed (inscription), directions to the pharmacist or other dispenser (subscription), directions to the patient that must appear on the label, the prescriber's signature, and, in some instances, an identifying number.

128 Prophylactic. (1) Preventing the spread of disease. (2) An agent that prevents the spread of disease.

129 Pure Food and Drug Act. Passed in 1906, this was the first federal legislation regulating the quality of medicine.

130 Receptors. A specific nerve ending that binds with a specific type of molecule.

131 Reflex. The involuntary functioning or movement of any organ or part of the body in response to a particular stimulus. The function or action occurs immediately, without the involvement of the will or consciousness.

132 Relaxant. A generic name that is given to any drug that causes a reduction of muscle tension.

133 Resistance. A force or a situation that opposes movement or change. Also the natural or acquired ability to ward off disease.

134 Respiratory depressant. A drug or agent that directly or indirectly restricts or diminishes the action of ventilatory muscles.

135 Respiratory stimulant. A drug or agent that initiates or increases the activity of pulmonary muscles.

136 Salicylates. Any of several widely prescribed drugs derived from salicylic acid. Salicylates exert analgesic, antipyretic, and anti-inflammatory actions. The most important is acetylsalicylic acid, or aspirin. Sodium salicylate has also been used systemically, and it exerts similar effects. Many of the actions of aspirin appear to result from its ability to inhibit cyclo-oxygenase, a rate limiting enzyme in prostaglandin biosynthesis. Aspirin is used in a wide variety of conditions, and, in the usual analgesic dosage, it causes only mild adverse effects. Severe occult gastrointestinal bleeding or gastric ulcers may occur with frequent use. Large doses taken over a long period can cause significant impairment of hemostasis. Occasionally, an asthma-like reaction is produced in hypersensitive individuals. Because of ready availability of aspirin, accidental and intentional overdosage is common. symptoms of salicylate intoxication include tinnitus, gastrointestinal disturbances, abnormal respiration, acid-base imbalance, and central nervous system disturbances. Fatalities have occurred from ingestion of as little as 10 to 30 grains of aspirin in adults or as little as 4 ml of methyl salicylate in children. In addition to aspirin and sodium salicylate, which are used topically as a counterirritant in ointments and liniments. Methyl salicylate can be absorbed through the skin in amounts capable of causing systemic toxicity. Another salicylate, salicylic acid, is too irritating to be used systemically and is used topically as a keratolytic agent, such as for removing warts.

137 Sedative. (1) Of or pertaining to a substance, procedure, or measure that has a calming effect. (2) An agent that decreases functional activity, diminishes irritability, and allays excitement. Some sedatives have a general effect on all organs; others affect principally the activites of the heart, stomach, intestines, nerve trunks, respiratory system, or vasomotor system. Barbiturates and nonbarbiturate sedatives, such as carbromal, chloral hydrate, ethinamate, furazepam, glutethimide, and various minor tranquilizers, are used to induce sleep, reduce pain, facilitate the induction of anesthesia, and treat convulsive conditions, anxiety states, and irritable bowel syndrome.

138 Seizure. See Convulsion.*

139 Shock. An abnormal physiologic state; the first phase of the body's alarm reaction to trauma. The common clinical signs of shock include reduced cardiac output, circulatory insufficiency, tachycardia, hypotension, restlessness, pallor, and diminished urinary output. Shock often results from severe tissue damage and may be primary, secondary, or hemorrhagic.

140 Solute. A substance dissolved in a solution.

141 Solution. A mixture of two or more substances dissolved in another substance. The molecules of each of the substances disperse homogenously and do not change chemically. A solution may be a gas, a liquid, or a solid. Compare colloid,* suspension.

142 Solvent. Any liquid in which another substance can be dissolved. Informally, the term is used to refer to organic liquids like benzene, carbon tetrachloride, and other volatile petroleum distillates that when inhaled can cause intoxication as well as damage to mucous membranes of the nose and throat and the tissues of the kidney, liver, and brain. Repeated, prolonged exposure can result in addiction, brain damage, blindness, and other serious consequences, some of them fatal.

143 Spansule. A term describing a time released encapsulated drug whose action occurs over a prolonged time period.

144 Spastic. Of or pertaining to spasm or other uncontrolled contractions of the skeletal muscles.

145 Specificity. The ability of a test to identify only those who do not have a disease. Also the ability of a drug or agent to act on a certain type of tissue or nerve ending.

146 Stereoisomerism. The relationship between different compounds whose atoms are bound together in the same sequence with the difference being in spatial positions of the atoms.

147 Steroids. Drugs that have anti-inflammatory action, immunosuppressive activity, and antiarrhythmic potential. (See also Unit 22.1.)

148 Suspension. (1) A liquid in which small particles of a solid are dispersed, but not dissolved, and in which the dispersal is maintained by stirring or shaking the

---

*See Mosby's medical, nursing, & allied health dictionary, ed 3, St Louis, 1990, The CV Mosby Co.

mixture. If left standing, the solid particles settle at the bottom of the container. (2) A treatment, used primarily in spinal disorders, consisting of suspending the patient by the chin and shoulders. (3) A temporary cessation of pain or of a vital process.

149 Sympathomimetic. A pharmacologic agent that mimics the effects of stimulation of organs and structures by the sympathetic nervous system by occupying adrenergic receptor sites and acting as an agonist or by increasing the release of the neurotransmitter norepinephrine at postganglionic nerve endings. Various sympathomimetic agents are used as decongestants of nasal and ocular mucosa, as bronchodilators in the treatment of asthma, bronchitis, bronchiectasis, and emphysema, and as vasopressors and cardiac stimulants in the treatment of acute hypotension and shock; they are also used for maintaining normal blood pressure during operations under spinal anesthesia. Drugs in this group include cyclopentamine, dobutamine, dopamine, ephedrine, isoproterenol, levarterenol, metaraminol, metaproterenol, mephentermine, methoxamine, methoxyphenamine, naphazoline, phenylephrine, phenylpropanolamine, propylhexedrine, protokylol, pseudoephedrine, terbutaline sulfate, tetrahydrozoline, tuaminoheptane, xylometazoline, and epinephrine, a synthetic isomer of the hormone secreted by the adrenal medulla. Adverse effects of sympathomimetic drugs may be nervousness, severe headache, anxiety, vertigo, nausea, vomiting, dilated pupils, glycosuria, and dysuria.

150 Synapse. (1) The region surrounding the point of contact between two neurons or between a neuron and an effector organ, across which nerve impulses are transmitted through the action of a neurotransmitter, such as acetylcholine or norepinephrine. When an impulse reaches the terminal point of one neruon, it causes the release of the neurotransmitter, which diffuses across the gap between the two cells to bind with receptors in the other neuron, muscle, or gland, triggering electrical changes that either inhibit or continue the transmission of the impulse. Synapses are polarized so that nerve impulses travel in only one direction; they are also subject to fatigue, oxygen deficiency, anesthetics, and other chemical agents. (2) To form a synapse or connection between neurons. (3) (in genetics) To form a synaptic fusion between homologous chromosomes during meiosis. Kinds of synapses include axoaxonic synapse, axodendritic synapse, axodendrosomatic synapse, axosomatic synapse, dendrodendritis synapse. (Compare Ephapse.*)

151 Syndrome. A complex of signs and symptoms resulting from a common cause or appearing, in combination, to present a clinical picture of a disease or inherited abnormality. (See also specific syndromes.)

152 Synergy. The process in which two organs, substances, or agents work simultaneously to enhance the function and effect of one another. Also called synergism.

153 Synthetic. Of or pertaining to a substance that is produced by an artificial rather than a natural process or material.

154 Syrup. Any sweet solution used as a vehicle for medication.

155 Tachyphylaxis. (1) (in pharmacology) A phenomenon in which the repeated administration of some drugs results in a marked decrease in effectiveness. (2) (in immunology) Also called mithridatism. Rapidly developing immunity to a toxin owing to previous exposure, such as from previous injection of small amounts of the toxin.

156 Therapeutic index. Ratio of effective drug concentration and drug toxicity.

157 Tolerance. The ability to endure hardship, pain, or ordinarily injurious substances like drugs without apparent physiologic or psychologic injury. A kind of tolerance is work tolerance.

158 Tonus. (1) The normal state of balanced tension in the tissues of the body, especially the muscles. Partial contraction or alternate contraction and relaxation of neighboring fibers of a group of muscles hold the organ or the part of the body in a neutral, functional position without fatigue. Tone is essential for many normal body functions, like holding the spine erect, the eyes open, and the jaw closed. (2) The state of the tissues of the body being strong and fit.

159 Topical. (1) Of or pertaining to the surface of a part of the body. (2) Of or pertaining to a drug or treatment applied topically.

160 Toxicity. (1) The degree to which something is poisonous. (2) A condition that results from exposure to a toxin or to toxic amounts of a substance that does not cause adverse effects in smaller amounts.

161 Undesired effect of a drug. An action by a drug or agent that is not the intended action. It may or may not be harmful to the patient.

162 Universal antidote. A mixture of 50% activated charcoal, 25% magnesium oxide, and 25% tannic acid, formerly thought to be useful as an antidote for most types of acid, heavy metal, alkaloid, and glycoside poisons. It is now believed that the mixture is no more effective than activated charcoal given with water.

163 Untoward effect of a drug. A side effect of a drug regarded as harmful to the patient.

164 Vasoconstrictor. (1) Of or pertaining to a process, condition, or substance that causes the constriction of blood vessels. (2) An agent that promotes vasoconstriction. Cold, fear, stress, and nicotine are common exogenous vasoconstrictors. Internally secreted epinephrine and norepinephrine cause blood vessels to contract by stimulating adrenergic receptors of peripheral sympathetic nerves. Other endogenous vasocon-

---

*See Mosby's medical, nursing, & allied health dictionary, ed 3, St Louis, 1990, The CV Mosby Co.

strictors are angiotensin, which is formed in the blood-through the action of renin, and antidiuretic hormone, which is secreted by the pituitary. Adrenergic sympathomimetic drugs cause some degree of vasoconstriction, and several of these agents are used for this action in maintaining blood pressure during anesthesia and in treating pronounced hypotension resulting from hemorrhage, myocardial infarction, septicemia, sympathectomy, or drug reactions. Among these therapeutic agents are methoxamine hydrochloride, metaraminol bitartrate, and levarterenol (norepinephrine).

165 Vasodilator. (1) A nerve or agent that causes dilation of blood vessels. (2) Pertaining to the relaxation of thesmooth muscle of the vascular system. (3) Producing dilation of blood vessels. Vasodilators are a recent, important addition to the treatment of heart failure. Included are hydralazine, nitroglycerin, nitroprusside, and trimethaphan. They have proved very useful in the treatment of acute heart failure in myocardial infarction, in cases associated with severe mitral insufficiency, and in heart failure resulting from myocardial disease.

166 Vial. A glass container with a rubber stopper that is used to hold a number of doses of a drug.

2.2 Some common abbreviations employed in prescription orders (Table 15-1)

3.0 CONTROL OF DRUGS
3.1 Agencies involved in the control of drugs

1 Federal Drug Administration (FDA). Controls the overall manufacture and sale of drugs.

2 Regulations under which the FDA implements their authority:

  a The Federal Food, Drug, and Cosmetic Act of 1938 made it mandatory that manufacturers perform toxicity tests in laboratory animals before seeking FDA approval for a drug.

  b The Durham-Humphrey Amendment of 1952 allowed the FDA to determine which medications could be dispensed only by a physician's order.

  c The Drug Abuse Control Amendment of 1965 provided strict control over the manufacture, distribution, and sale of barbiturates, amphetamines, and other drugs that affect the CNS.

3 Federal Trade Commission (FTC). Jurisdiction over advertising of nonprescription drugs. Their primary concern is protection of the public against false advertising.

4.0 DRUG INFORMATION SOURCES
4.1 Drug publications

1 The *Pharmacopeia of the United States (USP)* was the first published in 1820. It is updated every 5 years and is the "bible" for information regarding safe dosage ranges for drugs.

2 The *National Formulary (NF)* is similar to the *USP*, although drugs are explained in more detail.

3 The *Physician's Desk Reference (PDR)* is a yearly publication printed by the pharmaceutical companies with updated information on their products, i.e., dose, effects, action, side effects, indications, and contraindications.

TABLE 15-1 Abbreviations used in prescription orders

Abbreviation	Derivation	Meaning
aa	ana	of each
a.c.	ante cibum	before meals
ad lib.	ad libitum	as freely, or as often, as is desired
aq. (dest)	aqua (destillata)	water (distilled)
b.i.d.	bis in die	twice a day
c̄	cum	with
caps.	capsula	capsule
comp.	compositus	compound
dil.	dilutus	dilute
d.t.d.	dentur tales doese	give as many doses as indicated by the number
disp.	dispensa	dispense
elix.	elixir	elixir
ext.	extractum	extract
et	et	and
F or ft.	Fac. or fiat	make; let be made
flext.	fluidextractum	fluid extract
g	gramma	gram
gr.	granum	grain
gtt.	gutta	a drop
h.	hora	hour
M	misce	mix
noct.	nox, noctis	night
no.	numerus	number
non rep.	non repetat	do not repeat
o	omnis	every
o.d.	omni die	every day
o.d.	oculus dexter	right eye
o.h.	omni hora	every hour
o.s.	oculus sinister	left eye
pil.	pilula	pill
p.c.	post cibos	after meals
p.o.	per os	by mouth
p.r.n.	pro re nata	literally, as the occasion arises; occasionally; when it seems to be desirable or necessary
q. or qq	quaque	every
q.h. or qqh	quaque hora	every hour
q. or q.d.	quaque die	every day
q.i.d.	quater in die	four times a day
q.s.	quantum sufficit	a sufficient amount
℞	recipe	to take
s̄	sine	without
S or sig.	signa	write (on the label)
s.o.s.	si opus sit	if needed
sol	solutio	solution
sp.	spiritus	spirit
ss	semis	half
stat.	statim	immediately
syr.	syrypus	syrup
tab	tabella	tablet
t.i.d.	ter in die	three times a day
tr.	tinctura	tincture
ut dict.	ut dictum	as directed

4.2 Naming drugs

The following methodology is followed in naming drugs:

1 The official name (generic or *chemical* name). The name listed for the drug in the *USP* or *NF*. This name refers to a class of drugs and does *not* link the drug with a particular manufacturer. These can be found in the *PDR* yellow section.

2 The USAN or United States Adopted Name is the name given to a drug by a council.

3 The *proprietary* or *trade* name is the brand name assigned to a drug by the manufacturer. The name is always capitalized (whereas the nonproprietary or generic name begins with lower case letters. These are found in the PDR pink section.)

4.3 Common respiratory therapy drugs.

1 Using the *PDR* one can easily look up the *brand* names of the following drugs.

Generic name	Brand name
a Racemic epinephrine	Micronefrin, Vaponefrin
b Isoproterenol	Isuprel
c Cromolyn sodium	Intal, Aarane
d N-acetyl-L-cysteine	Mucomyst
e Isoetharine	Bronkosol

2 Use the *PDR* to look up the *generic* names and manufacturer of the following drugs.

Brand name	Generic name
a Bricanyl	Terbutaline sulfate
b Albuterol	Salbutamol
c Decadron	Dexamethasone sodium phosphate
d Pavulon	Pancuronium
e Anectine, Quelicin	Succinylcholine chloride

5.0 DRUG EFFECTS
5.1 Factors influencing drug effect

1 Dosage. Strength of the drug.

2 Time. Frequency and length of exposure to a drug.

3 Weight, age, sex. Relationships exist between the mass of drug use and the mass of tissue through which the drug will be distributed and diluted.

4 Metabolism rate. Toxic effects can occur whenever a drug is administered in amounts that are not metabolized before another dose is given. This condition is referred to as *cumulative toxicity*.

5 Combined action of two or more drugs in the body, e.g., additive 1 + 1 = 2.

a It is important to note that the effect of a dose of a drug may be increased or decreased by another drug the patient is receiving.

b This action may be planned and desirable or not planned and dangerous.

c Drugs that act *together* to bring about a desired effect are *synergistic,* e.g., 0 + 1 = 2.

d Synergistic drugs can become *toxic* when calculated dosages are reached in the body.

e Drugs that cause opposing effects are *antagonists*. Antagonists sometimes are given to cancel the undesired effects of another drug.

f Drugs can be given in combination to bring about effects that are the sum of the effects that each drug would cause separately. This effect is additive and desired when planned. NOTE: Drugs given in combination can cause a stronger effect than if the drugs were given separately. This is called *potentiation* and may be either desirable or dangerous, e.g., 1 + 1 = 3.

g Respiratory care personnel must be aware of all drugs that they administer in order to recognize and hopefully avoid undesired reactions in the patient.

6.0 DRUG METABOLISM
6.1 Factors determining drug metabolism

1 Critical concentration. Drug dosage required to get the desired change at the desired action site.

2 Lipid solubility/ionization. Substances that are soluble in lipids (such as alcohol) rapidly pass through the mucosal surface of the stomach and intestine. Substances that are not readily soluble in lipids are not easily absorbed and usually will remain at the site of injection for long periods of time. Sulfonamides, for example, are not absorbed by the stomach and pass into the gut. Antibiotics, such as streptomycin and neomycin, must be given by injection because of the fast absorption by the intestinal mucosa.

3 Drugs administered parenterally include drugs given by any route other than external. These are rapidly absorbed, with the rate directly related to the method of administration, e.g., subcutaneously, intramuscularly, or intravenously.

4 Inhalation. The second most rapid route of absorption is through deposition of a drug into the alveoli. The speed of absorption of a drug into the bloodstream from the alveoli is based on diffusion that occurs because of the proximity of the pulmonary capillaries to the alveolar membranes.

5 Age frequently makes a difference in the way a patient responds to a drug. For example, newborn infants require smaller doses than would be indicated by their size and body weight because they have not yet developed mechanisms to metabolize and excrete the drugs. In adults, similar reactions may occur if the patient lacks certain enzymes required for drug detoxification. Other patients may have an acquired tolerance to the drug so that larger doses are required to gain the desired effect.

7.0 DRUG ACTION
7.1 Theories

Drugs cause effects by:

1 Combining with cellular sites (receptors)

2 Interacting with cellular enzyme systems

3 Altering the physiochemical properties of outcellular membranes and intracellular structures.

7.2 Drug receptor theory

1 Drugs are thought to combine with chemical groups that have an affinity for the drug on or in a cellular structure.

2 It is believed that drug molecules are attracted to and fit into a cell's receptor sites, much as a key fits into a lock.

3 This combination stimulates or depresses the action potential of this cell. For example, acetylcholine is a natural body chemical that combines with receptors in the membranes of muscle and nerve cells that are specifically designed to receive it.

4 Combining acetylcholine with choline-receptive substances in the muscle initiates changes that trigger nerve cells to make the muscle contract.

5 Synthetic drugs that resemble acetylcholine will fit the same receptor site and cause the same action. This type of drug is called an *agonist*.

6 Not all agonists cause a pharmacologic action.

7 If another drug complex is present at the cell, the agonist may, in fact, serve as an antagonist to a natural agonist.

7.3 Role of enzymes

1 Enzymes are molecules that control all chemical reactions occurring within the cell.

2 Each enzyme controls only one reaction acting with one specific molecule (substrate).

3 Drugs that affect an enzyme must resemble the substrate.

4 Enzymes receive and react to drugs using the lock and key receptor theory, much the same as cells.

5 The active site of an enzyme can receive a substrate and convert it into a new chemical substance.

6 The new chemical substance produced by the enzyme will serve as a substrate for other enzymes through a series of chemical reactions.

7 This mechanism frees the initial enzyme to react with another molecule, etc.

8 Natural chemicals are kept from combining with a cell or enzyme because of the presence of a foreign (synthetic) chemical that has filled the lock) in the treatment of cancer and in the prevention of other undesirable cellular activities. This response is known as *competitive inhibition*.

9 Drugs that alter the inner and outer function of the cell membrane are still under development and are beyond the scope of consideration of this module.

8.0 ADMINISTRATION OF DRUGS
8.1 Routes of administration

1 Topical. Placed directly onto a surface.

2 Oral. Taken by mouth.

3 Rectal. Placed into the rectum.

4 Sublingual. Placed under the tongue.

5 Parenterally. Injected.
  a Intradermally
  b Subcutaneously
  c Intramuscularly (IM)
  d Intravenously (IV)

6 Inhalation. Inhaled into the lungs as a gas, aerosol, or powder.

8.2 Factors determining the route of administration.

1 The reason one selects a specific route of administration will depend on:
  a Intended action site for the drug.
  b Desired time delay before drug action occurring.
  c Length of time drug action should continue.
  d Availability of administration site.

2 For the factor of desired time delay before drug action occurs, one would select *intravenous* as being the fastest and *inhalation* as a second fastest route for obtaining systemic response to a drug.

9.0 HEALTH CARE TEAM RESPONSIBILITIES IN ADMINISTRATION OF DRUGS
9.1 General responsibilities

1 The responsibilities of the physician in drug administration include:
  a *All* drugs given by respiratory care personnel must be prescribed by a physician.
  b Prescriptions must be recorded and signed in the patient's chart by the physician. In extenuating circumstances, a technician may initially act on a physician's verbal order to provide emergency treatment, provided a witness is present and the order is written as soon as the emergency is over. Many hospitals use *standing orders,* written orders, and protocols that are agreed on by the medical staff as appropriate treatment for patients with specific pulmonary problems.

2 The registered nurse's responsibilities include:
  a In the absence of the physician, the nurse is responsible for all drugs administered to the patient.
  b The nurse must also secure a written prescription for the administration of drugs.

3 The role of respiratory care personnel includes:
  a Respiratory care personnel are responsible to the physician and registered nurse for proper administration of all drugs.
  b Technicians may be responsible to the registered therapist for administration of drugs.

10.0 ADMINISTRATION OF DRUGS BY TECHNICIANS
10.1 Principles to be observed by respiratory care personnel while administering drugs

1 Give only drugs that are prescribed.

2 Have a written order for all patient treatments.

3 Never carry out an order unless it is clearly understood.

4 Always know the drug to be given.

5 Know the average dose.

6 Understand the method of administration.

7 Know and recognize the desired effect.

8 Know and recognize the symptoms of an overdose and

other untoward effects and be prepared to take appropriate action.

9 Administer the drug to the patient on time.

10 Provide the patient with necessary instruction for safe and correct administration of the drug.

11 Contact supervisor/nurse if a patient refuses drug or is resistant.

12 Never give a drug that has been premixed by someone else.

13 Never give a drug that is out of date or appears altered.

14 Never give a drug from an unmarked container.

15 Never leave open drug containers on a tray or table.

16 Never return a drug to a container once it has been poured or drawn.

17 Use clean equipment to administer a drug. Report any errors or adverse effects immediately.

18 Chart all treatment according to departmental practice.

11.0 CORRECT PREPARATION AND ADMINISTRATION OF DRUGS
11.1 Guidelines for preparation

The following guidelines are examples of general rules that should be followed when preparing drugs for administration:

1 Drugs should be administered only by the person who prepares them.

2 Check order in department.

3 Verify order in patient's chart and review other pertinent data, e.g., patient history, diagnosis, laboratory tests, x-ray examinations, and current treatment.

4 Never administer a medication that has changed color, consistency, or odor or that is out of date.

5 Use a sterile syringe to withdraw medications from a sterile bottle in lieu of a medicine dropper.

6 Use only one syringe per medication.

7 Always clean the outside of the container with alcohol swab before inserting a needle to withdraw the medication.

8 If unit dose medication vials are used, always empty a vial once it is opened.

9 If a unit dose is too strong for a patient, the remaining medication can be withdrawn into a labeled syringe and capped for another patient, provided it is used immediately and is the prescribed dosage.

10 Never leave medications opened to the environment or left out where they can be picked up by an unauthorized person.

11 Never add medication to a container that holds unused medication.

12 Always store unused medications according to manufacturer's recommendations.

13 Always dispose of used needles and syringes according to department policy and procedure. Increased concern over illegal drug use and cross contamination of AIDS and other infections have caused health care agencies to adopt special handling precautions. Avoid accidental needle sticks!!

12.0 ADMINISTERING AEROSOLIZED DRUGS
12.1 Using a nebulizer to deliver medication

1 As previously stated, the inhalation of drugs, with subsequent deposition in the lungs, is the second most rapid route of administering medication. It takes less than 1 second for inhaled aerosols to cross the blood-gas barrier of the lung and enter the pulmonary circulation. As with the intravenous route, drugs administered via inhalation cause rapid response. Therefore any inhaled medication that is not sterile and of the proper dosage can be extremely dangerous.

2 The following general principles should be considered when nebulizing drugs:

a Nebulizers deposit aerosols generated from the solution in the nebulizer container.

b Solutions to be nebulized must be of the proper strength for the length of the prescribed treatment.

c Fresh medications should never be passed into a container holding used medications.

d A change in nebulizers *may* cause a different drug response for a given dose because of the variance in aerosol density and particle size from one unit to another, e.g., from a pneumatic nebulizer to an ultrasonic nebulizer.

e In prolonged nebulizer treatments involving medications, care must be taken to prevent reconcentration of the drug in the nebulizer container during the process of the treatment. This occurs because of the difference in vaporization between the solute and the solvent. As the solvent evaporates, the solute becomes increasingly more potent.

f As a result of the effects of condensation, heated aerosol and gas should not be mixed with cooled aerosol and gas unless a change in the deposition site is desired.

g For maximum drug effect from aerosol therapy, a patient must use proper breathing techniques.

h Before administering medications by way of a nebulizer, the clinician must know and recognize the desired and possible untoward effects of the drug.

13.0 ORDERS FOR AEROSOL DRUG THERAPY
13.1 The physician's order

1 A properly written medical order is the legal starting point for all respiratory care. The order should be comprehensive enough to define the boundaries of the therapy as well as the expected outcomes. However, it should be general enough to allow the clinician the latitude necessary to select the best technique and equipment for the desired outcome.

2 The written order for aerosol drug therapy should contain:

a Name of the medication

b How it is to be administered (route)

c Volume to be administered

d Drug concentration to be administered

e Duration of treatment

f Frequency of treatments

g Any special precautions/directions

h Number of shifts or days that the treatment is to be given

14.0 METHODS FOR DISPENSING DRUGS

14.1 Drawing a solution with a needle and syringe

1 Procedure 15-1, which is included at the end of this module, may be used as an example of how to use a needle and syringe to withdraw a solution from a vial and ampule without contaminating the solution.

2 Remember to properly dispose of the used needle/syringe once the procedure has been completed.

14.2 Dispensing a drug using a unit dose vial

1 Procedure 15-2, which is included at the end of this module, is an example of how to dispense a measured amount of solution into a container without contaminating the solution.

2 Do not save partially empty vials for subsequent use. The medication is contaminated and the dose may be inaccurate.

15.0 MATHEMATIC CONCEPTS AND PRINCIPLES FOR DOSAGE CALCULATION

15.1 Need for accurately calculating dosages

1 An accurate measurement of drug concentrations is one of the most important functions performed by respiratory care personnel when dealing with medications.

2 The administration of an inaccurate drug dosage is potentially *dangerous* to the patient and is also illegal.

3 The use of metered dosage containers by many departments has reduced, but not eliminated, the need for this competency by all respiratory personnel.

4 Calculations of drug dilutions and the conversion of measurements from the metric to the apothecary system is not difficult, provided the student has mastered basic mathematical skills in working with decimals, multiplication, division, and solving an equation for an unknown.

NOTE: If a student is weak in these areas, it is recommended that he or she acquire instruction or complete one of many self-development texts on this subject before beginning this unit of instruction.

15.2 Terminology and principles for calculating dosage

1 Ratio and percentage strengths

a Ratio strength. The expression of the number of parts of solute to the total number of parts of solution.

- For solid in liquid. The number of grams (g) of solute in the total number of milliliters (ml) of solution.
- For liquid in liquid. The number of milliliters of solute (the liquid in least concentration) in the total number of milliliters of solution. Example: 1:2000.

NOTE: Ratio strength is usually written so that the first member of the ratio (the numerator when the ratio is expressed as a common fraction) is one, as in the previous example.

b Percentage strength. The expression of the number of parts of solute in 100 parts of solution. This is similar to ratio strength as a percentage is the ratio of the number of parts of solute to 100 parts of total solution.

- For solid in liquid. the number of grams of solute in 100 ml of solution.
- For liquid in liquid. the number of milliliters of solute (the liquid in least concentration) in 100 ml of solution.
- For solid in solid. The number of grams of solute in 100 g of mixture.

2 Conversion from ratio strength to percentage strength

a Convert ratio strength (e.g., A:B), to a common fraction (e.g., A/B).

b Equate the common fraction with X/100 (e.g., A/B = X/100).

c Solve equation for X.

For example: What is the percentage strength of a 1:4000 solution?

- 1:4000 is 1/4000
- 1/4000 is X/100%
- X = (1) (100%)/4000
- X = 100%/4000
- X = 0.025%

3 Conversion from percentage strength to ratio strength

a Drop the percent sign from the percentage.

b Form a common fraction by dividing by 100.

c Express the common fraction as a ratio.

For example: What is the ratio strength of a 5% solution?

- 5% becomes 5
- 5 divided by 100 is equivalent to 5/100
- 5/100 is equivalent to 5:100
- NOTE: The first number of a ratio is usually expressed as the number one (1). To achieve this, divide both sides of the ratio by the first number.
- Therefore (5/5):(100/5) is equivalent to 1:20.

4 Calculations involving the use of percentage

a Determine the quantity of solute based on the percentage strength of the solution.

b Since percentage strength is the number of parts of solute per 100 parts of solution, i.e., number of parts of solute/number of parts of solution, the amount of solute contained in a given number of parts of solution can be calculated by the use of ratio and proportion.

FOR EXAMPLE: How many grams of a solute are in 10 ml of solution if the solution is a 5% solution?

- 5% = 5/100
- X/10 ml = 5 g/100 ml
- X/10 ml = 5 g/100 ml
- X = (5 g) (10 ml)/100 ml
- X = 50 g/100
- X = 0.5 g

Check:
- Is 0.5 g per 10 ml equivalent to 5%?
- $0.5/10 \times 100\% = 5\%$

5 Determine the percentage strength based on the quantity of solute in the solution

  a This procedure is also based on ratio and proportion. FOR EXAMPLE: 20 ml of a solution contains 5 g of solute. What is the percentage strength of the solution?
- $5 \text{ g}/20 \text{ ml} = X/100 \text{ ml}$
- $X = (5 \text{ g}) (100 \text{ ml})/20 \text{ ml}$
- $X = 500 \text{ g}/20$
- $X = 25 \text{ g}$

  b Since the percentage strength of a solution is the number of parts (grams) in 100 parts (grams) in 100 parts (milliliters) of solution, the percentage strength of the above solution is 25%, i.e., 25 g of solute per 100 ml of solution.

    Answer. 25%

6 Calculations involving the use of ratio strength

  a The only difference between problems using percentage strength and ratio strength is that conversion of the ratio strength to a percentage strength may be necessary; such a conversion was considered earlier in this presentation.

  b NOTE: Although some persons prefer to make this conversion, it is not necessary to do so in solving the problem, as will be shown in the following examples.

    EXAMPLE: How many grams of solute are contained in 50 ml of a solution having a ratio strength of 1:2000?
- $1:2000 = 1 \text{ g}/2000 \text{ ml}$
- $X/50 \text{ ml} = 1 \text{ g}/2000 \text{ ml}$
- $X = (50 \text{ ml}) (1 \text{ g})/2000 \text{ ml}$
- $X = 50 \text{ g}/2000$
- $X = 1 \text{ g}/40$
- $X = 0.025 \text{ g}$

    Check:
- Is 0.025 g per 50 ml equivalent to 1:2000?
- $0.025/50 = 1:2000$

    EXAMPLE: What is the ratio strength of a solution if 250 ml of the solution contains 2 g?
- $2 \text{ g}/250 \text{ ml} = 2:250$
- $2:250 = (2/2):(250/2)$
- $(2/2):(250/2) = 1:125$

15.3 Calculating dosages for infants and children

1 Infants and children are not just small adults and, in most cases, cannot tolerate adult dosages for drugs.

2 The following formulae can be used to adjust adult dosages for use by infants and children:

  a Young's rule uses child's age in years for children 2 to 12 years old.

$$\frac{\text{Age of child}}{\text{Age of child} + 12} \times \text{Adult dose} = \text{Child's dose}$$

  b Clark's rule uses the child's weight.

$$\frac{\text{Weight of child in pounds}}{150 \text{ (Average adult weight)}} \times \text{Adult dose} = \text{Child's dose}$$

  c Fried's rule uses age in months (used for children under 2 years).

$$\frac{\text{Age in months}}{150} \times \text{Adult dose} = \text{Infant dose}$$

  d Cowling's rule uses age at next birthday.

$$\frac{\text{Age next birthday}}{24} \times \text{Adult dose} = \text{Child's dose}$$

16.0 INDICATIONS, CONTRAINDICATIONS, DOSAGES, AND EFFECTS OF DRUGS USED IN RESPIRATORY CARE

16.1 Pharmacologic basis of drug action

The living body and each of its cells are the site of countless chemical reactions that go on continuously and endlessly. When a drug enters a living system, its millions of molecules immediately begin to react with those of the body's cells. Some of the drug molecules react with those of the living tissues in ways that change the functioning of the cells—that is, they produce pharmacologic effects.

No drug can produce an effect that the body is incapable of producing with its natural enzymes. The pharmacologic effects produced by a drug vary with the drug absorption, distribution, metabolism, and excretion.

1 *Drug concentration.* For a drug to produce its pharmacologic effects, it must reach a certain critical concentration in the fluids around the cells that are capable of responding to the drug. When the drug reaches this level in the reactive tissues, it brings about changes in cellular function. The rate of biochemical and physiologic activity is altered by the presence of the drug. Factors affecting drug concentration include:

  a Amount of drug administered

  b Extent and rate of drug absorption

  c Distribution of the drug following absorption

  d Binding of and localization of the drug

  e Rate of inactivation

  f Rate of excretion

2 *Drug absorption.* The term absorption refers to what happens to a drug from the time it enters the body until it enters the circulating fluids. The rate of absorption largely determines the latent period between administration and onset of action. Also, the rate of absorption determines the dosage and influences the route of administration used. Factors influencing the absorption of drugs include:

  a Physiochemical action.

  b Drug solubility. Drugs given in solution are more rapidly absorbed than those given in solid form.

  c Concentration of the drug. Drugs administered in high concentrations are absorbed more rapidly.

  d Circulation to the site of absorption. Increasing circulation by massage, application of heat locally, or administration of vasodilators, increases absorption.

Conversely, decreasing circulation decreases absorption.

   e Area of absorbing surface. Increasing the area of absorption increases the rate of absorption.

   f Route of administration. This is the most important factor, for it largely determines the area of absorption, e.g., intravenous administration has a larger area of absorption than intramuscular injection.

3 *Distribution.* After a drug is absorbed or injected into the bloodstream, it can enter or pass through various fluid compartments of the body, e.g., plasma, interstitial fluid, transcellular fluids, and cellular fluids. Some drugs accumulate in various areas of the body other than the site of action; these areas are referred to as storage depots.

4 *Storage depots.* The importance of storage depots is that these areas may rapidly accumulate the drug, removing it from the circulation and therefore preventing the drug from exerting its effect. As important is the fact that these sites then serve as reservoirs of the drug, slowly releasing the drug back into the circulation. This slow releasing of the drug can provide for extended durations of action from some drugs following a "priming" dose.

   a Plasma proteins. Some drugs have a great affinity for the proteins of the blood and may become bound. Although this does not result in removal of the drug from the circulation, it prevents the release of the drug from the circulation to the site of action; therefore the plasma proteins can be regarded as storage depots. Since the binding is a reversible one, i.e., the bound drug will be released as free drug as the free drug is removed from the circulation, this depot can result in extended durations of action.

   b Neutral fat depots. Some drugs possess a very high lipid (fat) solubility and therefore accumulate in the body's fat. Since fat may compose 50% of the obese person's body weight and as much as 10% of a person's weight after starvation, it should be evident that fat can serve as extremely large depots of certain drugs which possess a high lipid solubility, such as thiopental, an ultra-short-acting barbiturate that is used widely as an anesthetic in surgery.

5 *Redistribution.* Drugs are primarily terminated in their action by biotransformation (metabolism) or excretion; however, inactivation can result from redistribution of the drug from the site of action to other tissue.

   a Biotransformation, or metabolism, is a process that allows the body to convert drugs to a form that can be rapidly removed from the body. This usually involves converting a lipid-soluble drug (usually a weak organic acid or base), which is generally rapidly reabsorbed from the renal tubules, to a more polar compound, which is reabsorbed less. The polar compound is less able to bind proteins, is less able to be stored in fat depots, and is less able to penetrate cell membranes. Therefore the drug is usually inactivated by this biotransformation. Some metabolites are active, however, and their action is terminated by further metabolism or by excretion. It should be noted that it is the metabolites of some drugs, not the drugs themselves, that are responsible for the action of the drugs.

   b The primary site of biotransformation is the *liver.* Other sites include the plasma, the kidney, and other tissues.

   c The process of biotransformation is dependent on the presence of enzymes (organic compounds, frequently proteins, capable of accelerating or producing by catalytic action some change in a substrate for which they are often specific). The most prominent group of enzymes are the hepatic microsomal enzymes.

6 The factors affecting drug-metabolizing enzymes include:

   a Administration of various drugs and hormones

   b Age

   c Sex

   d Strain

   e Temperature

   f Nutritional status

   g Pathologic state

7 Excretion is another important route of drug elimination by the body.

8 The routes of excretion are:

   a Renal

   b Fecal

   c Mamillary

   d Pulmonary

   e Perspiratory

   f Salivary

9 Of these routes of excretion, the *renal* route is the most important one, because it accounts for most drug excretion.

16.2 Physiologic basis of drug action

1 The drugs discussed in this section are ones that act primarily by affecting the functioning of nervous tissue. The most important agents of this type are the ones that are able to penetrate the blood-brain barrier and exert their effects on the brain and spinal cord or what is called the central nervous system (CNS).

2 Drugs that interfere with the functioning of the CNS may affect only a single activity, such as the perception of pain; however, they are more likely to have multiple effects because the various parts of the CNS are functionally interrelated so that stimuli that affect one area also affect others.

3 Before discussing the various types of centrally acting drugs, one should first review those aspects of the anatomy and physiology that are most pertinent to an understanding of the actions of drugs on this complex system. (See Module Four.)

4 The structural unit of the nervous system is the *neuron,* or nerve cell. The neuron is made up of a cell body with thin threadlike projections branching from its surface called dendrites. The dendrites *receive* signals from many other interconnecting neurons. Another projection on the nerve cell body is a more elongated process that does not branch until it comes close to other neurons—this is an axon. An axon *transmits* messages to dendrites. Such functions between the axon of one neuron and the dendrites of another neuron are called *synapses*.

5 Drugs affect nerve cell function by increasing or reducing the responsiveness of nerve impulse conduction at the synapse. Nerve impulses can either be excitatory or inhibitory in nature, thus maintaining a state of homeostasis. Many centrally-acting drugs exert their effects by altering the balance between the excitatory and the inhibitory impulses. They may do so by increasing either excitatory or inhibitory activity, or by blocking nerve impulses of one or the other.

6 The CNS is made up of the brain and spinal cord. Some of the primary functions of the CNS include:
 a Sensory functions
 b Motor (somatic) activity
 c Regulation of autonomic functions
 d Memory and association

7 The CNS can be divided into:
 a The somatic nervous system
 b The autonomic nervous system

8 The autonomic nervous system is further divided into the:
 a Parasympathetic nervous system
 b Sympathetic nervous system

9 The five parts of the brain and a brief description of each follows.
 a Cerebrum
  • Largest portion of the brain
  • Represents 7/8 of the total weight of the brain
  • Contains nerve centers governing all sensory and motor activities, as well as for the exercise of reason, memory, and intellegence
 b Cerebellum
  • Regulates skeletal muscle tone
  • Maintains balance and equilibrium
  • Maintains posture
  • Coordinates voluntary muscle movements
 c Midbrain
  • Contains nuclei for certain auditory and visual reflexes
  • Overall, serves as conduction pathways between the spinal cord and other parts of the brain
 d Pons
  • Transmits ascending and descending fibers to higher or lower levels of the nervous system
  • Is the origin of several cranial nerves
  • Contains the apneustic and the pneumotaxic centers
 e Medulla oblongata
  • Is point of origin for several cranial nerves that govern such vital functions as the action of the heart, respiration, etc.
  • All pathways between the brain and spinal cord pass through the medulla

10 Since the complicated nerve pathways involved in the control of many functions are still not completely mapped out, it is not surprising to realize that we cannot fully explain how drugs exactly affect the CNS. Nonetheless, we can make some general comments about the nature of drug actions on the CNS. Nervous tissue is characterized by *excitability,* and drugs may act by altering such nerve cell irritability. The state of excitability of various nerve cells at any moment in time is the sum of excitatory and inhibitory stimuli impinging simultaneously on the cell. Drug molecules can be considered a form of foreign intervention that alters the precarious balance between these excitatory and inhibitory influences that normally determine the degree of central neuronal excitability.

11 Drugs may be general in their action or selective (as general anesthetics vs. tranquilizers). CNS drug effects are based on the dosage of the drug administered.

12 Broadly speaking then, drugs may first be classified as central stimulants or depressants. Each of these may, in turn, be subdivided on the basis of whether their actions affect the entire CNS or act on various sites.

13 Stimulation of the CNS may lead to hyperexcitability, convulsions and death. Depression of the CNS may lead to sedation, hypnosis, anesthesia, coma, and death. The drugs capable of depressing all nervous tissue are never given or deliberately used in doses that would knock out nerve centers completely. Fortunately, the medullary centers (those centers that control heart beat and breathing) are the last to go.

14 Certain CNS depressants that have a general action may seem to be causing stimulation. Alcohol may, for example, appear to be producing excitement. This stimulation results from the depressant action on inhibitory centers in the brain. As a result, the areas with decreased inhibitory control may send out excitatory impulses at a more rapid rate. Such "pseudostimulation" accounts for the uninhibited behavior of the individual intoxicated by alcohol.

15 Thus, depending on the dose, the general depressant drugs can cause every degree of depression from light sedation to deep coma. The general depressants, therefore, are commonly classified as:
 a Sedatives
 b Hypnotics
 c General anesthetics

16 Secondary pharmacologic actions of these drugs may include:
 a Anticonvulsant activity
 b Muscle relaxation
 c Analgesia

17 Sedatives are drugs that produce mild drowsiness while reducing restlessness. They are often given during the day to calm the tense, anxious patient without seriously interfering with his ability to function normally.

18 Hypnotics are drugs that reduce sensitivity to pain by inhibiting nerve impulses, causing partial or complete unconsciousness. Massive amounts of these drugs can lead to coma and death.

19 Sedative-hypnotics have a selective activity on the reticular formation in the brainstem. Small doses deactivate this area that is important in maintaining consciousness and wakefulness.

20 Anesthesia is partial or complete loss of sensation with or without loss of consciousness, which may occur as a result of disease, injury, or administration of a drug. An analgesic is a drug that produces insensitivity to pain.

17.0 MEDICATIONS THAT CAUSE RESPIRATORY DEPRESSION

17.1 Barbiturates

The following units cover the drugs with which the respiratory therapy practitioner should be familiar since he/she will encounter their use daily. Many of these drugs will cause respiratory depression and, for that reason, they are of special importance.

1 The barbiturates are by far the most important class of sedative-hypnotics. Hundreds of these substances have been synthesized, but only a couple dozen derivatives are in common use today.

2 The various barbiturates differ mainly in the speed of the onset of effects and in the duration of action. How fast and how long a particular barbiturate acts depends on how the body handles it after it has been administered and absorbed into the systemic circulation. Drugs of rapid onset (thiopental sodium [Pentothal] and secobarbital [Seconal]) pass the blood-brain barrier more readily than the slow-acting drugs (phenobarbital).

3 The slow-onset drugs have a longer duration of action, because they are excreted slowly, unchanged by the kidneys. The quick-acting barbiturates wear off rapidly, because they soon leave the blood-brain barrier and are distributed to other areas, primarily the liver, for detoxification.

4 Barbiturates may be useful in modifying general changes in physiologic functions caused by anxiety, such as:
  a Cardiac palpitations
  b Increased blood pressure
  c Difficulty in breathing
  d Epigastric pain
  e Diarrhea
  f Dullness, fatigue, sleepiness
  g Restlessness
  h Insomnia

5 The barbiturates have little direct effect on relaxing smooth visceral muscles of the gastrointestinal tract. However, anxiety reduction is beneficial in peptic ulcers and anxiety-related gastrointestinal problems.

6 Barbiturates may reduce a patient's reaction to stressful situations and therefore may be helpful also in allergic disorders.

7 Two major considerations of barbiturate usage are that:
  a They may be habit-forming (addictive). Withdrawal from barbiturate addiction can be fatal if not handled under medical supervision.

  b They are poor analgesics.

8 Side effects are relatively few; but in some patients, they may produce drowsiness, lethargy, and headache. They should be carefully used in liver or hepatic disorders. The use of alcohol with barbiturates has been responsible for many drug overdoses and deaths.

9 The general *classifications of barbiturates* and some general characteristics of each are included here.
  a The characteristics of *long-acting* barbiturates are:
    • Stable in body fluids
    • Excreted unchanged by the kidneys
    • Slow onset (1-2 hours)
    • Long-lasting (24-36 hours)
    • Their uses include:
      – Continuous mild sedation
      – Control of moderate hypertension
      – Suppression of epilepsy
    • Examples of long acting barbiturates include:
      – Barbital (Veronal)
      – Phenobarbital (Luminal)
  b The characteristics of *intermediate-acting* barbiturates are:
    • Onset—1 hour
    • Duration—12 hours
    • The uses include:
      – Relief of insomnia
      – Reduction of anxiety
    • An example of an intermediate-acting barbiturate is:
      – Amobarbital (Amytal)
  c The characteristics of *short-acting* barbiturates are:
    • Rapid onset (20-30 minutes)
    • Duration of 6 hours
    • Rapid distribution in fat depots
    • 75% decomposition in the liver
    • Examples of short-acting barbiturates are:
      – Pentobarbital (Nembutal)
      – Secobarbital (Seconal)
  d The characteristics of *ultrashort-acting* barbiturates are:
    • Usually given IV
    • Effective in 30 seconds
    • Duration of less than 30 minutes
    • Uses include:
      – IV anesthesia (induction)
      – Anticonvulsants
    • Examples of ultrashort-acting barbiturates include:
      – Thiopental (Pentothal)
      – Thiamylal (Surital)
      – Methohexital (Brevital)

10 *Nonbarbiturate sedative-hypnotics.* These are older, less expensive drugs with somewhat less reliable effects. Some hypnotics, such as methaqualone, are of relatively recent discovery. They are sometimes used for patients allergic to barbiturates. Some general drugs included in this category are:
  a Chloral hydrate
    • Produces sedation, sleep, or anesthesia, depending on dose

  • Effective, inexpensive, causes stomach upset
 b Glutethimide (Doriden)
 c Methyprylon (Noludar)
 d Ethchlorvynol (Placidyl)
 e Methaqualone (Quaalude)
 f Ethanol
 g Bromide
 h Paraldehyde

17.2 Tranquilizers

1 Tranquilizers are also known as *psycholeptic* or *ataractic* agents and produce a state of "peace of mind." Tranquilizers are divided into major and minor categories. Major tranquilizers are usually used to treat psychotic patients and minor tranquilizers are used more as adjuncts to temporary stressful situations and treatment of neurotic behavior and anxiety. These do not produce sleep and coma as readily as the barbiturates, but some can be *more addictive* and prone to abuse. Some general uses of the tranquilizers include:
 a Treatment of neuroses/psychoses
 b Treatment of vomiting
 c Hypotensive and antihistaminic effects
 d Treatment of dyskinesia
2 The first drugs to produce an important impact in the care of psychiatric patients were the *rauwolfia alkaloids.* Used in India for years, they were first used routinely in the United States in the 1950s. Today they are used to treat hypertension. The rauwolfia alkaloids, particularly *reserpine,* from the Indian snakeroot plant *(Rauwolfia serpentina),* have many side effects, such as:
 a Nasal congestion
 b Fatigue, drowsiness
 c Headache
 d Dizziness
 e Nausea
 f Bizarre dreams
3 The *phenothiazines,* a major tranquilizer group, were developed in France and put in general use in this country during the mid-1950s. They are capable of causing many pharmacologic effects besides sedation. Chlorpromazine and other phenothiazines are in widespread use in the treatment of the mentally ill. These psycholeptic drugs are responsible for many former mental patients being able to live normal lives and for drastic reductions in the number of institutionalizations. Some of the actions that are clinically useful include:
 a Reduction of schizophrenic episodes
 b Motor sedation
 c Control of nausea and vomiting
 d Antipruritic (itching control)
 e Antitussive responses
4 Some examples of the phenothiazines are:
 a Chlorpromazine (Thorazine)
 b Triflupromazine (Vesprin)
 c Prochlorperazine (Compazine)
 d Thioridazine (Melleril)

5 Some *adverse* reactions of the phenothiazines include:
 a Parkinsonism. Muscular tremors, rigidity, etc.
 b Dyskinesias. Sudden contractions of muscles resembling convulsive seizures (these adverse reactions are controlled by benztropine [Cogentin] and diphenhydramine hydrochloride [Benadryl]).
 c Allergic skin reactions. Photosensitivity.
 d Liver disorders (especially with Thorazine) and jaundice.
 e Agranulocytosis. A blood disorder characterized by low white cell counts.
6 Another major tranquilizer group is the *butyrophenones,* which are of recent introduction into the United States. Examples are:
 a Haloperidol (Haldol)
 b Droperidol (Inapsine)
7 The minor tranquilizers do not cause the kinds of autonomic nervous system imbalances often seen with use of the major tranquilizers. These are primarily antianxiety agents and are used more frequently in the general population. Diazepam (Valium), recently accused of being prescribed to the point of abuse, is the most often ordered drug in the United States. Although these drugs are labeled as minor agents, when taken in sufficient dosages they can be addictive and even lethal.
8 Some examples of these minor tranquilizers are:
 a Meprobamate (Equanil, Miltown), which relaxes skeletal muscle spasm and tension; used in the treatment of arthritis.
 b Hydroxyzine (Atarax, Vistaril), which also has antihistaminic effects, antiemetic effects, and antispasmatic effects to relieve gastrointestinal smooth muscle spasm.
 c Chlordiazepoxide (Librium).
 d Diazepam (Valium).
 e Mephenesin (Tolserol).

17.3 Narcotics (analgesics)

1 A true *analgesic* is a drug that acts centrally to relieve pain, but without causing loss of consciousness.
2 Analgesics are divided into two classes.
 a Those relieving mild-to-moderate pain.
 b Those that overcome severe pain.
3 The patent analgesics can be broadly subdivided into:
 a The organic opiates (morphine).
 b The synthetic opiate analgesics.
4 A *narcotic* (opiate) is capable of producing CNS depression, including respiratory depression, and must be given cautiously. The most widely used narcotic analgesic is *morphine,* after Morpheus, the Greek god of dreams. The patient may still perceive severe pain but may not mind the pain, even if aware of it, as morphine interferes with nervous pathways.
5 Some of the effects of morphine include:
 a Raising the patient's pain perception threshold.
 b Reduction of anxiety and fear of pain.
 c Production of sleep in the presence of severe pain.
6 Small doses of morphine depress the cough reflex center and may be useful for patients with broken ribs or

bronchial carcinoma in which pain and coughing occur together. However, morphine also depresses respiration and therefore must be used with caution.

7 The side effects of morphine may include the following.

a Drowsiness, nausea, vomiting, constipation.

b Bronchoconstriction in patients with asthma and emphysema.

c An increase in intracranial pressure that may contraindicate its use in head trauma cases.

d Venous pooling that leads to a decreased cardiac output and blood pressure; cautious use is recommended in shock patients.

e Depression of respiratory center response to hypercapnia and hypoxia, which may then result in Cheyne-Stokes respirations and circulatory collapse.

f Addition. NOTE: Narcotic effects are reversible with naloxone.

8 *Codeine* was the second drug isolated from opium. Although best known as an additive to cough syrups, it has pain reducing abilities but requires higher doses than morphine. Some characteristic features of codeine include:

a Weaker than morphine.

b Requires a dose about 6-10 times for same analgesic effect.

c Less depressing to respirations.

d Less addictive.

e Is of value as an analgesic and antitussive.

f No value as a respiratory depressant for controlling ventilation.

9 The third, and perhaps the most infamous, of the opium derivatives is *heroin*. This unit will not address the obvious addictive qualities and social destabilization caused by heroin.

10 *Synthetic* (man-made) opiates frequently encountered in medical situations are:

a Hydromorphone (Dilaudid)

b Meperidine (Demerol)

c Methadone (Dolophine)

d Fentanyl (Sublimaze)

e Oxycodone hydrochloride

11 The synthetic narcotics are generally considered safer analgesics without the severe side effects of morphine and codeine. The synthetics produce less euphoria and are considered somewhat less addictive. They also produce less drowsiness, dizziness, and disorientation. For this reason, they are ordered more frequently for ambulatory patients.

12 Some specific characteristics of a synthetic narcotic, meperidine (Demerol), are as follows.

a 1/10 as potent as morphine.

b Not as euphoric.

c Less depressing to respiration.

d Used postoperatively following chest and upper abdominal surgery.

e Used for obstetrical analgesic to minimize fetal depression.

f Capable of muscle relaxation.

13 The *attenuated* narcotics are less potent pain relievers and have far less addictive properties. Examples are:

a Propoxyphene (Darvon)

b Ethoheptazine (Zactane)

c Dextromethorphan (Romilar)

14 Non-narcotic analgesics are:

a Pentazocine (Talwin)

b Levoprome (Methotrimeprazine)

17.4 Narcotic antagonists

1 In acute narcotic overdose, the primary direction of management is to combat respiratory depression and/or respiratory arrest.

2 Narcotic antagonists are used to reverse the effects of narcotics. They are not stimulants, but compete with the narcotic molecules for cellular receptors in drug-depressed neurons.

3 Examples of antagonists are:

a Nalorphine (Nalline)

b Levallorphan (Lorfan)

c Naloxone (Narcan)

4 The antagonists also possess some analgesic properties, but much less than the narcotics.

18.0 CNS DEPRESSANTS
18.1 Use of CNS depressants in respiratory therapy

1 Central nervous system depressants are used in respiratory care to relieve anxiety, restlessness, and pain in patients who:

a Are intubated

b Are being mechanically ventilated

c Have tracheostomies

d Are receiving continuous oxygen therapy

2 These drugs eliminate or depress the patient's tendency to resist therapy and, as such, facilitate ventilator control.

3 Some patients must have their respiratory drive significantly reduced in order for them to be treated effectively with mechanical ventilation and measures such as positive end expiratory pressure (PEEP).

4 Situations that need to be closely monitored when using these drugs include:

a Hypotension

b Hypoventilation

c Respiratory depression/respiratory arrest

19.0 ANESTHETIC DRUGS
19.1 Anesthetic drugs and patient care in respiratory therapy

1 It has been established that the fears a patient has preoperatively influence his recovery period after anesthesia. Since this is true, it is important that all personnel be aware of these fears so that one may care for the patient with a better understanding of his emotional state.

2 The following are some of the most common fears that influence postanesthesia recovery.

a Fear of going to sleep and not waking up.

b Fear of the unknown.

c Fear that the anesthetic will not relieve the pain and that he/she will still hurt.

d Fear that he/she will be extremely nauseated and vomit and might choke to death after anesthesia.

e Fear that he/she will talk and reveal facts that he/she does not wish known.

f Fear that after receiving a spinal anesthetic he/she will become paralyzed.

g Fear of repetition of a previous bad experience with an anesthetic.

3 Respiratory care personnel should have a basic understanding of the stages of anesthesia so that they may better understand the patient's mental processes and physical actions as he/she returns to consciousness.

a Stage I. Extends from the beginning of the administration of an anesthetic to the beginning of the loss of consciousness.

b Stage II. Often called the stage of excitement or delirium, extends from the loss of consciousness to the loss of eyelid reflexes. If the patient is very apprehensive or was not given premedication correctly or on time, this stage, usually of short duration, may last longer. The patient may become markedly excited and struggle, shout, talk, laugh, or cry. The nurse or therapist in the recovery room may find that some patients, recovering from the effects of general inhalation anesthesia, pass through Stage II again before becoming fully conscious and are very noisy and restless.

c Stage III. The stage of surgical anesthesia, extends from the loss of the lid reflex to cessation of respiratory effort. The patient is unconscious, his muscles are relaxed, and most of his reflexes have been abolished.

d Stage IV. The stage of overdosage or the stage of danger. It is a complicated respiratory and circulatory failure. Death will follow unless the anesthetic is immediately discontinued and artificial respiration given.

4 Respiratory care personnel also should be knowledgeable about the different types of anesthetics administered to patients.

5 The first category of anesthetics is *inhalation anesthesia*. This type of anesthesia is produced by having a patient inhale the vapors of certain liquids or gases. Oxygen is usually given with these anesthetics. These gases can be administered either by mask or through an endotracheal tube.

a Ether. This gas is rarely given because of its low flash point when mixed with oxygen. It is an excellent muscle relaxant and is still used in surgery requiring maximum relaxation of the patient.

b Nitrous oxide. This gas is nonirritating and nonflammable. It is always given with oxygen in proportionate amounts. It is a very weak anesthetic, however, and must be given in conjunction with other agents. It is relatively inexpensive compared with other agents. An excessive amount of this gas could possibly be given without enough oxygen in proportion. This is very detrimental to patients with cardiovascular or respiratory diseases, as they cannot tolerate the lack of oxygen.

c Cyclopropane. This gas is highly flammable and *explosive*. It is no longer used in the operating room at most hospitals, but may still be used in the delivery room. It produces unconsciousness quickly, and patients recover quickly (about 10 minutes after the gas is stopped). It also produces adequate relaxation for most abdominal surgery. It has been established that this gas does cause increased cardiac irritability and tends often to cardiac patients. Pulse rate and rhythm must be checked often for any irregularities. Vomiting often occurs after this anesthetic. No adrenalin may be given to patients who have had cyclopropane.

d *Halothane* (Fluothane). This gas is highly potent. It is flammable but nonexplosive. It is easily inhaled and usually administered through special vaporizers with nitrous oxide and oxygen. Sodium pentathol is usually given beforehand. This gas is nonirritating and does not cause laryngospasm or irritate the pulmonary tract. Induction and recovery is generally rapid. Halothane can depress the circulation when high concentrations are given. Gastrointestinal discomfort in the postanesthesia period is minimal compared with other agents.

e Penthrane. This gas is nonexplosive and noninflammable. Induction with penthrane is prolonged so sodium pentathol is usually given beforehand. This gas seldom causes nausea and is believed to be extremely low in toxicity. It does, however, have a very long-lasting effect. It is eliminated very slowly from the body through the kidneys and cannot be given to patients with kidney disorders.

f Chloroform. This gas is not used at most hospitals. It is very *toxic* and has a narrow margin of safety. A very small amount can cause death.

6 The second category of anesthetics is *intravenous anesthesia*. These drugs are either injected directly or added through the IV line.

a *Sodium pentathol*. This produces unconsciousness quickly and recovery is rapid. It is used mostly for brief minor procedures and to produce sleep before an inhalation anesthesia is used. Laryngospasm is likely. One must watch for restlessness, apprehension, stridor, retraction of soft tissues about the neck, and cyanosis. Personnel should also watch for signs of depressed respirations (shallow and slow) and also a generalized muscle twitching. The cause of this twitching is not known.

b General anesthesia. This is simply inhalation anesthesia with intravenous supplements. These can be sodium pentathol, curare, succinylcholine chloride (Anectine), pancuronium bromide (Pavulon), morphine, meperidine (Demerol), or fentanyl citrate (Innovar). This type of anesthetic can cause depressed respirations and hypotension, or it may cause hypertension if the patient is in pain.

   c Brevital. This drug is a very short-acting barbiturate. It is sometimes used for quick induction or to relax a patient before emergency intubation. It is not used very often because it can cause severe hiccups.

   d Ketamine HCL (Ketaject). This is known as a disassociative anesthesia. It is a rapid-acting general anesthesia that produces a state of profound analgesia. Pharyngeal and laryngeal reflexes are normal. Skeletal muscle tone is normal or slighly enhanced. The cardiovascular and respiratory systems are stimulated. Following the administration of Ketamine HCL, blood pressure and pulse rate are usually moderately and temporarily increased. Loud noises should be avoided around these patients. Postoperative confusional states may occur, and respiratory depression may occur with overdosage.

   e Fentanyl citrate (Innovar). This drug is a combination of a narcotic analgesic fentanyl (Sublimaze) and a neuroleptic (tranquilizer), droperidol (Inapsine). This drug produces a state termed "neuroleptanalgesia." This is characterized by general quiescence, reduced motor activity, and profound analgesia. Compete loss of consciousness usually does not occur. The incidence of postoperative pain and emesis may be reduced. Other CNS depressant drugs will have additive or potentiating effects with fentanyl citrate; therefore, the administration of CNS depressants and fentanyl citrate should be monitored carefully. When the patient is receiving these drugs concomitantly the dose of fentanyl citrate required may be less than usual. Postoperative narcotics and other depressants should be given in reduced doses, as low as one fourth or one third of those usually recommended. The most adverse reactions reported to occur with fentanyl citrate are respiratory depression, apnea, muscular rigidity, and hypotension. If severe hypotension occurs and is persistent, the possibility of hypovolemia should be considered.

7 *Infiltration anesthesia* is the third type of anesthesia. These agents include local anesthetics such as:

   a Procaine

   b Tetracaine (Pontocaine)

   c Dibucaine (Nupercaine)

8 When these drugs are absorbed into the bloodstream, they cause stimulation or depression of the CNS, depending on the dosage.

9 Epinephrine may be added to the solution of local anesthetic to produce vasoconstriction in the area of the injection.

10 *Spinal anesthesia* is the fourth type of anesthesia. It is also called a saddle block-type of anesthesia and is given in the subarachnoid space where it acts on the nerves as they emerge from the spinal cord. Depending on the area of anesthesia desired, the injection is made through the second, third, or fourth interspace of the lumbar vertebrae.

11 After a patient has received this type of anesthetic, he should be kept flat in bed for 6 to 12 hours. He may have a pillow under his head. Severe headaches have been known to follow spinal anesthesia if the patient has his/her head greatly elevated.

12 Following a spinal anesthetic, the nurse must watch for signs of respiratory or circulatory depression. The patient should not be placed in shock position for 1 hour following surgery unless ordered by the anesthesiologist.

13 The fifth type of anesthesia is a form of spinal anesthesia called *caudal block* or *epidural*. Also known as conduction anesthesia, it is injected in the caudal canal or the epidural space lying below the cord and affects the nerve trunks that supply the body from the umbilicus to the toes. These patients should be treated as if they had a general anesthetic rather than a spinal anesthetic. Their blood pressure should be monitored carefully.

20.0 CNS STIMULANTS
20.1 Use of CNS stimulants

1 Many natural and synthetic substances can excite CNS cells into increased activity. Such drug-induced central stimulation is manifested in many ways. Excitation of some brain cells results in only an increased alertness, whereas stronger stimulation may trigger massive convulsive spasms followed by a period of postconvulsive depression.

2 The various kinds of central stimulants are divided mainly on the basis of the several types of clinically significant activity that they tend to promote most prominently and include:

   a Those that stimulate psychomotor activity. Various kinds of cerebral cortical functions.

   b Those that cause convulsive activity. The convulsants.

   c Those that act mainly as respiratory stimulants. The so-called analeptics.

3 The naturally occuring stimulants are:

   a Caffeine (coffee, cocoa, cola nut)

   b Nicotine (tobacco)

   c Theobromine (cocoa, chocolate)

   d Theophylline (tea)

   e Cocaine (coca plant)

4 The synthetic stimulants were first discovered in the 1920s when a man-made substitute for the naturally occurring sympathomimetic, ephedrine, was being investigated in the United States. Examples:

   a Amphetamine (Benzedrine)

   b Methamphetamine (Methedrine)

   c Dextroamphetamine (Dexedrine)

5 The synthetic stimulants, like heroin, are among the most abused of our useful pharmaceutical products.

6 It is now recognized that there are only two valid uses for the amphetamine family: the treatment of narcolepsy, a very rare condition, and the treatment of hyperkinesis in children. Their appropriate use in weight reduction is negligible and ineffective beyond short-term usage.

7 The respiratory stimulants act mainly as brainstem stimulants in two ways:

a Small doses stimulate the vital centers located in the medulla oblongata. They tend to increase the sensitivity of the respiratory center neurons to the carbon dioxide that has built up to abnormal blood levels during the patient's period of depression.

b Somewhat larger doses stimulate the reticular activating system in a manner that may alter EEG activation and result in clinical arousal from states of drug-induced depression.

8 When this class of drug is administered in doses needed to produce arousal, the stimulating actions of these drugs spread to other parts of the nervous system. Such generalized central stimulation can cause various adverse reactions such as:

a Respiratory difficulties such as cough, hiccup, laryngospasm, bronchospasm, and dyspnea.

b Cardiovascular complications such as irregular heart rhythms and the elevation of blood pressure.

c Motor system stimulation marked by muscular twitching and even massive convulsive spasms.

9 Some respiratory stimulant drugs include:

a Doxapram (Dopram)

b Ethamivan (Emivan)

c Nikethamide (Coramine)

10 Other respiratory stimulants and their actions are presented in Table 15-2 below.

21.0 ANTIBIOTIC MEDICATIONS

21.1 Antibiotics

1 Antibiotic. Chemical substances produced by microorganisms (or chemically related to microbial products) that inhibit growth of or destroy other microorganisms. NOTE: There are also anti-infective agents produced by chemical synthesis. Anti-infective agents are sometimes confused with antibiotics. Anti-infective agents are also called antibacterial and can be bacteriostatic or bactericidal.

2 Terminology denoting the spectrum of antibiotic activity follows.

a Narrow-spectrum. Denotes that the drug is effective against only a few species of microbes (e.g., the majority of the penicillins are effective against only gram-positive bacteria).

b Intermediate-spectrum. Denotes, as the name implies, that the drug is effective against a number of species of microbes, greater than narrow, but less than broad-spectrum.

c Broad-spectrum. Denotes that the drug is effect against a large number of microbes (e.g., the tetracyclines are effective against gram-positive and gram-negative bacteria, rickettsiae, some large viruses, etc.).

d Superinfection. An overgrowth of nonsusceptible organisms, including fungi, usually caused by antibiotics.

3 The general adverse reaction to antibiotics include:

a Hypersensitivity
• Anaphylaxis, which may include laryngospasm and shock.
• Serum sickness—arthritic-type pains, fever, skin rash with severe itching, and respiratory embarrassment.

b Gastrointestinal reactions
• Nausea, vomiting, diarrhea
• Glossitis, stomatitis

c Skin
• Skin rash
• Photosensitivity (especially with tetracyclines)

d Hematopoietic
• Thrombocytopenia (platelet deficiency)
• Agranulocytosis

4 Topical application and inhalation of antibiotics produce more sensitization than the other routes of administration; therefore these two routes of administration are not often used today.

5 The type of infecting organism determines the type of antibiotic to be used. Ideally, all antibiotics prescribed would be selected from results of a culture and sensitivity study.

6 Antibiotics have been used in situations other than the treatment of infections. Tetracycline has been used in the diagnosis of malignancies. Some antibiotics are used in the treatment of neoplastic diseases (squamous cell carcinoma of the lung—bleomycin).

21.2 Specific antibiotics

1 Penicillin. The first antibiotic, and the antibiotic of choice against those infective organisms that are susceptible to it.

TABLE 15-2 Respiratory stimulants

Drug	Action	Used for/to
Doxapram	Analeptic stimulates by direct medullary action	Drug overdose, poisoning respiratory failure
Salicylates	Stimulates medullary respiratory center	Increase ventilatory rate and death
Narcan	Narcotic antagonist	Reverse respiratory depression caused by morphine
Naltrexone	Narcotic antagonist competitive binding at opioid receptor site	Reverse respiratory depression caused by IV opioids and analgesics
Progestins	Crosses blood-brain barrier; specific action site unknown	Stimulation of respiration
Dextroamphetamine	Direct respiratory center	Stimulation of respiratory rate and tidal volume

a Advantages of penicillin are:
- Practically non-toxic
- Many years of clinical experience
- Bactericidal

b Disadvantages of penicillin are:
- Narrow-spectrum
- High incidence of allergic reactions
- Destroyed by the enzyme, penicillinase
- Susceptible to destruction by acid

2 Cephalosporins

a These antibiotics, although closely related chemically to penicillin, are obtained from different sources.

b Cephalosporins are bactericidal, and, with few exceptions, they are broad-spectrum antibiotics.

c The classification of cephalosporins into their three generations is presented in Unit 2.0.

d Expanded-spectrum penicillins are:
- Ampicillin
- Amoxicillin
- Carbenicillin
- Mezlocillin
- Piperacillin
- Ticarcillin

e Semisynthetic penicillins used for infections caused by staphylococci that are resistant to penicillin are:
- Dicloxacillin
- Methicillin
- Nafcillin
- Oxacillin

3 Tetracyclines

a These are bacteriostatic, broad-spectrum antibiotics.

b Adverse effects are:
- Photosensitivity
- Tooth enamel dysplasia and inhibition of growth or deformities of bones in children
- Depressed plasma prothrombin activity

c Tetracyclines must *not* be taken with antacids containing aluminum, calcium, or magnesium. Also, some foods and dairy products may interfere with absorption of the antibiotic.

4 Chloramphenicol. This antibiotic is bacteriostatic and perhaps has the broadest spectrum of activity. It is not widely used because of the possible risk of causing fatal blood dyscrasias, one of which is aplastic anemia.

5 Erythromycin. This is very similar in spectrum to penicillin and can be used for patients who are allergic to penicillin. It is bacteriostatic. It has recently had an increase in use for infections caused by *Legionella pneumophila*.

6 Streptomycin

a Unlike penicillin, this drug is not destroyed by bacteria or other enzymes.

b Streptomycin is bacteriostatic for susceptible organisms in low concentrations and is bactericidal at higher levels.

c Streptomycin is effective against gram-positive organisms, but is most widely used against gram-negative bacteria.

d A weakness of streptomycin is that bacteria rapidly develop resistance to it.

e Adverse reactions to streptomycin include hypersensitivity with associated allergic reactions and toxicity manifested by vertigo and loss of balance.

7 Neomycin sulfate

a Neomycin is an antibiotic that is not destroyed by bacteria or their enzymes and that is stable and active in alkaline solutions.

b Neomycin exhibits activity against gram-positive and gram-negative organisms.

c Because of its potential toxicity, it is rarely used today.

8 Vancomycin

a Vancomycin is a bactericidal antibiotic active only against gram-positive cocci.

b Its major clinical use is in the treatment of severe infections caused by methicillin-resistant staphylococci.

9 Kanamycin. This is a bactericidal antibiotic effective against some gram-positive and gram-negative organisms.

10 Gentamicin. This bactericidal antibiotic is effective against gram-negative organisms. Gentamicin is an aminoglycoside antibiotic. Other recently released aminoglycoside antibiotics include tobramycin and amikacin.

22.0 STEROID MEDICATIONS
22.1 Drugs that affect metabolism (steroids)

1 The adrenal glands consist of two intermingling glands, the *adrenal cortex* and the *adrenal medulla*. The *adrenocorticosteroids* are hormones secreted by the *cortex* that function in metabolism regulation and water and electrolyte balance. NOTE: the *adrenal medulla* secretes the naturally occurring sympathomimetics, epinephrine and norepinephrine.

a One class of the adrenocorticosteroids is the *glucocorticoids*. Glucorticoids stimulate gluconeogenesis as discussed in the sections that follow.

b Natural glucocorticoids, cortisol and hydrocortisone, affect metabolism directly as the body's metabolic demands, or "stress" levels, rise.

c Conditions that result in changing levels of glucocorticord levels are:
- Hyperadrenalism (Cushing's syndrome)—an excess level.
- Hypoadrenalism (Addison's disease)—a deficient level.

d Systemic effects produced by glucocorticoids include:
- Gluconeogenesis. The production of glucose from amino acids derived from the breakdown of proteins. This breakdown in protein results in protein loss, which causes muscle wasting and weakness.
- Osteoporosis. A reabsorption of calcium from the bone that results in "softening of the bones." This can result in the bones becoming brittle with an increased risk of fracture.

- Increased production and deposition of fat. This can result in "moon face" or "buffalo hump," as the excess fat is deposited in the tissues of the head and trunk. These are symptoms of Cushing's syndrome.
- Impairment of the immunologic response. Inactivation of circulating antibodies, by preventing the antigen-antibody response. However, they also lower one's resistance to infection. The glucocorticoids may be useful for patients receiving organ transplants or in treating severe allergies.
- Decreased inflammation. Decrease in the local vascular congestion and cellular infiltration that is a natural response to injury or infection. In addition, they inhibit deposition of fibrous tissue. Because of these effects, these agents are used to control the adverse effects of inflammation. However, they also facilitate the spread of infection by interfering with the process of "localization." This can be serious for the patient with quiescent tuberculosis.
- Increased gastric acidity. Increased production of gastric acid that can worsen an existing ulcer or result in the formation of a previously nonexisting ulcer.
- Increased blood pressure. Used in shock when sympathomimetics are not effective.

2 Adrenocorticotropic hormone (ACTH). This is the hormone secreted by the anterior pituitary gland that stimulates the adrenal cortex to release glucocorticoids. It is used therapeutically under several circumstances.

a A risk involved in prolonged glucocorticoid therapy is atrophy of the adrenal cortex. This is the result of a feedback mechanism that may inhibit further release of natural glucocorticoids.

b The usual route of administration is oral or sometimes parenteral. Dexamethasone (Decadron) is sometimes used by the inhalation route. It must be remembered that when used by inhalation, this agent can produce the systemic effects discussed previously. The value of the drug by this route is disputed. There is definite danger in a patient's self-medication with such a drug because of intentional or accidental overdosage.

c The glucocorticoids are used in treating respiratory diseases because of their antiinflammatory effect and their antifibrinogenic effect.

3 Prostaglandins. The prostaglandins are a group of pharmacologically active lipids that are widely distributed in mammalian tissues and body fluids. The modern prostaglandin era began in the mid 1950s with the isolation of prostaglandin E (PGE) and $PGF_{2\alpha}$ by 1962.

a At the same time the modern era of prostaglandins was developing, the biologic role of cyclic 3,5 adenosine monophosphate (AMP) was being established.

b Cyclic AMP has been described as a "second messenger" in many biologic systems. It so happens that prostaglandins often affect the enzyme, adenyl cy-

clase, and so may also modify cyclic AMP-mediated systems.

c It is currently thought that the prostaglandins are not stored, but are rapidly synthesized in response to various stimuli including electrical nerve stimulation, treatment with chemical histamine releases, tissue injury by ischemia, trauma, burn, and osmotic shock.

d The lung parenchyma is a rich source of prostaglandins making available comparatively large amounts of $PGF_{2\alpha}$ and lesser amounts of PGE_2; conversely, PGE_2 predominates over $PGF_{2\alpha}$ in the bronchi. PGE_1 has been shown to have bronchodilating effects. PGE_2 and PGE_2 aerosol reverse bronchoconstriction caused by histamine, acetylcholine, serotonin, bradykinin or anaphylaxis. $PGF_{2\alpha}$ is a potent bronchoconstrictor of human bronchial muscle. PGE_1 decreased pulmonary artery pressure and increases cardiac output and heart rate when given intravenously.

e In studies performed, there was an associated small decrease in arterial oxygen saturation, implying that there is also arterial venous shunting resulting in abnormal ventilation-perfusion relationships when PGE_1 was given.

f Studies on the action of prostaglandins on bronchial smooth muscle have demonstrated that $PGF_{2\alpha}$ inhibits catecholamine and theophylline-induced relaxations of that tissue in several species, including man. PGE_1 is a bronchodilator and has been shown to be five times more potent than isoproterenol and may be of therapeutic value in bronchial asthma.

g A comparison of the effect of isoproterenol and PGE_1 on the heart rate shows that isoproterenol by aerosol elicits a 7% increase in heart rate, whereas PGE_1 elicited only a 2% increase in heart rate when administered by aerosol. In this regard, prostaglandins of the E series have potential therapeutic value in bronchial asthma because of their metabolism in the lung when administered by aerosol.

23.0 ANTIHISTAMINES
23.1 Histamine reaction and treatment

1 Drugs that compete with histamine for cellular binding sites, and therefore block histamine from attaching to its effector sites, are antihistamines.

2 Mast cells of the blood and tissues contain large amounts of histamine, which they apparently synthesize and release only when they are disintegrated or participate in allergic reactions. This cellular damage is usually the result of the antigen-antibody reaction, which causes mast cells to release histamine and other agents. The foreign invader (antigen) sensitizes the cells, which in turn produce an antibody to that antigen. This reaction is also discussed in Module Eight.

3 Another agent, called slow-reacting substance of anaphylaxis (SRS-A) or leukotrienes, has potent bronchoconstricting activity on human bronchi and may be released from mast cells with histamine. SRS-A activity

has been recently shown to be secondary to leukotrienes. Antihistamines do *not* block the action of SRS-A.

4 Histamine may also be released by the use of morphine, d-tubocurarine (curare), MAO inhibitors, and other organic bases.

5 The release of histamine has the following effects.
   a Contraction of the smooth muscle of the bronchioles, vascular system, intestines, uterus, etc.
   b Dilation and increased permeability of the capillaries and swelling of the skin and mucous membranes.
   c Stimulation of the lacrimal, nasal, pulmonary, and digestive secretions.
   d Action on the nerve endings of the skin, producing pain and itching.

6 Histamine is rapidly inactivated in the body by enzymes such as *histaminase,* which is found in most body tissues, but in largest amounts in the kidney and intestines.

7 When tissues are depleted by histamine, it is rapidly replenished by *histidine,* an essential amino acid. Cortisone prevents the replenishment of histamine.

8 Reactions of antihistamines are:
   a Anticholinergic activity that promotes the drying of secretions and causes mucous plug formation. Dryness of the mucous membranes in the mouth and nasal passages may also occur.
   b CNS depression resulting in sedation and drowsiness may or may not disappear within a few days.
   c Excitation of the CNS rarely occurs in adults but may be seen in children at ordinary dosages. This may be manifested by insomnia and agitation, and at toxic levels, convulsions may precede coma.
   d Use in patients with narrow-angle glaucoma is discouraged since antihistamines may increase intraocular pressures.
   e Paradoxic bronchospasms may occur.

9 Examples of antihistamine drugs effective in the symptomatic treatment of seasonal allergic rhinitis, vasomotor rhinitis, and anaphylactic reactions (adjunctive to epinephrine and cortisol) are:
   a Chlorpheniramine (Chlor-Trimeton)
   b Diphenhydramine (Benadryl)
   c Promethazine (Phenergan)
   d Pyrilamine maleate (used in many brands)
   e Tripelennamine (Pyribenzamine)
   f Brompheniramine (Dimotane)

24.0 AUTONOMIC NERVOUS SYSTEM
24.1 Action of the autonomic nervous system

1 The sympathetic division of the autonomic nervous system is the branch that leaves the CNS through a thoracolumbar outflow, i.e., from the *thoracic* and *lumbar* segments of the spinal cord.

2 The sympathetic branch is concerned with the "fight, fright, and flight" response, that is:
   a Mobilization of the body's energy stores.
   b Increased blood flow through certain body structures (for example, the heart) at the expense of other body structures (the abdominal organs).
   c Exhibition of signs of alarm and excitement.

3 The parasympathetic division of the autonomic nervous system is the branch that leaves the CNS through a craniosacral outflow, i.e., from the lower *brainstem* and the *sacral* area of the spine.

4 The parasympathetic branch is concerned with:
   a Conservation of energy
   b Elimination of body wastes
   c Restoration of body resources
   d Protection (e.g., pupil constriction)

5 The autonomic (occasionally referred to as involuntary, vegetative, or visceral) nervous system is concerned with the maintenance of constancy of the internal environment or homeostasis of the organism.

6 The body structures innervated by the autonomic postganglionic fibers are: smooth muscle, cardiac muscle, and glands.

7 There are two main motor divisions to the autonomic nervous system: the sympathetic (adrenergic-thoracolumbar) and the parasympathetic (cholinergic-craniosacral) divisions.

8 Most organs or systems (effectors) receive innervation from both these divisions. Generally, but not always, the two divisions are qualitatively opposed in their action on a given effector.
   a Afferent (sensory) fibers. Afferent fibers carry impulses from the sensory organs to the spinal cord and ultimately to the brain.
   b Efferent (effector) fibers. Efferent fibers carry impulses (that originate by the afferent impulse reaching the cerebrum) from the spinal cord to the effector organs, muscles, or glands.

9 Nearly all organs supplied with autonomic nerves receive innervation from two sources, one from the *sympathetic (adrenergic)* and one from the *parasympathetic (cholinergic)*.

10 This double nerve supply is frequently mutually antagonistic; for example, the parasympathetic vagi inhibit the heart, the cervical sympathetics accelerate it.

11 In most instances, the relationship between the nerves from this double supply should be looked on as complementary rather than antagonistic. For example, the filling of the urinary bladder is made possible by the sympathetic; the emptying is controlled by the parasympathetic.

12 The parasympathetic predominates in resting conditions, for the most part, and serves to maintain a relatively constant internal environment; the sympathetic is usually activated by emergency situations and serves to protect the relative constancy of the internal environment (e.g., body temperature, blood flow).

13 While the autonomic nervous system serves to maintain the internal homeostasis of the body, the *somatic* nerves innervate the skeletal muscles that adjust the body as a whole to the external environment.

14 The somatic nerves innervating the skeletal muscles

make direct connection between these organs and the central nervous system. The somatic (voluntary) nervous system motor nerves liberate acetylcholine at the preganglions and at the myoneural junction.

15 At the ganglia, preganglionic nerves of both the autonomic and the voluntary system liberate acetylcholine (all preganglionic nerves are cholinergic), but the character of the acetylcholine ganglionic receptors is different from those in the neuroeffectors, so that the two types of receptors are not blocked by the same drugs.

16 The opposite of the two divisions of the autonomic nervous system reflects the fact that the chemical substances (mediator, transmitter, or neurohumor) liberated by the postganglionic nerve terminals are *not* the same for the two divisions.

17 The neurohumoral transmitter in the sympathetic branch is *acetylcholine* in the preganglionic fiber and *norepinephrine* in the postganglionic fiber with the exception of the sweat glands and certain blood vessels that are innervated by the sympathetic nerves, but liberate acetylcholine at the endings of the postganglionic fibers.

18 In the sympathetic system, the ganglia are most often located near the spinal cord as a member of the paravertebral "chain ganglia" (short preganglionic fibers; long postganglionic fibers).

19 This branch is characterized by convergence, i.e., many preganglionic fibers innervate one ganglion, and by divergence, i.e., many postganglionic fibers leave from one ganglion.

20 The effect of acetylcholine is of short duration as a result of the action of an enzyme, *cholinesterase,* which results in the cleavage of the ester bone of acetylcholine to yield choline, a much less active cholinergic agent. Although this enzyme is found throughout the body (cholinesterase in the circulation instantaneously destroys acetylcholine when the latter is injected intravenously), the enzyme is responsible for destruction of the transmitter in the junctional cleft—rapidly terminating the transmitter's (acetylcholine) effect.

21 In the sympathetic (adrenergic) system there are two main types of receptors:

a Alpha receptors. The *alpha adrenergic receptors* elicit smooth muscular stimulation and some intestinal relaxation, adrenergic sweating, adrenergic salivating, and lipolysis. Generally, the alpha receptor is excitatory, i.e., vasoconstriction. Norephinephrine is primarily an activator of alpha receptors, as is phenylephrine.

b Beta receptors. The *beta adrenergic receptors* elicit smooth muscle relaxation everywhere, except possibly in some veins; they also cause stimulation of the heart and glycolysis. The beta receptors may be subdivided into two divisions designated as $beta_1$ and $beta_2$ receptor sites. A few sympathomimetic drugs have a preferential affinity for $beta_1$ and a weak affinity for $beta_2$ receptor sites or vice versa.

22 Generally the $beta_2$ receptors are inhibitory in action,

causing relaxation of vascular and bronchial smooth muscle and resulting in vasodilation of pulmonary and skeletal muscle blood vessels and bronchodilation.

a $Beta_1$ adrenergic receptor sites. $Beta_1$ receptor sites are located in the cardiac muscle and in certain blood vessel muscle cells. $Beta_1$ activation results in increased rate and force of cardiac contraction and is thought to cause dilation of coronary blood vessels.

b Epinephrine has both alpha and beta receptor stimulatory activity. However, when given by aerosol, epinephrine elicits a relatively greater $beta_1$ activity than it does $beta_2$.

c $Beta_2$ adrenergic receptor sites. $Beta_2$ receptor sites are located in the bronchi and vascular bed. $Beta_2$ activation results in bronchodilation and vasodilation of pulmonary blood vessels as well as some skeletal blood vessels.

d Salbutamol for example, is the classic $beta_2$ receptor activator, showing little, if any, $beta_1$ activity. Terbutaline sulfate (Bricanyl) shows greater $beta_2$ activity—but in general exhibits epinephrine-type side effects. More detail on beta-receptor drugs will be given un Unit 28.6.

23 To understand the mechanism of action of some of the adrenergic (sympathomimetics) drugs, it is necessary to understand what causes a termination of action of norepinephrine. Norepinephrine's duration of action is considerably longer than that of acetylcholine, because the norepinephrine is not rapidly destroyed by enzymes, but is taken back into the nerve fiber from which it was released. It is this "reuptake" that results in the termination of norepinephrine's effect. Monoamine oxidase (MAO) and catechol-o-methyltransferase (COMT) are the two enzymes basically responsible for termination of norepinephrine activity. MAO is located within the adrenergic neuron that oxidatively deaminates norepinephrine to the inactive dihydroxymandelic acid.

24 Elsewhere in the body, especially in the liver and kidney, MAO similarly oxidizes circulating norepinephrine. COMT, at the neuroeffector junction (and elsewhere, especially the liver and kidneys), methylates norepinephrine, giving rise to the metabolite normetanephrine.

25 In the effector cell, COMT and mitochondrial MAO terminate norepinephrine activity.

26 NOTE: Some drugs list a precaution against the concurrent use with MAO inhibitors. The MAO inhibitors are a class of drugs primarily used as antidepressants and CNS stimulants that act by bringing about an increase in levels of serotonin, norepinephrine, and epinephrine. Their primary danger in use with other CNS drugs is that they inhibit the detoxification of such agents as amphetamines and barbiturates. Examples are: (see Module Five, Unit 3.3)

a Iproniazid (Marsilid)

b Isocarboxazid (Marplan)

c Phenelzine (Nardil)

24.2 Classification of drugs affecting the autonomic system

1 *Parasympathomimetics* (cholinomimetics, cholinergics)

  a Direct-acting. These elicit their effects by combining directly with the receptors of effector tissue (methacholine chloride, edrophonium chloride, etc.).

  b Indirect-acting. These elicit their effects by displacing neuronal acetylcholine, which subsequently attaches to receptors and produces the pharmacologic response.

  c Parasympathetic enzyme inhibitors. These inhibit the action of cholinesterase (neostigmine methylsulfate, pyridostigmine bromide).

2 *Parasympatholytics* (cholinergic blocking agents, anticholinergics)

  a Ganglionic blockers. These block the effect of acetylcholine at the ganglia (trimethaphan camsylate).

  b Effector blockers. These block the effect of acetylcholine at the effector organ (atropine).

3 *Sympathomimetics* (adrenomimetics, adrenergics)

  a Direct-acting. These elicit their effects by combining directly with the receptors of effector tissue (norepinephrine bitartrate).

  b Indirect-acting. These elicit their effects by displacing neuronal norepinephrine, which subsequently attaches to receptors and produces the pharmacologic response (amphetamines).

  c Sympathetic enzyme inhibitors. These inhibit the action of MAO and COMT.

4 *Sympatholytics* (adrenolytics, alpha and beta adrenergic blocking agents)

  a Alpha blockers. These block the alpha response to norepinephrine (phentolamine, phenoxybenzamine HCl).

  b Beta blockers. These block the beta response to norepinephrine (propranolol).

25.0 CARDIAC RELATED DRUGS (see also Module Twenty-one)

25.1 Types of cardiac related drugs

1 *Digitalis* and related drugs act on the heart and circulation.

  a Digitalis has several actions on the heart, but most important of these is its ability to *increase* the strength of the heartbeat. This ability to make the myocardium contract more forcefully is demonstrated most clearly in patients with congestive heart failure.

  b Other drugs such as the *sympathomimetics* also strengthen the heartbeat, yet these adrenergic drugs are *contraindicated* for most cardiac patients because they force the heart to work too hard, causing it to pound, race, and demand more oxygenated blood than the coronary vessels can deliver.

  c Digitalis, on the other hand, *slows* the heartbeat as it strengthens it. The heart muscle fibers contract more fully and more efficiently so that each systolic contraction drives a greater amount of blood out of the heart, without consuming more oxygen.

  d The strengthening action of digitalis on the contractions of the weakened, hypodynamic heart usually produces prompt and dramatic relief from symptoms of congestive heart failure. The improved circulatory competence is apparent, in part, by desirable changes in the rate, rhythm, and size of the heart itself.

  e Benefits of better circulatory function are also observed in the kidneys, lungs, and other organs.

2 *Antiarrhythmic drugs*

  a *Automaticity, rhythmicity, conductivity,* and *contractility* are intrinsic physiologic properties of cardiac tissue.

  b Cardiac arrhythmias constitute one of the most serious and alarming conditions encountered in medical practice.

  c A number of therapeutic measures are available for control of cardiac arthythmias. Treatment selection is based on the urgency of the situation, the etiologic or potentiating factors, and the nature of the specific arrhythmia.

  d Initial effects should always be directed toward correcting such factors as hypotension, shock, pulmonary edema, etc. Pressor drugs such as metaraminol are particularly useful for this purpose.

  e *Isoproterenol* (Isuprel), a beta drug, is effective in terminating ventricular tachycardia in the presence of advanced atrioventricular block. In primary heart block, isoproterenol is also an effective agent for stimulating the activity of the higher pacemaker centers.

  f *Procainamide* (Pronestyl) depresses the irritability of the ventricular muscle. It is less toxic and produces less central nervous system stimulation than other drugs. It is used in the treatment of ventricular and atrial arrhythmias and in decreasing the incidence of extrasystoles.

  g *Lidocaine* is effective in the treatment of ventricular arrhythmias, particularly those associated with acute myocardial infarction. By reducing the irritability of the myocardium, it terminates ventricular tachycardia and suppresses multiple ventricular extrasystoles.

  h *Phenytoin* (Diphenylhydantoin, Dilantin) is effective in suppressing frequent premature contractions and paroxysmal ventricular and supraventricular tachycardia. It may also reduce the ventricular rate in patients with atrial flutter or fibrillation but rarely does conversion occur.

  i These drugs are often classified by groups*:

    • Group I: procainamide, quinidine, and disopyramide

    • Group II: phenytoin and lidocaine

    • Group III: propranolol

    • Group IV: bretylium

---

*Campbell JW and Frisse M, editors: Manual of medical therapeutics, ed 24, Boston, Little, Brown & Co Inc.

• Group V: verapamil

j Drugs in Group III are the beta blocker drugs: Group IV contains bretylium, which is currently used more frequently for dysrhythmia, and group V contains the calcium channel blocker drugs.

3 *Coronary vasodilator drugs*

a Drugs that dilate the coronary arterioles are not usually very effective for relieving the pain of an acute coronary occlusion; however, they are often quite useful for helping to overcome *anginal* attacks. These drugs are thought to act mainly by relaxing spasms of the coronary arterioles. The resulting dilation of these vessels is believed to bring a better flow of blood to the hypoxic myocardial tissues.

b Some of these drugs include nitrates and nitrites that:
• Relax smooth muscle fibers
• Decrease blood pressure
• Increase local blood flow

c Examples of these drugs include:
• Amyl nitrite
• Nitroglycerin
• Pentaerythritol tetranitrate (Peritrate)
• Isosorbide dinitrate (Isordil)
• Papaverine
• Dioxyline phosphate (Paveril)

4 *Antihypertensive drugs*

a Antihypertensives are drugs used to control high blood pressure.

b The drugs used for hypertension act either on the nervous system or directly on the heart and blood vessels to lower blood pressure. The various kinds of antihypertensive drugs include:
• The rauwolfia alkaloids (reserpine [Serpasil])
• The sulfonamide diuretics (chlorothiazide [Diuril])
• The ganglionic blocking agents (guanethidine sulfate [Ismelin])
• Antiadrenergic agents such as methyldopa (Aldomet) and clonidine (Catapress)
• Alpha-adrenergic blocking agents such as phenoxybenzamine (Dibenzyline), phentolamine (Regitine), and prazosine (Minipress)
• Beta-adrenergic blocking agents, such as propranolol (Inderal), nadolol (Corgard), metoprolol (Lopressor), atenolol (Tenormin), timolol (Blocadren), and pindolol (Visken)
• Nonadrenergic vasodilating agents such as hydralazine (Apresoline) and minoxidil (Loniten)
• Angiotensin II—blocking agents such as captopril (Capoten)

5 *Antihypotensive drugs*

a The infarcted heart may pump less blood than normal into the aorta. Since adequate coronary circulation depends on perfusion from the aorta, this drop in cardiac output may interfere still further with cardiac action, thus setting off a vicious cycle that may cause cardiogenic shock.

b The drugs most commonly employed for raising blood pressure and increasing cardiac efficiency are

levarterenol bitartrate (Levophed), metaraminol bitartrate (Aramine), dopamine HCl (Intropin), and mephentermine sulfate (Wyamine). These adrenergic drugs are said to precipitate fewer arrhythmias than other agents of this class.

26.0 DIURETIC DRUGS
26.1 Action of diuretic drugs

1 Diuretics are defined as drugs that cause an *increased* output of urine. Most diuretics also do more than this. By aiding the renal excretion of electrolytes or dissolved salts, these agents can also alter the chemical composition of blood and body fluids.

2 This property of diuretics allows them to be used clinically for counteracting edema.

3 When the kidneys are capable of functioning, diuretic drugs can act to influence the processes of glomerular filtration, tubular reabsorption, and tubular secretion to produce a copious flow of urine.

4 The most effective diuretic drugs are those that alter tubular reabsorption, such as the organic mercurials and sulfonamides.

5 It is thought that the sulfonamides inhibit the enzymes that produce the energy needed to reabsorb filtered ions from the tubular fluids. The tubular epithelial cells then fail to pull back some of the sodium (for example) in the glomerular filtrate, and these ions pass on to the collecting tubules, carrying with them the water that would otherwise have been reabsorbed into the blood and would have leaked into the tissue spaces.

6 Tubular secretion can also be altered by drugs with a resultant removal of excess sodium and water. For example, drug-induced inhibition of the enzyme, carbonic anhydrase, results in decreased production and secretion of hydrogen ions by the renal tubular epithelial cells.

7 When fewer hydrogen ions are available to be exchanged for sodium ions, the water-trapping sodium winds up in the urine instead of moving back into the blood and the fluids in the extravascular tissue spaces.

8 The simultaneous loss of bicarbonate ions and retention of chloride causes a relative loss of fluid from the tissues.

9 Glomerular filtration may be increased by drugs that bring an increased amount of blood to the capillary filter beds. Sodium and chloride ions, when they are delivered to the tubules in amounts exceeding the reabsorption capacity of the lining cells, are passed on into the collecting tubules, carrying water along with them in a copious urine flow.

10 Drugs of the *xanthine* class are thought to act, in part, by increasing the amount of blood filtered by the glomeruli. This may be the result of their heart-stimulating action and the consequent circulatory improvement, or it may be a result of direct dilation of renal arterioles.

11 The *diuretics* are divided into the following classes:

a The organic mercurials
• Merethoxylline (Dicurin)

- Mercaptomerin (Thiomerin)
  b The sulfonamides/thiazides
  - Chlorothiazide (Diuril)
  - Furosemide (Lasix)
  - Hydrochlorothiazide (Hydrodiuril)
  c Carbonic anhydrase inhibitors
  - Acetazolamide (Diamox)
  d Xanthines and cytosines
  - Dyphylline (Neothylline)
  - Oxtriphylline (Choledyl)
  - Theobromine
  - Theophylline
  e Miscellaneous
  - Mannitol (Osmitrol)
  - Calcium chloride
  - Ammonium chloride
  - Spironolactone (Aldactone)
  - Ethacrynic acid (Edecrin)

27.0 XANTHINES

27.1 Action and use of xanthines

1 The xanthines are *alkaloids* found in coffee (caffeine), tea (theophylline), and cocoa (caffeine and theobromine).

2 Caffeine, theophylline, and theobromine are *methylated xanthines* and are also referred to as the *methylxanthines*.

3 They stimulate the CNS, act on the kidney to produce diuresis, stimulate cardiac muscle, and relax smooth muscle, especially bronchial muscle. The relative strength of each xanthine is shown in Table 15-3 (1 is most active, 3 is least active).

4 In addition, the xanthines inhibit *phosphodiesterase.* This phosphodiesterase inhibition is credited with increasing the body's store of cyclic adenosine 3', 5', monophosphate (3', 5', cAMP) which, in turn, produces bronchial dilation.

5 Cellular action of xanthines. Methylxanthines, particularly theophylline, are competitive inhibitors of the cyclic nucleotide phosphodiesterase, an enzyme that catalyzes the conversion of 3', 5', cAMP to the inactive 5' adenosine monophosphate.

6 3', 5', cAMP concentrations are thus elevated in some tissues following exposure to methylxanthines.

7 The elevated tissue levels of 3', 5', cAMP result in an inhibition of muscular contraction, although the mechanism of this action has *not* yet been clearly established. (The elevated 3', 5', cAMP caused by epinephrine's action on the enzyme adenyl cyclase is used to explain epinephrine's mode of action; therefore any substance that causes an elevation of 3', 5', cAMP may produce a synergistic effect when used together.) For this reason, theophylline, in combination with ethylenediamine, may be given together with epinephrine or beta$_2$ bronchial dilators.

8 *Aminophylline* is a combination of 85% theophylline and 15% ethylenediamine. Ethylenediamine is thought to be inert therapeutically, but a pharmaceutical neces-

TABLE 15-3 A comparison of the strength of methylxanthines

	Caffeine	Theophylline	Theobromine
CNS and respiratory stimulation	1	2	3
Heart stimulation	3	1	2
Coronary stimulation	3	1	2
Smooth muscle relaxation	3	1	3
Skeletal muscle stimulation	1	2	3
Diuresis	3	1	2

sity used to facilitate the solution of the poorly soluble theophylline.

a Aminophylline's pharmaceutical actions are:
- Increased depth and rate of ventilation
- Increased cardiac output
- Increased renal blood flow
- Bronchial dilation

b Aminophylline causes bronchial smooth muscle to relax. For this reason, it is of considerable therapeutic value in the treatment of bronchial asthma.

c Preparations of aminophylline come in 2 ml (500 mg) IM ampules; 10 ml (250 mg) and 20 ml (500 mg) aqueous solution for IV injection; as tablets; and as suppositories.

d It is *not* given as an aerosol.

9 *Oxtriphylline* (Choledyl) is a salt of theophylline formed by choline cations replacing hydrogen atoms in theophylline.

a It is more stable, better absorbed from the gastrointestinal tract, and less irritating to the gastric mucosa than aminophylline.

b Oxtriphylline's actions include increases in cardiac output and vital capacity.

c It is available in 100 mg and 200 mg tablets and as a 100 mg/5 ml elixir.

d It is *not* given as an aerosol.

10 *Dyphylline* (Lufyllin) is a natural derivative of theophylline, stable in gastric juices.

a It produces less gastric irritation than most theophylline compounds.

b Its actions include those of other theophylline compounds.

c Dyphylline is available in 200 mg tablets and 250 mg/1 ml, 2 ml ampules for injection.

d It is *not* given as an aerosol.

11 *Caffeine and sodium benzoate.* Caffeine, being poorly absorbed, is mixed with the therapeutically inert sodium benzoate in equal measures.

a Its actions include:
- Stimulation to ventilation
- An antidote in dangerous cases of alcohol poisoning
- Powerful CNS stimulation

b Caffeine is indicated in the following:
- Some forms of migraine and headache
- CNS stimulation following nervous exhaustion
- A diagnostic test for gastric hydrochloric acid secretions

c It is available as 500 mg/2 ml ampules for injection.

d It is *not* given as an aerosol.

28.0 RESPIRATORY CARE PHARMACOLOGY
28.1 Classification

1 Respiratory care medications are classified as follows.

a Antibiotics. Agents used as an adjunct to systemic, antimicrobial therapy.

b Antifoamant. An agent (alcohol) used to modify surface tensions of pulmonary fluids.

c Antihistamines. Agents that reduce allergic reactions and therefore reduce effects such as sinus and nasal drainage, mucosal irritation, sneezing, and cough. Many antihistamines also have a mild sedative effect.

d Antitussives. Agents that act on the central nervous system or peripherally in the body to reduce the cough reflex and/or the need to cough.

e Bronchodilators. Agents used to increase the lumen of the airway by relaxing spasms of the smooth bronchial muscle fibers.

f Detergents/wetting agents. Used to reduce surface tension and viscosity of tenacious sputum, thereby facilitating mucokinesis.

g Enzymes. Agents used to depolymerize DNA and used where there is an accumulation of purulent sputum.

h Expectorants. Agents that act systemically to modify the production and viscosity of pulmonary fluids.

i Mucolytics. Agents effective in breaking up mucoproteins responsible for the viscosity of sputum.

j Steroids. Agents used for their potent antiinflammatory and antifibrotic effects in acute and chronic obstructive diseases and resistant allergies of the respiratory tract.

k Vasoconstrictors/decongestants. Agents that relieve congestion by causing a contraction of the muscle fibers of the arterioles and small arteries, thereby reducing blood flow to the affected area and lowering the hydrostatic pressure that permits fluid to move into the tissues.

l Miscellaneous. Agents that do not fit the above categories.

2 Most of these drugs can be administered topically to the tracheobronchial tree by aerosol. Those drugs that are not given by aerosol are usually given in conjunction with the aerosolized medications.

3 The clinician should memorize the particulars on each of the following drugs since they form the basis of pulmonary disease treatment.

4 The specific drugs in the following units will be listed with their action, use, average dosage (subject to the ordering physician), cautions, side effects, and storage particulars, where relevant.

a Each will be listed according to its use, e.g., an expectorant, bronchodilator, etc.

b Some of the drugs listed have already been covered in some detail in other units in this module.

28.2 Antibiotics/anti-infectives

NOTE: Delivering antibiotic agents topically by aerosolization is a point of controversy in some parts of the country. Dosages have not been clearly established. The dosages recommended in this unit are average adult doses and are sometimes given by diluting in 3 to 5 ml of normal saline and nebulized 2 to 4 times daily. Refer to the *Physicians' Desk Reference* for further details.

1 Amphotericin B (Fungizone). Although not an antibacterial, amphotericin B is frequently used in respiratory therapy in similar circumstances. It is used in cases of *fungal* infection, particularly against *Aspergillus* mycetoma and *Coccidioides immitis*.

a Since Amphotericin B is poorly absorbed after oral ingestion, it is generally given parenterally. The most common route of administration is intravenous injection. Amphotericin is not nebulized, but may be instilled directly into the trachea, usually via an endotracheal or tracheal tube and sometimes through an indwelling transtracheal catheter.

b Average maintenance dosage is 0.4-0.7 mg/kg/day.

2 Carbenicillin (Geopen and Pyopen). This is a penicillin derivative that has been used against gram-negative organisms in the lungs. It is particularly effective against *Pseudomonas* organisms. It can be nebulized in a dose range of 10 to 20 mg. Recent studies have shown ticarcillin, a carbenicillin derivate, to have greater anti-*Pseudomonas* activity. Both should be given with a synergistic antibiotic, such as gentamicin, to prevent the emergence of resistant strains.

3 Chloramphenicol (Chloromycetin). This is a powerful agent against gram-positive and gram-negative organism; it is recommended only for serious infections. It has been proved effective against:

a *Salmonella* species

b *Hemophilus influenzae*

c *Rickettsia*

d Lymphogranuloma—psittacosis group

e Gram-negative organisms (various), causing bacteremia and meningitis

4 Colistin (Coly-Mycin). This drug has been proved effective against *Pseudomonas aeruginosa*. It is *not* generally for nebulization.

5 Gentamicin (Garamycin). This is a broad-spectrum aminoglycoside considered very effective against *Pseudomonas aeruginosa* and *Klebsiella*.

• Dosage range is 40 to 120 mg parenterally.

6 Kanamycin (Kantrex). An aminoglycoside that has an antimicrobial range narrower than that of gentamicin.

• Microorganisms not responsive to this antibiotic include *Pseudomonas* and *Streptococcus*. It is active in vitro against the following:

– *Stephylococcus aureus*

– *Hemophilus influenzae*

– *Escherichia coli*

– *Enterobacter* species

– *Klebsiella pneumoniae*

– *Serratia marcescens*

– *Proteus* species

7 Neosporin. A combination of polymyxin B, bacitracin, and neomycin. Considered too toxic for systemic use, it has been used successfully as a topical antibiotic, especially in its ointment forms. Neosporin ointment is frequently used to apply tracheostomy dressings.

28.3 Antifoamants

1 Ethyl alcohol
   a Action. It breaks down frothy material by reducing the surface tension of the secretions and destablizing bubbles.
   b Use. Acute pulmonary edema.
   c Dosage. None set, usually 3 to 5 ml per aerosol treatment. Intermittent positive pressure breathing (IPPB) may also be used to deliver the aerosol as the positive pressure is said to aid the treatment of pulmonary edema. A 30% to 50% solution is recommended. NOTE: 100% proof vodka is 50% ethyl alcohl and is suitable for use.
   d Precautions. None significant, may be irritating to oral-nasal mucosa. Do *not* give methyl or isopropyl alcohol.
   e Side effects. Mouth dryness, mucosal irritation, alcohol intoxication.

28.4 Antihistamines

1 Antihistamines are used frequently in respiratory disorders and conditions. They are *not* to be nebulized.
2 They are used to relieve the symptoms of cold, allergy, sinusitis, and related illnesses.
3 There are four major types of antihistamines:
   a Ethylenediamines
     • Diphenylpyraline hydrochloride (Hispril)
     • Pyrilamine maleate (contained in Triaminic)
     • Tripelennamine hydrochloride (Pyribenzamine)
   b Ethanolamines
     • Carbinoxamine maleate (contained in Rondec-DM)
     • Diphenhydramine hydrochloride (Benadryl)
     • Doxylamine succinate (contained in Bendectin)
   c Propylamines
     • Brompheniramine maleate (Dimetane)
     • Chlorpheniramine maleate (Chlor-Trimeton)
     • Dexbrompheniramine maleate (Disomer)
     • Dexchlorpheniramine maleate (Polanil)
     • Dimethindene maleate (Triten)
     • Triprolidine hydrochloride (Actidil)
   d Phenothiazines
     • Methdilazine (Tacaryl)
     • Promethazine hydrochloride (Phenergan)
     • Trimeprazine (Temaril)

28.5 Antitussives

1 Antitussives, as the name implies, work against cough. They do so in two ways: *centrally,* by depressing the cough reflex in the medulla of the brain; and *peripherally,* by any of the following ways:
   a "Soothing" the tracheal and respiratory mucosa
   b Aiding in the expulsion and removal of mucus
   c Providing humidity
   d Relaxing bronchial constriction
2 Centrally acting antitussives are either narcotic or nonnarcotic. Examples are as follows:
   a Narcotic (opium derivates and synthetic)
     • Morphine
     • Codeine
     • Ethylmorphine hydrochloride (Dionin)
     • Dihydrocodeinone bitartrate (contained in Citra Forte)
     • Hydromorphone hydrochloride (Dilaudid)
   b Non-narcotics
     • Dextromethorphan hydrobromide (used in many brands)
     • Levopropoxyphene (Novrad)
     • Noscapine (contained in Conar)
3 Peripherally acting antitussives work by several methods, which include bronchodilators (Unit 28.6) and wetting agents/detergents (Unit 28.7). The following antitussives are of the demulcent and anesthetic types.
   a Demulcents
     • Acacia
     • Eucalyptus
     • Glycerin
     • Horehound
     • Licorice
     • Menthol
     • Propylene glycol
     • Wild cherry
   b Anesthetics
     • Benzocaine (used in many brands)
     • Benzonatate (Tressalon)
     • Chlophedianol hydrochloride (Ulo)
     • Dimethoxanate hydrochloride (Cothera)
     • Pipazethate (Theratuss)

28.6 Bronchodilators

Bronchodilators are of two types: *sympathomimetic agents* and xanthine derivatives. In this unit, the sympathomimetic drugs will be discussed in detail, since they are most frequently delivered by respiratory care personnel.
1 Atropine (anticholinergic bronchodilator)
   a Action
     • Reduces secretions. Atropine inhibits secretions of nose, mouth, pharynx, and bronchi, and by reducing fluid volume, increases viscosities.
     • Bronchodilation. Blocks cholinergic constricting influences on bronchial muscle; atropine potentiates beta adrenergic dilation and increases airway lumen.
   b Use
     • Relieves symptoms of the common cold.
     • Is sometimes used before surgery to reduce bronchial secretions.
     • Prevents atrial bradycardia.
   c CAUTION: The patient with thick secretions before administration of this drug faces an increased risk of developing mucous plugging and obstruction.

2 Cyclopentamine (Aerolone Compound)

a Action
- Also contains isoproterenol hydrochloride
- Bronchodilation

b Use
- Asthma
- Bronchospastic disorders

c Dosage
- Used in a similar manner as epinephrine, 1:100.
- Six to twelve inhalations, once a day, will usually bring relief. Several cases may require more frequent dosing.

d Cautions
- Used with caution in patients with hypertension, hyperthyroidism, and cardiac disease.

e Side effects
- Tachycardia, nervousness, dizziness, palpitation

3 Ephedrine (Bronkotabs)

a Action
- Vasoconstriction
- Bronchodilation

b Use
- Asthma
- Bronchospastic disorders

c Dosage
- Not given by inhalation
- Oral dose—25 to 50 mg every 3 to 4 hours

4 Epinephrine hydrochloride (Adrenaline 1:1000, 1:100 solution)

a Action
- Potent bronchodilator
- Vasoconstrictor
- Bronchial gland suppression

b Use
- Asthma
- Bronchospastic disorders

c Dosage (NOTE: May be given by inhalation or parenterally, with rapid action either way.)
- Inhalation dose—0.25 to 0.5 ml of 1:100 in 3 to 5 ml diluent.
- Patient inhales once or twice; allow 1 to 2 minutes between inhalations to prevent overdosage.
- NOTE: Rinsing the mouth after inhaling epinephrine will prevent the sensation of dryness.
- When given by subcutaneous or intramuscular injection, solution strengths of less than 1:1000 should be used to avoid necrosis resulting from vasoconstriction.

d Cautions
- Excessive use leads to increasing tolerance.
- Effects, although rapid, are generally short-term.
- Do not use if brown or discolored. Do not use with metals; it is unstable at room temperature.

e Side effects
- Hypertension, anxiety, restlessness, headache, dizziness, palpitation, weakness, tremor.
- Generally subside rapidly after epinephrine is discontinued.

5 Ethylnorepinephrine hydrochloride (Bronkephrine)

a Action
- Bronchodilation
- Beta-active (few vasopressor effects)

b Use
- Asthma
- Bronchospastic disorders

c Dosage
- It is *not* given as aerosol.
- 0.5 to 1.0 ml subcutaneous or intramuscular injection for adults.

d Cautions
- It should not be used with patients who have cardiovascular disease, history of stroke, or coronary artery disease.

e Side effects
- Blood pressure changes, palpitation, headache, dizziness, nausea

6 Isoetharine (Bronkosol)

a Action
- Bronchodilation
- Primarily a $beta_2$ stimulant with mild $beta_1$ and slight alpha effects

b Use
- Asthma
- Bronchospastic disorders

c Dosage
- 0.25 to 0.5 ml of 1:100 in 2 to 5 ml normal saline given per nebulizer.
- May be given every 4 hours as needed; do *not* give continuously.

d Cautions
- Dosage should be carefully adjusted in patients with hyperthyroidism, hypertension, acute coronary disease, limited cardiac reserve, and sensitivity to sympathomimetic amines.

e Side effects
- Tachycardia, palpitation, nausea, headache, nervousness, tingling of extremities, insomnia, dizziness

7 Isoproterenol hydrochloride (Isuprel)

a Action
- Bronchodilator
- Bronchial muscle relaxation
- $Beta_2$ stimulant

b Use
- Asthma
- Treatment of epinephrine-fast patients with asthma
- Bronchospastic disorders

c Dosage
- It can be given intravenously and sublingually.
- 0.25 to 0.5 ml of 1:200 solution diluted with 2 ml of normal saline for inhalation.
- Give every 3 to 4 hours, as needed. *Never* give continuously.

d Cautions
- It should not be given concomitantly with epinephrine.

- It is not to be given to patients with pre-existing cardiac arrhythmias.
- It may turn pink or brown when left standing.

e Side effects
- Tachycardia, anginal pain, palpitation, dizziness, tingling of extremities, shock

8 Metaproterenol sulfate (Metaprel)

a Action
- Bronchodilation

b Use
- Asthma
- Bronchospastic disorders

c Dosage
- May be given orally in tablet form.
- Uses aerosol metered-dose device—two to three inhalations are taken every 3 to 4 hours.
- Inhalation dose—0.2 to 0.3 ml of 5% solution in 3 ml normal saline.

d Cautions
- It should be given with caution to patients with hypertension, coronary artery disease, congestive heart failure, hyperthyroidism, and diabetes.

e Side effects
- Nervousness, tremor, nausea, vomiting, tachycardia, palpitation, "bad taste" in mouth

9 Methoxyphenamine hydrochloride (Orthoxine)

a Action
- Bronchodilation

b Use
- Asthma
- Bronchospastic disorders

c Dosage
- Oral dosage only
- 50 to 100 mg every 4 hours

d Cautions
- Similar precautions as with metaproterenol

e Side effects
- Similar side effects as metaproterenol

10 Pseudoephedrine (Sudafed) (See Unit 28.12)

11 Racemic epinepherine (Vaponephrine)

a Action
- Relaxes bronchial smooth muscle
- Reduces bronchial edema by vasoconstriction

b Use
- Asthma
- Bronchospastic disorders
- Croup
- Glottic edema

c Dosage
- 0.25 to 0.5 ml of 2.25% solution in 3 to 5 ml normal saline.

d Cautions
- For aerosol use only.
- Store in refrigerator once opened.
- Do not use if discolored or if precipitate forms.
- Use with caution in patients with hypertension, cardiovascular disease, etc.

e Side effects
- Nervousness, restlessness, tachycardia, hypertension

12 Salbutamol (Albuterol)

a Action
- Derivative of isoproterenol
- Preferential $beta_2$ stimulant with very little $beta_1$ activity
- Slower metabolism than other adrenergic agents, giving it prolonged action

b Use
- Asthma
- Bronchospastic disorders

c Dosage
- Oral dosage available.
- Available in a metered-dose pressurized aerosol.
- Approximate dose is 200 µg, with 2 to 4 mg received in a day's time.

d Cautions
- Negligible

e Side effects
- Negligible

13 Terbutaline sulfate (Bricanyl)

a Action
- Bronchodilation
- Derivative of isoproterenol
- Sympathomimetic amine with preferential $beta_2$ activity

b Use
- Asthma
- Bronchospastic disorders

c Dosage
- Oral dose—2.5 to 5 mg tablet three times a day.
- Inhalation dose—1.0 to 2.0 ml of 0.1% solution in 2.0 ml normal saline.
- May also be given by subcutaneous injection.

d Cautions
- Similar to those of metaproterenol

e Side effects
- Similar to those of metaproterenol.

14 Theophylline ethylenediamine (Aminophylline)

a CNS stimulation, respiratory stimulation, smooth muscle relaxation, diuresis, coronary artery stimulation, skeletal muscle stimulation (See Unit 27.1).
- Bronchodilation

b Use
- Asthma
- Diffuse bronchospasm

c Dosage
- Same as IV preparation often requiring 0.5 to 0.7 gm. Aminophylline given as aerosol may lead to erratic dosages and is considered noneffective.

d Side effects
- Headache, nausea, dizziness, hyperventilation, and hypotension, although rare.

28.7 Detergents/wetting agents

1 Distilled water U.S.P. (sterile)

a Action

- Assists in liquefaction of viscid sputum
- Adds humidity to respiratory tract
b Use
- When viscid sputum interferes with effective expectoration
- When dry gases delivered to the respiratory tract must be humidified
- To dilute/mix other medications
c Dosage
- It can be used continuously or as an intermittent therapy.
d Cautions
- It must be sterile.
- The use of aerosol mists with neonates and infants should be carefully monitored to avoid possible overhydration.
- Distilled water is hypotonic to body tissues and may produce local irritation and coughing.
e Side effects
- None significant
2 Normal saline solution (0.9% sodium chloride)
a Action
- Same as distilled water
b Use
- Same as distilled water
c Dosage
- Same as distilled water
d Cautions
- It must be sterile.Same as distilled water, with the exception that normal saline is isotonic, not hypotonic and compatible with body tissue.
e Side effects
- None significant
3 Hypotonic saline solution (0.45% sodium chloride).
a Action
- Greater distribution in distal airways making it more effective for loosening secretions in small airways.
b Use
- Used for people on salt-restricted diets.
c Dosage
- 0.45% NACL
d Cautions
- It must be sterile.
- Hypotonic particles grow smaller as they osmotically give up water to the surrounding gas molecules (see Module Twelve).
e Side effects
- None significant.
4 Hypertonic saline solution
a Action
- Water is osmotically drawn out of surrounding gas and surface mucosa thereby aiding in sputum production of a patient with a nonproductive cough.
b Use
- Sputum induction
c Dosage
- 1.8 to 10%

d Cautions
- Aerosol is irritating and may produce undesired bronchospasm as well as production of cough. In patients with large amounts of retained secretions care must be taken to assist the patient should a bronchotic effect occur (see Module Twelve).
e Side effects
- Bronchospasm with increased airway resistance.
5 Sodium bicarbonate
a Action
- Raises pH of sputum, resulting in a decrease in viscosity
- Hypertonic solutions may have a bronchorrheic effect promoting expectoration
b Use
- To improve mucokinesis
- To improve the mucolytic actions of acetylcysteine
c Cautions
- Concomitant bronchodilators (acid solutions) undergo rapid breakdown in an alkaline pH; therefore the solution should be given immediately after mixing.
d Side effects
- Bronchospasm and coughing may occur with higher concentrations.

28.8 Enzymes

NOTE: The use of enzymes in the respiratory tract is no longer recommended. This unit is included as a historical reference, rather than as a guide for therapy.
1 Pancreatic dornase (Dornavac)
a Action
- Derived from beef pancrease
- Reduces tenacity and viscosity of mucopurulent pulmonary secretions
- Breaks down deoxyribonucleoprotein (DNA) material in purulent mucus
b Use
- Bronchiectasis
- Necrotizing pneumonias
2 Trypsin (Tryptar)
a Action
- Derived from beef pancreatic trypsin
- Reduces tenacity and viscosity of mucopurulent pulmonary secretions
- Digests mucoprotein material in mucus
b Use
- Bronchiectasis
- Necrotizing pneumonias

28.9 Expectorants

1 Acetylcysteine (See Unit 28.10)
2 Ammonium chloride (Benylin)
a Composition
- Benadryl 12.5 mg
- Ammonium chloride 125 mg
- Sodium citrate 50 mg
- Choroform 20 mg
- Methol 1 mg

b Action
  - Increased ciliary transport
  - Expectorant

c Use
  - Increase mucokinesis
  - Improve efficiency of cough

d Dosage
  - As per manufacturer's recommendation, depending on how ammonium chloride is compounded with other drugs

e Cautions
  - None significant

f Side effects
  - None significant

3 Guaifenesin (Robitussin 2/G)

  a Action
  - Vagal stimulation and direct bronchial gland stimulation resulting in mucokinesis

  b Use
  - Expectorant
  - Improve efficiency of cough

  c Dosage
  - As per manufacturer's recommendations

  d Cautions
  - None significant

  e Side effects
  - Cerebral depression and vomiting may occur with large dosages

4 Iodide—saturated solution of potassium iodide (SSKI)

  a Action
  - Stimulation of gastropulmonary vagal reflex, thus activating submucosal bronchial glands
  - Direct bronchial gland stimulation
  - Enhances breakdown of mucoprotein
  - May stimulate ciliary activity
  - May have an anti-inflammatory effect

  b Use
  - Improved mucokinesis

  c Dosage
  - 5 to 10 drops in H_2O or fruit juice (to mask bitter taste) 3 to 4 times daily

  d Cautions
  - Thyroid function may be adversely affected

  e Side effects
  - Nausea, vomiting, and diarrhea
  - Serum-sickness, which may consist of acneform eruptions, fever lymph node enlargement, and upper airway edema
  - Chronic toxicity may develop with long-term usage

5 Ipecac (Phenergan Expectorant)

  a Action
  - Stimulation of gastropulmonary vagal reflex

  b Use
  - Most common used as an emetic agent
  - At smaller doses, may be used as a mucokinetic

  c Dosage
  - 0.5 to 2.0 ml 3 to 4 times daily

d Side effects
  - In smaller doses, nausea and vomiting are usually not a problem

28.10 Mucolytics

1 Acetylcysteine (Mucomyst)

  a Action
  - Breaks down the disulfide bonds in mucus
  - Reduces the viscosity of thick, tenacious mucus

  b Use
  - Cystic fibrosis
  - Bronchiectasis
  - Pulmonary infection

  c Dosage
  - May be nebulized or instilled directly in trachea
  - Available in 10% or 20% solutions
  - 1 to 3 ml may be nebulized three to four times a day
  - Many physicians who order this drug insist that it be diluted further to 5% or to an even weaker solution; the manufacturer does not believe this further dilution is necessary

  d Cautions
  - It is irritating to mucosal tissues; rinsing the mouth after treatments may be useful.
  - It does not stand well after opening; keep bottle closed and refrigerated after opening; discard unused portions after 48 hours.
  - It reacts irreversibly with metals and rubber; rinse equipment well after use.
  - It is incompatible with tetracycline, oxytetracycline, and erythromycin; do not give these combinations concurrently.

  e Side effects
  - Bronchospasm. If this occurs, discontinue therapy immediately and administer a sympathomimetic bronchodilator (isoproterenol) by aerosol inhalation; acetylcystine is frequently ordered in combination with isoproterenol or isoetharine to prevent bronchospasm
  - Mucosal irritation

2 Sodium bicarbonate (see Unit 28.7)

3 Carboxymethylcysteine (Mucodyne)

  a Actions
  - Direct stimulation of bronchial glands to decrease the viscosity of secretions rather than directly disrupting disulfide bonds

  b Use
  - Cystic fibrosis
  - Chronic bronchitis
  - Bronchiectasis

  c Dosage
  - Suitable for oral or inhalational administration
  - 3 g daily

  d Side effects
  - After oral therapy, mild gastrointestinal disturbances, palpitations, and dizziness may occur

4 Dithiothreitol (Cleland's reagent)

  a Action

    • Similar to acetylcystine, resulting in liquified secretions

  b Use

    • At present, this sulfhydryl compound has not been proved clinically useful.

5 Tyloxapol (Alevarie) (see Unit 28.7)

6 Sodium bicarbonate (see Unit 28.7)

7 Sodium chloride (see Unit 28.7)

8 Terpin hydrate

  a Action

    • Similar to guaifenesin

  b Uses

    • Probably ineffective for mucokinesis in conventional dosages

    • May be considered a "flavoring agent" when combined with other expectorants

  c Dosage

    • 5 ml by oral administration (85 mg)

28.11 Steroids (see also Unit 22.1)

1 Steroids, by their anti-inflammatory action, may afford dramatic relief from bronchial edema when used judiciously for short intervals.

2 They have been proved of value in acute asthma attacks and in relieving symptoms of asthma. However, their use is *not* to be taken lightly. When used for the treatment of asthma that is uncontrolled by other measures, most patients, once on corticosteroids, will have to remain on them indefinitely.

3 Dosage depends on the route of administration; many steroids are given orally, intravenously, or by aerosol inhalation. The following steroids are shown with equivalent milligram dosage:

a Cortisone	25.00 mg
b Hydrocortisone	20.00 mg
c Prednisolone	5.00 mg
d Prednisone	5.00 mg
e Methylprednisolone	4.00 mg
f Triamcinolone	4.00 mg
g Paramethasone	2.00 mg
h Betamethasone	0.75 mg
i Dexamethasone	0.75 mg

4 The following steroids are used especially as aerosols, usually delivered in metered-dose aerosol devices; not all are available in the United States.

  a Dexamethasone (Decadron)

  b Prednisolone (Hydeltrasol)

  c Beclomethasone diproprionate (Beclotide)

  d Triamcinolone acetonide (Kenalog)

  e Flunisolide

28.12 Vasoconstrictors/decongestants

1 The vasoconstrictor drugs work by their sympathomimetic effects. By constricting (shrinking) the blood vessels in the nasal mucosa, swelling, and edema are reduced , offering dramatic relief (see the box that follows).

Vasoconstrictor and drying agents

SYMPATHOMIMETIC AGENTS	ANTICHOLINERGIC AGENTS
a Cyclopentamine HCl (Clopane)	**a** Isopropamide
b Ephedrine sulfate	**b** Methscopolamine bromide
c Epinephrine HCl (Adrenalin)	**c** Belladonna
d Naphazoline HCl (Privine)	**d** Atropine
e Oxymetazoline HCl (Afrin)	**e** Scopolamine
f Phenylephrine HCl (Neo-Synephrine)	
g Phenylpropanolamine HCl (Propadrine)	
h Propylhexedrine (Benzedrex)	
i Pseudoephedrine HCl (Sudafed)	
j Racemic epinephrine (Vaponephrine)	
k Tetrahydrozoline HCl (Tyzine)	
l Tuaminoheptane (Tuamine)	
m Xylometazoline HCl (Otrivin)	

---

2 Some of these drugs are anticholinergics and are used for their drying effect on the mucosa. (See the box that follows and Unit 28.6, "Atropine.")

3 The vasoconstrictors, notably phenylephrine hydrochloride, are sometimes used in conjunction with other bronchodilators. However, their primary use is for nasal decongestion. If given as an aerosol, the dosage of Neo-Synephrine is 2 ml of 0.25% solution. Do *not* give continuously.

4 Care must be taken with sympathomimetic vasconstrictors since a "rebound reaction" can occur with overuse. This is a *reflex* swelling of the mucosa that follows a period of constriction of the blood vessels.

28.13 Miscellaneous respiratory drugs

1 Cromolyn sodium (Intal). This drug is unique in that it may be inhaled as a powder as well as in solution, and although it is used for asthma attack prevention, has absolutely no effect once an attack is underway.

  a Action

    • Inhibits the degranulation of mast cells sensitized as a result of exposure to specific antigens

    • Inhibits release of histamine from within the sensitized mast cell

  b Use

    • Reduces occurrence of severe bronchial asthma attacks

    • No role in the treatment of asthma attacks, especially status asthmaticus

c Dosage
  • Powdered form—1 capsule delivered to the lungs through a special inhaler, four times a day
d Contraindications
  • Patients who have shown hypersensitivity to it: patients with hepatic or renal function failure
e Side effects
  • Urticaria or maculopapular rash, which clears after drug is discontinued
  • Occasional cough or bronchospasm after inhalation

29.0 DRUGS USED IN CARDIOPULMONARY EMERGENCIES
29.1 Emergency drug list

1 The following drugs are normally found on emergency carts. Although they are *not* usually administered by respiratory care personnel, knowledge of their actions may assist the practitioner in understanding the treatment of the patient in emergency situations and in recognizing normal/abnormal responses.
2 Each drug will be listed by its generic and brand name and by a short description of its use during emergency situations. The most common drugs are:
  a Metaraminol bitartrate (Aramine): A vasopressor used in situations of acute hypotension.
  b Mephentermine sulfate (Wyamine). A vasopressor used in situations of acute hypotension; may prevent arrhythmias induced by cyclopropane and halothane anesthesia.
  c Levarterenol (Levophed). A vasopressor used in situations of acute hypotension.
  d Sodium bicarbonate U.S.P. A base buffer used to counteract acute acidosis.
  e Methoxamine hydrochloride (Vasoxyl). A vasopressor, used in situations of acute hypotension; also used to maintain blood pressure during spinal anesthesia.
  f Lidocaine (Xylocaine). A local anesthetic used in emergencies to reduce cardiac irritability and reduce premature ventricular beats, arrhythmias, etc.
  g Calcium chloride U.S.P. A salt used to restore electrolyte balance.
  h Epinephrine (Adrenalin). Injected directly into the heart to increase heart rate and cardiac output.
  i Mannitol. Used as a diuretic.
  j Urea (Ureaphil). Used as a diuretic.
  k Furosemide (Lasix). Used as a diuretic.
  l Pancuronium bromide (Pavulon). A neuromuscular blocking agent used to temporarily paralyze a patient to prevent resistance during intubation, mechanical ventilation, etc.
  m Succinylcholine chloride (Anectine). A neuromuscular blocker.
  n Isoproterenol hydrochloride (Isuprel). A bronchodilator and cardiac stimulant used with heart block and cardiac standstill.
  o Lanatoside C (Cedilanid). A digitalis derivative used

in cases of congestive heart failure, atrial flutter, atrial fibrillation, atrial tachycardia.
  p Digoxin (Lanoxin). A digitalis derivative used in cases of congestive heart failure, atrial flutter, atrial fibrillation, atrial tachycardia.
  q Procainamide hydrochloride (Pronestyl). Depresses irritability of the heart to electrical stimulation; used for ventricular arrhythmias and tachycardia.
  r Dopamine hydrochloride (Intropin). Catecholamine precursor of norepinephrine; increases cardiac output.

30.0 APPLYING KNOWLEDGE OF DRUGS
30.1 Summary

1 The drugs presented in this module are those most frequently encountered by respiratory care personnel.
  a Those presented in Units 28.1 to 28.13 are used by most respiratory care personnel. For this reason the practitioner *must be knowledgeable* in their administrations and their actions.
  b Respiratory care personnel are becoming more involved in critical care and should be aware of all drugs that the patient may be receiving. Failure to recognize a drug can result in a situation where a respiratory therapy drug is given to a patient who should not receive the drug as a result of changes in his clinical condition or because he is already receiving a drug that would react to the respiratory medication.
  c The drugs presented in Units 30.2 to 30.4 demonstrate clinical application of drugs used in respiratory care.

30.2 Bronchospasm

1 Bronchospasm may be defined as a spasmodic contraction of bronchial smooth muscle.
2 It is usually caused by antigen antibody reaction, inhalation of irritants, infection, psychologic stress, mechanical irritation of the airways, exercise and/or extreme changes in temperature of inhaled gases.
3 Bronchospasm manifests itself in people with COPD such as asthma, bronchitis, emphysema and with other conditions such as cystic fibrosis where airway secretions are trapped.
4 It is estimated that approximately 17 million patients suffer from COPD in North America. Most of these patients will receive treatment for bronchospasm sometime during the course of their disease.
5 Drugs most commonly used in the treatment of bronchospasm are presented in Table 15-4 on the next page.
6 A legend describing beta$_1$ and beta$_2$ actions used for interpreting the Table follows.

Legend of Actions

beta$_1$—	myocardial contractions
	cardiac rate
beta$_2$—	bronchdilation
	vasodilation
	secretion of glucagon
	potassium production

TABLE 15-4 Nebulized drugs used in the treatment of bronchospasm and bronchial inflammation

Drug (Generic name)	Preparation	Typical dose Adult (mg or mcg as indicated)	Action site	Onset (min)	Duration (hr)	General side effects
Albuterol	MDI	0.18 (2 puffs)	β_1+ $<\beta_2$	15	3-4	Sympathomimetics NOTE: (Use package insert or reference book for specifics on each drug.)
Bitolterol mesylate	MDI	0.74 (2 puffs)	β_1+ $<\beta_2$	3-4	5-8	
Epinephrine*	MDI SVN	.20 (6-4 puffs) 1:100 or 2.25%	$\alpha+$ β_1+ β_2	3-5	1-3	Headaches Tremors Tachycardia Vasoconstriction Dizziness
Isoproterenol*	MDI SVN	0.16 (2 puffs) 0.625	β_1+ β_2	2-5	.5-2	
Metaproterenol	MDI SNV	1.3 (2 puffs) q. 3.4 hrs max 12 daily 15.0	β_1+ $<\beta_2$	1-5	3-4	
Isoetharine	MDI SVN	0.68 (2 puffs) 5.0	β_1+ $<\beta_2$	1-6	1-3	
Ephedrine*	SVN	25 tid	$\alpha+$ β_1+ β_2	3-6	1	
Terbutaline	MDI SVN	2.4 (2 puffs) 2	β_1+ $<\beta_2$	5-30	3-6	
Pirbuterol mesylate	MDI SVN	0.4 (2 puffs) 0.2 q. 4-6 hr	β_1+ $<\beta_2$	5	5	Anticholinergics Increased heart rate Urinary retention Dry mouth Psychosis Seizures Blurred vision
Ipratropium bromide	SVN	40-80 2 puffs (36 μg) 4 × daily	Site specifically inhibits vagally mediated reflexes	15	4-6	
Atropine sulfate	SVN	0.025 mg/kg in 3-5 ml diluent 3 × daily	Muscarinic receptors + mast cells	2-5	4-5	Corticosteroids NOTE: These drugs are not bronchodilators and should not be used for rapid relief of bronchospasm. Sore throat Decreased resistance to infection. Myopathy Bronchospasm
Beclomethasone dipropionate	MDI	2 puffs (84 μg) 3-4 × daily	Bronchial mucosa	3-5	3-15	
Flunisolide	MDI	2 puffs (500 μg) 2 × daily	Bronchial mucosa	6	1-2	Mast-cell stabilizer NOTE: Not to be used as a bronchodilator. It may induce or worsen existing bronchospasm. Bronchospasm Unaphylate reaction Dizziness Heakache Rash Nausea
Triamcinolone acetonide	MDI	2 puffs (500 μg) 2 × daily	Bronchial mucosa	60		
Cromolyn sodium	MDI	800 (2 inhalations q.i.d)	Mast cell	10-15	4-6	

*NOTE: First generation bronchodilators are readily metabolized by enzymes and therefore are not as long acting as newer beta₂ agonists.
SVN = small volume hand held nebulizer; MDI = metered dose inhaler.

30.3 Mucus control

A healthy lung may produce up to 100 ml of mucus daily and diseased lungs up to 1000 ml daily. Sites involved in the production of bronchial secretions include:

Goblet cells
Bronchial glands
Submucal vessels
Clara cell and type II alveolar cells
Epithelial microvilli
The removal of retained secretions is a primary concern

TABLE 15-5 Mucokinetic agents for nebulization

Drug class	Typical agent	Expected action
Diluent	Water, saline (0.9%, 0.45% sodium bicarbonate (2% to 7.5%)	Adds water to secretion.
Surfactants	Wetting agents, detergents (sodium bicarbonate, propylene glycol, glycerin)	Reduces tenacity (sticking to bronchial surface) and viscosity of secretions.
Mucolytics	a. Proteolytic enzymes (Dornase, Trypsin, Streptodonase) b. Thiol compounds (Acetylcysteine, Dithiothreitol)	Breakdown of microprotein structure of mucus.
Bronchorrheics	Hypertonic saline (1.8% to 10%)	Increased osmotic potential in mucus (draws water from cells into mucus).
Mucoregulators	5—carboxymethylayoteine (NOTE: Investigative; used in foreign countries)	Causes mucus glands to alter viscous structures of muscus to less viscous mucoproteins.

of respiratory care personnel. Drugs used in various modalities to assist in the removal of secretions are listed in Table 15-5.

Mucokinetic agents is a general term classifying many drugs that interact with secretions by adding water topically and internally, causing breakdown of mucoprotein structures or by altering the viscous secretions of bronchial glands for less viscous glycoproteins. Drug classes, typical agents, and expected actions are shown in Table 15-5.

30.4 Pharmacologic management of asthma

The etiology, pathogenesis, and social and economic impact of asthma was presented in Module 8, Unit 23.10.

This unit will focus on various drugs that are used for the treatment of asthma. The drugs covered in this unit are typical of the agents used to treat bronchospastic disease and other types of chronic obstructive conditions.

Asthma is a disease characterized mainly by bronchospasm but also involves inflammatory responses that play a key role in the pathophysiology of severe cases. A reduction in the mortality of asthma patients probably will depend on therapeutic measures that prevent and manage the inflammatory response and control bronchospasm.

Since the late 1970s clinicians have noted that the immediate hypersensitivity response in an acute asthma attack marked by bronchospasm is followed by an inflammatory phase known as the pulmonary late-phase response or late asthmatic response. Pathologic changes in severe asthma include:

Bronchial inflammation
Eosinophilic infiltration
Desquamation of ciliated epithelium

Traditional pharmacologic therapy to treat asthma has utilized beta adrenergic agents and methylxanthines with corticosteroids used primarily as a final resort to control airway resistance. The problem with this approach is that an asthma reaction occurs in two phases:

Immediate spasmogenic phase. A recurring phase with an increase in airway resistance that appears at least 2 hours after the initial reaction to an antigen. Treatment of the initial phase reaction by bronchodilator therapy may relieve symptoms only to have them reappear. The second phase is the treatment of the late phase response.

After exposure to an antigen, histamine, neutrophils,

and eosinophils are immediately released. It is the activity of these three mediators that generate and amplify the last phase inflammatory response now considered to be an important pathogenic factor in asthma.

The following medications are suggested as a graded therapy approach to the treatment of asthma. These medications were presented in Table 15-4.

Step I therapy for asthma

Patients who benefits from Step I care are those with mild, intermittent asthma whose disease flares seasonally, For such patients, inhaled beta adrenergic agents continue to constitute first line therapy.

Inhaled bronchodilators are also used during exacerbations of asthma when Step II agents - aerosol corticosteroids fail to prevent acute attacks.

1 Beta adrenergic agents. The route by which beta adrenergic agents are given greatly influences their efficacy and side effects. In general, inhalation through a metered dose inhaler (MDI) provides the most efficient and rapid means of relieving acute symptoms. Orally-administered beta$_2$ agonists take up to 2 hours for maximum effects; consequently, this route is of limited value in reversing acute symptoms. Subcutaneously administered sympathomimetic agents have a greater tendency to produce such effects as headaches, tremors, and tachycardia and are no more effective than inhaled sympathomimetics. For these reasons, inhaled sympathomimetics are preferred over oral and subcutaneous bronchodilators.

The prototype of the beta adrenergic bronchodilators, epinephrine, stimulates alpha$_1$, beta$_1$, and beta$_2$ receptors. Ephedrine and isoproterenol are also potent stimulators of both beta$_1$ and beta$_2$ adrenergic receptors. The use of these three agents in the management of asthma is limited by their potential to cause an array of undesirable clinical effects, including vascoconstriction, cardiac stimulation, and muscle tremors. In addition, the first generation drug isoetharine has less beta$_2$ mediated side effects than the other first generation bronchodilators, which have a relatively short duration of action. Thus, their use has been eclipsed by newer and more beta$_2$-specific inhaled bronchodilators. Unlike the endogenous catecholamines, such as epinephrine, which are readily metabolized by enzymes, newer

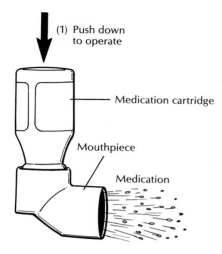

(1) Push down to operate

Medication cartridge

Mouthpiece

Medication

FIGURE 15-1 Typical metered dose aerosol unit.

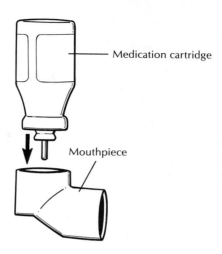

Medication cartridge

Mouthpiece

FIGURE 15-2 Assembly of a metered dose aerosol unit.

beta$_2$ agonists have been designed to better withstand enzymatic degradation. The second generation beta$_2$ agonists are therefore longer acting than first generation bronchodilators.

Adrenergic agents with beta$_2$ receptor specificity include metaproterenol, terbutaline, albuterol, bitolterol, and pirbuterol. These agents are also preferred to first generation bronchodilators because they cause less cardiac stimulation and are more potent. They also are longer acting and therefore may be especially useful for nocturnal asthma. Efficacy and duration of action of these new bronchodilators are similar.

  a Metaproterenol, the time-honored drug in this class, is principally a beta$_2$ adrenergic agonist. Inhalation of metaproterenol has little effect on the beta receptors in the heart. The onset of action with inhaled metaproterenol is about 5 minutes, and bronchodilating effects last up to 4 hours. This agent also has the advantage of being relatively inexpensive.

Metaproterenol is available in several forms, including syrup, tablets, metered dose inhaler, nebulized solution, and a single nebulized solution in saline. The metered dose inhaler contains 225 mg of the drug; 0.65 mg is nebulized per dose. This drug is administered in 2 to 3 deep inhalations every 3 to 4 hours. When the total daily dose exceeds 12 inhalations Step II agents should be used to decrease inflammation. A greater number of inhalations can be used as Grade 3 agents are used to decrease inflammation.

  b Terbutaline, a beta$_2$ selective agonist, can be administered orally, subcutaneously, and by inhalation. Its chemical structure, and thus its clinical effects, are similar to those of albuterol and pirbuterol.

  c Albuterol, another potent selective beta$_2$ adrenergic agonist, can be administered orally or by inhalation.

  d Bitolterol, another beta$_2$-specific agonist, has an effect that is similar to that of albuterol. After inhalation, bitolterol is activated primarily by lung esterases to coltertol, an active catecholemine. Its du-

ration of action is approximately 5 to 8 hours, which makes it especially useful for patients with noctural asthma. Bitolterol is generally well tolerated and appears to produce few cardiovascular effects. It is available as an MDI, which contains 370 mg per inhalation. For patients over the age of 12, the usual dosage is 2 to 3 deep inhalations administered 1 to 5 minutes apart.

  e Pirbuterol recently became available in this country. Its chemical structure is similar to that of terbutaline and albuterol; thus, it has the same pharmacologic properties and clinical effects as these agents. However, it appears to have a somewhat longer effect.

2 Problems with beta adrenergic therapy. There are two major stumbling blocks in beta adrenergic therapy. Perhaps the most important is improper use of the MDI (Fig. 15-1). The MDI is convenient for ambulatory patients who can learn to use the device properly, and it is particularly useful in preventing bronchospasm caused by exercise. It is crucial, however, to watch the patient using his or her MDI to make sure it is assembled correctly and that the canister is well shaken (Figs. 51-2 and 15-3), and that the patient holds the mouthpiece of the actuator 4 cm in front of his mouth (Fig. 15-4). Watch the patient slowly exhale and then discharge the inhaler while deeply inhaling. Finally, check to see whether the patient holds his breath for 10 seconds before exhaling.

Many patients are unable to master the technique. The most common problem is failure to coordinate discharge with inspiration. Spacer devices or specially designed chambers have been designed to overcome this difficulty (Fig. 15-5). (See also Module 12, 5.2.)

The second problem with beta adrenergic agents is underdosing. These agents are often taken in doses too small to provide effective symptomatic relief. If the full benefit of an inhaled bronchodilator is not promptly appreciated, several inhalations, 3 to 4 puffs within 10 minutes, may be particularly helpful.

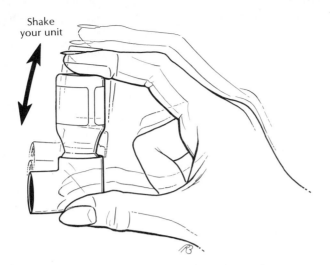

FIGURE 15-3 Shaking the unit before inhalation.

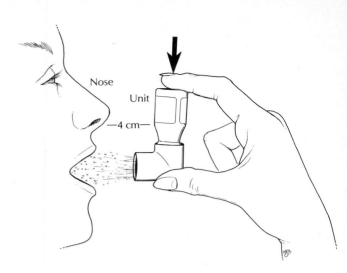

FIGURE 15-4 Taking a "puff" of medication from an MDI positioned approximately 4 cm from opened mouth.

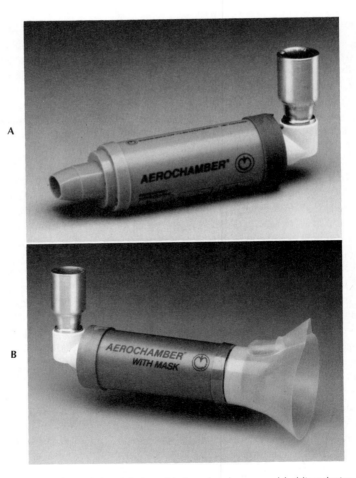

FIGURE 15-5 A, Metered dose inhaler with Aerochamber aerosol holding device. **B,** Aerochamber with pediatric mask. (Courtesy Monaghan Medical Corporation, Plattsburgh, New York.)

3 Anticholinergic agents. When a properly administered beta agonist agent does not afford prompt, effective relief from bronchospasm, adjunctive use of an inhaled anticholinergic agent is indicated to quell acute symptoms. Anticholinergic agents produce bronchodilation by inhibiting the release of tonic acetylcholine from nerves in the airway.

These drugs are generally less effective than beta agonists in controlling bronchospasm due to asthma, however, and are better used as first-line agents in patients with bronchospasm predominatly associated with chronic bronchitis or emphysema. Nevertheless, there is some evidence that beta sympathomimetics and anticholinergics are more effective than the use of beta sympathomimetics alone in asthma and that anticholinergics can be used in conjunction with Beta sympathomimetics to enhance the clinical effects of therapy without an increase in toxicity.

  a Ipratropium bromide is a quaternary ammonion anticholinergic agent that causes bronchodilation by inhibiting vagally-mediated bronchoconstriction. The onset of bronchodilation after ipratropium administration is slower than beta sympathomimetics. However, the effect is prolonged. When administered by aerosol, ipratropium significantly increases forced expiratory volume in one second.

The initial adult dose is 40 to 80 mg. The duration of action of this agent is about 6 hours. Even when given in high doses, inhaled ipratropium seems to have no discernible effect on mucus production or clearance or sputum viscosity. The lack of systemic effect is partially the result of the fact that this drug is not well absorbed from the respiratory tract.

  a Theophylline is not usually regarded as a first-line agent in the management of asthma. However, theophylline can be used as an adjunct to Step I therapy, particularly for patients who are already taking this medicaiton and are tolerating the medication well.

Use of theophylline must be individualized in patients whose asthma is not adequately controlled with inhaled beta agonists and either cromolyn and/or inhaled corticosteroids. The risk-to-benefit ratio of theophylline must be weighed carefully in those patients for whom this agent is prescribed. Despite its narrow therapeutic index, theophylline can be useful for managing noctural asthma. If used, theophylline levels should be drawn to decrease the likelihood of toxicity.

Step II therapy for asthma

Agents used for Step II treatment of asthma protect against and/or manage the late-phase inflammatory response with few side effects. With the exception of those patients with mild, intermittent asthma whose occasional asthma attack is controlled with beta-sympathomimetic agents, most patients with asthma are likely to benefit from Step II care.

Suitable candidates for aerosol corticosteroid therapy, the mainstay of Step II care, are those who depend regularly on inhaled bronchodilators to control acute attacks of asthma. Daily use of an aerosol corticosteroid can decrease the frequency of acute exacerbations and thereby reduce the need for bronchodilators. Administration of these agents, if necessary in doses double to triple those usually recommended, may decrease inflammation to such an extent that Step III agents are seldom or never needed except in the most severe asthmatic patient.

  4 Aerosol corticosteroids. The pharamacologic effect of corticosteroids is to stimulate the production of lipocortin, an intracellular protein, which prevents cleavage of arachidonic acid from its parent phospholipids. This, in turn, inhibits the synthesis of prostaglandins and leukotrienes that cause mucus secretion, vascular permeability, and smooth muscle spasm.

Formulations of inhaled corticosteroids currently available in this country include beclomethasone dipropionate, flunisolide acetate, and triamcinolone acetonide. These agents are particularly effective in the management of chronic asthma since they inhibit the late-phase inflammatory response and decrease airway reactivity.

  a Beclomethasone can be given in daily doses of 2 puffs per day or 36 mg 4 days a day.

  b Flunisolide is given in daily doses of 2 puffs per day, 500 mcg. 2 times daily.

  c Triamcinolone is 2 puffs or 500 mcg. 2 times daily. Recent data indicate that triamcinolone may be particularly helpful for patients who cough in response to other aerosol corticosteroids.

When taken in adequate doses, inhaled corticosteroids can decrease the frequency of acute asthma exacerbations. However, the dosage at which these agents are usually taken is often too low to prevent acute attacks. Thus, when the clinical response is inadequate (as determined by serial measurements of peak flow), the dosage should be increased up to three times the usual amount to afford maximum protective effect. In adults, significant adrenal suppression should not occur in doses two to three times the usual dose.

Compliance with a regimen of aerosol corticosteroids can be a problem, because these agents do not immediately relieve symptoms, as do the inhaled bronchodilators. It is therefore important that patients learn the therapeutic expectations involved in using corticosteroids.

It is emphasized that aerosol corticosteroids can markedly ameliorate symptoms related to inflammation and thus may reduce the number of acute attacks. Inhaled corticosteroids are associated with relatively few side effects. These effects are limited to oral candidiasis, hoarseness, sore throat, and dysphonia.

The use of a spacer device helps to decrease the risk of oropharyngeal candidiasis and may increase the efficacy of these agents.

  5 Cromolyn sodium therapy should be considered for every patient with asthma. This agent may inhibit mediator release from effector cells, including mast cells and basophils. It may also block phosphorylation of a membrane protein that is necessary for mediator release.

Cromolyn sodium is particularly useful for young patients and for those whose asthma is precipitated by allergens or exercise. It is administered prophylactically against flare-ups of asthma; the agent decreases the severity of the early and late phase inflammatory response. It may also facilitate withdrawl from oral or inhaled corticosteroids.

Cromolyn comes in an MDI and in a capsule form that is filled with a powder and inhaled with a special device. For most patients, the daily dose is 2 puffs 4 times daily. Because clinical effects of cromolyn may not be apparent for 2 to 4 weeks, a 4- to 6-week trial of prophylactic therapy is recommended.

If asthma is not controlled by the combined use of Step I and Step II agents, a one-time trial of theophylline is recommended. This agent may prove to be a useful adjunct to Step II agents, and, in some patients, may help to avoid Step III agents, systemic corticosteroids.

Step III therapy for asthma

Step III agents, oral or intravenous corticosteroids are reserved for patients with severe exacerbations that are not controlled by Step I and II agents. Patients must be taught to self-administer oral corticosteroids when asthma symptoms are not responding to bronchodilators and inhaled corticosteroids. During a severe attack, oral prednisone may be given in doses as high as 30 to 60 mg each morning for up to 2 weeks. Peak flow rates are monitored daily as the prednisone is gradually tapered.

After the disease is under control, aerosol therapy (for those not already using a Step II agent) as determined by an absence of symptoms and stable peak flow rates can be started as the oral agent is withdrawn. When aerosol corticosteroids do not adequately control the disease and oral agents must be taken, one may consider giving prednisone along with daily doses of inhaled steroids.

About half of all asthma patients who depend on oral corticosteroids can be treated with alterate day therapy. This regimen may avoid adrenal suppression in some patients. If asthma flares, the dose can be increased temporarily or daily therapy reinstituted. It is probably prudent to avoid long-acting oral preparations like dexamethasone and triamcinolone. In the rare patients who require daily therapy, complications associated with use of these agents can be pronounced. For these patients, shorter-acting agents can be given at more frequent intervals.

Side effects associated with systemic corticosteroids are common. After only a few days of high dose therapy, moon facies, mood changes, fluid retention, and gastrointestinal upset may develop. Long-term administraton can result in hypertension, adrenal insufficiency, aseptic necrosis, and osteoporosis with bone fractures. Thus, every attempt must be made to wean patients from oral to inhaled corticosteroids.

To avoid the side effects of prednisone, a higher dose of inhaled steroids can be used as explained earlier. The higher dose of inhaled steroids should be used before an increase in asthma symptoms. The increased dose is signaled by a drop in the peak flow measured by the patient or by an increase in the need for aerosolized bronchodilator.

PROCEDURE 15-1

Drawing medication

No.	Steps in performing the procedure
1	The practitioner will use a needle and syringe to withdraw medication. Collect necessary materials: **1.1** Sterile 5 ml syringe with needle **1.2** Alcohol swab **1.3** Multidose-type vial of sterile distilled water **1.4** Appropriate labeling materials
2	Wash hands.
3	Use alcohol swab to clean top of vial.
4	Pull syringe plunger out to 2 ml mark.
5	Remove needle guard.
6	Insert needle into vial.
7	Push syringe plunger all the way forward.
8	Invert vial and syringe.
9	Withdraw 2 ml of distilled water.
10	Withdraw needle from vial.
11	Replace needle guard without contaminating needle.
12	Label syringe according to hospital policy.
13	Dispose of the syringe:* **13.1** Eject the distilled water. **13.2** Break needle by holding needle guard and bending needle back and forth until it breaks. **13.3** Dispose of the broken needle in an appropriate container. Do *not* put into trash can. **13.4** Break the syringe plunger (depending on brand) by pulling halfway out of syringe barrel and breaking in two. **13.5** Dispose of the broken syringe in an appropriate container.

*If this procedure is different from hospital's policy, always follow the procedure recommended in the hospital.

PROCEDURE 15-2

Using a unit dose medication container

No.	Steps in performing the procedure
1	The practitioner will use a unit dose medication container to add sterile distilled water to a small volume nebulizer. Collect necessary materials: **1.1** 5 ml unit dose container of sterile distilled water **1.2** Small volume nebulizer
2	Wash hands.
3	Depending on the brand of unit dose container: **3.1** Break off the top without contaminating the vial's contents. **3.2** Add 3 ml of the sterile distilled water to the nebulizer vial.
4	Dispose of the remaining 2 ml of distilled water and the opened vial in an appropriate container.

BIBLIOGRAPHY

Austin FK and Orange RP: Bronchial asthma: the possible role of the chemical mediators of immediate hypersensitivity in the pathogenesis of subacute chronic diseases, Am Rev Respir Dis 15:3, 1976.

Bone RC: Step care for asthma, JAMA 260:543, 1988.

Burton GG, Gee BN, and Hodgkin JE, editors: Respiratory care: a guide to clinical practice, Philadelphia, 1977, JB Lippincott Co.

Civetta JM: Intensive care therapeutics, New York, 1980, Appleton-Century-Crofts.

Evans R et al: National trends in the morbidity and mortality of asthma in the United States, Chest 91:658, 1987.

Holgate ST: The role of medicators and inflammation in asthma, J Respir Dis 8:20, 1987.

Jenkins CR et al: Ipratropium bromide and fenoterol by aerosolized solution, Br J Clin Pharmacol 14:113, 1982.

Jenne JW: The clinical pharmacology of bronchodilators, Basics of R.D., New York, 1977, American Lung Association.

Kaliner MA: The late-phase reaction and its clinical implications, Hosp Pract 22:73, 1987.

Katzung BG, editor: Basic and clinical pharmacology, Los Altos, 1982, Lange Medical Publications.

Kirby RR and Civetta JM: The Hyland symposium: point-counter-point: factors in pulmonary edema, Crit Care 7:83, 1979.

Kirkpatrick CH: Steroil therapy of allergic diseases, Med Clin North Am 57:1309, 1973.

Larsen GL: The pulmonary late-phase response, Hosp Pract 22:155, 1987.

Lehnert BE and Schachter EN: The pharmacology of respiratory care, St Louis, 1980, The CV Mosby Co.

McFadden ER Jr: Pathogenesis of asthma, J Allergy Clin Immunol 73:413, 1984.

Nelson RP and Lockey RF: Current treatment for patients with severe asthma, J Respir Dis 9:29, 1988.

Newhouse MT and Dolovich NB: Control of asthma by aerosols, N Engl J Med 315:870, 1986.

Pingleton WW et al: Oropharyngeal candidiasis in patients tested with triamcinolone acetonide aerosol, J Allergy Clin Immunol 60:245, 1977.

Rau JL: Respiratory therapy pharmacology, Chicago, 1978, Year Book Medical Publishers, Inc.

Reed CE: New therapeutic approaches in asthma, J Allergy Clin Immunol 77:537, 1986.

Shim CS, William MH Jr: Cough and wheezing from bachomethasol aerosol are absent after triamcinolone acetonide, Ann Intern Med 106:700, 1987.

Spearman CB, Sheldon RL, and Egan DF: Egan's fundamentals of respiratory therapy, ed 5, St Louis 1990, The CV Mosby Co.

Wilson MC, Larsen GL: Gaining control over the last asthmatic response, J Respir Dis 7:51, 1986.

Physical assessment

1.0 CHEST PHYSICAL ASSESSMENT
1.1 Need for chest physical assessment

Respiratory care personnel are rapidly expanding their clinical roles and the manner in which they interact with the patient, physician, and other members of the health team.

1 In this changing role, they are expected to do a great deal more than "just work with equipment."

For example, they should be participating in the patient interview and development of the patient's medical history. In this capacity they are also performing physical assessment of the chest and other primary clinical assessment procedures, such as bedside pulmonary function evaluation.

2 Physical assessment is one of the most useful skills to be mastered by the clinician because it allows detection of problems and initiation of appropriate action before more serious developments can occur.

3 It also increases the practitioner's contribution to better patient care through his or her understanding and performing physical assessment as a means of evaluating the patient's response to medical treatment.

4 Physical assessment skills *cannot* be learned primarily from a textbook. For proficiency, a variety of clinical experiences that can be applied to various patient care situations must be acquired.

5 Although it would be desirable to understand the knowledge and skills required to perform physical assessment of the total patient, respiratory care personnel are presently expected to be primarily knowledgeable about *chest physical assessment,* which is the focus of this module.

2.0 TERMINOLOGY AND DEFINITIONS
2.1 Glossary of terms and definitions associated with chest assessment

1 Adventitious sounds. Abnormal breath sounds for a particular area of the chest.
2 Amplitude. Loudness or intensity of sound.
3 Anterior and posterior axillary lines (Fig. 16-1, *A*). Imaginary lines extending on either side of the midaxillary line, further dividing the lateral chest into anterior and posterior planes.
4 Bronchial sounds. Loud sounds that have a blowing quality, similar to air moving through a pipe.
5 Chest auscultation. Use of the aided or unaided ear to listen for the presence, absence, and quality of sounds occurring within the chest during the breathing cycle.
6 Costal angle. The angle formed by the intersection of the lower rib cage with the sternum (see Fig. 16-1, *B4*).
7 Crackles. Fine, dry, crackling sounds heard primarily during inspiration in particular lung pathologies.
8 Dullness. A short, nonmusical sound indicating airless tissue such as occurs in atelectasis, over the spinal column, heart, or abdominal viscera.
9 Duration. Length of time a sound is heard.

10 Evaluation. Determining the efficiency of a treatment, equipment, medication, or other activity to achieve desired outcomes or to assess the patient or situation according to preset standards or experience. Nursing texts describe evaluation as a five-step process. This process begins with a determination of whether the therapy goals are being met and concludes with evaluating impact of the care on the patient and family.
11 Examination. An investigation of the patient in order to identify problems and other situations influencing his or her care.
12 Flatness. Absolute dullness (lack of resonance or tympany) such as occurs after the percussion of a large muscle mass or in pleural effusion or hemothorax.
13 Fremitus. A term describing vibrations felt by the hand placed against the chest wall.
14 Frequency. Pitch or tone of a sound.
15 Manubrium sterni junction (Louis's angle). A point that is used for counting ribs because the superior border of the second rib joins the sternum at this point (see Fig. 16-1, *B1*). Ribs are counted along the midclavicular line *(2)*.
16 Midaxillary line. Imaginary lines extending vertically from the top of the axillae to the bottom of the chest, dividing the lateral chest in anterior and posterior portions (see Fig. 16-1, *B6*).
17 Midclavicular lines. Imaginary lines beginning at the midpoint of the clavicles and extending through the chest from top to bottom on either side of the sternum (see Fig. 16-1, *B2*).
18 Midspinal line. An imaginary line that runs from top to bottom through the middle of the spine (see Fig. 16-1, *C7*).
19 Midsternal line. An imaginary line drawn through the sternum and extending from the top to bottom of the chest (see Fig. 16-1, *B5*).
20 Palpation. Using the fingers of palm of the hand to feel sound as a vibration.
21 Percussion. Striking the chest to generate sound that will vary in loudness and quality because of underlying pathology.
22 Physical. Literally defined as a naturally occurring event or entity. In this module "physical" also refers to examining a patient to discover any abnormal conditions.
23 Position (in respiratory cycle). A sound heard during inspiration or exhalation; beginning, middle, or end of each phase.
24 Resonance. A long, clear, low-pitched sound indicating a normal air-tissue ratio.
25 Rhonchi (sing. *rhonchus*). A better term is wheezes; musical sounds of low or high pitch that may be heard on inspiration or exhalation in cases with elevated airway resistance. Wheezes are continuous sounds; crackles are discontinuous.
26 Scapular lines. Imaginary vertical lines that are drawn through the inferior angles of the scapula on either side of the spine (see Fig. 16-1, *C8*).

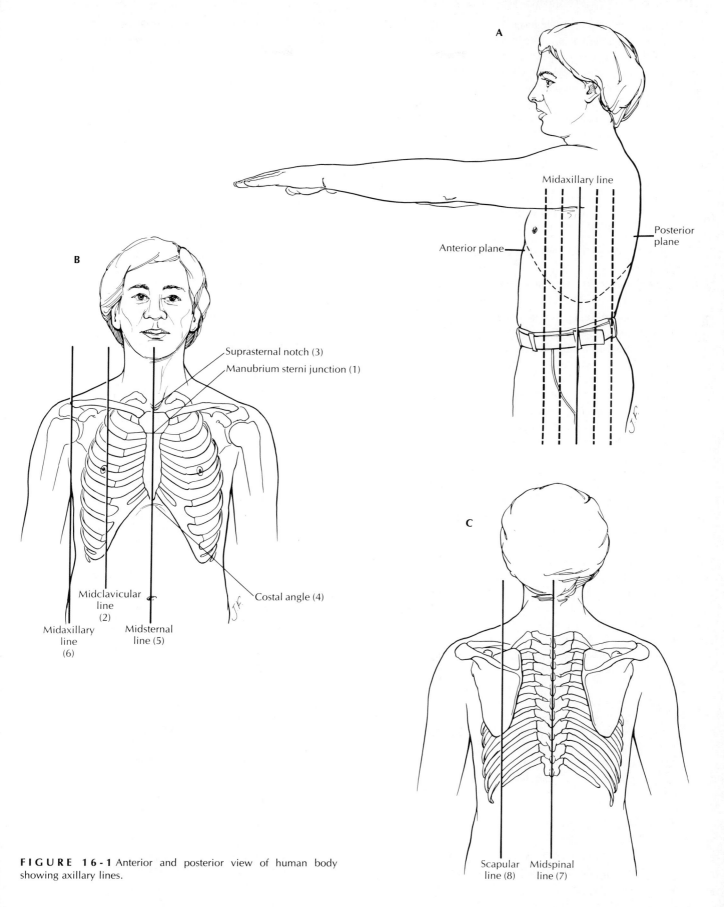

FIGURE 16-1 Anterior and posterior view of human body showing axillary lines.

27 Sound. A period fluctuation of pressure that can be heard. It is characterized by frequency, amplitude, duration, and position of the respiratory cycle.

28 Suprasternal notch. A depression located at the superior aspect of the manubrium (see Fig. 16-1, *B3*). This notch is used when palpating location of the trachea.

29 Topographic landmarks. External anatomic features of the chest that can be used to pinpoint underlying structures.

30 Tympany. A bell-like "hollow" sound indicating excessive air-to-tissue ratio such as occurs in emphysema, hyperinflation, lung cavities, and pneumothorax.

For additional information on bronchopulmonary anatomy, see Modules Four and Eight.

3.0 PROCEDURE FOR PHYSICAL EXAMINATION OF THE CHEST

3.1 General steps involved in performing physical examination of the chest

1 Many inexperienced respiratory care personnnel assume that *auscultation* should be the first and most important step in examination of the chest. This usually is *not* the case, because a good physical examination should include:
a Patient interview—questioning
b Inspection—looking
c Palpation—feeling
d Percussion—thumping
e Auscultation—listening

2 The clinical evaluation of the respiratory system is similar to that of any other organ system. It includes:
a A *history* focusing on cardinal respiratory symptoms.
b A *review* of symptoms from other organ involvement that may influence respiratory disorders.
c An *examination* and simple *bedside pulmonary function* test performed by the interviewer.

3 The participation of respiratory care personnel in the physical examination process will vary from one medical situation to another, as well as from one hospital to another. For example, if the first contact with the patient is on the medical unit, a patient history probably would already have been performed by the admitting physician. If this were the case, the practitioner should carefully review the patient's history and workup by the admitting physician. The patient interview could then be omitted, unless clarification of information is required or specific questions need to be answered.

The following units assume that the patient has *not* been previously interviewed and will therefore require a complete workup.

4.0 CONDUCTING A GOOD PATIENT INTERVIEW

4.1 Purpose of the patient interview

1 The overall purpose of the patient overview is to accumulate as much *verbal* and *visual* data as possible from the patient regarding the medical problem.

2 The patient should be encouraged to provide as much unsolicited information as possible without direct questioning. The clinician should be an *active listener, not an interrogator*.

3 The *main points* that must be answered before the conclusion of an interview are:
a The major symptoms (complaints)
b The time, mode of onset, and duration of the first symptom
c The chronologic sequence of subsequent symptoms
d Current status of the medical problem

4 The symptoms most closely associated with respiratory diseases are:
a Dyspnea or labored breathing
b Cough, sputum/hemoptysis
c Chest pain

5 The *cardinal signs/symptoms* of pulmonary disease include:
a Respiratory distress
b Respiratory rate
c Depth of breathing
d Rhythm of breathing
e Signs of respiratory failure, such as hypercapnia, hypoxia, cyanosis, polycythemia, digital clubbing, and hypertrophic pulmonary osteoarthropathy

4.2 Conducting the patient interview

1 Conducting the patient interview is the *first step* in gathering information about the patient and developing a thorough medical history.

Before seeing the patient, the interviewer should review any available information about the patient, e.g., charts from previous admissions.

2 The *second step* is to establish an environment for the patient that is as nonthreatening and as comfortable as possible.
a This environment includes privacy and quietness of the room, soft yet adequate lighting, a comfortable temperature for someone who is disrobed, location and comfort of furniture, and the interviewer's own appearance, demeanor, and attitude.
b The approach to the patient must take into account special problems frequently involved with respiratory patients. For example, one such problem is the fact that many respiratory diseases may be considered "self-caused" by the patient who smokes or works in a hazardous environment. The interviewer must not let personal feelings for this situation influence the rapport and trust level that must be developed between the clinician and the patient.
c The clinician *must* reflect patience, understanding, and a sincere desire to help the patient, regardless of the patient's attitude and level of cooperation.
d The interview technique should involve enough questions to probe specific areas of concern but should be open enough to allow the patient to volunteer information about his or her condition and to ask questions of the interviewer (see Module Eight for a sample of typical questions). Being a *good listener* is

an important aspect of conducting a thorough patient interview.

e The interviewer must feel comfortable and be able to put the patient at ease when responding to different types of situations that may arise during the interview. For example:

Patient's attitude	Interviewer's response
Periods of silence	Analyze it, assess it, use it.
Talkativeness	Direct as necessary to the interview.
Fear	Be supportive.
Anger/hostility	Accept as a symptom.
Depression	Recognize limits of questioning.

3 The interviewer should accurately record the information given during the interview with as much objectivity as possible, since the physician will interpret this information along with laboratory data to reach a diagnosis. The interviewer should also use a standardized format for gathering information for the patient history, use terminology that can be easily and clearly defined at a subsequent date, and avoid using personal shorthand or definitions that may be open to misinterpretation.

4 Fig. 16-2 is an example of a checklist format incorporating the nine cardinal signs and symptoms of respiratory disease. This format may be used as a guide to obtaining a thorough patient history. When using the checklist for data gathering, the practitioner should be as thorough as possible and note as much information as possible about each clinical category.

5 A thorough *physical examination* should be coordinated with the history-taking process. Frequently, it is desirable to ask questions and examine the patient simultaneously. The examination, like the history, should be organized and standardized to include:

a Inspection
b Palpation
c Percussion
d Auscultation

6 A chest radiograph and simple bedside pulmonary function testing are frequently included as a routine component of a pulmonary physical examination.

Procedure 16-1 (at the end of this module) may be used as a guide for conducting a patient interview.

5.0 SIGNS OF PULMONARY DISEASE BASED ON EXTERNAL APPEARANCES ON THE CHEST
5.1 Inspecting the chest

1 The examination should be standardized and organized into a *systematic routine* that is followed with each patient. Most examiners *begin their assessment at the periphery* of the chest and work from top to bottom. Special attention is directed toward explaining and documenting abnormal findings for subsequent, in-depth investigation.

a Physical examination of the chest begins with a thorough inspection of the chest area.
b This inspection involves a systematic process of

Clinical indicator — **Explanation of event (when, where, why)**

1 Cough pattern
 a Day or night
 b During the interview
 c Abrupt change
 d Subtle (chronic)
2 Sputum production
 a Change in volume
 b Color
 c Odor
 d Thickness
 e Time of expectoration
3 Bleeding (hemoptysis)
 a Bloody
 b Mixed
 c Volume: minimal or gross amount
4 Chest pain
 a Site (pleural, tracheobronchial, neuromuscular, cardiovascular)
 b Emotional
5 Dyspnea (classify as 1 to 4 with patient at rest)
 a Acute
 b Paroxysmal
 c Chronic
6 Wheezing
 a Diffuse
 b Local
 c Stridor
7 Infection
 a Fever, chills, shakes, signs, sweats
 b Loss of appetite, malaise
8 Voice change
9 Exposure to pulmonary irritants
 a *Smoking history:* dose per day, type of tobacco product, filtered or not, inhaled or not, duration and present habit
 b *Family history:* (note hereditary traits) list allergies, asthma, sinusitis, COPD, cystic fibrosis, cancer, sickle cell anemia, pulmonary emboli, and restrictive disease
 c *Social and working history:* industrial exposure (time, dose, chronicity of exposure) location of living or traveling arrangements

FIGURE 16-2 Checklist format incorporating the nine cardinal signs and symptoms of respiratory disease. May be used as a guide to obtain a patient history.

looking at the chest and should be performed with the patient seated and clothing removed to the waist (Fig. 16-3). The patient who is unable to sit in a chair should be placed in the Fowler's position in bed.

2 Initially, the examiner should evaluate the overall appearance of the chest by comparing any findings to known anatomic landmarks and lines of reference.

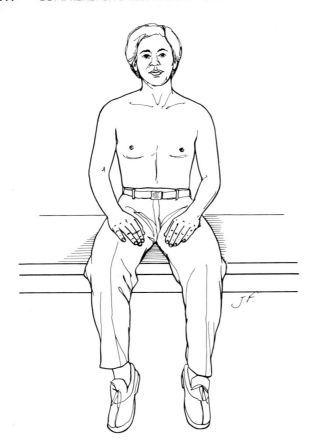

FIGURE 16-3 Patient should be seated with clothing removed to the waist for a chest inspection.

3 Skin color, temperature, and condition should be noted along with any scars, bruises, or discoloration.

4 The depth, rate, and regularity of breathing should be assessed and compared to norms for the patient's age and current activity level.

5 The chest size and shape should be compared to norms, especially changes in the anteroposterior (AP) diameter, which is indicative of obstructive lung diseases.

6 Chest symmetry (how one side compares to the other) should be evaluated by observing the patient's breathing. This observation should be made from different angles as the examiner moves to different positions around the patient.

NOTE: Standing directly in front of the patient is the best position to determine equal movement by both sides of the chest.

7 Any deformities of the bone structures of the chest and/or spine should be noted. These include kyphoscoliosis, barrel chest, pectus excavatum, and others, which will be discussed later in the module.

8 The work of breathing should be estimated by determining whether or not the accessory muscles of breathing are being used and to what degree (see Module Four, Units 15.1 through 16.3).

Ask yourself the following questions as breathing is observed*:

a Does the chest move appropriately to the inspiratory effort exerted?

b Does it move symmetrically?

c Is there a lag on one side during inspiration?

d Are the accessory muscles of inspiration and exhalation used?

e What is the shape of the chest?

f Are the chest, ribs, or spine deformed?

g What is the respiratory rate?

h Is the breathing pattern regular or irregular?

• If irregular, is it Cheyne-Stokes respiration, Biot's breathing, etc.?

i Is the volume of air moved with each breath (V_T) normal for the patient's age, size, and circumstances?

j What is the breathing process: eupnea, dyspnea, tachypnea, hyperpnea, Kussmal's respiration, etc.?

k What is the inspiratory to expiratory ratio (I:E)? Is it normal, i.e., 1:1.5-2.0? Is inspiration longer than exhalation? Is it equal? Is expiration prolonged?

5.2 Abnormalities of the rib cage and spine

When inspecting the chest, the examiner should do the following†:

1 Compare the shape of the patient's chest and spine to that of normal bony structures. For inspection of the posterior chest, the patient should be sitting, leaning slightly forward; for the anterior chest, recumbent.

When sitting or lying, the patient should be relaxed, with upper clothing removed so that the anterior and posterior chest is exposed and accessible for viewing.

2 Initially, observe the *overall appearance* of the chest by comparing it to a normal size and shape for a particular age-group and sex. For example, infants and children normally have a chest that presents a circular or cylindric configuration as compared to an adult's, which is not rounded except in certain diseases such as emphysema.

3 Note symmetry of chest movement during breathing. A good rule of thumb is to use the patient as his or her own control and compare the movement of one side of the chest to the other.

4 Note the muscles involved in breathing.

5 Compare the *AP diameter* to the lateral diameter of the chest to normal. The ratio of AP to lateral diameter should be no more than 5:7 and usually as 1:2, except as altered by disease.

6 To examine for possible spinal deformity (Fig. 16-4) see that the patient is sitting straight or standing erect.

a Check for *kyphosis*. This is a deformity resulting in a

---

*See Module Six, Units 4.4 and 4.5, for a review of breathing patterns and terms.

†Procedure 16-2 may be used for conducting chest inspection. The reader is encouraged, if it is possible, to observe a physician performing chest inspection and a patient interview.

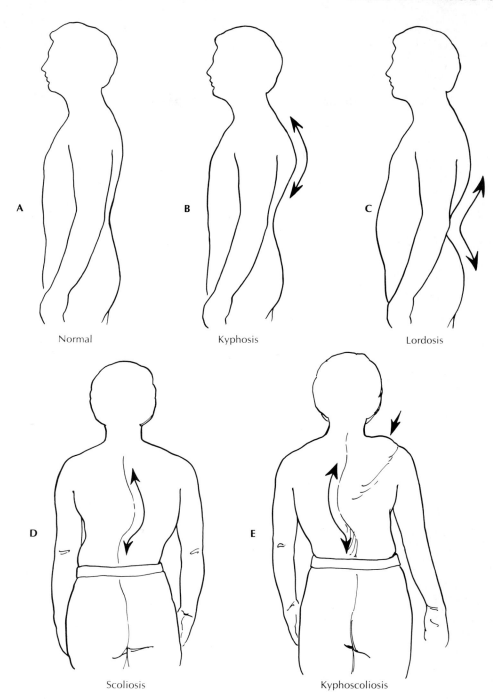

A   Normal

B   Kyphosis

C   Lordosis

D   Scoliosis

E   Kyphoscoliosis

FIGURE 16-4 Patient should be sitting straight or standing erect to examine for spinal deformity.

backward curve of the spine, causing a humpback appearance *(B)*. If the curvature is angular, it is called *gibbous* (not shown). Kyphosis may be caused by degenerative bone change or age, or it may be associated with chronic obstructive disease.

b Check for *lordosis*. Lordosis describes a backward curvature of the lumbar spine resulting in a swayback appearance *(C)*. It is usually not directly connected with respiratory problems. Indirectly, misalignment may cause the thorax to assume a fixed

expiratory position that infringes on effective ventilation.

c Check for *scoliosis*. This is a lateral curvature of the spine *(D)*. This condition causes a rotation of the vertebral bodies, resulting in a flattening of the ribs anteriorly and a bulging of the chest posteriorly. Severe cases can interfere with pulmonary mechanics and with proper ventilation.

d Check for *kyphoscoliosis (E)*, a combined deformity caused by scoliosis (lateral curvature) *(D)* and ky-

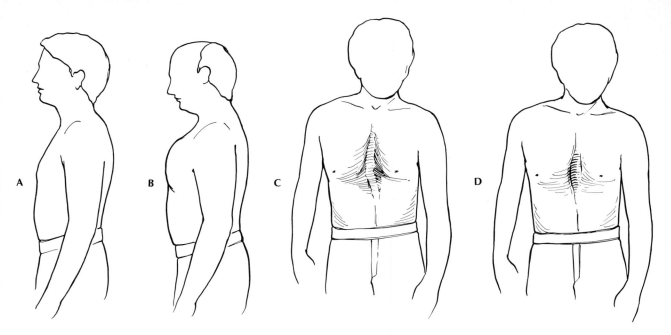

FIGURE 16-5 Abnormalities of the rib cage. **A,** Normal chest. **B,** Barrel chest. **C,** Pigeon breast. **D,** Funnel chest.

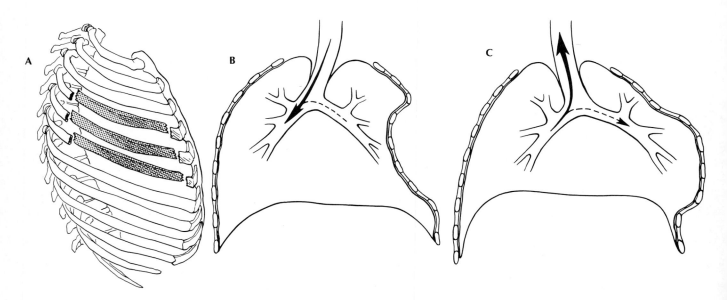

FIGURE 16-6 Paradoxical breathing. **A,** Flail chest injury. **B,** Inspiration. **C,** Exhalation.

phosis *(B)*, or humpback. This condition is best observed by inspecting the patient's back for a lateral bending of the spine as evidenced by different shoulder heights. For example, the right scapula is higher than the left because there are flared interspaces between the ribs on the right side. This lateral curvature of the spine combined with the humpback may distort the lungs, restrict lung volumes, and hinder effective alveolar ventilation.

e Check for *barrel chest* (Fig. 16-5, *B*). This is a condition usually caused by underlying chronic obstruc-

tive lung disease. The chest becomes shaped as though the patient is in a constant state of inspiration, i.e., ribs upward and outward. During inspiration the chest moves as a unit with very little lateral expansion of the chest wall. This condition increases the patient's work of breathing and results in a decreased effectiveness of the chest.

f Check for *"pigeon breast" (C)* and *"funnel chest" (D)*. Observe the relationship of the sternum to the rest of the chest (Fig. 16-5). An anteriorly displaced sternum may cause pigeon chest, or a depression in

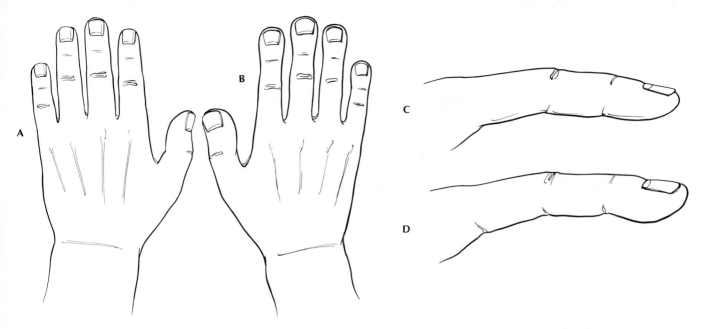

FIGURE 16-7 Digital clubbing. **A,** Normal. **B,** Clubbing. **C,** Normal angle. **D,** Loss of angle.

the sternum may cause funnel chest. Funnel chest may be a genetic condition, or it may possibly be acquired under certain conditions of long standing, e.g., "cobbler's disease." Severe funnel chest may infringe on movement of the lungs and cause decreased lung volumes.

7 Check for *localized flattening* of the chest wall. This condition usually is caused by underlying lung disease, such as fibrosis or long-standing lung collapse.

8 Check for *paradoxical breathing.* This condition is easily identified by the fact that the chest moves "in" on inspiration and "out" on exhalation, i.e., the opposite of what should be occurring. This type of movement may involve the whole chest or any portion where there are two or more ribs fractured, ventral and dorsal. This type of breathing frequently occurs with flail chest injury (Fig. 16-6, *A*) and can cause *pendelluft respiration* (Fig. 16-6, *B* and *C*). When this occurs, a volume of gas moves from one lung to the other during inspiration and exhalation (like a pendulum) instead of in and out of the lungs. This condition causes inadequate alveolar ventilation and can result in hypoxemia and CO_2 buildup.

9 Check for related peripheral signs of lung disease. Long-standing lung disease is reflected by digital clubbing, which is a change in the shape of the tips of the fingers and toes (Fig. 16-7, *A* and *B*). There is a loss of the angle between the nail and the dorsum of the terminal phalanx, and the skin at the base of the nail appears shiny with the tactile appearance of a sponge when gentle pressure is applied (Fig. 16-7, *C* and *D*).

6.0 PALPATION OF THE CHEST
6.1 Concepts involved in palpation of the chest

1 Palpation is the process of using the sense of touch to feel physical signs. It involves feeling for skin temperature, the presence or absence of moisture, motion of the chest, use of the chest, use of the ventilatory muscles, points of tenderness, presence and quality of vibrations, and any crepitus from subcutaneous emphysema.*

2 Palpation, like any other clinical skill, requires that the clinician understand what is normal and abnormal so that a discriminiation of the physical signs and interpretations of the findings can be made.

3 With palpation, the hands are placed flat on the chest to assess its movement and to detect vibratory sensation.

4 Four different techniques can be used to palpate different aspects of the external chest (Fig. 16-8). For example, the fingertips best detect texture; the back of the hand is the most temperature-sensitive.

5 The term "fremitus" means vibration. *Tactile fremitus* is the sense of vibration in the hand when it is laid on the chest and the patient speaks. Fremitus is said to feel like a cat purring. A soft touch usually yields good results.

---

*Procedure 16-3 may be used for practicing palpation of the chest on another person. The reader is encouraged to observe a physician palpate the chest of a patient with a known consolidation and, if possible, practice this technique under the direction of the physician.

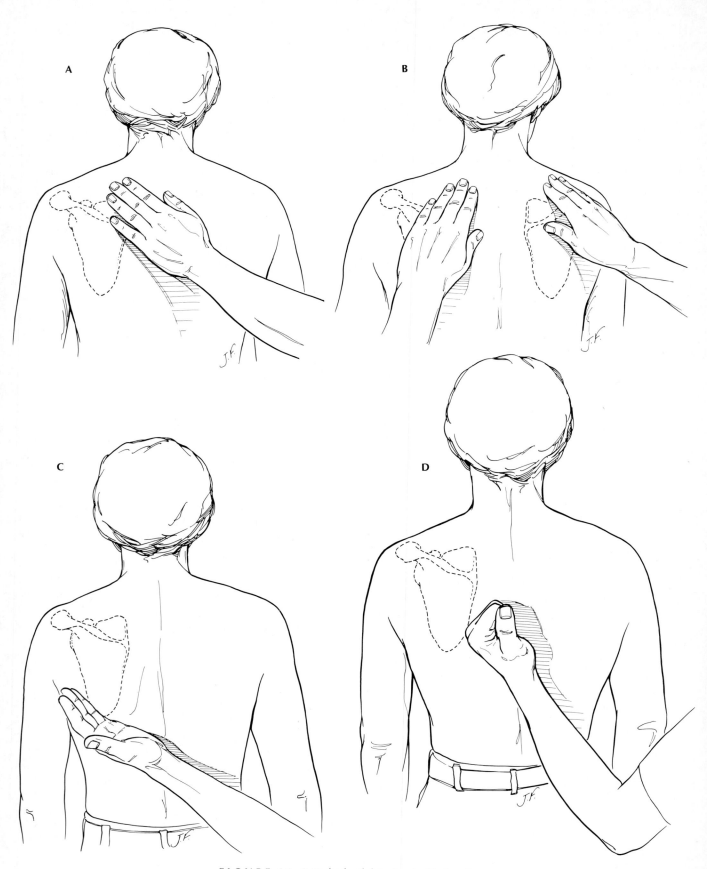

FIGURE 16-8 Methods of detecting tactile fremitus.

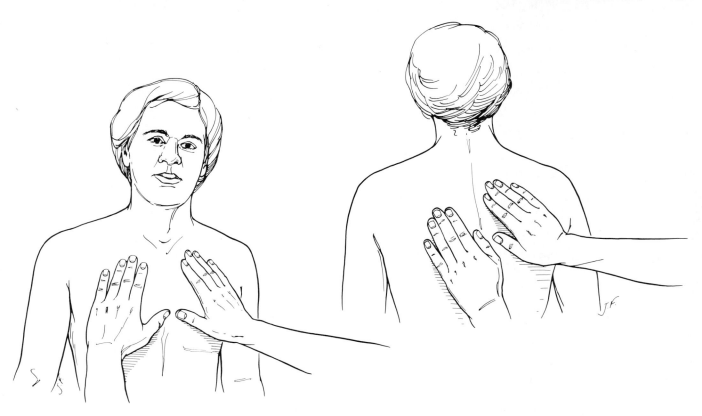

FIGURE 16-9 Anterior and posterior placement of hands to detect bilateral changes in fremitus.

6 The methods of detecting fremitus involve:
a The palm of the hand flat on back or chest (see Fig. 16-8).
b The fingertips of both hands against the skin *(B)*.
c The ulnar side of the hands open against the chest *(C)*.
d The ulnar side of the closed fist against the chest or back *(D)*.

7 Theoretically, fremitus is caused by sounds transmitted from the larynx downward into the bronchi of the lungs. These sounds cause a vibration of the chest wall, known as vocal fremitus, which when felt is called tactile fremitus.

8 To elicit fremitus, the patient should be asked to repeat phrases such as "ninety-nine," "one," or "blue moon." As sounds are made, the examiner routinely checks and compares positions *anteriorly* and *posteriorly* on the patient's chest using the ball of one hand only.

9 *Bilateral position* should be checked and compared for changes in fremitus as the examiner gently but firmly places his or her hands over the chest at specific locations, anteriorly and posteriorly, as indicated by Fig. 16-9.

10 The key to palpation is to recognize *diminished tactile fremitus* that occurs whenever some interposing substance isolates the examiner's hand from the vibrations sent out by the underlying lung. Vibrations are decreased by fluid, pneumothorax, atelectasis, or abnormal tissue masses.

11 The *position of the mediastinum* is also determined by palpation. Normally, the trachea rests in a midline position. In diseases such as pulmonary collapse or fibrosis, the trachea is pulled toward the involved side of the chest. This is opposite from the movement caused by a tension pneumothorax or hemothorax, which forces the trachea away from the involved side.

12 The position of the *trachea* is determined in a patient who is sitting or recumbent by pressing the tip of a fully extended index finger into the suprasternal notch (Fig. 16-10, *A* and *B*). Once it is positioned, the finger is gently pressed downward toward the cervical spine on one side of the notch and then the other. If the trachea is midline, the probing finger will contact only soft tissue. If not, the finger will contact the trachea on the side to which it has shifted.

13 The position of the *apical pulse* also should be determined. Displacement of the pulse beat from its normal position can indicate a mediastinal shift resulting from intrathoracic disease, which causes the heart to move toward the lesion. The normal position for the apical beat is medial to the midclavicular line in the fifth intercostal space (Fig. 16-11). To locate the apical pulse, the lower side of the chest is palpated with the palm of the hand, which is moved progressively from the midaxillary line toward the sternum until the heartbeat is felt *(A* and *B)*. A fingertip of the right hand is placed over the pulsation, and its position is noted by using the left hand to count the rib spaces down from the sec-

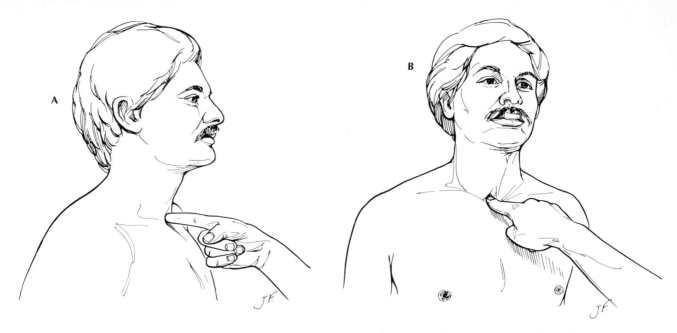

FIGURE 16-10 Detecting the position of the trachea by pressing index finger into suprasternal notch.

ond rib intercostal spaceuntil the level of the right fingertip is reached.

14 An estimated position and movement of the *diaphragm* can be assessed by palpating the posterior area of the back. The level of the diaphragm can be assessed on each side by using the ulnar side of the extended hand held parallel to the expected level of the diaphragm. The hand is then progressively moved downward until no fremitus is felt, which indicates the resting level of the diaphragm. This is repeated for each side of the chest (see Fig. 16-8, *C*). The diaphragm is normally higher on the right side, although abnormally high levels may indicate atelectasis, pleural effusion, or other intrathoracic disease.

15 Movement and symmetry of the *upper and middle lobes* can be assessed by palpation of the superior aspect of the anterior chest. The theory is that diminished distensibility may be one of the earliest clinical signs of underlying pulmonary disease. Chest movement can be assessed by spreading the hands over the area to be evaluated (Fig. 16-12). While the patient breathes quietly, palms and finger surfaces are firmly fixed to the chest wall by pressure so that the skin of the chest is stretched toward the middle of the chest. The thumbs are brought together so that they touch in the middle of the chest during exhalation *(A)*. The patient is then requested to take a deep breath. As inspiration progresses, the examiner's hands and thumbs will move away from each other *(B)*. In the healthy chest the movement of the hands should be equal on both sides.

16 A similar technique can be used to assess excursion of the midthorax *(C and D)*, the posterior thorax *(E and F)*, and the costal margins *(G and H)*. This technique can be used to assess chest movement over the upper lobes anteriorly, the middle lobe and lingual, and posterior lower lobes.

7.0 PERCUSSION OF THE CHEST

7.1 Concepts involved in percussion of the chest

1 Percussion is the process of *listening* to sound produced by tapping on areas of the body, with either the hand or an instrument.

2 The pitch of the sound produced by percussion is determined by the ratio of tissue containing air to solid tissue.

  a Tissue that has *good aeration* will produce a low-pitched resonant sound when the area is struck.

  b *Poorly aerated tissues* or solids will produce a dull, flat note.

3 The sequence for percussion usually begins over healthy tissue and progresses to suspect areas. The best technique is to move the pleximeter (finger on the chest) slowly and continuously through the anterior and posterior aspects of the chest covering the *apex to the base* of each lung (Figs. 16-13 and 16-14).

  If the apex of the lung is the suspected area of involvement, an exception to this sequence is recommended, and the base should be percussed initially.

4 It is essential that percussion be performed in a systematic way and that the percussion sound heard on one side of the chest be compared with that on the corresponding location on the opposite side (see Fig. 16-13).

NOTE: The pitch of the percussion is not the only important consideration. The *intensity* and *duration,* as well as quality, should be considered.

  As previously noted, tones caused by percussion vary in sound characteristics, depending on the amount of air and solid underneath.

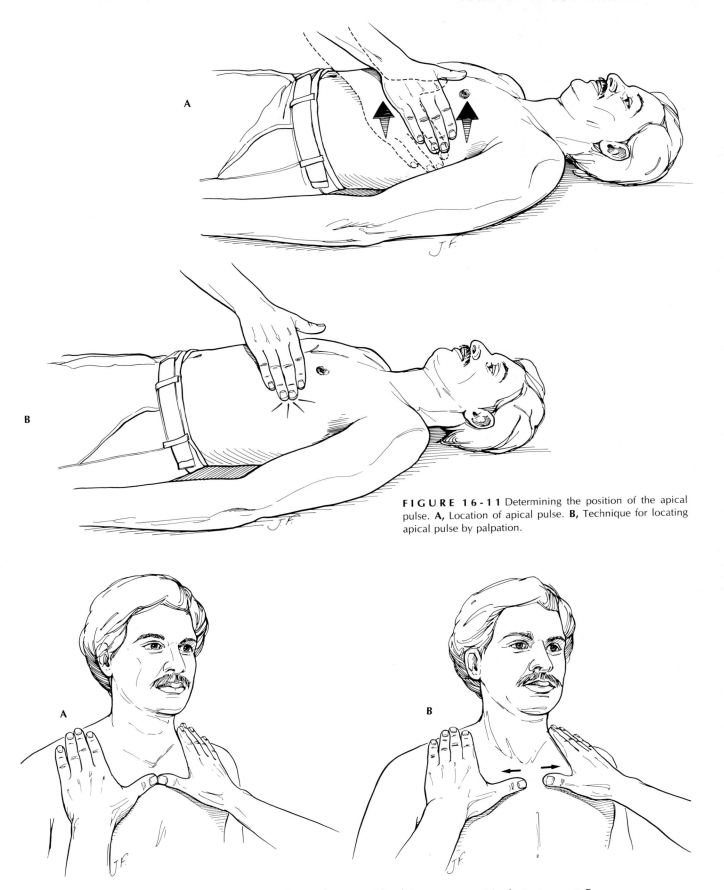

FIGURE 16-11 Determining the position of the apical pulse. A, Location of apical pulse. B, Technique for locating apical pulse by palpation.

FIGURE 16-12 A, Expiration. Proper placement of hands to assess symmetric chest movement. B, Symmetric movement during inspiration.

Continued.

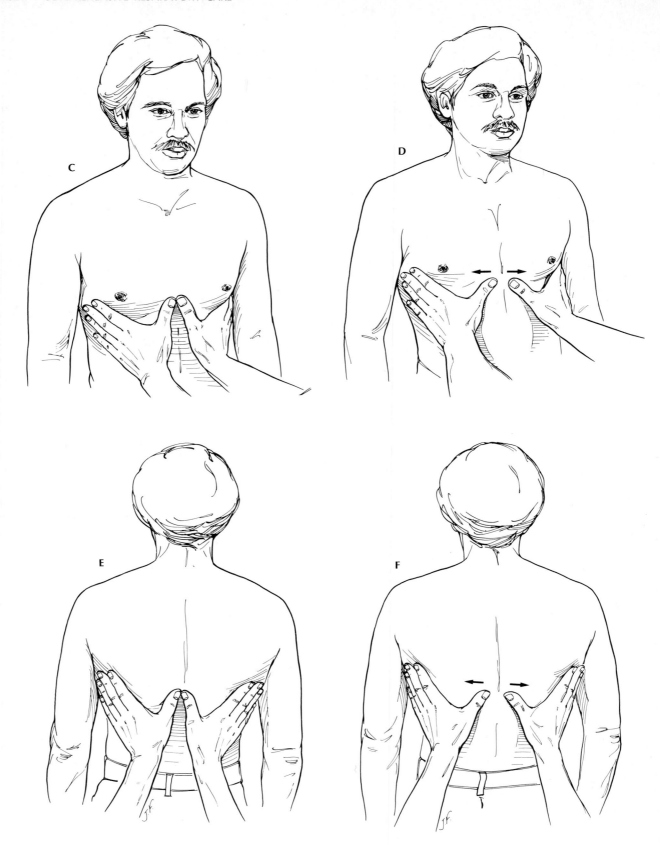

FIGURE 16-12, cont'd. C, Assessing excursion of midthorax expiration. **D,** Inspiration.
E, Posterior thorax expiration. **F,** Inspiration. **G,** Costal margins expiration. **H,** Inspiration.

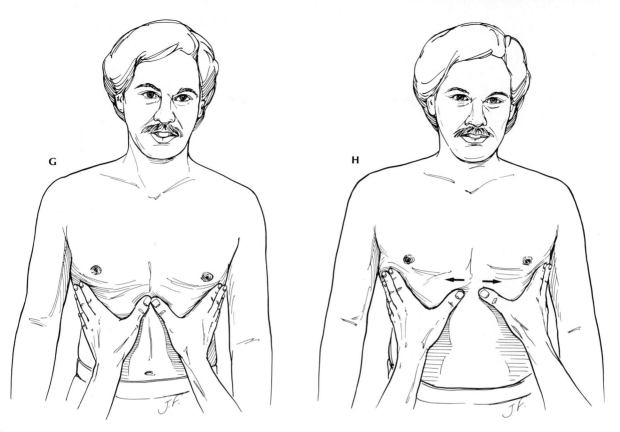

FIGURE 16-12, cont'd For legend see opposite page.

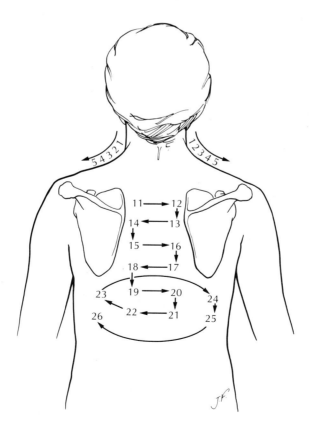

FIGURE 16-13 Technique for percussion of posterior chest.

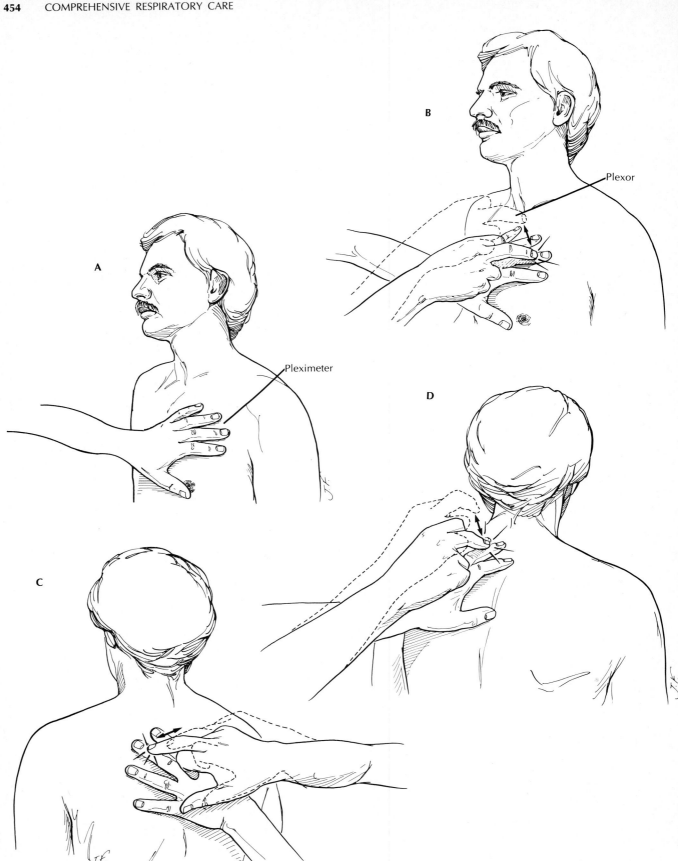

A

Pleximeter

B

Plexor

C

D

FIGURE 16-14 Technique for percussion of anterior and posterior chest.

5 There are five basic percussion notes, each designating different densities of tissue underneath.

  a *Flatness* (absolute dullness) is the term indicating large amounts of solid material. It is a short "dead" sound, as would be heard when percussing a water barrel or water container.

  b *Dullness* is the less dense term from flatness. Between flat and normal lung tissue sound (resonance), it is softer, higher pitched, and shorter in duration than normal resonance. It resembles a "thud." A sense of increased resistance is often left with little or no vibration.

  c *Resonance* is the sound produced by normal lung tissue (not at the apices). It is easily heard, sustained, and low in pitch. This is the basis for determining the other sounds of quality, and only experience can really convey what this sound is like.

  d *Hyperresonance* is of lower pitch, well-sustained, and of a "booming" quality. It may normally be heard in children.

  e *Tympany* is a musical "drumlike" sound heard in the air-filled stomach and abdomen, but it always abnormal if heard in the chest.

6 Percussion is of two types: *mediate* (direct) and *immediate* (indirect).

  a Immediate percussion refers to striking the chest with the flat of the hand or tip of the fingers. It is rarely used.

  b Mediate percussion is the act of striking the finger fixed on the chest (pleximeter) with a percussion hammer or finger (plexor).

7 If the finger is used for percussion of the chest wall, the middle finger of one hand is pressed *firmly* against the chest, parallel to the ribs (in the intercostal spaces).

8 The palm of the hand near the chest should be *off* the skin (see Fig. 16-14, *A* and *B*). The other fingers are preferably held off the skin but may be lightly touching it if the fingers are apart and the same technique is used consistently.

9 Important considerations involved in percussion include:

  a Keeping the percussing finger bent at a right angle.

  b Using as much force as necessary to elicit sound.

  c Using wrist action, not the elbow, to move the striking finger.

  d Using a quick, "piano-hammer" type blow to cause the tip of the middle finger of the right hand to strike the middle finger of the left hand just behind the nail.

10 Positioning the patient for percussion is important. Best results are obtained if the patient is sitting upright for percussion of the lung apices and posterior lung. Proper body support should be used to ensure patient comfort and safety. For maximum results, percussion should be performed only when the patient's muscles are relaxed. Tense muscles decrease the resonant note and may cause a misinterpretation of the sound.

11 If the patient cannot sit up, it is best to position the patient on one side and then the other to examine the posterior chest. Note that while the patient is lying on the side, the area of the lung compressed near the mattress will reflect a dull resonance.

12 Diaphragmatic movement (excursions) can be assessed by percussion over certain areas of the patient's back between the inspiratory and expiratory phases of the breathing cycle. This assessment should be performed while the patient is sitting straight. Other percussion techniques of the back should be performed with the patient bent forward with arms crossed to separate the scapulae (see Fig. 16-14, *C* and *D*).

13 Common mistakes include applying the whole hand over the area to be percussed, which dampens the resonant note, and striking the pleximeter finger too hard. In most instances a soft touch and a soft impact render the best response. It is important to realize that percussion sounds do not penetrate more than 4 to 5 cm below the surface and therefore are not useful in locating deep lesions or other complications.

Procedures 16.4 and 16.5 may be used for performing mediate percussion.

8.0 RECOGNIZING NORMAL AND ABNORMAL BREATH SOUNDS

8.1 Auscultation of the chest

1 Auscultation, along with the patient history and chest radiograph, compose the core of a pulmonary evaluation.

2 Auscultation can provide very useful information regarding lung function. Basically, it is the process of listening to sounds produced by the body itself.

3 Like percussion, auscultation is of two types:

  a Intermediate: use of the unaided ear against the area to be examined.

  b Mediate: use of a stethoscope to pick up and transmit sounds to the examiner's ear.

4 Many inexperienced practitioners are awed by a stethoscope. They feel it is magical and will make sounds louder, thus allowing them to hear and recognize sounds they would otherwise miss.

This is not necessarily the case, for a stethoscope only transmits *unamplified* sounds to the ear.

5 Most stethoscopes are equipped with a bell and a diaphragm. The bell is used to pick up very low-pitched sounds such as certain heart murmurs. The diaphragm picks up low-pitched, as well as high-pitched sounds, and is generally used for examining the chest. A general discussion on the stethoscope is presented in Module Six.

6 The stethoscope chest piece should be clean and hand-warmed before it is placed against the patient's skin.

Once the chest piece is positioned, it must be held firmly and stationary in the area auscultated. Any movement will produce extraneous sounds that may be misinterpreted as breath sounds.

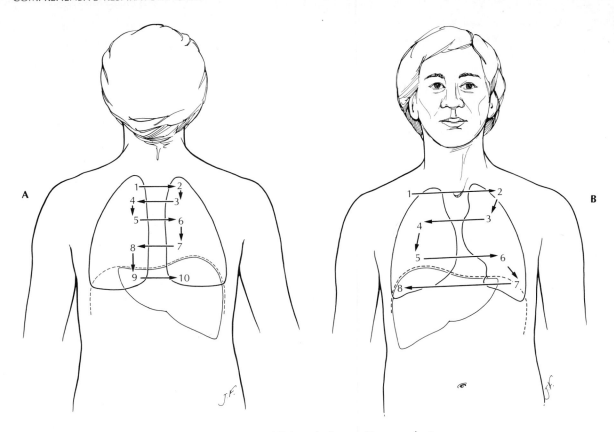

FIGURE 16-15 Auscultation positions on chest.

7 If the diaphragm is used, it must be held tight against the bare skin for best results. If placed over hair areas, it is best to moisten the hair to reduce extraneous sounds.

8 Positioning the patient for auscultation is basically the same as that for percussion.

The sitting position is preferred although the supine patient can be examined, provided the examiner is aware that the posterior lung fields are obscured. In these cases it is best if help is acquired in helping the patient sit up in bed. If this is not possible, the patient should be positioned first on one side and then the other while the upper lung and subsequent areas are auscultated.

9 During auscultation of the chest, the area to be examined *must be bared*. This should be accomplished as modestly as possible, especially with the female patient.

a Have the patient breathe deeply in and out with *mouth open* to minimize nasal and throat sounds. Listen to a *full* breathing cycle (inspiration and expiration) at each location.

b Work from *top* to *bottom* of the chest while comparing the sounds heard on one side to those heard at the same location on the opposite side.

c Auscultate posterior chest areas first and then the anterior chest according to the positions presented in Fig. 16-15, *A* and *B*.

10 In addition to positioning of the patient, the room must be quiet. The examiner must concentrate only on the sounds heard, and the patient must be constantly instructed as to desired breathing patterns.

Procedure 16-6 may be used for auscultating the posterior and anterior chest with a stethoscope.

8.2 Interpretation of breath sounds

The beginner need not become overwhelmed by the long list of terms used to describe auscultatory findings. It is more important to learn to differentiate between the *presence* and *absence* of sounds in an area and the difference between *normal* and *abnormal* breath sounds.

It is recommended that the reader practice listening for normal breath sounds on himself or herself and on another person.

NOTE: It is important during this initial learing period to work with an experienced clinician until normal sounds for specific locations can be recognized and agreement can be reached as to what is a normal versus abnormal sound.

1 One way of learning to differentiate between normal and abnormal sound is to use a teaching stethoscope (one with a single chest piece but two sets of earpieces), which enables the reader and partner to listen simultaneously to a sound. Still another method is to use a separate stethoscope but have the experienced partner assist the reader in placing the stethoscope and identifying normal breath sounds.

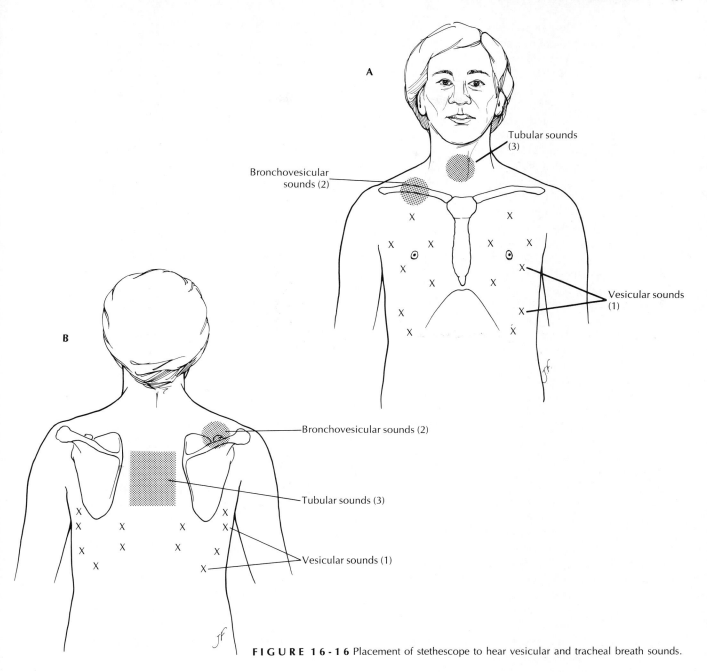

Bronchovesicular
sounds (2)

Tubular sounds
(3)

Vesicular sounds
(1)

Bronchovesicular sounds (2)

Tubular sounds (3)

Vesicular sounds (1)

FIGURE 16-16 Placement of stethoscope to hear vesicular and tracheal breath sounds.

Normal breath sounds are a reflection of the noise created by air as it passes through the larynx. This sound varies in *intensity* (loudness) and in *rhythm,* depending on the distance between the stethoscope and the larynx. Normal breath sounds are categorized as vesicular and tracheal (bronchial) breathing.

Vesicular breathing is described as a gentle rustling sound, much like the rustling of leaves in a gentle breeze, and is heard over the entire chest wall except for the right supraclavicular area, where *bronchovesicular* sounds are present. It is loudest during inspiration and quickly diminishes and disappears early during exhalation. Exhalation is normally heard for about one third the length of time as inspiration.

a Place the stethoscope chest piece over the axillary region of your own chest or a partner's, and listen for vesicular breath sounds (Fig. 16-16, *A* and *B* *[1]).* Vesicular sounds are normal and should be easily heard throughout the chest but especially in areas close to central airways.

b Place the stethoscope chest piece over the right supraclavicular region of your own or a partner's chest, and listen for bronchovesicular breath sounds (Fig. 16-16, *A* and *B [2]).* These normally occur in this region because of the close proximity of the bronchi of the apex of the right lung to the surface of the chest.

Tubular breath sounds (also known as bronchial

sounds) (see Fig. 16-16, *A* and *B*) are louder and higher pitched than bronchovesicular sounds and appear to be closer to the ear. These sounds are normally heard over the trachea and main stem bronchi (Fig. 16-16, *A* and *B* [3]). Bronchial sounds are identified as having inspiratory and expiratory notes that are equal in pitch, loudness (intensity), and duration and separated by a *period of silence.*

- Bronchovesicular and bronchial sounds are very similar except that there is *no pause* between inspiration and exhalation in bronchovesicular sounds.
- Bronchial sounds are *not* normal when heard in other areas of the lung. They usually indicate consolidation, collapse, or fibrous disease. These types of pathologies result in an increased transmission of sounds from the large airway to the periphery.

c Place the stethoscope chest piece over your own trachea or your partner's and listen for tubular (bronchial) breath sounds (see Fig. 16-16, *A* and *B [3]*).

2 Abnormal sounds include the following:

a *Adventitious breath sounds,* such as crackles, wheezes, and pleural rubs, are caused by the presence of disease, foreign materials, or Glasgow's sign.

b *Crackles (rales)* are discrete, disconnected, bubbling, or crackling sounds that are heard most clearly during inspiration. Coarse rales are caused by an excessive amount of fluid, such as pulmonary edema, and may be heard with the unaided ear. Edema may actually be seen spilling from the patient's nose, mouth, or tracheal tube. Rale-like sounds can be created by rolling dry hair strands together close to the ear.

- Descriptive terms for crackles include crepitant, sonorous, small, medium, moist, or dry. Crackles are probably caused by the sudden equalization of pressure within airways during inspiration.

c *Wheezes* are low- or high-pitched musical sounds that may occur on inspiration or exhalation. The pitch of the wheezes will vary according to the degree of narrowing and the location of the partial obstruction. Generally, inspiratory wheezes are lower in pitch than expiratory wheezes because of the higher airway resistance that usually occurs with exhalation.

- Descriptive terms for wheezes include high-pitched, sibilant, musical, low, and sonorous.

d *Pleural friction rub* is an abnormal creaking, grating, or clicking sound caused by the friction that occurs between layers of pleura as they attempt to slide one over the other during the breathing process. Pleural rubs occur during both inspiration and exhalation and are generally localized to the involved area of the chest. Pleural rubs are frequently associated with *pleurisy,* causing the patient to experience a great deal of pain throughout the breathing process. Pleural rubs are most frequently heard in the lower regions of the chest and very seldom occur in the upper areas.

e A *splash* is the sound made by air and fluid in the pleural space. This sound can be detected by gently shaking the thoracic cage.

8.3 Bronchophony and egophony

Voice sounds (resonance) used in conjunction with auscultation can assist the examiner in identifying the presence of thickening of tissues and consolidation within the chest cavity. Words such as "one, one, one," "blue, blue, blue," or "ninety-nine" can be used.

1 The technique of using voice sounds in the presence of altered pathology is called *bronchophony.*

a Spoken words are transmitted loudly, but indistinctly, through the chest wall when heard through a stethoscope.

b Bronchophony is normal in areas between the scapula and sides of the sternum (where bronchovesicular breath sounds are common) but abnormal in other locations. This technique is most useful for evaluating areas that have bronchial breath sounds.

c Increases in loudness combined with an increased voice clarity indicate peripheral consolidation or peribronchial edema.

2 *Egophony* is a term describing an increased amplitude and transmission of low-frequency spoken sounds resulting in a change of the sound to the listener. For example, a low-frequency spoken *e* in the presence of segmental or lobar consolidation will sound like a higher frequency *a* with a nasal tone when heard through a stethoscope.

Whispered voice sounds also can be used to detect the absence or presence of segmental or lobar consolidation. In the healthy lung whispered sounds are *not* heard. Whispered *pectoriloquy* is an increase in the loudness of the whispered sentence so that it is clearly heard through the stethoscope placed over a specific area of the chest.

8.4 Other abnormal sounds heard through a stethoscope*

1 *Cogwheel breathing.* Breath sounds that have numerous interruptions or pauses between inspiration and exhalation. This breathing pattern is frequently associated with tuberculosis and is heard in the apical regions of the lung.

2 *Succussion sounds.* Splashing sounds caused by air and fluid in an enclosed cavity or when the bowel has herniated through the diaphragm.

3 *Coin-click sounds.* Metallic, bell-like sound produced by striking the edge of one coin against another, which is held flat against the patient's chest while sounds are auscultated by a stethoscope placed on the opposite chest wall.

8.5 Pulmonary conditions causing abnormal breath sounds

Abnormal bronchial breath sounds are heard in patients with severe consolidation or cavitation of lung tissue.

1 Sounds such as crackles are usually caused by fluid or secretions in the alveoli and air passages.

2 Wheezes are caused by situations of increased resistance to airflow into or out of the lungs and indicate

---

*The reader is encouraged to make rounds with an experienced practitioner to listen to the breath sounds discussed in this module.

T A B L E 1 6 - 1 Identification of pulmonary condition by physical assessment

Pulmonary condition	Inspection	Palpation	Percussion	Auscultation
Atelectasis with open bronchus (pneumonia)	Decreased excursion on side, "grunting," lying on side of disease	Increased tactile fremitus	Decreased resonance	Bronchial breath sounds, right, vocal fremitus increased
Atelectasis with obstructed bronchus (tumor)	Decreased excursion on side, tracheal shift to side affected	Decreased tactile fremitus	Decreased resonance	Decreased breath sounds, vocal fremitus decreased
Pneumothorax (collapsed lung)	Trachea shifted away from side affected	Decreased tactile fremitus	Increased resonance	Decreased breath sounds, vocal fremitus decreased
Hydrothorax	Trachea shifted away from side affected	Decreased tactile fremitus	Decreased resonance	Decreased breath sounds, rales above, bronchial breathing above, vocal fremitus decreased
Obstructed airways	Prolonged expiration, pursed-lip breathing, "grunting"	Decreased tactile fremitus	Increased resonance	Decreased breath sounds, expiratory wheezes, vocal fremitus decrease
Asthma	Prolonged expiration, pursed-lip breathing, "grunting" (in acute episode)			
Upper airway: crushed trachea, secretions	Stridor, rib retraction on inspiration			Tracheal noises, inspiratory and expiratory
Flail chest	Paradoxical motion on side, tracheal shift during respiration	Pain on side (rib fracture), tactile fremitus variable	Decreased resonance	Decreased breath sounds on side, vocal fremitus variable

partially obstructed small-to-medium size airways.

3 Pleural rubs are identified by a creaking leathery sound. These sounds are caused by inflammation of the pleurae.

4 Bronchophony is caused by consolidation in the periphery of the lung.

Table 16-1 presents additional pulmonary conditions and correlated effects as detected by physical examination of the chest.

A summary of the various types of breath sounds, their causes, and their location is presented in Table 16-2.

Procedure 16-7 may be used for performing a complete chest physical assessment, incorporating patient interview, inspection, palpation, percussion, and auscultation on another student and, with supervision, on selected patients.

9.0 ROENTGENOGRAPHY AS A USEFUL DIAGNOSTIC TOOL

9.1 Development of x-ray photography (roentgenography)

1 The development of roentgenography was closely related to experimentation with electrical current. Sir William Crookes, an English physicist, discovered that application of a high voltage current to the sealed electrodes of a glass vacuum tube caused an invisible radiation that produced a ghostly glow where it struck the glass.

a This cathode-ray tube led to additional experiments so that in 1895 Wilhelm Roentgen, a German physicist, discovered that cathode rays, after striking a metal target and being reflected, give rise to radiation. In 1901 Roentgen received the first Nobel prize in physics for his findings.

b Characteristics of these rays of radiation were that they exposed photographic plates, were not affected by a magnet, and could penetrate objects. Because of their mysterious nature, the new rays were named "x-rays" after the algebraic unknown factor x. Since their discovery, x-ray beams have been used in industry and in medicine as a method of identifying internal structures.

2 X-ray film is a photographic film mounted on a metal plate that is positioned so that the x-ray beam will pass through the object and strike the plate, exposing the film. The greater the strength of the beam, the darker the x-ray film. Application of this principle explains light and dark contrasts seen on a roentgenkymogram (x-ray film).

a As the x-ray beam passes through the various body structures, it is partially absorbed before it reaches the film plate. The degree to which it is absorbed by each structure varies the strength of the beam, causing it to expose the film plate accordingly. This varying intensity causes the film to form light and dark images much like an object casts a shadow when it blocks the sun.

b The difference between a shadow and x-ray image is that in the case of the x-ray image, the greater the exposure, the less dense the structure; the stronger the x-ray beam, the darker the image on the film.

9.2 Useful radiologic terms

1 Angiography. A procedure in which a radiopaque substance is injected into the blood so that it can be traced through the pulmonary circulation during exposure to

TABLE 16-2 Various breath sounds

Breath sounds	Description	Mechanism	Location	Pathology
Tracheobronchial	E louder than I; general background rumble with spitting overlay	Air turbulence in trachea	Sternum, parasternal, mid-scapular	Normal
Bronchial	E louder than I; generally less amplitude (softer than tracheal B.S.)	Air turbulence in large bronchi	Parasternal, midscapular	Normal*
Normal vesicular	I louder than E; rustle of leaves in a tree	Air vortex (swirls) in smaller airways	Diffus—peripheral	Normal
Diminished vesicular	Same as vesicular but decreased loudness	Air vortex (swirls) in smaller airways	Local to pathology	Decreased local ventilation; pleural effusion or pneumothorax
Harsh vesicular	Same as vesicular but increased loudness and more spitting noises	Air vortex (swirls) in smaller airways; also question of secretions in airway	Local to pathology	Consolidation—may be incomplete
Bronchovesicular	Both bronchial and vesicular together, I and E have *equal* loudness	Increased conduction of bronchial sounds	Local to pathology	Consolidation—may be incomplete
Amphoric breathing	Hollow reverberating quality but with high pitched (ringing) overtones	Air flow in airways near stiff-walled cavity	Local to pathology	Cavity

ADVENTITIOUS BREATH SOUNDS

Crackling	Short, burst of noise, primarily in I	Popping of bubbles and/or opening of small airways	Local to pathology—mostly at bases	Fibrosis, CHF, pulmonary edema, alveolar protenosis, peripneumonic
Fibrotic	High frequency (like hair rubbing together)			
Peripneumonic and CHF	Medium frequency			
Pulmonary edema	Low frequency (both I and E)			
Wheeze	Prolonged sound—E more than I but can be both; often musical. The higher pitched are from smaller airways	Air current at point of airway bifurcation	Local to pathology	Airway constriction
Rub	Low pitched, duration is very specific—often at end inspiration	Pleural surfaces rubbing together	Local to pathology	Pleural inflammation or mass

Modified from Mitchell RS and Olson DE: History and physical examination in patients with pulmonary problems, unpublished manuscript, 1979.
E, Expiration; I, inspiration; B.S., breath sounds; CHF, congestive heart failure.
*When this sound is conducted to peripheral lung fields, it is termed "bronchial breathing" and strongly suggests consolidation.

x-rays. This test helps identify the presence or absence of pulmonary emboli.

2 Anteroposterior (AP). Describes the route of the x-rays through the chest from *front to back*.

3 Bronchography. The use of radiopaque substances that are injected directly into the lung before taking an x-ray film. This technique clearly shows the patency of bronchial branching.

4 Bronchoscopy. Direct visual inspections of the trachea and bronchi using a rigid bronchoscope or a smaller and more flexible fiberoptic bronchoscope.

5 Bullae (blebs). Air-filled, dark areas (radiolucent) surrounded by normal tissue.

6 Cavity. A dark spot surrounded by lighter tissue, usually indicating a lung abscess.

7 Consolidation. Well-defined light areas in the lung field, usually caused by pneumonia or other related fluids.

8 Homogenous density. A term describing thick masses such as a tumor, blood, or fluid in the chest.

9 Infiltration. A general term describing spotted or diffuse white areas in a lung field. These infiltrated areas are usually caused by disease or irritation.

10 Interstitial density. A thickening appearance of the interstitial tissue of the lung, which has a cobweb appearance or that of ground glass.

11 Lateral (right or left). Describes x-rays that pass from one side of the chest to the other, causing a lateral (side) view of the chest on film.

12 Nodule. A term describing an individually clustered or a single isolated circular density.

13 Pleural density. A term describing thickening of the pleura caused by fluid, inflammation, or trauma.

14 Posteroanterior (PA). Describes the route of the x-rays through the chest from *back to front*.

15 Radiodensity. A term describing the opposite effect of

radiolucency, i.e., dense shadows that appear whiter on film.

16 Roentgenogram. The formal term for x-ray.

17 Stereoscope films. Simultaneous pictures of the lung, allowing the viewer to see the image as three-dimensional.

18 Tomogram. A special x-ray procedure involving radiographing a single plane whose thickness can be varied. This allows specific identification of structures or objects at different levels within the lung, which is not possible using a standard x-ray technique.

19 Translucency (radiolucency). A term describing the depth to which x-rays are able to penetrate the chest.

9.3 The use of roentgenography for chest examination

1 The chest is an ideal region for x-ray examination because air-filled lungs offer little resistance to the x-ray beam, therefore exposing the film and creating very clear dark images. These relatively dark shadows can be easily contrasted to the lighter images caused by the soft tissues and bones of the thoracic wall, the heart, great vessels, and diaphragm.

2 Before studying a chest radiograph, one should understand how to determine the degree of film darkness in terms of *density* and the appearance and location of the heart and lungs in a normal film.

9.4 Determining degrees of film darkness in terms of densities

1 Although already presented, the following terms are specifically useful when describing the degree of darkness in a radiograph.

　a *Radiolucent* is a term meaning the x-rays pass through the material, causing the x-ray film to appear darker in these exposed areas.

　b *Radiopaque* is a term relating to material that absorbs or will *not* allow passage of x-rays, causing the film to appear light (white).

2 Densities of tissues range from most radiolucent to radiopaque, including *air density* (radiolucent), *fat density* (medium radiolucency), *water density* (skin, heart tissue), *bone* (calcium), which is radiopaque, and *metal* which is the most radiopaque.

10.0 PROPER POSITIONING
10.1 Positioning the patient for roentgenograms

1 Roentgenograms are taken of the patient in different positions. A *standard* chest film is taken at a distance of 6 feet from the front of the upright patient during a *maximum* inspiration. The x-rays penetrate the chest from back to front.

　This position is called the *posteroanterior* (PA) view (Fig. 16-17, *A*, p. 462).

2 For a portable film at the bedside, an *anteroposterior* (AP) view (Fig. 16-18 on p. 464) is usually taken at a shorter distance. This produces a better contrast of the shadows of the thoracic cage and mediastinum than does a standard film.

3 Under certain situations, a right or left lateral film may also be taken to give the viewer a more isolated image of the right or left lung (Fig. 16-19 on p. 465). At least two different views are required to allow better viewing of the superimposed structures within the chest and to better pinpoint specific lesions.

4 It is important that the patient's body is in a straight position. Otherwise the trachea may appear deviated to one side or the other and thus mistakenly suspected of abnormality. If the patient is positioned properly (i.e., straight position), the distance between the ends of the clavicles and the spinal column will be equal when the film is viewed (see Figs. 16-17, *A* and 16-18).

5 It is also important that the film be taken during a maximum inspiration. Films taken during exhalation will appear cloudy and may give appearance of disease that is *not* present.

　An inspiratory film should show the lung well-aerated and the diaphragm descended to about the tenth rib level.

11.0 PROCEDURES FOR REVIEWING CHEST FILMS
11.1 Reading chest films*

1 A review of considerations regarding the reading of chest films includes the following principles:

　a *Lungs* with air have the *least* density and appear black, or nearly so.

　b Areas of the lung without air, or with lesions, will appear lighter than uninvolved well-aerated areas.

　c *Tissue structures* such as the heart, blood vessels, mediastinum, lymph nodes, and the diaphragm absorb some x-ray but allow more to pass than do bones, causing a gray shadow on the film.

　d Structures that are the *most dense* block or absorb most of the x-ray and therefore do not expose the film. This causes the images of these structures to appear whiter on the developed film.

　　• *Bones* are very dense, impeding the passage of x-ray and appearing white on the film.

　　• Metal appears the whitest. This may be densities resulting from surgical clips or wire, dental fillings, or jewelry.

2 The *first step* in reading a radiograph (see Fig. 16-17, *D*) is to verify the patient's name and number, which usually appear on one corner of the film *(1)* and on the folder containing the film.

3 The *second step* is to place the film on the viewing screen so that when the viewer faces the film, the right side of the patient's chest will be to the viewer's left and the left side of the patient's chest to the viewer's right *(2)*.

　The left side of the chest is easily identified because the major portion of the heart lies to the left *(3)*. Also, the film is usually marked with the letters *L* or *R*, indicating the right or left side of the patient.

---

*The reader is encouraged to obtain a *normal PA chest film* to view while studying this section.

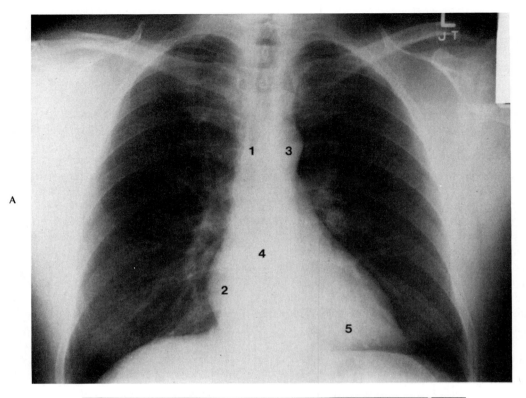

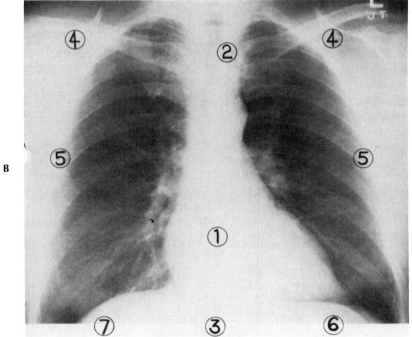

FIGURE 16-17 Positioning of patient for posteroanterior (PA) chest roentgenogram.

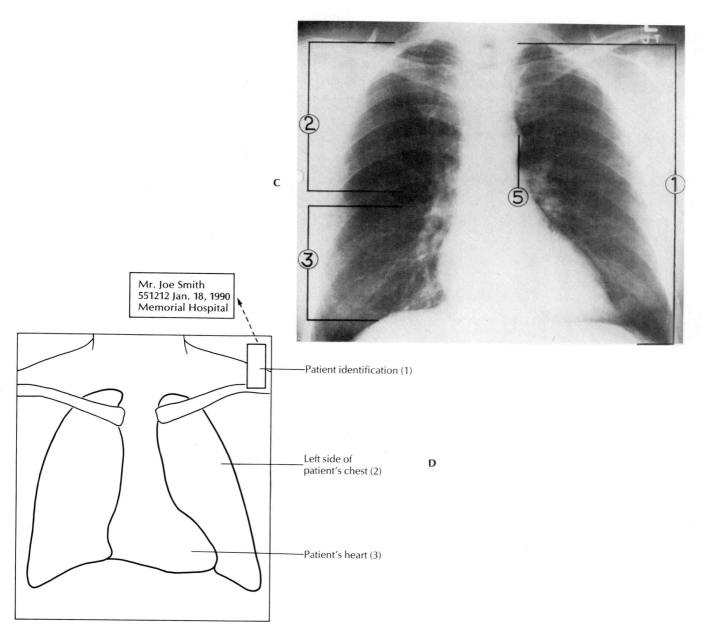

C

D

Mr. Joe Smith
551212 Jan. 18, 1990
Memorial Hospital

Patient identification (1)

Left side of
patient's chest (2)

Patient's heart (3)

FIGURE 16-17, cont'd For legend see opposite page.

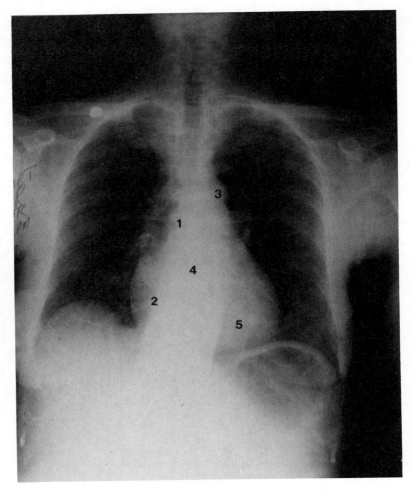

FIGURE 16-18 Positioning of patient for anteroposterior (AP) chest roentgenogram.

4 The *third step* is to identify and distinguish basic soft tissues of the chest surrounding the bony thorax and to inspect the white bony structures of counting ribs and looking for fractures, deformities, or lesions. Lung fields, pleurae, the heart, and mediastinal areas should also be examined.

  a Identify specific soft tissue shapes such as breast shadows (female) and each side of the diaphragm.

  b Note any abnormalities, and describe them according to location, density, size, shape, and influence on the lung and related structures.

5 The sequence of examination of an x-ray film will vary from one viewer to another. However, the most important aspect is that one use the same pattern of reviewing all films. In summary, the following simple viewing sequence may be useful for the beginning practitioner:

  a Soft tissues
  b Thoracic cage
  c Diaphragm
  d Mediastinum
  e Lung fields

11.2 Looking at soft tissues of the external chest

1 Soft tissue outside the thoracic cage can cause shadows that may confuse the viewer who is not aware of their normal presence.

2 Most of the shadows caused by external soft tissue can be easily traced as extending beyond the thoracic cage. These tissues include muscles of the chest, the breasts, and nipple shadows.

3 Breast markings are most easily distinguished on the lateral film.

11.3 Looking at the thoracic cage

1 The bony thorax should be examined for evidence of spinal deformity and/or any differences in the pattern of the rubs on either side.

2 Bones should be examined for signs of trauma, fractures, or erosion. Erosion can be caused by pressure exerted on the bone by tumors, osteomyelitis, or from enlarged arteries such as the aorta.

3 The ribs and clavicles should appear white but somewhat lighter than the heart or other tissue structures of the chest.

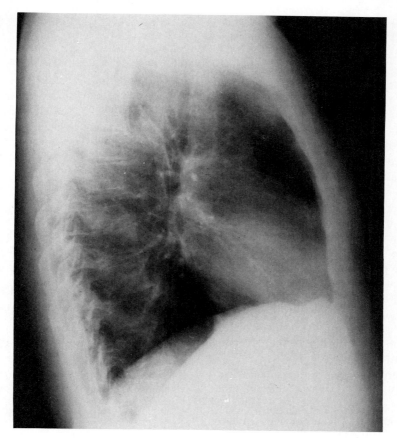

F I G U R E   1 6 - 1 9 Positioning of patient for lateral chest roentgenogram.

11.4 Assessing the diaphragm

1 In a posteroanterior (PA) film, the diaphragm should appear as a rounded and domed white shadow at about the level of the anterior end of the sixth rib. This shadow is not caused by the diaphragm but by air or another contrast medium that may be on either side of it.

2 Both hemidiaphragms (right and left side) should be compared for height, contour, and sharpness of their angles to the verticle chest wall and any unusual structures that may indicate a hernia or growth. The angles of the diaphragm may be obscured by pleural effusion. Specific medical conditions may cause one hemidiaphragm to lie abnormally high when compared to the other.

3 Note that the dome of the diaphragm on the right side normally rests 1 to 2 cm higher than the left during all phases of respiration. Elevation of one hemidiaphragm can be caused by lung collapse, abscess, damage to the phrenic nerve, spinal misalignment, or even gas in the stomach.

4 Other diseases, such as emphysema, may cause the diaphragm to appear flattened throughout the respiratory cycle, indicating restricted diaphragmatic movement.

11.5 Assessing the mediastinum

1 The mediastinum (containing the heart and great vessels) is denser than the surrounding aerated lungs and does not allow passage of as much x-ray. Thus this area appears as gray shadow on the x-ray film.

2 When looking at the mediastinum, the viewer first notes the position and width of the trachea. Normally, the trachea is midline at the top and a little to the right at its base. Misalignment of the trachea may result from growths or intrathoracic pressure caused by a tension pneumothorax.

3 The heart's position, width, contour, and size are compared to the inner thoracic diameter.

4 The cardiac shadow on an anteroposterior (AP) or posteroanterior (PA) film should be seen as a white structure in the midline of the chest, with the left heart borders easily determined.

5 Assessment of hypertrophy (enlargement) of the heart is dependent on the film quality and the position in which it was taken. For example, a portable film, an AP film, or one not at full inspiration will exaggerate heart side. In a good PA film taken on an erect patient, the horizontal width of the base of the heart should be less than one half the width of the chest.

6 The cardiovascular silhouette is composed of the pericardial, cardiac, great vessel, and mediastinal structures. It normally varies greatly in size and shape (but not in position) among different patients.

7 The main mass of the heart rests to the left of the midline of the chest, although this varies according to the size of the patient. For example, tall, thin patients usually have a narrow heart, centrally located, whereas short, fat people usually have a horizontally located heart with a pronounced left border.

8 The borders of the heart shadow (see Figs. 16-17, *A*, and 16-18) are outlined on the right by the superior vena cava in the upper thorax *(1)*, by the right atrium in the lower half *(2)*, by the aortic knob *(3)*, main pulmonary artery trunk in the middle *(4)*, and the left ventricle below *(5)*. The left atrium lies just below the shadow caused by the pulmonary artery trunk.

9 On an AP film taken at full inspiration, a diagnosis can be confirmed by fluid levels, lung markings, and heart size.

10 As previously stated, a normal heart size should be less than one half the width across the chest. More than this is usually indicative of heart failure, in which case the lung will appear hyperinflated (chronic obstructive pulmonary disease—COPD) with very dark densities and decreased vascular markings, or the lung will have more water density, noted as a butterfly-shaped central whiteness of infiltrates in the lung fields.

11.6 Assessing lung fields

1 In a posteroanterior (PA) chest film (see Fig. 16-17, *B*) the heart *(1)*, vertebrae *(2)*, and areas below the diaphragm *(3)* should appear white.

2 The clavicles *(4)* and ribs *(5)* should be white but somewhat lighter than the heart *(1)*, stomach *(6)*, and liver *(7)*.

3 In Fig. 16-17, *C*, the lungs *(1)* appear dark with apical areas *(2)* having fewer vascular markings (white streaks) than the bases *(3)*.

4 The carina *(4)* is often visible at about the level of the fourth vertebra, which is near the area of the aortic knob *(5)* of the heart.

5 Note that lung density should appear equal on both sides. Lung fissures are not normally visible. Under some conditions, the right transverse fissure may be visible in the right upper lobe. The azygous vein may resemble a fissure as it crosses the lung field.

6 Bronchi are not usually visible in a standard chest film beyond the point of the main stem bronchi. Pulmonary veins and lymphatics vary in size and sharpness. Background lung density is normally a result of the presence of blood in the pulmonary capillaries, whereas larger vessels cause visible lung markings.

7 The hili or lung roots are poorly defined in the superior central portion of the lung fields. The hilar markings are comprised of the pulmonary blood vessels, the bronchi, and lymph nodes.

8 The lung pleurae normally do not cast a shadow except

when there is inflammation or excess fluid between them.

11.7 Artifacts that influence chest films

1 As in an electrocardiogram (ECG), chest films may have artifacts that can distract and mislead a viewer into making a false diagnosis.

2 Common artifacts include:
   a Hair or braids overlapping pulmonary apices
   b Shadows caused by breast nipples
   c Clothing
   d Metal objects
   e Warts
   f Marks caused by improper film handling
   g Incomplete film development
   h Opaque media in or under the radiographic table

12.0 SIGNS OF CARDIOPULMONARY DISEASE THAT MAY APPEAR ON CHEST FILMS

12.1 Air bronchogram

1 The *air bronchogram sign* appears on films as black tubular bronchi.

2 Normally, bronchi are *not* visible because they are air-filled and do not present enough density to block or absorb x-ray beams.

3 As the bronchi become filled with water, blood, or other fluids and infiltrates, they become more dense and create a white-to-gray shadow on film. This allows the viewer to differentiate between bronchi containing pneumonia, infarcts, pulmonary edema, bronchiectasis, and other causes that increase bronchial density and are not visible in healthy structures.

12.2 Signs of cardiopulmonary disease: the cardiac silhouette sign

1 The silhouette sign results when a border of the heart, aorta, or diaphragm comes into contact with a condition causing increased fluid density to the degree that it obliterates that portion of the structure's silhouette.

2 For example, the heart border is adjacent to the right middle lobe, lingula, and anterior basal segments of the lung. Collapse of all or any one of these lung areas could create a density similar to the water density of the heart.

3 The even density (i.e., lack of contrast) would obscure one of the heart borders and make it difficult to see where the heart ends and lung tissue begins. This would indicate that an area of diseased lung is present in that specific location.

12.3 Changes caused by atelectasis and pneumothorax

1 Collapse of alveoli can be caused by many different types of medical complications. Collapse may be of small areas, a segment, or a whole lobe or lung (Fig. 16-20).

2 Atelectasis is derived from the Greek, meaning "imperfect expansion." Medically, it is applied to conditions

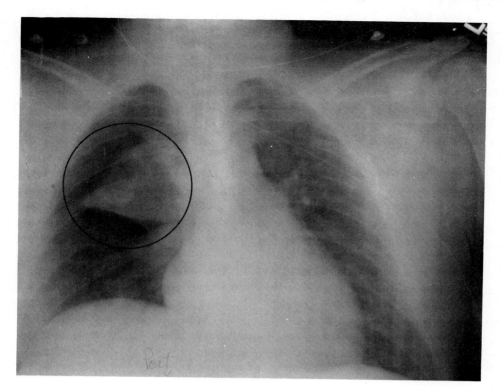

F I G U R E   1 6 - 2 0 Chest radiograph showing atelectasis.

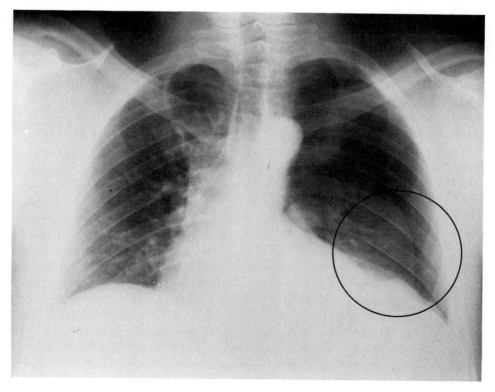

F I G U R E   1 6 - 2 1 Chest radiograph showing a pneumothorax.

where alveoli in specific areas of the lung have become airless and collapsed.

3 Pneumothorax means free gas within the pleural space, which is normally airless. Air in this space causes pressure on adjacent lung tissues with subsequent incomplete expansion (Fig. 16-21).

4 Atelectasis and pneumothorax can be caused by the obstruction of air passages, compression of alveoli, and contraction of alveoli.

5 Collapse of an airless lung lobe or segment would appear on film as a white density (see Figs. 16-20 and 16-21). If air is trapped within the collapsed space, the film, because of decreased density of air, should present very dark areas with no vascular markings in the involved areas.

6 Diseases that can cause atelectasis or pneumothorax are:

  a Mucus-producing diseases, combined with restrictive or obstructive pathologies
  b Pneumonitis, pneumonia
  c Asbestosis, silicosis

12.4 Changes caused by respiratory distress syndrome

1 Respiratory distress syndrome (RDS) involves a plate-like or miliary atelectasis that neither appears immediately on chest radiograph nor, on treatment, shows immediate improvement in the patient's condition.

2 As atelectasis worsens, a fluffy and cottonlike appearance occurs in the lung. This indicates that lung areas have collapsed and that measures need to be taken to prevent further alveolar collapse if the patient is to improve.

13.0 IDENTIFICATION OF SPECIAL SITUATIONS
13.1 Identifying critical situations by roentgenogram

1 Respiratory care personnel are not required or expected to diagnose cardiopulmonary conditions through roentgenography. However, it is reasonable to expect the ability to look at a chest film and quickly and accurately identify the following:

  a A normal chest—PA view (see Fig. 16-17, *B*).
  b A normal lateral chest (see Fig. 16-19).
  c Atelectasis (see Fig. 16-20).
  d A pneumothorax (see Fig. 16-21).
  e A misplaced tracheal tube (see Fig. 16-22).
  f Acute pneumonia (see Fig. 16-23).
  g Pulmonary edema (see Fig. 16-24).
  h Respiratory distress syndrome (not shown).
  i Aspiration of foreign objects (not shown).

2 The reader is encouraged to attend x-ray rounds or to study texts showing radiographic plates until familiarity is attained in recognizing the most common types of pulmonary conditions as diagnosed by roentgenogram.

3 Procedures 16-8, 16-9, and 16-10 may be used for interpreting chest films.

14.0 OTHER MEASURES USED IN CHEST PHYSICAL EXAMINATION (See Module 28 for more details on these and other patient monitoring devices)

14.1 Noninvasive measure of oxygenation: oximetry

1 The development of more responsive, accurate, smaller, and less expensive *oximeters* has increased their popularity as a practical means of measuring in vivo oxygen saturation.

Ear oximetry and pulse oximeters have proven to be a reliable method of evaluating arterial oxygenation under both stable and changing clinical conditions.

2 Clinical applications for oximeters include:
  a Exercise studies.
  b Sleep apnea studies.
  c Routine measurement of the benefits of supplemental oxygen.

3 In the clinical setting the earlobe or finger is used primarily as the site of attachment for the oximeter. The oximeter is calibrated and a periodic or continuous determination of oxygen saturation may be taken.

4 Oximeters determine oxygen saturation by measuring the light transmitted or reflected by oxygenated versus reduced hemoglobin at specific wave lengths.

  a The maximum difference between saturated and reduced hemoglobin occurs at a wavelength of approximately 650 nanometers (nm) at the *isosbestic* point (approximately 810 to 815 nm); a measurement of the light absorbed is independent of the degree of oxygenation.
    • This point is used by most oximeters as the zero or reference point.
  b The oximeter measures blood at 650 nm and compares it to this isosbestic point. The difference between the two readings yields a value that correlates with degree of oxygen saturation.

14.2 Transcutaneous measurements

Another noninvasive method of determining O_2 saturation and CO_2 levels is through the use of transcutaneous (tc) (cutaneous) monitors.

For many years it has been known that oxygen and carbon dioxide diffuse across the skin barrier into the surrounding atmosphere. In addition, with maximum hyperemia, transcutaneous oxygen tension ($Ptco_2$) and $Ptcco_2$ correlate closely with arterial oxygen tension (Pao_2) and $Paco_2$ in patients with adequate blood flow states.

1 In the early 1970s researchers developed special electrodes that were attached to the skin for the purpose of capturing O_2 and CO_2 molecules at the skin's surface.

  a These special electrodes work in a manner that is similar to the traditional Clark electrode except for the fact that they continuously heat the skin underneath the area of the contact to approximately 44° C.
  b Increased surface temperature causes increased capillary blood flow to the area with a corresponding increase in gas diffusion to the skin's surface.
  c Diffusion of the O_2 and CO_2 molecules into the electrode causes an electrical charge that is transmitted to a recorder and reported as Po_2 and Pco_2 values.

2 The steps involved in a typical tc electrode/monitor assembly follow:

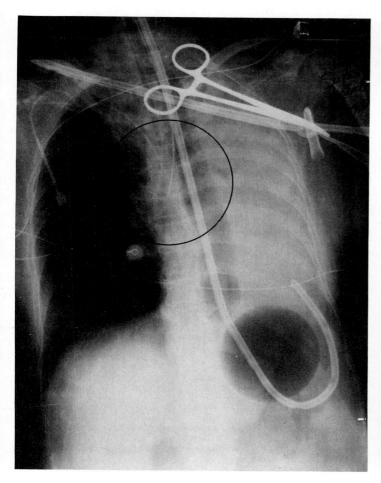

FIGURE 16-22 Chest radiograph showing a misplaced tracheal tube.

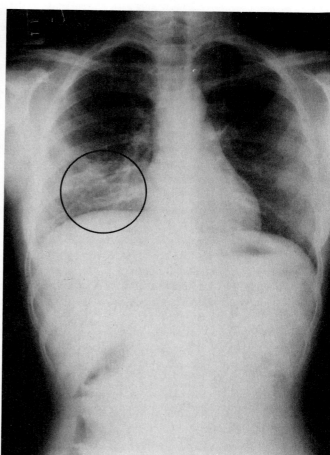

FIGURE 16-23 Chest radiograph showing acute pneumonia.

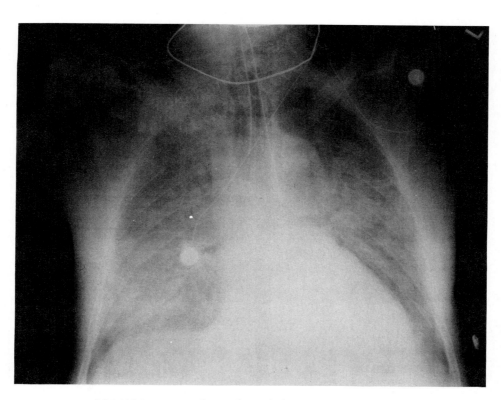

FIGURE 16-24 Chest radiograph showing pulmonary edema.

Step 1 The electrode is attached to the skin.

Step 2 The electrode is heated to approximately 44° C, and the heat stimulates nerves that dilate blood vessels under the skin.

Step 3 O_2 and CO_2 molecules disperse from the capillaries across the skin and into the electrode.

Step 4 An electrical current is created and sent to the monitor as an electrical signal that is read as $Ptco_2$ and/or $Ptcco_2$.

3 The major problem encountered with the use of tc monitors is the *inaccuracy* of $Ptco_2$ and $Ptcco_2$ in patients who are hemodynamically unstable.

In this situation blood is shunted away from the cutaneous circulation resulting in abnormally low transcutaneous values when compared to arterial blood gas samples.

4 Clinical applications for tc monitoring include:

a Use as a continuous noninvasive method for rapidly identifying shock and hypoxia.

b Substituting for repetitious arterial blood gas sticks in hemodynamically stable patients after a baseline has been established.

c Monitoring O_2 and CO_2 levels in patients during transport to and from hospitals.

d Monitoring O_2 and CO_2 levels in patients during exercise testing.

PROCEDURE 16-1

Conducting the patient interview

No.	Steps in performing the procedure
	The practitioner will demonstrate appropriate techniques in conducting the patient interview.
1	Review patient's chart.
2	Prepare the environment for optimum conditions.
	2.1 Select a quiet area.
	2.2 Adjust temperature for comfort of disrobed patient.
	2.3 Provide for patient privacy.
	2.4 Provide comfortable seating or lying facilities for the patient to allow you 360-degree access to the patient.
	2.5 Assist patient in acquiring a comfortable position.
	2.6 Position lighting so that patient can clearly see you.
3	Wash hands.
4	Identify patient by wrist band.
5	Introduce yourself to the patient.
6	Gather history:
	6.1 Use nondirect questions to allow patient to volunteer information.
	6.2 Use direct questions to clarify information or gather details.
	6.3 Ask questions to elicit psychosocial history.
	6.4 Assure and comfort patient as needed.
7	Take notes (do not distract from interview).

PROCEDURE 16-2

Inspecting the chest for signs of pulmonary disease

No.	Steps in performing the procedure	No.	Steps in performing the procedure
1	The practitioner will inspect the patient for external signs of pulmonary disease. Review patient's chart.	10	Check skin. Note:
2	Prepare the environment for optimum conditions.		**10.1** Color
	2.1 Select a quiet area.		**10.2** Vascularity
	2.2 Adjust temperature for comfort of disrobed patient.		**10.3** Lesions
	2.3 Provide for patient privacy.		**10.4** Edema
	2.4 Provide comfortable seating or lying facilities for the patient to allow you 360-degree access to the patient.		**10.5** Moisture
			10.6 Temperature
			10.7 Texture
			10.8 Turgor
	2.5 Position lighting so that you can clearly see the patient.		**10.9** Condition of nails
		11	Inspect patient's neck. Note:
			11.1 Engorgement or visual pulsation of veins
3	Wash hands.		**11.2** Distention of jugular vein on exhalation
4	Identify patient by wrist band.	12	Inspect patient's extremities. Note:
5	Introduce yourself to the patient.		**12.1** Clubbing of fingers and toes
6	Familiarize the patient with assessment procedure.		**12.2** Ankle edema
7	Position patient in sitting position (unless contraindicated).	13	Inspect patient's chest. Note:
			13.1 Chest symmetry
8	Conduct general survey of patient. Note:		**13.2** Angle of ribs
	8.1 State of health		**13.3** Muscle development
	8.2 Signs of distress (shortness of breath during talking)		**13.4** Chest proportions
			13.5 Respiratory movement
	8.3 Posture	14	Evaluate movement of chest and related structures.
	8.4 Motor activity and gait		**14.1** Identify abdominal breathing (mainly in men/children).
	8.5 Dress/grooming/personal hygiene		**14.2** Identify costal breathing (mainly in women).
	8.6 Mannerisms		**14.3** Check symmetry of movements for upper lobes.
	8.7 Attitude		
	8.8 Speech		**14.4** Check symmetry of movement for middle and lingular lobes.
	8.9 Mental alertness		**14.5** Check symmetry of movement for lower lobes.
9	Check vital signs:		
	9.1 Pulse		
	9.2 Respiratory rate (also note rhythm and depth)		
	9.3 Blood pressure		

PROCEDURE 16-3

Palpation of the chest

No.	Steps in performing the procedure	No.	Steps in performing procedure
	The practitioner will palpate the chest for skin temperatures, presence or absence of moisture, motion, use of ventilatory muscles, points of tenderness, presence and quality of vibrations and crepitus.	12	Palpate for position of trachea. 12.1 Position patient sitting, looking straight ahead. 12.2 Place index finger in suprasternal notch. 12.3 Compare space between right side of trachea and left side for equality. 12.4 Note any deviations.
1	Review patient's chart.		
2	Prepare the environment for optimum conditions. 2.1 Select a quiet area. 2.2 Adjust temperature for comfort of disrobed patient. 2.3 Provide for patient privacy. 2.4 Provide comfortable seating or lying facilities for the patient to allow you 360-degree access to the patient. 2.5 Position lighting so that you can clearly see patient.	13	Identify areas of chest pain. Palpate by starting away from the pain and working toward the site.
		14	Evaluate movement of chest and related structures. 14.1 Identify abdominal breathing (mainly in men/children). 14.2 Identify costal breathing (mainly in women). 14.3 Check symmetry of movements for upper lobes. 14.4 Check symmetry of movement for middle and lingular lobes. 14.5 Check symmetry of movement for lower lobes. 14.6 Examine action of the diaphragm. 14.7 Evaluate diaphragm or costal margins.
3	Wash hands.		
4	Identify patient by wrist band.		
5	Introduce yourself to the patient.		
6	Familiarize the patient with assessment procedure.		
7	Position patient in sitting position (unless contraindicated).	15	Examine chest for vocal fremitus, posterior chest. 15.1 Begin with the back (Fig. 16-25). 15.2 Position patient in sitting position with upper body bent slightly forward and arms folded across chest, with forearms resting on thighs. 15.3 Place the ball (palm of the hand at base of fingers) over each area of the chest according to the sequence in 16-25 while asking the patient to speak "ninety-nine," "one, one, one," or "one, two, three," at each new position. 15.4 Ask patient to speak louder if fremitus is faint.
8	Check vital signs: 8.1 Pulse 8.2 Respiratory rate (also note rhythm and depth) 8.3 Blood pressure		
9	Check skin. Note: 9.1 Color 9.2 Vascularity 9.3 Lesions 9.4 Edema 9.5 Moisture 9.6 Temperature 9.7 Texture 9.8 Turgor 9.9 Condition of nails	16	With patient sitting and back exposed, estimate level of the diaphragm on both sides of back. 16.1 Use ulnar side of extended hand. 16.2 Place hand below posterior tips of scapula (Fig. 16-26). 16.3 Move hand downward until fremitus disappears. 16.4 Note this point as diaphragmatic level.
10	Inspect patient's neck: Note: 10.1 Engorgement or visual pulsation of veins 10.2 Distention of jugular vein on exhalation		
11	Inspect patient's chest. Note: 11.1 Chest symmetry 11.2 Angle of ribs 11.3 Muscle development 11.4 Chest proportions 11.5 Respiratory movement		

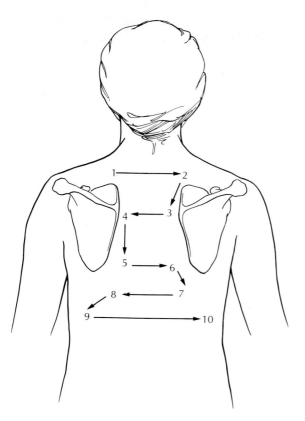

FIGURE 16-25

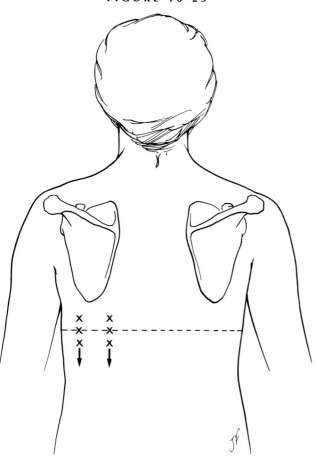

FIGURE 16-26

Performing mediate percussion

No.	Steps in performing the procedure
	The practitioner will demonstrate proper mediate percussion technique.
1	Spread apart the fingers of the left hand above the surface to be percussed.
2	Hyperextend the middle fingers of the left hand (pleximeter finger).
3	Place the distal phalanx and joint of the pleximeter finger lightly on the skin.
4	Avoid contact of surface with any other part of the hand.
5	Position right forearm close to the left hand.
6	Bend the hand upward at the wrist.
7	Partially flex the right middle finger.
8	Use wrist action to strike the pleximeter finger with the tip of the right middle (plexor finger).
9	Strike pleximeter finger at base of terminal phalanx or at interphalangeal joint.
10	Once contact is made with pleximeter finger, quickly remove plexor finger.
11	Stroke one or two blows at a point before moving.
12	Use only wrist to generate finger movement.
13	Identify and discuss the quality, duration, intensity, and pitch of each percussion note.

PROCEDURE 16-5

Percussing the chest

No.	Steps in performing the procedure	No.	Steps in performing the procedure
	The practitioner will position the patient and use mediate percussion to identify areas of consolidation or changes in density in patients with known lung involvement.	10	Inspect patient's chest. Note: **10.1** Chest symmetry **10.2** Angle of ribs **10.3** Muscle development **10.4** Chest proportions **10.5** Respiratory movement
1	Review patient's chart.	11	Evaluate movement of chest and related structures.
2	Prepare the environment for optimum conditions. **2.1** Select a quiet area. **2.2** Adjust temperature for comfort of disrobed patient. **2.3** Provide for patient privacy. **2.4** Provide comfortable seating or lying facilities for the patient to allow you 360 degree access to the patient. **2.5** Position lighting so that you can clearly see patient.		**11.1** Identify abdominal breathing (mainly in men/children). **11.2** Identify costal breathing (mainly in women). **11.3** Check symmetry of movement for upper lobes. **11.4** Check symmetry of movement for middle and lingular lobes. **11.5** Check symmetry of movement for lower lobes. **11.6** Examine action of the diaphragm. **11.7** Evaluate diaphragm or costal margins.
3	Wash hands.	12	Percuss the posterior chest wall.
4	Identify patient by wrist band.		**12.1** Place the patient in a slightly bent forward position with back exposed and arms crossed in front of chest (see Fig. 16-14).
5	Introduce yourself to the patient.		**12.2** Percuss across the tops of each shoulder and then down the back according to the sequence in Fig. 16-13.
6	Familiarize the patient with assessment procedure.	13	Identify the level of the diaphragm using percussion.
7	Position patient in sitting position (unless contraindicated).		**13.1** Position the patient sitting erect with back exposed.
8	Check vital signs: **8.1** Pulse **8.2** Respiratory rate (also note rhythm and depth) **8.3** Blood pressure		**13.2** Hold pleximeter finger parallel to expected border of diaphragmatic dullness. **13.3** Percuss in 5-cm intervals downward on each side until dullness is reached during quiet respiration (Fig. 16-26).
9	Check skin. Note: **9.1** Color **9.2** Vascularity **9.3** Lesions **9.4** Edema **9.5** Moisture **9.6** Temperature **9.7** Texture **9.8** Turgor **9.9** Condition of nails		**13.4** Note level of the diaphragm by comparing between level of dullness on full expiration to full inspiration (normal 5 to 7 cm).

PROCEDURE 16-6

Auscultating the chest

No.	Steps in performing the procedure	No.	Steps in performing the procedure
	The practitioner will position the patient and use auscultation to identify sounds of a pathologic nature in patients with known lung involvement.	11	Evaluate movement of chest and related structures.
1	Review patient's chart.		**11.1** Identify abdominal breathing (mainly in men/children).
2	Prepare the environment for optimum conditions.		**11.2** Identify costal breathing (mainly in women).
	2.1 Select a quiet area.		**11.3** Check symmetry of movements for upper lobes.
	2.2 Adjust temperature for comfort of disrobed patient.		**11.4** Check symmetry of movement for middle and lingual lobes.
	2.3 Provide for patient privacy.		**11.5** Check symmetry of movement for lower lobes.
	2.4 Provide comfortable seating or lying facilities for the patient to allow you 360-degree access to the patient.		**11.6** Examine action of the diaphragm.
			11.7 Evaluate diaphragm or costal margins.
	2.5 Position lighting so that you can clearly see the patient.	12	Auscultate the posterior chest.
3	Wash hands.		**12.1** Seat patient erect with back exposed.
4	Identify patient by wrist band.		**12.2** Instruct patient to breathe deeply and slowly with mouth open.
5	Introduce yourself to the patient.		**12.3** Systematically place the stethoscope to examine the lung apices and the posterior chest (Fig. 16-27).
6	Familiarize the patient with assessment procedure.		
7	Position patient in sitting position (unless contraindicated).	13	Auscultate the lateral chest.
			13.1 Seat patient erect and expose upper chest.
8	Check vital signs:		**13.2** Have patient raise arms.
	8.1 Pulse		**13.3** Using stethoscope, compare breath sounds heard on one side of the chest to those heard on the opposite side, according to the sequence and locations in Fig. 16-28.
	82. Respiratory rate (also note rhythm and depth)		
	8.3 Blood pressure	14	Auscultate the anterior chest.
9	Check skin. Note:		**14.1** Seat patient erect and expose the anterior chest.
	9.1 Color		**14.2** Use stethoscope to auscultate the anterior chest according to the sequence and locations in Fig. 16-15.
	9.2 Vascularity		
	9.3 Lesions		**14.3** Compare breath sounds heard on one side of the chest to those heard in similar locations on opposite side of the chest.
	9.4 Edema		
	9.5 Moisture		
	9.6 Temperature		
	9.7 Texture		
	9.8 Turgor		
	9.9 Condition of nails		
10	Inspect patient's chest. Note:		
	10.1 Chest symmetry		
	10.2 Angle of ribs		
	10.3 Muscle development		
	10.4 Chest proportions		
	10.5 Respiratory movement		

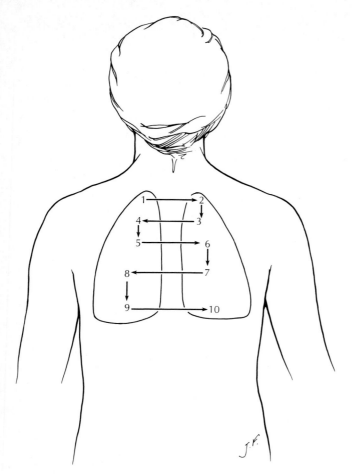

FIGURE 16-27

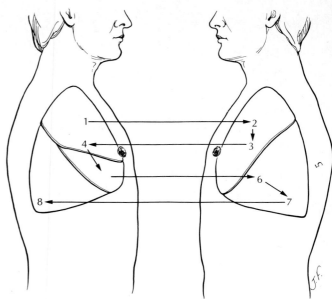

Right lateral   Left lateral

FIGURE 16-28

PROCEDURE 16-7

Performing physical assessment of the chest

No.	Steps in performing the procedure	No.	Steps in performing the procedure
	The practitioner will inspect the ambulatory patient for signs of pulmonary disease, using visual and tactile techniques.	14	Inspect patient's eyes. Note:
			14.1 Color
1	Review patient's chart.		**14.2** Presence of engorged veins
2	Prepare the environment for optimum conditions.		**14.3** Swelling of optic discs
	2.1 Select a quiet area.		**14.4** Pupils for reaction
	2.2 Adjust temperature for comfort of disrobed patient.	15	Inspect patient's neck. Note:
			15.1 Engorgement or visual pulsation of veins
	2.3 Provide for patient privacy.		**15.2** Distension of jugular vein on exhalation
	2.4 Provide comfortable seating or lying facilities for the patient to allow you 360-degree access to the patient.	16	Inspect patient's extremities. Note:
			16.1 Clubbing of fingers and toes
			16.2 Ankle edema
	2.5 Assist patient in acquiring a comfortable position.	17	Inspect patient's chest. Note:
			17.1 Chest symmetry
	2.6 Position lighting so that patient can clearly see you.		**17.2** Angle of ribs
			17.3 Muscle development
3	Wash hands.		**17.4** Chest proportions
4	Identify patient by wrist band.		**17.5** Respiratory movement
5	Introduce yourself to the patient.	18	Palpate for position of trachea.
6	Familiarize the patient with assessment procedure.		**18.1** Position patient sitting, looking straight ahead.
7	Gather history:		**18.2** Place index finger in suprasternal notch.
	7.1 Use nondirect questions to allow patient to volunteer information.		**18.3** Compare space between right side of trachea and left side for equality.
	7.2 Use direct questions to clarify information or gather details.		**18.4** Note any deviations.
		19	Identify areas of chest pain: Palpate by starting away from the pain and working toward the site.
	7.3 Ask questions to elicit psychosocial history.	20	Evaluate movement of chest and related structures.
	7.4 Assure and comfort patient as needed.		**20.1** Identify abdominal breathing (mainly in men/children).
8	Take notes (do not distract from interview).		
9	Position patient in sitting position (unless contraindicated).		**20.2** Identify costal breathing (mainly in women).
			20.3 Check symmetry of movements for upper lobes.
10	Conduct general survey of patient. Note:		
	10.1 State of heath		**20.4** Check symmetry of movement for middle and lingular lobes.
	10.2 Signs of distress (shortness of breath during talking)		
			20.5 Check symmetry of movement for lower lobes.
	10.3 Posture		**20.6** Examine action of the diaphragm.
	10.4 Monitor activity and gait		**20.7** Evaluate diaphragm or costal margins.
	10.5 Dress/grooming/personal hygiene	21	Examine chest for vocal fremitus, posterior chest.
	10.6 Mannerisms		**21.1** Begin with the back (see Fig. 16-25).
	10.7 Attitude		**21.2** Position patient in sitting position with upper body bent slightly forward and arms folded across chest, with forearms resting on thighs.
	10.8 Speech		
	10.9 Mental alertness		
11	Check vital signs:		**21.3** Place the ball (palm of the hand at base of fingers) over each area of the chest according to the sequence that follows, while asking the patient to speak "ninety-nine," "one, one, one," or "one, two, three," at each new position.
	11.1 Pulse		
	11.2 Respiratory rate (also note rhythm and depth)		
	11.3 Blood pressure		
12	Check skin. Note:		**21.4** Ask patient to speak louder if fremitus is faint.
	12.1 Color	22	With patient sitting and back exposed, estimate level of the diaphragm on both sides of back.
	12.2 Vascularity		
	12.3 Lesions		**22.1** Use ulnar side of extended hand.
	12.4 Edema		**22.2** Place hand below posterior tips of scapula (see Fig. 16-26).
	12.5 Moisture		
	12.6 Temperature		**22.3** Move hand downward until fremitus disappears.
	12.7 Texture		
	12.8 Turgor		**22.4** Note this point as diaphragmatic level.
	12.9 Condition of nails		
13	Check head. Note:		
	13.1 Condition of hair.		
	13.2 Diseases or injuries to the scalp, head, or face		

This performance evaluation procedure is expanded beyond the scope of a normal rating scale, so that it can be used for detailed instruction and evaluation.

Continued.

PROCEDURE 16-7—cont'd

Performing physical assessment of the chest

No.	Steps in performing the procedure	No.	Steps in performing the procedure
23	Percuss the posterior chest wall.	28	Examine the anterior chest. Note:
	23.1 Place the patient in a slightly bent forward position with back exposed and arms crossed in front of chest (see Fig. 16-14).		**28.1** Deformities
			28.2 Muscles used for breathing
			28.3 Symmetry of breathing
	23.2 Percuss across the tops of each shoulder and then down the back according to the sequence in Fig. 16-13.	29	Palpate anterior chest for:
			29.1 Tenderness
24	Identify the level of the diaphragm using percussion.		**29.2** Respiratory excursion
	24.1 Position the patient sitting erect with back exposed.		**a** Place thumbs along each costal margin.
			b Rest hands along lateral rib cage.
	24.2 Hold pleximeter finger parallel to expected border of diaphragmatic dullness.		**c** Slide hands medially to raise a skin fold between two thumbs.
	24.3 Percuss in 5-cm intervals downward on each side until dullness is reached during quiet respiration, according to Fig. 16-26.		**d** Ask patient to take a deep breath.
			e Assess divergence of thumbs as chest expands for equality and range of movement.
	24.4 Note level of the diaphragm by comparing between level of dullness on full expiration to full inspiration (normal 5 to 7 cm).	30	Check anterior chest for vocal fremitus.
			30.1 Place patient in an erect position, and expose the anterior chest.
25	Auscultate the posterior chest.		**30.2** Place the ball (palm of the hand at base of fingers) over each area according to the following sequence and locations in Fig. 16-27.
	25.1 Seat patient erect with back exposed.		
	25.2 Instruct patient to breathe deeply and slowly with mouth open.		**30.3** Have patient speak "ninety-nine," "one, one, one."
	25.3 Systematically place the stethoscope to examine the lung apices and the posterior chest according to Fig. 16-27.		**30.4** Note areas of dullness.
		31	Percuss the anterior chest.
26	Assess the lateral chest by percussion.		**31.1** Use mediate percussion to assess corresponding areas of the anterior chest according to the sequence and locations in Fig. 16-19.
	26.1 Place patient erect in an erect position with upper chest exposed.		
	26.2 Have patient raise arms above head.		**31.2** Compare sounds heard on one side of the chest to those heard at the corresponding site on the opposite side.
	26.3 Percuss the lateral chest by comparing one side to the same location on the opposite side according to the following sequence and the location in Fig. 16-28.	32	Auscultate the anterior chest.
			32.1 Seat patient erect, and expose the anterior chest.
27	Auscultate the lateral chest.		**32.2** Use stethoscope to auscultate the anterior chest according to the sequence and locations in Fig. 16-15.
	27.1 Seat patient erect, and expose upper chest.		
	27.2 Have patient raise arms.		**32.3** Compare breath sounds heard on one side of the chest to those heard in similar locations on opposite side of the chest.
	27.3 Using stethoscope, compare breath sounds heard on one side of the chest to those heard on the opposite side, according to the following sequence and the locations in Fig. 16-28.		

PROCEDURE 16-8

Interpretation of chest films (posteroanterior)

No.	Steps in performing the procedure
	The practitioner will study posteroanterior (PA) x-ray films of the chest until he or she can identify a normal film from an abnormal film.*
1	Secure a normal PA chest film.
2	Identify patient name and number.
3	Locate and turn on view box.
4	Place film correctly on view box surface.
	4.1 Patient's left side is to viewer's right.
	4.2 Diaphragm is toward base of film.
5	Observe any grossly abnormal dark or light areas.
6	Systemically point out and assess normality of:
	6.1 Soft tissues of the chest
	6.2 Bony thorax
	6.3 Diaphragm
	6.4 Med[ia]stinum and its structures
	6.5 Lung fields
7	Observe symmetry and proper position of the:
	7.1 Trachea
	7.2 Heart
	7.3 Mediastinum
	7.4 Lung fields
	7.5 Hilar areas
8	Check heart for size.
9	Check for silhouette sign.
10	Check lung field for presence of abnormal air, tissue, infiltrates.
11	Check pleura for inflammation, fluid, air.
12	Check for shading of normal areas of the lung.
13	Check and compare diaphragm for:
	13.1 Normal shape
	13.2 Height of hemidiaphragms
	13.3 Any tissue abnormality
	13.4 Clarity of borders
14	Check for signs of aspiration.
15	Check for position of artificial airway.
16	Draw an accurate conclusion as to patient's condition, based on chest film.

*All findings should be discussed with your preceptor or medical advisor.

PROCEDURE 16-9

Interpretation of chest films (anteroposterior)

No.	Steps in performing the procedure
	The practitioner will study anteroposterior (AP) x-ray films of the chest until he or she can identify a normal film from an abnormal film.
1	Secure a normal AP chest film.
2	Identify patient name and number.
3	Locate and turn on view box.
4	Place film correctly on view box surface.
	4.1 Patient's left side is to viewer's right.
	4.2 Diaphragm is toward base of film.
5	Observe any grossly abnormal dark or light areas.
6	Systematically point out and assess normality of:
	6.1 Soft tissues of the chest
	6.2 Bony thorax
	6.3 Diaphragm
	6.4 Medinastinum and its structures
	6.5 Lung fields
7	Observe symmetry and proper position of the:
	7.1 Trachea
	7.2 Heart
	7.3 Mediastinum
	7.4 Lung fields
	7.5 Hilar areas
8	Check heart for size.
9	Check for silhouette sign.
10	Check lung field for presence of abnormal air, tissue, infiltrates.
11	Check pleura for inflammation, fluid, air.
12	Check for shading of normal areas of the lung.
13	Check and compare diaphragm for:
	13.1 Normal shape
	13.2 Height of hemidiaphragms
	13.3 Any tissue abnormality
	13.4 Clarity of borders
14	Check for signs of aspiration.
15	Check for position of artifical airway.
16	Draw an accurate conclusion as to patient's condition, based on chest film.

PROCEDURE 16-10

Interpretation of chest films (lateral)

No.	Steps in performing the procedure
	The practitioner will study lateral x-ray films of the chest until he or she can identify a normal film from an abnormal film.
1	Secure a normal lateral chest film.
2	Identify patient name and number.
3	Locate and turn on view box.
4	Place film correctly on view box surface.
5	Observe any grossly abnormal dark or light areas.
6	Systematically point out and assess normality of:
	6.1 Soft tissues of the chest
	6.2 Bony thorax
	6.3 Diaphragm
	6.3 Mediastinum and its structures
	6.5 Lung fields
7	Observe and note proper position of the:
	7.1 Trachea
	7.2 Heart
	7.3 Mediastinum
	7.4 Lung fields
	7.5 Hilar areas
8	Check heart for size.
9	Check lung field for presence of abnormal air, tissue, infiltrates.
10	Check pleura for inflammation, fluid, air.
11	Check for shading of normal areas of the lung.
12	Check diaphragm. Note:
	12.1 Normal shape
	12.2 Any tissue abnormality
	12.3 Clarity of borders
13	Check for signs of aspiration.
14	Check for position of artificial airway.
15	Draw an accurate conclusion as to patient's condition, based on chest film.

BIBLIOGRAPHY

Beachy P and Whitfield JM: The effect of transcutaneous PO_2 monitoring on the frequency of arterial blood gas analysis in the newborn with respiratory distress, Crit Care Med 9:584, 1981.

Cobal L et al: Factors affecting heated transcutaneous PO_2 and unheated transcutaneous PO_2 in preterm infants, Crit Care Med 9:298, 1981.

Findley LJ and Sahn SA: The value of chest roentgenograms in acute asthma in adults, Chest 80:535, 1981.

Greenspan GH et al: Trancutaneous noninvasive monitoring of carbon monoxide tension, Chest 80:442, 1981.

Kram HB and Shoemaker WC: Use of transcutaneous O_2 monitoring in the intraoperative management of severe peripheral vascular disease, Crit Care Med 11:482, 1983.

Martin J et al: Factors influencing pulsus paradoxus in asthma, Chest 80:543, 1981.

McDowell JW et al: Follow-up evaluation of transcutaneous PO_2 monitoring before and after adult exercise testing, Respir Care 26:963, 1981.

Monaco F, Nickerson BG, and McQuitty JC: Continuous transcutaneous oxygen and carbon dioxide monitoring in the pediatric ICU, Crit Care Med 10:765, 1982.

Rebuck AS, Chapman KE, and D'Urzo A: The accuracy and response characteristics of a simplified ear oximeter, Chest 83:860, 1983.

Severinghaus JW: Transcutaneous blood gas analysis: the 1981 Donald F. Egan lecture, Respir Care 27:152, 1982.

Shoemaker WC and Vidyasagar D, editors: Transcutaneous O_2 and CO_2 monitoring of the adult and neonate (symposium issue), Crit Care Med 9:693, 1981.

Yahav J, Mindorff C, and Levison H: The validity of the transcutaneous oxygen tension method in children with cardiorespiratory problems, Am Rev Respir Dis 124:586, 1981.

Intermittent positive presssure breathing

On completion of this module the reader will be able to:

1.1 Present background material on intermittent positive pressure breathing* (IPPB) therapy.

1.2 Explain what is meant by IPPB therapy.

2.1 Draw an example of a typical IPPB cycle using an x-y graph.

2.2 Explain various points of the graphic representation as it relates to the breathing cycle.

3.1 Give examples of persons and events directly or indirectly involved in the development of IPPB therapy in medicine.

4.1 Describe indications for IPPB therapy.

4.2 Describe contraindications for IPPB therapy.

5.1 Support the nine considerations given as criteria for assessing a patient for IPPB therapy.

5.2 Explain measurements of the lung as a practical means for evaluating the need for and the effectiveness of IPPB therapy.

6.1 Differentiate the characteristic components of a properly written medical order for IPPB.

7.1 Instruct a patient in IPPB, using the suggested format.

7.2 Modify therapy techniques according to changing patient needs.

7.3 Describe proper breathing techniques for IPPB therapy.

8.1 Chart properly the techniques for IPPB therapy.

9.1 Explain terms and principles related to operation of IPPB machines.

10.1 Show how basic gas flow principles can be applied to operation of most IPPB devices.

11.1 Diagram and explain the function of various types of valves and breathing circuits in IPPB devices.

11.2 Describe gas flow through a standard Bird respirator circuit.

12.1 Distinguish the most important characteristics of the Bennett and the Bird series of IPPB devices.

13.1 Describe major specifications related to the Bennett PR-2 respirator.

13.2 Operate a Bennett PR-2 respirator according to the outlined steps.

14.1 Operate the Bird Mark-7 respirator according to the outlined steps.

15.1 Point out potential hazardous situations that could develop from IPPB therapy.

16.1 Give IPPB treatments to himself or herself, to other students, and to patients according to recommended techniques.

17.1 Differentiate among various causes of machine malfunction, and initiate corrective action.

18.1 Clean IPPB devices according to recommended techniques.

1.0 IPPB THERAPY
1.1 HISTORY OF IPPB THERAPY

1 Since 1950 the IPPB machine, more than any other single device, has served both as a developmental *and* a detrimental force in respiratory care and pulmonary medicine. Unfortunately, like so many other medical procedures, the use and development of the technique far exceeded the accumulation of data to objectively prove its therapeutic worth.

2 Consequently, in May 1974, at the Temple University Conference Center at Sugarloaf, Pennsylvania, a conference was held on the *scientific basis of respiratory therapy.* This conference, sponsored by the American Thoracic Society through a grant from the National Heart and Lung Institute (NHLI), was attended by respresentatives from the various professional associations and other groups involved in the treatment of lung disease.

The primary objectives of the meeting were:

a To assess existing data concerning the efficacy of various modes of respiratory therapy treatment in patients with stable chronic obstructive pulmonary disease (COPD).

b To indicate what additional data are needed to more adequately assess various modes of treatment.

c To make these findings available to NHLI and to the community of pulmonary scientists in order to stimulate appropriate investigations.

3 As a result of this conference, the NHLI *funded* clini-

---

*Referred to throughout this model as IPPB. See the Bibliography at the end of this module, especially (1) Spearman, Sheldon, and Egan and (2) McPherson, sources for some of the material in this module, which provides useful reference materials.

cal research projects to investigate the need for and efficacy of various respiratory therapy modalities, including oxygen therapy and IPPB.

In November 1979 a second conference was held on the *scientific basis of in-hospital respiratory therapy.* This conference was sponsored by the same groups as the first conference, and participation was by invitation only. Again, attendees represented the various medical and allied health professional associations interested in respiratory therapy.

The objectives of the second conference were similar to those of the first, with the focus on *in-hospital* respiratory therapy. The areas studied at the second conference were oxygen therapy, aerosols and humidity therapy, mechanical aids to lung expansion, and physical therapy.

The primary problems addressed at this conference were:

a Indiscriminate use of oxygen therapy.

b Lack of agreement as to specific guidelines for prescribing, administering, or assessing efficacy of these modalities.

c Problems with two rigid guidelines that could deny treatment to those who may need it.

  • As a result of this conference, still other studies were funded to further investigate IPPB, sleep apnea, and the benefits of humidity and aerosol therapy.

4 In September 1983 a third conference was sponsored by American College of Chest Physicians in Chicago, Illinois, to study the current and future status of oxygen therapy. The five specific areas studied were:

a Oxygen side effects and toxicity.

b The scientific basis for oxygen therapy.

c Criteria for institution and duration of oxygen therapy.

d Oxygen delivery systems.

e Monitoring oxygen therapy.

  • At this conference practitioners representing various medical and allied health associations presented papers and held workshops where they developed specific recommendations for basic and applied research in each of the five areas addressed.

5 The importance of these three conferences cannot be understated because they have influenced and will continue to influence current and future use of respiratory therapy in the areas studied.*

Respiratory therapy was represented at all but the first conference by appointees from the American Association for Respiratory Care (AARC). It is the responsibility of each respiratory care practitioner to study the results of these conferences, which have begun to establish and will continue to develop a scientific basis for respiratory care.

a IPPB was singled out as a primary example of medi-

cal overuse that has little objective data concerning its efficiency. Therefore it was implied that the use of IPPB should be controlled and reduced, if not eliminated, as a viable treatment technique.

  • Since these conferences, supporters and opponents of IPPB have researched the literature for previous studies to prove their points, with little objective documentation for either side.

b Subsequently, the use of IPPB has been greatly reduced, and alternate techniques—such as deep breathing exercises, incentive spirometry, and other techniques—have been substituted, with just as little objective data available for documented efficiency of these products. Although the opponents of IPPB argue that these techniques are *cheaper,* there is no evidence that they are better (or in fact as good for the patient) than IPPB.

The question regarding the best methods for helping the patient to take deep breaths, to deposit aerosol, to promote bronchial clearance (hygiene), and to control elevated carbon dioxide is still debated and left to the wisdom of the prescribing physician. The following units of instruction provide information regarding the indications, contraindications, and techniques for administering and evaluating IPPB as a treatment modality.

1.2 Definition of IPPB

1 IPPB is one of those terms that can mean different things depending on the situation. For example, generically it may be described as an artificial method of producing and delivering a positive gas pressure to the airway to assist in or cause inhalation to occur.

2 Exhalation begins and continues from the time the positive pressure is interrupted until the next positive pressure breath is generated. This sequence of delivering a positive pressure breath followed by exhalation (no positive pressure) describes a sequence of intermittent positive pressure breathing.

3 Another definition of IPPB describes it as a pneumatically cycled *device* (respirator) that is used to deliver inspiratory positive pressure breaths as a short 15- to 30-minute treatment.

4 Still another definition of IPPB describes it as a 15- to 30- minute *treatment,* usually given for the purpose of delivering an aerosol and/or hyperinflating the lung.

5 No matter when the term IPPB may be used, the practitioner must *not* think of IPPB as a means of prolonged or continuous ventilation, a procedure that requires much more advanced skills and equipment.

2.0 PRESSURE, FLOW, AND VOLUME TRACINGS
2.1 Graphing gas pressure, flow, and volume

1 Diagrammatically, gas pressure, flow, and volume can be dynamically recorded electronically or mechanically as a movement of a gradually increasing and decreasing line on a chart or oscilloscope (television-type screen) as the patient inhales or as a ventilator cycles on and off.

---

*The proceedings of these conferences were published in *American Review of Respiratory Disease, Chest, Respiratory Care* and other professional journals.

2 The shape of the line pattern (tracing) created by the patient or ventilator reflects the gas pressure flow or exhaled volume of the patient or of the ventilator. This tracing can be used for evaluation of the patient's breathing function or operational characteristics of each type of ventilator.

2.2 Applying the graph to an IPPB graph

1 Fig. 17-1 represents a typical x-y graphic scale that is used to record various components of ventilation on an oscilloscope (i.e., *pressure, flow,* and/or *volume*).

2 As the patient inhales, the attached ventilator cycles "on" and a line pattern appears on the screen of the oscilloscope—baseline *(1)*—and moves upward, as inspiration continues, to a *maximum* point on the *y* axis. This point represents maximum peak pressure, flow, or volume *(2)*.

3 When the ventilator cycles "off," the patient exhales, and the line pattern moves back toward the baseline *(3)*, where it remains until another inspiration occurs.

4 A downward deflection from baseline *(4)* usually represents a *subambient* respiratory maneuver by the patient or ventilator. This type of situation can occur as the patient begins *inspiration,* causing a subambient pressure in the airway, or it can be triggered by a ventilator that is mechanically causing subambient (negative) pressure to be created during the expiratory phase.

3.0 DEVELOPMENT OF IPPB

3.1 Events and persons involved in the medical development of IPPB

1 Mouth-to-mouth breathing was the earliest recorded method of positive pressure breathing. This occurrence was mentioned first in *The Bible* (Elisha used it to revive a child).

2 In 1934 pressure breathing with oxygen was used under continuous pressure by Poulton in England to treat pulmonary edema.

3 During World War II, IPPB was developed for use by pilots required to fly in high altitudes. One of the earliest examples of these units was the Bennett BX-1, developed at Wright's Field in 1945.

4 In 1946 Motley and associates treated with IPPB ten patients in circulatory failure and coma.

5 In 1947 fifteen cases of pulmonary edema were reported healed with IPPB treatment of coal miners with emphysema and fibrosis.

  a In 1947 Motley outlined requirements for the ideal ventilator based on the research conducted by him and his associates.

  b In 1947, Cournand, Motley, Werko, and Richards published a study on the effects of IPPB on hemodynamics. An ideal pressure pattern was described as a type III Cournand pattern in which the expiratory time was as long as or exceeded the inspiratory inspiration time, resulting in a low mean mask pressure.

6 In 1948 Motley, Lang, and Gordon first used IPPB aerosol to treat patients with chronic lung disease.

7 In 1950 Motley and associates were among the first to report arterial blood gas analysis before and after IPPB.

8 In 1951 IPPB aerosol was routinely used as a means of treatment for chronic lung disease.

9 In 1952 Engstrom developed a volume-type intermittent positive pressure ventilator to provide continuous ventilation to polio victims.

10 From 1951 to 1974 the use of IPPB in the United States to treat all types of respiratory problems was widespread and frequent. It was estimated that the use

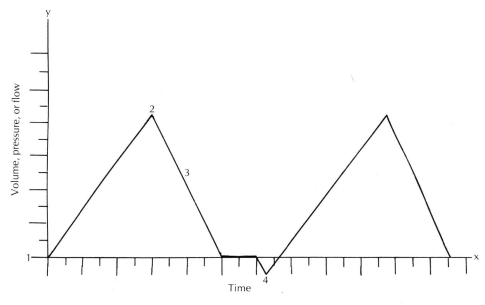

FIGURE 17-1 Graphic representation of IPPB ventilatory cycle.

of IPPB alone cost the federal government billions of dollars for Medicare and Medicaid reimbursement.

11 In 1974, at the Sugarloaf Conference (cosponsored by the National Institutes of Health [NIH]), a small group of investigators from various professional medical associations gathered to report on the various respiratory therapy modalities used in home care. IPPB became the focus of this group and led to the funding of a series of studies by NIH to investigate the efficacy of this treatment.

12 From 1975 to date IPPB has been used more discriminatingly and, in many instances, is being replaced by incentive breathing devices and breathing exercises.

4.0 INDICATIONS AND CONTRAINDICATIONS FOR IPPB THERAPY

4.1 Indications for IPPB therapy treatment

The following list is based primarily on *subjective opinions* regarding the need for IPPB as a short-term treatment. Unfortunately, clinical and scientific data are still not available to support the efficacy of IPPB in treating these conditions. Thus these indications for prescribing IPPB (and expected outcomes from the treatment) remain unproved. (See the chapter on IPPB in Spearman.)

1 *Acute or chronic hypoventilation.* A properly administered IPPB treatment, in most instances, will provide *increased tidal breaths* in those patients who are unable, because of altered chest bellows action, central nervous system (CNS) involvement, or drug depression, to provide adequate volumes (12 to 15 ml/kg) on their own. The question of relevancy arises in considering whether the provision of increased volumes for short periods of time (10 to 20 minutes), with little or no continued support between treatments, provides any real clinical benefits.

2 *Atelectasis.* In delivering intermittent elevated airway pressure, with or without controlled expiratory patterns, to open and stabilize atelectatic areas, the following questions are usually asked:

a Is the airway pressure normally employed during an IPPB treatment sufficient to open atelectatic areas?

b If sufficient pressure is used, will it result in *overdistention* of the nonatelectatic areas, with possible rupture of alveolar blebs?

c Does the *intermittent administration* of positive pressuring during inspiration prevent atelectatic areas from recollapsing during the expiratory phase of the breathing cycle?

d If IPPB is given with oxygen, will the removal of nitrogen from alveoli with subsequent elevated O_2 levels cause more atelectasis as a result of the *oxygen absorption theory?* (See Spearman's discussion of atelectasis.)

3 *Reduced cough.* Increased tidal breaths and a vital capacity of greater than *35% of the predicted* value should enable the patient with a reduced mechanical lung function to generate an expiratory peak flow rate of *greater* than 150 L/min necessary to produce an ef-

fective cough. This benefit is still under investigation, although it is documented that the IPPB will produce an increased tidal volume in many patients who are unable to generate adequate lung volumes. To be effective as a cough-producing mechanism, sufficient airway pressure must be generated, gas flow patterns must be controlled, and the patient must cooperate by following proper coughing instructions.

4 *Increased airway resistance.* IPPB alone does not reduce airway resistance. It may, in fact, increase airway resistance in the chronically obstructed patient who attempts to *forcefully exhale* increased lung volumes, which are delivered with the assistance of the IPPB machine. Other studies have shown that excessive gas flow rates or airway pressures may cause a reflex constriction of bronchial airways, resulting in an increase in airway resistance. IPPB may be beneficial in treating elevated airway resistance if it is used as a vehicle for delivering bronchodilators or other bronchoactive drugs to the sites of increased resistance. A major problem usually experienced with this approach is that tidal volumes, gas flow patterns, respiratory frequency, nebulizer production, and other variables must be rigidly controlled to prevent undesired systemic responses.

5 *Increased work of breathing.* IPPB can reduce the work of breathing, provided it is *properly* administered using adequate tidal volumes (12 to 15 ml/kg), that the inspiratory and expiratory flow rates are controlled based on the patient's total airway resistance, and that adequate humidification is provided to prevent a humidity deficit.

NOTE: IPPB can actually *increase* the work of breathing if:

a The ventilator setting is *not* sensitive enough to respond to the patient's inspiratory efforts.

b The flow rate is adequate to satisfy the patient's inspiratory demands.

c The tidal volume is inadequate to provide sufficient alveolar ventilation.

d Adequate time is not allowed for complete passive exhalation to occur.

6 *Accumulation of secretions.* IPPB is given to promote the clearance of airway secretions by delivery of aerosol to the obstructed areas and promotion of a productive cough. It has been generally established that IPPB is of some benefit in helping a patient remove secretions only if the patient is incapable of naturally producing an effective cough in the first place.

7 *Pulmonary congestion.* IPPB therapy may be of benefit in acute situations involving pulmonary edema. The benefits from IPPB include:

a Elevation of airway pressures to reduce the alveolar-capillary pressure gradient.

b Reduction of blood flow to the pulmonary capillaries by increasing the effect of transmural pressures on blood flow returning to the right side of the heart via the superior/inferior vena cavae.

c Increased arterial oxygen tension (Pao_2) as a result

of an elevated fraction of inspired oxygen (FIo_2), combined with increased lung volumes.

   d Possible reduced surface tensions in extreme situations by the administration of a 20% ethyl alcohol solution as an aerosol. This aerosol reduces the surface tension of the primary protein-based edema, which causes the frothy bubbles to dissipate. A reduction in pulmonary edema increases the alveolar surface available for ventilation and facilitates removal of the edema by reabsorption into the capillary circulation and through other lung clearance mechanisms. The use of ethyl alcohol remains controversial.

4.2 Contraindications for IPPB therapy

IPPB therapy is contraindicated in the following conditions:

  1 *Tension pneumothorax* without a chest tube in place (Fig. 17-2). An opening in the lung *(1)* will cause gas to pass into the intrapleural space *(2)*. Without a chest tube in place, the gas volume and subsequent pressure will continue to build with each breath, causing pressure outside the lung to prevent the inflation of the affected lung *(3)*. Uncorrected, this will cause the lung, and eventually the heart and great vessels of the chest, to be pushed out of position away from the affected side, interfering with cardiac output and ventilation *(4)*.

  2 *Pulmonary hemorrhage.* Elevated airway pressures may increase bleeding.

  3 *Active tuberculosis.* Administration of positive pressure may spread infection to other areas of the lungs.

  4 *Hyperventilation.* A patient who is hyperventilating may increase the level of hyperventilation when using a mechanical device. Hyperventilation can cause tissue hypoxia, depletion of potassium stores, and acute respiratory alkalosis.

  5 *Increased intracranial pressure.* Further pressure increases may occur and compromise closed head injuries.

  6 *Decreased cardiac output.* According to Cournand's work, IPPB may cause a further reduction in cardiac output by creating an external force on the great vessels of the chest, restricting return of venous blood to the right side of the heart.

  7 *Uncooperative patient.* It is doubtful that IPPB is beneficial in cases in which the patient is resisting the pressure generated by the machine. Most pressure-positive pressure-cycled devices will not deliver adequate tidal volumes under these circumstances, which may result in hypoventilation. IPPB should never be forced on the unwilling or uncooperative patient. Treatments given with masks to a resistant patient may cause patient exhaustion, gastric distension, and regurgitation of stomach contents, resulting in possible aspiration pneumonia.

  8 *Evidence of air trapping.* In situations involving air trapping in the lungs, IPPB may compound the problem by sequentially increasing inspiratory volumes without allowing adequate time for exhalation to occur. This situation can lead to accidental increased functional residual capacity (inadvertent or iatrogenic positive end expiratory pressure [PEEP]), causing adverse cardiac responses as a result of reduced cardiac output.

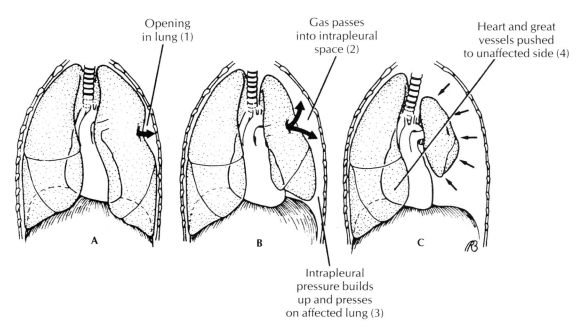

Opening in lung (1)

Gas passes into intrapleural space (2)

Heart and great vessels pushed to unaffected side (4)

Intrapleural pressure builds up and presses on affected lung (3)

FIGURE 17-2 Tension pneumothorax. **A** and **B,** An opening in the lung causes air to pass into the intrapleural space. **C,** Pressure builds, causing the affected lung to be compressed and the heart and great vessels to be pushed out of position.

9 *Improper prescription or supervision.* IPPB should not be given without a properly written medical prescription and constant supervision by qualified respiratory care personnel. For maximum benefits, patients *should never be left alone* during IPPB treatments for numerous reasons, including:

  a Syncope (fainting), resulting from decrease in blood flow to the brain.
  b Pneumothorax.
  c Cardiac involvement, because of infringement on cardiac output or changes in blood gases.
  d Undesirable reactions to drugs being aerosolized.
  e Improper breathing patterns or tidal volumes may negate any expected benefits from the treatment.

  If an IPPB treatment is to be effective, the patient must be constantly coached and the machine adjusted to compensate for the patient's changing airway conditions.

10 Availability of a more economical but equally effective method. The use of IPPB as a treatment has been greatly reduced because of alternative methods for helping patients increase their tidal volumes. *Incentive spirometry,* combined with breathing exercises, has been shown to prevent and reduce atelectasis in patients who are physically capable of generating elevated tidal volumes without mechanical assistance.

5.0 ASSESSING THE NEED FOR IPPB
5.1 Assessing the patient for IPPB

In assessing a patient for an IPPB treatment, the following considerations are important:

1 The *physiologic* and *pathologic rationale* for IPPB. Will it accomplish what is expected?
2 Any contraindications to IPPB:
  a Low blood pressure
  b Pulmonary bleeding
  c Pneumonthorax without a functioning chest tube
  d Tracheoesophageal fistula
  e Bullous disease
3 The patient's vital signs and the possible deleterious effects of IPPB.
4 The attitude and physical ability of the patient to cooperate.
5 Special needs of patient:
  a Positioning
  b Ventilator attachments
  c Assistance from another therapist in order to carry out the treatment
6 The effects of prescribed drugs on patient—awareness of any potential untoward (harmful) side effects of drug.
7 Whether or not another method would be better and less expensive for the patient.
8 Which IPPB machine would do the best job on the basis of flows, pressure limits, fraction of inspired concentration of oxygen (FIo_2) ranges, sensitivity, humidification, nebulization, and monitoring capabilities.
9 The capability of personnel to carry out orders.

5.2 Practical measurements for determining need for IPPB

1 One method for determining whether or not IPPB will improve a patient's alveolar ventilation is to compare the patient's lung volumes with IPPB to what he or she is capable of generating by spontaneous ventilation. (For details regarding measurement of lung volumes, see Module Fifteen.)
2 Methods for assessing the benefits of IPPB to achieve improved lung volume include:
  a 10% or greater vital capacity than that achieved by the patient during spontaneous efforts.
  b 10% or greater increase in inspiratory capacity than that achieved by the patient with spontaneous efforts.
  c Tidal volume greater than that achieved by the patient's breathing spontaneously.

These criteria also may be used to estimate how large a tidal volume should be delivered to provide an effective IPPB treatment.

6.0 WRITTEN MEDICAL ORDER FOR IPPB
6.1 Criteria for a medical order

1 IPPB, like all drugs, must be given according to a physician's prescription.

  A medical order should give directions as to what to do; when to do it; how to do it (i.e., what equipment, drugs, how long); and what precautions or special procedures are to be applied.

2 A *properly* written IPPB treatment order normally contains the following information:
  a Type of treatment.*
  b Treatment objectives.
  c Equipment, including method of connecting patient to the ventilator.*
  d Frequency of treatment.
  e Medication and/or humidity instructions should contain:
    • Type
    • Dosage
    • Instructions
    • Oxygen percentage
    • Physiologic indicators
    • Device*
    • Temperature
    • Percent or output volume in humidity
  f Length of treatment
  g Treatment pressure limits or other specific instructions, such as tidal volumes, FIo_2, peak pressures, chest physical therapy, deep breathing and coughing.
  h Special correlated instructions, such as:
    • Suction—as needed (PRN)*
    • Chest physical therapy*
    • Emergency action (standing orders)*
    • Alternatives to IPPB

---

*In some hospitals the items with an asterisk are chosen by the practitioner on the basis of standing orders or previous agreement with the medical staff.

7.0 TECHNIQUES CONCERNING IPPB TREATMENT

7.1 Suggested format for patient instruction

There are currently two methods for administering an IPPB treatment.

1 The first and most frequently used method is the *passive technique* in which the *ventilator performs the work* of pushing air into the lungs during inspiration. Exhalation is passive. The key to this type of treatment is for the patient to relax and let the machine do the work.

2 The second method for administering an IPPB treatment is the *active technique* in which the patient *actively inspires with the ventilator* as the positive pressure breath is being delivered. This technique is used most frequently as a deep breathing maneuver for patients who may be restricting chest movement because of postsurgical pain.

The following scenario is *one* approach for instructing the patient on how to take a passive IPPB treatment. It is imperative that the physician, the nurse, or you *explain the need* for the treatment and, before bringing the equipment to the bedside, answer any questions the patient may have.

Once you enter the room, you should position the machine so the patient can see it and you as you explain the procedure. Do not let the patient hold the mouthpiece or mask at this point. Then say to the patient:

"Mr. (or Ms.) _____, the following instructions will help you understand more about the [name the IPPB machine] and how you should use it. Please let me complete my instructions, and then I'll answer any questions you may have about the treatment."

You would then proceed to instruct the patient slowly and carefully on the following points:

"Please seal your mouth firmly around the mouthpiece." (Point it out.)

"Initially, I will need to hold your nose closed with a nose clip." (Demonstrate how it works.) "Eventually, you will learn to breathe on the machine without it. If you are a nose breather, you may feel a little short of breath initially, but this will disappear when you begin breathing on the machine."

"You will start the machine by taking a slight breath; that is, 'sip' on the mouthpiece."

"When you do this, the machine will come on, and you will hear this noise and will feel air going into your chest." (Turn machine on.)

"When this occurs, relax and let the machine fill your lungs until it turns off." (Cycle machine off.)

"Hold your breath for 1 to 3 seconds to help spread and deposit the medicine you will be inhaling. Then exhale slowly."

"When you breathe out, your efforts should be relaxed, and the gas in your chest will go out through the mouthpiece [or mask]. Be sure and allow time for your chest to empty before you take another breath."

Give the exhalation valve assembly to the patient and proceed:

"Do you have any questions?"

"If not, let's try one breath to make sure you understand the procedure." (Be sure the pressure and flow rate are low enough so as not to frighten the patient.)

Once the patient is able to use the machine, the practitioner should coach the patient and adjust pressure and gas flow to achieve desired results.

7.2 Points to remember about IPPB treatments

1 The machine must be *sensitive enough* to respond to the patient's slightest inspiratory effort. One method of observing sensitivity is to note the movement of the pressure manometer needle on the face of the machine (Fig. 17-3, *1*). Movements of the needle to indicate efforts of more than -2 cm H_2O pressure, as the patient attempts to take a breath, would indicate that the machine is *not* sensitive enough *(2)*.

2 A *tight seal* must be maintained at all times between the patient and the apparatus. Leaks may occur at tubing junctions, around the patient's mouth, through the nose, or around the fit of a mask. In most IPPB machines, a leak in the system will result in the machine *not* turning off after an inspiration is begun (pressure-limited type).

3 A *suitable control pressure and flow* should be selected that will not overinflate or underinflate the patient's lungs, resulting in unnecessary apprehension. Most patients can tolerate an initial positive pressure of 10 to 15 cm H_2O without experiencing apprehension. A desired tidal volume can be determined by using a spirometer-type device to measure exhaled volumes.

4 The patient must *relax* and let the respirator do the majority of the work of breathing. An uncooperative or apprehensive patient will cause the machine to cycle off prematurely once an inspiration has begun. Note the patient's position during the treatment. A slouched position will hamper diaphragmatic movement, resulting in smaller lung volumes.

5 The *nebulizer must be functioning properly,* and there must be an adequate quantity of medication. If a nebulizer is functioning, a mist can be seen during inspiration.

6 *Tidal volume must be greater* than what the patient can achieve breathing spontaneously, as measured by a spirometer.

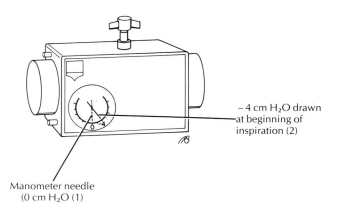

-4 cm H_2O drawn at beginning of inspiration (2)

Manometer needle (0 cm H_2O (1)

FIGURE 17-3 Pressure manometer on Bird Mark 7 face shows needle at rest (O cm H_2O) and during initiation of inspiration (-4 cm H_2O).

7 The practitioner should observe the patient, monitor the pulse, and make treatment adjustments as indicated by the treatment. An increase in the pulse of *20 beats/minute or greater* usually requires that the treatment be interrupted until the supervisor or nurse in charge is contacted, and modifications can be made in the treatment medication.

8 The practitioner should be aware that the obese patient will have difficulty in accepting an effective IPPB treatment unless care is taken to minimize the restriction of the chest by the stomach. If it is possible for these patients to stand during treatment, the results are better.

7.3 Breathing patterns for IPPB treatment

1 The lung is comprised of millions of small compartments (alveoli) interconnected by small and large airway passages. For this reason the lung does not fill or empty simultaneously. The pressure required to open the lung (critical opening pressure) and the point at which the lung unit closes (critical closing pressure) will vary from patient to patient and from breath to breath in the same patient. To obtain maximum alveolar ventilation and gas distribution, different gas flows and pressure patterns must be established for each patient.

2 A typical breathing pattern for an *obstructed patient* would be:

a Slow inspiration to preset pressure limit

b Breath held for 1 to 3 seconds

c Slow exhalation to baseline

NOTE: Exhalation should *not* be forced to the residual volume level.

d If the patient is unable to hold his or her breath (pause at the end of inspiration), an expiratory retard may be used, with a physician's order, to slow exhalation and create a more balanced internal to external airway pressure, preventing early airway collapse and gas trapping. Expiratory retard usually is achieved by placing a cap with small holes over the exhalation post of the exhalation valve. Patients with chronic obstruction pulmonary disease (COPD) have learned to create an anatomic retard by pursing their lips during exhalation or by whistling.

8.0 CHARTING AN IPPB TREATMENT

8.1 Proper charting procedure for IPPB therapy treatment

When the practitioner charts an IPPB treatment, the following information should be recorded, in ink:

1 The date

2 The time the treatment was started and finished

3 What was given

4 How it was given (method, technique, device used)

5 Length of treatment

6 Patient's response to the treatment (especially changes possibly caused by IPPB)

7 Special techniques that were used (instructions to the next practitioner)

8 Notations to the physician (suggestions, observations)

9 Who gave the treatment (full name and credentials)

10 Recommendations for discontinuing therapy, when indicated

9.0 IPPB TERMS AND PRINCIPLES

9.1 Terminology related to the operation of IPPB machine

1 Assist mode. A ventilator that is set to aid the spontaneously breathing patient by delivering a positive pressure breath during inspiration. The patient *must initiate* each breath whenever a ventilator is set to assist breathing.

2 Assist/control mode. A ventilator that is set to aid the spontaneously breathing patient who is breathing at a desired rate and volume. If the patient should stop breathing spontaneously or if the tidal volume becomes inadequate, the ventilator will automatically "take over" and control (breathe for) the patient. Most ventilators used for continuous ventilation have the capability of being operated in both the assist and control modes.

3 Breathing circuit. The external tubing and accessories that connect the ventilator to the patient.

4 Constant. A continuous action, regardless of internal and external influences. Ventilator performance may be identified as pressure, flow, or volume constant.

5 Control mode. A ventilator that is set to breathe for patients who are unable to maintain an adequate rate and depth of ventilation on their own.

6 Controls. Knobs or levers used to operate the ventilator. Although the function of most controls of various brands of ventilators are similar, the movement to activate the control will vary and should be understood before attempting to operate a ventilator on a patient.

7 "Cycle the machine." A phrase meaning to turn the ventilator to an "on" or "off" function.

8 Cycling valve. A device that causes gas to flow from the ventilator during inspiration and closes, stopping gas flow, for exhalation.

9 Expiratory valve. A device in the breathing circuit that closes at the end of exhalation and during inspiration to form an airtight system for positive pressure to be delivered to the patient. This valve subsequently opens during exhalation to permit the patient to exhale into the room or a spirometer rather than back into the ventilator (one-way valve).

10 Flow controlled. A flow-controlled device is one in which the flow rate is manually set by the operator.

11 Flow rate. Speed of gas movement between two points as caused by a pressure difference. Other things held constant the greater the pressure difference, the higher (faster) the gas flow. Gas flow is usually expressed as the volume (liters) of gas that moves from one point to another in a given period of time, usually per minute (L/min, lpm) or per second (L/sec).

12 Flow variable. A device in which the flow rate changes automatically to compensate for changes in distal airway pressure.

13 Generator. A device that produces some product or outcome, such as flow or pressure. The performance of ventilators is classified according to constant flow or pressure generators.

14 Pressure. Force generated to provide gas flow from a region of higher pressure at the machine to one of lower pressure in the patient's airway.

15 Pressure limit. Maximum pressure that can be achieved during inspiration.

16 Resuscitator. A device or person that intervenes to provide emergency life support to a patient whose heart and/or lungs have failed. A mechanical pulmonary resuscitator differs from a ventilator in that, normally, it is used for a short period of time (less than 1 hour) and therefore does *not* have the accessories needed for long-term ventilation.

17 "Trigger the machine." A phrase meaning to turn the ventilator to the "on" function.

18 Ventilator (respirator). A mechanical device used to deliver artificial breaths to a patient.

19 Ventilator classification. A verbal description of how a ventilator will function, based on evaluation of various criteria, such as pressure, flow, volume, resistance, and compliance.

10.0 IPPB DEVICES
10.1 Applying gas flow concepts to the operation of various types of IPPB devices

1 The delivery of intermittent positive pressure gas to a patient's airway (Fig. 17-4) is a relatively simple technology requiring a pressure source (usually 45 to 55 psig) *(1)* and a valve that opens and closes to block the expiratory port *(2)*. This valve can be as simple as placing a finger over the expiratory port (Fig. 17-5), or it can be complex, i.e., blocking the port with an electronic or a mechanical valve. When the device is in operation, during the inspiratory phase one end of the T is attached to the patient (see Fig. 17-5, *1*). The other end

is opened to the flowing gas source *(2)*. The third side or expiratory side (port) of the T is occluded *(3)*, causing the flowing gas under pressure to enter the patient *(4)*. Gas will continue to flow into the patient until:

a The expiratory side is opened.

b Pressure in the tubing system equals the source pressure.

c Pressure source is interrupted.

2 When gas flow is interrupted for any reason, gas pressure will be released and expiration will begin. Most ventilators and IPPB machines function by some variation of this principle. The following units present examples of various types of IPPB machines and a general description of how they function.

11.0 BASIC COMPONENTS OF IPPB MACHINES
11.1 Valves and breathing circuits

The respirators (ventilators) discussed in the following units represent three different types of devices selected primarily because of differences in valve function. These IPPB machines are primarily used to deliver 10- to 20-minute therapy treatments with nebulization; they are not for continuous ventilation, even though some of the units have this capability. Most IPPB devices incorporate the following *generic* components in one form or another:

1 *Gas pressure source.* The source gas for most ventilators is generated by a cylinder, wall piping system, or air compressor, powering the ventilator at 45 to 55 psig. If a reducing valve is used, it must be calibrated to deliver 45 to 55 psig without a flowmeter. Attachment to the ventilator is made directly from the outlet of the reducing valve to the ventilator via a high-pressure hose.

2 *Main control valve.* This valve is usually located inside the ventilator housing to the ventilator and serves the primary function of starting and stopping gas flow through the ventilator.

a Fig. 17-6 shows a ceramic switch (slide valve) like

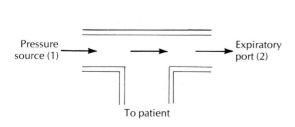

FIGURE 17-4 An IPPB device in its simplest form consists of a T-shaped tube with a gas pressure source at one end, an expiratory port at the other end, and the patient breathing tube between them. Blockage of the expiratory port will cause air to flow to the patient.

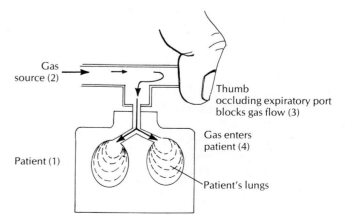

FIGURE 17-5 Simple IPPB device. Finger is used to block expiratory port and then inflate lungs.

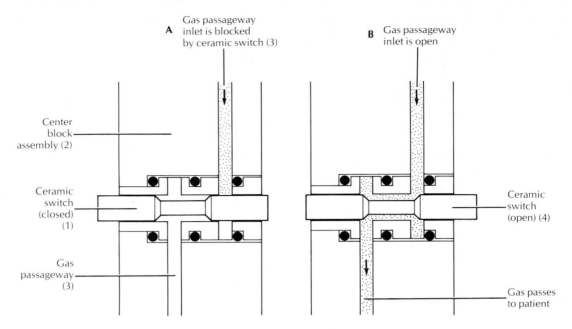

FIGURE 17-6 Ceramic switch assembly as seen in Bird Mark series. **A,** Gas flow is blocked by switch. **B,** Gas passageway is open for gas flow. (Courtesy Bird Corp, Palm Springs, Calif.)

the one used in the Bird Mark series of ventilators. This ceramic switch *(1)* is located in a center block assembly *(2)* (Bird Mark 7). The block assembly contains hollow passages or tubes through which gas is directed to perform various functions of the ventilator *(3)*. The switch moves *(4)* back and forth to open and close the valve.

Communication channels connect the ambient and pressure sides of the ventilator, which are separated by a rubber diaphragm. Increases or decreases in pressure cause the diaphragm to extend or relax, and thus the ceramic switch slides back and forth, opening or closing a channel located on the switch. (See McPherson for a complete explanation of the Bird ventilator.)

b Fig. 17-7 shows the Bennett valve system comprised of an adjustable pressure-regulating device, which is manually turned by a control knob *(1)* to reduce the source pressure from 45 to 55 psig to cm H_2O pressure as it leaves the reducing valve *(2)*. The drum valve (Bennett valve) *(3)* blocks the gas pressure *(4)* (cm H_2O) until it is rotated open *(5)* by the patient's inspiratory effort or automatically by a ventilator control. When the drum is rotated counterclockwise, an orifice (hole) through the valve center *(6)* is aligned with the block gas pressure. Once alignment occurs, gas passes through the valve and flows to the patient until the drum closes. The gas pressure generated at the patient is preset with the control knob *(1)*.*

c Fig. 17-8 shows a solenoid control valve that is both electrically and mechanically operated to open and close to provide gas flow to the patient. This valve will be explained in more detail because it is used in most electrically operated ventilators, including the Bennett MA and 7200 series, the Bourns BEAR, the Siemens Servo, and others, including many high-frequency ventilators.

A solenoid valve is comprised of two chambers (see Fig. 17-8, *A* and *B*) separated by a movable diaphragm *(1)*. To operate the valve, a control knob *(2)* is rotated to the right, putting pressure via a spring on the diaphragm *(3)*. The diaphragm rests against an electrical switch *(4)* in the "off" position. Source gas pressure at 45 to 55 psig is blocked from chamber *B* by a metal gate valve *(5)*. In the "assist" phase, when the pressure in chamber *B* is *reduced* by some action at the outlet *(6)*, such as a patient initiating a breath, the diaphragm moves down toward the reduced pressure area and contacts another electrical switch *(7)*.

This completes an electrical circuit to charge a core magnet *(8)*. The metal gate valve is attracted upward *(9)*, and gas enters chamber B until the pressure in chamber *B* pushes the diaphragm up and away from the switch *(7)* to close the valve *(4)*. When this occurs, the valve remains closed until the pressure in chamber *B* once again is reduced, and the process begins anew.

This process can be as rapid or as slow as the gas pressure is increased and decreased in chamber *B*. Opening and closing of the solenoid is usually coordinated with the inspiratory and expiratory needs of the patient. In high-frequency ventilators the sole-

---

*See McPherson for additional information on the theory of operation for the Bennett respirator series.

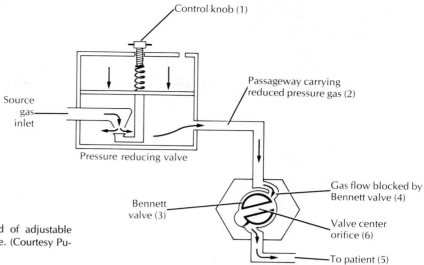

Control knob (1)

Passageway carrying reduced pressure gas (2)

Source gas inlet

Pressure reducing valve

Bennett valve (3)

Gas flow blocked by Bennett valve (4)

Valve center orifice (6)

To patient (5)

FIGURE 17-7 Bennett valve system comprised of adjustable pressure-regulating device and the Bennett drum valve. (Courtesy Puritan-Bennet Corp, Los Angeles, Calif.)

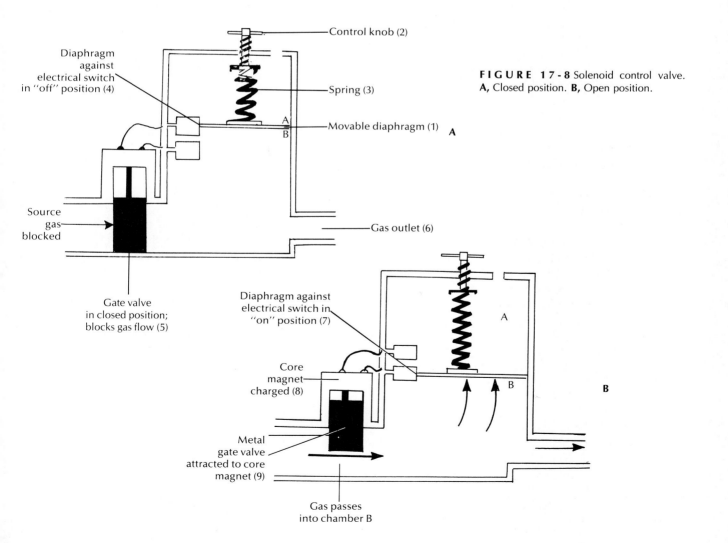

Control knob (2)

Diaphragm against electrical switch in "off" position (4)

Spring (3)

Movable diaphragm (1)   **A**

FIGURE 17-8 Solenoid control valve. **A**, Closed position. **B**, Open position.

Source gas blocked

Gas outlet (6)

Gate valve in closed position; blocks gas flow (5)

Diaphragm against electrical switch in "on" position (7)

Core magnet charged (8)

Metal gate valve attracted to core magnet (9)

Gas passes into chamber B

B

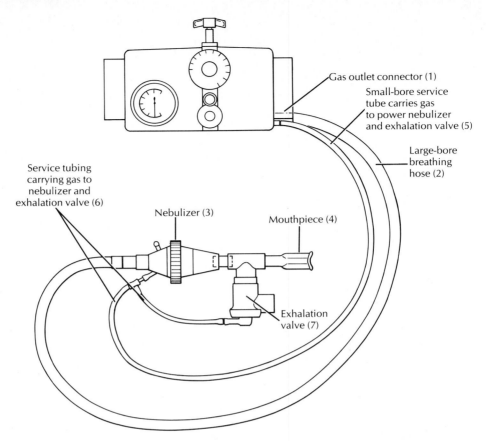

Gas outlet connector (1)

Small-bore service tube carries gas to power nebulizer and exhalation valve (5)

Large-bore breathing hose (2)

Service tubing carrying gas to nebulizer and exhalation valve (6)

Nebulizer (3)

Mouthpiece (4)

Exhalation valve (7)

FIGURE 17-9 Bird Mark 7 breathing circuit. (Courtesy Bird Corp, Palm Springs, Calif.)

noid may open and close at a rate greater than 1000 cycles per minute.

3 *Breathing circuit.* The breathing circuit provides the connection between the ventilator and the patient. It will vary in name, size, shape, color, and component parts, depending on the ventilator. Regardless of the brand of ventilator, most breathing circuits usually will include some variation of the components as shown in Fig. 17-10. Typical *standard* breathing circuits for IPPB machines are presented in Figs. 17-9 and 17-10.

a Bird Mark 7 respirator. The breathing circuit in Fig. 17-9 is attached to the ventilator by a male connector inserted into the gas outlet side of the ventilator cabinet *(1)*. A large-bore breathing hose *(2)* carries gas to a nebulizer *(3)* and to a mouthpiece *(4)*. A smaller tube (service tube) *(5 and 6)* supplies a flow of gas to power the nebulizer and to close the exhalation valve *(7)* during inhalation.

b Bennett PV-3P (see Fig. 17-10) shows a breathing circuit with more components than are standard with most IPPB circuits. A breathing circuit is attached to the ventilator at the gas outlet located on the bottom of the ventilator head *(1)* via a large-bore breathing tube *(2)*, connecting to a manifold containing a nebulizer *(3)* and exhalation valve *(4)*. Another large

tube attaches the expiratory port *(5)* of the exhalation valve to a spirometer *(6)* via a hollow metal tube *(7)*. The small tubes serve other components, such as the exhalation valve *(8)*, the nebulizer *(9)*, and the reset on the spirometer *(10)*.

4 *Automatic cycling control.* May or may not be present on IPPB therapy devices. It is used to cycle the machine automatically should the patient stop breathing and require controlled ventilation. This control is *not* normally used during routine therapy.

11.2 Gas flow through a standard Bird respirator circuit

Fig. 17-11 *(A and B)* on p. 494 diagrammatically illustrates gas flow through a standard Bird breathing circuit.

1 During inspiration, gas passes across the slide valve *(1)* and leaves the ventilator via a small-bore service hose *(2)* at an accelerated rate. This gas arrives first to power the nebulizer *(3)* and seats the exhalation valve by generating a gas pressure above the diaphragm *(4)*.

The main flow of gas flows by passing through the larger-bore main breathing tube *(5)* where it goes to the patient.

2 During exhalation the main valve in the ventilator is closed *(6)*, and gas flow is blocked to the breathing circuit.

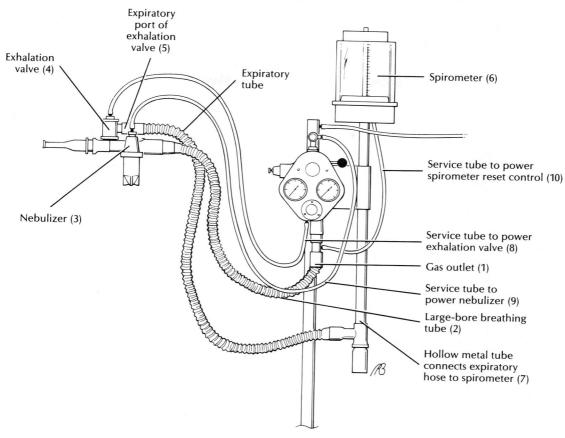

FIGURE 17-10 Bennett breathing circuit. (Courtesy Puritan-Bennett Corp, Los Angeles, Calif.)

When this occurs, the nebulizer stops operating, and the pressure above the exhalation diaphragm is vented, allowing the patient to exhale *(7)*. Most breathing circuits operate in a manner similar to this, whether operating on a therapy machine or a continuous ventilator.

3 Information important to the respiratory care practitioners includes:

a Knowing how to disassemble and reassemble any breathing circuits (for cleaning and service) they may be using.

b Avoiding the belief that disposable circuits are better or that they are used by all hospitals. Under Medicare's proposed payment system for reimbursement to hospitals, departments may return to decontaminating and reusing permanent circuits.

c Being especially aware of the need for secure connections and the position of valves, rubber gaskets, and other components whenever any breathing circuit is used.

12.0 OPERATIONAL CHARACTERISTICS OF TYPICAL IPPB THERAPY DEVICES
12.1 Characteristics of the Bennett and the Bird series

The distinguishing feature of the Bennett respirator series is the Bennett valve used in conjunction with an adjustable pressure regulator. This valve was invented by Dr. Ray Bennett in 1945 for use in high-altitude military air-

craft. Since then, it has been perfected for medical applications. The Bennett valve is flow-sensitive (i.e., open and closes to automatically increase or decrease flow rates in response to changes in resistance to the flowing gas as the tidal volume is being delivered). For this reason, Bennett IPPB therapy devices do not have separate flow controls. The adjustable regulator is called a mixing regulator because it can mix room air and pure oxygen. The regulator is located inside the Bennett cabinet and allows the operator to set positive pressure limits from 0 to 45 cm H_2O by turning a control knob located on the front of the cabinet. This pressure limit establishes the maximum pressure gradient (difference) that causes gas to flow through the Bennett valve when it is open to the patient's airway. As pressure builds in the patient's airway, the pressure gradient is decreased and the valve will rotate closed. The point at which the gas flow ceases is the *terminal flow*.*

1 Bennett respirators (ventilators) used for IPPB therapy include:

a Pneumatically powered units
  • Model TV-2P
  • Model PV-3P
  • Model TV-4
  • Model TO-2

---

*See McPherson (Index) for additional details regarding operation of the Bennett valve.

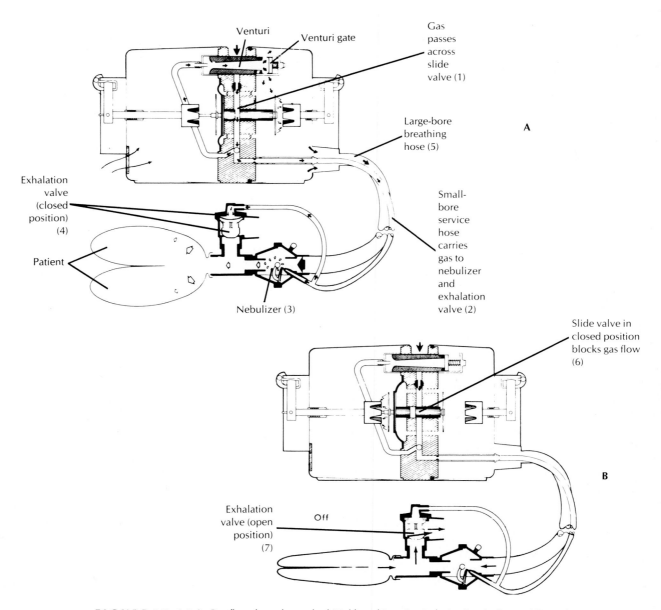

FIGURE 17-11 A, Gas flow through standard Bird breathing circuit during inspiration and **B,** expiration. Pre-1976 Mark 7. (Courtesy Bird Corp, Palm Springs, Calif., which now holds all rights to Bird 3-M Corp. [Minneapolis] equipment mentioned throughout this text.)

- Model PR-1*
- Model PR-2*
  b Electrically powered units using air compressors:
  - Models TA-1, TA-1B
  - Models AP-4, AP-4B
  - Models AP-5, AP-5B
2 Technical specifications for various Bennett IPPB units include:
  a Model TA-1 and 2, hand-held IPPB devices (Fig. 17-12):
  - Self-contained 115-volt compressor controlled by off/on knob on front of cabinet *(1)*.
  - Adjustable pressure range +10 to 30 cm H_2O by knob on front of cabinet *(2)*.
  - Adjustable flow to 85 L/min, preset at factory.
  - Sensitivity control unnecessary, since flow is continuous; occlusion of manual finger-operated valve provides positive pressure *(3)*.
  b Model AP-4 or AP-5, self-contained compressor-driven unit (see McPherson AP series):
  - Self-contained electrical compressor powered by off/on switch located on front of cabinet.
  - Pressure limits adjustable 0-45 cm H_2O by rotation of control knob.
  - Maximum flow rate of 85 L/min as determined by opening/closing of flow-sensitive Bennett valve.
  - Terminal flow preset at 4 L/min.
  - Nebulizer drive gas: maximum 6.5 psig or 8 L/min as regulated by nebulizer control valve.
  - Internal safety release: 7.5 psig.
  - Pressure that is being delivered appears on mask-pressure manometer.
  c Model TV-2P or PV-3P (see McPherson therapy models):
  - Powered by gas cylinder or wall service gas source. Incorporates Bennett flow-sensitive valve.
  - Air dilution or 100% FI_{O_2} selection option.
  - Constant drive nebulization with flow rate set by control.
  - Automatic cycling unavailable.
  - Sensitivity factory set at 1 cm H_2O; not adjustable.
  d Model TV-4 same as model TV-2P, but without 100% oxygen option.
3 The Bird respirators (ventilators)** used for IPPB therapy include:
  a Mark series
  - Mark 7, Mark 7A
  - Mark 8, Mark 8A[†]
  - Mark 10
  - Mark 14
  - Mark 1
  b Other Bird models

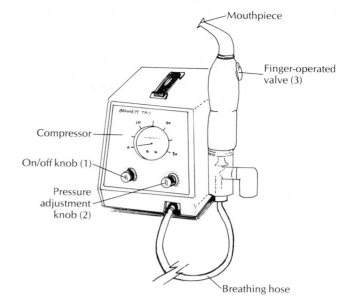

FIGURE 17-12 Model TA-1 hand-held IPPB device consisting of gas compressor providing continuous flow and breathing unit with manual finger-operated valve to provide positive pressure. (Courtesy Puritan-Bennett Corp, Los Angeles, Calif.)

- Portabird
- Minibird II
- Therapybird
4 The Bird Mark 7 respirator functions as follows (Fig. 17-13 shows a component description):
  a The oxygen from a 50 psig source enters the center body of the inlet assembly *(1)*.
  b The left side body is the ambient compartment *(2)*, and the right side body is the pressure compartment *(3)*.
  c Room air enters through a metal filter *(4)* to be mixed with the 100% oxygen. Gas that is to be delivered to the patient leaves the pressure compartment at the mainstream breathing hose connection *(5)*.
  d Gas used to drive the nebulizer and operate the exhalation valve leaves the pressure compartment *(6)*.
  e The adjustable flow rate is set with a dial control *(7)*, the sensitivity is adjusted with a rotary push-pull lever *(8)*, and the pressure is adjusted with a similar lever *(9)*.
  f A "push-pull" selector *(10)* allows the use of either 100% oxygen or air-mix for therapy gas.
  g The unit can be turned "on" (cycled) manually with the hand timer rod *(11)* or operated automatically with the pneumatic expiratory timer control *(12)*.
  h The system pressure is read on the pressure manometer *(13)*.

---

*These ventilators have automatic cycling capability and may be used for continuous ventilation as well as IPPB therapy.

**See McPherson for details on specifications of each Bird model.

†Manufactured but not sold in the United States.

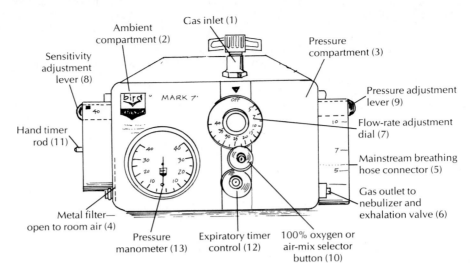

FIGURE 17-13 Components of Bird Mark 7 ventilator. (Courtesy Bird Corp, Palm Springs, Calif.)

13.0 OPERATION OF THE BENNETT MODEL PR-2 RESPIRATOR

13.1 Specifications for the Bennett PR-2 respirator (ventilator)

The Bennett PR series 1 and 2 are very popular devices for use in providing IPPB therapy.

1 The performance characteristics of the PR-1 and PR-2 devices are the same, with the following exceptions:
  a Peak flow rates are greater in the PR-2 because of a terminal flow control (12 to 15 L/min additional).
  b Peak flow rates can be adjusted on the PR-2 by rotating a choke valve, which forces gas leaving the Bennett valve to pass through a restricting orifice.
  c An expiratory timer control on the PR-2 allows the operator to prolong expiratory time and directly alter the patient's inspiratory to expiratory breathing ratio (I:E ratio).
    NOTE: This adjustment is used only when the respirator is used as a controller.
  d As negative-pressure control is provided with the PR-2, allowing the operator to create a subambient condition during the expiratory phase. This control is *not* used during IPPB therapy.
2 The Bennett PR-2 respirator is used as an example because it incorporates all the major features of the other Bennett units.* Performance data include:
  a Positive/negative phase ventilator.
  b Maximum pressure (45 cm H_2O at 40 to 70 psi) service pressure.
  c Maximum flow without accessories—110 L/min at 45 cm H_2O.
    • Inspiration nebulizer additional—20 L/min on maximum.
    • Terminal flow additional—12 L/min on maximum142 L/min total flow is available.
  d At 20 cm H_2O pressure: 100 L/min is available.
  e Flow into the exhalation diaphragm: 0.5 L/min to close the valve during inspiration.
  f A change from air-mix to 100% gas: drops total flow to the patient approximately 15% at any set pressure. This can be dangerous unless compensated for because it causes a decreased minute ventilation.
  g A decrease of peak flow via the control drops total patient flow as much as 84%. For example, at 20 cm H_2O pressure and air dilution, total flow is about 90 L/min. If peak flow is decreased, the total flow will decrease to 15 L/min.
  h Maximum cycling rate: 50 cycles/min at factory preset I:E ratio.
    • I:E ratio preset 1 to 1.5.
  i Sensitivity preset: pressure adjustable from −0.5 cm H_2O to −1 cm H_2O.
  j Terminal flow: 1 L/min.
  k Negative pressure: 0 to −6 cm H_2O.
  l Assisted inspiration: begun via pressure drop; ended via pressure buildup.
  m Control mode-inspiration begun via time; ended via elapsed time interval or pressure limit.
  n Bennett valve assembly:
    • Valve clearance—valve and face plate 0.001 inch each end, or total 0.002 inch.
    • Upper rubber bumper—adjusted so that peak flow is 75 L/min at 20 cm H_2O on 100% gas.
    • Lower bumper—controls sensitivity and terminal flow or pressure release on exhalation.

---

*The reader may find it helpful to have a Bennett unit available for reference while studying the material presented here.

13.2 General instructions for operation of the Bennett PR-2 respirator

To complete this unit of instruction the reader will need a Bennett PR-2 ventilator, a 50 psig gas source, and a test lung. The instructions presented in this section are general. More specific detail can be obtained from review of the PR-2 operator's manual. Refer to Fig. 17-14 while following these instructions.

NOTE: The patient should not be attached until all controls have been adjusted and the respirator checked for proper operation with a test lung.

1 Operation of assisted mode.
   a Connect the unit to a 45 to 55 psig gas source, either air or oxygen.
   b Turn all controls to "off."
   c Establish patient's tidal volume by turning control pressure *(1)* until desired level is read on the control pressure manometer *(2)*.
   d Select either 100% O_2 or air-mix by pushing in or pulling out dilution control located on the side of the cabinet *(3)*.
   e Rate control *(4)* should be turned to the right or "off" if the patient is breathing on his or her own (assisting).
   f Deliver aerosol (drugs). Turn inspiration nebulizer control *(5)* one full turn counterclockwise. Leave expiration nebulizer *(6)* control "off" unless patient has small tidal volumes, as in pediatric cases.
   g Determine inspiratory effort. Set sensitivity control *(7)*. This control establishes the amount of inspiratory effort a patient must generate before the machine cycles "on." Adjust by occluding end of breathing tube and turning sensitivity control counterclockwise until the machine begins to cycle "on" and "off" spontaneously (chatter). When this occurs, slowly turn control clockwise until chattering ceases. The manometer needle *(8)* will stop moving.
   h Shorten inspiratory time or compensate for a small-system gas leak. Turn terminal flow control *(9)* counterclockwise as patient inhales. This additional flow of gas combines with main gas flow coming from Bennett valve to generate desired system pressure. The greater the gas flow, the quicker the preset control pressure is reached and the shorter is inspiration. A small-system gas leak can be compensated for by opening the terminal flow control during inspiration until the respirator cycles "off."
   NOTE: Do *not* use terminal flow to compensate for a poor mouthpiece or mask fit.
   i Establish gas flow rate. Rotation of the peak flow control *(10)* serves to "dampen" (reduce) gas flow velocity by causing gas leaving the Bennett valve to pass across a variable orifice (hole).
   NOTE: Rotation of the peak flow control clockwise will decrease tidal volumes. This control is used to cause a more gradual rise of airway pressure to cause better distribution across airway obstructions.
   j During IPPB in an assisting patient, rate control *(4)*,

expiration time control *(11)*, and negative pressure control *(12)* should be "off."

2 Operation of controlled mode.
   If the patient is not ventilating adequately in terms of rate or depth, controlled ventilation is indicated. For administering IPPB therapy to the controlled patient, machine operation is the same as for assisted mode except:
   a Turn sensitivity control *(7)* to "off."
   b Adjust rate cycling control *(4)* clockwise until the machine cycles at the desired frequency.
   CAUTION: When used as a controller, the PR-2 is *time* cycled and will cycle "off" and "on" even if it is *not* attached to the patient. In this mode, one cannot rely on the sound of operation as an indicator that the patient is being ventilated. For this reason, *disconnect alarms* should always be used when the PR-2 is functioning as a controller.

The reader may wish to practice with a Bennett PR-2 testing his or her own lung, using all controls until familiarity with their actions are attained.

14.0 OPERATION OF THE BIRD MARK 7 RESPIRATOR
14.1 General instructions

The Bird Mark 7 respirator is presented as an example of the Bird Mark series because all models in this series use the basic Mark 7 design and operational characteristics, although maximum pressure limits and peak flow rates will vary, depending on the model.

The reader should refer to Fig. 17-15 on p. 499 while studying the following general operating instructions. More specific details can be obtained from the operator's manual.
NOTE: Use a test lung to practice adjustment of the respirator.

1 Bird Mark 7 performance data
   a Size: 5 inches $\times$ 5 inches $\times$ 8 inches
   b Weight: 6 pounds
   c Materials
      • Center body: forged aluminum
      • End compartments: transparent molded high-impact plastic
   d Power source: compressed air or oxygen at 50 psig $\pm$5 psi
   e Inspiratory pressure limit: adjustable from 5 to 60 cm H_2O (4 to 44 mm Hg)
   f Inspiratory flow rate: adjustable from 1 to 80 L/min
   g Assisted starting effort (sensitivity): -0.01 to -5 cm H_2O
   h Manual cycling: push/pull control rod
   i Inspired oxygen percentage: push/pull knob (assuming 100% oxygen as source gas)
      • Pulled out: 40% to 90% oxygen (air-mix)
      NOTE: FIO_2 will vary as Venturi opens/closes with changing resistances.
      • Pushed in: 100% oxygen
   j Expiratory time: variable during assisted operation and timed during controlled operation (0.5 to 15 seconds)

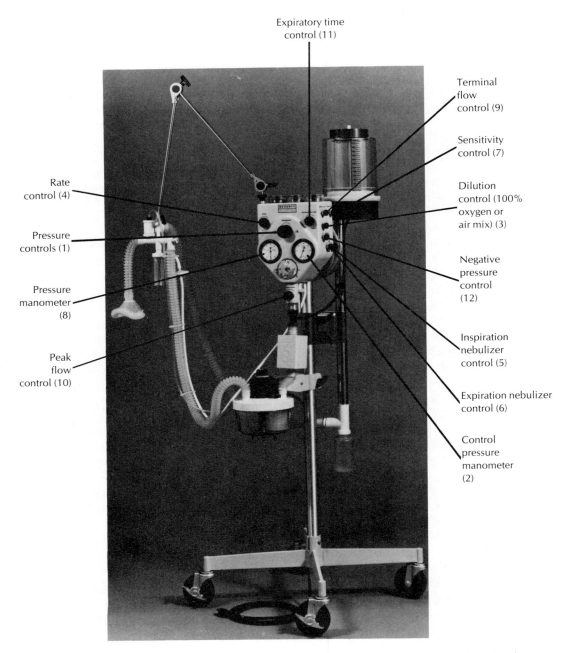

Expiratory time
control (11)

Terminal
flow
control (9)

Sensitivity
control (7)

Rate
control (4)

Dilution
control (100%
oxygen or
air mix) (3)

Pressure
controls (1)

Pressure
manometer
(8)

Negative
pressure
control
(12)

Inspiration
nebulizer
control (5)

Peak
flow
control (10)

Expiration nebulizer
control (6)

Control
pressure
manometer
(2)

F I G U R E   1 7 - 1 4 Components of Bennett PR-2 ventilator. (Courtesy Puritan-Bennett Corp, Los Angeles, Calif.)

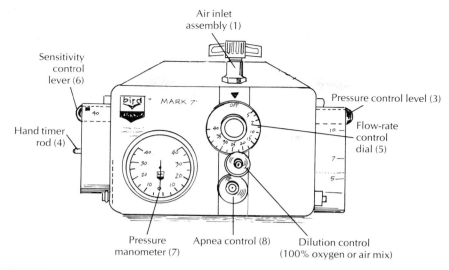

FIGURE 17-15 Operation of Bird Mark 7 ventilator. (Courtesy Bird Corp, Palm Springs, Calif.)

k Exhalation valve: nonrebreathing

l Safety entrainment valve: spring-loaded to entrain ambient compartment gas at -2 cm H_2O pressure

2 Operation of the Bird Mark 7 respirator in the assist mode (see Fig. 17-15)

a Connect Mark 7 to a gas pressure source, either air or oxygen, via the inlet assembly *(1)*.

b Attach a standard breathing circuit with a test lung attached to the patient connector at the end of the breathing circuit.

c Select either 100% oxygen or air-mix. Push air-mix control for 100% oxygen, and pull out for air mixing.

NOTE: FIO_2 is not specific and will vary from 40% to 90% oxygen, depending on gas flow rate, cycling pressure, airway potency, and patient variables.

d Adjust tidal volume. Set approximate inspiratory pressure limits by adjusting the pressure arm *(3)*. Use the manometer for accuracy.

e Manually cycle the respirator "on" by pushing in the red control rod *(4)*.

f Adjust inspiratory time. Once the inspiratory pressure limit is determined, inspiratory time is set by turning the *flow rate control (5)* counterclockwise. Adjustment should be made only during the *inspiratory* cycle so that an adequate I:E ratio and tidal volume can be established. Flow rate should be increased during inspiration until desired inspiratory time is reached, as indicated by the ventilator cycling *off*.

NOTE: Adjustment of pressure and flow will determine the patient's tidal volume in a leak-proof system. The Bird Mark 7 will not function unless the flow control is opened, allowing gas to flow to the ceramic switch.

g The apnea control *(8)* should be in the "off" position (clockwise) unless the patient needs controlled ventilation.

3 Operation of Bird Mark 7 respirator in the control mode

a If controlled ventilation is needed, controls are set for assist and the apnea control is opened (counterclockwise) until the desired cycling rate is obtained. NOTE: The Bird respirator is pressure-cycled, which means it will not cycle "off" unless the preset pressure is reached during inspiration, even though it will cycle "on" by a pneumatic timer (expiratory time control). *Disconnect alarms* should always be used when the Mark 7 is functioning in the control mode.

b A patient's chest excursion and measured exhaled tidal volumes must be used as ventilation indicators. However, actual adequacy of ventilation can only be assessed through analysis of arterial blood gases.

15.0 HAZARDS OF IPPB

15.1 Potentially hazardous situations related to the administration of IPPB therapy

The following hazards of IPPB administration should be taken into account.*

1 Hyperventilation. Respiratory alkalosis, caused by increased tidal volume and breathing frequency, can result in a decreased serum potassium ion (K^+) and increased cardiac irritability. Clinically, hyperventilation can cause muscle tremors, dizziness, tingling and numbness of extremities, and muscular spasms of the hands and feet.

2 Hypoxemia. IPPB can increase cellular hypoxia because of increased work of breathing and increased shunt.

---

*See Spearman's discussion of techniques of IPPB administration.

3 Tension pneumothorax. Elevated airway pressures, combined with a patient's uncontrolled cough, may cause rupturing of blebs in a patient's lung.

4 Hypoventilation. IPPB can cause hypoventilation in a patient who is uncooperative and in situations in which the practitioner is not aware of what constitutes an adequate tidal breath.

5 Hyperoxygeneration. Most oxygen-powered therapy machines are not capable of accurately delivering low concentrations of oxygen. Percentages of 40% to 90% oxygen may cause apnea in a CO_2 retainer.

6 Decreased cardiac output. Decreased venous return may be caused by use of excessive positive pressure combined with prolonged inspiratory times.

7 Gastric insufflation. Abdominal distension with or without subsequent nausea and vomiting may occur wherever airway pressures exceed 25 cm H_2O.

8 Adverse reaction to drugs. If nebulization is used, the patient may exhibit systemic side effects such as tachycardia, arrhythmias, nervousness, or nausea from aerosolized drugs.

9 Emotional reaction. Patient may be afraid of IPPB and/or experience claustrophobia because of mask, mouthpiece, or nose clip. Other patients may grow to depend on IPPB almost to the point of addiction.

10 Misuse. Perhaps the greatest hazard is the administration of IPPB by inexperienced personnel. This situation causes most of the aforementioned hazards.

16.0 ADMINISTERING AN IPPB THERAPY TREATMENT
16.1 Recommended techniques

1 Administering an effective IPPB treatment entails more than merely the operation of a machine. It requires a proper prescription by the physician, a thorough review of the patient's record by the practitioner, selection of appropriate equipment, a positive treatment environment for the patient, the development of rapport between the patient and practitioner, and careful instruction of the patient before and during the treatment.

2 After each treatment, patient progress should be evaluated in terms of projected goals as established by the physician and the practitioner before beginning therapy. IPPB treatments require constant attention of the practitioner, who must be continuously present during the treatment. Changes in the patient's response to therapy will require that appropriate modifications be made in the machine to provide the most effective combination of airway pressures, respiratory volumes, and flow rates.

3 A typical IPPB procedure checklist is included in Unit 17.1. For more information on giving an IPPB treatment, see Spearman's discussion of the technique of IPPB administration.

17.0 MACHINE MALFUNCTION
17.1 Recognizing problem areas

The following situations are most frequently the cause of malfunctions in pressure preset IPPB devices such as the ones described in this module. The following checklist may be used to identify and to correct the malfunction by placing a check in the space that best fits the malfunction and its solution.

Problem 1 The machine won't turn on even though the patient is assisting.
___ a Check the pressure manometer on the cabinet of the IPPB machine. If the pressure needle is moving into the negative area more than -2 cm H_2O, adjust the sensitivity control so that the machine is more sensitive.
___ b If the pressure needle is not moving, check the breathing circuit for a major leak; i.e., a disconnected tubing or an open exhalation valve.
___ c Check your gas supply for 50 psig pressure.
___ d Remove the machine from the patient and manually cycle the machine to "on." Check adequacy of gas flow, then occlude patient manifold to cause machine to cycle to "off."

Problem 2 The machine won't cycle to exhalation.
___ a Check for a leak in the system; check all connections, including tightness of patient's lips on the mouthpiece or fit of the nose clip. If a face mask is used, check for a leak around the mask.
___ b Check the exhalation valve to make sure it is sealing during the inspiratory phase. If a spirometer is being used, it will record a gas volume during inspiration if the exhalation valve is not sealing properly.
___ c Check for a sticking Bennett valve or Bird ceramic switch.

Problem 3 The machine rapidly cycles itself "on" and "off," even though the patient is attempting to breathe slowly.
___ a Check the sensitivity control and decrease sensitivity.
___ b Check the automatic cycling control and make sure it is "off."
___ c Check the pressure manometer. If the pressure needle moves rapidly up to cycling pressure and then down as the machine cycles "off," check for an occluded breathing tube, or check to see if the patient is occluding the mouthpiece with his or her tongue.

Problem 4 The pressure manometer needle is very slow returning to baseline after inspiration has ended.
___ a Check for a sticking exhalation valve.
___ b Check for a retard device on the exhalation valve.
___ c Check for a sticking spirometer.

Problem 5 Very little gas flow is coming out of the machine even though the flow control is all the way open.
___ a Check the gas source for 50 psig.
___ b Check to see if the inlet filter on the IPPB machine is clean.
___ b Check to see if the inlet filter on the IPPB machine is clean. This filter is usually located at the point where the high-pressure hose enters the machine.
___ c Check for an occluded breathing hose.
___ d Check for a major gas leak.

Problem 6 No mist is coming out of the nebulizer.

___ **a** Check for gas flow to the nebulizer.

___ **b** Check the solution level in the nebulizer.

___ **c** Check to see if the nebulizer is positioned properly.

___ **d** Check to see if the capillary tubes are open and positioned in the solution.

___ **e** Check to see if the nebulizer jets are open.

Problem 7 The patient is not getting a large enough tidal volume.

___ **a** Check the power source for 50 psig.

___ **b** Check the pressure adjustment; increase if needed.

___ **c** Check flow rate; increase or decrease as needed.

___ **d** Check the patency of all tubes.

___ **e** Check all connections for leaks.

___ **f** Check the exhalation valve to see if it is closing.

___ **g** Check to make sure the patient is not fighting the machine.

18.0 PROPER CLEANING PROCEDURE FOR IPPB DEVICES

18.1 Recommended techniques

The cleaning procedure for IPPB devices is similar to that of any respiratory care equipment.

1 It is especially important that each patient have his or her own personal breathing tube assembly, including hose, exhalation manifold, mouthpiece, and nose clip or face mask.

2 Many hospitals use disposable setups that are discarded on a routine basis and after each patient's treatment has been discontinued. As previously mentioned, this procedure may change as hospitals economize as a result of the prospective payment system for reimbursement.

3 The steps involved in cleaning follow:

  a Remove all equipment that may have been in contact with the patient's exhaled air.

  b Discard all disposable items.

  c Thoroughly wash and disinfect all reusable equipment.

  d A mainstream humidifier and its tubing, if used, should be removed daily and disinfected.

  e Wash the external cabinet and other parts of the IPPB machine to remove any dust and lint.

  f Remove any bacteria filters, and autoclave at least weekly.

  g Remove the main valve and inlet filter from the IPPB machine weekly. Clean both parts with alcohol or other suitable cleaning agent and dry thoroughly.

  h Store all equipment in a dust-free container, and cover the IPPB machine when it is not in use.

4 Clean IPPB devices according to hospital procedure.

BIBLIOGRAPHY

Burton GG, and Hodgkin JE, editors: Respiratory care: a guide to clinical practice, ed 2, Philadelphia, 1984, JB Lippincott Co.

DeTrozer A and Deisser P: The effects of intermittent positive pressure breathing on patients with respiratory weakness, Am Rev Resp Dis 124:132, 1981.

Gold MI: IPPB therapy, a current overview, Respir Care 27:586, 1982.

Indihar FJ, Forsberg DP, and Adams AB. A prospective comparison of three procedures used in attempts to prevent postoperative pulmonary complications, Respir Care 27:564, 1982.

McPherson SP: Respiratory therapy equipment, ed 4, St Louis, 1990, The CV Mosby Co.

O'Donohue BA, Peterson J, and Cane RD: Complication of mechanical aids to intermittent lung inflation, Respir Care 27:467, 1982.

Spearman CB, Sheldon RL, and Egan DF: Egan's fundamentals of respiratory therapy, ed 5, St Louis, 1990, The CV Mosby Co.

Incentive spirometry

1.0 INCENTIVE SPIROMETRY AND SUSTAINED MAXIMAL INSPIRATION

1.1 The use of incentive devices

Since 1975 alternative methods have emerged to replace intermittent positive pressure breathing (IPPB) treatments as a means of increasing a patient's lung volume. These methods include breathing exercises combined with chest physical therapy and incentive spirometry.

1 *Incentive spirometry (IS) or sustained maximal inspiration* (SMI) involves the use of a device that encourages a patient to make a larger-than-normal inspiratory effort and establish a breathing incentive.

  a This approach involves patients mentally and physically in their own recovery and is generally less expensive and yet, in most instances, as effective as IPPB therapy.

  b Incentive devices reward patients by letting them see their own progress through the use of visual indicators such as colored light displays, the suspension of colored ping-pong balls in a hollow tube, expanding bellows, flowing liquids, or electronic digital readouts. These visual rewards correlate numerically on the device to document a patient's inspired volumes.

2 The physiologic basis for these maneuvers is to persuade the patient to produce a SMI for a given period of time. This approach results in the generation of increased negative transpulmonary pressures and increased tidal volumes for the primary purpose of opening and stabilizing atelectatic areas of the lung against recurrent atelectasis.

1.2 Terminology and concepts

The following terms and concepts relate to sustained maximal inspiration and to clinical application.

1 Atelectasis. Collapsed alveoli, which may occur after illness or surgery because of secretions blocking communicating air passages, or hypoventilation during illness or surgery. It may be caused by monotonous tidal

volumes of the same depth in the spontaneously breathing or mechanically ventilated patient.

2 Incentive spirometry (IS). A reward system to encourage patients to take deep breaths.

3 Sustained maximal inspiration (SMI). The goal of incentive spirometry.

4 Valsalva's maneuver. Rapid increase of intrapulmonic pressure as a result of forcing exhalation against one's closed glottis. This effect causes a decreased venous return to the right side of the heart and, subsequently, a decrease in cardiac output. Clinical signs include disappearance of pulse, pounding sensation in the head, vertigo, and, eventually, fainting.

2.0 PREVENTING AND TREATING ATELECTASIS
2.1 Traditional approaches

1 At the beginning of this century it was surgically noted that the lung would "pop out" of the opening in the chest of patients with an open chest wound who performed a Valsalva's maneuver. It was incorrectly reasoned that a postoperative procedure that duplicated this expiratory straining would "pop out" or open areas of atelectasis in the closed chest.

2 In 1918 Harkin developed the "blow bottle" to replace the wind instruments he had been giving patients postoperatively to practice blowing (a noisy process!).

  a Collapsed alveoli, however, seem to be best expanded by generating large *negative* pleural pressures or by delivering positive pressures into the airway by intermittent positive pressure breathing (IPPB).

  b Unfortunately, blow bottles (or similar techniques) seemed to *compress* the lung by generating high positive intrapleural pressures. This caused further airway collapse, especially in the sick lung.

3 Frequently used expiratory maneuvers included:

  a *Induced cough.* Use of *indwelling intratracheal catheter* as a route for introducing irritants such as distilled water or normal saline to cause a cough.

  b *Blow bottles.* Forceful exhalation into a tube and bottle system, which generates enough pressure to cause water to flow from one bottle to the other, is supposed to create a back pressure sufficient to open atelectatic area. This is not so. As the patient exhales, the intrapleural pressure exceeds the alveolar pressure, and expansion cannot occur. Forced exhalation against resistances can, in fact, *cause* atelectasis as the intrapleural pressures consistently rise above alveolar pressure, causing airways to collapse (Fig. 18-1).

  c *Blow glove.* A clumsy, homemade device made from a plastic 60-ml syringe barrel, a rubber glove, and a rubber band. The back pressure developed is supposed to work like the blow bottles. Unless the glove is reversed first, the patient usually gets little from this treatment except "a lung full of talcum powder" (Fig. 18-2). Amazingly, this device is still used in some areas of the country. A commercial version of the blow glove is the plastic mouthpiece (Fig. 18-3) with an adjustable expiratory retard. Its effectiveness

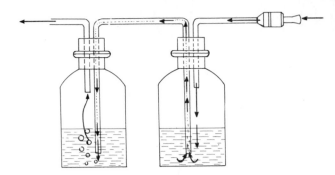

FIGURE 18-1 Blow bottles. Forceful exhalation into a tube and bottle system causes water to flow from one bottle to the other.

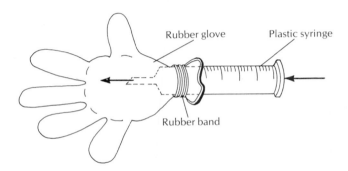

Rubber glove   Plastic syringe

Rubber band

FIGURE 18-2 Blow glove.

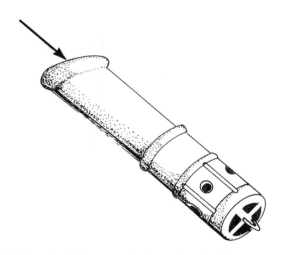

FIGURE 18-3 Plastic mouthpiece with adjustable expiratory retard.

rivaled the blow bottles as an alternative to IPPB because the procedure was less expensive and in most cases clinically as effective.

d *CO$_2$ induced hyperventilation.* Physiologically more sound than expiratory maneuvers because tidal volumes can be increased two or three times the normal resting level in most patients.

NOTE: CO$_2$ breathing can result in hypercapnia and hypoxia unless it is carefully controlled.

- One major disadvantage in the use of CO$_2$ for the treatment of atelectasis is that if the CO$_2$ levels rise, the patient usually increases *rate* more than *depth* of ventilation (minute ventilation) in an effort to "blow off" the accumulating CO$_2$.
- Devices used for CO$_2$ treatments include inhalation of 95% oxygen and 5% CO$_2$, using a nonrebreathing face mask, and use of rebreathing devices such as paper bags and long rebreathing tubes (Fig. 18-4). With any CO$_2$ rebreathing system, care must be taken to control CO$_2$ buildup and possible hypoxia.

3.0 INDICATIONS AND CONTRAINDICATIONS FOR INCENTIVE SPIROMETRY (IS)

3.1 Indications

The indications for IS are very similar to those for IPPB therapy, as presented in Module Seventeen.

1 Prevention of postoperative complications. Estimates suggest that pulmonary complications account for 2% to 3% of the overall morbidity following surgery involving general anesthesia. The primary purpose of incentive breathing programs is to help open closed alveoli, facilitate the cough reflex, help mobilize secretions, and prevent hyperventilation in the cooperative and physically capable patient.

2 Preoperative cleanup. Incentive techniques may be useful in strengthening pulmonary muscles, increasing voluntary ventilation, and generally improving "bronchial toilet" techniques before surgery.

3 Psychologic support. Involves patients mentally and physically in their own recovery process. This is especially useful in situations in which there are limited numbers of qualified persons to provide more sophisticated therapy or costs are prohibitive for the use of expensive medical equipment such as IPPB machines.

3.2 Contraindications

Contraindications for IS are similar to those for IPPB, as presented in Module Seventeen.

Uncooperative or physically disabled patients. Incentive spirometry is useful only when the patient is able to follow directions to generate an ideal inspiratory maneuver, i.e., a high alveolar-inflating pressure for durations of 5 to 15 seconds. Uncooperative patients, or patients with mental or central nervous system (CNS) disorders, are not generally good candidates for IS. Patients who are physically unable to generate large enough tidal volumes (12 to 15 ml/kg) are also not good candidates for IS.

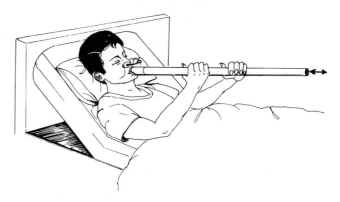

FIGURE 18-4 Rebreathing tube. Used to increase level of inspired CO$_2$.

4.0 TECHNIQUES FOR INSTRUCTING A PATIENT TO USE INCENTIVE DEVICES TO GENERATE SUSTAINED MAXIMAL INSPIRATION (SMI)

4.1 Primary considerations

Patients can be instructed in generating SMI with or without the assistance of an incentive device.

1 Incentive devices, however, do enable the practitioner to preset goals (desired lung volumes) and to see when they are achieved by the patient. Of equal or perhaps even greater importance, incentive spirometry allows the patient to participate in and see his or her own progress.

a With the use of an incentive device, the manufacturer's instructions should be followed.

b In addition, the patient should be coached to inspire *slowly* (200 ml/sec) to generate the *largest* possible tidal volume for 6 to 10 repetitions and to prolong inspiration for as long a period as possible (5 to 15 seconds).

2 Benefits derived from SMI are the result of increased tidal breaths and sustained inhalation. This sustained pressure from a prolonged inhalation allows times for generation of pressure gradients in slow-filling lung units to open and stabilize atelectatic areas.

5.0 INCENTIVE DEVICES

5.1 Functional characteristics

Since there are many different models of incentive spirometers, the following are examples of some units that use various physiologic and technical bases for their functions:

1 *Bartlett-Edwards* incentive spirometer (Fig. 18-5) functions as follows:

a A movable piston *(1)* enclosed in a cylinder *(2)* with a built-in leak in the bottom of the piston *(3)*.

b The patient is connected to the unit via a corrugated hose *(4)* and a mouthpiece *(5)*.

c When the patient takes a maximum inspiration, air is evacuated from the space above the piston *(6)*, and the piston rises as a result of the pushing effect of the atmosphere across the lower portion of the piston *(7)*.

d As the piston rises, it strikes the bottom of a volume indicator rod *(8)*. The distance this rod protrudes from the top of the spirometer indicates the volume and is set by an adjustable nut *(9)*.

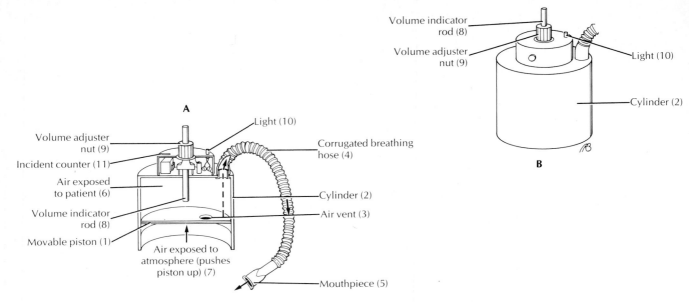

A

Volume adjuster nut (9)
Incident counter (11)
Air exposed to patient (6)
Volume indicator rod (8)
Movable piston (1)
Light (10)
Corrugated breathing hose (4)
Cylinder (2)
Air vent (3)
Air exposed to atmosphere (pushes piston up) (7)
Mouthpiece (5)

Volume indicator rod (8)
Volume adjuster nut (9)
Light (10)
Cylinder (2)

B

FIGURE 18-5 Barlett-Edwards incentive spirometer. **A,** Internal components. **B,** External components.

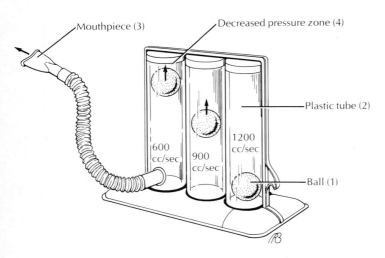

Mouthpiece (3)
Decreased pressure zone (4)
Plastic tube (2)
1200 cc/sec
600 cc/sec
900 cc/sec
Ball (1)

FIGURE 18-6 TriFlo II Incentive Deep Breathing Exerciser.

e When the rising piston strikes the bottom of the volume rod, a battery-powered light is illuminated *(10)* and an incident counter records the effort *(11)*. The light will remain on as long as the patient continues to inhale, holding the piston against the volume rod.

f The object is to have the patient *obtain the preset volume limit* and to *keep the light illuminated* for as long as possible by a sustained inspiratory effort against a preset leak *(3)* vent in the cylinder.

2 *TriFlo II* Incentive Deep Breathing Exerciser (Fig. 18-6) functions as follows:

a Round ping-pong-type colored balls of different weights *(1)* are contained in individual but interconnecting clear plastic tubes *(2)*.

b As the patient inhales through the mouthpiece *(3)*, a pressure gradient is created above each ball *(4)*, causing gas to flow into the chamber of the lightest ball first.

c When this ball reaches the top of the chamber and the patient continues to inhale, a second ball is pushed upward by room air flowing into the chamber.

d Since this process continues, the amount of gas volume being moved per second can be estimated by observing the position of each ball in the clear tube.

e The object of this exercise is to have the patient generate enough inspiratory effort to *support the balls*, correlated to the desired tidal breath as indicated by markings on the plastic cylinder. As with other incentive devices, the inspiratory effort should be slow and continuous to allow maximum lung volume with equal distribution of lung pressure.

f It is possible to reduce the degree of difficulty of raising the balls by tilting the plastic housing off the horizontal, but by doing so, the amount of volume generated as the balls are raised will also be reduced.

3 *Spirocare* Incentive Breathing Exerciser (Fig. 18-7) functions as follows:

a An electronic spirometer *(1)* incorporates different-colored light sequences *(2)*, which are matched to pre-established breathing goals.

b A disposable flow tube *(3)* is inserted into a holder *(4)*, which incorporates a laser beam to measure the revolutions per minute of a disk that spins inside the disposable flow tube as the patient inhales.

c The revolutions per minute (rpm) of the spinning disk are correlated to the liters per minute (L/min) gas flow and recorded by the control box as the number of breaths (goals) performed versus number of goals achieved *(5)*.

d The object of this device is to help motivate the patient to produce a desired tidal breath as set by the light sequence and to hold each breath for a desired time of 5 to 15 seconds.

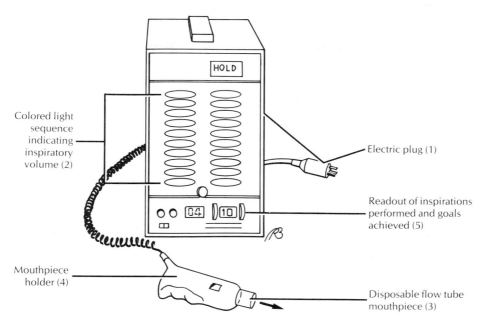

Colored light sequence indicating inspiratory volume (2)

Electric plug (1)

Readout of inspirations performed and goals achieved (5)

Mouthpiece holder (4)

Disposable flow tube mouthpiece (3)

FIGURE 18-7 Spirocare Incentive Breathing Exerciser.

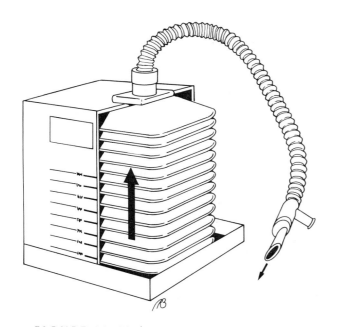

FIGURE 18-8 Volume Incentive Breathing Exerciser.

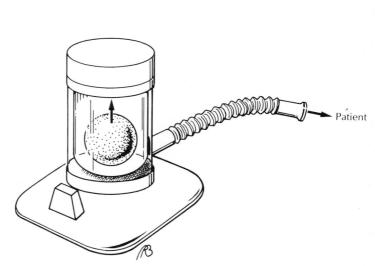

Patient

FIGURE 18-9 Incentive device and lung exerciser.

4 Other brands of incentive devices, shown in Figs. 18-8 through 18-11, incorporate similar principles to those used by the units described in *1* through *3*. They illustrate the progression of devices from those depending basically on mechanical technology to a blending of mechanical function with microprocessors.

a Fig. 18-8 represents a volume incentive breathing exerciser for performance of SMI and maximum tidal volume achieved.

b Fig. 18-9 illustrates a unit that can be used as an incentive device as well as a lung exercise for strengthening thoracic muscles. The unique inner chamber design creates a fixed-resistance to air flow that must be overcome by the patient as he or she inhales in an attempt to support the ball off its base.

c Fig. 18-10 shows an incentive unit with variable resistances to air flow. The incentive is to elevate the ball against increasing levels of resistance that can be preset with a control knob.

As resistance is increased, increased patient effort and inspiratory air flow must be generated to raise and maintain the ball off its base.

d Fig. 18-11 shows an electronic unit that can be used for bedside pulmonary function screening as well as for incentive applications. The unit measures forced vital capacity (FVC), forced expiratory volume at 1

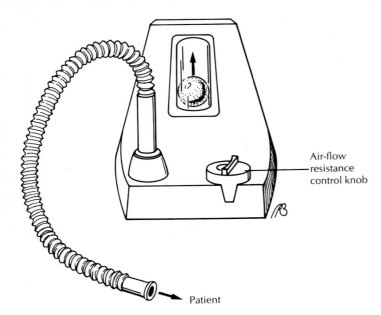

FIGURE 18-10 Incentive unit with variable resistance to air flow.

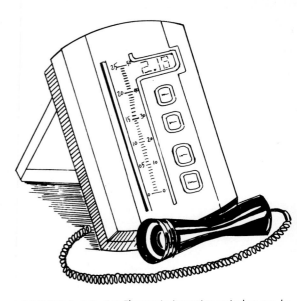

FIGURE 18-11 Electronic incentive unit that can be used for bedside pulmonary function screening.

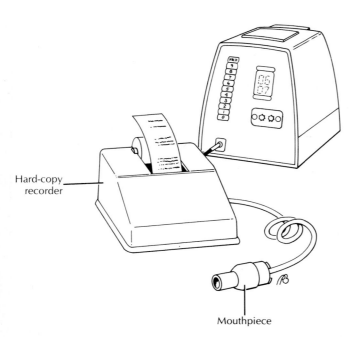

FIGURE 18-12 Computerized incentive spirometer with hard copy readout.

second (FEV_1), peak flow rates, and displayed inspiratory efforts.

e Fig. 18-12 shows a marriage of incentive spirometry with computer technology for better monitoring and documentation of patient performance. The hard-copy recorder enables the practitioner to establish a permanent record of a patient's progress while receiving incentive spirometry.

6.0 USING VARIOUS INCENTIVE DEVICES TO GENERATE SUSTAINED MAXIMAL INSPIRATION (SMI)

6.1 General steps

The practitioner should:

1 Before attempting to use an incentive spirometer, read the operator's instructions provided with the unit by the manufacturer.
2 Set incentive lung volumes based on the physician's prescribed limits.
3 When setting visual rewards, always set realistic, achievable goals initially and increase the level by 200 ml until the patient reaches the desired tidal volume.
4 Be sure that the patient understands the use of the device and does *not* attempt to achieve incentives by blowing into it instead of inhaling through it.
5 Stress the importance of achieving incentives and *coughing* to clear any secretions.
6 Have the patient splint any surgical incisions that may be stressed as a result of the exaggerated inspiratory effort.
7 Instruct and observe the patient in the proper use of inspiratory muscles.
8 Routinely check on the patient and coach him or her to continue SMI treatments.

Procedure 18-1 may be used for giving instruction on the use of incentive spirometry.

PROCEDURE 18-1

Use of the incentive spirometer to cause sustained maximal inspiration

No.	Steps in performing the procedure
	The practitioner will demonstrate knowledge of the use of the incentive spirometer.
1	Verify physician's order.
2	Review chart for patient history and other relevant data.
3	Gather appropriate incentive device, complete with:
	3.1 Breathing tube
	3.2 Mouthpiece
	3.3 Nose clips
4	Wash hands.
5	Identify patient and introduce yourself.
6	Set up incentive device including desired volume. Note that desired volume, if adjustable, should be set so patient can read incentives.
7	Check vital signs, which may include:
	7.1 Chest auscultation
	7.2 Tidal volume
	7.3 Vital capacity
	7.4 Peak flow rate
	7.5 Pulse
8	Explain procedure to patient.
9	Demonstrate technique to patient by taking and holding breath. (Do not, of course, use the patient's device.)
10	Explain and demonstrate proper breathing technique as follows:
	10.1 Increase inspiration slowly and gradually (200 ml/sec) until desired lung volume is reached or goal indicator is reached.
	10.2 Continue inspiration for 5 to 15 sec to ensure maximum inflation.
	10.3 Repeat exercise 6 to 10 times, or as prescribed.
	10.4 Emphasize visual incentive mechanism.
	10.5 Attempt successively larger breaths.
11	Instruct patient in proper coughing technique.
12	Recheck vital signs.
13	Wash hands.
14	Chart treatment: goals achieved, repetitions, cough results, etc.

BIBLIOGRAPHY

Bartlett RH et al: The physiology of yawning and its application to postoperative care, Lung Forum 21:222, 1970.

Colgan FJ, Mahoney PD, and Fanning GL: Resistance breathing (blow bottles) and sustained hyperinflations in the treatment of atelectasis, Anesthesiology 32:543, 1970.

Ingram RH Jr: Mechanical aid to lung expansion, Am Rev Respir Dis 122(2):23, 1980.

Martin RJ, Roger RM, and Grant BA: The physiologic basis for the use of mechanical aids to lung expansion, Am Rev Respir Dis 122(2):105, 1980.

McPherson SP: Respiratory therapy equipment, ed 4, St Louis, 1990, The CV Mosby Co.

Spearman CB, Sheldon RL, and Egan DF: Egan's fundamentals of respiratory therapy, ed 5, St Louis, 1990, The CV Mosby Co.

Pulmonary drainage procedures

On completion of this module the reader will be able to:

1.1 Explain how pulmonary drainage and related modalities became a respiratory care procedure.

1.2 Describe various principles and techniques of pulmonary drainage and related modalities.

1.3 Explain the rationale for pulmonary drainage.

2.1 Point out indications for pulmonary drainage based on clinical situations.

2.2 Point out contraindications for pulmonary drainage based on clinical situations.

3.1 Describe clinical situations and conditions requiring modified pulmonary drainage programs.

4.1 Outline general considerations to be followed when planning a pulmonary drainage program.

5.1 Appraise the patient's ability to tolerate a pulmonary drainage program using physical assessment criteria.

6.1 Relate general requirements for pulmonary drainage.

7.1 Create a schedule for a good pulmonary program by considering external factors that may interfere with the patient's schedule.

7.2 Explain deep cough techniques to patients.

7.3 Use performance evaluation records (procedures) to properly instruct a patient in coughing.

7.4 Rearrange and modify a pulmonary drainage program according to the patient's tolerances.

7.5 Establish priorities for draining areas of the lung.

7.6 Explain procedure for a pulmonary drainage program if affected areas are generalized.

8.1 Point out locations of lung segments, using diagrams, lung models, and another person.

9.1 Position bed and patient for maximum pulmonary drainage of all segments for generalized secretions throughout the lung.

10.1 Relate need for loosening secretions as an important part of a pulmonary drainage program.

10.2 Explain clapping (percussion) technique.

10.3 Describe precautions to be followed when using clapping.

10.4 Perform clapping on another person using various pulmonary drainage positions.

11.1 Explain vibration.

11.2 Describe precautions to take when using vibration.

11.3 Perform vibration on another person, using various pulmonary drainage positions.

12.1 Plan a typical pulmonary drainage program for a patient with generalized secretions, using respiratory care adjuncts, positioning, clapping, vibration, deep breathing, and cough techniques.

13.1 Explain the possible need for mechanical devices to supplement a pulmonary drainage program.

14.1 Describe the special positions and techniques used in delivering postural drainage, clapping, and vibration in neonates and children.

1.0 PULMONARY DRAINAGE PROGRAM

1.1 Pulmonary drainage as a respiratory care modality

1 Chest physical therapy (also called chest physiotherapy and pulmonary drainage) procedures were historically performed only by physical therapists and nurses.

Since the early 1970s, respiratory care personnel began to incorporate pulmonary *drainage procedures* and *breathing exercises* as techniques for airway maintenance.

  a A major concern was to help patients, in or out of the hospital, to provide their own airway care.

  b The scope of this care included educational and psychologic preparation of the patient (and eventually, the family) in the removal and control of airway secretions and elimination or reduction of ineffective respiratory movements.

  c These techniques were initially employed in hospital patient care areas in conjunction with other respiratory care modalities, but they rapidly spread to outpatient and home care applications.

2 Pulmonary drainage procedures are frequently used synonymously to mean "pulmonary rehabilitation." This is *not* the case, even though pulmonary drainage procedures do comprise an important portion of pulmonary rehabilitation.

This module presents techniques to assist repiratory care personnel in planning and performing pulmonary drainage, coughing, clapping (percussion), and vibration.

Clapping and vibration will be discussed after pulmonary drainage, even though they are frequently used *together* to loosen, mobilize, and remove secretions.

1.2 Principles and techniques of pulmonary drainage

1 The objectives of pulmonary drainage are to:
   a Liquefy viscous secretions in conjunction with aerosol therapy.
   b Loosen tenacious secretions.
   c Remove accumulated secretions.
2 Pulmonary drainage moves secretions by applying the theory of gravity settlement and the fact that liquids flow "downhill."

   To accomplish effective pulmonary drainage, the secretions must be *thin* enough to flow. This can be accomplished by *topically* exposing the airway secretions to liquefying agents, by adding water (i.e., humidity), or by increasing available cellular fluid through increasing the patient's fluid intake.
3 Pools of thickened secretions may become encrusted and adhere to each other and the adjacent pulmonary surfaces.

   Many of these secretions can be loosened by applying vibration or percussion to the external chest over the affected area.
4 *Vibration* involves manually or mechanically shaking the involved chest area during *exhalation*. Gentle vibrations are transmitted from the surface to the underlying tissues and airways as the patient exhales.
5 *Percussion* (clapping or cupping) involves manually or mechanically establishing vibrations of varying intensities and frequencies that are caused by carefully delivering blows to the chest wall over the affected area. The force of the methodically delivered impacts starts vibrations that are transmitted to underlying secretions in much the same manner as a tuning fork can generate and transmit waves through a container of water. This technique is also referred to as the "ketchup bottle" theory. Experience with ketchup teaches one that the bottle must be inverted, and blows must be delivered to its bottom to cause the ketchup to flow.
6 A primary consideration is that loosened secretions *must* be rapidly moved toward the proximal airways and eventually toward the pharynx or another exit route such as a tracheostomy tube. Stagnant loosened secretions may cause transient hypoxia and dyspnea as they move into major bronchi. Should this situation develop, the treatment of choice is to administer oxygen, maintain ventilation, and continue vigorous removal of the mobile secretions by positioning, coughing, and, when necessary, administering suction.

1.3 Rationale for pulmonary drainage procedures

1 Pulmonary drainage is a procedure to aid in lung ventilation and pulmonary hygiene by removing accumulated secretions that cause increased airway obstruction, resistance, and infection.

2 Pulmonary drainage is especially useful because it can be implemented with minimal equipment, and it allows the patient to become involved in his or her own care.

2.0 EVALUATING CLINICAL SITUATIONS FOR PULMONARY DRAINAGE

2.1 Indications for pulmonary drainage procedures

1 Secretions. Excessive production of or failure to remove secretions because of increased viscosity or ineffective cough can result in decreased ventilation of the lung, increased incidence of infection, atelectasis, and pulmonary shuntlike situations. Pulmonary drainage can remove secretions, reduce incidence of infection, and promote airway patency.
2 Restrictive diseases. Decreased effective ventilation (maximum voluntary ventilation [MVV] less than 33%) and expiratory gas flow rates (maximum expiratory flow rate [MEFR] less than 200 L/min) because of poor chest mechanics will result in an ineffective cough to remove secretions.
3 Aspiration. Patient positioning combined with humidity, vibration, percussion, and vigorous coughing may be beneficial in the removal of aspirated materials, such as gastric contents and foreign bodies.
4 Prophylactic care. Pulmonary drainage routines in patients expressing diminished tidal volumes (less than 10 ml/kg body weight), a vital capacity (VC) less than 0.6 L, or an MVV less than 33% of that predicted may prevent accumulation of secretions and decrease complications.

2.2 Contraindications for pulmonary drainage procedures

1 Abscess. Excessive flooding of air passages with secretions, and resultant asphyxiation, can occur if an abscess is ruptured during a drainage routine.
2 Severe airway resistance. Mobilization of secretions can result in transient increased airway resistance. In severe cases increased resistance may be sufficient to prohibit effective alveolar ventilation.
3 Rib fracture. Severe pain, combined with the potential puncture of a lung surface by protruding bone fragments, prohibits pulmonary drainage and percussion.
4 Hemoptysis. Bleeding from the lung is a contraindication for any procedure that could aggravate the condition and intensify the hemorrhaging. This includes intermittent positive pressure breathing (IPPB) treatments, breathing exercises, pulmonary drainage, and percussion procedures.
5 Diaphragmatic disorders. Diaphragmatic hernia, or other conditions involving the diaphragm, usually prevents the use of extreme pulmonary drainage procedures.
6 Head trauma and increased cranial pressure. Pulmonary drainage with "head down" position should *not* be used.
7 Hypertension and other cardiac disorders that are position-sensitive.

3.0 EVALUATING CLINICAL SITUATIONS FOR MODIFIED PULMONARY DRAINAGE
3.1 Conditions requiring modified programs

1 Hypoxia. Supplemental oxygen via nasal cannula may be indicated. Special care must be taken *not* to use a mask or other device that would obstruct the face and serve as a potential reservoir for loosened secretions or regurgitated stomach contents.

2 Cardiac patients. Cardiac patients should be handled with extreme care, and special attention should be given to vital signs, ECG, and hypoxia level.

3 Exhaustion. Programs for physically weakened or disabled patients must be planned so that the length of the treatment is tempered to the tolerance level of each patient. One approach is to establish a split program if multiple positions are required.

4 Pain. Severe pain of any nature is detrimental to the establishment of a good breathing pattern. Pain *associated* with breathing is especially prohibitive to adequate ventilation because patients will voluntarily restrict (splint) their chest bellows action to reduce the pain. Patient positioning, placement of pillows, blanket rolls, and the use of hands as splints will help patients control the pain during pulmonary drainage procedures.

5 Postoperative condition. Postoperative pulmonary complications are most common in patients who cannot generate an effective cough. Working with the postoperative patient requires understanding, patience, and the ability to recognize and modify treatments to the patient's physical limitations, especially if the incision involves or is closely related to respiratory muscles. Patients with potential postoperative complications should receive *preoperative* instruction in drainage positions and methods for protecting the surgical wound site against pain and accidental trauma.

6 Tracheostomy. Patients with a tracheostomy, with or without mechanical ventilation, require special handling because in most cases they cannot generate effective coughs and therefore cannot remove their own secretions. Before pulmonary drainage is performed, these patients should be informed about the suctioning technique and how they should cooperate. They should also be counseled as to possible feelings they may experience as the secretions are mobilized, including dyspnea. If the tracheostomy tube is cuffed, proper procedures for handling a cuffed tube should be followed, including suctioning *above* and *below* the cuff before deflation. Respiratory care personnel should be aware that these patients cannot talk.

7 Disoriented patients. Unconscious or disoriented patients frequently require pulmonary drainage because of an inability to clear their own secretions. These patients are difficult to work with and require modification of positions to ensure their safety as well as adequate draining. Pillows, sandbags, and restraints are frequently used to guard patients against falling or striking their bodies against hard objects.

8 Obese patients. Morbidly obese patients are rarely able to be placed in any position but supine and semi-Fowler's. Modified turning techniques may be the only positions available for therapy.

4.0 PULMONARY DRAINAGE PROGRAM PLANNING
4.1 General planning considerations

1 Frequency of treatment. Should be performed 3 to 4 times daily according to physician's order.

2 Coordination of treatment. Should be adjusted to patient's special needs and, when possible, given in conjunction with other treatments that provide a *synergistic* effect.

3 Length of treatment. Should be adjusted to patient's needs, although the treatment should *not* generally exceed 30 minutes. Maximum effort should be directed to draining regions containing the most accumulated secretions.

4 Time of treatment. Always performed before meals or ½ to 1 hour after meals.

5 Level of hypoxia. Patients must *not* become more hypoxic as a result of the procedure. Thus some general rules should be followed.

  a If the patient is receiving oxygen therapy, it should be continued, even if the modality must be modified (e.g., mask changed to cannula during the program).

  b If the patient has borderline hypoxemia, supplemental oxygen should be prescribed, especially during periods when coughing is encouraged.

  c If arterial blood gases are available and arterial oxygen tension (Pao_2) is less than 60 torr in room air, supplemental oxygen is probably indicated to prevent hypoxia.

6 Humidity therapy. If humidity therapy is to be administered, it should be given *15 to 20 minutes* before the pulmonary drainage procedures.

7 Intermittent positive pressure breathing (IPPB) therapy. If IPPB is ordered, it should be given before pulmonary drainage procedures except in situations in which patients are unable to generate adequate ventilation to produce a cough without assistance. If percussion or vibration is used in conjunction with IPPB, it should be applied only during exhalation. After drainage procedure, IPPB can be administered to relax the patient by relieving transient shortness of breath and to generate elevated tidal volumes, according to prescription.

8 Patients who are unable to raise and expectorate secretions that have been loosened by pulmonary drainage procedures may require mechanical suctioning. This procedure is discussed in detail in Module Twenty.

5.0 APPRAISING PATIENT'S ABILITY TO TOLERATE PULMONARY DRAINAGE
5.1 Physical assessment criteria for initiating program

Assessment is an important part of the program. The following factors should be noted.

1 Patient's position. A clinician should be aware that changing a patient's position can cause drastic changes

in the patient's vital signs and laboratory values. For example, changing a patient's position from supine to prone position alone can cause arterial oxygen tension (Pao_2) to change as much as 47 torr. This is an extreme example. Most studies indicate either little or no drop in Pao_2 or an actual increase during pulmonary drainage (i.e., changes associated with pulmonary drainage maneuvers).

2 Vital signs. Before pulmonary drainage procedures a patient's vital signs must be taken and recorded for subsequent reference. When checking the patient, the following should be noted.

a Blood pressure (BP) should not be high or low for patient's age, weight, and sex, unless the condition has been noted in patient's chart.

b BP should not change more than ±10 torr during the course of treatment.

c Pulse should be within acceptable ranges for age and sex, unless exceptions are noted in patient's chart.

d Pulse should *not* increase to 120/min or remain elevated over a 20-minute period.

e Respirations will usually increase as secretions are mobilized. An increase in frequency should not exceed 10/min during treatment.

3 Skin. Note the color, temperature, and feel. Drastic changes in color (i.e., presence of cyanosis) may indicate hypoxia or restricted circulation. Skin temperature changes may occur as a result of exposure to environmental influences and blood perfusion to the area. A sudden cooling of the skin may indicate restricted circulation or a drop in blood pressure. The presence of moisture on the skin is normal in some areas of the body but abnormal in others. The presence of a cool, clammy, pale skin could indicate that the patient is in shock.

4 Cough. The generation of an effective cough is a primary consideration of all patients receiving pulmonary drainage. The patient's ability to generate an effective cough depends on his or her pulmonary function, especially ability to produce expiratory flow. Pretreatment assessment should include measurement of:

a Maximum expiratory flow rate—should be greater than 150 L/min.

b Inspiratory force—should be greater than −20 torr.

c Vital capacity—should be greater than 1.5 L.

- If values are less than these indicated, the patient probably will have difficulty in producing an effective cough without mechanical assistance.

5 Level of consciousness. A patient's mental alertness should be noted before treatment. If any sudden changes occur in the patient's level of consciousness, the procedure should be halted and the physician and nurse notified.

6.0 REQUIREMENTS FOR A PULMONARY DRAINAGE PROGRAM

6.1 General requirements

1 Medical prescription. Pulmonary drainage and associated modalities and treatments should be given only with a properly written medical order. A medical order normally contains the following:

a Lung areas to be drained

b Length of treatment

c Frequency of treatment

d Related modalities such as vibration, percussion, and breathing exercises

e Supportive equipment/medication, such as oxygen and nebulization

f Special precautions such as undesirable positions, tracheostomy care, wound precautions, vital sign limits, and suctioning directions

2 Required equipment. The equipment available and on hand before beginning treatment should include:

a Positioning surface (bed or table)

b Disposable tissues

c Emesis basin

d Suctioning equipment

e Sputum cup for collection

f Pillows

g Sphygmomanometer and stethoscope

h Container for disposable tissues

i Towels

j Any special equipment, such as oxygen therapy devices, vibrators, or percussors

3 Methods for elevating patient's hips. The various methods for elevating a patient's hips for creating a postural drainage position include:

a Special table or bed

b Hospital bed

c Chair or blocks to elevate foot of bed

d Pillows or other bulky padding

e Jack used under foot of bed

7.0 SCHEDULING A PULMONARY DRAINAGE PROGRAM

7.1 Considering the major components

1 For best results the routine should be performed 2 to 3 times daily

2 The program should begin in the morning when the patient awakes, especially if the patient has been exposed to high-humidity therapy overnight.

3 Postural drainage should follow intermittent positive pressure breathing (IPPB), incentive (deep) breathing, or high-humidity therapy.

4 The program should be scheduled so that the patient has physical stress periods during the afternoon.

5 The schedule should be planned so that the drainage program occurs before meals or ½ to 1 hour after meals.

7.2 Procedure for controlled cough and expectoration

1 Coughing is defined as a violent expiratory effort preceded by a preliminary inspiration. It begins with a forced exhalation against a closed glottis after a deep inspiration.

2 During the forced exhalation, both thoracic and intrapulmonary pressure rises sharply until the glottis is abruptly forced open. Simultaneously the trachea is

narrowed, which results in a very rapid gas flow from the lungs at approximately 500 miles per hour! This outward rush of air dislodges secretions and other substances that may be in the airway and causes them to move toward the pharynx.

3 This same principle is used in the *Heimlich maneuver* to forcefully remove food or other foreign bodies that may be causing an airway obstruction.

4 One should remember that the cough generates very high airway pressures that can damage the airway, rupture blebs in the lung, and interfere with cardiac output. If cardiac output is hindered, the patient may feel faint or, in fact, may "black out," resulting from a condition known as *syncope*.

5 Controlled coughing or aseptic suctioning should follow postural drainage in order to clear the secretions loosened by an ineffective cough.

6 It is important to remember that postural drainage is not always effective and in some instances is dangerous if the patient is unable to bring up secretions, either through cough, assisted cough, or suctioning. Often, a *combination* of the previous three modes may be necessary.

7 The cough procedure (as told to the patient) is as follows:

a Inhale slowly and fully before coughing.

b Keep your head slightly forward.

c Clasp your arms across your abdomen.

d Stick your tongue forward; give three sharp coughs without taking another breath.

e Press your arms into your abdomen as you cough. You should feel your abdominal muscles tighten each time you cough.

f Hold your breath for a moment after each coughing series, then breathe in gently to prevent sucking mucus back into your lungs.

8 If a patient has had abdominal or thoracic surgery, a pillow or the practitioner's hands splinting the incision site will make coughing easier and less painful.

9 Tracheal tickling may be required to elicit an effective cough for the infant or the patient who is unwilling to cough because of fear of pain. By applying manual pressure to the trachea above the manubrial notch, an artificial obstruction is created. This obstruction serves to trigger an involuntary cough reflex that overrides the patient's inhibition.

NOTE: This procedure should not be routinely carried out without the attending physician's permission.

10 Assisted coughing is used with patients suffering from neuromuscular deficits that render the cough mechanism ineffective (e.g., scoliosis, quadriplegia, paraplegia, Guillain-Barré syndrome, myasthenia gravis). The practitioner can substitute for weak intercostal and abdominal muscles and a paralyzed diaphragm by applying manual compression to the abdomen and lateral thorax at the exact instant the patient reaches peak inspiratory effort. This would be similar to a modified Heimlich maneuver.

11 Techniques to facilitate instruction of diaphragmatic breathing in preparation for coughing follow.

a A *sniff* is a diaphragmatic breath and a good way to teach the movement to any patient. It works especially well with children.

b *Panting* is a series of exhalations followed by a quiet inhalation. A sample teaching technique (as told to the patient) follows.
- Give single, short, sharp breaths out through your mouth by quickly squeezing your ribs down and in.
- Tighten your abdominal muscles at the same time—as if you were saying a deep "ha-ha-ha."

Panting can be used to:
- Move secretions higher in the tracheobronchial tree.
- Move secretions higher in the chest to assist a weak cough. A sudden exhalation tends to dislodge secretions along the wall of the airways and/or move already loosened particles.
- Initiate a cough. If inhalation proceeds in a quiet fashion, the next pant is often effective in continuing this upward motion of secretions and frequently triggers a productive cough.

7.3 Performance evaluation records

Procedures 19-1 through 19-5 may be used to assist a patient to cough under various circumstances.

7.4 Individual programming

The therapeutic program must be modified according to the individual patient's needs and tolerance.

1 The length and frequency of a program should be prescribed based on a physical evaluation of the patient. (Review Module Sixteen.)

2 The technician should modify time and frequency of the program if the patient becomes extremely fatigued or has major changes in vital signs, level of dyspnea, pain, or consciousness.

3 Drainage routines should be prescribed to concentrate efforts on drainage of areas with *greatest* amounts of accumulated secretions. This can be identified by auscultation, percussion, and chest radiographs.

4 The maximum length of time for any program should probably *not* exceed 30 minutes.

5 In extreme cases, the number of procedures per day should be increased rather than attempting to extend the time of each program, which can seriously fatigue the patient.

7.5 Localized lung drainage

Priorities should be established for draining specific areas of the lung.

1 Drain the involved areas of the lung first.

2 Choose an approach that will allow the patient to ventilate, using the good lung as secretions are mobilized in involved areas.

NOTE: These steps will serve as a precautionary mechanism to clear any secretions that may have been transposed to the good lung.

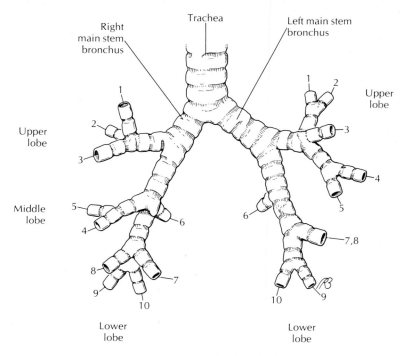

FIGURE 19-1 Tracheobronchial tree.

7.6 Procedure for removing generalized secretions

1 Drain the lower lobes first.
2 Drain the middle lobe and lingular region next.
3 Drain upper lobes last.

NOTE: This sequence is reversed in infants or patients who are primarily restricted to the prone or supine position.

8.0 LUNG SEGMENTS
8.1 Names and locations

Proper patient positioning for pulmonary drainage cannot be achieved until the respiratory care practitioner can visualize the locations of lung segments within the chest and how these segments are positioned to cause secretions to drain toward the trachea.

In addition to Figs. 19-1 through 19-10, it is recommended that the reader study a lung model (if available) with segments identified.

1 The *right* lung has three lobes. Each lobe is connected with its respective main stem bronchus.

The right bronchus divides into the upper lobe bronchus, which subsequently divides into the middle and lower lobe bronchi.

2 The *left* lung has two lobes that communicate with their main stem bronchus.

The left bronchus divides into upper and lower bronchi, which communicate with ten pulmonary segments. The lower part of the upper lobe serves the lingular segment.

3 The upper, middle, and lower lobe bronchi of the right lung subdivide to form *ten* bronchopulmonary segments.

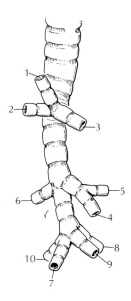

FIGURE 19-2 Position and numbers of segmental bronchi of right lung for anteroposterior and lateral views.

a The position and numbers of segmental bronchi of the right and left lungs for anteroposterior and lateral views are shown in Figs. 19-2 and 19-3. The position of each segment is that of a person standing in anatomic postion. The numbers identifying each bronchus correspond to the names listed in Table 19-1 for all segments in the anterior and lateral views.

b Topographicly, the lobes of each lung and their segments can be identified by approximating the location of underlying lobes to external anatomy.

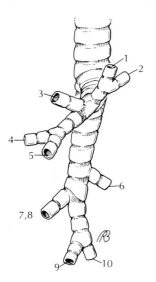

FIGURE 19-3 Position and numbers of segmental bronchi of left lung for anteroposterior and lateral views.

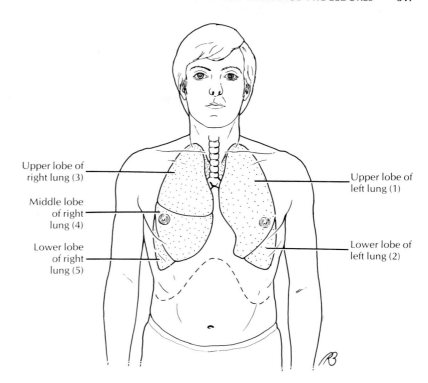

Upper lobe of right lung (3)

Middle lobe of right lung (4)

Lower lobe of right lung (5)

Upper lobe of left lung (1)

Lower lobe of left lung (2)

FIGURE 19-4 Lobes of lung as seen in anterior view of thorax.

TABLE 19-1 Names of lung segments in anterior and lateral views

Right lung segment of bronchus	Left lung segment of bronchus
Upper lobe	
1 Apical	
2 Posterior	Apical-posterior
3 Anterior	Anterior
Middle lobe	**Lingula**
4 Lateral	Superior
5 Medial	Inferior
Lower lobe	
6 Superior	Superior
7 Medial basal	
8 Anterior basal	Anterior basal
9 Lateral basal	Lateral basal
10 Posterior basal	Posterior basal

4 Fig. 19-4 represents a view of the anterior thorax.

  In this view, the upper lobe of the left lung *(1)* and the lower lobe of the left lung *(2)* can be approximated by comparing their location with the nipple and lower boundaries of the ribs. The right lung with its three lobes—upper *(3)*, middle *(4)*, and lower *(5)*—can be identified using the same topographic landmarks.

5 Fig. 19-5 represents a posterior view of the thorax. In this position only the upper and lower lobes of both the right *(1)* and left *(2)* lungs can be seen.

6 Fig. 19-6 shows a lateral view of the right thorax. In this position the upper *(1)*, middle *(2)*, and lower *(3)* lobes of the right lung can be seen.

7 Fig. 19-7 shows a lateral view of the left thorax. In this position both the upper *(1)* and lower *(2)* lobes of the left lung can be seen.

8 Clinically, it is extremely important that the clinician learn the bronchopulmonary segments by *number* and by *location*. This understanding will be applied to identification of mucus or secretions in specific locations and for positioning of the patient to achieve pulmonary drainage (Figs. 19-8, 19-9, and 19-10).

  Once the names and locations of lung segments have been memorized using the lung model and figures, the reader may find it helpful to use water-soluble pens to draw the approximate location of lung segments on another person's chest. This approach will enable the reader to relate the figures to the surface anatomy of the chest. This technique also enables the reader to visualize drainage of segments and lobes in various drainage positions.

9.0 POSITIONING PATIENTS FOR PULMONARY DRAINAGE OF ALL LUNG SEGMENTS
9.1 Generalized lung involvement

  When the lungs have generalized secretions, a complete drainage program should be implemented, using the following sequence of positions. Figs. 19-11 through 19-19 provide examples of anatomic positioning.

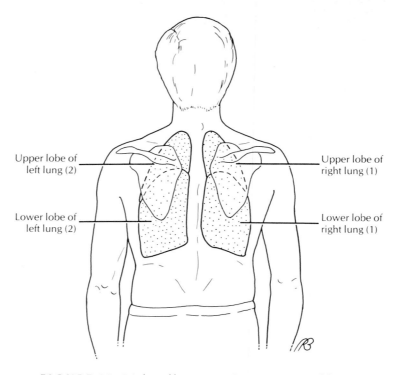

Upper lobe of
left lung (2)

Upper lobe of
right lung (1)

Lower lobe of
left lung (2)

Lower lobe of
right lung (1)

FIGURE 19-5 Lobes of lung as seen in posterior view of thorax.

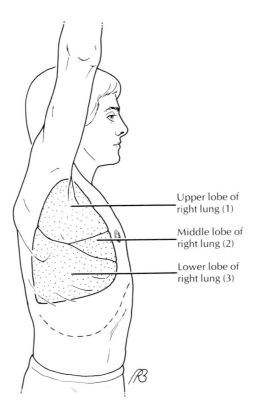

Upper lobe of
right lung (1)

Middle lobe of
right lung (2)

Lower lobe of
right lung (3)

FIGURE 19-6 Lobes of lung as seen in lateral view of
right thorax.

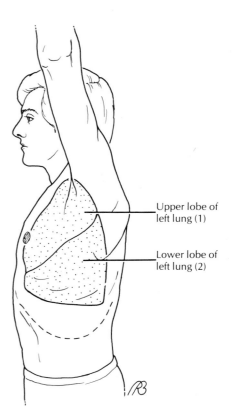

Upper lobe of
left lung (1)

Lower lobe of
left lung (2)

FIGURE 19-7 Lobes of lung as seen in lateral view of
left thorax.

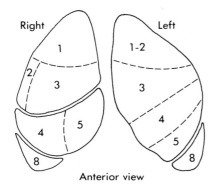

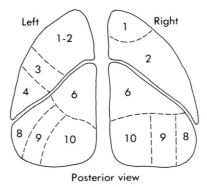

F I G U R E   1 9 - 8 Bronchopulmonary segments identified by number and location for anterior view of right and left lungs. (From Scanlan CL, Spearman CB, and Sheldon RL: Egan's fundamentals of respiratory care, ed 5, St Louis, 1990, The CV Mosby Co.)

F I G U R E   1 9 - 9 Bronchopulmonary segments identified by number and location for posterior view of right and left lungs. (From Scanlan CL, Spearman CB, and Sheldon RL: Egan's fundamentals of respiratory care, ed 5, St Louis, 1990, The CV Mosby Co.)

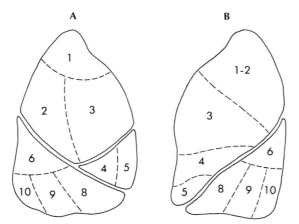

F I G U R E   1 9 - 1 0 Bronchopulmonary segments identified by number and location for lateral view of **A,** right and **B,** left lungs. (From Scanlan CL, Spearman CB, and Sheldon RL: Egan's fundamentals of respiratory care, ed 5, St Louis, 1990, The CV Mosby Co.)

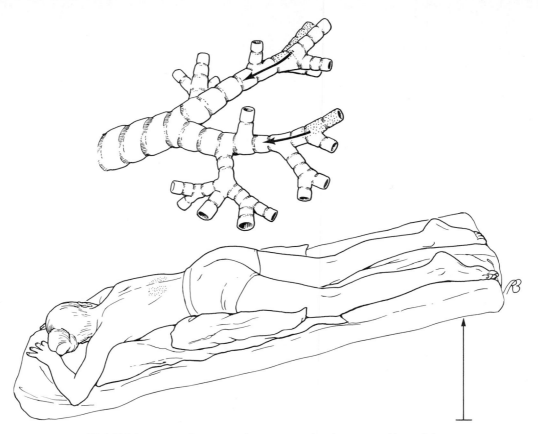

FIGURE 19-11 Position to drain posterior basal segment of lower lobe.

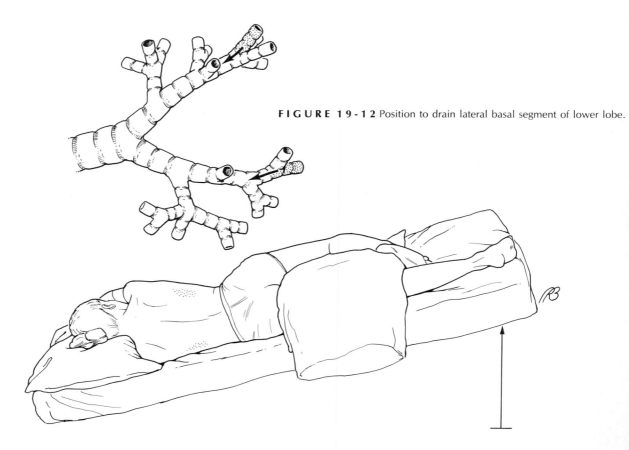

FIGURE 19-12 Position to drain lateral basal segment of lower lobe.

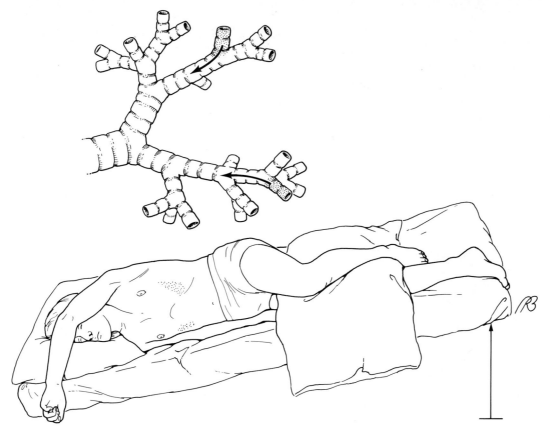

FIGURE 19-13 Position to drain anterior basal segment of lower lobe.

1 Drain lower lobes first.

  a *Posterior basal segment* (Fig. 19-11). Foot of table or bed elevated 18 inches or 30 degrees. Patient lies on abdomen, head down, with pillow under hips. Upper leg can be flexed over lower ribs close to spine on each side of the back.

  b *Lateral basal segment* (Fig. 19-12). Foot of table or bed elevated 18 inches or 30 degrees. Patient lies on abdomen, then rotates quarter turn upward. Upper leg may be flexed over a pillow for support. Clap or vibrate (if ordered) over uppermost portion of lower ribs.

  c *Anterior basal segment* (Fig. 19-13). Foot of table or bed elevated 18 inches or 30 degrees. Patient lies on side, head down, pillow under knees. Clap or vibrate (if ordered) over lower ribs just beneath axilla.

  d *Superior segment* (Fig. 19-14). Table or bed flat. Patient lies on abdomen with pillow under hips. Clap or vibrate (if ordered) over middle of back below tip of scapula on either side of spine.

2 Drain middle lobe second (Fig. 19-15)—*lateral and medial segment.* Foot of table or bed elevated 14 inches or 15 degrees. Patient lies head down on left side and rotates quarter turn backward. Pillow may be placed behind patient from shoulder to hip. Knees should be flexed. Clap or vibrate (if ordered) over right nipple area.

3 Drain upper lobes third.

  a *Lingular segment, superior and inferior* (Fig. 19-16). Foot of table or bed elevated 14 inches or 15 degrees. Patient lies head down on right side and rotates quarter turn backward. Pillow may be placed behind patient from shoulder to hip. Knees should be flexed. Clap or vibrate (if ordered) over left nipple area.

  b *Anterior segment* (Fig. 19-17). Table or bed flat. Patient lies flat on back with pillow under knees. Clap or vibrate (if ordered) between clavicle and nipple on each side of the chest.

  c *Apical segment* (Fig. 19-18). Table or bed flat. Patient leans back on pillow at 30-degree angle. Clap or vibrate (if ordered) over area between clavicle and top of scapula on each side (shoulder).

  d *Posterior segment* (Fig. 19-19). Table or bed flat. Patient leans over folded pillow at 30-degree angle (may also lean over pillow placed over the back of a chair). Clap or vibrate (if ordered) over upper back on each side.

Procedure 19-6 may be used as a guide for performing postural drainage procedures.

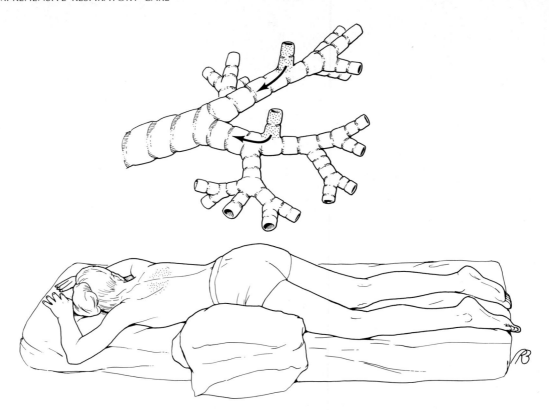

FIGURE 19-14 Position to drain superior segment of lower lobe.

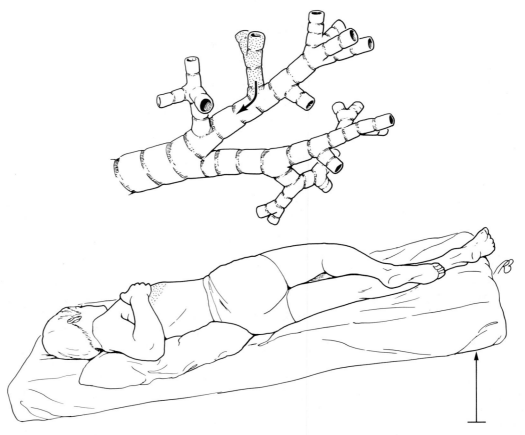

FIGURE 19-15 Position to drain lateral and medial segments of middle lobe.

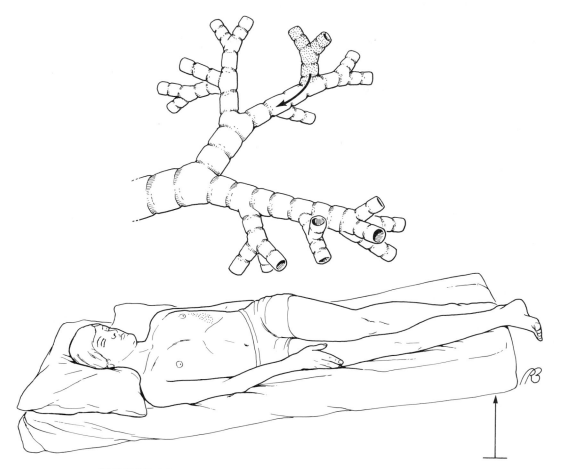

FIGURE 19-16 Position to drain superior and inferior lingular segment.

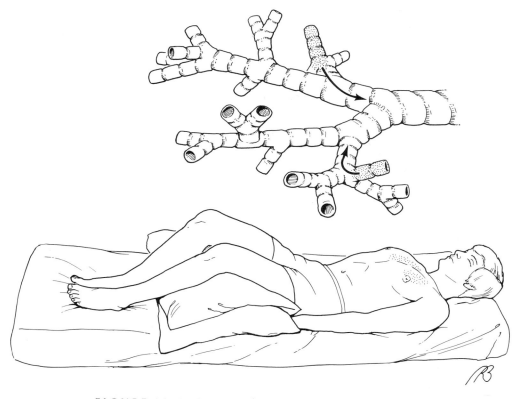

FIGURE 19-17 Position to drain anterior segment of upper lobe.

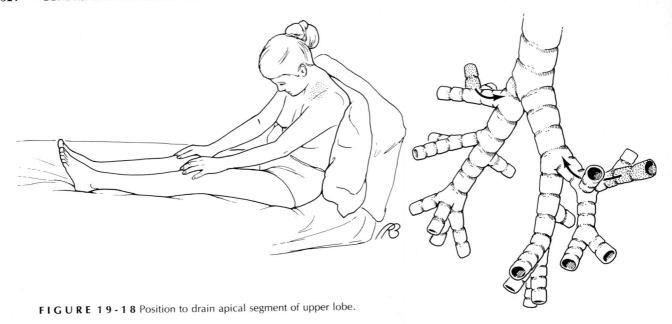

FIGURE 19-18 Position to drain apical segment of upper lobe.

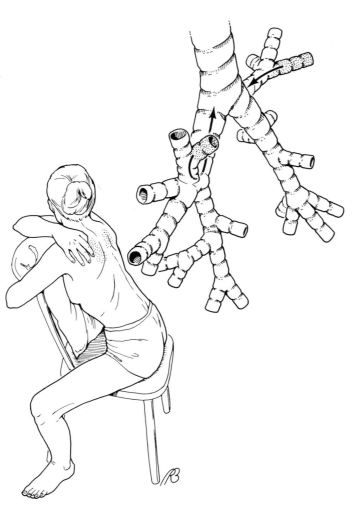

FIGURE 19-19 Position to drain posterior segment of upper lobe. Some authors believe that eleven rather than eight positions are necessary for draining specific conditions. However, this procedure increases the length of treatment, and it may unnecessarily fatigue the patient.

10.0 CLAPPING (PERCUSSION) AS AN ADJUNCT TO PULMONARY DRAINAGE

10.1 Lossening lodged secretions

1 The composition of mucus is primarily a protein base combined with tracheal debris and fluids.
2 As fluids are evaporated from the exposed surface of mucus, they become *viscous* and *tenacious,* often lodging in the airways.
3 Before pulmonary drainage can be effective, secretions must be dislodged and sufficiently liquefied to move in response to gravity.
4 Liquefaction of secretions can be accomplished by topical deposition of water, by increasing humidity in the airway, and internally by increasing fluid intake.

10.2 Clapping (percussion or cupping) technique

1 Secretions can be dislodged by applying clapping (cupping) and vibration to the external chest wall *adjacent* to the underlying site of accumulated secretions.
2 *Clapping* is the process of alternately but rhythmically striking the external chest with one cupped hand and then the other.
3 Forming the hand in the shape of a cup (Fig. 19-20) creates an air pocket that traps air between the hand and external surface as the hand strikes the chest. Percussive force is generated by compression of the air, which causes vibrations to be transmitted to the underlying bronchi to dislodge accumulated secretions. As previously stated, this action is similar to striking the bottom of a ketchup bottle in order to get the ketchup to flow.
4 Properly shaped hands and force of impact will result in a characteristic hollow *popping* sound as the hands strike the surface of the chest.
5 Improperly striking the chest with *flattened* hands

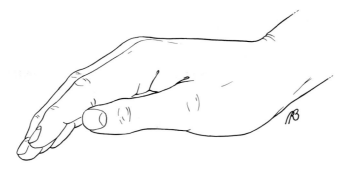

F I G U R E   1 9 - 2 0 Cup-shaped formation of hand for chest clapping.

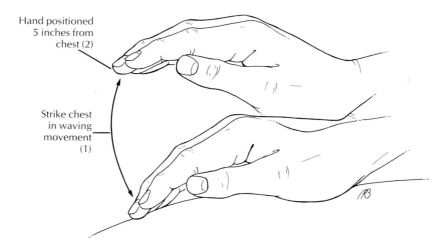

Hand positioned
5 inches from
chest (2)

Strike chest
in waving
movement
(1)

F I G U R E   1 9 - 2 1 Movement of cupped hand at wrist to percuss chest.

rather than cupped, or with the palms of the hands, will result in a *slapping* sound.

CAUTION: This technique is ineffective and may sting the patient's skin or cause injury to the patient, depending on the force of the impact of the hand on the chest.

6 Proper impact force and rhythm can be generated by alternately flexing and extending the wrists to strike the chest in a movement similar to a *waving* gesture (Fig. 19-21, *1*).

7 When clapping, the hands should be positioned 5 inches from the chest *(2)*.

8 The rhythm, frequency, and impact of the clapping can be rapid or slow. The object is to establish a technique that will be effective to generate *vibrations* that will carry to the underlying secretions.

It is important to point out that mucus is most effectively moved when the frequency of percussion is maintained between 25 to 35 Hz. This frequency is beyond the capabilities of most practitoners using manual methods.

9 Clapping is normally performed in conjunction with pulmonary drainage positions and should be applied for 5 to 7 minutes in *each* position.

10.3 Precautions when administering clapping

1 Clapping should *not* be performed without a medical order.

2 Clapping should *not* be applied to the bare skin, over buttons or other hard objects, or over clothing seams. Bare skin needs to be covered with a *light* cloth or bath towel. This also preserves the modesty and dignity of the patient.

3 Clapping or undue pressure should be avoided in areas near surgical wounds.

4 If the patient complains of a stinging sensation of the skin during clapping, or if the skin becomes red, the position of the hand and force of impact should be corrected.

5 Clapping should *not* be performed directly over or immediately adjacent to the spine, kidneys, or sternum. Efforts should be made to avoid striking the female's breasts. If the patient has large, pendulous breasts, the

breast may be gently held out of the way and clapping applied to the correct adjacent area.

NOTE: Male practitioners should use a folded towel to hold the breast out of the way.

6 Attention should be given to the patient's respiratory and general condition throughout the procedure. Any acute changes should be assessed and handled according to indicated procedures. Refer to the ECG monitor if one is available.

7 Relative contraindications are:
 a Thoracic or abdominal trauma
 b Acute medical/surgical emergencies
 c Acute local pain
 d Complications such as empyema, pleural effusion, pneumothorax, and hemoptysis (depending on the cause)
 e Abscess

10.4 Demonstration of clapping technique

Procedure 19-7 may be used as a guide for performing clapping technique with the patient in various postural drainage positions.

11.0 VIBRATION AS AN ADJUNCT TO PULMONARY DRAINAGE

11.1 Vibration to dislodge and mobilize secretions

1 Normally, shaking or vibration is performed after clapping, while the patient is still in a pulmonary drainage position.

2 Vibration is a subtle yet effective shaking that is applied to the chest through the practitioner's *arms* and *hands* (Fig. 19-22).

3 Vibration is performed only during *exhalation.*

4 The patient must inhale through the nose and exhale slowly through *pursed lips,* as though attempting to whistle.

5 The practitioner takes a position adjacent to the patient so that direct access can be attained to the area to be vibrated.

6 With the arms held *straight* and the hands placed one on top of the other over the segment to be drained, the practitioner generates gentle vibration movements.

11.2 Precautions when performing vibration

1 Vibration should *not* be performed without a medical order.

2 Care must be taken not to shake too hard on the chest, especially in areas near surgical wounds.

3 Vibration should be subtle, *not* vigorous enough to move the patient's body.

4 Refer to Unit 10.3 for precautions with regard to the female breast.

5 The patient's respiratory and general status must be continually assessed and corrective action taken if acute changes occur.

6 Refer to Unit 10.3 for relative contraindications.

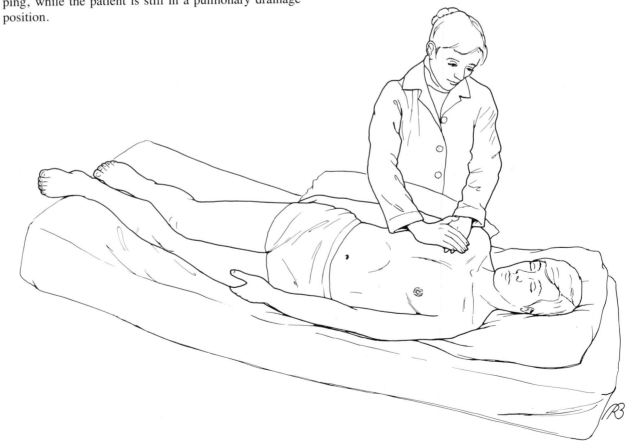

FIGURE 19-22 Chest vibration.

11.3 Demonstration of vibration technique

Procedure 19-7 may be used as a guide for performing vibration on patients in various postural drainage positions.

12.0 LOOSENING, MOBILIZING, AND REMOVING SECRETIONS

12.1 Typical pulmonary drainage routine for generalized secretions

A typical drainage routine* may include the following:
1 Prior humidity therapy by aerosol or ultrasonic generator.
2 Intermittent positive pressure breathing (IPPB), with or without bronchodilators and/or mucolytic agents.
3 Pulmonary drainage of all positions with clapping and vibration over those areas with the most involvement.
  NOTE: When clapping and vibration are used, it may be useful to interchange vibration with clapping and deep coughing while the patient is in a drainage position.
  a 5 to 7 minutes clapping per position
  b Deep breathing of patient, with vibration on exhalation only
  c Deep cough technique between positions
4 Deep breaths, sustained maximum inspiratory (SMI), or IPPB with coughing, as indicated, after pulmonary drainage therapy.
  NOTE: When secretions are mobilized, they *must* be removed. If the patient is comatose and unresponsive and/or unable to cough effectively, the secretions should be removed by tracheal suctioning.

13.0 SUPPLEMENTING A PULMONARY DRAINAGE PROGRAM

13.1 Mechanical devices

1 Several types of mechanical devices can be used to imitate manual percussion (clapping) and produce very efficient vibration. Mechanical tables can also position the patient with little or no effort on the patient's part.
2 The primary *advantage* of any mechanical device over manual techniques is that the device does not tire and will continue to deliver consistent rates, rhythm, and force of impact.
3 Mechanical devices are only as good as the practitioner directing their use and should be used to complement rather than replace the practitioner.
4 One major *disadvantage* of mechanical devices is that they do not allow the personal contact and assessment that is a part of "hands on" therapy. Also, when improperly used and directed, electrical devices can be dangerous. Some devices feature a "thumping" intensity that can actually injure the patient.
5 Mechanical percussors are able to deliver an energy frequency well within the range of 25 to 35 Hz, previously described as optimal for the movement of mucus toward the proximal airway.

6 An example of a mechanical percussor is the G5 Vibramatic unit (Fig. 19-23, *A* and *B*). The advertised feature of the unit is the fact that it incorporates a *direction*-stroking percussion apparatus *(1)*, which loosens the secretions and directionally moves them toward the upper airway. A variable speed output control *(2)* sets the rate of percussion in cycles per second (cps), and an automatic timer turns the unit off after a preset time *(3)*.

To use the G5 Vibramatic the practitioner plugs the unit into an electrical outlet, turns on the switch, and sets the percussion rate at 20 to 60 cps. The cushioned application is then held over the area to be percussed until desired results are produced or a preset time is achieved. The impact of the applicator foot is preset so that the patient receives a constant force and rate of percussion.

Still another example of an adult mechanical percussor is the Vibracare Unit. The primary difference between this unit and the Vibramatic percussor described earlier is its size. The Vibracare is small, weighing less than 37 oz, and is self-contained so that a cabinet is not required (Fig. 19-24, *A* and *B*).

Again, an advantage to a mechanical percussor is the consistency of the rate and impact of percussion, which are controllable constants no matter the length of the treatment.

14.0 SPECIAL SITUATIONS

14.1 Positions and techniques for neonates and children

Neonates and children are *not* small adults and cannot be treated medically as if they were.
1 Because of differences in the size of airways, in respiratory rates and tidal volumes, and in ability to cooperate and because of less cartilage support of the airways, neonates and children require *special* techniques and treatments.
  NOTE: Airway patency is a special problem in infants and small children not only because of their relatively small airways, but also because their compliant chests are not as capable of generating a cough as the adult's.
2 Fig. 19-25, *A* to *J* illustrates special pediatric positions for postural drainage. Positions for the neonate and very small infants can be adapted from the adult and child positions, using folded towels or pillows to achieve the desired angle.
3 Clapping, obviously, cannot be performed with the adult hand in treating small children and infants. Unfortunately, a commercial pediatric "cupper" or percussion aid is currently unavailable. Many pediatric and neonatal units develop their own versions of these manual clapping aids by jerry-building with available materials.
  a One such device is the rubber-lined bell on a stethoscope chest piece. This bell, when used gently, produces a very efficient "pop," but must be handled with care because of its metal construction.
  b Another popular homemade device uses a Puritan-

---

*All therapeutic routines must be ordered by a physician.

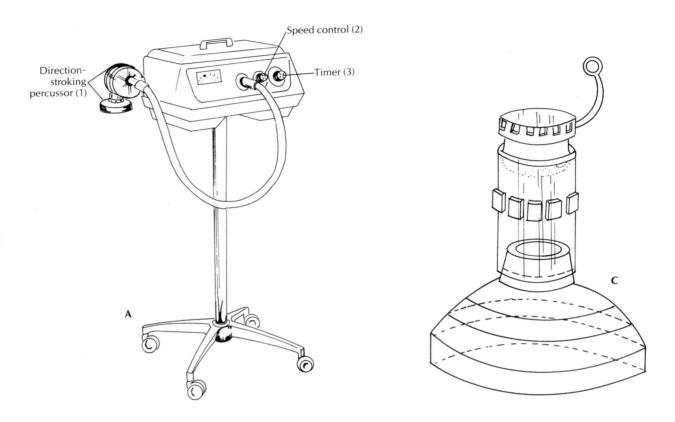

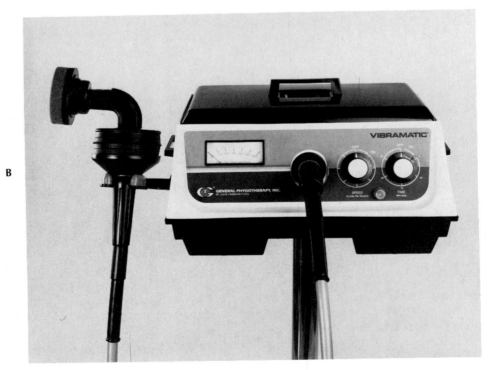

FIGURE 19-23 A and **B,** G5 Vibramatic mechanical percussor. (Courtesy General Physiotherapy, Inc, St Louis.) **C,** Manual clapping aids used to percuss infants and small children.

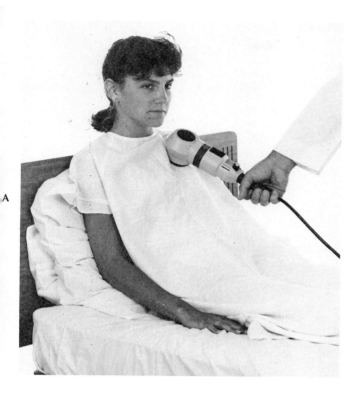

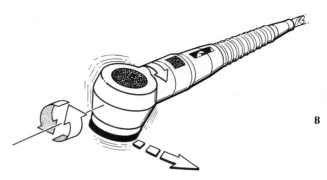

FIGURE 19-24 A and **B,** Vibracare self-contained hand-held mechanical percussor (Courtesy General Physiotherapy, Inc, St Louis.)

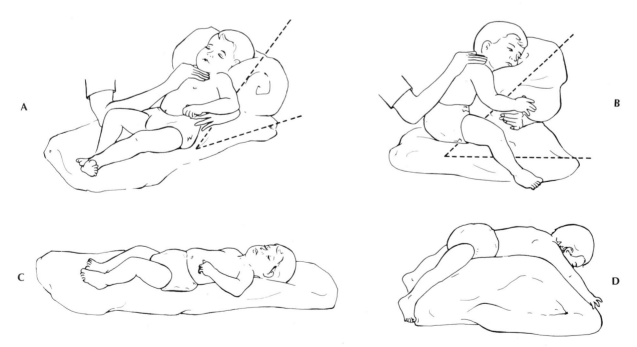

FIGURE 19-25 Positions for pulmonary drainage in infants. **A,** Apical segment. **B,** Posterior segment. **C,** Anterior segment. **D, E,** and **F,** Superior segment. **G** and **H,** Anterior basal segments (*H* lying on right and left sides). **I,** Lateral basal segment (lying on right and left sides). **J,** Posterior basal segment. (From Crane L: Physical therapy for the neonate with respiratory disease. In Irwin S and Tecklin JS: Cardiopulmonary physical therapy, ed 2, St Louis, 1990, The CV Mosby Co.)

Continued.

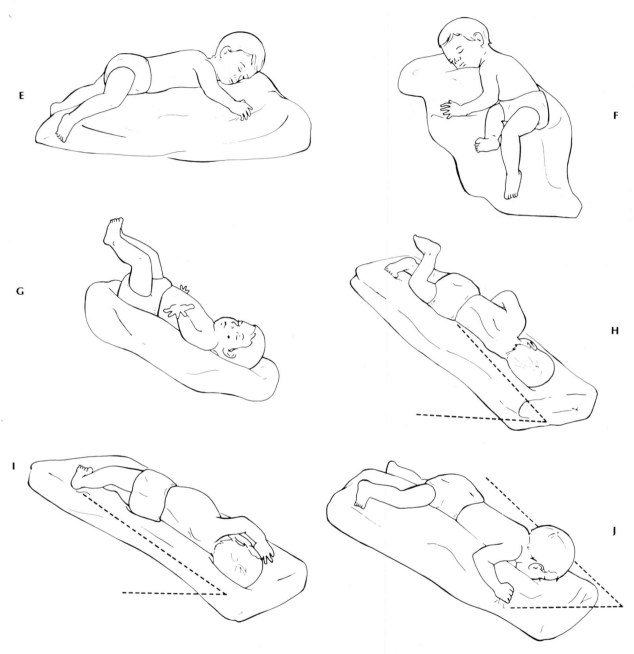

FIGURE 19-25, cont'd. For legend see opposite page.

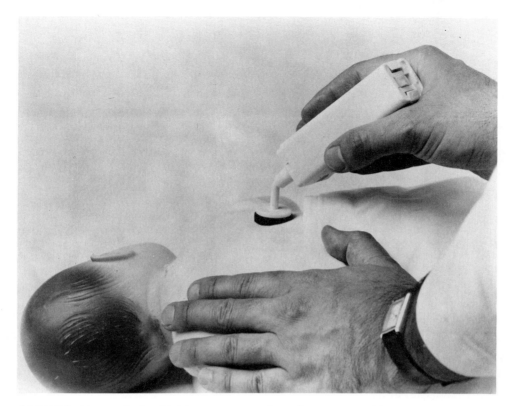

FIGURE 19-26 The hand-held Neo-Cussor Mechanical percussor used for infants and neonates. (Courtesy General Physiotherapy, Inc, St Louis.)

Bennett infant mask, a Bird 15-mm adapter, and a Bird stopper cap (see Fig. 19-23, *C*).

c General Physiotherapy has recently made available a Neo-Cussor that is battery-operated and small enough to fit inside infant environmental chambers.

The unit has disposable applicators that are used for directional-stroking or vibration (Fig. 19-26).

Additional details concerning special neonatal and pediatric techniques are presented in Module Twenty-six, Pediatric Respiratory Care.

PROCEDURE 19-1

Instruct patient (without a surgical incision) to perform deep cough from a sitting position

No.	Steps in performing the procedure
	The practitioner will demonstrate ability to instruct patient in this procedure.
1	Check medical order.
2	Greet patient and verify patient's identity.
3	Wash hands.
4	Instruct patient as to necessity of performing a deep cough.
5	Reassure patient that a controlled cough is not as painful as a spontaneous cough.
6	Position patient in sitting position in a chair, with forearms resting on top of thighs and feet placed firmly on floor. Modify position as needed.
7	Instruct patient to take 4 to 6 slow deep breaths using diaphragm and/or costal breathing.
8	Instruct patient to hold deep breath before initiating cough.
9	Instruct patient to lean forward in a flexed position, pushing diaphragm upward as forced contraction of expiratory muscles causes glottis to open, followed by a cough.
10	Instruct patient to direct cough into a tissue or away from you, but not to block the cough.
11	When relevant, instruct patient on how to collect a sputum sample with a minimum of contamination.
12	Instruct patient on how to dispose of expectorated sputum.
13	If single cough is ineffective, instruct patient to use double cough technique (i.e., cough staging, deep breaths, and cough, followed by a second cough) without a breath in between efforts.
14	Instruct patient on ineffectiveness of progressive efforts beyond two coughs.
15	Instruct patient to take a deep breath, cough, and refill lungs, using most effective inspiratory muscles.
16	Evaluate patient's level of dyspnea and modify coughing routine if necessary.
17	Evaluate effectivness of cough by listening to patient's chest and upper airway.
18	Wash hands.
19	Chart therapy, noting items such as sputum color, smell, consistency, and volume raised.

PROCEDURE 19-2

Instruct patient (with muscle weakness from a surgical incision) to perform a deep cough from a sitting position

No.	Steps in performing the procedure
	The practitioner will demonstrate ability to instruct patient in this procedure.
1	Check medical order.
2	Greet patient and verify patient's identification.
3	Wash hands.
4	Explain necessity for coughing.
5	Explain coughing procedure, including "staged cough."
6	Explain/demonstrate how incision can be protected against pain during coughing.
7	Seat patient in dangling position on bed or on a seat with no backrest. Modify position as needed.
8	Approach patient from behind.
9	Encircle arms around patient.
	9.1 Place hands gently on either side of incision.
	9.2 Hold forearm against lateral chest wall for support of sides.
	9.3 Stabilize anterior chest wall by retropressure of hands.
10	Instruct patient to cough as gentle pressure is applied to all areas of contact.
11	If patient is unable to maintain independent sitting position:
	11.1 Approach patient from front.
	11.2 Place arms around patient's chest, with hands on patient's back.
	11.3 Rest hands on top of each other on patient's back, if desired.
	11.4 Pass forearms firmly against lateral chest wall to provide side support.
	11.5 Hold patient for anteroposterior support.
12	Instruct patient to cough so that it is directed away from you, while gentle pressure is applied at all contact points.
13	Instruct patient to cough, using staging technique.
14	Instruct patient in ineffectiveness of progressive efforts beyond two coughs.
15	Instruct patient to take a deep breath after cough and refill lungs, using most effective inspiratory muscles.
16	Evaluate patient's level of dyspnea and modify coughing routine.
17	Evaluate effectiveness of cough by listening to patient's chest and upper airway.
18	Wash hands.
19	Chart therapy, noting items such as sputum color, smell, consistency, and volume raised.

PROCEDURE 19-3

Instruct patient (with surgical incision) to provide support for incision during deep cough

No.	Steps in performing the procedure
	The practitioner will demonstrate ability to instruct patient in this procedure.
1	Check medical order.
2	Greet patient and verify patient's identification.
3	Wash hands.
4	Explain necessity for coughing.
5	Explain coughing procedure.
6	Explain/demonstrate how patient can protect incision against pain and possible injury by using a cloth band or towel.
	6.1 Position patient in seated position on bed or chair.
	6.2 Direct patient to encircle lower chest with towel or other soft material, forming a band.
	6.3 Direct patient to grasp ends of towel with *opposite* hands (crossing arms).
	6.4 Direct patient to pull inward on towel as cough is generated.
7	Explain how incision can be protected without band.
	7.1 Direct patient to flex body slightly forward.
	7.2 Direct patient to cross arms across chest over pillow or blanket pad.
	7.3 Direct patient to press inward with arms as cough is generated.
8	Instruct patient to direct cough into a tissue or away from you, but not to block the cough.
9	When relevant, instruct patient on how to collect a sputum sample with a minimum of contamination.
10	Instruct patient on how to dispose of expectorated sputum.
11	If single cough is ineffective, instruct patient to use double cough technique (i.e., cough staging, deep breaths, and cough, followed by a second cough) without a breath in between efforts.
12	Instruct patient on ineffectiveness of progressive efforts beyond two coughs.
13	Instruct patient to take a deep breath, cough, and refill lungs, using most effective inspiratory muscles.
14	Evaluate patient's level of dyspnea and modify coughing routine if necessary.
15	Evaluate effectiveness of cough by listening to patient's chest and upper airway.
16	Wash hands.
17	Chart therapy, noting items such as sputum color, smell, consistency, and volume raised.

PROCEDURE 19-4

Instruct patient (with thoracotomy incision) to perform deep cough, using assisted protective technique

No.	Steps in performing the procedure
	The practitioner will demonstrate ability to instruct patient in this procedure.
1	Check medical order.
2	Greet patient and verify patient's identification.
3	Wash hands.
4	Explain necessity for coughing.
5	Explain coughing procedure.
6	Explain/demonstrate how incision can be protected against pain and possible injury.
	6.1 Place patient in seated or semi-Fowler's position.
	6.2 Position yourself in front of patient, but on side opposite the incision.
	6.3 Encircle one arm around patient's chest, resting it along the path of the incision.
	6.4 Encircle other arm around chest from unoperated side.
	6.5 Place hand *lateroposteriorly* on the chest, just below the incision.
	6.6 Apply gentle pressure with the arms and hands to provide support.
	6.7 Support anterior and posterior chest with your own body.
	6.8 Instruct patient to cough, using proper technique, while supportive pressure is applied to all contact points.
7	Instruct patient to direct cough into a tissue or away from you, but not to block the cough.
8	When relevant, instruct patient on how to collect a sputum sample with a minimum of contamination.
9	Instruct patient on how to dispose of expectorated sputum.
10	If single cough is ineffective, instruct patient to use double cough technique (i.e., cough staging, deep breaths, and cough, followed by a second cough) without a breath in between efforts.
11	Instruct patient on ineffectiveness of progressive efforts beyond two coughs.
12	Instruct patient to take a deep breath, cough, and refill lungs, using most effective inspiratory muscles.
13	Evaluate effectiveness of cough by listening to patient's chest and upper airway.
14	Evaluate effectiveness of cough by listening to patient's chest and upper airway.
15	Wash hands.
16	Chart therapy, noting items such as sputum color, smell, consistency, and volume raised.

PROCEDURE 19-5

Instruct patient (with thoracotomy incision) to perform deep cough using self-administered protective technique

No.	Steps in performing the procedure	No.	Steps in performing the procedure
	The practitioner will demonstrate ability to instruct patient in this procedure.		7.2 Position patient to use weight of arms and hand pressure on rolled pillows to support incision during cough.
1	Check medical order.		
2	Greet patient and verify patient's identification.	8	Instruct patient to direct cough into a tissue or away from you, but not to block the cough.
3	Wash hands.		
4	Explain necessity for coughing.	9	When relevant, instruct patient on how to collect sputum sample with a minimum of contamination.
5	Explain coughing procedure.		
6	Explain/demonstrate how patient can protect incision against pain and possible injury by using a towel or other soft material.	10	Instruct patient on how to dispose of expectorated sputum.
	6.1 Assist patient to form a sling, using soft material.	11	If a single cough is ineffective, instruct patient to use double cough technique, (i.e., cough staging, deep breaths, and cough, followed by a second cough,) without a breath in between efforts.
	6.2 Assist patient to cover incision with sling by placing material over shoulder on unoperated side, using opposite hand.		
	6.3 Instruct patient to use opposite hand to wrap sling around the incision, passing the ends under the arm of the operated side.	12	Instruct patient on ineffectiveness of progressive efforts beyond two coughs.
		13	Instruct patient to take a deep breath, cough, and refill lungs, using most effective inspiratory muscles.
	6.4 Show patient how to hold sling firmly against chest with hand as cough is generated.	14	Evaluate patient's level of dyspnea and modify coughing routine, if necessary.
7	Explain and demonstrate how incision can be self-supported using pillows.	15	Evaluate effectiveness of cough by listening to patient's chest and upper airway.
	7.1 Position patient so that rolled pillows are pressed against incision with patient's own body weight.	16	Wash hands.
		17	Chart therapy, noting items such as sputum color, smell, consistency, and volume raised.

PROCEDURE 19-6

Positioning patient for pulmonary drainage of all segments*

No.	Steps in performing the procedure	No.	Steps in performing the procedure
	The practitioner will demonstrate ability to instruct patient in positioning.	10	Position bed/patient for drainage of lower lobes:
1	Check medical order.		**10.1** Posterior basal segment (see Fig. 19-11).
2	Read chart for other relevant data, such as physical history, patient progress notes, arterial blood gases (ABGs), and chest radiograph.		**10.2** Lateral basal segment (see Fig. 19-12).
			10.3 Anterior basal segment (see Fig. 19-13).
			10.4 Superior segment (see Fig. 19-14).
3	Assemble appropriate equipment, such as:	11	Encourage and instruct patient on how to cough in each position.
	3.1 Blankets	12	Continually assess patient's tolerance of each position.
	3.2 Pillows		
	3.3 Sputum cup	13	Position bed/patient to drain right middle lobe (see Fig. 19-15).
	3.4 Disposable tissues		
	3.5 Blood pressure manometer/stethoscope	14	Position bed/patient to drain upper lobes:
	3.6 Special oxygen therapy equipment		**14.1** Lingular segment—superior/inferior (see Fig. 19-16)
4	Greet patient and verify patient's identification.		
5	Wash hands.		**14.2** Anterior segment (see Fig. 19-17).
6	Explain procedure to patient.		**14.3** Apical segment (see Fig. 19-18).
7	Instruct patient in deep cough techniques.		**14.4** Posterior segment (see Fig. 19-19).
8	Check and record vital signs and other assessment observations.	15	Return patient and bed to normal position.
		16	Disconnect any special therapy.
9	Administer any special treatment, such as aerosol or oxygen therapy, allowing appropriate treatment time before positioning patient.	17	Encourage patient to deep breathe and cough.
		18	Recheck vital signs.
		19	Offer patient fluids if allowed.
		20	Discuss treatment with patient; answer questions.
		21	Wash hands.
		22	Chart procedure, noting patient's progress, any adverse responses, special modification, instructions to next clinician, sputum color, smell, consistency, and volume raised.

*Use Figs. 19-11 through 19-19 as a guide for this exercise.

PROCEDURE 19-7

Clapping/vibration of the chest

No.	Steps in performing the procedure	No.	Steps in performing the procedure
	The practitioner will demonstrate ability to instruct patient in clapping/vibration of the chest.		**15.3** Use alternate flexation/extension of wrist on each arm to establish clapping motion.
1	Check medical order.		**15.4** Establish desired:

2	Read chart for other relevant data, such as physical history, patient progress notes, ABGs, and chest radiograph.		**a** Rate
			   b Rhythm
			   c Force of impact

3	Assemble appropriate equipment, such as:	16	Perform clapping for 3 minutes over each segment.
	3.1 Blankets	17	Interrupt clapping after 3 minutes and perform vibration.
	3.2 Pillows		**17.1** Position yourself to gain direct access to chest area.
	3.3 Sputum cup		**17.2** Extend arms straight.
	3.4 Disposable tissues		**17.3** Place hands one on top of the other over chest area to be vibrated.
	3.5 Blood pressure manometer/stethoscope		**17.4** Generate gentle vibrations to the chest via the hands by causing the arms to shake.
	3.6 Special oxygen therapy equipment	18	Instruct patient to cough after vibration and deep breathing.
4	Greet patient and verify patient's identification.	19	Return to clapping for another 3 minutes.
5	Wash hands.	20	Perform vibration for second time as patient is instructed to exhale after a deep inspiration.
6	Explain procedure to patient.	21	Encourage patient to cough and expectorate secretions, using proper technique.
7	Instruct patient in deep cough techniques.	22	Reposition patient as clapping and vibration are applied to involved segments.
8	Check and record vital signs and other assessment observations.	23	Continually assess patient's tolerance of drainage position of clapping/vibration.
9	Prepare bed/patient for postural drainage in concurrence with clapping/vibration.	24	Modify program with patient; answer any questions.
10	Administer any special treatment, such as aerosol or oxygen therapy, allowing appropriate treatment time before positioning patient.	25	Recheck vital signs.
11	Use stethoscope to pinpoint affected areas.	26	Wash hands.
12	Position patient to gain maximum access to affected areas.	27	Chart procedure, noting patient's progress, any adverse responses, special modification, instructions to next clinician, sputum color, smell, consistency, and volume raised.
13	Remove heavy clothing from area to be clapped, and place a hospital gown or soft cloth over area.		
14	Position yourself for maximum accessibility.		
15	Use proper clapping technique.		
	15.1 Form hand into cupped shape.		
	15.2 Place hands within 5 inches of chest.		

BIBLIOGRAPHY

Buscaglia AJ and St Marie MS: Oxygen saturation during chest physiotherapy for acute exacerbation of severe chronic obstructive pulmonary disease, Respir Care 28:1009, 1983.

Denton R: Bronchial secretions in cystic fibrosis: the effects of treatment with mechanical percussion vibration, Am Rev Respir Dis 86:41, 1962.

Flower KA et al: New mechanical aid to physiotherapy in cystic fibrosis, Br Med J 2:630, 1979.

Harris JA and Jerry BA: Indications and procedures for segmental bronchial drainage, Respir Care 20:1164, 1975.

Holody B and Goldberg HS: The effect of mechanical vibration physiotherapy on arterial oxygenation in acutely ill patients with atelectasis or pneumonia, Am Rev Respir Dis 124:372, 1981.

Indihar FJ, Forsberg DP, and Adams AB: A prospective comparison of three procedures used in attempts to prevent postoperative pulmonary complications, Respir Care 27:564, 1982.

Mackenzie CF et al, editors: Chest physiotherapy in the intensive care unit, Baltimore, 1981, Williams & Wilkins.

Pania D, Thomson M, and Phillipakos D: A preliminary study of the effect of a vibrating pad on bronchial clearance, Am Rev Respir Dis 113:92, 1976.

Radford R et al: A rational basis for percussion-augmented mucociliary clearance, Respir Care 27:556, 1982.

Tyler ML: Complications of positioning and chest physiotherapy, Respir Care 27:458, 1982.

Airway management

8.8 Point out the parts of a tracheostomy tube.

8.9 Distinguish between the types of special tracheostomy tubes based on their different functions.

9.1 Explain the need for respiratory care personnel to be able to suction an airway.

9.2 Describe the circumstances requiring one to suction an airway.

9.3 Differentiate between the types of suctioning techniques.

9.4 Discuss the principle of suctioning devices.

9.5 Describe criteria for a functional suction system.

9.6 Justify the necessity for selecting the proper size and type of suction catheter.

9.7 Identify the equipment necessary to carry out a sterile suctioning procedure.

9.8 Discuss possible hazards and complications from transtracheal suctioning.

9.9 Perform sterile endotracheal suctioning according to a recommended general procedure.

9.10 Perform oropharyngeal or nasopharyngeal suctioning according to a recommended general procedure.

10.1 Discuss the rationale for the insertion of an esophageal obturator airway.

10.2 Identify general concerns in placing the esophageal obturator airway.

10.3 Identify the steps in placing the esophageal obturator airway.

1.0 AIRWAY MANAGEMENT

1.1 The role of the clinician in airway management

1 The various structures composing the cardiopulmonary system have been presented in Modules Four and Eight. It is recommended that the reader review the specific units dealing with the airway in these modules before proceeding with this module. In addition, the first units of this module will serve as a review of those anatomic structures that are most frequently associated with life-threatening airway management problems. These include the pharynx, larynx, trachea, and main stem bronchi.

2 The more distal airway passages are not usually the site of obstruction from foreign objects unless it is liquid or gas. Even then, the obstruction is usually the result of associated bronchospasm caused by a foreign agent and not the agent itself.

3 Module Twenty will present airway management problems and techniques for alleviating these problems when they occur in the upper airway, as well as present identification methods and techniques for recognizing and controlling lower airway obstructions. The emphasis of this module will be "how to"—how to recognize a problem and how to eliminate it. This module, therefore, presents some of the most critical clinical skills necessary for respiratory care personnel. This is be-

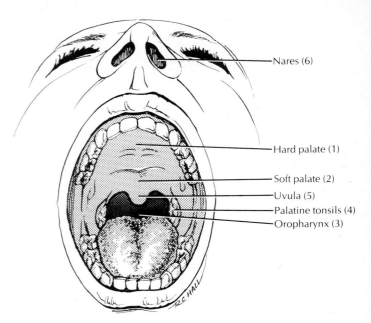

FIGURE 20-1 Upper airway structures visible through open mouth.

cause airway difficulties, especially blockages, can cause death if they are not quickly recognized and resolved.

4 The following statements indicate the need for respiratory care personnel to become expert "airway managers":

a Recognizing the need for and providing a patent airway is one of the most fundamental yet important skills a clinician must acquire.

b Without an adequate airway, the patient will eventually die as a result of hypoventilation.

c To recognize airway obstruction, one need only to look, listen, and sometimes feel for indications of air movement.

d Once airway obstruction is determined, the quickest and least traumatic method of providing a patent airway should be employed. This does *not* necessarily require the use of any mechanical aids. In many instances repositioning of the patient's head and jaw is sufficient. If positioning is not effective, other procedures must be quickly employed.

e In cases of acute airway obstruction, the clinician has from 4 to 6 minutes to remove the obstruction before the patient experiences permanent brain damage and/or death.

f As in most medical techniques, the clinician should employ the quickest and simplest corrective action first and then select more complicated alternatives only if the airway is not successfully provided.

1.2 Structures of the upper airway

1 Fig. 20-1 illustrates the view that would be seen if one looked into an open mouth. The hard palate *(1)* and soft palate *(2)* can be seen in the upper portion of the

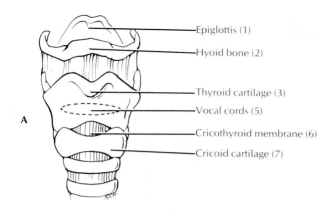

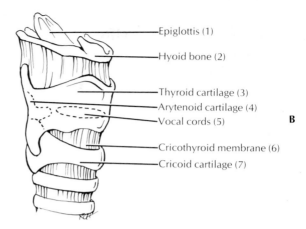

FIGURE 20-2 Larynx. Anterior **A,** and lateral **B,** view.

oropharynx, with the soft midline uvula *(5)* hanging to its posterior. The oropharynx *(3)* and the palatine tonsils *(4)* can be seen below and behind the palate.

4 The nares *(6)* can be seen from this view with the nasopharynx lying directly behind them. The nasopharynx is not visible; however, it lies directly above the oropharynx.

5 Additional information concerning the anatomic structures can be found in Modules Four and Eight.

1.3 Anatomic structures surrounding the larynx*

1 Anatomic structures that compose the larynx or are located close to the larynx (see Fig. 20-2, *A* and *B*) are the epiglottis *(1)*, hyoid bone *(2)*, thyroid cartilage *(3)*, arytenoid cartilage *(B, 4)*, vocal cords *(5)*, cricothyroid membrane *(6)*, and cricoid cartilage *(7)*.

2 The *hyoid bone (2)* is responsible in part for suspension of the epiglottis. Note that the vocal cords are lying directly below the epiglottis and can be seen *(5)* in an open position. This bone is the anatomic landmark for locating the cricothyroid membrane, which is penetrated for insertion of a tube during cricothyroidotomy.

3 The *cricoid cartilate (7)* is the first ring of the trachea and is responsible for preventing collapse of the upper trachea during breathing.

4 The *thyroid cartilage (3)* serves as a protective covering over the larynx and is often referred to as the "Adam's apple."

1.4 Anatomic structures of the larynx as viewed through a laryngoscope*

1 Fig. 20-3 is a laryngoscopic view of the larynx of a patient seen in a supine position with the epiglottis *(1)* protruding toward the observer. The vocal cords *(2)* are

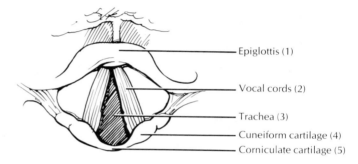

FIGURE 20-3 Structures of the larynx as viewed through a laryngoscope.

open, and the trachea *(3)* can be seen directly below the cords.

2 The cuneiform *(4)* and corniculate cartilage *(5)* are easily visible from this view.

2.0 AIRWAY MAINTENANCE

2.1 Anatomic structures and their effects on airway maintenance

1 The position of the head and neck has a direct relationship for maintaining the patency of the airways. This is especially true with comatose or unconscious patients (Fig. 20-4, *A* through *C*). When the head is flexed, the ability of the airways to remain open may be compromised by causing the soft tissue of the airway to "drop back," narrowing the position diameter of either the nasopharynx *(1)*, oropharynx *(2)*, or hypopharynx *(3)* (see Fig. 20-4, *B*).

2 When the head is *extended*, a straight-line relationship exists between the oropharynx and the larynx, making it the optimum position for clearance of the upper Airway or intubation. It is also the position that the head and neck are placed in when the head-tilt maneuver is performed to open an airway or to prevent airway ob-

---

*Additional information concerning the surrounding anatomy of the larynx may be found in Module Eight.

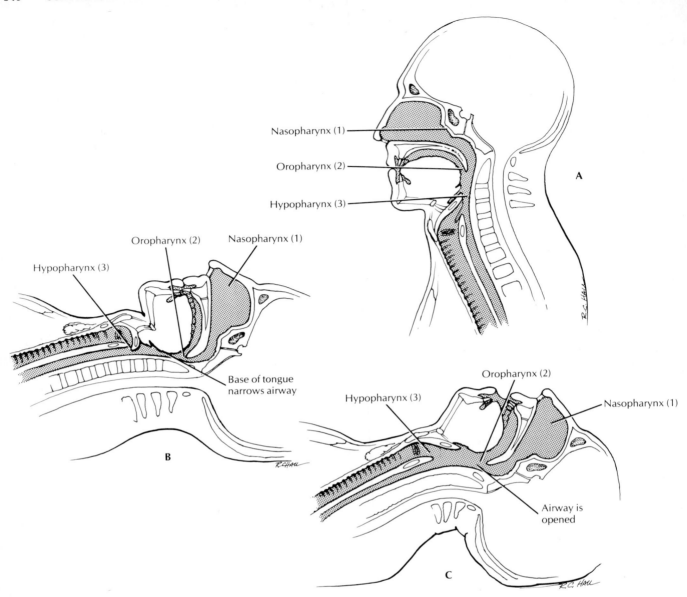

FIGURE 20-4 View of upper airway when head is in **A,** upright, **B,** flexed, and **C,** extended positions.

struction when the patient is asleep or unconscious (see Fig. 20-4, *C*).

3.0 AIRWAY OBSTRUCTION

3.1 Primary causes of airway obstruction

1 Blockage of the *nasopharynx, oropharynx,* and *hypopharynx*
2 Anatomic displacement of the tongue and other soft tissues of the hypopharynx
3 Aspiration of solid, liquid, or gaseous objects or agents
4 Trauma to the airway by crushing or penetrating injuries
5 Obstruction by mucus
6 Obstruction by tumors or other growth
7 Spasm caused by foreign objects or agents
8 Obstruction caused by improperly placed artificial airways

3.2 The nasopharynx

1 The nasopharynx is a cavity that, as seen through the open mouth, begins with the external nares and extends posteriorly to the region adjoining the oral cavity.
2 The nasopharynx is composed of bone and soft tissue.
3 The mucous membrane of the nose is formed by soft tissue called the *pharyngeal tonsil.*
4 In the young child this tissue can become enlarged, causing *adenoids,* which can block the airway and create an emergency situation that requires intubation.

3.3 The oropharynx

1 The oropharynx begins with the area that can be seen through the open mouth and extends posteriorly to the area above the epiglottis. (Fig. 20-1 depicts the view that would be seen as one looks into the open mouth.)
2 The *hard (1)* and *soft (2) palates* can be seen in the up-

per portion of the oropharynx, with the soft *uvula (5)* hanging midline and to the posterior.

3 The *oropharynx (3)* and the *palatine tonsils (4)* are shown below and behind the palate.

4 The *nares (6)* are also shown in this figure, although the nasopharynx is not visible.

5 If desired, the reader may use a flashlight to identify each of the above structures in the mouth of another person.

6 In children, the palatine tonsils can become so enlarged that they converge, blocking the airways and making emergency tracheal intubation very difficult.

7 The base of the tongue begins just above the opening to the larynx and is attached to the epiglottis of the larynx by three folds.

8 Structurally, the base of the tongue is irregular and has a tendency to extend into the airway.

9 The oropharynx is a continuation of the nasopharynx above and the hypopharynx below.

3.4 The hypopharynx

1 The *hypopharynx* extends from the epiglottis to the opening of the esophagus.

2 The epiglottis covers the opening to the larynx and soft tissues of various cartilages of the larynx from the anterior wall of the hypopharynx.

3 This is the region most frequently involved in airway obstruction, usually as a result of relaxation of the base of the tongue into the hypopharynx, blocking the air passage.

3.5 Soft tissue obstruction of the airway

1 In the unconscious or comatose patient the muscles holding the tongue in position (out of the airway) are relaxed. When this occurs, especially in the supine patient, the base of the relaxed tongue and other soft tissues of the hypopharyngeal region drop backward into the airway, causing partial or complete blockage. (See Fig. 20-4, the flexed position.)

2 This occurrence can be manifested by something as simple as snoring or as critical as interruption of gas passage into and out of the lungs.

3 Other causes of soft tissue obstruction include cysts, tumors, and other growths extending into the airway. These growths usually manifest themselves with elevated airway resistance, causing increased work of breathing or feelings of fullness in the area of the growth. Pain usually is not a reliable warning sign, because it may not appear until the lesion has caused significant tissue damage.

4 X-ray examination is usually *not* diagnostic, unless a soft tissue study is performed using a radiopaque dye.

3.6 Airway obstruction caused by aspiration

1 *Aspiration* is defined as the accidental inhalation of a foreign substance into the airway.

2 Contrary to common belief, foreign substances are *not* usually aspirated into the distal regions of the lung.

3 Most aspirated substances cause immediate and severe spasm to the larynx, trachea, and bronchus. These foreign substances usually are lodged between the vocal cords, in the trachea, or in a main stem bronchus.

4 Solid objects that are aspirated and pass through the vocal cords usually lodge themselves in the right main stem bronchus.

5 Aspirated gases or liquids may be an exception to the rule regarding depth of aspiration, although in *near* drownings, when the patient remains conscious, less than 75 ml of liquid is usually found in the patient's lungs. It is only *after* the victim loses consciousness and the airway's protective mechanisms fail that the lungs are flooded.

6 In gas inhalation the protective bronchial spasm may be immediate, (e.g., in smoke inhalation).

7 The bronchi may not show severe damage or spasm for periods up to 72 hours. This is sometimes called the *silent period,* following a victim's exposure to caustic fumes; it is also a dangerous period for near-drowning victims.

3.7 Airway obstruction caused by trauma

1 Injuries to the upper airway are a cause for immediate concern and action.

2 *Crushing injuries* caused by impaction of the nose, mouth, larynx, or trachea into an object, or vice versa, can cause hemorrhage into the airway, creating a situation for possible aspiration of blood and other foreign matter into the lungs. In addition, if the larynx or trachea is crushed, the airway may be immediately obstructed or subsequently become obstructed because of swelling. For example, if the hyoid bone is fractured, the upper portion of the trachea has a tendency to collapse inward in response to the decreased pressure caused by inspiratory efforts.

3 Crushing injuries are treated as *emergencies* and will probably require intubation, cricothyroidotomy, or a tracheostomy.

4 Injuries caused by penetrating objects can be as serious as crushing injuries and should also be treated as emergencies.

5 Penetrating injuries are especially dangerous, not only because of the hemorrhage and possible collapsed airway, but also because of the possibility of *subcutaneous emphysema.*

6 Subcutaneous emphysema is the presence of air in the tissues lying underneath the wound site. This in itself may not be serious unless it continues and involves the head, neck, chest, and even abdominal structures. If the air moves into (dissects) the mediastinum (pneumomediastinum), it may rupture the pleura and cause a *pneumothorax,* which can be fatal if not quickly resolved.

3.8 Airway obstruction caused by mucus or other body fluids

1 It is almost ironic that one can die from asphyxia as a result of obstruction caused by the abnormal presence

of the body's own fluids, such as mucus, blood, or gastric contents, in the airway.

2 The airway has very effective physiologic protective mechanisms (depending on the location of the foreign substance), such as reflex spasm, the sneeze, the cough, constant movement of cilia, peristalsis of the smaller bronchioles, and even phagocytosis at the alveolar level.

3 Unfortunately, even these protective mechanisms are not sufficient to protect the airway from the aspiration of large amounts of fluids or copious volumes of mucus and other secretions.

4 Airway secretions, especially mucoid types, are sticky and tend to accumulate in pools or pockets along the airway system, with the greatest accumulation occurring at the site of an irritation or infection. The greatest dangers from accumulated secretions are:
a Infection—with subsequent production of still more secretions and airway involvement.
b Airway obstruction—may be partial and cause diminished gas flow to the areas distal to the obstruction and increased work of breathing. Complete obstruction may occur and cause cessation of gas flow to the distal regions. If the obstruction is in a main bronchus or lobe, a total lung can be involved. If smaller bronchi are involved, then smaller lung areas will be isolated, usually causing atelectasis and, eventually, infection.

5 Secretions are primarily fluid (water) by volume, containing smaller amounts of lung debris and/or cellular matter. For this reason, secretions are normally moved toward the proximal airway on a blanket of serous fluid by the cilia. If the airway becomes dehydrated, the secretions lose their fluid volume to the passing gases and become sticky plugs. Dehydration of the airway occurs because of the inhalation of unhumidified gases or inadequate fluid intake by the patient. Pooled secretions that become lodged within the airway are said to be *inspissated* or impacted.

6 Besides the inherent complications of atelectasis, the greatest danger from inspissated secretions are that they potentially can become dislodged and move from one location in a minor bronchiole to block a major bronchiole. This situation can cause severe airway obstruction manifested by acute dyspnea, hypoxemia, and other events, leading to respiratory distress and/or failure.

3.9 Airway obstruction caused by spasm

1 Beginning with the larynx, the airway protects itself by the stimulation of abundant numbers of vagal nerve endings. Stimulation of this nerve causes a cough reflex that usually expels any foreign substance.

2 The cough reflex is located in the laryngeal area and at the level of the carina.

3 It must be remembered that if a cough is artificially caused by stimulation of the vagus nerve with a catheter or other object, the heart and respirations may be simultaneously slowed as a result of vagal interaction and possibly adversely affect the patient.

4 Once an aspirant passes through the larynx it usually proceeds through the trachea and lodges either at the carina or in the right main stem bronchus.

5 If the aspirant is small enough, it can pass into the smaller bronchi or bronchioles, where it will usually lodge before reaching the alveoli. The exceptions to this are liquids or toxic gases.

6 Like the larynx, the bronchi are richly endowed with nerves that respond from exposure to foreign substances. The speed and magnitude of response will depend on the toxicity and volume of the aspirant. The response may be instantaneous, such as occurs in chlorine gas inhalation, or delayed, as in cases of smoke inhalation.

7 The aspiration of gastric contents (pH 2.5) is one of the most damaging insults to the airway, resulting in a chemical burn of the mucosa and subsequent pneumonitis. This type of injury may be localized or may involve the entire airway stem.

8 Airway spasm caused by aspiration can cause acute dyspnea and other symptoms manifested by respiratory failure.

4.0 DETERMINING THE ABSENCE OR PRESENCE OF AIRWAY OBSTRUCTION
4.1 Signs of airway obstruction

1 Airway obstruction manifests itself by visual, audible, and tactile signs, depending on the location, severity, and type of obstruction.

2 The visual signs of airway obstruction are:
a An increased rate of breathing
b Gasping efforts
c Exaggerated use of the muscles of inspiration
d Retraction of soft thoracic tissues during inspiratory attempts
e Cyanosis, diaphoresis
f Signs of fear, anxiety, thrashing of arms and legs
g Unconsciousness

3 The presence or absence of vocal sounds may be important indicators of airway obstruction.

4 A complete absence of sounds and gas flow combined with exaggerated inspiratory attempts indicates *complete* airway obstruction. This is an *emergency* situation.

5 If the airway obstruction is *partial* and occurs in the upper airway, the patient will probably make some of the following audible sounds:
a Crowing
b Gasping
c Snoring
d Stridor
e Gurgling
f Wheezes
g Rales
h Rhonchi

6 If the airway obstruction is partial and if it is located in the lower airways, the patient will demonstrate wheezes, rales, and rhonchi on auscultation.

7 Diminished or abnormal breath sounds, combined with diminished chest excursion, probably indicates bronchial obstruction and/or consolidation of lung tissue.

8 Tactile signs of airway obstruction and respiratory distress include:

   a A rapid pulse (greater than 120 beats/min)

   b A very slow pulse

   c An irregular pulse

   d Clammy, wet skin

9 Obviously, airway obstruction, depending on its degree, should be handled minimally as a critical situation and in most cases as an emergency.

4.2 Circumstantial signs of airway obstruction

1 Airway obstruction can be suspected based on the circumstances under which the patient was initially seen, (e.g., eating, drinking).

2 Physical evidence can also be used to lead one to suspect airway obstruction: for instance, reddening or swelling in the area of the trachea, soot around the mouth or nostrils, vomitus in the mouth, etc.

3 A rapid questioning of someone near the victim may expedite the decision to initiate one type of treatment vs. another.

5.0 ELIMINATING AIRWAY OBSTRUCTION

5.1 Selecting the most proper method of correcting airway obstruction

1 The method selected to correct an airway obstruction should be simple, quick, and effective.

2 For example, the Heimlich maneuver would probably be the initial method of choice for a complete airway obstruction.

3 Care must be taken that the "cure" does not cause more trauma than the initial problem. For example, attempting to pass a nasotracheal tube in a patient whose nasal passages are partially blocked will damage the mucosa of the nose and may cause profuse bleeding. This possibly may be avoided if the clinician uses an orotracheal tube or provides an airway by simple hyperextension of the neck.

4 In most cases the Heimlich maneuver should be performed before other methods are attempted.

5.2 Development and use of the Heimlich maneuver

1 In June of 1974, *Emergency Medicine* published a description of a new technique that would save the life of a person whose airway is obstructed by food or another type of foreign object.

2 The technique was developed by Henry J. Heimlich, MD, who is a professor of advanced clinical sciences at Xavier University in Cincinnati.

3 The Heimlich maneuver, as it was later named by the American Medical Association, uses the air that is trapped in the chest at the time of the obstruction as the medium to remove the obstruction. The force necessary to compress the air and blow out the obstructing object is supplied by external compression of the lungs by a rescuer. Since 1974, the Heimlich maneuver has been credited with saving over 3000 lives.

4 The primary advantages of the maneuver are:

   a It can be performed with no equipment.

   b It can be performed on choking victims of all ages and can also be self-administered.

   c It can be performed while the victim is standing, sitting, or lying down.

   d It causes none-to-minimum trauma to the victim if it is properly applied.

5 The Heimlich maneuver is the preferred method for clearing an obstruction from the airway.

6 Backslapping techniques should *not* be used because it wastes valuable time and can cause the aspirated object to become more tightly and deeply impacted.

7 The *general* steps involved in performing a Heimlich maneuver are:

   a Recognize that life-threatening choking is occurring.

   b Clear the mouth of any foreign objects (Do not probe into the pharynx because it can force the object tighter.)

   c Position the victim so that you can properly place your hands on the individual's epigastrium and provide the necessary inward and upward thrusts.

8 The theoretic basis for the Heimlich maneuver is that as the diaphragm is moved quickly upward by the rescuer's thrusts to the epigastrium, residual lung volume is compressed, causing a rapid rise of air pressure behind the obstruction, causing it to "pop" from the airway, much as the cork pops from a champagne bottle.

9 Studies have shown that air flows of approxiamtely 205 liters per minute (L/min) at approximately 31 mm Hg can be generated by the maneuver. It is this flow of air that provides the force necessary to remove the occluding object.

5.3 Specific steps in performing a Heimlich maneuver

1 Recognize a choking victim. The audible, visual, and tactile signs of airway obstruction are presented in Procedure 20-1 at the end of this module and in Unit 4-1.

   a The primary sign of choking in the conscious victim is clutching of the throat while making attempts to talk, combined with a look of panic (Fig. 20-5). The victim may run and attempt to resist assistance until overcome by asphyxia. Attempts should be made to calm the victim so that the maneuver can be immediately performed.

   b In the unwitnessed situation one may need to use the circumstances surrounding the victim as an indication that choking is the cause of unconsciousness.

   c Location of the victim near an eating place may be a sign that the victim became embarrassed and left the table only to collapse in the hallway.

2 Quickly question witnesses who may have viewed the episode.

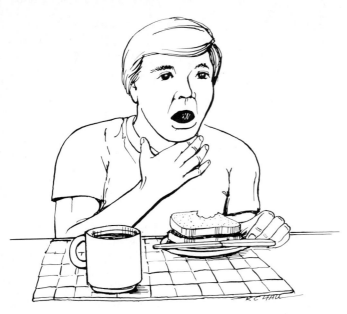

FIGURE 20-5 Victim indicating primary signs of choking.

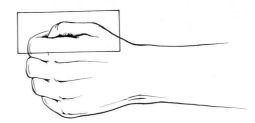

FIGURE 20-6 To perform Heimlich maneuver, make a fist so that knob is formed by thumb and index finger.

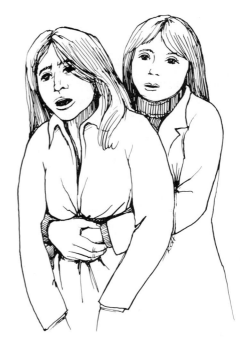

FIGURE 20-7 Standing behind victim, place fist with thumb against abdomen, slightly above navel and below ribcage.

3 Quickly position the victim for the maneuver.
  a Make a fist so that a knob is formed by the thumb and index finger (see Fig. 20-6).
  b Standing behind the victim, place your fist with the thumb against the victim's abdomen, slightly above the navel and below the rib cage (see Fig. 20-7).
  c Grasp your fist with your free hand and press it up and into the abdomen with a quick upward thrust (see Fig. 20-8).
4 This procedure can be performed while the victim is standing or sitting. In either case, stand behind the victim with your arms wrapped around the victim's waist (see Figs. 20-9 and 20-10).
5 Place the victim who has fallen flat on his or her back so that the head is straight and facing up. The head and neck must be positioned properly or the airway may be distorted, which would reduce the effectiveness of the Heimlich maneuver.
6 Place yourself astride the victim's hips, and place the heel of one hand on the abdomen, slightly above the navel and below the rib cage. Place the free hand over the first hand and press the heel of the hand up and into the victim's abdomen with a quick upward thrust (see Fig. 20-11).
7 If the victim is a small child at least 1 year old, the maneuver is performed the same as it is on an adult.
  NOTE: Subdiaphragmatic thrusts are not recommended for infants less than 1 year old because of the potential for intra-abdominal injury. In these victims a combination of back blows and chest thrusts is recommended by the American Heart Association. (See Fig. 20-12, A through C).
8 If the infant is less than 1 year old, a series of back blows and chest thrusts are alternately performed in lieu of the adult-type Heimlich maneuver.

9 In order to perform a back blow maneuver, the infant is picked up and cradled in one hand by the rescuer, making sure the infant's head is supported by holding its jaw.
10 The infant is then placed in a head-down position by the standing rescuer by resting his or her forearm on his or her thigh. (Fig. 20-12, A).
11 With the free hand opened and with fingers together, the rescuer delivers *four* back blows by striking the heel of the hand forcefully high up on the infant's back, between the shoulder blades. (Fig 20-12, A).
12 If the obstruction is not removed, the rescuer places his or her free hand on the infant's back, so the infant is cradled between the resducer's hands.
  While making sure that the infant's head and neck are supported, the infant is turned over and rested on the rescuer's thigh with its head positioned lower than its chest.
13 Then the rescuer, using two fingers, performs four chest thrusts in the same location as would be used for external chest compression. (Fig. 20-12, B).

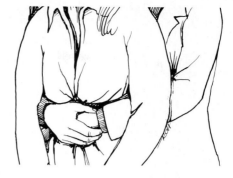

FIGURE 20-9 Heimlich maneuver with victim standing.

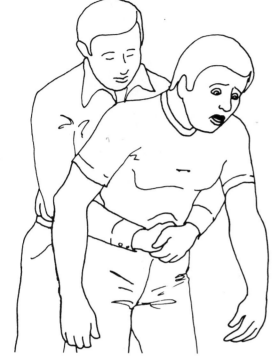

FIGURE 20-8 Grasp fist with free hand. Press up and into abdomen with quick upward thrust.

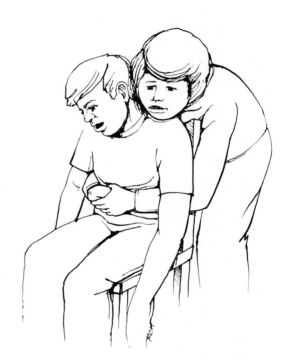

FIGURE 20-10 Heimlich maneuver with victim sitting.

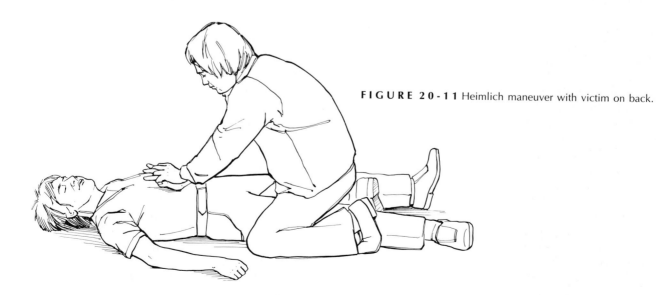

FIGURE 20-11 Heimlich maneuver with victim on back.

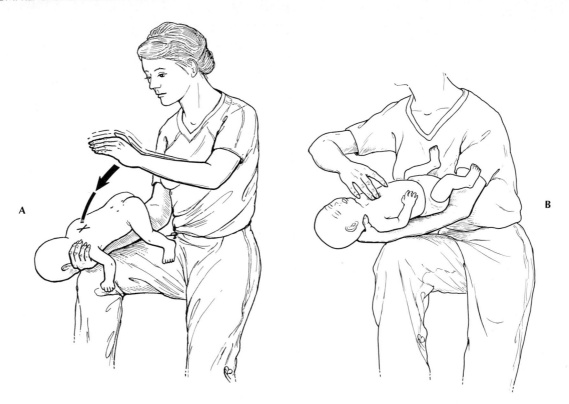

FIGURE 20-12 A, Positioning infant for back blows. Heel of hand strikes forcefully between shoulder blades. **B,** Two fingers are used to perform chest thrusts in same location as for external chest compression.

14 If the obstruction is not cleared, the rescuer opens the infant's mouth and checks for the obstruction.

15 If an obstructive substance is seen, it is removed and an attempt is made to deliver a resuscitative breath.

16 If this effort is unsuccessful, the infant is again carefully turned to the head-down position with head and neck support and four more back blows are delivered, using the same technique as described before.

17 This routine of *four back blows, plus four chest thrusts, plus mouth check, plus four back blows,* etc. is continued until help arrives.

18 With larger infants, the rescuer may find it easier to sit or kneel, using the thighs for support. The infant is placed in a head-down position and supported in the same manner as when the standing technique is used.

19 Continue airway clearance efforts until the object is removed. Usually this is recognized by a loud noise, as the object pops from the airway, a gasp for air by the victim, and presence of the object. Remember that if the victim is *still not* breathing, *immediate* steps must be taken to begin life support measures, such as cardiopulmonary resuscitation (CPR).

20 Procedures 20-1, 20-2, and 20-3, which are included at the end of this module, may be used practicing controlled thrust maneuvers on another person. If one is alone, a modified Heimlich maneuver can be self-administered by placing oneself over a fixed edge, such as the back of a chair, and pressing the abdomen into

the edge with a firm quick movement (Fig. 20-13).

21 The Heimlich maneuver may also be self-administered by placing your own hands into the abdomen and performing a quick inward and upward thrusts, as though it were on someone else (Fig. 20-14).

22 Readers are encouraged to practice performing the Heimlich maneuver (gently) on themselves, using the chair and regular fist technique according to Procedure 20-14.

23 For greater details and proficiency, the reader is referred to CPR courses offered by the American Heart Association and American Red Cross.

5.4 Selecting the best technique for correcting airway obstruction

1 The techniques for removing airway obstructions extend from simple body positioning for partial obstructions to performing the Heimlich maneuver, or as extreme a measure as an emergency incision into the trachea. Always attempt to use the simplest, quickest, and most effective procedure available.

2 Unconscious or comatose patients who are placed in the supine position frequently experience airway obstruction caused by the base of the tongue dropping back into the airway.

3 In order to clear an obstruction caused by a flaccid tongue blocking the hypopharyngeal region, one would need to move the tongue forward by displacing the

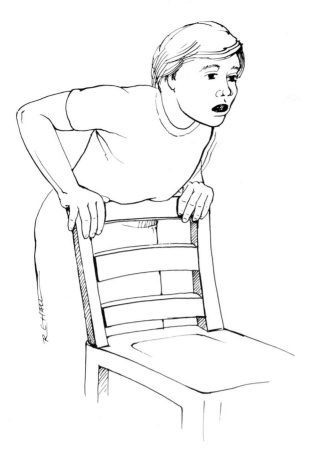

FIGURE 20-13 Self-administration of the Heimlich maneuver using the back of a chair.

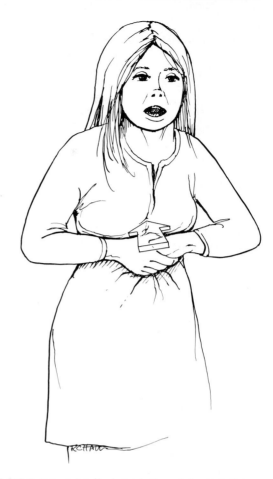

FIGURE 20-14 Self-administration of the Heimlich maneuver while standing. *Arrow* indicates direction of exerted pressure.

mandible forward. This can be accomplished by:

  a Hyperextending the neck by tilting the head backward, according to Procedure 20-5.

  b Using the chin-lift method, according to Procedure 20-6.

  c Using manual pressure at the angles of the jaws (jaw thrust), according to Procedure 20-7.

4 Once the obstruction has been cleared, the airway patency must be maintained to prevent the obstruction from recurring.

5 Techniques for maintaining an open airway in a patient in the supine position include elevating the patient's shoulders (especially with infants) and insertion of an artificial airway.

5.5 Use of artificial airways to prevent obstruction

1 An artificial airway is defined as a tube or tube-like device that is inserted through the nose, mouth, or into the trachea to provide an opening for ventilation.

2 The different types of artificial airways include:

  a Oropharyngeal airways (Fig. 20-15)

  b Nasopharyngeal tubes (Fig. 20-16)

  c Orotracheal tubes (Fig. 20-17)

  d Nasotracheal tubes (Fig. 20-18)

  e Esophageal obturator airways (Fig. 20-19)

  f Cricothyroid tubes (not shown)

  NOTE: The structure, the indications for, the hazards involved, and the techniques for insertion of individual tubes are discussed in the following units.

3 The indications for use of each of these devices will vary, depending on the patient's physical and physiologic condition, although general indications include:

  a Relieving airway obstruction

  b Maintaining an airway

  c Facilitating tracheobronchial clearance

  d Facilitating artificial ventilation

4 It is important to reemphasize the fact that the clinician should select the *simplest, quickest,* and most *effective* technique to relieve an airway obstruction.

5 The methods described thus far employ the use of *anatomic positioning* as a means of providing and maintaining an open airway in the unconscious patient.

6 Other methods incorporate the insertion of artificial airways through the mouth (oropharyngeal tube) or nose (nasopharyngeal airway) (Figs. 20-15 and 20-16).

7 Artificial airways are uncomfortable and can be traumatic to the patient. For this reason, they should be used only if simple anatomic positioning does not work or if someone is unavailable to constantly monitor the unconscious patient who may against experience airway difficulty.

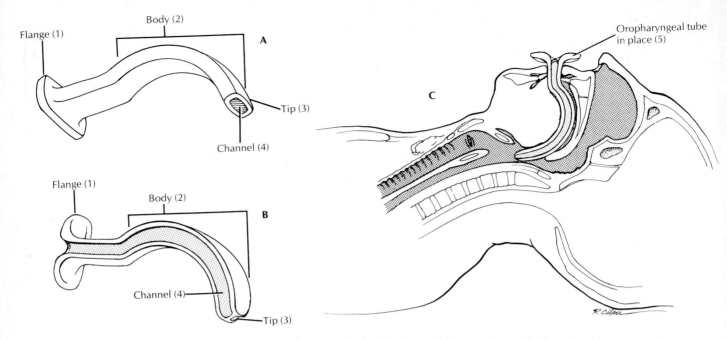

FIGURE 20-15 Oropharyngeal airways. **A,** Guedel airway. **B,** Berman airway. **C,** Airway in place.

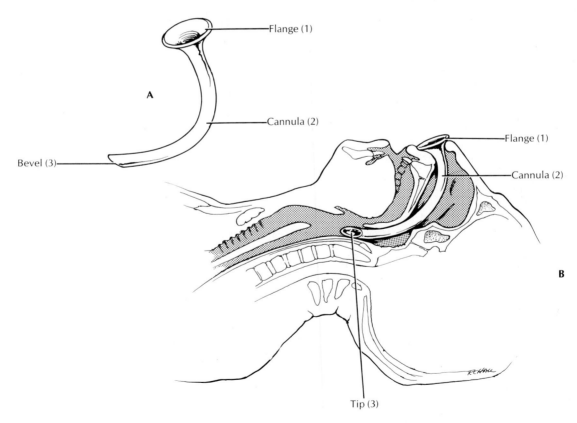

FIGURE 20-16 Nasopharyngeal airways. **A,** Parts of airway. **B,** Airway in place.

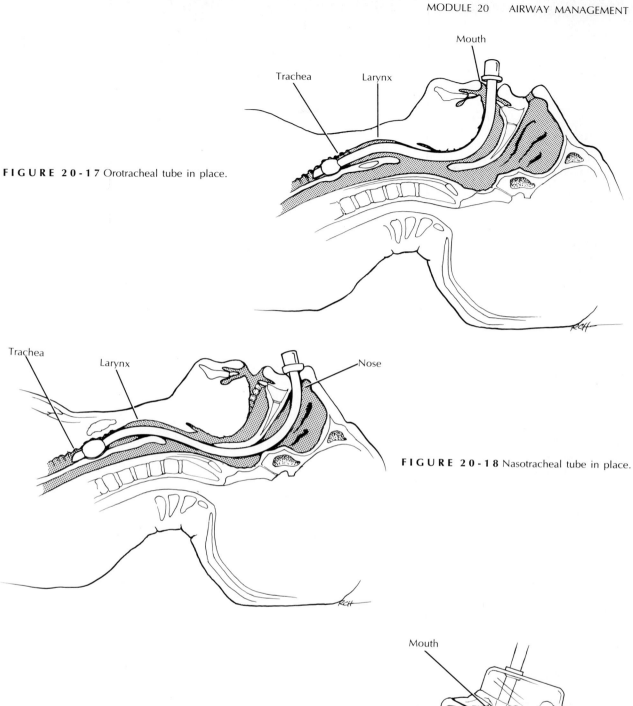

FIGURE 20-17 Orotracheal tube in place.

FIGURE 20-18 Nasotracheal tube in place.

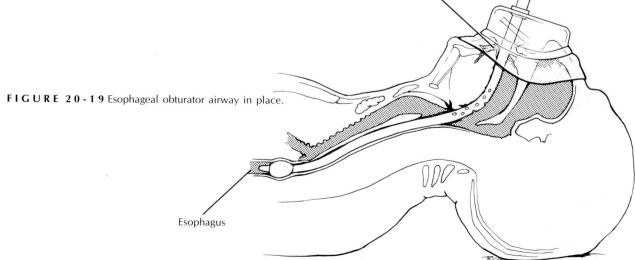

FIGURE 20-19 Esophageal obturator airway in place.

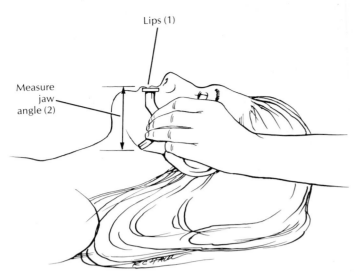

FIGURE 20-20 Determination of proper sized oropharyngeal airway.

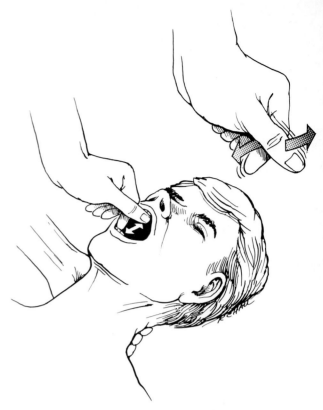

FIGURE 20-21 Opening patient's mouth using crossed-finger technique.

8 Oropharyngeal airways are usually made of plastic or rubber (Fig. 20-15). As their name implies, they are inserted through the open mouth, with the posterior tip resting in the patient's pharynx.

9 The oropharyngeal airway is placed over the tongue and shaped so that the curvature of the airway forces the patient's tongue forward, away from the posterior pharyngeal wall, the most common site of airway obstruction (see Fig. 20-15, C).

10 The parts and functions of the airway are (Fig. 20-15):
   a The flange (1) protrudes from the mouth and rests against the lips to prevent aspiration into the airway.
   b The body (2) determines the length of the airway over the tongue.
   c The tip (3) determines the depth of the airway tip toward the base of the tongue.
   d The channel (4) allows passage of a suction catheter through the center of the Guedel airway (A) or down the side channels in models such as the Berman oropharyngeal airway (B).

11 Oropharyngeal airways are available in different sizes: usually premature, infant, child, and small, medium, and large adult.

12 Care must be taken to select a proper size airway according to the patient's size. Insertion of an airway that is too small is not effective and can result in airway obstruction. One that is too large can cause impaction of the epiglottis by the tip of the airway.

5.6 Selecting an oropharyngeal airway

1 When selecting an oropharyngeal airway, one should measure the airway by placing it along side the patient's face (see Fig. 20-20).

2 The flange of the airway should be approximately at the patient's lips (1) and the tip of the airway should rest at the angle of the jaw (2).

3 The tip of the airway that is too large will extend beyond the angle of the jaw.

4 An airway that is too small will not reach the angle of the jaw.

5.7 Inserting the oropharyngeal airway

1 The oropharyngeal airway should *only* be placed in an *unconscious* patient. A conscious patient will resist the airway and may vomit as a result of stimulation of the *gag reflex*.

2 The steps for inserting an oropharyngeal airway are as follows:
   a Select a proper size airway.
   b After removing any foreign substances in the mouth, place the patient in a supine position.
   c Hyperextend the patient's neck; the mouth should fall open.
   d Open the victim's mouth using the *crossed-finger* technique (Fig. 20-21). This gives the clinician more leverage to open a tightly closed mouth.
      • The crossed-finger technique consists of crossing the thumb and index finger and putting them between the victim's lips in the corner of the mouth.
      • Next, cross the thumb under the index finger for the best leverage.
      • Brace the thumb and finger against the upper and lower teeth.
      • Push the thumb and index finger apart to separate the jaws.

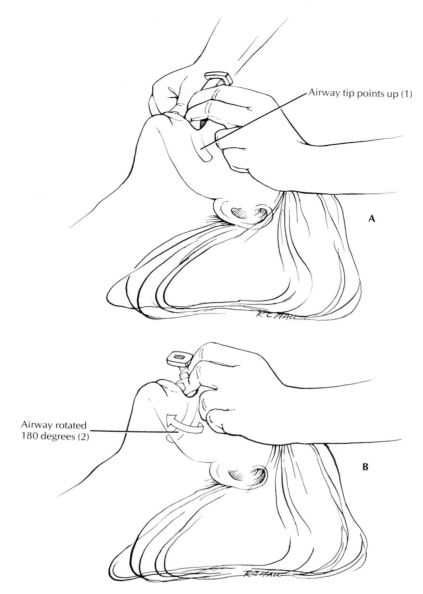

Airway tip points up (1)

A

Airway rotated
180 degrees (2)

B

F I G U R E 2 0 - 2 2 Inserting the oropharyngeal airway. **A,** Place airway in open mouth with tip facing up. **B,** Rotate airway 180 degrees.

NOTE: This technique involves great care to prevent injury to the fingers if the patient should be having seizures.

e Insert the airway over the base of the tongue (Fig. 20-22) with the tip up *(1),* toward the roof of the patient's mouth, until it passes the uvula.

f Rotate the tip 180 degrees, so that the tip is pointed down toward the pharynx and the airway is cleared *(2).*

g Recheck the size and position of the airway by noting whether or not the flange of the airway is resting against the patient's lips. If the airway flange is not resting against the lips, it is improperly placed or is the wrong size.

h Secure the airway in place with tape placed along the chin and cheek.

3 Procedure 20-8 may be used for opening the mouth of an unconscious patient.

4 Key points of inserting an oropharyngeal airway follow.

a The patient should be unconscious.

b The practitioner must select a proper size airway.

c The practitioner should use a proper insertion technique, making sure the tongue is not pushed into the airway as the artificial airway is placed.

5 Procedure 20-9 may be used for insertion of an oropharyngeal airway.

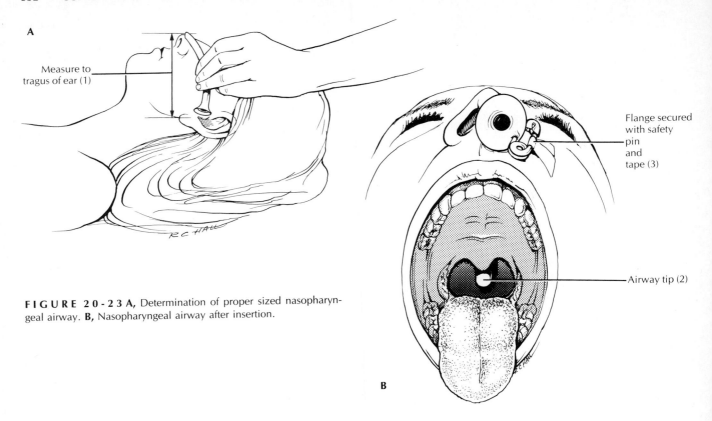

FIGURE 20-23 A, Determination of proper sized nasopharyngeal airway. **B,** Nasopharyngeal airway after insertion.

5.8 Hazards when using an oropharyngeal airway

1 The greatest potential hazard is that the airway is not effective in preventing airway obstruction.
2 The patient must *not* be allowed to gag or otherwise fight the airway.
3 The roof of the mouth can be lacerated as the airway is inserted.
4 The base of the tongue may be pushed into the oropharynx, actually blocking the air passage during insertion of the oropharyngeal airway.
5 The airway may be too large, causing impaction of the epiglottis into the larynx; or the airway may be too small; this is ineffective or may be aspirated into the airway.

6.0 THE NASOPHARYNGEAL AIRWAY
6.1 Inserting a nasopharyngeal airway

1 The nasopharyngal airway is a soft rubber catheter that is passed through the nose. The tip of the airway extends into the area separating the base of the tongue and the posterior wall of the pharynx (Fig. 20-16).
2 The nasopharyngeal airway serves the same function as the oropharyngeal airway, although unlike the oropharyngeal airway, it can be tolerated by the *conscious patient.*
3 It is especially useful for establishing an airway in patients suffering from soft tissue obstruction who have jaw injury or are experiencing spasm of the jaw muscles and trismus (lockjaw).

6.2 Parts of nasopharyngeal airway

1 The flange *(1)*. Helps prevent the tube from slipping into the airway.
2 Cannula *(2)*. Hollow shaft that admits air to the patient's lungs.
3 Bevel *(3)*. Opening at the distal end of the tube.

6.3 Inserting the nasopharyngeal airway

1 The technique for inserting a proper size airway is similar to that of the nasal catheter.
2 Select a proper size tube as measured by placing the tube from the tip of the patient's nose, with the distal end extended along the cheek (Fig. 20-23), *A* and *B*), to the tragus of the ear *(1)*.
3 Lubricate the airway with a water-soluble gel and insert it through the patient's most patent (open) nostril.
4 The tip of the inserted airway should be seen resting posterior to the base of the tongue *(2)*.
5 Secure the flange of the airway in place by inserting a safety pin through an exposed corner of the flange and taping it in place *(3)*.
6 Procedure 20-10 may be used for insertion of a nasopharyngeal airway.

7.0 TRACHEAL INTUBATION
7.1 Indications for endotracheal tubes

1 The airway devices discussed in the previous units may or may not be used strictly in emergency situations.
2 This is *not* the case when anticipating the passage of a

tube into a patient's trachea. This procedure, although relatively simple to perform, may become complicated by other factors; and for this reason, intubation should be considered only as an alternative to other less dramatic methods for establishing an airway. Endotracheal tubes are also used to correct for an obstruction that has already occurred and to serve as a secure and functional connection for mechanical ventilation (see Figs. 20-17 and 20-18).

3 Tracheal intubation, therefore, is most frequently used in conditions of, or leading to, respiratory failure, such as:

a Trauma to the airway or chest

b Neurologic involvement from drugs, myasthenia gravis, poisons, etc.

c Cardiovascular involvement leading to CNS impairment from strokes, tumors, trauma, infection, pulmonary emboli

d Pulmonary impairment from aspirants, infections, tumors, trauma, pneumonia, poisons, pneumothorax, chronic obstructive pulmonary disease, surgery, bronchiectasis

e Cardiopulmonary arrest

As with other airways, one must evaluate the patient's condition, circumstances, and available equipment before selecting a specific route for tracheal intubation. *Tracheal tube* is a generic term for endotracheal, which refers to *any tube* that is inserted into the trachea, regardless of its route of entry.

7.2 Routes for tracheal intubation

1 Tracheal intubation provides an immediate airway for the patient who is not physically able to provide or maintain his or her own airway. It provides a convenient and effective point for connecting a device to deliver artificial ventilation, allows a convenient route for suctioning the airway, and, if the tube is cuffed, prevents accidental aspiration of stomach contents or other foreign substances by the patient.

2 The trachea can be intubated using the four routes that follow.

a Mouth

b Nose

c Laryngeal opening

d Tracheal opening (tracheotomy)

3 The oral route is normally the easiest and most frequently used for tracheal intubation. Using a laryngoscope, one can easily visualize the glottis by inserting the laryngoscope blade into the mouth and visualizing the trachea by direct observation. NOTE: The oral route may not be the route of choice in patients who have trauma injuries to the mouth.

4 Specific steps involved in passing an orotracheal tube are presented in Procedure 20-13 at the end of this module.

5 Skill should be obtained in passing an orotracheal tube by practicing on a manikin or cadaver or by working with anesthesiologists in surgery.

6 The nasal route is more difficult to use for intubation than the oral route.

7 The nasal route requires that the tracheal tube be inserted into a nostril, passed through the nasal cavity, nasopharynx, oropharynx, and trachea.

8 This route requires the use of a longer and more flexible tracheal tube. It also requires that the tube be initially passed through the nose by touch. The tube cannot be seen until it has entered the oropharynx. At this point, the trachea can be visualized and tubed with the aid of a laryngoscope and with forceps.

9 In some instances of trauma, the entire procedure must be carried out without the aid of a laryngoscope (blind intubation).

10 Nasotracheal tubes are generally tolerated better by the conscious patient than orotracheal tubes. In some instances, the patient is even able to eat when the nasotracheal tube is used.

11 Specific steps for passing a nasotracheal tube using the blind technique and under direct vision are presented in Procedures 20-14 and 20-15.

12 Proficiency in passing a tube can be acquired by practicing on a manikin or cadaver or by arranging to work with the anesthesiologist in surgery.

7.3 Comparing the various routes of tracheal intubation

The decision to use one route of tracheal intubation compared with another is based on the following considerations.

1 Orotracheal and nasotracheal tubes should be removed as soon as their indication is over; tracheostomy should *not* be performed just because an arbitrary time interval has passed; complications of tracheostomy are greater than those of endotracheal intubation.

2 Oral intubation is usually the method of choice in emergencies that do not involve trauma to the mouth or mandible. Trauma may prevent proper anatomic positioning of the airway and complicate or prevent an intubation attempt.

3 A nasotracheal tube is generally tolerated better by the conscious patient who would otherwise fight an orotracheal tube.

4 A nasotracheal tube is more difficult to pass and may result in immediate or subsequent bleeding if the nasal mucosa is injured during the intubation process.

5 A *tracheotomy* is a surgical procedure that opens an incision (tracheostomy) through the anterior tracheal wall (Fig. 20-24, *A*). A tracheostomy tube is then placed through the incision and secured in place by ties that extend around the patient's neck (Fig. 20-24, *B* and *C*).

6 There have been reports of patients who have been intubated for periods of longer than 1 month without notable trauma to the airway. Orotracheal or nasotracheal intubations of this length of time are usually the result of the attending physician's wishing to avoid the risks of a surgical procedure and complications of a tracheostomy.

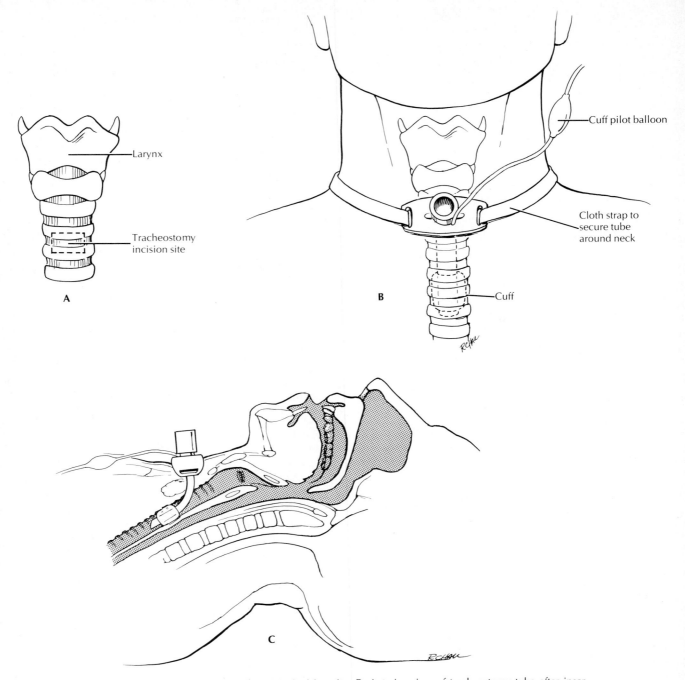

Larynx

Tracheostomy incision site

A

Cuff pilot balloon

Cloth strap to secure tube around neck

B

Cuff

C

FIGURE 20-24 A, Tracheotomy incision site. **B,** Anterior view of tracheostomy tube after insertion. **C,** Lateral view of tracheostomy tube after insertion.

7 A tracheotomy is performed for the same reason as those given for a nasal or oral intubation. In addition, a tracheotomy is indicated whenever the obstruction is above the level of the trachea and prevents the passage of an oral or nasal tube.

8 A tracheotomy, because it bypasses the anatomic structures of the upper airway, is said to reduce anatomic deadspace and the work of breathing of an adult patient in respiratory failure. However, it should be noted that in newborns, bypassing the glottis with a tracheotomy or an endotracheal tube causes the arterial oxygen tension (Pao_2) to *drop*. This finding is attributed to the elevated functional residual capacity (FRC) level in the newborn that was caused by the airway obstruction itself.

9 A *cricothyroidotomy*, as mentioned previously, is an *emergency* procedure that requires that an opening be made through the circothyroid membrane (Fig. 20-25). This procedure should be performed only in a life-or-death situation in which time is of the essence. The technique can be performed using any sharp object, provided a large enough opening is made into the tra-

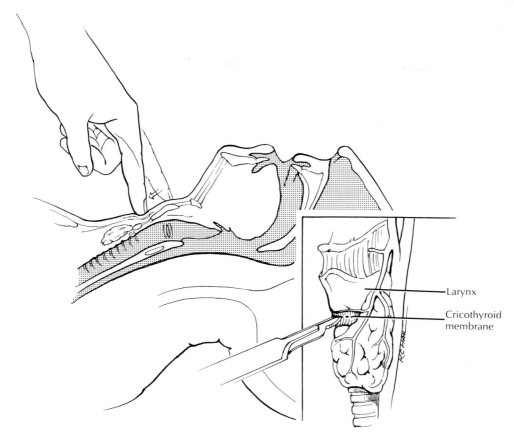

FIGURE 20-25 Cricothyroidotomy.

chea to allow the patient to maintain adequate ventilation. It is doubtful that a 14- to 16-gauge needle will serve this purpose in the adult patient, although this technique is recommended in some texts.

10 It is stressed that a cricothyroidotomy should not be performed by respiratory care personnel except in a life-or-death situation requiring an immediate airway opening.

7.4 Parts of an endotracheal tube

Refer to Fig. 20-26, *A,* for the following explanations.

1 The proximal end *(1)* protrudes from the mouth or nose and has a standard 15-mm male adapter inserted into the end of various attachments.

2 The curve of the tube *(2)* determines the angle of the tube once it is in place in the trachea.

3 The bevel *(3)* is the opening at the distal end of the tube. A tube may have a right- or left-facing bevel. Adult endotracheal tubes have another hole adjacent to the one at the tip *(3A)*. This extra hole ensures airflow in left and right directions at the carina and also provides a "back-up" opening for airflow, should the distal hole become clogged with secretions.

4 The angle of the bevel *(4)* is usually 45 degrees. In large tubes it may be 30 degrees.

5 The cuff *(5)* is an inflatable "balloon" that presses against the tracheal walls to prevent air leakage and pressure loss from the lung and the aspiration of secretions into the lung.

6 The cuff is left "flat" or deflated until after the tube is inserted into the trachea. The cuff is then inflated via a filling tube *(6),* which is attached to the endotracheal tube.

7 A pilot balloon *(7)* indicates whether or not the cuff contains air. NOTE: Contrary to popular belief, it is almost *impossible* with today's low-pressure cuffs to determine "how much" pressure is actually in the cuff. A properly fitted endotracheal tube with a properly inflated cuff (see Unit 7.6) will reveal very little "pressure" in the pilot balloon. The pilot balloon should serve only as an indication of whether the cuff is "up" or "down" or if cuff leaks are occurring.

8 Some brands have specially designed pilot balloons that vent excess pressure from the cuff or prevent excess amounts of air from being injected into the cuff.

9 The one-way valve *(8)* is used on most brands to accept a syringe tip to allow air to be injected into the cuff and then seal against leaks when the syringe is removed.

NOTE: Some brands to not have valves, and other means of "clamping" the filling tube must be used. Hemostats, unless fitted with plastic or rubber cushions,

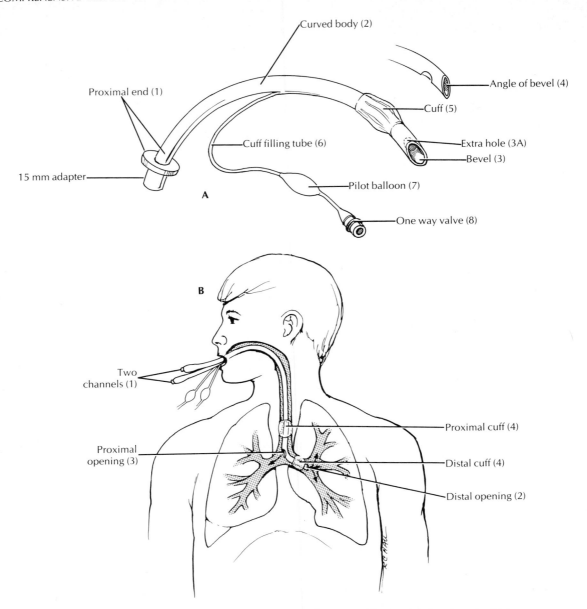

FIGURE 20-26 A, Parts of an endotracheal tube. **B,** Double-channeled endotracheal tube.

when clamped on the filling tube, will eventually cut into the tube and should not be used routinely.

10 Cuffs may be used on orotracheal, nasotracheal, and tracheostomy tubes.

11 When inflating a cuff, the following physiologic effects of applying pressure to the tracheal wall must be considered.

  a The blood vessels of the tracheal wall will *occlude* as pressure is applied to the cuff.

  b The intra-arterial vessels occlude at 30 to 35 mm Hg pressure; the venous vessels occlude at 18 to 20 mm Hg; and the lymphatic channels occlude at 5 to 8 mm Hg.

  c When these vessels are occluded, perfusion to the compressed area is diminished or ceases and damage to the tissue (necrosis) begins. Care must be taken to

keep inflating pressures less than 25 mm Hg.

12 A special double-cuffed tube (not shown) is available for use in patients suspected of having tracheal tissue trauma. This tube has two cuffs, one above the other, that can be alternately inflated. This varies the pressure site and minimizes trauma from pressure necrosis.

13 Another special type of tracheal tube (Fig. 20-26, *B*), originally described by Carlens, has *two* channels for ventilation, with independent connections to each *(1)*. One channel opens at the distal end of the tube *(2)*, and the other opens along the side of the tube proximal to the more distal opening in the other channel *(3)*. Two cuffs *(4)* are located so that the right and left lung can be preferentially ventilated, depending on which channel is used.

    For example, if the right-hand channel is attached to

the ventilator with the cuff inflated, only the right main stem bronchus will be ventilated. The left-hand channel is open and can be attached to another ventilator, resulting in ventilation of both lungs using two separate units. This type of tube is also used when pulmonary lavage is performed (one lung is flooded while the other is being ventilated).

14 A similar double-lumen tube is used for *high-frequency jet ventilation*. This tube also has two channels, one for inspiration and one for exhalation. The inspiratory channel is smaller than the expiratory channel so that expiratory resistance is minimized, thereby reducing or eliminating gas trapping that normally occurs with this type of ventilation.

15 The esophageal obturator airway is another special type of airway that will be discussed in Unit 10.1.

7.5 Types of tracheal tube cuffs

1 Research has shown that the most desirable cuff will provide a maximum airway seal with minimum tracheal wall pressure. The *optimum cuff* should have a sealing pressure of less than 15 mm Hg.

2 Functionally, most cuffs will seal at less than 25 mm Hg and will have an overall *inflated resting volume* of 2.5 cm (this means that 2.5 cm of cuff surface area is resting against the tracheal wall).

3 Three types of cuffs are currently being used on tracheal tubes and are classified according to the amount of air pressure it takes to cause them to seal the tracheal wall (Fig. 20-27).

4 The *low-volume–high-pressure cuff (A)* is an old design type. The small size of the cuff (and therefore limited contact with the tracheal wall) requires that as much as 40 mm Hg air pressure be injected before an effective seal is made. For the most part, this type of cuff is not desirable.

5 The *high-volume–low-pressure cuff (B)* has replaced the high-pressure style cuff mentioned in no. *4*. This new type of cuff has a relatively large inflation volume that requires less filling pressure to obtain a seal (less than 25 mm Hg). Note the shape of the cuff. The cylindric shape offers more surface area to contact the tracheal wall and allows the pressure to be distributed over a large area. CAUTION: This "advantage" can become a greater disadvantage when excess pressures are used; the greater surface area causes damage over a larger portion of the tracheal wall.

6 The third type of cuff uses no air injection at all. The *Kamen-Wilkinson cuff (C)* consists of air-filled foam cells and is "inflated" in its relaxed state. To insert the tube, one evacuates the air with a syringe *(1)*, causing the cuff to deflate *(2)*, and inserts the pilot port stopper *(3)* to prevent the reentry of air. After insertion, the pilot port is opened *(4)*, and air will reenter the cuff to expand it *(5)*. This cuff maintains very low pressures because the inflation is more than atmospheric pressure.

NOTE: It is very important to choose the proper size

tube, because air should *not* be injected into the cuff to "force" a seal against the tracheal wall.

7 Another type of cuff is a variation of the high-volume–low-pressure cuff. It is called a "floppy" cuff. The cuff material fits very loosely around the tube, thus allowing greater volume and a greater surface pressure for contact with the tracheal wall.

8 A historical note should be made at this point. At one time when tracheal tubes were made of metal or of rigid, reusable rubber, they were used over and over again and the cuffs were removable. This is because the cuffs always failed before the tubes did and it made replacement easier. A detailed description of "slide-on" cuffs will not be made in this text, except to say that they also "slid-off" and that they frequently did so while they were in use. Obviously, they should not be used unless other permanent fixed cuffs are not available.

7.6 Inflating the tracheal cuff

1 The most important consideration when inflating the cuff of a tracheal tube is to provide a *maximum* seal with *minimum* pressure.

2 Cuff inflation pressures can be determined by using the *minimal occlusion volume* (MOV) technique, the *minimal leak volume* technique (MLV), or by *actual measurement* of the intracuff pressure using a pressure manometer.

3 MOV is based on the theory that a patient *cannot* make vocal sounds when a cuff is sealed, preventing air from passing across the vocal cords. It also is based on the concept that positive pressure cannot escape from the airway if the cuff is sealed.

4 MOV means that a cuff is slowly inflated only until vocal sounds cease or air is not heard rushing past the cuff during a positive pressure inflation (delivered by a ventilator or a manual resuscitator bag).

5 Procedure 20-11 may be used for inflating cuffs using MOV.

6 Inflating a cuff using the MLV technique requires that the cuff be inflated to the point of complete occlusion and then deflated until a very *small* leak is heard escaping around the tube. This leak can be determined by listening for vocal sounds, auscultating the larynx, or noting a decrease in the delivered volume of a ventilator. NOTE: Care must be taken when using this technique *not* to create a leak that will allow aspiration of foreign substances or reduce the delivery of a required tidal volume from a mechanical device. Do *not* perform this procedure on a patient unless you have been trained.

7 Procedure 20-12 may be used for inflating cuffs using the MLV technique.

8 Inflating a cuff using a pressure monitor is an easy technique that requires the use of a pressure monitoring device connected in line with the cuff.

9 A pressure monitor (Fig. 20-28) may be purchased from several sources, or one can be made according to the procedure in Fig. 20-29.

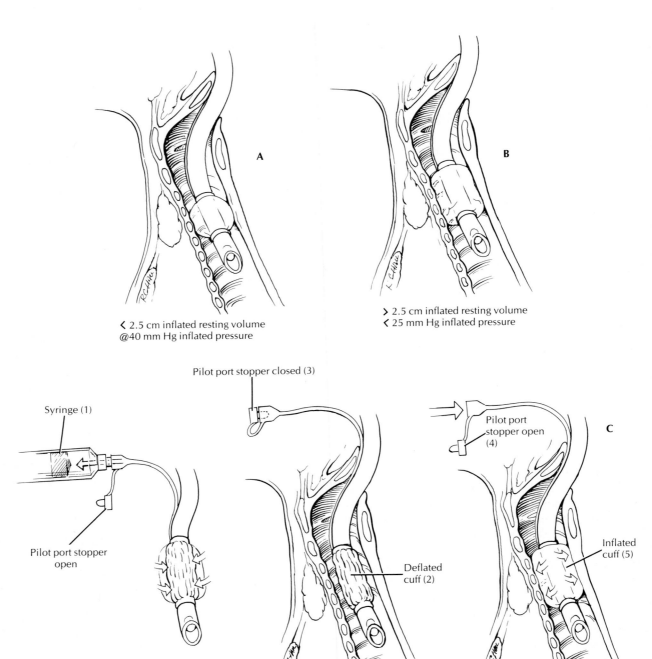

A

⟨ 2.5 cm inflated resting volume
@40 mm Hg inflated pressure

B

⟩ 2.5 cm inflated resting volume
⟨ 25 mm Hg inflated pressure

Pilot port stopper closed (3)

Syringe (1)

Pilot port stopper
open

Deflated
cuff (2)

Pilot port
stopper open
(4)

C

Inflated
cuff (5)

FIGURE 20-27 A, Low-volume–high-pressure cuff. **B,** High-volume–low-pressure cuff.
C, Kamen-Wilkinson cuff.

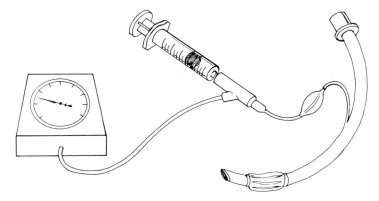

F I G U R E 2 0 - 2 8 Measuring cuff pressure by way of in-line pressure monitor.

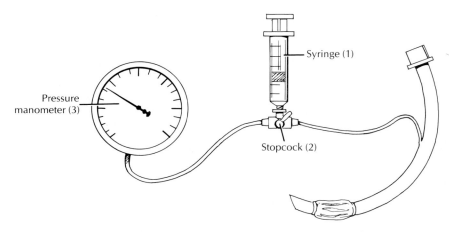

F I G U R E 2 0 - 2 9 Measuring cuff pressure by way of homemade pressure monitor.

10 In Fig. 20-29, air in 1 milliliter (ml) increments is injected into the cuff by the syringe *(1)*.

11 After each 1-ml injection, the stopcock *(2)* is reversed and the pressure is measured on the manometer *(3)*. The manometer from any pressure or volume ventilator can be used.

12 Using the MOV technique with the manometer will help assure the practitioner that minimal occlusion pressure is used and that this pressure does *not* exceed 25 mm Hg.

13 The cuff pressure should be monitored routinely because of changes in cuff volume, resulting from small leaks and pressure expansion according to Charles' and Boyles' laws. NOTE: This is especially significant if the patient is moved from one altitude to another without environmental pressurization.

7.7 Hazards of tracheal tubes and cuffs

1 Specific hazards from tracheal tubes include infection, dehydration, obstruction, trauma, tissue stenosis and necrosis of the trachea.

2 The danger from infection is *always* a potential problem. It is caused by insertion of a contaminated tube into the trachea or improper care once the tube is placed.

3 Dehydration of the airways occurs because any artificial airway bypasses the natural anatomic route for air to be warmed and humidified.

4 Obstructions can occur from mucous plugs developing in the airway and becoming lodged in the tube. This type of hazard occurs indirectly as a result of poor humidification and poor tube care. Obstructions at the distal end of the tube can also occur as a result of encrustation resulting from the tube having been left in place too long.

5 During the intubation process, teeth may be dislodged and membranes traumatized. It is possible for the laryngoscope blade to perforate the tissue of the mouth, esophagus, or larynx. The tracheal tube itself, with improper handling, can cause severe damage to the larynx and vocal cords. Other assorted hazards of intubation include:

a Accidental intubation of the esophagus or right main stem bronchus

b Bronchospasm, laryngospasm

c Cardiac arrhythmias resulting from stimulation of the vagus nerve

d Aspiration pneumonia resulting from vomiting during the intubation process

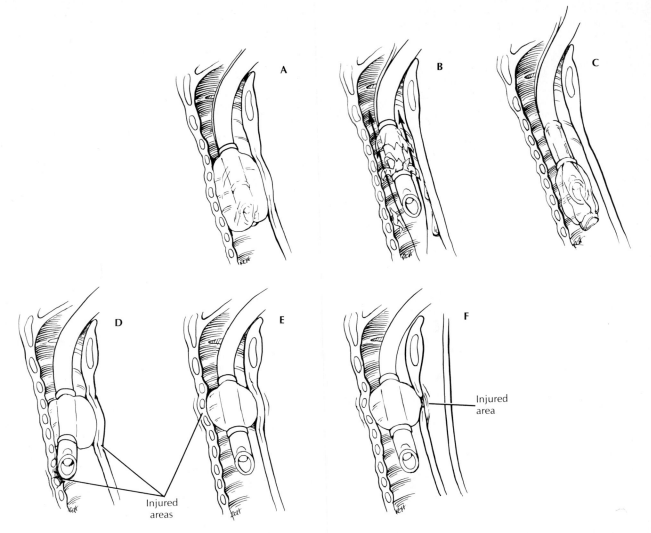

FIGURE 20-30 Hazards of tracheal tube cuffs. **A,** Cuff overinflation and distension over tube end. **B,** Cuff rupture. **C,** Cuff slippage. **D,** Uneven inflation. **E,** Cuff overinflation causing tracheal stenosis and necrosis. **F,** Tracheoesophageal fistula.

e Later complications, which may include:
  • Paralysis of the tongue
  • Broken or loosened teeth
  • Ulceration of the mouth
  • Respiratory tract infection
  • Paralysis of the vocal cords
  • Tracheal stenosis

6 Fortunately, tracheal stenosis and necrosis are seen much less frequently today as a result of better care and better materials. However, whenever ischemia occurs in the tracheal wall as a result of cuff pressure, the possibility for necrosis exists. Once necrosis occurs, there is very little that can be done for the patient except extensive and complicated reconstructive surgery to the trachea (segmental resection and anastomosis). Another cause of stenosis and necrosis is erosion of the tracheal wall by the tip of the tube.

7 Not a direct danger from tubes, but one that needs consideration, is the *psychologic* problem that exists with intubated patients. Patients cannot talk and cannot usually swallow, even though they may be perfectly alert. Alternative means of communication ("magic slates," "talking boards," and writing materials) will offset this problem to some extent. Great patience and care are called for when dealing with the intubated patient.

8 Other isolated tube problems result from movement by the patient. They include:

  a Traumatic or accidental extubation. Extubation with the cuff inflated occurs as a patient is being moved about on the bed by poorly trained hospital personnel or as a direct result of the patient pulling the tube out with his or her own hand.

  b Right main stem intubation may occur due to tube slippage as a result of improper securing of the tube's proximal end.

  c Pressure necrosis and erosion from the tube and tissue contact points.

9 Some of the additional hazards, although rare (Fig. 20-

30), that can result from problems with the cuff are:

a Cuff overinflation and distension over the end of the tube *(A)*

b Cuff rupture, which allows foreign matter to enter the lungs and positive pressure to escape *(B)*

c Cuff slippage over the end of the tube *(C)* (very rare with today's tubes)

d Uneven cuff inflation, which causes the tip of the tube to erode the tracheal wall *(D)*

e Cuff overinflation, which causes tracheal stenosis and necrosis *(E)* and possibly a tracheoesophageal fistula *(F)*

7.8 Monitoring a patient with tracheal intubation

1 The clinical signs of tracheal tube complications may be as minor as a sore throat and croup or as traumatic as a complete airway obstruction.

2 Tube complications can be prevented by alert personnel who recognize the fact that a sore throat, bleeding, inspiratory stridor, or tracheal malacia can occur during or following tracheal intubation.

3 Routine checks must be conducted to evaluate whether or not the tube is in its proper position, with the distal tip just above the carina. This can be assessed by auscultating the chest for bilateral breath sounds, proper care to the proximal end of the tube, and by chest x-ray examination.

4 More details on tube positioning and care will follow in the next unit.

7.9 Preventing tracheal damage

1 Tracheal tubes, directly or indirectly, cause trauma of varying degrees to the airway. The extent of the trauma depends on the:

a Intubation technique

b Size of the tube

c Composition of the tube

d Location of the tube

e Length of intubation

f Type of cuff

g Pressure in tube cuff

h Tracheal tube care

i Activity of the patient

2 Postextubation complications will vary from patient to patient, and the extent of the symptoms will depend on the extent of the trauma. In addition to sore throat and croup, which are common, postextubation problems may include:

a Granuloma

b Vocal cord paralysis

c Mucosal damage

d Laryngeal and/or tracheal stenosis

3 Good tube care technique includes acute awareness of the following items.

a Measure cuff pressure. Keep cuff pressure below 24 mmHg.

b Maintain aseptic conditions. Dressings around tra-

cheostomy sites should be changed frequently (every 4-6 hours).

c Provide good oral hygiene. Clean the patient's mouth with a standard mouthwash or use lemon-glycerin swabs. Clean well around the tube if it is an oral one. Apply lotion to the lips to prevent cracking and splitting. Keep the mouth suctioned.

d Clean the tube. If the tube is disposable, keep the tube, as well as the patient, suctioned as necessary. If the tube is a metal type, remove and clean the inner cannula (if available) at least every 8 hours and as needed to prevent plugging.

e Provide proper humidification. Since a tracheal tube bypasses normal warming and humidification, these must be provided. Approximately 75% of all body humidity is normally added by the time inspired air has reached the main bronchi. Therefore air reaching the lungs through a tracheal tube will cause dehydration and resultant reduction of ciliary activity, secretion movement, and increased mucus production, unless additional humidity is provided.

f Provide effective airway clearance. Use the patient's cough mechanism whenever possible. If the patient is not responsive or is unable to generate an effective cough, suctioning may be required. Suctioning technique is covered later in the module.

g It was once considered necessary to routinely deflate cuffs every 2 hours or so to "re-establish circulation." This should *not* be done with modern low-pressure cuffs. Cuff pressures less than 25 mm Hg should not seriously hamper circulation. Routine deflation encourages aspiration, cuff overinflation, filling valve damage, and possible lethal disruptions to mechanical ventilation.

The boxed material contains a checklist for preventing tracheal damage.

8.0 ENDOTRACHEAL AND TRACHEOSTOMY TUBES
8.1 Composition of tracheal tubes

1 Tracheal tubes are constructed of metal, natural rubber, polyvinyl chloride (PVC), and silastic materials (silicone rubber, nylon, and Teflon).

2 The key to selecting a tracheal tube is to pick a tube that will cause the least tissue reaction, yet still maintain its shape and lumen as it warms to body temperatures.

Preventing tracheal damage—patient rounds checklist

_____	1	Measure cuff pressure (<25 mm Hg)
_____	2	Maintain aseptic conditions around tube
_____	3	Provide good oral hygiene
_____	4	Clean the tube and inner cannula
_____	5	Provide proper warmed humidification
_____	6	Provide effective airway clearance
_____	7	Check tube restraints (ties)

3 Red rubber tubes kink easily and will become stiff with repeated use.

4 Plastic and synthetic tubes are usually more flexible and retain their shapes with repeated use.

5 Caution must be used to ensure that all tubes are marked "I.T./Z-79," which means they have been *implant-tested* for use in human tissue and conform to standards by the *International Z-79 Committee* for anesthesia tubes.

6 It should be noted that a tracheal tube must mold itself to the shape of the trachea, which is different from that of tracheostomy tubes. The amount of force required to shape a newly inserted tube varies and depends on the shape and material of the tube. Generally, red rubber tubes require more force than vinyl tubes.

8.2 Selecting a correct size tracheal tube

1 It is *critical* that a proper size tube be selected for intubation.

2 In order to select the proper size tube, one must match the length and outside diameter of the tube to the size of the patient.

3 The length of the tube must be sufficient to allow the end of the tube to reach the mid-tracheal area and to allow the proximal end to protrude far enough to be firmly secured and attached to ventilating or humidification devices. The tube moves as much as 2 cm up and down with extension and flexion of the head.

NOTE: A nasotracheal tube must be longer than an orotracheal tube. Most tracheal tubes are marketed in the nasal length and are shortened when used as an oral tube. Some hospitals and anesthesia departments keep a ready supply of precut tubes for oral intubation, but this is *not* recommended, since opening the packages to cut the tube contaminates their sterility.

4 The tube's outside diameter (OD) is critical because it determines the size of the inside diameter (ID). Remembering *Poiseuille's law,* resistance of gas flow through a tube varies inversely with the fourth power of the inside diameter of the tube. If one reduces the inside diameter of the tube by one half, the resulting airflow resistance will be 16 times greater. This situation may not be critical as long as the patient is on a mechanical ventilator and it is doing the work of breathing for the patient, except for the fact that the patient must *exhale* against this higher resistance under his or her own power. This situation is critical when the patient is on *intermittent mandatory ventilation (IMV)* or is on a T piece aerosol. In these cases, the patient must do most, if not all, of the work of breathing, and increased or abnormal resistance can actually cause respiratory failure.

5 One "rule of thumb" is to select a tube that has an outside diameter that matches the size of the adult patient's little finger.

6 There is also a "sex and age" quick-reference system that is discussed later in the unit.

7 The most exact method is to select *three* sizes, based

TABLE 20-1 Endotracheal tube size equivalents

Diameter sizing		Magill*	French*
Internal (mm)	External (mm)*		
2.5	4.0		12
3.0	4.5	00	12-14
3.5	5.0		14-16
4.0	5.5	0-1	16-18
4.5	6.0	1-2	18-20
5.0	6.5		20-22
5.5	7.0	3-4	22
6.0	8.0		24
6.5	8.5	4-5	26
7.0	9.0	5-6	28
7.5	9.5	6-7	30
8.0	10.0	7-8	32
8.5	11.5	8	34
9.0	12.0	9-10	36
9.5	12.5		38
10.0	13.0	10-11	40
10.5	13.5		42
11.0	14.5	11-12	42-44
11.5	15.0		44-46

*Since tube thicknesses vary from one style to another, the above is intended to serve as a guide only.

TABLE 20-2 Pediatric to adult endotracheal tube sizes

Age	Tube size (mm)	Suction catheter (French)
Premature	2.5	6
Newborn	3.0	6
6 mo	3.5	8
18 mo	4.0	8
3 yr	4.5	8
5 yr	5.0	10
6 yr	5.5	10
8 yr	6.0	10
12 yr	6.5	10
16 yr and small adult females	7.0	14
Adult females (average)	8.0	14
Adult males	9.0	14

on the patient's size, age, and sex, that can be determined by a chart. By choosing a tube size directly above and below the one that is "supposed" to fit, one can rule out wasting time at the time of intubation.

8 There are three tube size classifications:
  a Magill—obsolete, for the most part
  b French—becoming obsolete, but still used
  c Metric—found on almost all modern tubes

9 The French scale is based on the *circumference* of the tube. To convert from metric to French, multiply the metric outside diameter of the tube by 3.14 (or 3). A 6 mm tube is equal to an 18 French.

10 Tubes in the French system have mostly even numbers, which range from a size 12 for a newborn to a size 46 for a large adult.

NOTE: Suction catheters, as well as other medical tubing (urinary catheters, drains, chest tubes, etc.), are still sized according to the French system.

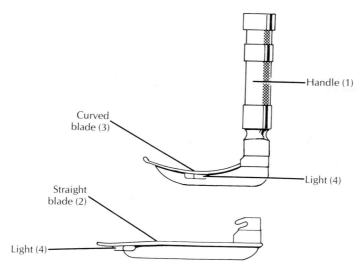

FIGURE 20-31 Laryngoscope showing straight and curved blades.

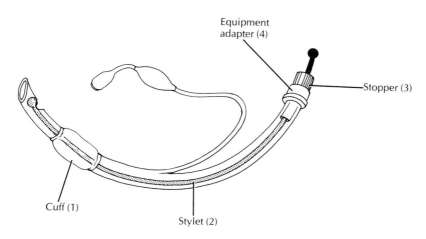

FIGURE 20-32 Tracheal tube.

11 Tubes in the metric system are listed by their *internal diameter* and range from 2.5 mm for newborns to 11.5 mm for large adults (see Table 20-1).

12 Table 20-2 gives an approximate "sex and age" reference to endotracheal tubes and gives corresponding suction catheter sizes.

13 Tracheostomy tubes are sized according to a somewhat different system (see Unit 8.8).

14 One *irresponsible* action a practitioner can take during intubation is to purposely choose a smaller size tube because "it is easier to get in."

8.3 Tracheal intubation equipment

Tracheal intubation can be a life-saving procedure in those patients who need an artificial airway as a result of anatomic obstruction in order to ventilate artificially and to protect the lungs from aspiration. Intubation should *not* be attempted unless one has the proper equipment and skill. Intubation should be performed quickly and nontraumatically, but should *not* be considered an *emergency* proce-

dure. That is to say, the practitioner should have all materials at hand and should proceed with deliberate technique to avoid trauma and unnecessary reintubation. The following items are required for passing an endotracheal tube and can be used as a checklist.

1 Laryngoscope (Fig. 20-31). This device is comprised of a handle *(1)* and blade *(2 and 3)* and is used to visualize the larynx and help guide the tube into position. Blades may be straight or curved. The different shaped blades displace the epiglottis in a different manner, but both allow direct observation of the larynx and vocal cords. A built-in light source *(4)* aids in the process.

2 Tracheal tube. Assorted cuffed tubes (Fig. 20-32) should be available, including one that has been sized for the patient. It may be made of various materials, but is usually a plastic or vinyl. The cuff *(1)* should be left deflated during insertion. The tube should be long enough, once secured, to rest slightly above the carina.

3 Stylet. A metal or vinyl-coated metal rod (Fig. 20-32, *2*) that is inserted into the tube to give it rigidity and to

adjust the angle of insertion if necessary. The stopper in the end *(3)* maintains its insertion length. The distal end of the stylet should never be allowed to protrude beyond the end of the tube. The stylet must be removed from the tube as soon as the tube is passed through the cords and before cuff inflation.

4 Water-soluble lubricant (K-Y jelly). This is used to lubricate the tube before insertion. It should always be sterile.

5 Adhesive tape. This is used to secure the proximal end of the tube once it is in place.

6 Bite block. This is used to prevent the patient from biting down on the endotracheal tube and damaging it or possibly occluding the airway. Many devices can be used as bite blocks, including:
   a Oropharyngeal airways
   b Tongue depressors, wrapped on the end with adhesive tape to form a "bite pad" or cushion
   c Commercially available plastic or rubber "blocks"; some simply keep the teeth apart and resemble rubber wedges

7 Suction equipment. Various suctioning equipment is necessary, including:
   a Assorted sizes of catheters
   b A metal (Yankauer) mouth suction tip
   c Suction device or vacuum pump, if wall suction is not available
   d Connecting hose to connect suction to catheters
   e Sterile gloves

8 Tracheal tube equipment adapters (15 mm), if not included with the tracheal tube (see Fig. 20-32, *4*).

9 Assorted oropharyngeal airways.

10 Manual resuscitator bag with mask. This is used to ventilate the patient before (and during, if necessary) the intubation attempt.
   NOTE: Manual resuscitator bags will be covered in detail in Module Twenty-three.

11 A syringe with a two-way stopcock. This is used to inflate the cuff once the tube is in place.

12 Oxygen. This is given to the patient via the resuscitator bag before, during, and after intubation.

13 Other materials, which are not absolutely necessary, include:
   a Tongue depressors.
   b Magill forceps. These are used to aid in nasal intubation.
   c Hemostat. The hemostat is used to clamp the filling tube if a one-way valve does not come with the tracheal tube.
   NOTE: Always cover the blades of the hemostat with catheter or other material to prevent cutting the filling tube once the hemostasis clamped in place.
   d Atomizer. This is used to spray a local anesthetic into the patient's pharynx.

8.4 Using the laryngoscope

1 The *laryngoscope* is one of the most valuable instruments used for the intubation process.

2 It is composed of two major parts—a blade and a handle.

3 The blades come in different sizes, ranging from sizes for infants to sizes for adults. The blades are also available in different shapes, ranging from straight blades (Miller blades) to variations of curved blades, such as the MacIntosh (see Fig. 20-31).

4 The *MacIntosh* blade (Fig. 20-33) is a popular blade because it offers a gentle curved surface on which to lift the tongue. It also has a spatula *(5)* and flange *(1)* that pushes the tongue to one side as the blade is inserted, allowing easier visualization of the larynx and vocal cords.

5 Blades are attached to the handles through the use of a hook and snap mechanism *(2)*. This system allows the user to quickly snap the blade into place by inserting the grooved base of the blade over the bar of the laryngoscope handle and lifting *(3)* up on the shaft of the blade to snap the base of the blade into place. Once the blade is connected, the lamp in the tip of the blade should light automatically *(4)*.

6 The blade has the following parts (Fig. 20-33).
   a The spatula *(5)*. The main shaft that manipulates the soft tissue of the lower jaw so that the epiglottis and larynx can be visualized.
   b The flange *(1)*. Projects from the leading edge of the spatula and serves to displace the tongue to one side of the mouth.
   c The tip *(6)*. Fits under the epiglottis and is used to elevate the epiglottis so that the glottis and larynx can be seen.

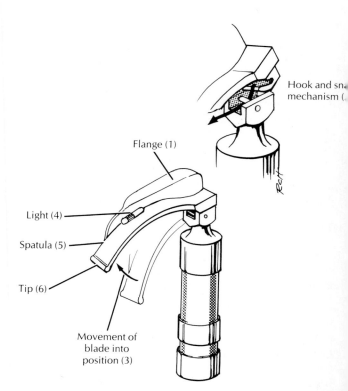

FIGURE 20-33 Parts of laryngoscope. MacIntosh blade.

d The lamp *(4).* Screws into the flange of the blade and provides illumination for the intubation procedure.

e The base. Contains the contact *(2)* that allows current to flow from the handle to the lamp and secures the blade to the handle.

7 The handle contains the batteries for powering the lamp located in the blade flange. An electrical connection is made between the blade and handle when it is snapped into place *(3).* The laryngoscope should be tested for operation before packaging and immediately before inserting the tube.

8 Each blade, curved or straight, has its own technique for displacing the epiglottis. See Fig. 20-34 *(A* and *B)*

and note the location of each laryngoscope blade tip relative to the epiglottis.

8.5 Intubating the trachea

1 The indications for tracheal intubation have been discussed previously.

2 Also discussed previously was the fact that endotracheal tubes can be used in lieu of tracheostomy tubes for periods of from 1 to 5 days with no notable damage to the trachea at the cuff or tube contact points.

3 It must be remembered that the intubation process must be quick and nontraumatic, because a patient's ventilation is compromised during this time interval.

4 For this reason, a patient should be *well ventilated* and

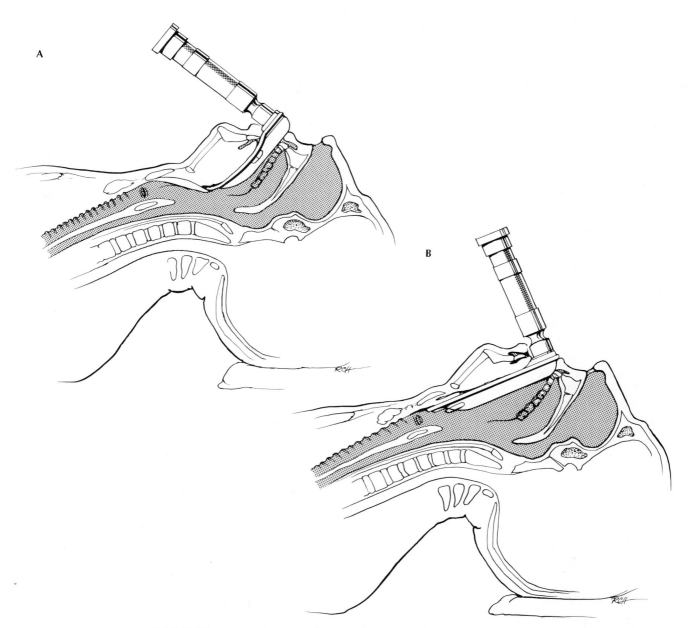

F I G U R E   2 0 - 3 4 Placement of **A,** curved vs. **B,** straight laryngoscope blade.

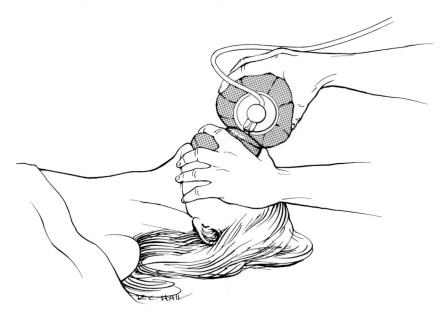

FIGURE 20-35 Ventilation using bag and mask.

oxygenated using a bag and mask or other methods before beginning the intubation process, and then reventilated, using oxygen, at least *every 15 to 20 seconds* if intubation is not successful with the first attempt.

5 In addition to time considerations, the mouth and upper airway must be cleared of vomitus and other substances that could be aspirated, before ventilation is begun.

6 Once the airway has been cleared and ventilation is maintained using a bag and mask, the intubation process can proceed.

7 Hospitals have varying procedures for intubating patients that must be followed. The following steps are general and can be used in lieu of a formal hospital procedure. A checklist featuring an outline of the steps is presented in the box.

  a Assemble and check equipment for ready operation (batteries, bulbs, correct tube sizes, etc.)

  b Clean the mouth and airways of secretions, vomitus, blood, etc., using the Yankauer tip and/or large bore suction catheters.

  c Place the patient on his or her back with the head straight and facing up.

  d Ventilate the patient with bag, mask, and airway with 100% oxygen (Fig. 20-35).

  e Select the proper size tube for age, size, and sex. Test the cuff for uniform inflation.

  f Insert the stylet into the tube and tighten plug in the proximal end of the tube so that the end of the stylet is no closer than ½ inch from the distal end of the tube (see Fig. 20-32). Shape the tube as necessary to allow for smooth passage through the cords.

  g Lubricate the tube with sterile water-soluble jelly.

  h Select the proper size laryngoscope blade, and attach it to the handle. Check the bulb operation (see Fig. 20-33).

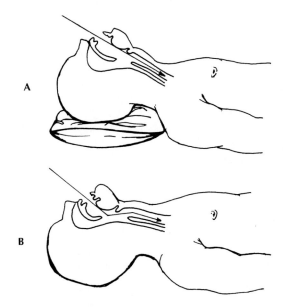

FIGURE 20-36 A, Correct preintubation head position. **B,** Incorrect preintubation head position.

  i Position the head and shoulders so that the patient's head is in the "sniffing" position (Fig. 20-36). The correct position *(A)* is accomplished by placing folded towels or blankets under the patient's head and neck, lifting the head about 2 inches off the level surface. The incorrect, flat supine position *(B)* illustrates the difficulty in seeing the cords. Hyperextending the head without the flexion of the cervical spine makes for a more difficult intubation.

  j A right-handed person would grasp the laryngoscope handle in his or her left hand and introduce the blade into the mouth, displacing the tongue to the patient's left and lifting the lower jaw until the

Checklist for intubation

____	1	Assemble and check equipment.
____	2	Clean the mouth of foreign material.
____	3	Place the patient in the proper position.
____	4	Ventilate the patient with 100% oxygen.
____	5	Select the proper size tube and check cuff.
____	6	Insert the stylet into the tube and lubricate.
____	7	Select the proper size laryngoscope blade.
____	8	Check the operation of the light bulb.
____	9	Position the patient's head in the "sniffing" position.
____	10	Displace the tongue with the laryngoscope.
____	11	Lift the tongue and jaw up and away at a 45-degree angle to visualize the vocal cords.
____	12	Use the free hand to guide the tube through the cords.
____	13	Remove the stylet.
____	14	Inflate the cuff.
____	15	Auscultate for bilateral breath sounds.
____	16	Secure the tube.
____	17	Connect the patient to the appropriate ventilation device.

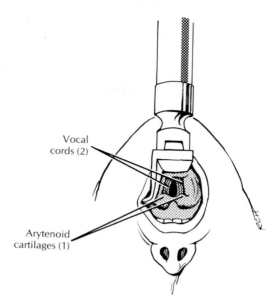

FIGURE 20-37 View of larynx through laryngoscope.

arytenoid cartilages *(1)* and the vocal cords *(2)* are visualized (Fig. 20-37).

- If a straight blade laryngoscope is used, lift the *tip* of the *epiglottis* (see Fig. 20-34, *B*) with the tip of the blade, and lift the laryngoscope handle upward and away at a 45-degree angle, until the cords are seen. Do *not* use the laryngoscope blade and handle as a fulcrum to pry the mouth open.
- If a curve blade is used, place the tip of the blade in the *vallecular* space above the epiglottis (see Figs. 20-34 and 20-38), and lift the handle upward and away at a 45° angle, until the cords are seen. As previously cautioned, do *not* use the laryngoscope blade and handle as a fulcrum. This will break teeth and damage tissue.

k Once the vocal cords are in view, insert the endotracheal tube with the right hand from the right corner of the patient's mouth (Fig. 20-37). Pass the tube alongside the right side of the pharynx and through the vocal cords above the arytenoid cartilages. Do *not* use the blade as a tube guide; it is meant as a visual guide. The tube will get in the way and you will not be able to visualize the cords.

l After the cuff has passed slightly beyond the cords and this is *visualized,* remove the laryngoscope and then the stylet, while holding the tube steady with the right hand.

NOTE: If you are left handed, reverse the instructions above. Left-handed blades are available for those unable to accomplish intubation from the right.

m Inflate the cuff using either the MOV or the MLV technique and ventilate the patient with 100% oxygen to check results. Watch the chest for bilateral movement and auscultate the patient carefully for bilateral breath sounds.

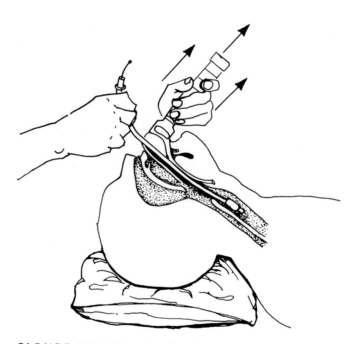

FIGURE 20-38 Insertion of tracheal tube using curved laryngoscope blade.

n If breath sounds are louder on one side than the other or absent on one side, the tube is probably in the right or left main stem bronchus.
- Deflate the cuff and carefully withdraw the tube a centimeter or so.
- Do not extubate the patient at this point.
- Reinflate the cuff, using proper technique.
- Auscultate again for bilateral breath sounds.

o Once the tube has been properly placed, secure it in place with adhesive tape. Procedures vary among hospitals, but the method illustrated in Fig. 20-39 *(A*

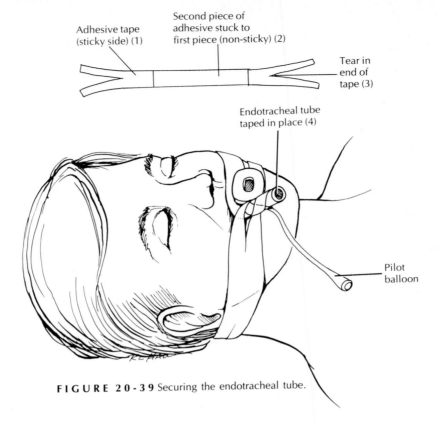

Adhesive tape (sticky side) (1)

Second piece of adhesive stuck to first piece (non-sticky) (2)

Tear in end of tape (3)

Endotracheal tube taped in place (4)

Pilot balloon

FIGURE 20-39 Securing the endotracheal tube.

and *B)* will secure a tube against accidental extubation and undue tube movement.

- Tear a length of 2-inch adhesive tape long enough to reach around the patient's neck *(1)*.
- Tear a shorter length of tape *(2)* and place the two sticky sides together *(1)* and *(2)*. This will eliminate the hair getting stuck in the tape.
- Slide the "harness" under the patient's neck and bring the two sticky ends toward the tube. Get a firm bond on the patient's cheeks. Tear as shown *(3)*.
- Wrap the torn ends around the tube from opposite directions. Cut or tear off excess.
- The taping shown *(4)* includes an oropharyngeal airway to serve as bite block and to facilitate oral care.

  NOTE: Commercial tube retainers are available from various sources that may be safer to use in situations in which unusual stress may be placed on the tracheal tube.

p Connect the patient to whatever device is appropriate: ventilator or aerosol "T."

q It is always a good idea to call for a chest x-ray examination to verify proper tube placement (2 cm above the carina).

8 Blind nasotracheal intubation is presented in Procedures 20-14 and 20-15 for the practitioner who may need or want this skill.

9 The use of short-term paralysis and/or anesthesia to allow for ease of intubation will not be discussed in this module. The interested reader may wish to contact an anesthesiologist to explain various drugs used in elective and emergency intubation.

10 If possible the reader is encouraged to "dress out" for surgery and observe the anesthesiologists and nurse anesthetists intubate under controlled conditions.

11 Take advantage of whatever opportunity presents itself to intubate a cadaver or surgical patient under the *direction* of an anesthesiologist or nurse anesthetist.

12 Procedure 20-13 can be used for passing an orotracheal tube.

13 Procedure 20-14 may be used for passing a nasotracheal tube.

14 The introduction of fiberoptics in 1968 for bronchoscopy was expanded during the 1970s to use for difficult intubations. Even though the technique for using fiberoptics to pass a tracheal tube has been well described, it has not gained widespread popularity because of the expense of the instrument and the general lack of experience in using fiberoptics for this purpose.

Types of patients and situations in which fiberoptics may be of benefit include patients with:

a Massive facial or neck trauma

b A small mouth opening

c Extreme cervical spine deformities

d Laryngeal growths

e Epiglottitis

f Tumor growths

g Short bull-like necks

The technique for passing a tracheal tube using fiberoptics is not discussed here. If more information is desired the reader is recommended to contact an anesthesiologist or pulmonologist who has used this technique or to refer to the bibliography following this module.

8.6 Rational for tracheotomy

1 Tracheostomy tubes ("trach tubes") have been used since 1871.
2 The first tubes were probably hollow reeds inserted into animals. These have evolved through the years into metal, rubber, and, currently, polyvinyl chloride (PVC) and other types of synthetics.
3 Tracheostomy tubes, as their name implies, are inserted into the trachea through an incision (stoma) made through the anterior portion of the throat. The incision procedure (tracheotomy) is made at a level approximately the width of one finger below the cricoid cartilage through the second, third, or fourth tracheal rings (see Fig. 20-24).
4 Tracheotomies were initially performed for glottic obstructions that could not be corrected with passage of an endotracheal tube.
5 Today tracheotomies are performed to:
  a Bypass upper airway obstruction
  b Provide an accessible route to the lower airway without interfering with the nose or mouth
  c Prevent aspiration of blood and other body fluids
  d Reduce anatomic deadspace (by approximately 50%)
  e Provide a functional attachment for prolonged mechanical ventilation and prevent the problems encountered when the patient has an orotracheal or nasotracheal tube.
  NOTE: Besides the above indications for a tracheostomy, it is important to point out that it also allows a patient to swallow, hence receive nourishment orally, which is *not* possible with translaryngeal intubation.
6 In summary, tracheostomy is performed in patients to prevent or treat long-term respiratory failure.

8.7 Hazards of tracheotomy

1 Tracheotomies are performed as elective or emergency procedures.
2 If the procedure is elective, it is performed in surgery under sterile conditions. If it is an emergency procedure, the procedure is performed under aseptic but not necessarily sterile conditions, usually at the bedside. There are few indications for emergency tracheotomies.
3 The most common complications resulting from a tracheostomy and their approximate time of onset are presented in Table 20-3.
4 A patient who has recently undergone tracheostomy should be observed closely for bleeding during the 24-hour period postoperatively.
5 During this 24-hour period the incision site should be checked for abnormal bleeding and any signs of subcu-

TABLE 20-3 Common complications resulting from a tracheostomy

Complication	Approximate time of onset
Postsurgical bleeding	Greatest problem within first 24 hr
Infection	Greatest problem after 48 hr
Mediastinal emphysema	Time is variable
Pneumothorax	Usually occurs during the procedure
Subcutaneous emphysema	Time is variable

taneous emphysema. Also, the inner cannula, if one is used, should be removed and cleaned as needed to prevent any accumulation of blood, which may clot and obstruct the tube.
6 A fresh tracheostomy tube should *not* be moved or changed during the first 36 hours after the procedure, because a firm *tract* through the opening made into the trachea has *not* yet formed. The fresh stoma may collapse, making intubation difficult. If extubation is required during this period it should be performed in surgery or with a full tracheostomy surgical tray on hand.

8.8 Parts of a tracheostomy tube

1 A tracheostomy tube is a hollow cannula that is inserted through an incision into the trachea.
2 Tracheostomy tubes come in various styles and are usually named after their developers:
  a Jackson—a silver tube with inner cannula and obturator
  b Engström—a silver tube with inner cannula
  c James—a red rubber tube with a cuff
  d Oxford—a latex tube with spiral reinforcement and cuff, without an inner cannula
  e Shiley—a plastic tube with inner cannula, obturator, and soft cuff
  f Lanz—a plastic tube with a soft cuff, pressure-regulating valve, and external balloon
  g Kamen-Wilkinson—a plastic tube with a foam-filled cuff that requires no air for inflation, no inner cannula
3 In Fig. 20-40 a plastic-type tracheostomy tube with a soft, large-volume–low-pressure cuff and external pilot balloon is shown. Other tubes may be made of rubber, silver, or a metal that is not reactive to tissue; their parts and their functions will be similar.
4 The *outer cannula (1)* forms the primary structural unit of the tracheostomy tube, with the cuff *(2)* and the flange *(3)* attached.
5 The *inner cannula (4)* is inserted into the outer cannula to provide a removable passageway that is easily cleaned while the patient continues to breathe through the outer cannula that is left in the trachea. This model uses a built-in 15-mm adapter *(5)* that locks into the outer cannula at *6*.
6 The *cuff (2)* is a balloon that is inflated with air once

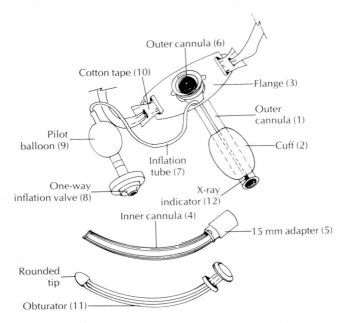

Outer cannula (6)

Cotton tape (10)

Flange (3)

Outer cannula (1)

Pilot balloon (9)

Cuff (2)

Inflation tube (7)

One-way inflation valve (8)

X-ray indicator (12)

Inner cannula (4)

15 mm adapter (5)

Rounded tip

Obturator (11)

FIGURE 20-40 Parts of a tracheostomy tube.

TABLE 20-4 Pediatric to adult tracheostomy tube sizes*

Jackson size	Internal diameter	External diameter	French size
00	2.5	4.5	13
0	3.0	5.0	15
1	3.5	5.5	16.5
2	4.0	6.0	18
3	4.5-5.0	7	21
4	5.5	8	24
5	6.0-6.5	9	27
6	7.0	10	30
7	7.5-8.0	11	33
8	8.5	12	36
9	9.0-9.5	13	39
10	10.0	14	42
11	10.4-11.0	15	45
12	11.5	16	48

*Tube sizes are approximate.

TABLE 20-5 Approximate tracheostomy tube sizes

Age	Jackson reference
Premature	000-00
Birth-6 mo	0
6-18 mo	1
18 mo to 4-5 yr	1-2
4-5 yr to 10 yr	2-3
10 yr to 14 yr	3-5
14 yr to adult	5-9

the tracheostomy tube is in place to prevent aspiration and to seal the area around the tube to prevent air leaks during mechanical ventilation.

7 The *inflation tube (7)* connects the cuff to a one-way inflation valve *(8)* into which a syringe is inserted and air is injected.

8 The *pilot balloon (9)* inflates as the cuff is inflated to indicate that air volume is present in the cuff *(2)*. The one-way valve holds the air in the cuff until it is opened by inserting the syringe tip.

9 The *flange (3)* is a protective plate that is attached to the proximal end of the outer cannula. The flange rests on the outer skin of the patient's throat and prevents the tube from accidentally being dislodged or slipping into the incision. It is held in place by two woven cotton tapes that are tied around the patient's neck.

10 The *obturator (11)* is used to aid insertion of the outer cannula into the tracheostomy and the trachea and to minimize trauma. Before insertion of the outer cannula into the stoma, the inner cannula is removed and replaced with the obturator. The rounded head of the obturator protrudes out the end of the outer cannula, making a smooth surface for insertion. Once insertion is made, the obturator is quickly pulled out and replaced with the inner cannula, which is "locked" into place.

11 The *x-ray indicator (12)*. Most tracheostomy tubes have a radiopaque line or marker on the distal end of the outer cannula that helps to locate the tube's position on x-ray examination.

12 Table 20-4 shows the relative sizes used in tracheostomy tubes. The Jackson size reference is based on the Jackson silver tacheostomy tube and is still used as a reference, although the Jackson tubes are no longer as popular as they once were.

13 Table 20-5 gives approximate tracheostomy tube sizing based on age.

8.9 Special tracheostomy tubes

1 The airways and tubes described in the previous units are used to provide an emergency airway and were not intended, for the most part, to be used for long-term care.

2 The following tubes are used during the postemergency period to allow the patient to eat or talk without compromising the stoma site for use as an emergency airway if it once again becomes necessary.

3 The *tracheostomy button* (Fig. 20-41) is a hollow plastic cannula *(1)* that is inserted through the stoma *(2)*, so that the distal end rests in the lumen of the trachea and the proximal end remains exposed.

   a Once the cannula is in place, the cap *(3)* is inserted into the cannula.

   b This blocks the lumen of the cannula and causes the flange *(4)* on the distal end of the cannula to spread open, securing the cannula in place.

   c When the cannula is capped, the patient has the function of his or her upper airway. If needed, the cap is removed and the tracheostomy airway is used.

4 The *Kistner tracheostomy tube* (Fig. 20-42) is a hollow plastic tube (cannula) *(1)* that has a flexible wall with a flange on the distal end *(2)* and a one-way valve on the proximal end *(3)*.

   a To insert the tube, a clamp is inserted past the one-

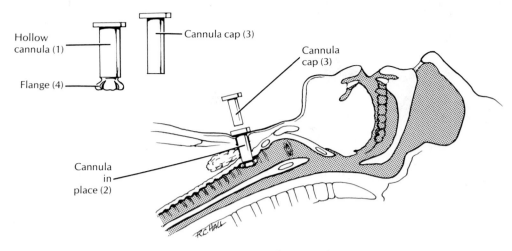

FIGURE 20-41 Tracheostomy button.

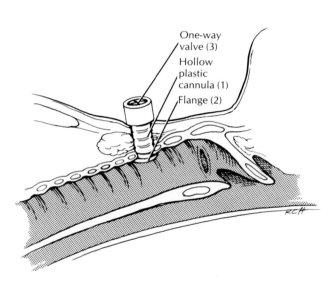

FIGURE 20-42 Kistner tracheostomy tube.

way valve to pinch the flanged portion of the tube together from the inside.

b Once inserted in the stoma, the clamp is released and the flange opens to secure the tube from within the lumen of the trachea.

c The one-way valve permits the patient to inhale through the tracheostomy stoma. During exhalation the one-way valve closes and permits normal exhalation and speech.

5 Speaking tracheostomy tubes have been used since the early 1970s. The earliest of these was the *Pitt Speaking Tracheostomy Tube* (Fig. 20-43).

a This system used a constant gas flow of compressed air at 4 to 6 liters per minute (L/min) *(1)* that could intermittently be delivered to the larynx by occluding one side of a simple Y connector *(2)*.

b The air rising through the vocal cords *(3)* allows the patient the ability, albeit limited, to speak.

c The tracheostomy cuff pressure *(4)* is controlled separately by normal means, shown here with a three-

way stopcock *(5)* and a pressure-monitoring manometer *(6)*.

6 The *Olympic Trach-Talk Tube* and *Communitrach 1* (not illustrated) are other models of speaking tracheostomy tubes. Like the Pitt, they are connected to a continuous gas flow that is directed up through the vocal cords.

7 More recent systems, such as the Venti-Voice Speech system by Bear Medical Systems Inc, incorporates electronics to operate the flow of gas and a voice generator to produce sounds. This system operates independently of the ventilator and may be operated with a head switch by quadraplegic patients.

8 The *fenestrated tracheostomy tube* is a special type of tube with a hole (fenestration) in the outer cannula (Fig. 20-44).

a With the inner cannula removed *(1)*, air can pass through the hole *(2)* toward the cords and pharynx.

b This two-way breathing encourages weaning from the tracheostomy tube and allows for some speech.

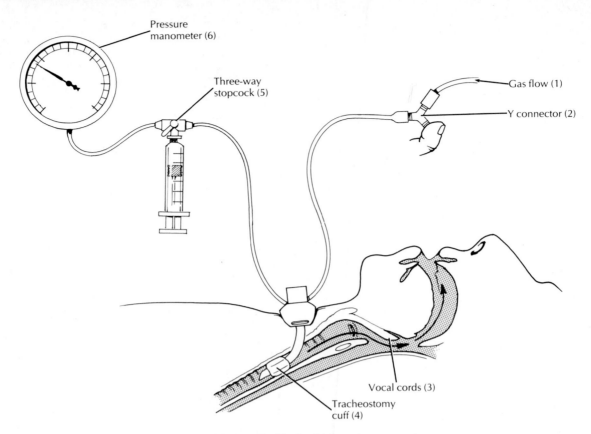

FIGURE 20-43 Pitt Speaking tracheostomy tube.

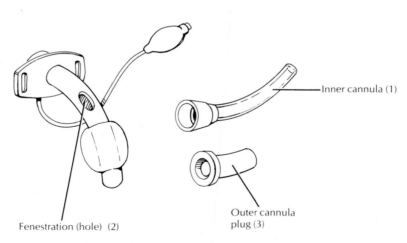

FIGURE 20-44 Fenestrated tracheostomy tube.

c To further the weaning process, the outer cannula can be capped using a plug *(3)* that is inserted in the proximal end of the outer cannula. This plugging forces all the ventilation through normal channels while leaving access for suctioning and, if needed, reintroduction of tracheostomy ventilation.

CAUTION: Precut, commercially fenestrated tracheostomy tubes may not have the fenestration properly lo-cated for the tracheal anatomy of all patients. Care must be taken to check that the fenestration is in fact open once the tube has been placed. A blocked fenestration in a capped tube with the cuff inflated will create a closed airway leading to asphyxiation of the patient. If the fenestration of the tube is not properly located, the practitioner should custom-cut a fenestration in a regular tracheostomy tube.

9.0 AIRWAY SUCTIONING

9.1 Principles of airway suctioning

1 The removal of airway substances using a suction device is a necessary but potentially hazardous procedure.

2 One must consider that vacuum pressures sufficient to remove mucus and other substances must also remove air containing oxygen from a patient who is probably already at best, borderline hypoxic.

3 Studies have shown that the removal of oxygen by suction for as short a period as 30 seconds to 1 minute can cause deadly hypoxia levels, resulting in premature ventricular contractions leading to cardiac fibrillation and cardiac arrest.

4 In addition, one must remember that the larynx and trachea are innervated by the vagus nerve, which when stimulated can cause lethal bradycardia, a drop in blood pressure, and decreased respiratory rates.

5 Suctioning can also cause trauma to the lining of the trachea as a result of the catheter adhering to the wall of the trachea, where it tears away delicate tissue as it is being withdrawn by the anxious clinician.

6 Having briefly mentioned the possible hazards, it is safe to say that the personnel responsible for airway care should be skilled in airway clearance procedures.

7 Respiratory care practitioners are earning more and more responsibility for the primary airway care of patients with acute and chronic pulmonary problems. It follows therefore that the suctioning procedure be included in routine respiratory bedside care.

9.2 Indications for endotracheal suctioning

1 The purpose of mechanical suctioning (aspiration) is to remove secretions or other substances from the trachea or main stem bronchi that cannot be naturally removed by the patient.

2 Normally there are five major reflexes located in the pharyngeal region that aid in the removal of secretions.
   a Swallowing
   b Gagging
   c Sneezing
   d Spasm
   e Coughing

3 Of these, coughing is the most common maneuver for removing secretions that might obstruct the airways.

4 To be effective, the *cough reflex* follows four stages or steps.
   a A large inspiration occurs (air behind the secretion or obstruction will help push it forward for clearance).
   b The glottis is closed.
   c Pressure is built up in the thorax by moving the diaphragm upward against the closed glottis and rapidly contracting the muscles of exhalation.
   d The glottis is opened suddenly, and an explosive release of air occurs that moves the secretion or obstruction.

5 Occasionally conditions will occur that will prevent the body from clearing its own secretions. These conditions include:
   a A decrease in the state of consciousness
   b Disease, especially of the nervous system
   c Poor pulmonary mechanics (i.e., restriction, fractured ribs, etc.)
   d Trauma (including surgery) to head, neck, or chest
   e Age extremes
   f Drug or alcohol sedation
   g Dehydration of the respiratory tract and resultant "mucous plugging"
   h Injury to the airway surface (i.e., hot gases, aspiration of stomach acid, etc.)

6 The signs of upper and lower airway obstruction are discussed in Unit 4.0. In review, it is important that the clinician note the following.
   a The patient's general appearance and behavior (i.e., restlessness, anxiety, pallor)
   b Change in vital signs (i.e., increased heart rate, respiratory rate, blood pressure, and possibly temperature)
   c Quality of breathing (i.e., breath sounds diminished, patient seems dyspneic, respirations labored, possible retractions)

7 Once a patient has exhibited these signs and symptoms and is unable to remove his secretions by another method (i.e., coughing), then suctioning the patient is indicated.

9.3 Types of suctioning techniques

1 Numerous suctioning methods are available to help the patient clear his or her secretions. These methods include:
   a Nasal suctioning. A catheter is introduced through the nose; the nasal and nasopharyngeal cavities are cleared.
   b Oral suctioning. A catheter is introduced into the mouth;
      the mouth and oropharyngeal areas are cleared.
   c Intratracheal suctioning. A catheter is passed into the trachea via the nose of mouth; the trachea is cleared.
   d Endotracheal suctioning. A catheter is passed through the tracheal tube; the tube and tracheobronchial areas are cleared.
   e Laryngostomy suctioning. A catheter is passed through the laryngectomy opening; the laryngeal region is cleared.
   f Tracheostomy suctioning. A catheter is passed through a tracheostomy tube; the tube and tracheobronchial areas are cleared.

2 The method chosen for a patient will depend on the patient's particular problem or situation. Also, it is helpful if the clinician knows the characteristics of the secretions being suctioned; some are more tenacious than others, some will be blood tinged, some will have odor, etc. These indicators may be useful in helping the physician evaluate the patient's status and whether or not suctioning is effective.

TABLE 20-6 Recommended amounts of negative pressure

Patient	Inches of H$_2$O	mm Hg
Infant	3-5	60-100
Child	5-10	100-120
Adult	7-15	120-150

NOTE: The American Heart Association recommends suction units that produce 30 L/min free airflow at the end of the delivery tube and 300 mm Hg when the tube is clamped.

9.4 Principles of suctioning devices

1 A suctioning apparatus creates a vacuum or negative pressure. This vacuum is achieved in a variety of ways by using different types of pump mechanisms. Today three basic pump types exist:
   a Diaphragm or oil-free pump
   b Piston
   c Rotary
2 The manometers that register the amount of negative pressure created also vary. One of the most common is the *wall suction manometer*. It is read in millimeters of mercury (Hg) pressure. Portable suction manometers indicate inches of H$_2$O. Depending on the patient's age, circumstances, and character of secretions, varying amounts of negative pressure are recommended (see Table 20-6).
3 Module Seven contains more information on vacuum pumps and piping systems.

9.5 Criteria for a functional suction system

1 Tracheal suction requires the use of a vacuum source that will generate between 80 to 120 mm Hg negative pressure.
2 Vacuum sources include electric suction pumps. Venturi-type injectors, and pipeline outlets that are connected to a central vacuum system.
3 When selecting a vacuum source, the primary considerations include:
   a Size of the unit. The unit must be able to evacuate up to 500 ml of liquid without interruption of operation for emptying.
   b Free airflow. The vacuum source must be able to generate a *free outflow* of 25 to 30 L/min.
   c Vacuum source. The vacuum source must be capable of removing at least 8 L/min.
   d Response time. A maximum suction force must be generated in 5 to 15 seconds.
   e Maximum pressure. A negative force of 80 to 120 mm Hg should be generated.
   f Suction tubing. The internal diameter of the tubing should be 6 to 8 mm, and the tubing should be limited to 3 feet in length.
   g Suction catheter. The catheter must be flexible to reduce tissue trauma and have a minimum of 2 holes, one at the tip and one located on the lateral wall above the tip.

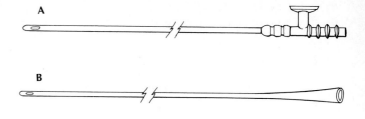

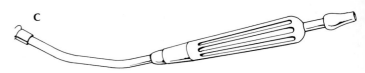

FIGURE 20-45 Types of suction catheters. **A,** Disposable, vented, polyvinyl chloride catheter. **B,** Nondisposable, nonvented rubber catheter. **C,** Yankauer-type tonsil suction.

9.6 Types of suction catheters

1 A variety of suction catheters are available.
2 The differences exist in the designs of the catheters and in their construction materials (Fig. 20-45).
   a Disposable, vented, polyvinyl chloride plastic catheter *(A)*
   b Nondisposable, nonvented, rubber catheter *(B)*
   c Metal, Yankauer-type tube. Commonly called a tonsil suction and used for oropharyngeal suctioning of thick and/or copious secretions *(C)*
3 When selecting a suction catheter, one should choose a catheter that is soft and pliable but not so soft that it will collapse inward when suction is applied.
4 The distal tip should be open and have smooth edges to prevent trauma.
5 Trauma can be further minimized by having at least two holes at the distal end. Various manufacturers have advertised catheters with a variety of tips, each designed to produce less tissue trauma than the competition. Examples are illustrated in Fig. 20-46, *A* through *F*).
6 Fig. 20-47 shows a thumb control valve. When the finger valve port is open (not occluded), room air is entrained through the catheter valve *(1)* and no suction should occur at the catheter tip *(2)*. All suction catheters should have this feature because it permits intermittent suction. To operate the valve (create action), one places one's thumb over the valve opening to create suction at the distal tip. Suction is stopped when the thumb is removed from the valve.

Care must be taken to select catheters with valve openings that do not allow suction to occur at the catheter tip when the valve is unoccluded. One way of testing this is to attach a sample catheter to an active vacuum source and submerge the tip into a glass of water. If water is drawn even partially up the catheter when the finger valve is unoccluded, the valve opening is *not* sufficient to prevent air (oxygen) from being removed from the airway during insertion of the catheter.

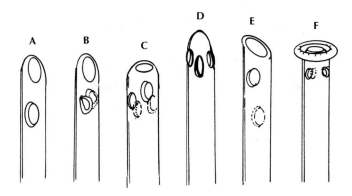

FIGURE 20-46 Suction catheter tips.

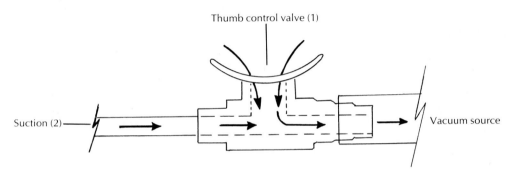

FIGURE 20-47 Suction catheter thumb control valve.

7 A suction catheter works because a drop in pressure occurs from the atmosphere to the tip of the catheter and then to the suction source. The pressure in the lungs during suction therefore is the same as that which exists at the tip of the catheter.

8 During suction, negative pressure is created only when the thumb control valve is occluded and air is flowing up the catheter.

  a This air comes from the lungs and from a free space between the suction catheter and the tracheal tube.

  b A suction catheter that is too large will fill this free space and all the air will come from the lungs.

  c When intratracheal suctioning is performed through the mouth or nose, most of the air comes from the lungs and some through the open mouth or opposite nostril.

9 This movement of air from the lungs may result in excessive depletion of air (and therefore oxygen), causing hypoxia and airway collapse with resultant atelectasis.

10 A general rule is to select a catheter that is approximately one half the size of the inner diameter of the tube into which it is to be inserted. Do *not* use a catheter that is more than two thirds the size of the inner diameter.

11 Most adults can be suctioned with a 14 French size catheter. Refer to Table 20-2 for a recommended list of tube sizes and corresponding suctioning catheter sizes.

9.7 Equipment for sterile suctioning technique

1 Normally, the respiratory tract below the larynx is sterile. To introduce a suction catheter into this area that is anything but *sterile* is doing the patient a great disservice.

2 To reduce the hazard of infection, sterile, disposable equipment and sterile technique should be used.

3 The following equipment is needed to carry out a sterile suctioning procedure:

  a Sterile disposable catheter; one with a multiple-hole tip and thumb valve.

  b Sterile disposable gloves for handling catheter.

  c Sterile water or normal saline to flush the catheter after use; a sterile container to hold the liquid.

  d A sterile disposable towel or paper sheet is convenient but not necessary.

  e A suction source, from either the wall or from an electrical vacuum pump, and a collection jar with connecting tubing.

  NOTE: Many commercial brands of sterile, suctioning "kits" are available.

9.8 Possible hazards and complications of transtracheal suctioning

1 The most common hazard and/or complication is *hypoxemia*. Hypoxemia may result from the removal of alveolar gas or the replacement of oxygen-enriched air with ambient air. This can lead to numerous cardiac problems, including arrhythmias or tachycardia.

2 Vagal stimulation may lead to *bradycardia, hypotension,* and *respiratory arrest.*

3 *Lung collapse,* as a result of poor technique, is another complication. This may be avoided by choosing a suction catheter that is no more than one half the inner diameter of the tracheal tube.

4 Tissue trauma may also occur. Vacuum pressure greater than 100 torr can destroy delicate mucosal tissues and denude the airways of cilia.

5 The introduction of contaminated catheters can cause serious and life-threatening complications, such as bacteremic and nonbacteremic pneumonias, in the compromised patient.

9.9 Performing tracheal suctioning*

1 Follow sterile technique at *all* times. The exception to this is a life-or-death situation in which times does not allow normal sterile routine to be followed.

2 Always hyperoxygenate the patient before the suctioning procedure.

3 Once a proper suctioning level of 80 to 120 mm Hg has been set, gently slide the catheter into place. *Never* jab or push against a resistance.

4 Insert the catheter until a *slight* obstruction is met, pull the catheter back about ½ inch, then apply suction. It is recommended that a patient's head be alternatively turned to the right to help direct the catheter into the left main stem branches and vice versa.

5 Pull the catheter out in one smooth motion, while rotating the catheter with the fingertips. Do *not* run the catheter in and out while applying suction.

6 Apply suction *intermittently* when withdrawing the catheter and *never* for longer than *15 seconds.* The total time from interruption of ventilation to return of ventilation should not take longer than approximately 20 seconds. This will reduce the hazards of hypoxia and tissue trauma.

7 Wait until at least five deep breaths have been taken and until vital signs return to normal after each procedure before repeating it. Studies have shown pronounced hypoxia to exist for periods up to 1 hour following a suctioning procedure.

8 If complications occur during the procedure, stop immediately and re-establish hyperoxygenation. Monitor the patient throughout the procedure, especially if an electrocardiogram (ECG) monitor is in use at the bedside.

9 After suctioning, hyperoxygenate the patient, preferably with positive pressure, if the patient is intubated. Be aware that patient receiving positive end expiratory pressure (PEEP) or constant positive airway pressure (CPAP) are especially vulnerable to suction-induced hypoxia because functional residual capacity (FRC) levels are acutely depleted during suctioning. Some PEEP and CPAP circuits have incorporated suction ports to minimize interruption of the elevated baseline during a suctioning procedure.

10 A note about suctioning and cuffs. *Always* suction *above* a cuff, using the oronasal suction, before deflating a cuff for any reason. This prevents built-up secretions from flooding the lower airways as the cuff is deflated. After suctioning the pharynx, discard the catheter and glove and use fresh sterile supplies before entering the tracheal tube.

11 If while suctioning the tracheal tube, you notice that oronasal suction is again needed, it is permissible to use the same catheter only if the order is tracheal tube first, oronasal second. *Never* introduce a catheter into a tracheal tube that has been in the mouth or nose.

12 Procedure 20-16 can be used for performing a sterile tracheal suctioning technique.

13 The fiberoptic bronchoscope is frequently used with or without intermittent positive pressure breathing (IPPB) or jet ventilation to remove copious amounts of secretions or tenacious aspirants that cannot be easily removed by standard tracheal suctioning technique. In difficult cases of tenacious and/or impacted secretions, a bronchopulmonary lavage of each lung may be performed using aliquots of saline solution passed through a Carlens catheter.

9.10 Oropharyngeal and nasopharyngeal suctioning

1 Patients will frequently have secretions and other substances that must be suctioned from the mouth and nose.

2 The procedure for aspirating these areas is similar to that for tracheal suction, except that the danger of inducing infection and hypoxia is not as great.

3 Nevertheless, sterile equipment and technique should be used for this procedure.

4 Procedure 20-17 can be used to perform oropharyngeal and nasopharyngeal suctioning.

10.0 THE ESOPHAGEAL OBTURATOR AIRWAY (EOA)
10.1 Insertion of an esophageal obturator airway

1 The esophageal obturator airway is a tubelike device that is placed *in the esophagus* to prevent stomach contents from entering the lungs while the patient is being artifically ventilated, usually with a resuscitator device and a mask.

The EOA was developed in 1973 by Dr. Don Michael as an alternative to tracheal intubation, which was restricted primarily to use by physicians. Since 1973, the literature has reported that millions have been safely intubated using an EOA. Ironically, the development and use of the EOA has pointed out that allied health personnel can be trained to make decisions about when to pass an artificial airway and about which

---

*The specific techniques for performing tracheal suctioning will vary from hospital to hospital. For this reason, the procedure that follows is offered as a general guideline. For more details, the reader is encouraged to refer to a hospital procedure manual.

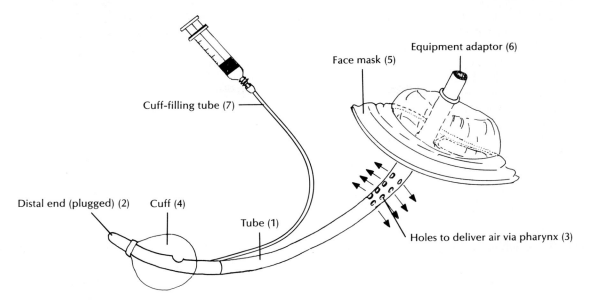

FIGURE 20-48 Parts of esophageal obturator airway.

type of airway is indicated for a particular situation.

In essence, the EOA has not limited the use of tracheal intubation but has given the practitioner still another choice for providing an artificial airway.

2 The parts of an EOA are shown in Fig. 20-48.

  a The EOA consists of a hollow tube *(1)* that is plugged on the distal end *(2)*.

  b Holes near the proximal end *(3)* allow air to be delivered to the patient's lungs via the pharynx.

  c A cuff *(4)* seals the esophagus and prevents stomach contents from passing up the esophagus.

  d The face mask *(5)* is placed over the patient's face to prevent air leaks. A ventilating device can be attached to the tube's proximal end *(6)*.

  e A filling tube *(7)* allows the cuff to be inflated with a syringe.

10.2 General concerns when placing the EOA

1 The EOA is placed in the esophagus (Fig. 20-49). The cuff must be passed *beyond* the carina before it is inflated. Inflation is via the filling tube and uses approximately 35 cc of air.

2 When the patient is being ventilated, care must be taken to ensure a *tight* fit of the mask. Leaks will result in inadequate ventilation.

3 Care must be taken to ensure that the tube is not accidentally placed in the trachea instead of the esophagus.

4 If an esophageal airway is available, have a clinician show it to you and, if possible, practice it on a cadaver.

10.3 Steps in placing the EOA

1 The following steps are a typical procedure for placing an EOA.

  a Assess the need for EOA vs. other methods.

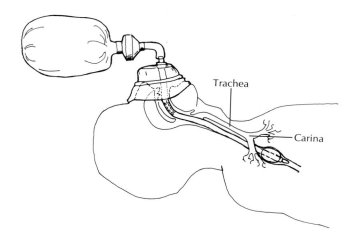

FIGURE 20-49 Proper placement of esophageal obturator airway.

  b Hyperventilate the patient's lungs four times.

  c Pull the jaw straight forward without hyperextension of the neck.

  d Insert the tube into the mouth and gently advance the tube behind the tongue and into the esophagus, following the natural curvature of the tube and anatomic passage.

  e Advance the airway until the mask is fitted firmly over the patient's face.

  f Hold the mask firmly on the patient's face.

  g Apply IPPB with a mechanical ventilator.

  h Check for chest movement during delivery of the positive pressure breath. If the chest does not rise, the tube may be in the trachea. If this is suspected, remove the airway, ventilate the patient, then re-attempt passing the airway.

i Once a chest rise is noted during the application of a positive pressure breath, the balloon (cuff) should be inflated with 35 ml of air.

j Remove the syringe from the filling tube valve.

k When removing the EOA, turn the patient to one side and deflate the balloon and withdraw the tube from the patient's throat. Use caution and be aware that the patient usually vomits at this point.

2 If desired, an endotracheal tube may be passed while the EOA is in place. This is accomplished by removing the mask from the EOA and passing the tracheal tube according to standard procedure.

Once the tracheal tube is in place and the cuff is inflated, the balloon in the EOA is deflated and the airway is removed.

3 Since its introduction in 1973, the EOA has experienced many modifications. These modifications are beyond the scope of this work, other than to point out that the practitioner should use judgment in selecting an airway and be proficient in its application before using it on patients.

4 Complications reported from the use of the EOA include:

a Accidental intubation of the trachea instead of the esophagus

b Esophageal laceration and perforation

c Aspiration of vomitus around the balloon

d Inability to properly seal the mask to achieve adequate ventilation

e Improper removal technique resulting in esophageal injury and/or aspiration of vomitus

PROCEDURE 20-1

Perform a Heimlich maneuver on an adult—standing

No.	Steps in performing the procedure
	The practitioner will recognize the signs of airway obstruction and perform a Heimlich maneuver on a standing adult (simulated victim).
1	Demonstrate the visual choking sign usually made by a victim.
2	Discuss other visual signs of choking: **2.1** Panic **2.2** Grasping inspiratory efforts **2.3** Cyanosis **2.4** Unconsciousness **2.5** Circumstances surrounding location of victim
3	Discuss audible signs of choking: **3.1** Complete obstruction (no sounds) **3.2** Partial obstruction (stridor, crowing, gasping)
4	Discuss tactile signs of airway obstruction: **4.1** Rapid, slow, and/or irregular pulse **4.2** Clammy, moist skin
5	Position yourself behind the victim and encircle victim's waist with your arms (see Fig. 20-9).
6	Make a "Heimlich fist" according to Figs. 20-6 through 20-8.
7	Place knob of fisted hand into victim's abdomen: **7.1** Above navel **7.2** Below xyphoid process
8	Press into victim's abdomen with quick upward thrust.
9	Repeat thrusts as necessary, as separate efforts.
10	Assess airway patency: **10.1** Patient begins to breathe. **10.2** Air movement is felt coming from mouth and nose. **10.3** Visual and audible signs of obstruction disappear.
11	Nonbreathing patients must be ventilated immediately using mouth-to-mouth or manual resuscitator methods.

PROCEDURE 20-2

Perform a Heimlich maneuver on an adult—sitting

No.	Steps in performing the procedure
	The practitioner will recognize the signs of airway obstruction and perform a Heimlich maneuver on a sitting adult (simulated victim).
1	Demonstrate the visual choking sign usually made by a victim.
2	Discuss other visual signs of choking: **2.1** Panic **2.2** Gasping inspiratory efforts **2.3** Cyanosis **2.4** Unconsciousness **2.5** Circumstances surrounding location of victim
3	Discuss audible signs of choking: **3.1** Complete obstruction (no sounds) **3.2** Partial obstruction (stridor, crowing, gasping)
4	Discuss tactile signs of airway obstruction: **4.1** Rapid, slow, and/or irregular pulse **4.2** Clammy, moist skin
5	Position yourself behind the victim and encircle victim's waist with your arms (see Fig. 20-10).
6	Make a "Heimlich fist" according to Figs. 20-6 through 20-8.
7	Place knob of fisted hand into victim's abdomen: **7.1** Above navel **7.2** Below xyphoid process
8	Press into victim's abdomen with quick upward thrust.
9	Repeat thrusts as necessary, as separate efforts.
10	Assess airway patency: **10.1** Patient begins to breathe. **10.2** Air movement is felt coming from mouth and nose. **10.3** Visual and audible signs of obstruction disappear.
11	Nonbreathing patients must be ventilated immediately using mouth-to-mouth or manual resuscitator methods.

PROCEDURE 20-3

Perform a Heimlich maneuver on an adult—supine

No.	Steps in performing the procedure
	The practitioner will recognize the signs of airway obstruction and perform a Heimlich maneuver on a supine adult (simulated victim).
1	Demonstrate the visual choking sign usually made by a victim.
2	Discuss other visual signs of choking: **2.1** Panic **2.2** Gasping inspiratory efforts **2.3** Cyanosis **2.4** Unconsciousness **2.5** Circumstances surrounding location of victim
3	Discuss audible signs of choking: **3.1** Complete obstruction (no sounds) **3.2** Partial obstruction (stridor, crowing, gasping)
4	Discuss tactile signs of airway obstruction: **4.1** Rapid, slow, and/or irregular pulse **4.2** Clammy, moist skin
5	Place victim on back: **5.1** Place yourself astride the victim's thighs, facing the victim (Fig. 20-11). **5.2** Place your palms, one on top of the other, between the xyphoid and the naval.
6	Press into victim's abdomen with quick upward thrust.
7	Repeat thrusts as necessary, as separate efforts.
8	Assess airway patency: **8.1** Patient begins to breathe. **8.2** Air movement is felt coming from mouth and nose. **8.3** Visual and audible signs of obstruction disappear.
9	Nonbreathing patients must be ventilated immediately using mouth-to-mouth or manual resuscitator methods.

PROCEDURE 20-4

Perform Heimlich maneuver on self

No.	Steps in performing the procedure
	The practitioner will simulate a self-administered Heimlich maneuver using hands and chair back or other appropriate surface.
1	Stand erect.
2	Make a "Heimlich fist" according to Figs. 20-6 through 20-8.
3	Place knob of fisted hand into abdomen: **3.1** Above navel **3.2** Below xyphoid
4	Press fist quickly upward (see Fig. 20-14).
5	Repeat as necessary.
6	If thrusts do not work and you are still alone: **6.1** Position yourself over the edge of a chair, railing, table, etc. **6.2** Compress abdomen by pressing down on the surface edge (see Fig. 20-13). **6.3** Repeat as necessary.

PROCEDURE 20-5

Using head-tilt/chin-lift method to open airway

No.	Steps in performing the procedure
	The practitioner will correct for airway obstruction by using the head-tilt method. CAUTION: This method is not used if the victim is suspected of or has a spinal injury.
1	Recognize visual signs of airway obstruction: **1.1** Increased rate of breathing **1.2** Grasping efforts **1.3** Exaggerated use of inspiratory muscles **1.4** Retraction of soft thoracic tissue during inspiration **1.5** Cyanosis
2	Recognize audible signs of airway obstruction: **2.1** No breathing sounds linked with exaggerated inspiratory efforts **2.2** Laryngeal sounds, such as snoring, crowing, gasping, stridor, gurgling, etc.
3	Attempt to arouse patient if unconscious ("shake and shout").
4	Position victim on back with face uwpard, call for help.
5	Use head-tilt/chin-lift method to open airway: **5.1** Position yourself to one side of victim's shoulders. **5.2** Place the other hand on the victim's forehead, with fingers together. **5.3** Apply firm backward pressure with palm to tilt head back. **5.4** Place fingers of other hand under bony part of lower jaw near the chin, lift to move the chin forward and almost close the teeth. **5.5** Make sure fingers do not press into soft tissue under chin. **5.6** Make sure mouth is not completely closed.
6	Assess airway patency: **6.1** Patient begins to breathe. **6.2** Air movement is felt coming from mouth and nose. **6.3** Visual and audible signs of obstruction disappear.
7	Nonbreathing patients must be ventilated immediately using mouth-to-mouth or manual resuscitator methods.

PROCEDURE 20-6

Using chin-lift method to open airway

No.	Steps in performing the procedure
1	The practitioner will correct for airway obstruction by using the chin-lift method. CAUTION: This method is *not* used if the victim is suspected of or has a spinal injury. Recognize visual signs of airway obstruction: **1.1** Increased rate of breathing **1.2** Gasping efforts **1.3** Exaggerated use of inspiratory muscles **1.4** Retraction of soft thoracic tissue during inspiration **1.5** Cyanosis
2	Recognize audible signs of airway obstruction: **2.1** No breathing sounds linked with exaggerated inspiratory efforts **2.2** Laryngeal sounds, such as snoring, crowing, gasping, stridor, gurgling, etc.
3	Attempt to arouse patient if unconscious ("shake and shout").
4	Position victim on back with face upward, call for help.
5	Use chin-lift method to open airway: **5.1** Position yourself to one side of victim's shoulders. **5.2** Place on head, with fingers together, on victim's forehead. **5.3** Place thumb of other hand inside victim's mouth and grasp chin with fingers. **5.4** Lift victim's chin upward, causing mandible to move forward, while applying gentle downward pressure on forehead with the other hand.
6	Assess airway patency: **6.1** Patient begins to breathe. **6.2** Air movement is felt coming from mouth and nose. **6.3** Visual and audible signs of obstruction disappear.
7	Nonbreathing patients must be ventilated immediately using mouth-to-mouth or manual resuscitator methods.

PROCEDURE 20-7

Using jaw-thrust method to open airway

No.	Steps in performing the procedure
1	The practitioner will correct for airway obstruction by using the jaw-thrust method. NOTE: Modifications of this technique can be used in cases of spinal injury. Recognize visual signs of airway obstruction: **1.1** Increased rate of breathing **1.2** Gasping efforts **1.3** Exaggerated use of inspiratory muscles **1.4** Retraction of soft thoracic tissue during inspiration **1.5** Cyanosis
2	Recognize audible signs of airway obstruction: **2.1** No breathing sounds linked with exaggerated inspiratory efforts **2.2** Laryngeal sounds, such as snoring, crowing, gasping, stridor, gurgling, etc.
3	Attempt to arouse patient if unconscious ("shake and shout").
4	Position victim on back with face upward, call for help.
5	Use jaw-thrust method to open airway: **5.1** Position yourself at the top of the victim's head. **5.2** Place the fingers of both hands behind the angles of the victim's mandible. **5.3** Lift the mandible forward by applying pressure with both hands at the mandible angles, while tilting head backward.
6	Assess airway patency: **6.1** Patient begins to breathe. **6.2** Air movement is felt coming from mouth and nose. **6.3** Visual and audible signs of obstruction disappear.
7	Nonbreathing patients must be ventilated immediately using mouth-to-mouth or manual resuscitator methods.

PROCEDURE 20-8

Open the mouth of an unconscious patient using crossed-finger technique

No.	Steps in performing the procedure
1	The practitioner will open the mouth of an unconscious patient, using the crossed-finger technique. Position the patient in supine position.
2	Wash hands.
3	Cross your thumb under your index finger (see Fig. 20-21).
4	Slip your crossed thumb and finger between patient's lips in the upper corner of the mouth.
5	Brace your thumb and finger against the front of the upper and lower teeth.
6	Push your fingers apart to open jaw: **6.1** Do *not* put your fingers behind teeth. **6.2** Apply even pressure when forcing jaws open.
7	Wash hands.

PROCEDURE 20-9

Insert an oropharyngeal airway

No.	Steps in performing the procedure
	The practitioner will select the proper size oropharyngeal airway and insert it in the unconscious patient. NOTE: A manikin or cadaver may be used for initial practice.
1	Recognize airway obstruction.
2	Wash hands.
3	Remove any dentures or foreign objects in mouth.
4	Position patient on back.
5	Select proper size airway:
	5.1 Place airway alongside patient's face.
	5.2 Determine proper length by noting extension of airway from center of mouth to angle of jaw (see Fig. 20-20).
6	Hyperextend patient's neck using head-tilt method.
7	Open patient's mouth using crossed-finger technique (see Procedure 20-8).
8	Hold patient's mouth open using crossed fingers.
9	Hold airway in other hand; insert it into mouth with tip pointed up toward roof of mouth.
10	Slide airway along roof of mouth, over tongue, until tip passed uvula. Do *not* force.
11	Rotate the airway 180 degrees into position with the tip pointed down into the pharynx. Take care not to lacerate the palate as the airway is rotated.
12	Note position of airway:
	12.1 Flange should be resting against the patient's lips; if beyond the lips, it is too large.
	12.2 Replace airway if it is too large or too small.
13	Assess patient's acceptance of airway (e.g., gagging or trying to "spit it out").
14	Assess effectiveness in relieving airway obstruction.
15	Airway may be secured by a piece of tape across the top of the flange. CAUTION: Do *not* occlude the air passage with tape.

PROCEDURE 20-10

Insert a nasopharyngeal airway

No.	Steps in performing the procedure
1	The practitioner will select the proper size nasopharyngeal airway and insert in the unconscious patient. NOTE: A manikin or cadaver may be used for initial practice. Collect necessary equipment:
	1.1 Various size nasopharyngeal airways
	1.2 Sterile, water-soluble lubricant
	1.3 Sterile gauze pads (4 × 4s)
	1.4 Tongue depressor
	1.5 Flashlight
2	Recognize airway obstruction.
3	Wash hands.
4	Remove any dentures or foreign objects in mouth.
5	Position patient on back.
6	Measure airway for proper size:
	6.1 Place airway alongside patient's face.
	6.2 Measure from tip of nose to tragus of ear plus 1 inch (see Fig. 20-23).
7	Place water-soluble lubricant on sterile gauze pad (4 × 4).
8	Coat the airway with the lubricant.
9	Select most patent nostril.
10	Gently slide airway in nostril, parallel to hard palate.
11	Check location of airway in pharynx with flashlight and tongue depressor.
12	Secure flange of airway according to Fig. 20-23.
13	Assess patient's acceptance of airway.
14	Assess effectiveness in relieving airway obstruction.
15	Check for excessive bleeding in nasal passage.

PROCEDURE 20-11

Inflate tracheal tube cuff using minimal occlusion volume (MOV) technique

No.	Steps in performing procedure
1	The practitioner will inflate a tracheal tube cuff using MOV technique on a tracheal tube that is already in place. Check patient's record for any special directions or complications related to tracheal tube or interrupting respiratory therapy.
2	Wash hands.
3	Introduce yourself to patient.
4	Verify patient's identification.
5	Explain procedure to patient.
6	Remove any oxygen or humidity tubing from tube.
7	Use aseptic oronasal pharyngeal suction technique to suction above cuff before deflating it.
8	Deflate cuff.
9	Have patient cough to raise secretions.
10	Use sterile tracheal suction technique to clear any secretions in the tracheal tube.
11	Insert tip of 10-ml syringe, filled with air, into filling tube valve.
12	Have patient phonate or use stethoscope over larynx to auscultate for breath sounds over vocal cords.
13	Slowly inject air until the point at which sounds cease over larynx.
14	Remove syringe tip, check pilot balloon to make sure that air is still in cuff.
15	Replace any oxygen or humidity tubing.
16	Observe patient for any untoward results from suctioning procedure.
17	Wash hands.
18	Chart procedure according to departmental policy.

PROCEDURE 20-12

Inflate tracheal tube cuff using minimum leak volume (MLV) technique

No.	Steps in performing the procedure
1	The practitioner will inflate a tracheal tube using MLV technique on a tracheal tube that is already in place. Check patient's record for any special directions or complications related to tracheal tube or interrupting respiratory therapy.
2	Wash hands.
3	Introduce yourself to patient.
4	Verify patient's identification.
5	Explain procedure to patient.
6	Remove any oxygen or humidity tubing.
7	Use aseptic oronasal pharyngeal suction technique to suction above cuff before deflating it.
8	Deflate cuff.
9	Have patient cough to raise secretions.
10	Use sterile tracheal suction technique to clear any secretions in the tracheal tube.
11	Insert tip of 10-ml syringe, filled with air, into filling tube valve.
12	Use syringe to inflate cuff, while auscultating over larynx, until sounds cease.
13	Slowly withdraw air from the cuff until a *small* leak is heard escaping through the larynx.
14	Remove syringe tip, check pilot balloon to make sure that air is still in cuff.
15	Replace any oxygen or humidity tubing.
16	Observe patient for any untoward results from suctioning procedure.
17	Wash hands.
18	Chart procedure according to departmental policy.

PROCEDURE 20-13

Passing an endotracheal tube under direct vision—oral

No.	Steps in performing the procedure	No.	Steps in performing the procedure
	The practitioner will, under direct supervision, select and pass an endotracheal tube of the oral-type in an adult patient. NOTE: This procedure should be taught by a physician, preferably an anesthesiologist, and practiced on a manikin or cadaver before working with patients.	15	Using either style blade, lift the laryngoscope up and away from you at 45 degree angle, in the direction of the operator's thumb (Fig. 20-38). Do *not* pull back toward you.
1	Justify need for endotracheal intubation.	16	Lift until the vocal cords are clearly seen. Gentle pressure may be applied with the free hand to the "Adam's apple" to aid in visualization.
	1.1 Prevent aspiration in unconscious patient	17	Place endotracheal tube in free hand:
	1.2 Provide route for artificial ventilation		17.1 With stylet in place
	1.3 Airway patency cannot be assured using simpler methods		17.2 With pretested cuff
2	Assemble and, where appropriate, test intubation materials:		17.3 With sufficient lubrication
	2.1 Proper size endotracheal tube and 15-mm adapter		17.4 With its curve to match laryngoscope (curve down)
	2.1 Stylet	18	Pass tube gently along side of mouth, down to and through vocal cords.
	2.3 Laryngoscope handle with proper size blade	19	Continue to insert tube until cuff is no longer visible past cords:
	2.4 10-ml syringe		19.1 In adults, if not cuffed, pass tip of tube 3 to 4 cm past cords.
	2.5 Water-soluble lubricant		19.2 In children under 6 months, if not cuffed, pass tip of tube no more than 1 cm past cords.
	2.6 Adhesive tape	20	Hold tube firmly in place with hand:
	2.6 Bite block		20.1 Withdraw laryngoscope
	2.8 Manual resuscitator with accessories		20.2 Withdraw stylet
	2.9 Magill forceps	21	Inflate cuff using either:
	2.10 Oxygen source and connecting tubing		21.1 MOV technique
	2.11 Oropharyngeal airways		21.2 MLV technique
	2.12 Suctioning equipment with accessories		21.3 Monitor cuff pressure (less than 25 mm Hg)
3	Wash hands.	22	If at *any* stage, intubation is unsuccessful:
4	Position patient for intubation according to Fig. 20-36, *A*.		22.1 Replace mask on patient's face.
	4.1 Place patient on back with face upward.		22.2 Ventilate and oxygenate with 100% oxygen.
	4.2 Slightly elevate head on a pad into "sniffing position."		22.3 Attempts without reoxygenation should last no longer than 15 seconds.
5	Place oropharyngeal airway, if necessary.	23	Auscultate chest for bilateral breath sounds, check lung bases as well as apices. Note bilateral chest expansion.
6	Ventilate and oxygenate patient with 100% oxygen using manual resuscitator, mask and airway.	24	Reposition tube if unequal sounds are heard or are absent.
7	Check laryngoscope to ensure proper operation.		24.1 Withdraw tube 1 to 2 cm if sounds are unequal.
8	With blade locked in place, grasp laryngoscope in one hand.		24.2 Remove tube immediately if esophageal intubation is suspected.
9	Use free hand to open patient's lips and move jaw.	25	Place bite block or oropharyngeal airway in mouth.
10	Insert blade along side of mouth, between teeth, to displace tongue.	26	Tape tube securely using around-the-head technique or an approved technique accepted at your hospital.
11	Advance blade inward and toward midline of the tongue.	27	Wash hands.
12	Advance blade and identify:		
	12.1 Base of tongue		
	12.2 Uvula		
	12.3 Epiglottis		
13	Once the epiglottis is seen, if a *straight blade* is used:		
	13.1 Advance so that blade tip barely passes epiglottis (see Fig. 20-34).		
	13.2 Do not advance too far; blade will go into esophagus.		
	13.3 Advance sufficiently so that tip of epiglottis does not slip off blade and cover glottis.		
14	Once the epiglottis is seen, if *curved blade* is used:		
	14.1 Advance blade tip into space between the base of tongue and epiglottis.		
	14.2 Lift the tip of the blade into this space (see Fig. 20-34).		

PROCEDURE 20-14

Passing an endotracheal tube using blind technique—nasal

No.	Steps in performing the procedure	No.	Steps in performing the procedure
	The practitioner will, under direct supervision, select and pass an endotracheal tube of the nasal-type in an adult patient. NOTE: This procedure should be taught by a physician, preferably an anesthesiologist, and practiced on a manikin or cadaver before working with patients.	9	Select nasal-length tube: **9.1** With pretested cuff **9.2** With sufficient lubrication (lidocaine jelly if available)
1	Justify need for endotracheal intubation: **1.1** Prevent aspiration in unconscious patient **1.2** Provide route for artificial ventilation **1.3** Airway patency cannot be assured using simpler methods	10	Introduce tube into patient's nose *parallel* to hard palate: **10.1** Withdraw tube and extend patient's head further if tube does not turn downward into pharynx.
2	Assemble and, where appropriate, test intubation materials: **2.1** Proper size endotracheal tube and 15-mm adapter **2.2** Stylet **2.3** Laryngoscope handle with proper size blade **2.4** 10-ml syringe **2.5** Water-soluble lubricant **2.6** Adhesive tape **2.7** Bite block **2.8** Manual resuscitator with accessories **2.9** Magill forceps **2.10** Oxygen source and connecting tubing **2.11** Oropharyngeal airways **2.12** Suctioning equipment with accessories	11	Close off other nostril and mouth so airflow will be directed through tube, causing audible airflow.
		12	Use airflow noise to continue to introduce tube. NOTE: The vocal cords are open during airflow. Do *not* push tube when there is no airflow.
		13	Recognize cough and/or outrush of air as indication of tracheal intubation.
		14	Withdraw tube completely. If airflow stops during intubation attempt: **14.1** Replace mask on patient's face. **14.2** Ventilate and oxygenate with manual resuscitator and 100% oxygen.
		15	Inflate cuff using either: **15.1** MOV technique **15.2** MLV technique **15.3** Monitor cuff pressure (less than 25 mm Hg)
		16	Auscultate chest for bilateral breath sounds, check lung bases as well as apices. Note bilateral chest expansion.
3	Wash hands.	17	Reposition tube if unequal sounds are heard or are absent: **17.1** Withdraw tube 1 to 2 cm if sounds are unequal. **17.2** Remove tube immediately if esophageal intubation is suspected.
4	Position patient for intubation according to Fig. 20-36, *A*. **4.1** Place patient on back with face upward. **4.2** Slightly elevate head on a pad into "sniffing position."		
5	Place oropharyngeal airway, if necessary.	18	Tape tube securely using around-the-head technique or an approved technique accepted at your hospital.
6	Ventilate and oxygenate patient with 100% oxygen using manual resuscitator, mask, and airway.		
7	Select most patent nostril.	19	Wash hands.
8	If available, spray nostril with vasoconstrictor spray (Neo-Synephrine, oxymetazoline).		

PROCEDURE 20-15

Passing an endotracheal tube under direct vision—nasal

No.	Steps in performing the procedure	No.	Steps in performing the procedure
	The practitioner will, under direct supervision, select and pass an endotracheal tube of the nasal-type in an adult patient. NOTE: This procedure should be taught by a physician, preferably an anesthesiologist, and practiced on a manikin or cadaver before working with patients.	10	Introduce tube into patient's nose *parallel* to hard palate: 10.1 Withdraw tube and extend patient's head further if tube does not turn downward into pharynx.
1	Justify need for endotracheal intubation: 1.1 Prevent aspiration in unconscious patient 1.2 Provide route for artificial ventilation 1.3 Airway patency cannot be assured using simpler methods	11	Once tube is in pharynx, insert laryngoscope.
		12	Insert blade along side of mouth, between teeth, to displace tongue.
		13	Advance blade inward and toward midline of the tongue.
2	Assemble and, where appropriate, test intubation materials: 2.1 Proper size endotracheal tube and 15-mm adapter 2.2 Stylet 2.3 Laryngoscope handle with proper size blade 2.4 10-ml syringe 2.5 Water-soluble lubricant 2.6 Adhesive tape 2.7 Bite block 2.8 Manual resuscitator with accessories 2.9 Magill forceps 2.10 Oxygen source and connecting tubing 2.11 Oropharyngeal airways 2.12 Suctioning equipment with accessories	14	Advance blade and identify: 14.1 Base of tongue 14.2 Uvula 14.3 Epiglottis
		15	Rotate proximal end of tracheal tube until tube is in midline of larynx.
		16	Advance tube into trachea until cuff disappears.
		17	Use Magill forceps, if necessary, to guide the distal end of tube through cords. The anesthesiologist will explain the use of this aid.
		18	Inflate cuff using either: 18.1 MOV technique 18.2 MLV technique 18.3 Monitor cuff pressure (less than 25 mm Hg)
3	Wash hands.	19	If at *any* stage, intubation is unsuccessful: 19.1 Replace mask on patient's face. 19.2 Ventilate and oxygenate with 100% oxygen. 19.3 Attempts without reoxygenation should last no longer than 15 seconds.
4	Position patient for intubation according to Fig. 20-36, *A*. 4.1 Place patient on back with face upward. 4.2 Slightly elevate head on a pad into "sniffing position."	20	Auscultate chest for bilateral breath sounds, check lung bases as well as apices. Note bilateral chest expansion.
5	Place oropharyngeal airway, if necessary.	21	Reposition tube if unequal sounds are heard or are absent. 21.1 Withdraw tube 1 to 2 cm if sounds are unequal. 21.2 Remove tube immediately if esophageal intubation is suspected.
6	Ventilate and oxgenate patient with 100% oxygen using manual resuscitator, mask and airway.		
7	Select most patent nostil.		
8	If available, spray nostril with vasoconstrictor spray (Neosynephrine, oxymetazoline).	22	Tape tube securely using around-the-head technique or an approved technique accepted at your hospital.
9	Select nasal-length tube: 9.1 With pretested cuff 9.2 With sufficient lubrication (lidocaine jelly if available)	23	Wash hands.

PROCEDURE 20-16

Perform tracheal suction using sterile technique

No.	Steps in performing the procedure	No.	Steps in performing the procedure
	The practitioner will perform tracheal suctioning under direct supervision and the aid of an assistant.		**12.2** Do *not* occlude thumb valve during insertion.
1	Check patient record for any special orders and/or complications of which to be aware.		**12.3** To direct catheter into left bronchus, patient's head should be turned to the right while inserting.
2	Collect suction equipment:		**12.4** To direct catheter into right bronchus, patient's head should be turned to the left while inserting.
	2.1 Sterile, disposable suction catheters		
	2.2 Sterile gloves		
	2.3 Sterile water or normal saline	13	Stop insertion when an obstruction is met or when the area to be suctioned is reached.
	2.4 Sterile basin	14	Occlude thumb control valve *intermittently* and withdraw catheter in one smooth, uninterrupted motion, rotating the catheter with fingertips as it is pulled out.
	2.5 Vacuum device with jar and collection tubing		
	2.6 Manual resuscitator with accessories		
	2.7 Oxygen source		
3	Obtain an assistant.		
4	Wash hands.	15	Do *not* apply suction for longer than 5 seconds at any time during the procedure. The entire procedure should *not* take more than 15 seconds.
5	Discuss procedure with patient. Reassure patient.		
6	Position patient for easy access and best results.		
7	Assemble suction equipment:	16	Constantly monitor patient during procedure; note ECG pattern if scope is available.
	7.1 Test vacuum device.		
	7.2 Open sterile water, pour some into basin.	17	After catheter is withdrawn, rinse with sterile water in the basin. Note the character of the secretions.
	7.3 Open sterile catheter package without contaminating catheter.	18	Ask the assistant to hyperinflate and oxygenate patient with manual resuscitator and 100% oxygen for 2 or 3 deep breaths.
	7.4 Open sterile glove package and don glove on dominate hand with contaminating glove.		
	7.5 Take catheter from opened package with gloved hand without contaminating catheter.	19	Reconnect patient to therapy equipment and wait at least 3 to 5 minutes before suctioning again, unless copious secretions are evident and blocking the airway.
	7.6 Hold suction collection tubing with ungloved hand and insert catheter with gloved hand without contaminating catheter.		
8	Grasp thumb control valve with ungloved thumb and hand, while holding catheter with gloved hand, and activate suction by occluding thumb valve.	20	Repeat steps 10 through 19 if additional suctioning is required. NOTE: A new sterile catheter should be used with each repetition.
		21	After the procedure is finished, coil the catheter in the gloved hand. Disconnect the thumb control valve from the suction collection tubing and pull the glove off, keeping the contaminated catheter inside the glove.
9	Check vacuum pressure by occluding catheter tip with gloved hand; note pressure and adjust with ungloved hand if necessary.		
10	Ask assistant to hyperinflate and oxygenate patient with manual resuscitator and 100% oxygen for 2 or 3 deep breaths.	22	Dispose of all contaminated equipment.
		23	Rinse the suction collection tubing again.
		24	Turn off vacuum device.
11	Ask assistant to remove manual resuscitator.	25	Assess the patient for untoward effects of the procedure.
12	Insert catheter, following natural "droop" into tracheal tube:	26	Wash hands.
	12.1 Insert using firm but gentle motion; do *not* force catheter.	27	Chart procedure according to departmental policy.

PROCEDURE 20-17

Perform oropharyngeal and nasopharngeal suctioning

No.	Steps in performing the procedure
	The practitioner will perform oropharyngeal and nasopharyngeal suctioning under direct supervision.
1	Check patient record for any special orders and/or complications of which to be aware.
2	Collection suction equipment:
	2.1 Sterile, disposable suction catheters
	2.2 Sterile gloves
	2.3 Sterile water or normal saline
	2.4 Sterile basin
	2.5 Vacuum device with jar and collection tubing
	2.6 Manual resuscitator with accessories
	2.7 Oxygen source
3	Wash hands.
4	Discuss procedure with patient. Reassure patient.
5	Position patient for easy access and best results.
6	Assemble suction equipment:
	6.1 Test vacuum device.
	6.2 Open sterile water; pour some into basin.
	6.3 Open sterile catheter package without contaminating catheter.
	6.4 Open sterile glove package and don glove on dominate hand without contaminating glove.
	6.5 Take catheter from opened package with gloved hand without contaminating catheter.
	6.6 Hold suction collection tubing with ungloved hand and insert catheter with gloved hand without contaminating catheter.
7	Grasp thumb control valve with ungloved thumb and hand while holding catheter with gloved hand; activate suction by occluding thumb valve.
8	Check vacuum pressure by occluding catheter tip with gloved hand; note pressure and adjust with ungloved hand if necessary.
9	Have patient take 6 to 8 deep breaths before suctioning, if the patient is conscious. If the patient is unconscious, use a manual resuscitator.
10	Insert the catheter into one nostril *parallel* to the hard palate, 4 to 6 inches.
11	Occlude the thumb control valve *intermittently* and withdraw the catheter.
12	Rinse the catheter with sterile water from the basin.
13	Repeat the procedure in the opposite nostril and/or mouth as necessary.
14	Reoxygenate following the procedure.
15	After the procedure is finished, coil the catheter in the gloved hand. Disconnect the thumb control valve from the suction collection tubing and pull the glove off, keeping the contaminated catheter inside the glove.
16	Dispose of all contaminated equipment.
17	Rinse the suction collection tubing again.
18	Turn off vacuum device.
19	Assess the patient for untoward effects of procedure.
20	Wash hands.
21	Chart procedure according to departmental policy.

BIBLIOGRAPHY

Acres JC and Kryger MH: Clinical significance of pulmonary function tests; upper airway obstruction, Chest 80:207, 1981.

American Heart Association: Standards and guidelines for cardiopulmonary resuscitation and emergency cardiac care, JAMA 255:2841, 1986.

Babinski MF et al: Animal and lung model studies of double-lumen tracheal tubes for high frequency ventilation, Respir Care 28:754, 1983.

Bishop MJ: Endotracheal tube lumen compromise from cuff overinflation, Chest 81:100, 1981.

Burton GG and Hodgkin JE, editors: Respiratory care; a guide to clinical practice, ed 2, Philadelphia, 1984, JB Lippincott Co.

Chatburn RL, McClellan LD, and Lough MD: A new patient circuit adaptor for use with high frequency jet ventilators, Respir Care 28:1291, 1983.

Demers RR: Complications of endotracheal suctioning procedures, Respir Care 27:453, 1982.

Handler SD et al: Unsuspected esophageal foreign bodies in adults with upper airway obstruction, Chest 80:234, 1981.

Heebink DM: Dr. Heimlich maneuvers again—this time with transtracheal oxygen therapy, Respir Care 27:1110, 1982.

Ishida T et al: Quantitative analysis of tracheal damage, Chest 11:283, 1983.

Jett JR, Cortese DA, and Dines DE: The value of bronchoscopy in the diagnosis of mycobacterial disease, Chest 80:575, 1981.

Keszler P and Buzna E: Surgical and conservative management of esophageal perforation, Chest 80:158, 1981.

Lundgren R, Haggmark S, and Reiz S: Hemodynamic effects of flexible fiberoptic bronchoscopy performed under topical anesthesia, Chest 82:295, 1982.

McPherson SP and Spearman CB: Respiratory therapy equipment, ed 4, St Louis, 1990, The CV Mosby Co.

Nakao MA, Killam D, and Wilson R: Pneumothorax secondary to inadvertent nasotracheal placement of a nasoenteric tube past a cuffed endotracheal tube, Crit Care Med 11:210, 1983.

Neff TA and Clifford D: A new monitoring tool—the ratio of the tracheostomy tube cuff diameter to the tracheal air column diameter (C/T ratio), Respir Care 28:1287, 1983.

Off D et al: Efficacy of the minimal leak technique of cuff inflation in maintaining proper intracuff pressures for patients with cuffed artificial airways, Respir Care 28:1115, 1983.

Simon RR and Brenner BE: Emergency crico-thyroidotomy in the patient with massive neck swelling, Part 1, anatomical aspects, Crit Care Med 11:114, 1983.

Simon RR, Brenner BE, and Rosen MA: Emergency cricothyroidotomy in the patient with massive neck swelling, Part 2, clinical aspects, Crit Care Med 11:119, 1983.

Smyth JA and Volgyesi GA: Simple device for measurement of mean airway pressure, Crit Care Med 11:130, 1983.

Snyder GM: Individualized placement of tracheostomy tube fenestration and in-situ examinations with the fiberoptic laryngoscope, Respir Care 28:1294, 1983.

Spearman CB, Sheldon RL, and Egan DE: Egan's fundamentals of respiratory therapy, ed 5, St Louis, 1990, The CV Mosby Co.

Stauffer JL and Silverstri RC: Complications of endotracheal intubation, tracheostomy and artificial airways, Respir Care 27:417, 1982.

Williams T and Thomas P: The diagnosis of pleural effusions by fiberoptic bronchoscopy and pleuroscopy, Chest 80:566, 1981.

Electrocardiogram recognition

On completion of this module the reader will be able to:

1.1 and **1.2** Explain the terms and concepts used in describing cardiac anatomy and function.

2.1 Point out the major divisions of the nervous system.

2.2 Discuss the functions of the autonomic nervous system.

2.3 Contrast the anatomy and physiology of the sympathetic and parasympathetic divisions of the autonomic nervous system.

2.4 Compare the sympathetic effects of alpha, beta$_1$, and beta$_2$ receptor sites.

2.5 Give an example of a drug in each of the following categories and summarize its actions with regard to the autonomic nervous system

    a Sympathomimetic

    b Parasympatholytic

    c Xanthine

2.6 Give examples of common cardiac drugs and explain their relationship to common respiratory therapy treatment drugs.

3.1 Name the chambers and valves of the heart.

3.2 Differentiate between systemic and pulmonary circulation.

3.3 Explain the relationship of systole and diastole to the cardiac cycle.

3.4 Name the three layers of the heart.

4.1 Trace the pathway of the coronary circulation system.

4.2 Explain the relationship between coronary circulation and the events of the cardiac cycle.

5.1 Name the two types of electric forces and explain their relationship to one another.

5.2 Explain the interaction of forces involved in maintaining a resting membrane potential.

5.3 Explain the relationship between coronary circulation and the events of the cardiac cycle.

5.1 Name the two types of electric forces and explain their relationship to one another.

5.2 Explain the interaction of forces involved in maintaining a resting membrane potential.

5.3 Explain the process involved in initiation of an action potential, including appropriate use of the vocabulary words "polarized," "depolarized," and "repolarized."

5.4 Differentiate between absolute refractory period and relative refractory period.

6.1 Name the structures of the cardiac conduction system.

6.2 Explain the influence of the autonomic nervous system on the cardiac conduction system.

7.1 Explain how the heart's electrical activity is transcribed onto an electrocardiogram (ECG).

7.2 Explain the use of ECG paper with regard to measurements of time and voltage.

8.1 Label each wave in a cardiac cycle in an ECG tracing of a normal pattern.

8.2 Determine whether the P-R interval and the QRS complex in a given ECG are of normal duration.

8.3 Name five possible causes of artifact on an ECG tracing.

8.4 List four steps in examining an ECG tracing.

9.1 Explain the normal correlation between the waves and intervals of an ECG pattern and events of the cardiac cycle.

10.1 Recognize the lethal arrhythmias, especially ventricular tachycardia, ventricular fibrillation, and ventricular standstill.

10.2 Discuss transvenous pacing and identify the characteristic spike of a cardiac pacemaker on an ECG strip or monitor.

10.3 Describe circumstances that mimic lethal arrhythmias.

10.4 Identify the difference between normal sinus rhythm and an abnormal ECG pattern.

11.1 Know the characteristic ECG changes associated with abnormal potassium and calcium levels.

12.1 Name seven risk factors in the development of coronary heart disease (or coronary artery disease) and the disease process of atherosclerosis.

12.2 Differentiate between angina pectoris and a myocardial infarction.

12.3 List the data necessary in diagnosing a myocardial infarction.

13.1 List the sources and types of information necessary to obtain from a patient's chart with regard to cardiac status before beginning prescribed respiratory care.

13.2 Explain the purpose of consulting other health care team members regarding patient condition before beginning the prescribed respiratory care.

13.3 List the direct patient observations necessary before beginning a respiratory care treatment.

13.4 Gather information pertinent to a patient's cardiac status according to standard procedure.

14.1 Compare benefits of resting versus stress ECG.

This module will begin with a review of necessary background information before proceeding to actual instruction in the interpretation of ECGs. The knowledge and skills gained will then be related to clinical practice situations.

1.0 CARDIAC ANATOMY AND PHYSIOLOGY

1.1 Terms and concepts

NOTE: It may be helpful if the reader has access to a medical dictionary such as *Mosby's Medical, Nursing, & Allied Health Dictionary** when studying this module.

The terms and concepts defined below are grouped according to the unit in which they will be discussed.

1 Medications and the autonomic nervous system (Unit 2.1)
  a Distal. Farther from any point of reference (i.e., at the far end from the center of the body).
  b Ganglion. Groups of nerve cells located outside the central nervous system (CNS).
  c Neuroeffector. The organ, gland, or muscle on which a nerve has influence, or on which it produces an effect.
  d Neurotransmitter. A substance released at the synapse of a neuron that induces activity in susceptible cells.
  e Postganglionic. Distal to a ganglion.
  f Preganglionic. Proximal to the ganglion.
  g Proximal. Nearest to the center of the body.
  h Synapse. The functional junction between two neurons, where a nerve impulse is transmitted from one neuron to another (neuron = nerve cell).

2 Chambers and valves of the heart (Unit 3.1)
  a Aortic valve. Guards the orifice between the left ventricle and the aorta.
  b Atrium. Upper chamber of the heart that receives blood and transfers it to the ventricle on the same side of the heart.
  c Mitral valve. The two-cusped structure (valve) between the left atrium and the left ventricle, sometimes called the "bicuspid valve."

  d Pulmonary valve. The pocketlike structure that guards the orifice between the right ventricle and the pulmonary artery.
  e Tricuspid valve. A three-cusped, one-way valve between the right atrium and right ventricle.
  f Ventricle. Lower chamber of the heart that receives blood from the atrium. The right ventricle then pumps blood to the pulmonary circulation, and the left ventricle pumps blood out to the aorta and the systemic circulation.

3 Circulatory systems (Unit 3.2)
  a Pulmonary system. Formed by the pulmonary artery, pulmonary veins, and all the vessels surrounding the alveoli in the lungs.
  b Systemic circulation. All the vessels of the body except the pulmonary vessels.

4 Cardiac cycle (Unit 3.3)
  a Diastole. The filling phase of the cardiac cycle; the passive state when blood is being received in the heart chambers.
  b Systole. Contraction of the muscles; active pumping by a heart chamber.

5 Layers of the heart (Unit 3.4)
  a Endocardium. The inner layer of the heart that lines the heart chambers; this layer is very thin.
  b Epicardium. The outer layer of the heart; this layer is also quite thin.
  c Myocardium. The actual heart muscle; it makes up most of the mass of the heart and is the middle layer.

6 Coronary circulation (Unit 4.1)
  a Coronary veins. Vessels that carry deoxygenated blood from the coronary circulation back to the right atrium.
  b Left coronary artery. One of the two main vessels; it serves the left side of the heart and has two main branches—the anterior descending artery and the circumflex artery.
  c Right coronary artery. One of the two main vessels; it serves the right side of the heart. Its two parts are the right main posterior descending coronary artery and the marginal artery.
  d Valsalva's sinus. An opening just beyond the aortic valve that is the entry to the coronary circulatory system.

7 Electric forces (Unit 5.1)
  a Charge. Electric energy occurring in two forms; it is designated arbitrarily as positive and negative.
  b Electricity. The class of physical phenomena arising from the existence and interaction of an electric charge.

8 Chemical principles (Unit 5.2)
  a Active transport. The movement of ions or molecules across the cell membrane and epithelial layers, usually against a concentration gradient, resulting directly from the expenditure of metabolic energy.
  b Concentration gradient. The tendency to move from an area of greater concentration to an area of lower concentration.

---

*Mosby's medical, nursing, & allied health dictionary, ed 3, St Louis, 1990, The CV Mosby Co.

c Diffusion. The movement of solute, solvent, and gas molecules in all directions in a solution or in both directions through a freely permeable cell membrane.

d Electrolytes. Particles that, when dissolved in solution, carry an electric charge. For example, $NaCL \rightarrow Na^+$ and Cl^-.

e Equilibrium potential. The dynamic balance between electric forces; measured in millivolts.

f Ion. An atom or group of atoms having a charge of positive (cation) or negative (anion) electricity by virtue of having gained or lost an electron and of forming one of the elements of an electrolyte.

g Resting membrane potential. The electrical difference across a cell membrane (measured in millivolts) when the cell is not physiologically active.

9 Action potential (Unit 5.3)

a Action potential. The rapid change of membrane potential; only nerve and muscle cells are capable of producing action potentials.

b Depolarize. The process or act of neutralizing polarity. The membrane potential is said to be depolarized when the membrane potential is less negative than the resting membrane potential, (i.e., closer to zero).

c Excitability. The property or capability of producing action potentials.

d Hyperpolarize. When the membrane potential is more negative than the resting level.

e Polarity. The condition of having opposite effects at the two extremities; with regard to the cell membrane, it refers to the condition of opposite sides of the membrane having opposite charges.

f Repolarize. Following depolarization, when the cell membrane moves back toward its resting potential.

10 Refractory periods (Unit 5.4)

a Absolute refractory period. The period of depolarization and repolarization of the cell membrane that takes place after excitation and during which the nerve or muscle fiber cannot respond to a second stimulus.

b Relative refractory period. The period of depolarization and repolarization of the cell membrane after excitation during which it can respond only to a strong stimulus.

c Threshold. The level that must be reached for an effect to be produced; the degree of depolarization that must occur before an action potential is fired.

11 Cardiac conduction system (Unit 6.1)

a Atrial conducting tracts. Pathways for impulses to travel from the sinoatrial (SA) node to the atrioventricular (AV) node.

b Atrioventricular node (AV node). Specialized tissue located at the base of the intra-atrial septum, near the tricuspid valve.

c Bundle branches (right and left). Conducting tissues that travel down the interventricular septum and out into the respective ventricles; divisions of the bundle of His.

d Bundle of His. The first conducting tract of the ventri-

cles; located immediately below the AV node.

e Purkinje fibers. A complex fiber network of conducting tissue that transmits impulses to the individual muscle fibers of the ventricles.

f Sinoatrial node (SA node). Specific group of cells located in the right atrium; the normal pacemaker of the heart.

12 Arrhythmias (Unit 10.1)

a Cardioversion. The application of a high-voltage shock of very brief duration through the chest wall. The purpose is to suddenly stop the chaotic electric activity within the heart in order to permit the heart's natural pacemaker to regain command so that the heart can once again function efficiently. It is used as a lifesaving emergency measure to terminate ventricular fibrillation (defibrillation) or as an elective or voluntary measure to convert certain atrial and ventricular tachyarrhythmias (cardioversion) to normal rhythm. The cardioversion may require about 7000 V. Because it is administered for such short duration, it does not injure the heart.

b Defibrillation. Emergency cardioversion (see *a*).

c Defibrillator. Device used to administer the electric shock in emergency cardioversion.

d Precordial shock. Cardioversion (see *a*).

13 Chemical imbalances (Unit 11.1)

a Diuretics. A classification of medications that increase urine excretion or the amount of urine. They are prescribed primarily to rid the body of excess fluid.

b Edema. Excess fluid accumulation in the tissues that causes swelling.

1.2 Glossary

Other terms encountered in discussions of the heart are listed here alphabetically.

1 Adams-Stokes syndrome. Sudden attack of unconsciousness, sometimes with convulsions, that may accompany heart block.

2 Adrenalin. One of the secretions of two small glands, called adrenal glands, located just above the kidneys. This secretion, which is also called epinephrine and which is sometimes prepared synthetically, constricts the small blood vessels (arterioles), increases the heart rate, and raises blood pressure. It is called a "vasoconstrictor" or "vasopressor substance."

3 Angina pectoris. Literally means "chest pain." A condition in which the heart muscle receives an insufficient blood supply, causing pain in the chest and often in the left arm and shoulder. Commonly results when the arteries supplying the heart muscle (coronaries) are narrowed by atherosclerosis (See definition of coronary atherosclerosis.)

4 Angiocardiography. An x-ray examination of the heart and great blood vessels that follows the course of an opaque fluid that has been injected into the bloodstream.

5 Anticoagulant. A drug that delays clotting of the blood. When given in cases of a blood vessel plugged up by a clot, it tends to prevent new clots from forming or the existing clots from enlarging, but it does not dissolve an existing clot. Examples are heparin and warfarin (Coumadin).

6 Antihypertensive agents. Drugs that are used to lower blood pressure, such as rauwolfia, reserpine, veratrum, hydralazine, and hezamethonium chloride.

7 Aortic insufficiency. An improper closing of the valve between the aorta and the lower left chamber of the heart that admits a back flow of blood.

8 Aortic stenosis. A narrowing of the valve opening between the lower left chamber of the heart and the large artery called the "aorta." The narrowing may occur at the valve itself or slightly above or below the valve. Aortic stenosis may be the result of scar tissue forming after a rheumatic fever infection, or it may have other causes.

9 Aortography. An x-ray examination of the aorta (the main artery conducting blood from the lower left chamber of the heart to the body) and its main branches. This is made possible by the injection of a dye that is opaque to x-rays.

10 Bacterial endocarditis. An inflammation of the inner layer of the heart caused by bacteria. The lining of the heart valves is most frequently affected. It is most commonly a complication of an infectious disease, operation, or injury.

11 "Blue babies." Babies that have cyanosis as a result of insufficient oxygen in the arterial blood. This often indicates a heart defect but may have other causes, such as premature birth or impaired respiration.

12 Bradycardia. An abnormally slow heart rate. Generally anything below 60 beats/min is considered bradycardia.

13 Cardiac cycle. One total heartbeat (i.e., one complete contraction and relaxation of the heart). In humans this normally occupies about 0.85 second.

14 Cardiac output. The amount of blood pumped by the heart per minute.

15 Carditis. Inflammation of the heart.

16 Carotid sinus. A slight dilation at the point where the internal carotid artery branches from the common carotid artery. The carotid arteries are those arteries that supply blood to the head and neck. The carotid sinus contains special nerve end organs that respond to a change in blood pressure by causing a change in the rate of heartbeat. External pressure on the carotid sinus (carotid massage) by stimulating some of the nerves in the sinus can also cause a drop in blood pressure and fainting.

17 Catheter. A diagnostic device used to take samples of blood or to take pressure readings within the heart chambers that might reveal defects in the heart. It is a thin tube of woven plastic or other material to which blood will not adhere. It is inserted in a vein or artery, usually in the arm, and threaded into the heart. The catheter is guided by the physician who watches the progress by radiographic means.

18 Catheterization. In cardiology the process of examining the heart by means of introducing a catheter into a vein or artery and passing it into the heart.

19 Cerebral vascular accident (CVA). Sometimes called "cerebrovascular accident," "apoplectic stroke," or simply "stroke." An impeded blood supply to some part of the brain, generally caused by one of the following four conditions:

a Formation of a blood clot in the vessel (cerebral thrombosis)

b Rupture of the blood vessel wall (cerebral hemorrhage)

c Obstruction of a cerebral vessel (cerebral embolism) by a piece of clot or other material from another part of the vascular system that flows to the brain

d Pressure on a blood vessel as by a tumor

20 Coarctation of the aorta. Literally a pressing together or a narrowing of the aorta, which is the main trunk artery and which conducts blood from the heart to the body. One of several types of congenital heart defects.

21 Commissurotomy. An operation to widen the opening in a heart valve that has become narrowed by scar tissue. The individual flaps of the valve are cut or spread apart along the natural line of their closure. This operation is often performed in cases of rheumatic heart disease. (See definition of mitral valvulotomy.)

22 Congestive heart failure. When the heart is unable to adequately pump out all the blood that returns to it, there is a backing up of blood in the veins leading to the heart. A congestion or accumulation of fluid in various parts of the body (lungs, legs, abdomen, etc.) may result from the heart's failure to maintain a satisfactory circulation.

23 Coronary atherosclerosis. Commonly called "coronary heart disease." An irregular thickening of the inner layer of the walls of the arteries that conduct blood to the heart muscle. The internal channels of these arteries (the coronaries) become narrowed, and the blood supply to the heart muscle is reduced.

24 Coronary occlusion. An obstruction (generally a blood clot) in a branch of one of the coronary arteries that hinders the flow of blood to some part of the heart muscle. This part of the heart muscle then dies because of lack of blood supply. Sometimes called a "coronary heart attack" or simply a "heart attack."

25 Coronary thrombosis. Formation of a clot in a branch of one of the arteries that conducts blood to the heart muscle (coronary arteries). A form of coronary occlusion. (See definition of coronary occlusion.)

26 Cor pulmonale. Heart disease resulting from disease of the lungs or the blood vessels in the lungs. This is a result of resistance to the passage of blood through the lungs, causing right-sided heart hypertrophy.

27 Decompensation. Inability of the heart to maintain adequate circulation, usually resulting in a waterlogging of tissues (edema). A person whose heart is failing to

maintain normal circulation is said to be "decompensated."

28 Dextrocardia. Two different types of congenital phenomena are often described as dextrocadia. The first is a condition in which the heart is slightly rotated and lies almost entirely in the right (instead of the left) side of the chest. The second is a condition in which there is a complete transposition; the left chambers of the heart being on the right side and the right chambers on the left side, so that the heart presents a mirror image of the normal heart.

29 Digitalis. A drug prepared from leaves of the foxglove plant *(Digitalis purpurea)* that strengthens the contraction of the heart muscle, slows the rate of contraction of the heart, and by improving the efficiency of the heart, may promote the elimination of fluid from body tissues.

30 Ductus arteriosus. A small duct in the heart of the fetus between the artery leaving the left side of the heart (aorta) and the artery leaving the right side of the heart (pulmonary artery). Normally this duct closes soon after birth. If it does not close, the condition is known as patent or open ductus arteriosus.

31 Electrolyte. Any substance that, in solution, is capable of conducting electricity by means of its atoms or groups of atoms and that in the process is broken down into positively and negatively charged particles. Examples, sodium or potassium.

32 Embolism. The blocking of a blood vessel by a clot or other substance carried in the bloodstream.

33 Endocarditis. Inflammation of the inner layer of the heart (endocardium) usually associated with acute rheumatic fever or some infectious agent.

34 Essential hypertension. Sometimes called "primary hypertension" and commonly known as "high blood pressure." An elevated blood pressure not caused by kidney or other evident disease.

35 Extrasystole. A contraction of the heart that occurs prematurely and interrupts the normal rhythm.

36 Fluoroscopy. The examination of a structure deep in the body by means of observing the fluorescence of a screen caused by x-rays transmitted through the body.

37 Foramen ovale. An oval hole between the left and right upper chambers of the heart that normally closes shortly after birth. Its failure to close is one of the congenital defects of the heart, called a "patent foramen ovale."

38 Gallop rhythm. An extra, clearly heard heart sound that, when the heart rate is fast, resembles a horse's gallop. It may or may not be significant.

39 Heart block. Interference with the conduction of the electrical impulses of the heart that can be either partial or complete. This can result in dissocation of the rhythms of the upper and lower heart chambers.

40 Hypertrophy. The enlargement of a tissue or organ as a result of an increase in the size of its constituent cells. This may result from a demand for increased work.

41 Hypothermia. The lowering of the body temperature (usually to 86° to 88° F in order to slow the metabolic processes during heart surgery. In this cooled state, body tissues require less oxygen.

42 Iatrogenic heart disease. Literally means "caused by the doctor." A patient's belief that he has heart disease implied from the actions, manner, or discussions of the physician or some member of the medical team.

43 Incompetent valve. Any valve that does not close tightly and that leaks blood back in the wrong direction; also called "valvular insufficiency."

44 Insufficiency. Incompetency. An improper closing of the valves that admits a back flow of blood in the wrong direction. Myocardial insufficiency is an inability of the heart muscle to do a normal pumping job.

45 Ischemia. A local, usually temporary, deficiency of blood in some part of the body. Often caused by a constriction or an obstruction in the blood vessel supplying that part.

46 Mitral insufficiency. An improper closing of the mitral valve between upper and lower chambers in the left side of the heart that admits a back flow of blood in the wrong direction. Sometimes the result of scar tissue forming after a rheumatic fever infection.

47 Mitral stenosis. A narrowing of the valve (called "bicuspid" or "mitral" valve) opening between the upper and the lower chamber in the left side of the heart. Sometimes the result of scar tissue forming after a rheumatic fever infection.

48 Mitral valvulotomy. An operation to widen the opening in the valve between the upper and lower chambers in the left side of the heart (mitral valve). Usually performed when the valve opening is so narrowed as to obstruct blood flow, which sometimes happens as a result of rheumatic fever.

49 Murmur. An abnormal heart sound, sounding like fluid passing an obstruction, heard between the normal "lub-dub" heart sounds.

50 Nitroglycerin. A drug (one of the nitrates) that relaxes the muscles in the blood vessels. Often used to relieve attacks of angina pectoris and spasm of coronary arteries; it is one of the vasodilators.

51 Noradrenalin. An organic compound that produces a rise in blood pressure by constricting the small blood vessels. Sometimes used in the treatment of shock; also called "norepinephrine" and "Levarterenol."

52 Pacemaker. A small mass of specialized cells in the right upper chamber of the heart that give rise to the electric impulses that initiate contractions of the heart. Also called "SA node of Keith-Flack." The terms "pacemaker," or more exactly, "electric cardiac pacemaker," or "electrical pacemaker" are applied to an electric device that can substitute for a defective natural pacemaker and control the beating of the heart by a series of rhythmic electric discharges. If the electrodes that deliver the discharges to the heart are placed on the outside of the chest, it is called an "external pacemaker." If the electrodes are placed within the chest wall, it is called an "internal pacemaker."

53 Palpitation. A fluttering of the heart or abnormal rate or rhythm of the heart experienced by the person himself.

54 Pancarditis. Inflammation of the whole heart including inner layer (endocardium), heart muscle (myocardium), and outer sac (pericardium).

55 Pericarditis. Inflammation of the thin membrane sac (pericardium) that surrounds the heart.

56 Phlebitis. Inflammation of a vein, often in the leg. Sometimes a blood clot is formed in the inflamed vein.

57 Rheumatic fever. A disease, usually occurring in childhood, that may follow a few weeks after a streptococcal infection. It is sometimes characterized by one or more of the following: fever, sore swollen joints, a skin rash, occasionally by involuntary twitching of the muscles (called "chorea" or "St. Vitus Dance") and small nodes under the skin. In some cases the infection affects the heart and may result in scarring the valves, weakening the heart muscle, or damaging the sac enclosing the heart.

58 Stasis. A stoppage or slackening of the bloodflow.

59 Stenosis. A narrowing or stricture of an opening. Mitral stenosis, aortic stenosis, etc., means that the valve indicated has become narrowed so that it does not function normally.

60 Stroke volume. The amount of blood that is pumped out of the heart at each contraction of the heart.

61 Tachycardia. Abnormally fast heart rate. Generally anything over 100 beats/min is considered a tachycardia.

62 Tetralogy of Fallot. A congenital malformation of the heart involving four distinct defects (hence, tetralogy). Named for Etienne Fallot, French physician who described the condition in 1988. The four defects are
  a An abnormal opening in the wall between the lower chambers of the heart
  b Misplacement of the aorta, "overriding" the abnormal opening, so that it receives blood from both the right and left lower chambers instead of only the left
  c Narrowing of the pulmonary artery
  d Enlargement of the right lower chamber of the heart

63 Thrombectomy. An operation to remove a blood clot from a blood vessel.

64 Thrombophlebitis. Inflammation and blood clotting in a vein.

65 Thrombosis. The formation or presence of a blood clot (thrombus) inside a blood vessel or cavity of the heart.

66 Thrombus. A blood clot that forms inside a blood vessel or cavity of the heart.

67 Vasoconstrictor. The vasoconstrictor nerves are one part of the involuntary nervous system. When these nerves are stimulated, they cause muscles of the arterioles to contract, thus narrowing the arteriole passage, increasing the resistance to the flow of blood, and raising the blood pressure. Chemical substances that stimulate the muscles of the arterioles to contract are called "vasoconstrictor agents" or "vasopressors." An example is epinephrine.

68 Vasodilator. Vasodilator nerves are certain nerve fibers of the involuntary nervous system that cause muscles of the arterioles to relax, thus enlarging the arteriole passage, reducing resistance to the flow of blood, and lowering blood pressure. Vasodilator agents are chemical compounds that cause a relaxation of the muscles of the arterioles. Examples of this type of drug are nitroglycerin, nitrites, thiocyanate, and many others.

2.0 EFFECTS OF THE AUTONOMIC NERVOUS SYSTEM AND OF COMMON RESPIRATORY THERAPY MEDICATIONS ON THE CARDIOPULMONARY SYSTEM

2.1 Divisions of the nervous system

A basic principle of the sciences is that energy can be changed from one form into another. For example, running water can be dammed and its energy used to generate electricity. In the body, energy is constantly being changed from one form to another (e.g., the electric impulses of the cardiac conduction system are changed into mechanical energy as they stimulate the heart muscle to contract, pumping blood out of the heart chambers). This unit will review the mechanisms involved in the *autonomic nervous system*, especially as it relates to the cardiopulmonary system.

1 The nervous system is very complex and has been divided into these major categories:
  a Central nervous system
    • Brain
    • Spinal cord
  b Peripheral nervous system
    • Sensory (afferent)
    • Motor (efferent)
    • Autonomic
      – Parasympathetic
      – Sympathetic

2 The brain and spinal cord together are called the "central nervous system" (CNS). All other nerves in the body have been labeled as the "peripheral nervous system." There are so many nerves performing such varied functions that they have been further subcategorized according to the function and the way they are structured.

3 The autonomic nervous system is one division of the peripheral nervous system. The autonomic system has been divided into the sympathetic and parasympathetic branches.

2.2 Functions of the autonomic nervous system

1 The autonomic nervous system is like an "automatic pilot." It runs the body's functions in a reflex manner and requires no conscious thought to do so. For example, it is not necessary to concentrate on breathing or digesting food. The autonomic system adapts to circumstances by balancing the opposing forces of the parasymethatic and sympathetic systems automatically.

2 The sympathetic system takes charge (i.e., has predominant influence) whenever there is danger (or anger, or excitement) as if preparing to fight an enemy or run from danger. The heart speeds up, digestion slows,

the blood pressure increases, and the bronchial muscles dilate and relax.

3 The parasympathetic system functions as the "at ease" system and has predominance during calmer times. It stimulates digestion, the heart slows to a normal rate, blood pressure is normal, and bronchioles constrict.

4 Many of the glands and smooth muscles of the body are innervated by both parasympathetic *and* sympathetic nerves, and the one that influences the gland or smooth muscle at any particular time depends on the circumstances (i.e., is the person relaxed or afraid?). Table 21-1 shows autonomic effects on various organs of the body and at different sites.

2.3 The comparative anatomy and physiology of the sympathetic and parasympathetic divisions of the autonomic nervous system (See also Module Four)

1 Sympathetic system

a The sympathetic nerves leave the spinal cord in the thoracolumbar region. The preganglionic fiber is short and synapses (connects) with a long postganglionic fiber. When the sympathetic nerve impulse reaches the ganglionic synapse, it causes acetylcholine to be released from small vesicles in the end of the preganglionic nerve.

b The acetylcholine crosses the synapse to the postganglionic fiber, initiating the action potential. When the impulse reaches the end of the postganglionic fiber that is the neuroeffector site (the destination of the sympathetic impulse—a smooth muscle or gland) norepinephrine is released.

c Norepinephrine and acetylcholine are called *neurotransmitters,* because they are chemical carriers of the impulse from one nerve to another.

2 Parasympathetic system.

a The parasympathetic nerves leave the spinal cord in the cranial region and in the sacral region, hence they are called "craniosacral" nerves. The preganglionic fiber is long, reaching almost to the neuroeffector site.

b At its synapse with the short postganglionic fiber, the ganglionic synapse, acetylcholine is the neurotransmitter—just as in the sympathetic branch. However, the neurotransmitter at the parasympathetic neuroeffector site is acetylcholine—unlike the sympathetic branch (Fig. 21-1).

2.4 Categories of sympathetic receptor sites

1 Sympathetic neuroeffector sites have been categorized acording to their reaction to several drugs as either alpha, $beta_1$, or $beta_2$. The classification is useful because it permits the practitioner to know *which* of the

TABLE 21-1 Autonomic effects

Organ	Parasympathetic effect	Sympathetic effect
Heart	Slowed rate, decreased force of atrial beat	Increased rate, increased force of beat
Coronary arteries	Constricted	Dilated
Bronchioles	Constricted	Dilated
Sweat glands	None	Profuse sweating
Kidney	None	Decreased output
Liver	None	Glucose released
Gut		
Lumen	Increased peristalsis, tone	Decreased peristalsis, tone
Sphincter	Decreased tone	Increased tone
Pupil of eye	Contracted	Dilated

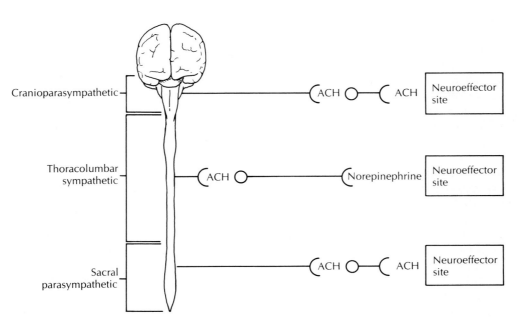

FIGURE 21-1 Sites of origin of sympathetic and parasympathetic divisions of the autonomic nervous system and their neurotransmitter substance.

sympathetic effects a particular drug will have on a patient according to its classification as having alpha, beta$_1$, and/or beta$_2$ effects.

2 Alpha receptors generally "excite" when they are stimulated by their sympahetic nerves (except the intestines).

3 Beta receptors generally relax the effector organ or site (except the heart).

  a Beta$_1$ receptors increase the rate and force of cardiac contraction.

  b Beta$_2$ receptors relax bronchial smooth muscle.

4 Table 21-2 presents autonomic nervous system effects on the cardiopulmonary system.

2.5 Examples of sympathomimetic, parasympatholytic, and xanthine drugs commonly used in respiratory care* (See also Module Fifteen)

1 Sympathomimetics

  a Isoproterenol (Isuprel). One of the purest beta stimulants (both beta$_1$ and beta$_2$). Administration results in bronchial smooth muscle relaxation, pulmonary vasodilation, and cardiac excitation. Hazards include an initial increase in blood pressure and tachycardia.

  b Metaproterenol sulfate (Alupent, Metaprel). An analogue of isoproterenol. It is $\frac{1}{20}$ to $\frac{1}{40}$ as strong, but it is primarily a beta$_2$ stimulator. Therefore it gives bronchodilation with minimum effect on the heart.

  c Terbutaline sulfate (Bricanyl, Brethine). Another analogue of isoproterenol. It is preferential beta$_2$ stimulant.

  d Isoetharine (Bronkosol). A preferential beta$_2$ stimulant. Isoetharine gives bronchodilation with minimum cardiac side effects. It is $\frac{1}{64}$ to $\frac{1}{16}$ as strong as isoproterenol with regard to its bronchial action, but it has 300 times *less* effect on the heart.

  e Albuterol (Proventil, Ventolin). A longer-acting, primarily beta$_2$ stimulator. It gives bronchodilation with minimum effect on the heart.

2 Parasympatholytics

  a Atropine. Atrophine blocks parasympathetic influence. It promotes bronchodilation by blocking parasympathetic influence rather than by stimulating sympathetic activity. It has commonly been used as a preoperative medication with the intention of drying the excessive secretions and combating bradycardia of anesthesia.

3 Xanthines

  a Theophylline ethylenediamine (aminophylline). This drug acts most predominantly in bronchial dilation, smooth muscle relaxation, cardiac stimulation, pulmonary vasodilation, and coronary vasodilation. it does not act directly on the beta receptors but rather interferes with the metabolism of the neurotransmitters.

---

*Review respiratory care drugs in Module Fifteen.

TABLE 21-2 Autonomic nervous system effects on the cardiopulmonary system

Site	Parasympathetic	Sympathetic
Heart	Decreased rate and force	Beta$_1$ increased force, conduction, and rate
Lungs		
Bronchial smooth muscle	Constricts	Beta$_2$ relaxes (dilates)
Circulation	Vasodilation	Alpha and beta
Bronchial mucous glands	Vagus secretion	
Systemic circulation		
Peripheral (dermal)	Vasodilation	Alpha constricts
Skeletal muscle		Beta dilates
Coronary		Beta dilates

2.6 Common cardiac drugs relevant to respiratory care

1 Digitalis preparations (digoxin [Lanoxin])

  a Digitalis is a pure cyrstalline glycoside that occurs in nature in the purple foxglove plant. The synthetic preparations decrease the undesirable side effects. Digitalis acts to decrease the heart rate and at the same time strengthen the force of each contraction. Although the complete mechanism of action is not understood, it is known that it slows the heart partly by raising the vagal tone (stimulating parasympathetic influence), increases the duration of the action potential, and slows the rate of impulse conduction from the SA to the AV node.

  b Digitalis is used in the treatment of heart failure and may be used in the treatment of atrial tachyarrhythmias such as atrial fibrillation and flutter.

  c Toxic levels (overdose) are reflected in exaggerations of the therapeutic effects—excessive slowing of heart rate and excessive slowing or blocking of impulse conduction (e.g., first-degree heart block). The medication is usually not given if the heart rate has been slowed to 60 beats/min. The pulse should be checked before administration of each scheduled dose.

    • Symptoms of digitalis overdose may be countered by administration of isoproterenol or atropine, if the situation indicates immediate action.

2 Quinidine (from quinine) and procainamide (from procaine)

  a These drugs bind to the cell membrane and prevent the ready movment of cations (such as sodium) across it. As a result, depolarization takes longer, and conduction of the action potential is slowed. The refractory period is also increased during repolarization because the drugs make it difficult for potassium to leave the cell.

  b Quinidine and procainamide also act as anticholinergics. The patient taking these medications may have an increase in heart rate, which is undesirable for patients with myocardial infarction, if he or she

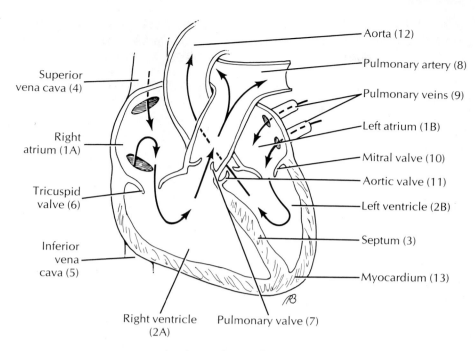

F I G U R E 2 1 - 2 Chambers, valves, and major blood vessels of the heart.

is not digitalized before these medications are begun. Starting quinidine administration after a patient is digitalized with digoxin can cause digitalis toxicity and should not be considered in such circumstances.

  c The effect of these drugs is to decrease the likelihood of ectopic beats. They are most useful in cardiac conditions characterized by very rapid ventricular rates.

  d Side effects of quinidine include ringing in the ears, blurring of vision, and gastrointestinal disturbances. Overdose can produce serious difficulties, such as AV block, reduced strength of contractions, and ultimately cardiac arrest.

3 Lidocaine hydrochloride (Xylocaine)

  a This drug is an antiarrhythmic, but it is also classified as a local anesthetic. It is used to prevent or treat ventricular tachycardia. Whenever dangerous premature ventricular contractions occur in the adult patient, a bolus of lidocaine (50 to 100 mg IV) is given and followed by a continuous IV infusion of lidocaine.

  b It has no effect on sodium transport during depolarization and no effect on conduction velocity. It enhances potassium escape from the cell during repolarization, thus shortening the refractory period.

  c CNS side effects from large doses of lidocaine over long periods of time (as in a cardiac care unit [CCU]) include convulsions and coma.

4 Propanolol (Inderal)

  a This drug has a beta-blocking effect. It decreases the force of heart contraction, thereby decreasing the work of the heart. For that reason, it has been used in the treatment of patients with angina pectoris.

However, it is contraindicated if the patient is suffering from heart failure.

  b It decreases automaticity and conduction velocity but shortens the refractory period. It is most useful in the treatment of supraventricular tachyarrhythmias that are not induced by digitalis.

5 Propanolol should be administered with caution in situations where patients are receiving other drugs, such as aerosolized atropine.

3.0 THE MECHANICAL SYSTEM OF THE HEART
3.1 The chambers and valves of the heart (Fig. 21-2 and Module Four)

1 The heart is divided into two separate sides—the right side, *A,* and the left side, *B.* Each side is further divided into an atrium and a ventricle *(1A/2A, 1B/2B).* The two sides are separated by a septum *(3).*

2 The right atrium *(1A)* receives deoxygenated blood (venous blood) from the body by way of the superior vena cava *(4)* and the inferior vena cava *(5).*

3 The right atrium pumps the blood through the *tricuspid valve (6)* and into the right ventricle *(2A).*

4 The right ventricle pumps blood out through the *pulmonary valve (7)* and into the pulmonary artery, which branches out to each lung *(8).* The blood then goes to the lungs where it is oxygenated. The oxygenated blood returns to the left atrium *(1B)* by way of left and right pulmonary veins *(9).*

5 The left atrium pumps blood through the *mitral valve (10)* and into the left ventricle *(2B).* The left ventricle pumps the oxygenated blood out through the *aortic valve (11),* into the aorta *(12),* and out through the rest of the body by the descending aorta.

3.2 Pulmonary versus systemic circulatory systems

1 The function of the atria is to receive blood into the heart; the function of the ventricle is to pump blood out of the heart.

2 The right side of the heart serves the *pulmonary circulatory system,* which is a relatively low-pressure system formed by the pulmonary artery, pulmonary veins, and the vessels surrounding the alveoli in the lungs.

3 The left side of the heart serves the *systemic circulation* and is made up of all the vessels in the body not included in the definition of pulmonary circulation.

3.3 Systole and diastole related to the cardiac cycle

1 Both atria contract at the same time, pushing blood into their respective ventricles. After the ventricles have received blood from the atria, they contract at the same time.

2 One sequence of both atria and then both ventricles contracting is a heartbeat, or one *cardiac cycle.*

3 Atrial systole occurs before ventricular systole. While the ventricles are contracting, the atria are in diastole, and when the atria are in systole, the ventricles are in diastole.

3.4 The three layers of the heart

1 The heart is located in the anterior inferior mediastinum, and in an adult, it weighs about 600 g (see Fig. 21-2).

2 The heart has three layers. The inner layer, the *endocardium,* forms a thin lining for all the chambers of the heart.

3 The middle layer, the *myocardium,* is the actual heart muscle and makes up most of the mass of the heart. The walls of the myocardium are thicker in the left ventricle than in the right *(13),* because more force is required to pump blood into the relatively high-pressure systemic circulation as compared to the shorter, relatively low-pressure pulmonary circulatory system.

4 The outer layer of the heart is the *epicardium,* which forms a thin covering.

5 There is also a thick, fibrous covering called the *pericardium,* which envelops about two thirds of the front of the heart. If it becomes inflamed, the process is called "pericarditis." In *cardiac tamponade* this area becomes filled with blood and eventually compresses and restricts the ability of the heart to contract and expand—a potentially life-threatening situation.

4.0 THE CIRCULATORY SYSTEM OF THE HEART

4.1 Coronary circulatory system

1 The heart muscle receives nutrition and oxygen through its own specialized circulatory system, the coronary circulatory system (Fig. 21-3).

2 Just beyond the aortic valve is an opening called "Valsalva's sinus" *(1).* The two main coronary arteries, the right coronary artery *(2)* and the left coronary artery *(3),* come off the aorta at that point. The pathway the main arteries travel after leaving Valsalva's sinus may differ somewhat in different people. The most common arrangement is presented here.

3 The left coronary artery divides soon after it leaves Valsalva's sinus into the anterior descending artery *(4)* and the circumflex artery *(5),* which travels posteriorly to anastomose (join) *(6)* the branches from the right coronary artery.

4 The right coronary artery sends it main stem branch, the posterior descending branch *(7),* around to the back of the right side of the heart, where it anastomoses

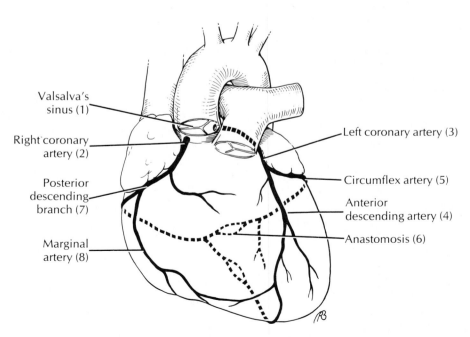

FIGURE 21-3 Coronary circulatory system.

with the circumflex branch *(6)*. A smaller branch of the right coronary artery is the marginal artery, which comes over toward the front of the right heart *(8)*.

5 The venous return of the coronary circulation returns to the right atrium by way of the coronary veins and the coronary sinus.

4.2 Relationship between the coronary and the cardiac cycle

1 When the ventricles contract (systole) the heart presses down on its own circulatory system, preventing free flow of blood through its own musculature. The rest of the body receives freshly oxygenated blood during this contraction.

2 However, the heart muscle itself must receive blood during diastole, when the heart is not contracting and is not squeezing its own blood vessels. If the heart is beating too fast for some reason, the diastolic time may not be long enough for the heart muscle to receive an adequate blood supply.

5.0 THE ELECTRIC FORCES INVOLVED IN MEMBRANE POTENTIALS
5.1 Electric forces

It is necessary to be familiar with some basic electric and chemical principles to understand how impulses are normally transmitted through nerves and muscles (in particular, along the cardiac conduction system and heart muscle) and then to understand how certain events can upset the normal process.

1 Electric charge is a fundamental property of matter. There are two types of electric charge—positive and negative—and they behave according to established principles.

2 *Like charges* repel one another, whereas *opposite charges* are attracted to one another (Fig. 21-4). In other words, positive charges repel positive charges, and negative charges repel negative charges. Positive charges are attracted to (pulled toward) negative charges.

3 The amount of pull or the degree of repulsion between two charges is a form of energy. The force exerted be-

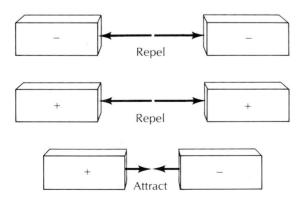

FIGURE 21-4 Like charges (+ to + or − to −) repel one another, whereas opposite charges (+ to −) are attracted to one another.

tween charges, either toward or away from one another, depends on the numbers of charged particles involved and the distance between them. The closer the charges are and the greater the number of charges, the greater the force.

5.2 Interaction of forces in a resting membrane potential

1 Please review the following definitions and concepts before proceeding with Unit 5.2.
a Diffusion. Movement of molecules from a source of high pressure to a lesser pressure across a fully permeable membrane.
b Concentration gradient. Difference in molecular number that exists between substances (liquid or gas) usually separated by a membrane.
c Active transport. movement of a substance across a membrane opposite to the concentration gradient.
d Electrolyte. Substances whose solutions conduct an electric current.
e Osmosis. Movement of the solvent from an area of high concentration (pressure) to an area of lower pressure across a semipermeable membrane. Also known as "diffusion" and "osmotic pressure." The molecular pressure gradient that exists between two substances separated by a membrane as a result of one side having a higher concentration of the substance than the other.

2 The inside of a cell differs in composition from the outside of the cell.

Ions	Extracellular concentration	Intracellular concentration
Sodium (Na^+)	150 mEq/L	15 mEq/L
Potassium (K^+)	5 m Eq/L	150 mEq/L

3 In view of the principles already reviewed, how is it that the cell maintains the extreme differences in ion concentrations on either side of its membrane?
a The cell membrane is 50 to 75 times more permeable to potassium (K^+) than to sodium (Na^+). This makes it easy for K^+ to enter the cell but difficult, although not impossible, for Na^+.
b Since the concentration of K^+ is so much higher inside the cell than outside, it would be expected that K^+ would tend to leave the cell along its concentration gradient, and, in fact, some K^+ does leave the cell. Since K^+ is positively charged and is added to the large concentration of positively charged NA^+ ions on the outside of the cell, the inside of the cell quickly becomes *negatively* charged in comparison with the outside of the cell.
c The K^+ ions are then attracted to the inside of the cell, according to the electric forces (opposites attract: positively charged K^+ is attracted to the negative charge inside the cell).
d The balance between the force of the concentration gradient and the electric force is called the *equilibrium potential*. When the number of ions in and out of the cell stabilizes and the forces are in balance, this is dynamic equilibrium. This equilibrium poten-

tial is measured electrically in millivolts.

e Na$^+$ is also positively charged and is also attracted to the relative negative charge inside the cell. However, Na$^+$ is prevented from entering along its concentration gradient or its electric attraction force because of the following:

• The cell membrane is structured so that it is difficult for Na$^+$ to enter.

• The cell membrane *activity transports* the small amounts of Na$^+$ that do enter it, back out again.

The "sodium pump" carries one escaped K$^+$ ion back into the cell in exchange for every Na$^+$ ion it pumps back out of the cell.

4 In summary, it may be said that the concentrations of intracellular and extracellular K$^+$ and Na$^+$ are maintained through the interaction of electric forces, chemical forces, and active transport. The resulting negative *resting membrane potential* is −80 to −90 mV.

5.3 Action potentials

1 A rapid change of membrane potential is called an *action potential*. A stimulus of some kind at the cell membrane causes a change in membrane permeability that results in a change in the membrane potential. Only nerve and muscle cells are capable of producing action potentials. This ability is called *excitability*. In addition to generating action potentials, these cells are able to transmit them along their surfaces.

2 Action potentials are the way nerve impulses travel and muscles contract. When the cell membrane is sufficiently stimulated the membrane permeability changes, thus allowing Na$^+$ to easily enter the cell along its concentration gradient and electric attraction. The influx of Na$^+$ into the cell changes the balance of ions so that opposite sides of the membrane are no longer polarized with opposite charges—they have been *depolarized* (they are no longer opposite) (Fig. 21-5, *1*).

3 In fact, so much Na$^+$ rushes into the cell that there is actually a temporary reverse in the charge of the inside versus the outside of the cell; the inside becomes positively charged with respect to the outside of the cell *(2)*.

4 Once the action potential (change in membrane potential) has occurred, the cell membrane quickly moves to regain its resting state. It begins, in other words, to *repolarize (3)*. The high levels of Na$^+$ in the cell as a result of the action potential stimulate the cell membrane to again "close its doors" to Na$^+$, preventing further influx. Also, the cell membrane increases its permeability to K$^+$ so that more K$^+$ leaves the cell. This makes enough K$^+$ available on the outside of the cell so that many Na$^+$ ions can be actively transported out through exchange for extracellular K$^+$.

5 There is a rebound effect as repolarization takes place. The cell actually overshoots a little and *hyperpolarizes (4)*. The inside charge of the cell may drop considerably before restablizing at its normal resting potential of −80 to −90 mV *(5)*.

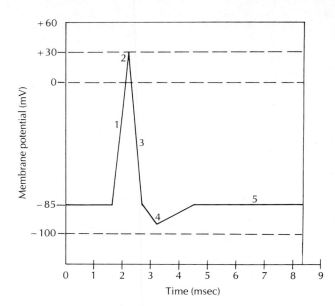

FIGURE 21-5 An action potential shows the electric charges in the cell membrane over time: depolarization, *1;* maximum depolarization at +30 mV, *2;* repolarization, *3;* hyperpolarization, *4;* normal resting potential, *5.*

6 An action potential begins in response to a stimulus, as stated earlier. However, not every stimulus causes an impulse to travel from cell to cell. The stimulus must be of sufficient strength before it will be effective in causing the cell to fire an action potential (Fig. 21-6). It is like squeezing the trigger of a gun—you either squeeze hard enough to fire it or it does not fire. Hence the "all or none" principle of action potentials.

7 The cell membrane has a *threshold (1)* (i.e., the point at which the stimulus is strong enough to cause an action potential). In most cells the stimulus must cause enough change in the membrane potential so that it is 5 to 15 mV more depolarized than it is at rest. In a human nerve cell the stimulus must bring the inside of the cell up to −60 mV to trigger an action potential.

5.4 Refractory periods

1 The cell membrane must recover from the transmission of one action potential before it can pass on another impulse. Similarly, a gun must be reloaded before it can be fired again. The recovery period, or reloading time, is called the *refractory period*.

2 There is an *absolute* refractory period that lasts about 1 msec after the peak of the action potential. During this period, no matter how strong the stimulus is, the membrane must wait before it can initiate a second action potential.

3 Following the absolute refractory period, before complete repolarization has occurred (the gun is only partially reloaded), there is a *relative* refractory period that lasts 10 to 15 msec. During that time a very strong stimulus can cause a second firing. Familiarity with these terms will be useful in discussion of cardiac arrhythmias later.

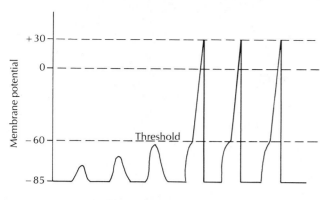

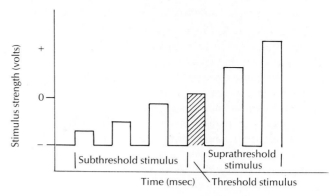

FIGURE 21-6 Cell membrane potential (electric charge) in relation to the strength of a stimulus (measured in volts). Stimulus must be of sufficient strength *(2)* to cause an action potential to be fired (threshold *1*). (Modified from Vander AJ, Sherman JH, and Luciano DS: Human physiology, ed 3, New York, 1980, McGraw-Hill Book Co, Inc.)

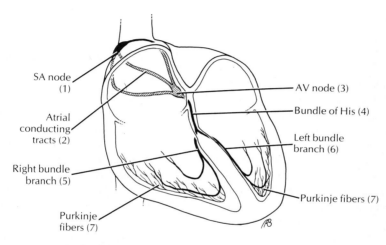

FIGURE 21-7 Cardiac electric conduction system.

6.0 THE ELECTRIC CARDIAC CONDUCTION SYSTEM
6.1 Structures

1 The pacemaker of the heart under normal circumstances is the *sinoatrial node* (SA node). It usually initiates impulses at a rate of about 75/min. All parts of the heart have the property of excitability and automticity and so could initiate their own action potentials (Fig. 21-7).

2 However, the inherent rate of SA node *(1)* is normally faster than other parts of the heart (see below), so it normally sets the pace.

3 After an impulse has been initiated by the SA node, the impulse travels down the *atrial conducting tracts (2)* (including Bacman's tract) to the *atrioventricular node* (AV node) *(3)*.

4 Pacemaker rates of various parts of the heart are given below:

Site	*Intrinsic pacemaker rate*
SA node	About 75/min
AV node	About 55/min
Bundle branches	About 40/min or less

5 From the AV node, the impulse progresses to the *bundle of His (4)*, which is the first part of the conduction system located in the ventricles (actually in the interventricular septum).

6 The bundle of His divides into the *right bundle branch (5)* and the *left bundle branch (6)*, which deliver the impulse to the right and left sides of the heart respectively.

7 The bundle branches further divide into a complex network of conducting fibers, the *Purkinje fibers (7)*, which transmit the impulses to the individual muscle fibers of the ventricles, causing them to contract.

8 As the impulse leaves the SA node the conduction system depolarizes, thus transmitting the impulse all along the conduction system and to the heart muscle, which also depolarizes and contracts. Depolarization is then followed by repolarization, a resting state that corresponds to diastole.

6.2 Influence of the autonomic nervous system on the heart

1 Although the SA node initiates its own action potentials (i.e., an intrinsic rhythm), the rate of firing is adjusted according to messages received from other parts of the body via the nervous system or blood (e.g., hormones and oxygen levels).

2 The autonomic nervous system is divided into the sympathetic and parasympathetic systems (see Unit 2.1). The parasympathetic nerve of influence in the case of the heart is the *vagus nerve*. Stimulation of the vagus nerve will cause the SA node to slow its rate of firing, thus slowing the heart rate. Stimulation of the sympathetic nerves (from excitement, anger, exercise) will cause the SA node to fire faster, increasing the heart rate. The AV node is influenced by these same nerves but to a lesser extent.

3 As the reader is aware from studying pharmacology, many medications used in respiratory care can cause increased heart rate by sympathetic stimulation.

7.0 PRINCIPLES OF ELECTROCARDIOGRAPHY

7.1 The electrocardiogram

1 The electric forces of the heart are transmitted outward from the heart and reach the surface of the body. Because of this, it is possible to detect and measure the electric activity of the heart. Sensors called *electrodes* are placed in direct contact with the skin, and the signals received are then transmitted to the cardiac monitor or electrocardiogram machine.

2 The signals are amplified and transformed so that the electric activity is represented as an electrocardiogram. The instrument that receives and transforms the signals is called the *electrocardiograph*. The actual recording of the electrical activity is the *electrocardiogram* (ECG).

3 The heart muscle and its electric activity exist in three dimensions. The electrodes can record electric activity in only one plane at a time. Similarly a camera can take a picture from only one angle at a time. A photographer must shoot pictures from several angles to get a complete picture of the subject. Likewise, the electrodes can be placed to obtain a picture of the electric activity of several planes of the heart.

4 There are *12 standard positions* for electrode placement. Each placement is referred to as a particular *lead*. If ECG recordings are obtained from all 12 positions, it is called a 12-lead ECG. Although a patient can be monitored for cardiac arrythmias through the use of only one position (lead), diagnosis of cardiac condition, such as the site of a myocardial infarct or ventricular hypertrophy, requires analysis of a complete 12-lead ECG (e.g., an electric picture from all angles).

5 The 12 leads are divided as follows:
  a Three standard limb leads—LL I, LL II, and LL III
  b Three augmental limb leads—AV_L, AV_R, and AV_F
  c Six precordial leads—V_1 through V_6

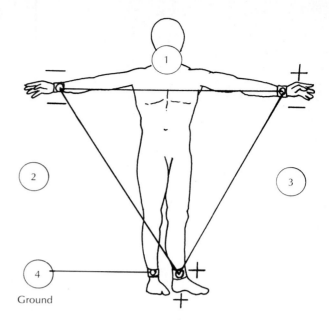

FIGURE 21-8 Placement of the three standard limb leads takes the shape of a triangle superimposed on the patient's body—the Einthoven triangle. Electrodes are placed on the right and left arms and the left leg. A ground is placed on the right leg *(4)*.

6 The *standard* limb leads are bipolar (i.e., they measure electric activity between two electrodes. One electrode is designated as the positive electrode, the other as the negative electrode. It is helpful to consider the three limb leads in the context of a triangle superimposed on the patient's body—*Einthoven's triangle* (Fig. 21-8).

7 Electrodes are placed on the right arm, left arm, and left leg. Limb lead I measures the electric potential between the right arm (designated as the negative electrode) and the left arm (positive) *(1)*. Limb lead II measures electric potential between the right arm (negative) and the left leg (positive) *(2)*. A modification of lead II is the lead most commonly used for continuous monitoring of arrhythmias. Limb lead III measures electric potential between the left arm (negative) and left leg (positive) *(3)*. A ground is placed on the right leg *(4)*.

8 The precordial leads and the augmented limb leads are unipolar (i.e., they measure the electric activity of the heart at the point directly beneath them). The precordial leads are numbered V_1 through V_6 (Fig. 21-9). They are most useful in determining the location of myocardial infarction.

9 The augmented leads will not be discussed in detail here, but additional information may be found in any standard text on electrocardiography.

10 The respiratory care practitioner will see the precordial (chest) leads often, and it is important to note that these leads are frequently misplaced. Unlike the arm and leg leads, they cannot be placed just anywhere. A distance of only ¼ inch (6 mm) will make a difference in the proper placement of chest leads (see Fig. 21-9).

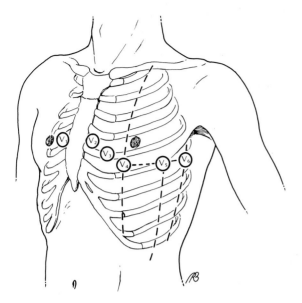

FIGURE 21-9 Placement of six precordial leads.

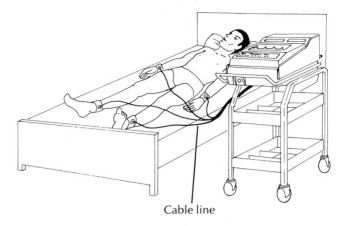

Cable line

FIGURE 21-10 To obtain an electrocardiogram, electrodes are strapped in the appropriate limb lead sites. Electrodes are connected by cables to an ECG machine.

a Lead 1. Placed at the *fourth* intercostal space at the *right* border of the sternum.

b Lead 2. Placed at the *fourth* intercostal space at the *left* border of the sternum.

c Lead 3. Placed in a straight line between lead 2 and lead 4.

d Lead 4. Placed at the midclavicular line and at the *fifth* intercostal space (should be over the heart's apex).

e Lead 5. Placed at the anterior axillary line level with lead 4 horizontally.

f Lead 6. Placed at the midaxillary line level with lead 4 and 5 horizontally.

11 Long-term or temporary electrodes may be used in obtaining an ECG. For temporary monitoring, conducting jelly is rubbed onto the skin. A small metal plate is rubbed over the jelly and then straped in the appropriate sites for limb leads. The rubbing of the jelly (or paste) and the electrode on the skin is to ensure a good connection (Fig. 21-10).

12 The plates are connected by cables to the electrocardiograph machine. For precordial leads a suction cup is placed over the jellied sites on the chest, and the cup is attached by a cable to the machine. Temporary monitoring, usually of limb lead II, is what is most often seen during cardiopulmonary resuscitation in the hospital.

13 A more permanent arrangement is used in the coronary care unit where there is a continuous monitoring for arrhythmias over several days (Fig. 21-11). Prepackaged electrodes, with conducting jelly in the center *(1)* and adhesive in a ring around the jelly *(2),* are usually used. The electrode *(3)* fits into the adhesive rings, and

the permanent cable can be snapped off or on. A modified limb lead II is most commonly seen.

a An electrode is placed at the upper right side of the chest (instead of on the right arm) as the negative pole *(4).*

b A second electrode is placed on the upper left side of the chest (instead of on the left leg) as the positive pole *(5).*

c A third electrode is used as a ground and can be attached in any convenient location *(6).*

d The electrode wires are connected to an oscilloscope that is similar to a television screen and that gives a continuous, moving picture of the ECG tracing.

14 Often there is a monitoring oscilloscope at the patient's bedside and at the nursing station. Usually a printed ECG readout can be obtained simply by switching on the electrocardiograph printer at the nurses' station without disturbing the electrodes or the patient in any way.

15 Both the patient's bedside monitor and the nursing station monitor are equipped with alarms for extreme heart rates. The machine is often set to alarm for rates below 60/min or above 100/min, but most can be adjusted to meet the needs of individual patients. (There can be problems with false alarms that will be explained in the next unit.)

16 There must be good skin contact to obtain a clear ECG. A person with a great deal of hair on his chest should be shaved in the spots where electrodes are to be placed. Also, the electrodes should be checked to be sure the conducting jelly has not dried out (if prepackaged electrodes are used), and all connections should be checked to be sure the cables are snugly in place.

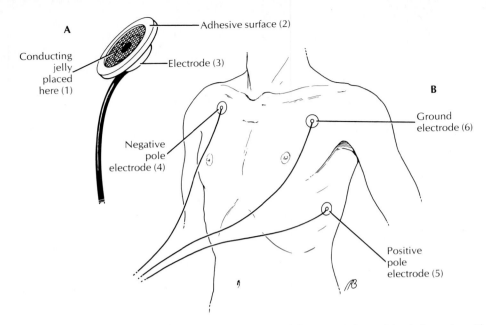

A

Adhesive surface (2)

Conducting
jelly
placed
here (1)

Electrode (3)

B

Ground
electrode (6)

Negative
pole
electrode (4)

Positive
pole
electrode (5)

FIGURE 21-11 Continuous monitoring of an electrocardiogram. **A,** Prepackaged electrodes with adhesive surface. **B,** Placement of electrodes on chest.

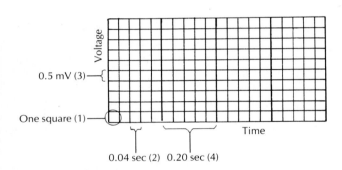

Voltage

0.5 mV (3)

One square (1)

Time

0.04 sec (2) 0.20 sec (4)

FIGURE 21-12 ECG paper measures time horizontally and voltage vertically.

R wave (4)

P wave (2)

T wave (6)

Baseline (1)

Q wave (3) S wave (5)

FIGURE 21-13 ECG measurement of a single cardiac cycle is represented by a series of waves named P, Q, R, S, and T.

7.2 Measurement of time and voltage

1 The ECG paper measures voltage and time. There are very small squares on the paper. Fig. 21-12 *(1)* is a magnified illustration measuring 1 mm². The horizontal direction of the paper measures time. Every small square represents 0.04 second *(2)*. The vertical direction measures voltage, with every small square representing 0.5 mV *(3)*.

2 There is a darkened line at every fifth small square to make counting time a little easier. The time between two darkened lines is (0.04 × 5) = 0.20 second *(4)*. Therefore counting the number of beats (cardiac cycles) in five of the darkened line spaces (1 second × 60) would give a 1-minute (60-second) heart rate.

8.0 A NORMAL ECG PATTERN
8.1 Recognizing a normal ECG pattern

1 If an ECG machine is turned on when it is not attached to anyone, the ECG paper will show only a straight

line (Fig. 21-13). That straight line is called the *baseline (1)*. When the electrodes are in place and an ECG tracing is being obtained, there are deviations recorded in a regular pattern above and below the baseline.

2 The positive deflections are those waves above the baseline *(2)*. Positive deflections indicate that the wave of depolarization in the heart is traveling toward the electrode.

3 Negative deflections are those waves below baseline; they indicate that the wave of depolarization is traveling away from the electrode *(3)*.

4 A single cardiac cycle is represented by a series of waves, named randomly as P, Q, R, S, and T. These waves are defined here.

a P wave. The first positive wave of the cardiac cycle *(2)*.

b Q wave. The first negative wave *(3)* in the cardiac cycle. It is sometimes absent, even in healthy people.

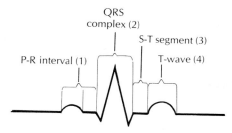

FIGURE 21-14 Measurement of the distance between different waves of the cardiac cycle.

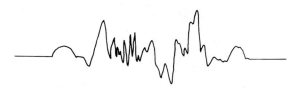

FIGURE 21-15 "Fuzzy" ECG tracing showing *artifact* (artificial movement caused by mechanical interference).

c R wave. The positive wave *(4)* that follows the Q wave (if there is one) or the first positive wave after the P wave.

d S wave. The negative wave *(5)* that follows the R wave.

e T wave. The positive wave *(6)* following the S wave and preceding the P wave of the next cardiac cycle.

5 *Exercise.* It is suggested that the reader obtain practice in recognizing normal ECGs by drawing a complete cardiac cycle and labeling the P, Q, R, S, and T waves accurately. It is further suggested that the reader obtain samples of normal ECGs (in lead II if possible) to study and practice labeling the waves.

8.2 Measurement of intervals

1 Measurement of the distance between different waves of the cardiac cycle indicates how long it takes the electric impulse to travel from one part of the heart to another. The distance from the beginning of the P wave through the end of the T wave would show how long it took for an impulse to travel through the whole heart (depolarize and repolarize) (Fig. 21-14).

2 The usual measurements of interest are as follows:

a P-R interval. Measured from the beginning of the P wave to the beginninig of the Q wave *(2)*. Measures the time it takes for the impulse to travel from the SA node through the AV node. Normal for adults is 0.12 to 0.20 second (three to five small squares).

b QRS complex. Measured from the beginning of the Q wave to the end of the S wave *(2)*. If there is no Q wave, measure from the beginning of the R to the end of the S wave. Indicates the time needed for depolarization of the ventricles. A normal time is less than 0.12 second (less than three small squares).

c S-T segment. Measured from the end of the S wave to the beginning of the T wave *(3)*. Represents the time it takes for ventricles to begin repolarization. (May be elevated above or below baseline in disease conditions.)

d T wave. From beginning to end of T wave *(4)*. Represents ventricular repolarization. If electric activity is disrupted as a result of muscle injury, the T wave may be a negative rather than positive deflection.

3 Note that atrial repolarization is *not* accounted for

among the waves of the cardiac cycle. Atrial repolarization occurs as the ventricles are depolarizing (i.e., during the QRS complex). Therefore the atrial repolarization is obscured (hidden) in the QRS complex.

4 *Exercise.* It is suggested that the reader complete the following exercise. Obtain an actual ECG tracing with a normal pattern. Measure the P-R interval and the QRS complex, determine the times, and decide whether the time intervals are within the normal range. Calipers, if available, or a specially calibrated ruler should be used.

8.3 Artifact

1 A number of events can interfere with recording of a clear ECG pattern. It is important to be able to distinguish *artifact* (mechanical interference causing artificial movements) that are recorded on the ECG, from true abnormalities in the ECG (Fig. 21-15).

2 Possible causes for fuzzy ECG tracings are mentioned here.

a Failure to use enough conducting jelly on the sensor; the jelly on the prepackaged electrodes may have dried out.

b Too much hair between the electrode and the skin (necessary to shave site to get good contact).

c Friction of electrode wires against sheets, bedrails, etc.

d Loose connection of electrode wires into main cable.

e Muscle movement (e.g., twitching, or the patient may just be scratching his or her nose).

3 Fig. 21-16, *A*, illustrates another instance of artifact. As mentioned earlier, the ECG monitor counts the R waves of each cardiac cycle to calculate heart rate. It is set to alarm with rates above or below preset limits. One can see that the machine could mistake high artifact caused by the patient's moving about for a series of R waves, calculate a high heart rate, and alarm. Likewise, if the electrode wires are disconnected accidentally or if an electrode fell off the patient, the ECG would show a straight line, and the monitor would alarm, reading "low heart rate," because it did not sense any R waves.

4 Another form of artifact is that caused by electric interference called "60-cycle interference" (Fig. 21-16, *B*).

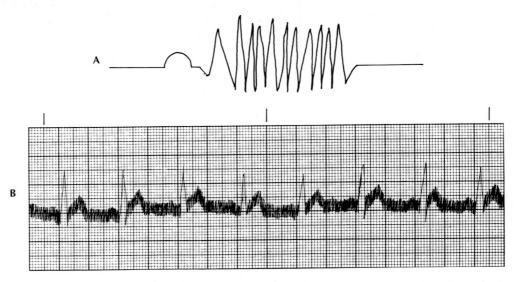

FIGURE 21-16 A, Artifact caused by patient movement. **B,** Artifact caused by 60-cycle interference. (From Wasserberger J, and Eubanks DH: Practical paramedic procedures, ed 2, 1981, St Louis, The CV Mosby Co.)

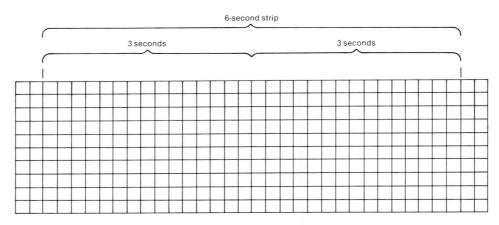

FIGURE 21-17 ECG paper marked off by small vertical lines every 3 seconds. Each small square equals 0.04 second.

5 It is always necessary to check a patient whenever an alarm sounds, since it may also be the result of a dangerous arrhythmia. The patient may be in serious trouble. *Never* take a cardiac monitor alarm for granted.

8.4 Four steps in examining an ECG

1 Once a clear ECG is obtained it should be studied in an orderly fashion. An ECG strip of at least 6 seconds is recommended.

A *Step one*

Calculate the heart rate. Most ECG paper is marked at the top at 3-second intervals with small vertical lines (Fig. 21-17). Count the number of cardiac cycles (or R waves) in a 6-second ECG srip and multiply by 10 to get the number of beats per minute. The rate can be classified as follows

1 Bradycardia—heart rate below 60/min
2 Normal—heart rate of 60 to 100 beats/min

3 Tachycardia—heart rate over 100 beats/min

B *Step two*

Determine the regularity of the R waves. A set of calipers is quite useful in this step (Fig. 21-18). Measure the distance beteen two consecutive R waves *(1)*. Then check the distance between the next pair of consecutive R waves without changing the calipers *(2)*. Check several consecutive pairs *(2 and 3; 4 and 5)* to determine if the distance between R waves is constant. If it is, then the rhythm is regular. The same method can be used to check the regularity of other waves also. This will be discussed later. If calipers are not available, a marked piece of paper can be used. Place it directly below or above the ECG pattern and mark the point of the R wave of two consecutive R waves on it. Then move the paper and check the marks with two other consecutive R waves *(6)*. The paper method is not as accurate but will give some ideas of the gross regularity or irregularity of the cardiac cycles.

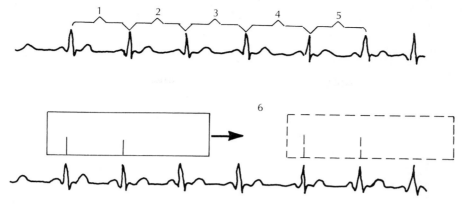

FIGURE 21-18 To determine regularity of heartbeat, measure the distance between consecutive R waves (*1* through *5*) with calipers. If calipers are unavailable, mark the distance of one set of consecutive R waves (*1*) and compare it to consecutive sets (*6*).

C *Step three*

Examine the P waves and the P-R interval. Check to see if there is a P wave before every QRS complex. Then measure the P-R interval for several cardiac cycles, and determine whether it is consistent. Observe whether the shape of the P waves is the same throughout the ECG strip. If the impulse for depolarization is consistently coming from the SA node, the P-R interval and shape of the P wave will vary little or none from cycle to cycle. If the P-R wave is longer than 0.20 second, the electric impulse is traveling slower than normal from the SA node through the AV node.

D *Step four*

Measure the duration of the QRS complex. The QRS complex reflects the time it takes for the ventricles to depolarize. If the QRS is wider than 0.12 second (three small squares), depolarization is occurring slower than normal (i.e., there is a conduction defect). This may be the result of poor blood supply to the cardiac conduction system or of an abnormal pathway of conduction resulting from an injury of the cardiac muscle.

■ ■ ■

If all of the above observations are found to be within normal limits, the ECG is said to show a *normal sinus rhythm.*

9.0 CORRELATING THE ECG PATTERN WITH CARDIAC ACTION

9.1 Correlation of conduction system and cardiac action

1 As the impulse travels from the SA node through the atrial muscles, it causes atrial systole. The impulse is delayed (travels more slowly) at the AV node to allow time for the ventricles to fill with blood before they contract. The impulse then continues through the bundle branches and the Purkinje fibers, causing ventricular systole. While the ventricles are contracting, the atria are in diastole and the atrial conduction system is repolarizing. Table 21-3 shows the conduction correlation.

TABLE 21-3 Conduction correlation

ECG	Electric conduction	Heart action
P-R interval QRS complex	SA node—AV node Bundle of His—Purkinje figers	Atrial systole Ventricular systole, atrial repolarization (atrial diastole)
T wave	Repolarization of ventricular conducting system	Ventricular diastole

10.0 LIFE-THREATENING ARRHYTHMIAS

10.1 Cardiac arrythmias

A number of arrhythmias will be described briefly in this unit. The arrhythmias most frequently seen by respiratory care practitioners are premature ventricular contraction (PVC), ventricular tachycardia (VT), ventricular fibrillation (VF), and ventricular standstill or ventricular asystole. All arrhythmias are presented assuming a limb lead II positioning of electrodes.

Deviations (arrhythmias) from a normal sinus rhythm may be classified according to the site or origin of the arrhythmia and by the mechanism of the disorder. The basic characteristics of 18 arrhythmias will be presented; identified as minor, major, or death-producing (lethal) arrhythmias, and comments will be made if appropriate.

The main sites of origin of arrhythmias are the SA node, the atria, the AV node, and the ventricles. The main mechanisms are as follows:

Tachycardia—rate over 100
Bradycardia—rate under 60 beats/min
Premature—occurring before it is due
Flutter—tremulous movement, extremely rapid but regular
Fibrillation—quivering, irregular
Defects in conduction

The name of each arrhythmia reflects its site of origin and the mechanism.

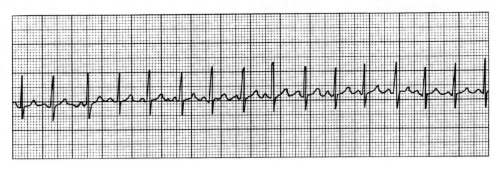

FIGURE 21-19 Sinus tachycardia. (From Wasserberger J and Eubanks DH: Practical paramedic procedures, ed 2, St Louis, 1981, The CV Mosby Co.)

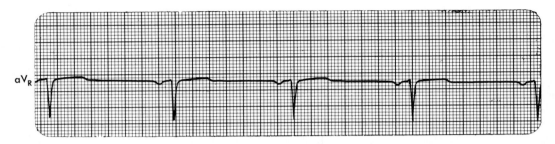

FIGURE 21-20 Sinus bradycardia. (From Goldberger AL and Goldberger E: Clinical electrocardiography: a simplified approach, ed 3, St Louis, 1986, The CV Mosby Co.)

1 Sinus tachycardia (minor arrhythmia) (Fig. 21-19)
  a Characteristics
    • Rate: 100 to 160 beats/min.
    • Rhythm: regular.
    • P wave/P-R interval: normal.
    • QRS complex: normal.
  b Comments: May be caused by increased sympathetic nervous activity (e.g., as a result of fear, anger, exercise, or medication). Treatment is according to the underlying cause. An elevated heart rate may overtax the heart if it has been damaged (e.g., following myocardial infarction).
2 Sinus bradycardia (minor arrythmia) (Fig. 21-20)
  a Characteristics
    • Rate: 40 to 60 beats/min.
    • Rhythm: regular.
    • P wave/P-R interval: normal.
    • QRS complex: normal.
  b Comments: May be the result of excessive parasympathetic influence. However, in conditioned athletes a slowed rate may reflect strong, efficient cardiac muscle. In other people the slow rate may be insufficient in meeting the body's needs. If the patient has symptoms (e.g., short of breath or abnormal beats), it may be treated with atropine, which blocks vagal influence, thereby giving more influence to the sympathetic control of the heart and increasing the rate.
3 Sinus arrhythmia (minor) (Fig. 21-21)
  a Characteristics

    • Rate: 60 to 100 beats/min.
    • Rhythm: slightly irregular, with R-R intervals varying more than 0.12 second from the longest R-R to the shortest R-R seen.
    • P-wave/P-R interval: normal.
    • QRS complex: normal.
  b Comments: The heart rate alternately increases and decreases. Usually the rate speeds with inspiration and slows with expiration. No treatment is necessary.
4 Sinoatrial arrest or block (minor)—"dropped beat" (Fig. 21-22)
  a Characteristics
    • Rate: usually normal, but may tend toward bradycardia if the dropped beat occurs to often.
    • Rhythm: regular, except when there is a dropped beat.
    • P wave/P-R interval: P wave present each time there is a cardiac cycle; P-R interval regular.
    • QRS complex: normal, when present.
  b Comment: May be caused by excessive vagal stimulation, excessive digitalis (medication), or insufficient oxygen supply to the SA node. Treament, if dropped beats are infrequent. If dropped beats occur often and if the patient is symptomatic, treatment is according to cause of the arrhythmia.
5 Premature atrial contraction (PAC)—if fewer than 6 beats/min, classified as minor arrhythmia; if more than 6 beats/min, classified as major arrhythmia (Fig. 21-23)

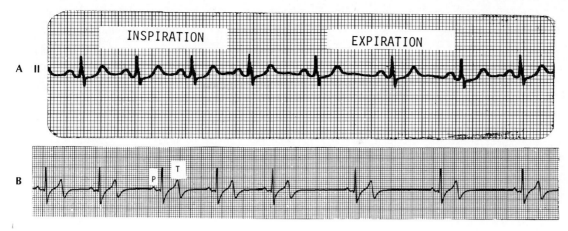

FIGURE 21-21 Sinus arrhythmia. **A,** Phasic. **B,** Nonphasic. (From Goldberger AL and Goldberger E: Clinical electrocardiography: a simplified approach, ed 3, St Louis, 1986, The CV Mosby Co.)

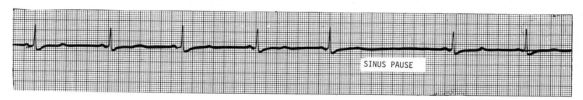

FIGURE 21-22 Sinoatrial arrest. (From Goldberger AL and Goldberger E: Clinical electrocardiography: a simplified approach, ed 3, St Louis, 1986, The CV Mosby Co.)

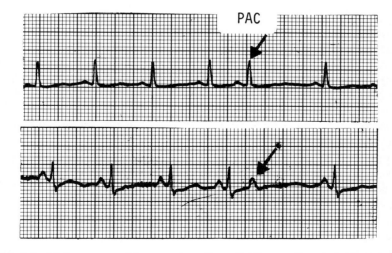

FIGURE 21-23 Premature atrial contraction. (From Goldberger AL and Goldberger E: Clinical electrocardiography: a simplified approach, ed 3, St Louis, 1986, The CV Mosby Co.)

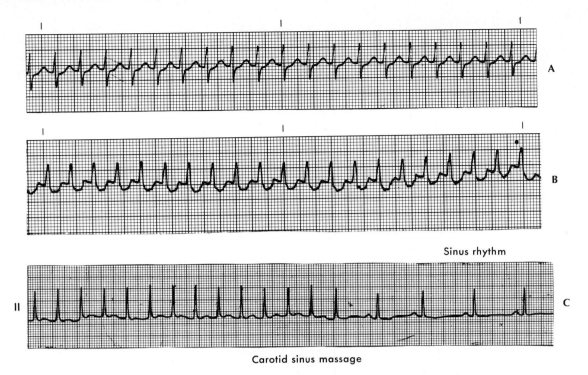

Sinus rhythm

Carotid sinus massage

F I G U R E   2 1 - 2 4 A, Paroxysmal atrial tachycardia (PAT) is a run of three or more consecutive premature atrial contractions. This strip shows PAT with rate of about 167 beats/min. Note marked regularity of rhythm. No P waves are visible. **B,** PAT with rate of about 200 beats/min. **C,** PAT treated with carotid sinus massage. The first 14 beats in this rhythm strip show PAT with rate of about 150 beats/min. Carotid sinus massage resulted in abrupt termination of the tachycardia, with appearance of normal sinus rhythm. (From Goldberger AL and Goldberger E: Clinical electrocardiography: a simplified approach, ed 3, St Louis, 1986, The CV Mosby Co.)

a Characteristics
  • Rate: usually normal.
  • Rhythm: regular, except for the early atrial beats
  • P wave/P-R interval: P waves and P-R interval normal except for the PACs. The PACs occur sooner than the next beat would be expected, the P waves look different than the normal beats, and the P-R interval is shorter (less distance between atrial muscle and AV node than between SA and AV nodes).
  • QRS complex: normal in all beats.
b Comment: PACs represent the spontaneous firing from an ectopic foci (abnormal spot) in the atria before the SA node. As a result the SA node is depolarized and cannot fire on schedule. The distance between regular beats will be the same as the distance between the PAC and the next regular beat. If there are more than six PACs per minute, they may be treated with medication.

6 Paroxysmal atrial tachycardia (PAT) (major) (Fig. 21-24, *A* through *C*)
a Characteristics
  • Rate: 140 to 250 beats/min.
  • Rhythm: regular
  • P wave/P-R interval: beats may be so close together that the P wave of one cardiac cycle may be hidden in the T wave of the preceding cycle. P

waves, if distinguishable, may be abnormally shaped. P-R interval is difficult to determine.
  • QRS complex: normal, or may be somewhat wider than normal.
b Comments: An atrial pacemaker outside the SA node becomes irritable and takes over at a fast rate. Every impulse is conducted. The degree of danger depends on how long the tachycardia lasts. (It may suddenly stop on its own.) It is not efficient over a long period of time, because the fast rate does not allow enough time for complete filling of the heart chambers before they are sent into systole. May be stopped with vagal stimulation via carotid massage, medication, and, in difficult cases, elective cardioversion.

7 Atrial flutter (major) (Fig. 21-25, *A* and *B*)
a Characteristics
  • Rate: ventricular rate may vary from 60 to 150 beats/min, depending on the number of atrial impulses conducted (allowed to pass) through the AV node. The atrial rate (number of P wave) is 250 to 400/min.
  • Rhythm: regular or irregular. If there is a pattern to how often the atrial impulss are conducted, the ventricular rate will be regular. For example, every second or third atrial impulse may be conducted.
  • P waves/P-R interval: regular, identical in appear-

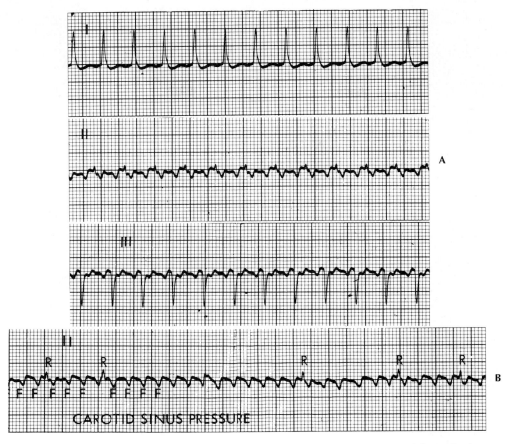

FIGURE 21-25 Atrial flutter. **A,** Note variable appearance of flutter waves in different leads. In lead I, flutter waves are barely apparent, and leads II and III show classic "sawtooth" waves. Ventricular rate is about 160 beats/min, and flutter rate is about 320 beats/min, so that atrial flutter with 2:1 conduction is present. **B,** Carotid sinus massage produces marked slowing of the ventricular rate by increasing vagal tone. (From Goldberger AL and Goldberger E: Clinical electrocardiography: a simplified approach, ed 3, St Louis, 1986, The CV Mosby Co.)

ance; there is a characteristic sawtooth pattern.

• QRS complex: normal.

b Comments: The pattern that results from the blocking of impulses is described as atrial flutter, with 2:1, 3:1, or 4:1 block. That means there are two, three, or four atrial impulses for every ventricular beat. In this arrhythmia the characteristic P waves may be referred to as "F" (flutter) waves. The arrhythmia can be identified only with an ECG. The potential danger depends on the degree of block in impulse transmission at the AV node and the resulting ventricular rate. Treatment could include cardioversion and medication, such as quinidine or digitalis (Unit 2.6).

8 Atrial fibrillation (major) (Fig. 21-26)

a Characteristics

• Rate: varies from under 100 to much faster, depending on the pattern of impulse conduction through the AV node.

• Rhythm: irregular in both atria and ventricles.

• P waves/P-R interval: indistinguishable.

• QRS complex: normal in shape.

b Comments: This arrhythmia represents a takeover by an irritable atrial pacer, which fires at a rate greater than 400 beats/min. The atrial muscles cannot respond at that rate and so are thrown into confusion, resulting in completely uncoordinated movement— quivering. The impulses are conducted at irregular intervals through the AV node, resulting in an irregular ventricular rate. The danger is in the fact that the atria do not effectively pump blood to the ventricles. This may cause the formation of clots in the atria and decreased blood supply to the cardiac circulation. It is treated with drugs (e.g., quinidine, digitalis; in resistant instances, with cardioversion).

9 AV nodal rhythm (major) (Fig. 21-27)

a Characteristics

• Rate: 40 to 60 beats/min.

• Rhythm: regular.

• P wave/P-R interval: abnormal. May occur before the QRS complex with shortened P-R interval; or within the QRS complex; so it is not visible.

• QRS complex; normal.

b Comments: Occurs when the rate of firing of the SA

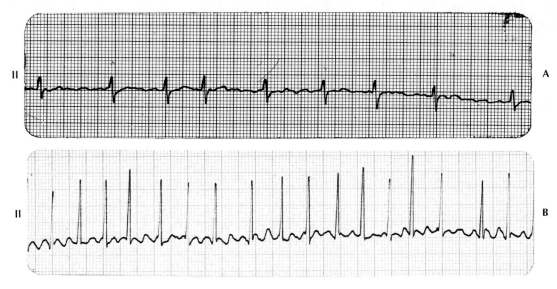

FIGURE 21-26 A, Atrial fibrillation. Note irregular undulation of baseline because of fibrillatory waves (F waves). There are no true P waves. Ventricular (QRS) rate is irregular. **B,** Rapid atrial fibrillation. Note coarse fibrillatory waves and rapid ventricular response. Patient had hyperthyroidism. (The commonly used term "rapid atrial fibrillation" is actually a misnomer since the word "rapid" refers to the ventricular rate, not the atrial rate. This is also true for the term "slow atrial fibrillation.") (From Goldberger AL and Goldberger E: Clinical electrocardiography: a simplified approach, ed 3, St Louis, 1986, The CV Mosby Co.)

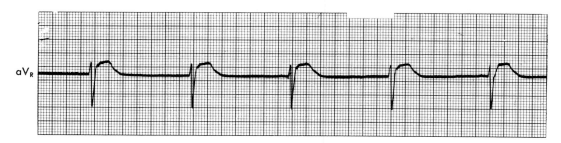

FIGURE 21-27 Junctional escape rhythm. AV nodal rhythm (major). (From Goldberger AL and Goldberger E: Clinical electrocardiography: a simplified approach, ed 3, St Louis, 1986, The CV Mosby Co.)

node (normally faster than the AV node) is depressed. For example, the SA may be slowed by vagal stimulation, too much digitalis, or an insufficient oxygen supply. Treatment is according to the cause and whether or not the patient has symptoms from the slow heart rate. Usually the SA node will take over again, once it begins to fire faster than the AV node (i.e., once the cause of slowed firing has been eliminated).

10 Premature AV nodal contractions (PNC)—if fewer than 6 beats/min, classified as minor arrhythmia; if more than 6 beats/min, classified as major arrhythmia (Fig. 21-28)

a Characteristics
- Rate: normal.
- Rhythm: regular except when a PNC occurs.
- P wave/P-R interval: normal in sinus beats. In PNC the P wave is either absent or may occur after the QRS complex. It may be a negative deflection, showing the backward depolarization of the atria

from the AV node upward. The P-R interval is normal in sinus beats. If there is a P wave in the PNC, the P-R interval will be very short.
- QRS complex: usually normal; may be widened in the PNC.

b Comments: PNCs occur as the result of irritability of the AV node. If the frequency of their occurrence increases, it may forewarn of more serious arrhythmias. If there are more than six PNCs per minute, it may be treated with medication (e.g., lidocaine).

11 First-degree heart (AV) block (major) (Fig. 21-29, *A* and *B*)

a Characteristics
- Rate: normal.
- Rhythm: normal.
- P wave/P-R interval: normal P wave; P-R interval over 0.20 second (only abnormality).
- QRS complex: normal.

b Comments: Lengthening of the P-R interval represents a delay in conduction of the impulse fired by

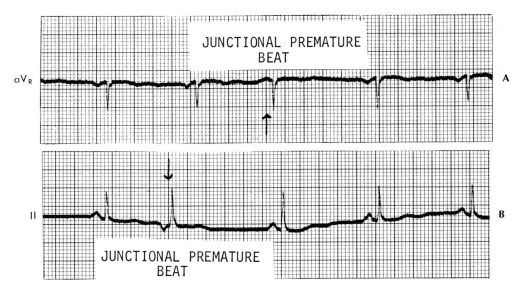

FIGURE 21-28 Junctional premature beats from same patient. Note retrograde P waves that are upright in lead AVR **(A)** and negative in lead II **(B)**, just the reverse of pattern seen with normal sinus rhythm. (From Goldberger AL and Goldberger E: Clinical electrocardiography: a simplified approach, ed 3, St Louis, 1986, The CV Mosby Co.)

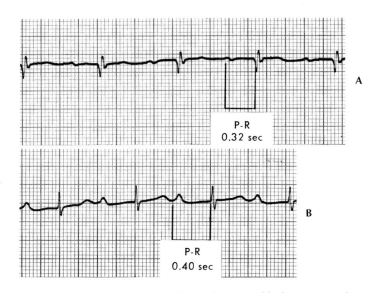

FIGURE 21-29 First-degree AV block. With first-degree AV block, P-R interval is uniformly prolonged above 0.2 second with each beat. **A** and **B** are from different patients. (From Goldberger AL and Goldberger E: Clinical electrocardiography: a simplified approach, ed 3, St Louis, 1986, The CV Mosby Co.)

the SA node through the AV node to the ventricles. This is dangerous because this slowed conduction is usually caused by ischemia of the AV node and may progress to the second- or third-degree block (see below). It may also be caused by certain medications (e.g., excessive digitalis).

12 Second-degree heart (AV) block (major) (Fig. 21-30, *A* and *B*)

  a Characteristics

    • Rate: the atrial rate may be normal, but the ventricular rate may be slow, as a result of failure of ev-

ery second, third, or fourth atrial impulse to pass through the AV node.

  • Rhythm: regular.

  • P waves/P-R interval: normal, but there are two, three, or four times as many P waves as QRS complexes. P-R interval is normal or prolonged, when conducted.

  • QRS complex: normal.

  b Comments: Usually is a progression from first-degree heart block. If the ventricular rate falls below 60 beats/min, a transvenous pacemaker (Unit 10.2)

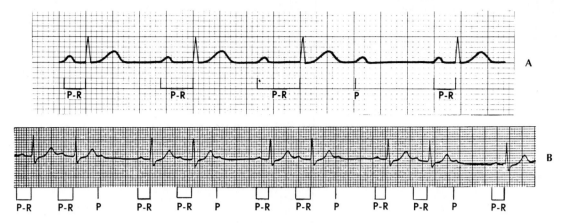

FIGURE 21-30 Wenckebach (Mobitz type I) second-degree AV block (major). (From Goldberger AL and Goldberger E: Clinical electrocardiography: a systematic approach, ed 3, St Louis, 1986, The CV Mosby Co.)

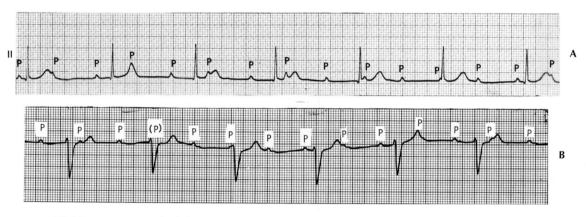

FIGURE 21-31 Third-degree (complete) AV block (major). (From Goldberger AL and Goldberger E: Clinical electrocardiography: a simplified approach, ed 3, St Louis, 1986, The CV Mosby Co.)

may be inserted on a standby basis. May progress to third-degree heart block.

13 Third-degree heart (AV) block (major) (Fig. 21-31, *A* and *B*)

 a Characteristics
 - Rate: atrial rate normal; ventricular rate less than 40 beats/min.
 - Rhythm: the atrial rate and ventricular rate are both regular, but they are independent of one another (e.g., the atrial rate might be 70 and regular, whereas the ventricular rate is 40 and regular; (remember, pulse is created by ventricular systole).
 - P wave/P-R interval: size and shape of P wave normal. P-R interval variable—cannot be definitely determined since none of the P waves is conducted through the AV node.
 - QRS complex: may be normal in appearance if the ventricles are being paced by a site just below the AV node. May be abnormally wide if the ventricles are being paced from a ventricular site.

 b Comments: Results from damage to the AV node,

(e.g., from ischemia [rarely, as a result of excessive digitalis]). Symptoms are the result of the slow ventricular rate and the consequent insufficient cardiac output. This may lead to fainting and heart failure. It is dangerous because it may warn of more dangerous, even lethal, arrhythmias. The main treatment is insertion of a transvenous cardiac pacemaker.

14 Bundle branch block (major)

 a Characteristics
 - Rate: normal.
 - Rhythm: regular.
 - P waves/P-R interval: normal.
 - QRS complex: widened over 0.12 second; abnormal shape.

 b Comments: May occur in either the right or left bundle branch of the ventricular conduction system. It represents a delay in conduction through one side, with the impulse reaching the "blocked" side by an other-than-normal route, which is slower. The widened QRS complex indicates the slowed ventricular depolarization. The site of the block can be identi-

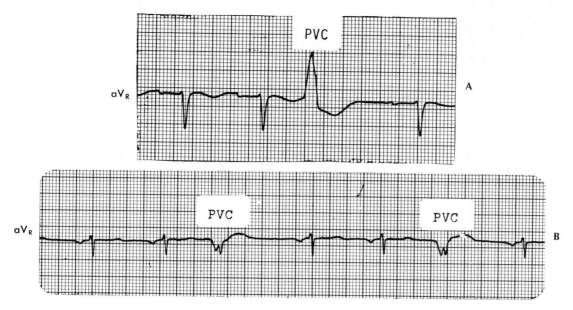

FIGURE 21-32 A, Premature ventricular contraction *(PVC).* **B,** Wide, aberrant PVC. (From Goldberger AL and Goldberger E: Clinical electrocardiography: a simplified approach, ed 3, St Louis, 1986, The CV Mosby Co.)

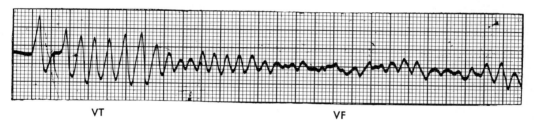

FIGURE 21-33 Ventricular tachycardia *(VT)* and ventricular fibrillation *(VF).* (From Goldberger AL and Goldberger E: Clinical electrocardiography: a simplified approach, ed 3, St Louis, 1986, The CV Mosby Co.)

fied by the shape of the QRS complex in a 12-lead electrocardiogram. The block in conduction is usually the result of tissue damage, as in a myocardial infarction, or scarring of the bundle branches. The slowed conduction can also be caused by too much quinidine or digitalis.

15 Premature ventricular contraction (PVC)—if fewer than 6 beats/min, classified as minor arrythmia; if more than 6 beats/min, classified as major arrhythmia (Fig. 21-32, *A* and *B*)

a Characteristics
- Rate: normal.
- Rhythm: regular, except for PVC.
- P wave/P-R interval: normal in sinus beats; not visible in the PVC.
- QRS complex: normal in sinus beats. Always widened and distorted in shape in PVC. Shape depends on the spot in the ventricle that initated the PVC.

b Comments: The time from the normal beat before the PVC and the normal beat after the PVC is twice the distance between two sinus beats. For example, there is a compensatory pause after the PVC, as if to get things back on schedule. PVCs are *especially*

dangerous in any of the following situations:
- There are more than 6/min.
- Every other beat is a PVC (bigeminy).
- The PVC occurs close to the T wave (relative refractory period) of the preceding beat: called the "R-on-T pattern." This could send the heart into ventricular tachycardia, a lethal pattern.
- The PVCs differ from one another in shape, indicating more than one irritable spot in the ventricles (multifocal PVCs).
- PVCs occur consecutively.

The primary treatment for PVCs is intravenous lidocaine.

16 Ventricular tachycardia (VT) (lethal) (Fig. 21-33)

a Characteristics
- Rate: 140 to 200 beats/min.
- Rhythm: regular.
- P waves/P-R interval: buried in QRS complex; cannot be identified (retrograde, or backward, conduction from ventricles to atria).
- QRS complex: wide complexes, identical in shape; looks like a series of unifocal PVCs.

b Comments: VT is usually preceded by signs of ven-

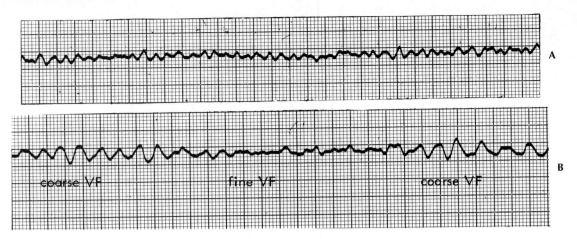

FIGURE 21-34 Ventricular fibrillation *(VF)*. **A,** Causing cardiac arrest. **B,** Producing coarse or fine waves. (From Goldberger AL and Goldberger E: Clinical electrocardiography: a simplified approach, ed 3, St Louis, 1986, The CV Mosby Co.)

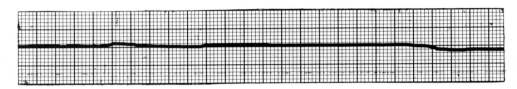

FIGURE 21-35 Ventricular standstill or ventricular asystole. (From Goldberger AL and Goldberger E: Clinical electrocardiography: a simplified approach, ed 3, St Louis, 1986, The CV Mosby Co.)

tricular irritability, such as increasing numbers of PVCs. VT requires emergency action. Patient is aware of palpitations when it begins and may experience chest pain, severe apprehension, nausea, and profuse perspiring. The VT may stop on its own, but even then there is a high probability that it will happen again—especially if the patient has had a myocardial infarction (MI). The arrhythmia is treated with large doses of intravenous lidocaine. If it does not stop, then immediate elective precordial shock is needed. The patient may become unconscious if VT continues unchecked and will die as a result of insufficient circulation. (The ventricles do not fill before contracting, and the atrial and ventricular systoles are uncoordinated because of the backward depolarization of the atria from the ventricles.) The patient may require cardiopulmonary resuscitation.

17 Ventricular fibrillation (VF) (lethal) (Fig. 21-34, *A* and *B*)

a Characteristics
- The ventricles are quivering in a bizarre, irregular manner as a result of depolarization. This pattern produces an ECG with no distinguishable P-Q-R-S-T configurations.

b Comments: In VF there is no effective pumping of blood out of the heart (i.e., circulation stops). Death will occur within minutes if the situation is not cor-

rected. The patient immediately becomes unconscious, and convulsions often occur as a result of inadequate circulation to the brain. There is no pulse or blood pressure. This arrhythmia may occur spontaneously (especially in a patient who has suffered a MI) or may be set off by the "R-on-T pattern," mentioned under PVCs. The only treatment for VF is *precordial shock.* It should be administered within 2 minutes of onset of VF. (Protocol concerning who is authorized to administer precordial shock varies from hospital to hospital. The method varies somewhat with the particular brand of defibrillator used.)

18 Ventricular standstill or ventricular asystole (lethal) (Fig. 21-35)

a Characteristics
- Rate: when ventricular standstill begins, the ventricles stop contracting. The SA node may continue to fire at a normal rate for a while.
- Rhythm: no heartbeat, once the ventricles stop.
- P wave/P-R interval: P waves for a while, with no QRS complexes.
- QRS complex: absent.
- The ECG rhythm will resemble small bumps on an otherwise straight line. If possible, it may help the reader to obtain the ECG strip of a terminally ill patient in a "dying heart" pattern.

b Comments: Ventricular standstill will result in sud-

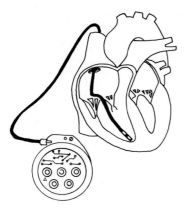

FIGURE 21-36 Transvenous pacing. Electrode introduced at peripheral vein and advanced through superior vena cava, through right atrium, and into right ventricle.

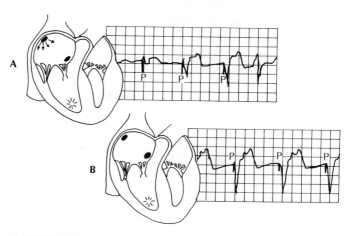

FIGURE 21-37 Pace generator can be set to fire continuously or only if needed.

den death, since the ventricles are responsible for maintaining circulation. Ventricular standstill is often preceded by third-degree heart block (see Fig. 21-31) or extreme bradycardia. Ideally, a standby transvenous pacer is already in place in response to the earlier warning arrhythmias and can be turned on when ventricular standstill occurs. However, the ventricles may begin to conduct again on their own without interference. In that case the person may have fainted or become dizzy as the ventricles stopped and will revive as they begin to contract again. Those episodes are called Adams-Stokes attacks.

The failure to conduct impulses in the ventricles may be the result of poor circulation to the ventricles or electrolyte imbalances. (Remember the role of electrolytes in transmission of action potentials.) Without an ECG the signs and symptoms of ventricular standstill are indistinguishable from those of ventricular fibrillation. If there is no standby pacer in place at the time of ventricular standstill, cardiopulmonary resuscitation is begun immediately. Defibrillation is *not* used. The physician may elect to try transthoracic pacing as an emergency measure.

10.2 Cardiac pacemakers

1 Transvenous pacing is the treatment of choice whenever the heart is *temporarily* unable to beat at a rate sufficient for circulatory needs. A pacing electrode is introduced at a peripheral vein and advanced through the superior vena cava, through the right atrium, and into the right ventricle (Fig. 21-36).

2 The electrode and the transvenous electrode are advanced under direct fluorscopic visualization. The electrode is positioned in contact with the endocardial surface of the right ventricle.

3 It is connected on the outside to a battery-operated pace generator. The desired rate is set on the pace generator, and it will fire at a certain rate continuously (fixed-rate firing) (Fig. 21-37, *A*). It can also be set to

fire only if needed (demand pacing) (e.g., if the heart rate slows below a specific rate, such as 55 or 60 beats/min [*B*]). The voltage necessary to stimulate a ventricular contraction is identified and also set on the pace generator.

4 The danger of a fixed-rate pacer is that the pacer may fire on the T wave (relative refractory period of one of the heart's own beats), throwing the heart into ventricular tachycardia—an iatrogenic "R-on-T" phenomenon.

5 Note the configuration of the ECG when the pacer is firing. A pacer spike (a straight line) is easily seen preceding each wide QRS complex: The QRS complex is wide because the pacer electrode is firing from the right ventricle, rather than from above the AV node. No P waves are visible for the same reason.

6 Indications for transvenous pacing include second- and third-degree heart block and ventricular standstill (Adams-Stokes episodes), or any other arrhythmias involving symptomatic bradycardia. If the arrhythmia in question proves to be chronic and is presumed to be permanent, then a permanent pacemaker is implanted surgically. The ECG tracing for a permanent pacemaker is the same as for a temporary pacemaker. The patient with a temporary pacemaker should be very still to avoid dislodging it.

7 Therefore always be sure to check whether a patient has a temporary or permanent pacemaker before beginning a respiratory therapy treatment. After the first few days after insertion of a permanent pacemaker, it is rather resistant to being dislodged.

10.3 Circumstances mimicking lethal arrhythmias

1 The reader is reminded that the ECG reflects the electric activity of the heart. It is by inference and observation of patient condition that the mechanical activity is correlated with the electric activity recorded on the ECG.

2 There are instances when electric activity continues af-

ter mechanical activity has stopped. That is called *electromechanical dissociation*. It is an extreme example of the clinical picture being far worse than would be expected on the basis of the ECG pattern. The impulses are still being sent, and the ECG may appear normal, but the heart muscle is not responding and circulation has stopped.

3 Other examples of confusion between the ECG pattern and the patient's condition follow. These examples point to the importance of always correlating patient condition with the ECG, rather than relying entirely on the ECG:

a Confusion between sinus tachycardia with bundle branch block versus ventricular tachycardia. The two arrhythmias would appear very similar, but the patient would likely be conscious in the first and in no immediate danger, whereas the second arrhythmia could be quickly lethal. The appearance of the patient is the clue. Additionally, vagal stimulation will slow the heart enough so that P waves are discernible if it is sinus tachycardia with bundle branch block but will have no effect on VT (vagal stimulation by way of carotid massage).

b Prolific artifact (e.g., the patient tries to scratch around the electrodes, which may cause skin irritation) versus ventricular fibrillation. On observing the patient you may find him or her completely undisturbed, sitting in bed reading. Of course the patient will appear much different with a real VF pattern.

c Disconnected leads versus ventricular standstill. Disconnected leads result in a straight line. Ventricular standstill *may* show a straight line or P waves only.

10.4 Procedure 21.1 included at the end of this module may be used as a guide for identifying a sinus rhythm from an abnormal ECG pattern

11.0 CORRELATING CHEMICAL IMBALANCES WITH ECG ABNORMALITIES
11.1 Chemical imbalances

1 Potassium (K^+)

a Normal: 3.5 to 5.0 mEq/L.

b Hypokalemia (below 3.5 mEq/L): most often, low levels of K^+ are the result of diuretic therapy without adequate replacement therapy. In other words, diuretics prevent excessive retention of fluid in the body by working to lose extra fluids through the kidneys. In the process, extra K^+ is lost in the urine.

c Low levels of K^+ are associated with cardiac irritability, usually manifested as PVCs and tachyarrhythmias. (A low K^+ level is especially dangerous if the patient is also medicated with digitalis.)

d Low levels of K^+ are also reflected in the ECG as depressed and shortened S-T segments and a prominent U wave (a small positive wave after the T wave and preceding the P wave of the next cycle).

e Hyperkalemia (above 5.0 mEq/L): high K^+ levels may be the result of disturbed renal function and

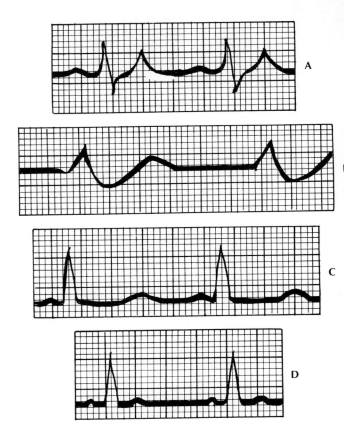

FIGURE 21-38 Electrocardiograms of patients with chemical imbalances. **A,** Hyperkalemia: mild case. **B,** Hyperkalemia: severe case. **C,** Hypocalcemia. **D,** Hypercalcemia.

consequent retention of K^+. The ECG shows a low P wave, prolonged P-R interval, prolonged QRS complex, and a tall, peaked, narrow T wave (Fig. 21-38). These ECG changes reflect conduction disturbances. In mild cases *(A)* the tracing resembles the illustration. In very extreme cases *(B)* the tracing is much different, with no P waves and a very wide QRS complex.

2 Calcium

a Normal: 9-11 mg % or 4.5 to 5.5 mEq/L.

b Hypocalcemia (below normal): calcium is very important in muscle function. Low calcium levels produce muscular irritability, tetany, and convulsions. The heart is affected in the form of a decreased ability to contract properly. The ECG shows prolonged S-T segment and Q-T interval and a flattened T wave (Fig. 21-38, *C*).

c Hypercalcemia (above normal): weakness is symptomatic of high calcium concentrations. The heart has decreased pumping strength, along with PVCs and idioventricular rhythms. The Q-T interval is shortened, the S-T segment is absent, and the T wave is close to the Q wave *(D)*.

12.0 DISEASES OF AND INJURIES TO THE HEART
12.1 Risk factors of coronary artery disease and atherosclerosis

1 Heart disease is the leading cause of death in the United States. The process leading to coronary heart disease (CHD; i.e., disease of the cardia circulatory system) is *atherosclerosis.* Atherosclerosis is a form of *arteriosclerosis,* commonly known as "hardening of the arteries."

2 Atherosclerosis refers to the arteriosclerotic process in which there are fatty deposits (especially cholesterol) on the inner layer of blood vessels. However, the term "atherosclerosis" is often used interchangeably with the word "arteriosclerosis," since atherosclerosis is the most common form of arteriosclerosis.

3 It is a *slowly* progressive disease that may start early in life. It can lead to heart attacks and strokes. As the disease progresses the walls of the arteries become roughened and thick. The arteries lose their elasticity; this is their ability to contract and expand. The arterial system is gradually narrowed, resulting in slow blood flow, and subsequently the vessel may be obstructed. This condition makes it easier for a clot to form; and once formed, a clot can travel to block circulation to the heart, brain, or other organs.

4 Atherosclerosis contributes directly to almost one million deaths yearly from heart attacks and strokes. In the past it was thought to be a disease Grandpa had in his 70s and 80s. However, during the Korean War, autopsies on supposedly normal soldiers in their 20s revealed some cases in which the atherosclerotic process had already reached advanced stages. Some of these 20-year-old soldiers had coronary arteries that were already 50% occluded.

5 Although not a common occurrence, autopsies performed on some high-risk children who have died in automobile accidents have revealed the beginnings of the atherosclerotic process. Evidence of atherosclerosis has even been found during autopsies on stillborn children. Atherosclerosis, a disease clinically associated with the aging process, may actually start at birth. It certainly is not considered part of the *normal* aging process.

6 The actual cause of CHD is unkown. At least 10 "risk factors" have been identified, however, as being associated with an increased chance of developing CHD.
   a Family history of CHD
   b Hypertension (high blood pressure)
   c High cholesterol levels
   d Gout
   e Diabetes
   f Being overweight
   g Cigarette smoking
   h Muscular body build, with heavy bones
   i Sedentary existence (i.e., life-style includes little or no exercise)
   j Aggressive, competitive personality (called a "Type A" personality)

7 Studies have shown that people who have a large number of these conditions at the same time are at high risk for developing CHD. Likewise, the fewer of these characteristics a person has, the less likely he or she is to develop CHD.

12.2 Angina pectoris

1 The atherosclerotic process may be quite advanced (i.e., the vessels quite narrow) before the person has signs or symptoms of the disease. If the vessels in the heart become so narrow that they are unable to carry sufficient blood to the heart to meet its needs, symptoms will appear. The classic symptom is *chest pain,* especially on exertion.

2 Chest pain of cardiac origin on exertion is called *angina pectoris.* The pain is the result of insufficient oxygen for the heart muscle—ischemia. (Similarly, if the leg muscles do not get enough blood supply, they begin to ache or cramp, causing leg pain.)

3 The pain of angina pectoris is most commonly located in the middle of the chest, but it may also shoot down one arm or up into the neck, jaw, or upper back. It is a steady pain and usually subsides with rest.

4 It is characteristically relieved by *nitroglycerin,* an oral vasodilator (opens up blood vessels temporarily) taken under the tongue and directly absorbed into the bloodstream. The nitroglycerin is believed to open the coronary vessels, thereby increasing the blood flow and oxygen supply, hence relieving the pain.

5 If angina pectoris worsens in time so that the pain is prolonged rather than of short duration on exertion, it is called *coronary insufficiency* or *preinfarction angina.* It represents a worsening condition.

6 If the artery to a part of the myocardium narrows and finally closes off completely (or is absolutely incapable of providing enough oxygen and nutrition to maintain a part of the myocardium), the part of the myocardium served by that vessel dies. The tissue death is called a *myocardial infarct (MI).* An MI is commonly called a "heart attack." (The general public may not distinguish between anginal episodes versus an MI when speaking of a "heart attack.") See Module Four, Unit 28.1.

7 In most cases the occlusion (blockage) occurs suddenly and may result in a heart that cannot work; the result is sudden death. However, death may not occur immediately but may still be a danger later, since arrhythmias may occur as a result of the damage.

8 The pain accompanying MI is characteristically a severe, crushing type. It is worse than the pain of angina. The person suffering MI will generally experience nausea, profuse perspiration, vomiting, and weakness soon after the pain begins. Additionally he or she will have a sense of impending doom and apprehension.

9 Not everyone who has MI will behave in this manner. The pain may resemble severe indigestion, or there may be only arm pain.

12.3 Diagnosis of a myocardial infarction

1 A myocardial infarction cannot be definitely diagnosed without the following data:

a An accurate history. Especially time of pain, type of pain, site of pain, and sensations (e.g., nausea) that accompanied the pain.

b Serial ECGs. That is, complete 12-lead ECGs over several days. If an infarct has been sustained, there will be gradual, characteristic changes in the ECG over time.

c Enzyme studies. When there is tissue death the deteriorating cells release certain enzymes into the blood. The blood concentration of three of these enzymes rise and fall in specific patterns over several days if there has been tissue death. The enzymes are listed here:
- Creatinine phosphokinase (CPK)—rises quickest after MI
- Serum glutamic-oxaloacetic transminase (SGOT)
- Lactic dehydrogenase (LDH)—rises on about the third day

2 Only after all these data are complete can a definite diagnosis be made regarding whether or not a person has suffered damage to the myocardium. Obviously the serial readings are not complete for several days. In the meantime the patient is *assumed* to have damage ("better safe than sorry") and treated accordingly in the coronary care unit.

3 The five major complications of a myocardial infarct are as follows:

a Arrhythmias (quite common after the MI)

b Acute heart failure

c Cardiogenic shock

d Thromboembolism (uncommon)

e Rupture of the left ventricle (uncommon)

4 Complications are less likely to occur after the first 5 days after the MI. It generally takes 6 to 8 weeks for the necrotic (dead) area of the myocardium to heal. At least the first 3 of those 6 to 8 weeks should be spent in the hospital setting. Years ago, post-MI treatment involved "rest and recovery." The current philosophy for post-MI therapy involves carefully graduated exercise that strengthens the undamaged heart muscle and develops collateral coronary blood circulation around the area of infarct.

13.0 IMPORTANCE OF CHECKING PATIENT CARDIAC STATUS BEFORE BEGINNING RESPIRATORY CARE TREATMENT

13.1 Checking the chart

Before beginning any respiratory care, the practitioner should check the chart for relevant information, consult with the nurse involved in the patient's care, and observe the patient directly. The following steps should be taken after receiving an order for a respiratory therapy treatment and before beginning administration of the prescribed treatment:

1 Check the admitting diagnosis. What brought the patient to the hospital?

2 Read the history and physical. It may describe problems (other than the primary problems for which the patient was admitted) that would have a bearing on the respiratory care. For example, a history of MI a year ago would warn of advanced coronary artery disease.

3 Check the problem list (if in use at the hospital). This may list problems that are new and therefore not in the initial history and physical. For example, a patient may have been admitted for gallbladder surgery, with no history of coronary problems, and then experienced chest pain during his or her recovery from surgery (angina?).

4 Check the results of laboratory tests, especially the electrolyte levels and, if performed, the blood gas analysis. Remember the effect of abnormal potassium and calcium levels on heart function and the effect of medications on electrolyte levels.

5 Medications. Especially check for cardiac drugs, diuretics, and oral bronchodilators. Consider the possibility of drug interactions.

6 ECG report. Especially relevant when there is a history of coronary disease, or an acute problem (e.g., suspected MI). An ECG is usually standard when surgery is scheduled on a patient over 30 to 35 years of age.

7 Vital signs over the last 24 hours. Include pulse, respiratory rate, and temperature (elevated temperature increases the heart rate).

8 Read the nursing notes and the doctors' progress notes over the last 24 hours, looking for new problems that are not mentioned in other places.

9 Consider whether there are any contraindications for the prescribed treatment or whether a different medication might be more beneficial or less hazardous for the patient.

13.2 Consulting the nurse and/or physician

1 After you have reviewed the relevant information on the chart, it is wise to identify the nurse involved in the care of the patient. There may have been recent events that have not yet been recorded on the chart that could influence the course of therapy.

2 Identify yourself to the nurse as the respiratory care practitioner assigned to provide treatment to the patient (name the patient and specify the treatment). Consult the nurse with regard to any uncharted events or circumstances that could have a bearing on the treatment prescribed. For example, Mr. Smith (the patient) may have had an episode of chest pain 10 minutes ago, and it may be necessary to delay the respiratory therapy treatment until the physician has been consulted.

3 On the other hand, you may have noted a contraindication to giving the respiratory therapy treatment prescribed and may wish to inform the nurse of the reason for the delay in treatment. You would then contact the physician who ordered the treatment to advise him of the problem or simply to suggest a more beneficial medication, and to receive his or her instructions.

13.3 Pretreatment patient observations

1 Observe the patient's general appearance; include observation of skin color and quality of respirations.
2 Introduce yourself to the patient and state the purpose of your presence.
3 Check the patient's pulse (apical and radial: compare the two to determine whether every apical beat is resulting in a pulse beat).
4 Listen to the patient's chest.
5 Ask the patient how he/she feels (if conscious). Is the patient feeling short of breath? Having pain? (Pain often renders the patient unable to cooperate with the treatment. Better to obtain relief from pain, if possible, before attempting a treatment.) Tired? Sleeping? (Weigh benefits of sleep versus necessity of treatment.) If it is decided to awaken the patient, wait until he/she is fully awake to begin the treatment.
6 Observe the bedside ECG monitor (if there is one). Other parameters relevant to the respiratory status and treatment of the critically ill patient are the central venous pressure and/or the arterial line or pulmonary wedge pressure.
7 Consider any contraindications to the prescribed respiratory therapy treatment.

13.4 Procedure 21-2 included at the end of this module may be used as a guide for gathering information pertinent to a patient's cardiac status.

14.0 TYPES OF ELECTROCARDIOGRAMS
14.1 Resting versus stress ECG

1 The *resting ECG* is the standard 12-lead assessment of the patient during inactivity. This test evaluates performance of the heart in a *static* condition and may not be useful in identifying abnormalities during periods of physical activity and stress.
2 The *stress ECG* may be one of two types.
   a Ambulatory ECG monitoring. A portable recorder is attached to the patient to record ECG activity as he/she conducts daily activities. The patient is instructed to simultaneously keep a log of activities so that activities can be matched to any abnormal ECG tracings.
   b Laboratory testing. Also called "stress testing." The stress ECG test is conducted in a laboratory under strenuous but controlled conditions. A treadmill or stationary bicycle is normally used to elicit maximum effort by the patient, and data are continuously recorded by a computerized ECG system. After the test the data are analyzed by the computer and used to determine fitness levels and coronary risk factors and to prescribe an exercise program.

PROCEDURE 21-1

ECG recognition: normal sinus rhythm versus abnormal pattern

No.	Steps in performing the procedure
1	The practitioner is provided with a clear, 6-second ECG strip and will carry out the following procedures: Calculate the heart rate. Determine whether it is **1.1** Bradycardia **1.2** Normal rate **1.3** Tachycardia
2	Determine the regularity of the cardiac cycles: regular or irregular?
3	Examine the P waves and P-R interval: **3.1** Description of P waves: shape, location with relation to QRS complex **3.2** P-R interval (in sec) **3.3** Determination: normal or abnormal
4	Duration of QRS complex: **4.1** QRS complex (in sec) **4.2** Shape: normal or abnormal
5	ECG recognition: **5.1** Is it a normal sinus rhythm? Yes or no? **5.2** Is it a lethal arrhythmia? Yes or no? If yes, which one? **5.3** Does the patient have a pacemaker? Yes or no?

PROCEDURE 21-2

Gathering information on a cardiac patient

No.	Steps in performing the procedure
1	The practitioner shall gather information pertinent to a patient's cardiac status before delivering respiratory therapy. From the chart: **1.1** Check the admitting diagnosis. **1.2** Read the history and physical. **1.3** Check the problem list (if applicable). **1.4** Check the results of appropriate laboratory tests. **1.5** Check the medication sheet/records. **1.6** Check the ECG report. **1.7** Check records of patient's vital signs over last 24 hours. **1.8** Read the nursing notes/physician's progress notes over last 24 hours. **1.9** Determine whether there are any contraindications for the prescribed respiratory therapy treatment. Also identify any reasons for caution, other alternatives for treatment, implications of data.
2	Consult the nurse and/or physician: **2.1** Introduce yourself to nurse, giving name, position. **2.2** Inform nurse of the prescribed treatment. **2.3** Consult nurse regarding any recent, uncharted changes in patient's condition. **2.4** Inform nurse of any concerns regarding appropriateness of the prescribed respiratory therapy treatment. **2.5** If indicated, consult physician regarding concerns (may be delayed until after direct patient observation).
3	Pretreatment patient observation: **3.1** Observe (and verbally describe to preceptor) patient's general condition, including skin color, quality of respirations, etc. **3.2** Introduce yourself to the patient; state purpose of visit. **3.3** Check the patient's pulse (apical and radial); note any discrepancy. **3.4** Listen to the patient's chest; describe findings. **3.5** Ask the patient how he/she feels (if conscious); proceed accordingly. **3.6** Observe the bedside monitor (if there is one); describe observations to preceptor accurately. **3.7** Consider any contraindications to prescribed treatment in view of the information from the chart, the consultation with the nurse/physician, and direct patient observation, and proceed with treatment or defer accordingly.

BIBLIOGRAPHY

Berne RM and Levy MN: Cardiovascular physiology ed 4, St Louis, 1981, The CV Mosby Co.

Blower MG and Smith RJ: How to read an ECG, ed 2, Oradell, N.J. 1977, Medical Economics Co.

Del Negro AA and Fletcher RO: Indications for and use of artificial cardiac pacemakers, Parts 1 and 2, Curr Probl Cardiol Oct-Nov, 1978.

DeSilva RA: Cardioversion and defibrillation, Am Heart J 100:881, 1980.

Dubin D: Rapid interpretation of EKGs, ed 3, Tampa, Fla., 1974, Cover Publishing Co.

Freeland JP: Defibrillation as a Heimlich maneuver, N Engl J Med 229:957, 1978.

Goldberger AL: Myocardial infarction: electrocardiographic differential diagnosis, ed 3, St Louis, 1984, The CV Mosby Co.

Goldberger AL: Recognition of ECG pseudoinfarct patterns, Mod Concepts Cardiovasc Dis 49:13, 1980.

Goldberger AL and Goldberger E: Clinical electrocardiography: a simplified approach, ed 3, St Louis, 1986, The CV Mosby Co.

Goldman MJ: Principles of clinical electrocardiography, ed 10, Los Altos, Calif, 1979, Lange Medical Publications.

Goodman SL: Prophylactic lidocaine in suspected acute myocardial infarction, J Am Coll Emerg Phys 8:221, 1979.

Guton AC: Textbook of medical physiology, Philadelphia, 1976, WB Saunders Co.

Hedges JR: Acute chlorine gas exposure, J Am Coll Emerg Phys 8:59, 1979.

Marriot JHL: Practical electrocardiography, ed 6, Baltimore, 1972, Williams & Wilkins Co.

Moorhead JM: Carbon monoxide and stress testing (letter), Chest 81:129, 1982.

Saimi M: A new method for evaluating anit-arrhythmic drug efficacy. Circulation 62:1172, 1980.

Standards and guidelines for cardiopulmonary resuscitation (CPR) and emergency cardiac care (ECG), JAMA 244:453, 1980.

Vos HP: The EKG—interpretation of common arrhythmias. Am Nurse Assoc 51:391, 1973.

Wasserberger J and Eubanks DH: Practical paramedic procedures, ed 2, St Louis, 1981, The CV Mosby Co.

Wellens JHH, Bar FW, and Lie KI: The value of the electrocardiogram in the differential diagnosis of a tachycardia with a widened QRS complex, Am J Med 64:27, 1978.

Willerson JT and Dehmer GJ: Exercise stress laboratories in the future; what should their capabilities be (editorial)? Chest 80:1, 1981.

Zema MJ et al: Electrocardiographic poor R-wave progression: correlation with postmortem findings, Chest 79:195, 1981.

Cardiopulmonary resuscitation

LEARNING OBJECTIVES

On completion of this module the reader will be able to:

1.1 Explain why cardiopulmonary resuscitation (CPR) is one of the most important skills available to a health care practitioner and a lay person.

1.2 Differentiate between the various levels of CPR certification by the American Heart Association (AHA).

2.1 Define the terms and definitions used in CPR.

2.2 Briefly describe the historical development of CPR.

3.1 Point out the value derived from participating in a CPR program.

4.1 Explain the various cultural influences relative to health care and CPR.

5.1 Describe the various physiologic events that influence function of the brain and heart after sudden death.

5.2 Defend expired air resuscitation as an effective method of alveolar ventilation.

5.3 Defend external cardiac compression as an effective method for causing circulation in the absence of a spontaneous heartbeat.

6.1 Point out the various performance standards for one- and two-person CPR in the adult and child.

7.1 Describe mechanical aids for practicing CPR.

7.2 Practice resuscitation with a CPR manikin or substitute.

8.1 Distinguish between clinical conditions that resemble a cardiopulmonary arrest and an actual cardiopulmonary arrest.

9.1 Explain the procedure for initiating emergency action once a cardiopulmonary arrest is identified.

9.2 Demonstrate correct CPR procedure for one rescuer.

9.3 Demonstrate correct CPR procedure for two rescuers.

10.1 Explain the steps presented for one- and two-rescuer CPR techniques.

11.1 Give examples of different self-inflating air-mask-bag units (manual resuscitators).

11.2 Describe the principles relative to the use of self-inflating manual resuscitators.

11.3 Explain general steps to be taken when preparing to use a self-inflating manual resuscitator.

11.4 Identify the component parts of a Laerdal resuscitation unit.

11.5 Explain the operation of the Laerdal resuscitation unit.

12.1 Demonstrate the operation of various self-inflating manual resuscitators.

12.2 Demonstrate proper technique for manually securing a face mask in place while using a self-inflating manual resuscitator.

13.1 Describe the use of the oxygen-powered resuscitator—demand valve.

14.1 Explain how mechanical cardiopulmonary resuscitators may be useful.

1.0 NEED FOR CPR SKILLS

1.1 General need for CPR

Cardiopulmonary resuscitation (CPR) is probably one of the most important skills that can be acquired by health care practitioners and by the general public. The uniqueness of CPR is that it is a life support activity that does *not* require special equipment or location to be performed effectively. It does require that the rescuer be proficient in CPR according to specific performance criteria. CPR is a combination of knowledge and skills that can be memorized and practiced, enabling one to react to an emergency in a methodic manner rather than in disorganized panic. It is important that CPR be initiated quickly and accurately, because time is the enemy of the victim, and cardiac compression, even when performed perfectly, is only 30% to 33% as efficient as the human heart.

1 Even though successful completion of this module will prepare the reader to perform at the *basic rescuer level*, it is recommended that the reader contact a local official of the American Heart Association or American Red Cross and enroll in a course leading to a certificate.

2 A certificate presented by either of these agencies is important documentation, should a question ever arise about one's competency to perform CPR.

1.2 Certification by American Heart Association

1 The American Heart Association in 1986 restructured its CPR course into two major levels: *basic life support* (BLS) and *advanced cardic life support* (ACLS).

2 Each of these levels has subcategories (levels) as outlined below:

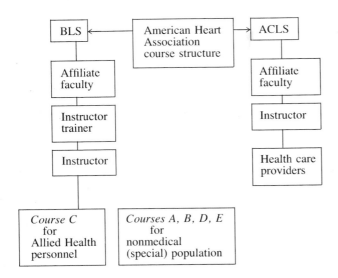

NOTE: BLS courses D and E are still under development.

3 When completed, course D will cover primarily prevention, pediatric CPR, and airway obstruction.

4 Course E will address the physically challenged population.

5 Courses A and B are first-level courses. These courses teach one to recognize a cardiopulmonary arrest and perform one-person CPR. The course takes approximately 4 hours to complete and is directed toward instructing the layperson.

6 The difference between BLS levels A and B is that level B is for laypeople with a specific interest in pediatric CPR.

7 The second level certificate is level *C,* which teaches one- and two-person CPR and treatment of obstructed airways and is directed more toward allied health personnel. This course takes approximately 8 hours to complete.

8 The third and highest level of noninstructor certification is the 2-day *Advanced Cardiac Life Support Course* (ACLS course). This course takes approximately 12 hours to complete and features advanced skills such as intravenous therapy, ECG interpretation, defibrillation, and intubation.

2.0 TERMS, DEFINITIONS, AND HISTORY AS RELATED TO CPR

2.1 Glossary of terms and definitions

1 Advanced cardiac life support (ACLS). Procedures and equipment used to stabilize a patient through definitive application of drugs, defibrillation, airway management, and transportation.

2 American Heart Association (AHA). A nonprofit agency devoted to educating the public about and supporting the treatment of heart and related organ disease. A local affiliate is probably listed in your phone book. The address of the national office is American Heart Association, 7320 Greenville Ave., Dallas, TX 75231; phone (214) 750-5362. Educational material and instructional aids are available from these agencies.

3 Artificial ventilation. A generic name given to various methods of artificially delivering a tidal volume to one who is *not* spontaneously breathing. Artificial ventilation can be delivered by expired air techniques, manual bag-and-valve units, and automatically cycling mechanical resuscitators and ventilators.

4 Backboard. Name given to a plywood or other rigid portable surface that is inserted under the bedridden patient before beginning CPR. The purpose of the board is to prevent the patient's body from being pushed into the mattress during external chest compression. The board ideally should be light, portable, and extend from the patient's shoulders to below the hips.

5 Bag-mask resuscitator. A general name given to an air-mask-bag unit (AMBU) that incorporates a nonrebreathing valve, a self-inflating bag, and a face mask. NOTE: These units can be used for resuscitation of patients with tracheal tubes by removing the face mask and attaching the resuscitator to the tracheal tube with a 15 mm OD adapter.

6 Basic life support (BLS). External cardiac compression combined with artificial ventilation. This is administered to sustain patients' vital functions until ACLS can be initiated or until patients are able to provide their own spontaneous life support.

7 Biologic death. A term describing the period of time after a cardiopulmonary arrest where cellular destruction is permanent and a patient who is resuscitated probably will experience brain and other tissue damage from hypoxia. CAUTION: The practitioner should *not* refrain from beginning CPR because 4 to 6 minutes may have elapsed since the arrest. Damage from tissue hypoxia is variable and depends on the patient's previous health, body temperature, and age. Successful resuscitations in children have been recorded after periods of up to 80 minutes under icy water.

8 Cardiac arrest. Cessation of an effective heartbeat as determined by absence of carotid or femoral pulse.

9 Cardiopulmonary arrest. Cessation of both breathing and effective heartbeat.

10 Head-tilt chin-lift maneuver. Replaces the previously recommended head-tilt/neck-lift method. Head tilt is accomplished by placing one hand on the victim's forehead and applying backward pressure to tilt the head back. The chin lift is completed by placing the fingers of the other hand under the bony part of the chin to lift it and bring it forward (see Module 20).

11 Circulation (perfusion). Movement of blood throughout the body.

12 Clinical death. A term describing the interval of time passing between the cessation of breathing and circulation and the beginning of biologic death (usually 4 to 6 minutes at normal temperature levels). Victims resuscitated *before* the beginning of biologic death usually do not suffer permanent brain damage because of hypoxia.

13 Emergency Medical Services (EMS). Consists of rescue personnel and local hospitals.

14 Emergency Medical Technician-Ambulance (EMT-A). The entry level allied health person who responds to emergency calls, provides basic emergency care at the scene, and transports the patient to the hospital.

15 Emergency Medical Technician-Paramedic (EMT-P). The advanced-level allied health person who responds to emergency calls, provides advanced emergency care (including IV infusion, defibrillation, intubation) at the scene, and transports the patient to the hospital.

16 External cardiac compression. The technique of compressing the external chest during cardiopulmonary resuscitation. This procedure causes blood to be pumped out of the heart as the compression is delivered.

17 Head-tilt maneuver. Tilting the patient's head backward while the patient is in a supine position. This technique is a means of opening the airway by lifting the base of the tongue off the airway leading to the trachea (see Module Twenty (and *10* above).

18 Heart attack. A general term used to describe a damaged heart muscle usually caused by blocked coronary blood vessels.

19 Heimlich maneuver. A technique of applying thoracic pressure to clear an airway obstructed by foreign matter (see Module Twenty).

20 Jaw-thrust maneuver. Alternate method of opening the airway. Used when the head-tilt/chin-lift does not work or if the patient has suspected neck injuries. The jaw thrust method requires that the rescuer lift the patient's jaw forward by applying pressure at the angles of the patient's mandible (see Module Twenty).

21 Myocardial infarction (MI). An abbreviation for a specific term describing death of heart tissue. An infarct is usually located in a specific area of the heart and is caused by blockage of coronary vessels to that area.

22 Mnemonics. Audible counts given by rescuers as they perform CPR as a means of coordinating key maneuvers during the resuscitation process. Mnemonics also allow national standards to be objectively evaluated during CPR exercises by trainers and instructors.

23 Mouth-to-mouth resuscitation. A method of expired air resuscitation where the rescuer exhales into the victim's mouth as the route of providing artificial ventilation to the victim.

24 Mouth-to-nose resuscitation. A method of expired air resuscitation where the rescuer exhales into the victim's nose as the route of delivering artificial ventilation to the victim.

25 Positioning the patient. A term referring to placement of the patient for CPR. It includes selecting a firm surface, placing the patient in a supine position, opening the airway, and positioning the rescuer for CPR.

26 Resuscitator. The instrument (person) used to revive one who is apparently dead.

27 Resuscitation. The act of reviving one who is apparently dead.

28 Respiratory arrest. Cessation of breathing or ineffective breathing.

29 Ventilator. Rescuer who provides mouth-to-mouth, mouth-to-nose, mouth-to-stoma, or bag adjunct breathing.

2.2 History of resuscitation

The history of expired air resuscitation is as long and as varied as there are books to report the findings. Therefore the following information represents only a summary of one version of the development of CPR. The purpose for this historical presentation is to help the reader understand the perspective that "there is nothing new under the sun."*

1 For the most part, resuscitation by respiratory methods was not practiced on humans until the eighteenth century. Resuscitation was practiced earlier on animals. Vesalius reported animal experiments as early as 1543.

a During the eighteenth century mouth-to-mouth respiratory resuscitation attempts were the most common method, with the first successful case reported in 1732.

b In the 1800s the medical profession regarded mouth-to-mouth methods as vulgar. However, the practice was continued by midwives on newborns.

c In the mid-1700s resuscitation methods utilized manipulations of the torso or the extremities. Variations of these methods continued until the late 1960s, when mouth-to-mouth resuscitation again became the method of choice.

2 Cardiac resuscitation progressed from open-chest methods in 1874 to the closed-chest technique in 1960.

a In 1874 Moritz Schiff, a graduate of the University of Gottingen, Germany, and professor of physiology at Florence, Italy, outlined the following procedure for *open cardiac massage:*

> If the thorax is opened and at the same time, air is insufflated into the lungs by rhythmical compression of the heart with the hands (care being taken in so doing not to interfere with the coronary circulation) and continue pressure of the abdominal aorta so as to bring the blood in greater quantity toward the head, it is possible to reestablish the heartbeat even up to a period of eleven and one-half minutes after the stoppage of that organ.

b In 1892 Maas, a German physician, performed one of the first successful cardiac resuscitations by closed-chest compression.

c In the 1950s open thorax heart massage was the method of choice, even though the survival rate was low (22%).

d In 1961 Jude, Kouwenhoven, and Knickerbocker reported in JAMA a 70% resuscitation rate after exter-

---

*Additional historical information and illustrations are presented in the August 1980 supplement to JAMA.

nal cardiac compression in 20 patients. In 1961 these men reported 24% long-term survival in 118 patients.

3.0 VALUE OF A CPR PROGRAM
3.1 Benefits from the CPR program

1 It is estimated that 35,000 heart disease victims die annually for lack of proper emergency medical care; 65% of these heart attack victims die within the first hour after the insult.

2 Undoubtedly, a good emergency medical program, including teaching BLS to citizens, will drastically reduce these statistics and allow as many as 30% of the heart attack victims to return to a productive life.

3 Other causes of sudden death include electric shock, drowning, anesthesia idiosyncracy, sensitivity reaction (bee stings), asphyxia, central nervous system (CNS) trauma, massive hemorrhage, and barbiturate overdose. Of these, death from heart attack and asphyxia (aspiration) are the most frequently encountered.

4 Today, because of advanced cardiopulmonary resuscitative technology, medical personnel must address the problem of assessing the value of performing resuscitation.

   a CPR should be *administered to anyone* dying suddenly and unexpectedly who can be restored to a useful existence.

   b Persons who are *not* usually resuscitated are listed here:

     • Patients with preterminal malignancies and chronic irreversible processes of liver, kidneys, lungs, heart, or brain.

     • Adults with no witnessed ventilation or circulation for 5 minutes at a normal environmental temperature

      NOTE: Children can tolerate hypoxia for longer periods of time at normal body temperature.

   c However, resuscitation should be attempted on *all* patients until specific orders not to start or to cease CPR are given directly by a physician.

4.0 CULTURAL INFLUENCES IN HEALTH CARE AND CPR
4.1 Cultural influences relative to health care and CPR

1 There are many cultural influences related to the delivery of health care in the United States, especially and specifically related to the delivery of CPR. In this culture we are basically a nontouching people. It is relatively unacceptable to touch other persons, and especially when administering CPR, the chest must be exposed to properly assess respirations, as well as properly assess excursion during chest compressions.

2 In some areas of the country there are people representing many different cultural backgrounds. These all affect the patients and their families' reaction to the "laying on of hands" necessary to the delivery any health care and especially the delivery of CPR.

3 Health care workers must assess their own feelings about hand-to-body contact, especially mouth-to-mouth contact. Each one must decide whether there is a conscious recognition of these feelings; for example, a man delivering mouth-to-mouth contact on another man is not an activity that normally occurs in the general population. Health care workers must recognize these feelings and deal with them in the manner most appropriate for themselves as individuals. It should also be noted that health alerts have been issued by some agencies expressing the possibility of contracting acquired immune deficiency syndrome (AIDS) from infected victims by mouth-to-mouth contact during CPR.

4 Many hospitals and prehospital emergency care agencies are using specially designed isolation valves to protect the rescuer from a risk of cross-contamination during exhaled air breathing. The Lifesaver isolation valve is an example of these units (Fig. 22-1, *A* and *B*).

5 With this unit as with the other brands, a series of measures are taken to protect the rescuer from accidental contact with a patient's vomit and/or exhaled air.

6 In this example the duckbill valve is a one-way valve that prevents exhaled air from being inhaled by the rescuer *(2)*. During exhalation gas passes around exhalation ports to the outside *(1)*.

7 Should the one-way valve fail, a fine-mesh bacteria filter prevents any of the victim's vomitus or other substance from reaching the rescuer *(3)*.

8 Many psychologic implications are associated with sudden death. Death in our culture is not generally discussed. There is a different treatment of death in our society than in many other societies and cultures.

9 For examples, an old-fashioned Irish wake is much more of a party, with much socialization, eating, drinking, and merriment, than the death and funeral process in the general population of the United States. Sudden death in particular is difficult not only for the health care worker to deal with in many situations but for the family as well. Understanding these feelings and dealing with them through whatever mechanism are beneficial.

   a Health care workers should examine their own feelings on death, the laying on of hands to other human beings, and dealing with a sudden-death patient who may not be successfully resuscitated, in spite of the proper procedures and efforts having been undertaken. Many people have strong feelings about dealing with sudden death in children. It is not uncommon to feel great emotional upheaval when a child dies, in spite of adequate resuscitation procedures and even though "everything was done that could have been done."

   b There is no shame in feeling sadness and showing emotion to the extent of crying with either the family or other workers over the untimely death of a patient. Often this facilitates resolution of feelings in the health care worker, as well as displaying an atti-

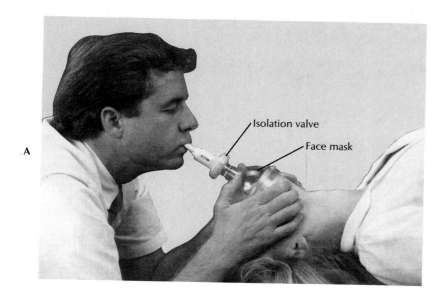
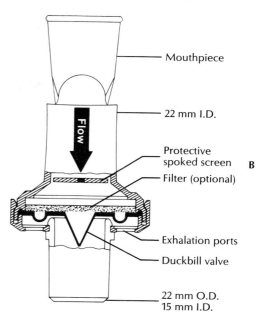

F I G U R E   2 2 - 1 A, Lifesaver isolation valve in use. **B,** Mechanics of isolation valve shows protective screen, filter, and one-way valve. (Courtesy Hudson RCI, Temecula, CA.)

tude of caring to the family, which will certainly help them.

10 The decision to initiate CPR in either terminally ill or "no code" patients does *not* rest with the health care worker but rather with a mutual decision arrived at between the physician and the patient and/or the family.

  a Occasionally there are patients in the hospital setting who are labeled "no codes." If this is the case, the proper procedure should be followed. The physician in charge of the patient should write an order on the chart indicating that no extensive resuscitation procedures will be initiated on the patient.

  b Unfortunately many physicians are hesitant to write this order on the chart and would rather communicate this information verbally to the nursing staff, and the nursing staff will often note on the Cardex (which is not part of the legal record) that the patient is a "no code." In the legal sense these patients should have resuscitation attempted regardless of the physician's verbal order. However, in reality and in practice it is not always attempted (see Module Two).

  c The entire question of *euthanasia* (i.e., "mercy killing") is more traumatic than simply making the decision not to begin resuscitation.

11 Outside the hospital setting, with the exception of obviously dead and hopeless patients (e.g., in a case of decapitation), resuscitation is always begun for a variety of reasons. Most specifically, a history is not usually available indicating that the patient does have a terminal illness or a physician is not usually present to make the decision whether or not to resuscitate.

12 Many seriously ill patients will have large numbers of family members present at all times. Therefore the health care worker is often placed in a position of having many observers present at the time of a cardiac arrest. Certainly family members should not remain in the hospital room or in the general vicinity during resuscitation; however, it is the responsibility of health care workers to communicate with the family. This is usually done by either the nurse or the physician, although others may be called upon if it will aid in the communication process.

5.0 PHYSIOLOGY OF SUDDEN DEATH, EXPIRED AIR RESUSCITATION, AND EXTERNAL CARDIAC COMPRESSION

5.1 Physiology of sudden death

1 Death is a physiologic and a biologic process that begins immediately after cessation of the heartbeat. Heart and/or respiratory arrest (clinical death) leads to permanent death (biologic death) unless delayed by effective CPR.

2 If respiratory arrest is *primary,* increasing hypoxia causes the pupils to begin dilation within approximately *45 sec,* followed by complete dilation after approximately *2 min.* If ventilation is returned within a 2- to 4-minute interval, a cardiac arrest probably can be averted. In research situations with animals the heart has continued to beat for as long as 8 to 10 minutes after cessation of ventilation.

3 If cardiac arrest is primary, the patient usually will experience gasping ventilations, followed by apnea within approximately *30 to 45 sec.*

4 When attempting to resuscitate a patient one must remember the general rule that a *hypoxic heart cannot be resuscitated.* This requires that one *always* initiate CPR by opening the airway and ventilating the patient before compressing the chest. Compressing the chest before ventilation would only circulate ineffective deoxygenated blood and waste valuable time.

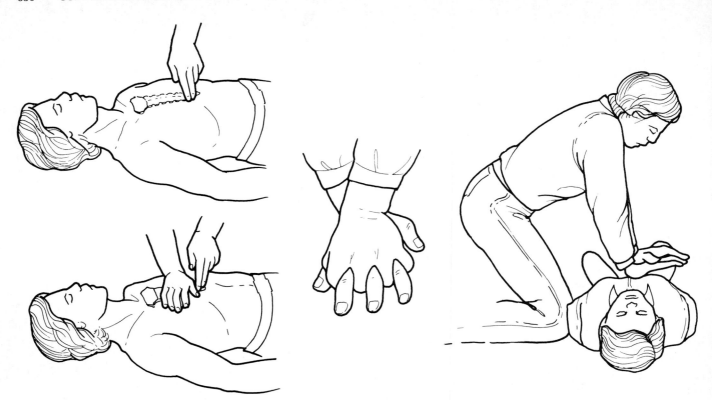

FIGURE 22-2 External cardiac compression on unconscious victim. (From Rosen P et al: Emergency medicine, ed 2, St Louis, 1988, The CV Mosby Co.)

5.2 Physiology of expired air resuscitation

The following is a simplified explanation of why one's expired breath can be effective in sustaining the oxygen (O_2) demands of another person. This explanation is calculated with a normal adult tidal volume of 500 ml.

1 Given a 500 ml tidal volume, the *first 150 ml* comes from the anatomic dead space of the rescuer. This volume of gas is equivalent to atmospheric gas or approximately 21% O_2 and less than 1% carbon dioxide (CO_2). Since it is delivered "first," the victim receives this as alveolar ventilation.

2 The *next 350 ml* exhaled by the rescuer represents the rescuer's alveolar ventilation, comprised of approximately 14% O_2 and 5.6% CO_2. Only 200 ml of this volume fills the patient's alveolar ventilation portion and the "last" 150 ml of the rescuer's 350 ml portion fills the victim's anatomic dead space and does not affect gas exchange at the alveolar level.

3 In this example the 500 ml of the exhaled gas volume used to resuscitate an arrested patient would consist of approximately 16% O_2 and 3.2% CO_2, instead of 20.9% O_2 and 0.03% CO_2.

4 It is important that one realize that the exhaled gas volume used to ventilate the patient can be brought closer to normal if the rescuer *increases the depth of his or her own tidal volume*, approximately 1½ times the normal volume. However, when performing expired air resuscitation the rescuer must also be aware that hyperventilation attempts can cause symptoms of dizziness and loss of consciousness. An unconscious rescuer is of no benefit to the patient!

5.3 Physiology of external cardiac compression

The following is a general explanation of how external compression works. It is recommended that the reader review anatomy of the heart from previous modules and in supplemental texts.

1 External cardiac compression describes the technique by which the rescuer places his or her hands on the sternum of the patient (Fig. 22-2). Circulation is generated when the rescuer compresses the sternum 1½ to 2 inches in the adult.

2 With each compression (downstroke) blood flows from the right side of the heart through the pulmonary artery into the lungs, where it is oxygenated by air that has been blown into the lungs by the rescuer (Fig. 22-3, *A*). Simultaneously blood goes from the left side of the heart through the aorta to the head via the carotid arteries and to the lower body via the descending aorta.

3 During relaxation (upstroke) blood flows into the right side of the heart (Fig. 22-3, *B*). As the chest reexpands from each compression, blood fills the right side of the heart via the superior and inferior vena cavae. Compression once again begins the circulatory cycle.

4 It is important that the chest compression cycle be *50% downstroke* and *50% upstroke,* and at a *proper rate* so that adequate time will be allowed for the blood to return to the heart before each compression.

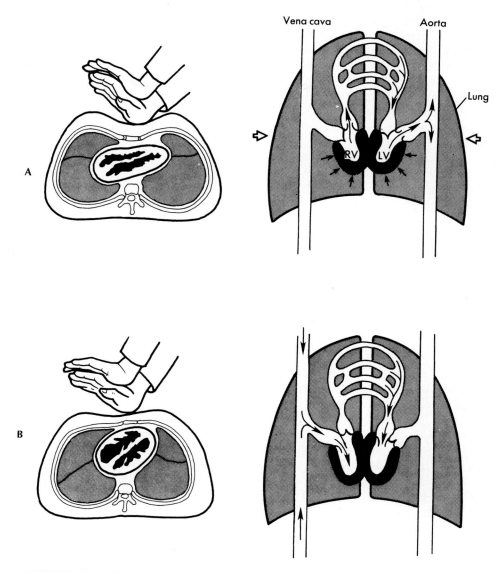

Vena cava

Aorta

Lung

RV LV

F I G U R E 2 2 - 3 External cardiac compression. **A,** Downstroke blood is forced to lungs and rest of body. **B,** Upstroke blood fills heart again. (From Rosen P et al: Emergency medicine, ed 2, St Louis, 1988, The CV Mosby Co.)

5 Time, force, and rhythm must be integrated to provide effective pumping action of the heart. This is true whether the heartbeat is self-generated or generated by cardiac compression.

6 Once started, the rhythmic compression and release of the chest result in a continuous blood flow that should not be interrupted for longer than 15 seconds at any given time.

7 It must be remembered that even when CPR is performed perfectly, it is only approximately 20% to 30% as effective as the patient's own efforts.

6.0 PERFORMANCE STANDARDS FOR CPR
6.1 Performance standards for CPR

The following information relates to standards that should be followed when performing CPR alone or with an assistant.

1 Ventilation—adult

  a During *one-person CPR* the patient is ventilated at 12 times per minute. This is the maximum rate that can be achieved, because the single rescuer must alternately switch from ventilation to compression.

  b This rate may seem low for an adult patient, but it is sufficient provided that adequate time (1 to 1.5 seconds) is allowed for each inspiration and the patient's chest rises.

  c During *two-person CPR* the ventilatory rate is 12 to 15 breaths per minute depending on whether or not the victim's airway is protected against aspiration with a cuffed endotracheal tube or esophageal obturator airway.

  d If the airway is protected, the patient may be ventilated in an asynchronous manner at a rate up to 15 times per minute. If one were to attempt to ventilate the untubed patient at this rate, the rapid inspiratory flow rate required would cause the airway pressure to exceed the esophageal opening pressure (approximately 25 cm H_2O) and air would be forced into the stomach.

  e A distending stomach may rupture, resulting in vomiting, and/or may force the diaphragm into the chest space, thus restricting lung inflation.

2 Ventilation—infant/child

  a The volume of air delivered to an infant or child is smaller than that given an adult, yet because the airways are smaller, more force may be required to make the chest rise. In an infant or child as with an adult, the breath should be delivered slowly, allowing 1 to 1.5 seconds for each inflation. Infants are especially vulnerable to gastic distension and care must be taken, as previously described, to avoid this situation.

  For an *infant* the ventilation rate is one breath every 3 seconds or 20 times per minute. For a *child* the rate is one breath every 4 seconds or 15 times per minute.

3 Circulation—adult

  a During *one-person CPR* the chest is compressed 80 to 100 times per minute.

  b The same rate is required for *two-person CPR*.

4 Circulation—infant/child

  a During one-person CPR in an infant the chest is compressed a minimum of 100 times per minute.

  b Two-person CPR is not required for an infant.

  c During one-person CPR of a child the chest is compressed 80 to 100 times per minute.

  d Two-person CPR usually is not required for a child. If the child is older than 8 years or is large for his or her age, two-person CPR may be used at the same rate as for an adult.

5 Ventilation-to-circulation ration—adult

  a The ratio of chest compressions to ventilations during CPR is very important to remember.

  b During one-person CPR the ratio is *15 chest compressions to 2 ventilations (15:2)* at a compression rate of 80-100 times/minute.

  c The ratio of chest compressions to ventilations during two-person CPR on an adult is *5 chest compressions to 1 ventilation (5:1)* at a rate of 80 to 100 times per minute.

6 Ratio of ventilation to compression—infants and children

  a The ratio of chest compressions to ventilation during one-person CPR on an infant is *5:1,* the same as two-person CPR on an adult, but the rate is at least 100 times per minute.

  b In order to perform CPR on an infant, one does *not* need to switch back and forth between ventilation and compressions as is required on an adult. This is because an infant is small enough so that the rescuer can perform mouth-to-mouth ventilation while simultaneously compressing the chest.

NOTE: Occasionally on larger children it will be necessary for two people to perform CPR, the same as for an adult, or a single person may perform CPR at the same ratio and using the same procedure as on an adult. On some children it may be necessary for the rescuer to compress the sternum using one hand instead of two as in the case of adults.*

More details on CPR are presented in Units 8 through 10 below.

7.0 PERFORMING CPR WITH MANIKINS AND RELATED MECHANICAL DEVICES

7.1 Mechanical CPR training aids

1 Before beginning this unit, learners are to obtain a training device for CPR practice. Manikins and other devices can be borrowed from the local heart association, police or fire department, Red Cross, public schools, or other public service organizations.

2 Two of the most popular devices are the Resusci-Anne and Recording Anne manikins, manufactured by the Laerdal Medical Corporation.

  a The Resusci-Anne is a life-size, lifelike manikin that allows direct mouth-to-mouth ventilation and bag-mask ventilation. External cardiac compression can also be done. Correct anatomic landmarks are also shown on the manikin chest.

  b The Recording Anne is similar to the Resusci-Anne but also features an ECG-type paper strip readout that prints a permanent record of the learner's efforts and shows whether their compressing strength and rate are adequate.

3 Laerdal also makes a Resusci-Baby for infant resuscitation practice and manikin heads for practicing tracheal intubation of both adults and infants.

4 A recent invention (Fig. 22-4) not only trains health workers to use proper chest compression technique but also can be used on a real patient's chest during an actual resuscitation attempt.

  a A rubber pad *(1)* is placed on a hard surface (or over the proper position on a patient's sternum).

  b The rescuer places his or her hands in the proper position on the rubber pad *(2)* and pushes down.

  c The compression pressure is read on the manometer *(3)* on either a force-in-pounds scale *(4)* or a scale showing general size ranges (e.g., child or small adult *[5]*).

  d The manometer also shows ineffective and excessive pressure ranges.

  e One manufacturer includes a battery-powered electronic timer that "beeps" in 60, 80, and 100/min rates to help with training or to time actual compressions.

5 Other manufacturers produce various training aids, but these will not be discussed because of space limitations.

---

*Refer to the JAMA August 1980 supplement for standards to use with infants and children.

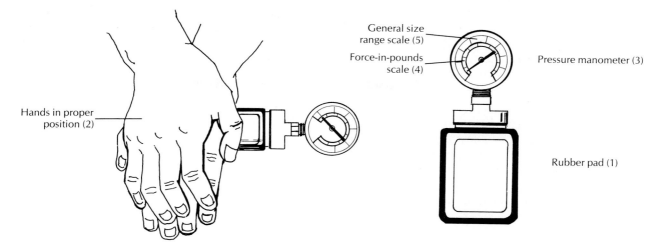

Hands in proper position (2)

General size range scale (5)

Force-in-pounds scale (4)

Pressure manometer (3)

Rubber pad (1)

FIGURE 22-4 Pressure manometer used to monitor health workers' chest compressions while performing CPR.

7.2 Resuscitation practice with manikins or substitutes

1 If manikins are used, it is recommended that they be checked for proper decontamination before their use.

In 1983 a Multidisciplinary Ad Hoc Committee for Evaluation of Sanitary Practices in CPR Training developed specific guidelines for preventing cross-infection from CPR training with manikins. The recommendations are available from the Centers for Disease Control, Atlanta, Georgia.

The use of 70% isopropyl alcohol is not sufficient in itself to prevent cross-infection from colds, hepatitis, and other pathogens. Persons with infections should *not* use the manikins. A typical routine service schedule for the Resusci-Anne is presented as Supplement 22-1 to this module.

2 If manikins are unavailable, CPR can be practiced with another person and imagination.

3 Role playing a cardiac arrest by having another person act the part of an unconscious victim is a desirable way of instructing arrest recognition, patient positioning, airway maintenance, and ventilation.

4 In the role-playing scenario the victim is unconscious and the rescuer follows the same techniques of recognition, positioning, opening the airway, and ventilation that would be used on a manikin.

5 This method of practice in many ways is more desirable than using a manikin, because it gives both the simulated victim and rescuer a different perspective of the psychologic and physiologic influences experienced during CPR. However, the role-playing method may create some resistance to the actual delivery of a mouth-to-mouth breath. If this is the case, a self-inflating manual resuscitator with a mask or disposable isolation valve unit can be used for ventilation. It will not harm people to be ventilated with a manual resuscitator provided they relax when the breath is delivered and excessive force is not used to empty the bag.

6 The location of proper hand positioning on a simulated victim's chest is easily taught by use of another person. The first step is to locate one's own sternal notch by moving one's hands along the sides of the ribs until the notch where the ribs meet the sternum is felt.

7 On the simulated victim, once the sternal notch has been located, final hand position is identified by placing two fingers on the sternal notch and then placing the heel of the appropriate hand in the middle of the sternum next to the two fingers.

8 CAUTION: In role-playing situations the sternum must not actually be compressed, because it could cause fractures, lung damage, or even cardiac arrest in a conscious person.

9 One can also practice actual compression at home by using a rigid suitcase that recoils once the side has been compressed. This approach allows one to practice body position, interlocking the fingers together, locking elbows, and performing compression with appropriate rate and rhythm. During compression rescuers should talk their way through the resuscitation effort for one- and two-person CPR by shouting compression counts and ventilation insertions as appropriate.

10 Practice for hand position and compression can also be obtained by using a cadaver, although none of these substitutes is as effective as a CPR manikin for instructional practices.

8.0 EVALUATION OF A PATIENT FOR CPR
8.1 Evaluating the patient for CPR

1 It is *dangerous* to perform CPR on someone who has an effective heartbeat and palpable carotid pulse. To prevent this accident a person must be able to distinguish between the various states and causes of unconsciousness that are not cardiac related. These include sleep, fainting, drug overdose, and coma caused by electrolyte imbalances.

2 Sleeping patients normally breathe more slowly and shallowly than when awake and can easily be mistaken as being in respiratory arrest.

3 A state of cardiopulmonary arrest is established by the following:

a *Level of consciousness.* Gently shake unconscious patients and call their names in an attempt to awaken them.

b *Absence of breathing.* Look and feel for chest motion, and listen at the patient's mouth and nose for sounds of air movement.

c *Absence of a pulse.* Feel for a carotid pulse using first one side of the neck, then the other. Do *not* feel for a carotid pulse on both sides of the neck simultaneously, because it may interrupt blood flow to the brain and cause unconsciousness and brain damage. If a pulse is *not* felt, the patient is in cardiac arrest.

4 Unconscious + no respirations + no carotid pulse = cardiopulmonary arrest.

5 If the patient is *not* in cardiopulmonary arrest, it is necessary for the rescuer to be able to assess whether or not the patient's pulse and respirations are *normal.* Unfortunately in medicine there are *no specific* normals—only ranges of normal.

a For example, the normal pulse range for a nonathletic adult can vary anywhere from 50 beats/min to 100 beats/min. Usually a rate below 60 beats is considered bradycardia. A rate above 100 beats is considered tachycardia.

b The normal pulse range for a child is 80 to 120 beats/min depending on the child's age. The younger the child, the faster the pulse rate, with a newborn having a normal range of 120 to 150. During crying or other intense activity the pulse rate may increase to 180 beats/min and during sleep may decrease to 70 to 90 beats/min.

c A normal range for adult respirations varies anywhere from 12 to 20 breaths/min. This range can fluctuate with activity, stress, and body temperature.

d A normal respiratory rate for a child can vary from between 20 to 35 breaths/min. Like the pulse, the younger the child, the faster the respiratory rate, with a newborn rate of 24 to 36 breaths/min.

e Systemic blood pressure in the adult is characteristically said to be normal at 120/80 mm Hg, although this also varies in adults and in children. In the newborn the blood pressure is 80/46 mm Hg at birth and gradually increases to 100/50 mm Hg by the tenth day.

9.0 EMERGENCY ACTION FOR ONE- AND TWO-PERSON CPR

9.1 Initiating emergency action

1 Once a cardiopulmonary arrest has been identified, the rescuer should immediately begin the "ABCs of resuscitation."

a **A**irway. Evaluate and open; check for spontaneous breathing and any signs of aspiration.

b **B**reathe. Breathe for the patient who is not breathing, breathing too shallowly, or too slowly.

c **C**irculate. Circulate blood by external chest compression if a carotid pulse is *not* present. Evaluate pulse for at least 10 to 15 seconds before beginning chest compression. CAUTION: Do *not* begin cardiac compression if a pulse is palpated.

2 The specific action to be taken by respiratory care personnel after determination of an arrest will vary from hospital to hospital. Employees should refer to the hospital or department policy and procedure manual on the details for answering an "emergency code."

9.2 BLS course A/B CPR study guide (one-person CPR)

1 The reader is encouraged to read CPR materials as provided by the AHA in addition to the information provided in this text.

2 If possible, the reader should complete one of the numerous courses offered by the AHA or American Red Cross for certification.

3 In any cardiac arrest situation, time and organization are very important. Standardized procedures, when followed, reduce wasted time by clearly indicating who does what, when, and how during the emergency. The steps involved in treating a cardiac arrest are clearly stated by most hospitals as a part of the department and/or hospital procedure manual.

4 A sample departmental procedure, "Initial Steps to Cardiopulmonary Resuscitation," is included as Supplement 22-2 at the end of this module as an *example* of a typical cardiac arrest procedure. This procedure shows the actions one should follow once an arrest has been identified in a hospital setting.

9.3 BLS course C (two-person CPR)

1 The use of a second person in a rescue attempt is advised for the following reasons:

a Allows the rescuers to perform CPR for a longer period of time

b Usually results in better technique

c Provides an option that will allow one rescuer to seek additional help if required

2 For this reason one should seek the assistance of another individual as quickly as possible. This must be accomplished without interrupting one-person CPR. Even if the second person is *not* familiar with CPR, this individual can observe the rescuer and quickly learn to provide the ventilation component. Remember, however, it is the trained individual's responsibility to ensure that the patient is receiving adequate ventilation and perfusion, even if it must be a single-rescue effort.

3 In most hospital situations two-person CPR will be used more frequently than one-person CPR. For this reason, readers are encouraged if possible to practice ventilating patients and compressing the chest so that they can switch with other rescuers as appropriate to the rescue effort.

4 When performing two-person CPR one person kneels close to the patient's side with one knee at the level of the head and the other knee at the level of the upper chest (Fig. 22-5).

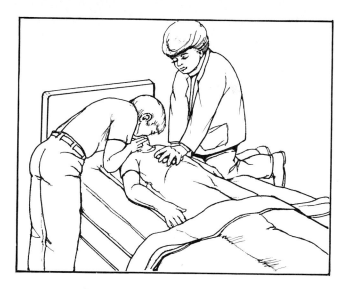

F I G U R E   2 2 - 5 Two-person CPR.

5   The second rescuer kneels alongside the patient's head on the opposite side of the patient from the rescuer performing cardiac compression.

6   In a two-person CPR routine the first rescuer continues to provide cardiac compression while the second rescuer enters the routine by delivering one ventilation at the end of 15 compressions. NOTE: The AHA has recently added another step at the point where the second rescuer enters the effort. Before beginning the ventilation the second rescuer must verify that the victim is actually pulseless (check the victim's pulse for 5 seconds) and in cardiac arrest (see Unit 10.1, *13*).

7   Ventilation is then interposed during the *upstroke* of each subsequent fifth compression. 1- to 1½-second-pause is allowed for each ventilation.

8   The cardiac compression rate is maintained at 80 to 100 compressions with two-person CPR and the compression-to-ventilation ratio becomes 5:1.

9   The person compressing the chest begins to count aloud, "1 one thousand, 2 one thousand, 3 one thousand, 4 one thousand, 5 one thousand," as a continuous process. A 1- to 1½-second pause is allowed at the end of the fifth compression for ventilation.

10 As previously explained, the pause for ventilation may be shortened or interposed with a pause if the patient's airway is protected from aspiration by a cuffed endotracheal tube.

11 After the first minute and every 4 to 5 minutes thereafter, CPR should be interrupted to check for a return of spontaneous breathing and a pulse for a maximum of 5 to 10 seconds.

12 If the rescuers tire and wish to change places, they should accomplish this without interruption. The person who is compressing the chest informs the ventilator of an intended switch by a verbal signal that replaces the count "1 one thousand, etc." with the mnemonic "*change* one thousand, 2 one thousand, 3 one thousand, etc."

13 Once the signal is given the ventilator gives a single breath after the fifth compression and turns to face the other rescuer. NOTE: This maneuver does not require the person to move to a different location.

14 The rescuer then locates the correct hand position on the patient's sternum with his or her index finger and middle finger and waits for the former chest compressor, who is *now* the ventilator, to signal the start of compressions.

15 The new ventilator is in position at the patient's head and now looks, listens, and feels for spontaneous breathing. At the same time the carotid artery is palpated for spontaneous pulse. This procedure should take a maximum of 5 to 10 seconds.

16 If no spontaneous pulse or ventilations are observed, the new ventilator gives one quick breath and states "*continue CPR,*" which signals the new compressor to begin compressions with "1 one thousand, etc."

10.0 ADEQUACY OF ONE- AND TWO-PERSON CPR
10.1 A cardiac arrest scenario

1   Use Fig. 22-6 *(A through L)* to visualize the action presented in the following scenario:

Mary Smith enters Mr. Jones' room for a routine O_2 check and greets him with the usual "good morning." Mr. Jones does *not* respond, and Mary notices he has a strange color and seems to be sleeping very soundly *(A)*.

(The patient who is unresponsive must be immediately evaluated to determine if cardiac arrest is present. The evaluation begins by observing the patient and noting that he appears to be unconscious.)

2   Mary places her hands on the shoulders of the patient and *shakes* gently, *calling* the patient: "Mr. Jones, Mr. Jones, are you awake?" *(B)*.

3   When there is no response or no movement on the part of the patient, Mary calls for *help* and then *places the patient on a hard surface* by either sliding him gently to the floor or by taking a backboard and placing it under the patient's trunk.

(In a hospital setting there is normally a procedure within the hospital to signal cardiac arrest. It may be an emergency announcement on the intercom; it may be "code blue," "Dr. Blue," or "code 99." Many other codes are used to announce over the intercom depending on the location. Many hospitals have a specific "code team" that responds to all cardiac arrests and assumes responsibility when they arrive. Some hospitals have a supervisory person who is the team leader of a code team. That person may be a physician, a nurse, a respiratory therapist, or an anesthesiologist, depending on the hospital.)

4   Once Mr. Jones is positioned, Mary immediately clears and opens his airway (see Module Twenty, Airway Management Techniques).

(This is done by placing one hand on the forehead and pushing back while using the other hand to lift up on the chin *[C]*. This position pulls the tongue up from

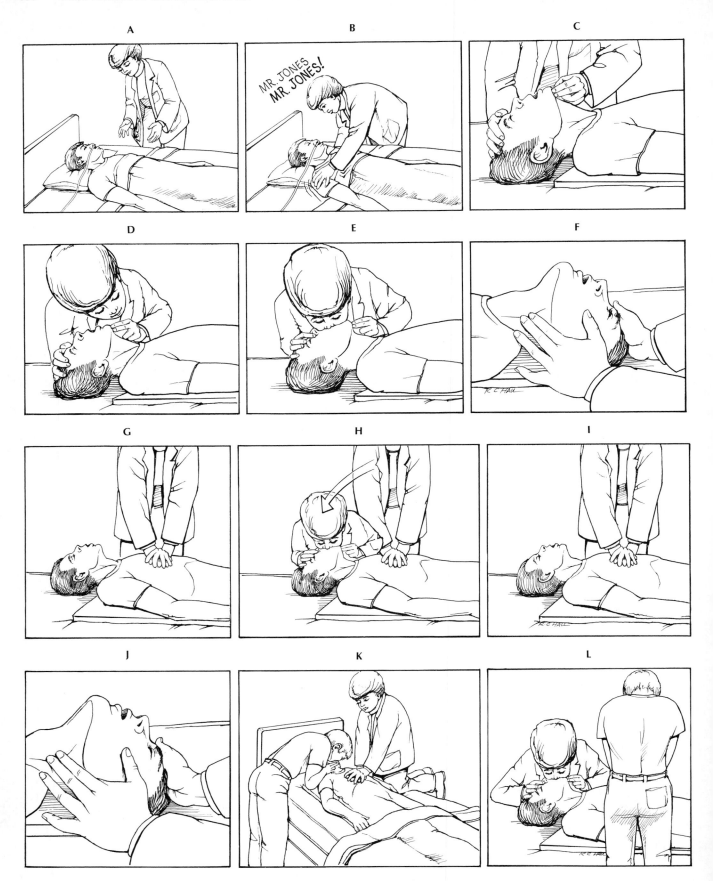

FIGURE 22-6 Cardiac arrest and CPR scenario.

the back of the throat, where it frequently blocks the airway in unconscious patients and is the most common cause of airway obstruction.)

5 Mary then assesses the patient for breathing signs (D).

(This is done by bending over the patient's face, looking at the chest and abdomen for movement, feeling with the side of the rescuer's cheek to determine if air is moving in and out of either the nasal passages or the oral passages, and, additionally, listening for breath sounds at the mouth and nose.)

6 Determining that there is no breathing, Mary administers four mouth-to-mouth ventilations (E).

(This is done by pinching the nose with the thumb and index finger. Mary then opens his mouth, takes a deep breath, and blows into the mouth of the patient with two deep, slow breaths. Each ventilation must be delivered with a separate breath from Mary, and take approximately 1-1½ seconds each.

7 After delivering the ventilations Mary then locates the carotid pulse (F).

(This is done by placing the index and middle fingers lightly on he voice box (larynx) and sliding the fingers around the side of the larynx to the area of the carotid pulse. This area must be palpated for a period of 5 to 10 seconds to determine if pulse is present. If the pulse is not present, the rescuer proceeds to initiate chest compressions.)

8 Mary positions herself alongside the patient opposite his nipple line and places her hands over his sternum (G).

(This is done by taking one hand and moving it along the side of the ribcage to locate the sternal notch area. After locating the sternal notch, two fingers should be placed upward on the sternum. The heel of the other hand is then placed directly on the centerline of the sternum, two fingers up from the sternal notch. The other hand is placed directly over the heel of the opposite hand, with the fingers entwined.)

(The heels of the hands are on the sternum, the elbows are locked, the shoulders are directly over the sternum, and a downward movement is begun to depress the sternum 1½ to 2 inches.)

(If the patient is still in the bed, it is necessary to either kneel on the bed beside the patient or stand on a stool beside the bed. The rescuer's shoulders must be located over the patient so that the elbows can be locked in a straight position.)

9 Mary counts out loud as 15 chest compressions are delivered, using the following mnemonic: "1 and 2 and 3 and 4 and 5 and 6 and 7 and 8 and 9 and 10 and 11 and 12 and 13 and 14 and 15."

10 At this point Mary leans (does not move her knees) rapidly back to the head, placing one hand on the forehead, the other hand under the chin, pinching the nose, and delivering two slow and deep mouth-to-mouth ventilations (H).

11 Mary then moves back to the chest again, locates the proper position for the heel of the hands, and again de-

livers 15 chest compressions (I) using the same mnemonic. The cycle is repeated at least three more times.

12 After 1 minute Mary stops for no more than 3 to 5 sec and checks the carotid pulse to ascertain if, in fact, there has been a spontaneous return of pulse (cardiac activity (J). (If the carotid artery remains pulseless, the cycle of alternate mouth-to-mouth ventilations and chest compressions is continued.)

While checking for the carotid pulse, Mary also leans over the body to look, listen, and feel for return of spontaneous breathing.

13 Another person, Joe, arrives. He is well trained in CPR and able to assist Mary. After positioning himself, Joe first checks for the carotid pulse being produced by Mary. He then asks Mary to stop compressions while he verifies that a pulseless state exists (5 to 6 seconds only). Satisfied that the patient is still in need of resuscitation, he enters resuscitation by delivering one quick breath and states "continue CPR." When the second rescuer enters into the resuscitation, Mary changes the mnemonic to the following: "1 one thousand, 2 one thousand, 3 one thousand, 4 one thousand, 5 one thousand." At the count of "5 one thousand" the second rescuer delivers one mouth-to-mouth ventilation (K). (Joe keeps one hand on the forehead of the patient, pinches the nose, and keeps his other hand under the patient's chin. Obviously, having two people kneeling in the same bed with a patient can be difficult [L]. The availability of a footstool cannot be overemphasized. The best position for the rescuers is to get the patient to the floor, but this is not always possible.)

14 As the CPR effort continues Mary tires of performing chest compressions and wishes to switch places with Joe, who is providing artificial ventilations. In order to coordinate the switch, she gives the following call in place of the regular mnemonic "1 one thousand, etc.": "change one thousand." This signal or call indicates that Mary is tiring and wishes to switch places with the rescuer giving the artificial ventilations. (Again, this is the call: "change one thousand, 2 one thousand, etc." This means the rescuer delivering the artificial ventilations will give two ventilations on the upstroke on the fifth compression, move from the head to the chest area, locate proper hand position, and wait for the verbal signal from the new ventilator to begin compressions. The new ventilator checks for spontaneous pulse and breathing for a maximum of 5 to 10 seconds and, if there are none, gives one breath and states "continue CPR.")

15 The new compressor begins "1 one thousand, 2 one thousand, etc." while delivering chest compressions. The new ventilator interposes a breath on the upstroke of the fifth compression, pausing for 1 to 1½ seconds for the breath to be delivered. (L).

16 The person delivering chest compressions is the person who must call out the mnemonic with each and every chest compression. REMEMBER: In two-person CPR the count consists of "1 one thousand, 2 one thousand, 3 one thousand, 4 one thousand, 5 one thousand."

17 During the administration of CPR it is important to monitor many techniques. One of them is to continuously observe that the chest wall is being depressed to a depth of 1½ to 2 inches. This is necessary to adequately squeeze the heart to pump blood to the vital organs. Additionally, ventilation should be delivered so that there is no leak. A good seal must be present, whether ventilations are delivered in mouth-to-mouth method or with a bag-mask resuscitator.

11.0 SELF-INFLATING MANUAL RESUSCITATORS

11.1 Air-mask-bag units

1 AMBU is an abbreviation for air-mask-bag unit, originally developed by Rubin in 1955 and registered as a trademark by the Air-Shields Corporation.

2 AMBU-type manual resuscitators refer to bag-and-valve devices that *self-reinflate* once they have been manually squeezed to provide a positive pressure tidal volume to the patient.

3 AMBU has come to mean *any* self-inflating air manual breathing unit. However, in the following units, manual resuscitator will be used in lieu of AMBU, which is a brand name. "Pulmonary resuscitator" is a generic term describing numerous manual and automatically cycling devices that are used to ventilate a patient, usually for a short period of time (30 minutes or less).

4 There are many different models of self-inflating manual resuscitators, which are manufactured by the following companies. These units differ in bag design and material of construction, as well as type of nonrebreathing and intake valves (Fig. 22-7).

  a Air Shields Corporation—AMBU unit *(A)*

  b Bird 3M Corporation—Air Bird unit *(B)*

  c Ohio Medical Products—Hope unit *(C)*

  d Puritan-Bennett Corporation—PMR unit *(D)*

  e Laerdal Corporation—Laerdal unit *(E)*

5 Rather than attempt to explain the operation of all of these units, the Laerdal adult model resuscitator will be used as an example in this module. The operation and features of this unit can be applied to understanding the operation of other self-inflating units.

6 The American Medical Association in its special issue of JAMA, "Standards and Guidelines for Cardiopulmonary Resuscitation and Emergency Care," made the following recommendations regarding criteria for a bag-mask unit:

  a A self-refilling bag that is easily cleaned and sterilized

  b A nonsticking valve system at 15 L of O_2 inlet flow per minute

  c No pop-off valve, including on pediatric models

  d Standard 15 mm/22 mm fittings

  e A system for delivery of high concentrations of O_2 through an ancillary oxygen inlet at the back of the bag or through an oxygen reservoir

  f A true nonrebreathing valve

  g Adequacy for practice on manikins

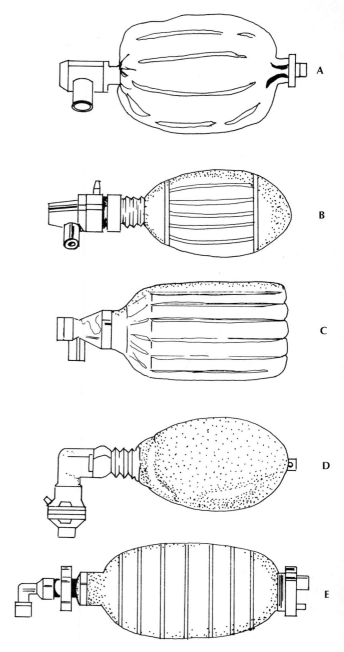

FIGURE 22-7 Manual resuscitator bags. **A**, AMBU. **B**, Air Bird unit. **C**, Hope unit. **D**, PMR unit. **E**, Laerdal unit.

  h Satisfactory performance under all common environmental conditions

  i Availability in adult and pediatric sizes

11.2 Guiding principles relative to use of self-inflating manual resuscitators

1 Regardless of the type of manual resuscitator, there are certain *principles* relative to their administration that should be followed:

2 Principle No. 1. In a pulmonary arrest situation, mouth-to-mouth or other methods of providing immediate ventilation should be initiated unless a manual resuscitator is readily available.

TABLE 22-1 Table of resuscitation bag evaluations

Manual resuscitator	Maximum stroke volume (ml)	Maximum cycling rate (breaths/min)	Maximum O_2% without reservoir	Maximum O_2% with reservoir	Overpressure relief (cm H_2O pressure)
AMBU	1240	69	76	93	85
Hope	1570	100	48	58	155
Puritan	1800	60	38		150
Laerdal	1100	70	35	95	65
Bird (Air Viva)	1380	50	38	86	75

3 Principle No. 2. With a manual resuscitator a leak-proof system must be maintained between the resuscitator and the patient.

4 Principle No. 3. Effective ventilation must be visually assessed by observing the patient's chest expansion during a manual inflation.

5 Principle No. 4. In nonintubated patients, care must be taken to protect the patient against possible regurgitation and aspiration of stomach contents.

6 Principle No. 5. A manual resuscitator must always be tested for correct operation before use on a patient.

7 Principle No. 6. Excessive flow rates or inflation pressures (greater than 25 cm H_2O) should not be used. They can cause distension of the stomach and/or excessive lung volumes, leading to possible barotrauma.

8 Principle No. 7. Self-inflating units refill from the atmosphere and cannot be used in smoke-filled or other air-polluted environments.

9 Principle No. 8. Supplemental O_2 must be added to the unit if the patient requires a fraction of inspired oxygen (FIO_2) greater than 0.21.

10 Principle No. 9. The FIO_2 of gases delivered by a manual resuscitator depends on the following:

a Stroke volume. The amount of volume squeezed between the thumb and all fingers out of the bag after full inflation of the bag. The larger the stroke volume, the larger the volume of O_2 that has to be used to refill the bag; the remaining volume entrained will be air, which will decrease the FIO_2.

b Refill time of the bag. The slower the bag refills with an O_2 flow, the smaller the amount of room air entrained, leading to a higher O_2 concentration. Refill time is controlled by a slow release of the hand.

c Rate. A fast ventilation rate will decrease the time available for the bag to refill, causing a decrease in O_2 concentration (a combination of *10a* and *10b*).

d Flow rate of O_2. The higher the flow rate of O_2 to the bag, the higher the concentration, provided items are not beyond normal design limits. CAUTION: The use of high O_2 flow rates (above 15 L/min) is not recommended without a special attachment, because it may interfere with the function of the valve in some units.

e The presence or absence of an O_2 reservoir bag. Table 22-1 illustrates the relationship between the tidal volume being delivered, the bag cycling rate, and

the flow of supplemental O_2 in determining the FIO_2 delivered to the patient using the adult 1600 ml Laerdal bag *without* an O_2 reservoir attachment. Similar performance tables should be examined on any manual resuscitator before it is purchased for use as an emergency device. O_2 percentages shown are not absolute and will differ according to the variables listed above.

11 Principle No. 10. Resuscitators with various size bags should be available for adult and pediatric use.

12 Principle No. 11. Relief ("pop-off") valves should be adjustable so that high airway pressure can be delivered when needed without the valve venting ("popping off") to the atmosphere. NOTE: Relief valves are not used except on pediatric and/or infant units.

13 The following manual resuscitator sizes are available from Laerdal. Other companies offer similar size selections.

a Adult—1600 ml bag for patients over age 10 years

b Child—500 ml bag for patients age 1½ to 10 years

c Infant—240 ml bag for newborns and infants to age 2 years

14 Principle No. 12. PEEP attachments should be available for use with patients who are not able to maintain adequate arterial oxygen tension (PaO_2) with a resuscitator without an attachment.

11.3 Preparing a self-inflating manual resuscitator for use

Before using a self-inflating manual resuscitator, the practitioner should take the following steps:

1 The patient must be positioned on the back, with the airway clear and head hyperextended to provide an open airway (refer to Module Twenty).

2 If a face mask is used, the proper size mask should be selected to fit the patient's face. In addition, the air-filled cushion should be inflated or deflated with the filling tube to achieve the best contour to the patient's face.

3 If a tracheal tube is in place, the mask should be pulled off the exhalation valve so that a 15 mm tube adapter can be inserted into the patient outlet of the valve housing.

If supplemental O_2 is to be added, an O_2 source with a flowmeter and delivery tube should be available.

Oropharyngeal airways should be available if a face mask is used for the resuscitation.

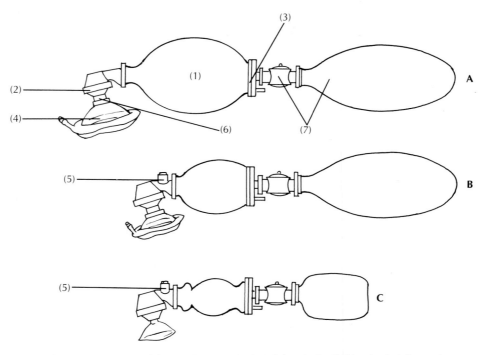

F I G U R E 2 2 - 8 Laerdal resuscitation unit. **A**, Adult unit. **B**, Child unit. **C**, Infant unit.

The breathing unit should be removed from its container and checked for proper valve operation by squeezing the bag and noting the rise and fall of the valves. Leaks should be identified by occluding the outlet port of the exhalation valve while squeezing the bag. If the bag collapses, there is a leak.

11.4 Components of the Laerdal resuscitation unit

1 The Laerdal self-inflating manual pulmonary resuscitator, which is available in adult, child, and infant sizes (Fig. 22-8, *A, B,* and *C*), incorporates the following components (according to Laerdal literature):

a A self-filling vinyl bag that can be folded for storage *(1)*

b An exhalation valve that *does not* jam with supplemental O_2 flows of 15 L/min, or at low temperature, or when foreign matter is aspirated into the valve housing *(2)*

c A disk membrane intake valve that allows easy entrainment of room air during bag reexpansion and addition of supplemental O_2 at flows to 15 L/min *(3)*

d A transparent plastic face mask with an air-filled or contoured resilent cushion to minimize leaks and maximize patient comfort *(4)*

e A preset 35 cm H_2O pressure-limiting valve ("pop-off") that can be finger controlled, on child and infant models only *(5)*

f Standard 15 mm/22 mm fittings to allow attachment of standard-size tube connectors and masks *(6)*

g A supplemental O_2 system that can be easily attached to the bag for delivery of FIo_2 greater than 0.65 *(7)*

h A special attachment to allow addition of PEEP or CPAP modification (not shown)

11.5 Operation of the Laerdal resuscitation unit

1 Inspiration

a The *ventilation bag* will automatically expand, once it is removed from its container, and reexpand after each squeeze (inspiration).

b When the ventilation bag is squeezed, positive pressure is generated inside the bag, causing the *lip-shaped* valve in the patient valve housing to open and allows gas to go to the outlet port. See the illustrations under "intake valve" and "patient valve."

c At the same time, when the bag is squeezed the disk membrane in the air-intake valve housing is pressed against its seat, preventing gas from flowing backward and leaking into the room.

d If the patient is breathing spontaneously (bag is not being squeezed), both the lip membrane and the disk membrane remain open to allow room air to flow through the unit to the patient.

2 Exhalation

a During exhalation a positive pressure caused by the exhaled gas closes the lip membrane of the patient valve, preventing a back flow of exhaled air into the ventilation bag. Simultaneously the external disk membrane in the air intake housing is lifted away from its seat by the inflow of air toward the decreased pressure gradient created by the expanding bag until the bag is full and the pressure equalizes, causing air entrainment to cease.

b If supplemental O_2 is being administered, it will mix

with the room air as it is entrained. Once the bag is fully expanded with room air and O_2, excess O_2 flow will be vented to the room through the open end of the intake valve.

3 If the O_2 reservoir assembly is used to provide a FIo_2 greater than 0.65, it is attached to the wide-bore connector in the rear of the intake valve.

   a The reservoir assembly consists of a valve unit and inflatable bag.

   b O_2 enters the reservoir assembly unit and the ventilator bag via the O_2 nipple of the intake valve during a patient's exhalation.

   c O_2 flow to the reservoir bag should be adjusted so that the reservoir bag *does not* completely collapse when the ventilation bag reexpands.

   d As the ventilation bag reexpands the complete expansion volume must come from the reservoir bag because the air intake vents on the ventilation bag are blocked by the wide-bore connector. If the O_2 flow to the reservoir bag is too low (indicated by a flat reservoir bag) for the patient's inspiratory demands, a safety air-entrainment valve opens in the O_2 valve housing, allowing room air to be entrained to supply the deficit between what is needed and what is being delivered.

4 If PEEP or CPAP (elevated baseline pressure) is required, a special *expiration diverter* can be attached to the nonrebreathing valve. This diverter directs exhaled gases through an inlet port, which can be used for attachment of a ventilation meter or elevated baseline modality (PEEP valve).

12.0 USE OF SELF-INFLATING MANUAL RESUSCITATORS

12.1 Using self-inflating manual resuscitators

1 The guiding principles presented in a previous unit established general rules that should be observed during use of a manual resuscitator.

2 Clinically it is most significant that the operator constantly assess the compliance of the patient's chest. This factor compared with other assessments, such as vital signs and level of consciousness, is a good indicator of whether or not the patient is improving or deteriorating. For example, a *decreasing* compliance, as signaled by an *increasing* airflow resistance as the operator squeezes the bag, probably indicates that the patient is deteriorating.

3 It is important that the clinician realize the limitations of any clinical assessment for predicting the effectiveness of ventilation. An accurate assessment of ventilation can be made only by analyzing arterial blood gases or, in some cases, through noninvasive methods such as transcutaneous monitoring devices.

4 Manual resuscitators are indicated in situations where short-term pulmonary ventilation is required. These include CPR efforts, transport of patients between points, hyperventilation techniques during suctioning, and, in emergencies, while the patient is being pre-

pared for attachment to a ventilator for continuous ventilation.

5 The hazards most frequently encountered when using manual resuscitators include the following:

   a Leaks around the face or tracheal tube that prevent proper lung inflation

   b Improperly functioning equipment because of missing parts, improper assembly, dirty and sticking valves

   c Poor ventilation technique by the operator, such as failure to empty the bag enough to deliver a functional tidal volume, too-rapid or too-slow breathing frequency, failure to maintain a patent airway, and pausing too long between breaths while other procedures are being delivered

   d Failure to recognize and properly handle tension pneumothorax, aspiration, or acute episodes of hypoxia

6 A method for assessing operation of a self-inflating manual resuscitator is included as Procedure 22-1 at the end of this module.

7 If possible, the reader is encouraged to practice using a manual resuscitator on a manikin, another person, and a patient according to Procedure 22-2, also included at the end of this module.

12.2 Applying a face mask

1 One of the most difficult skills to be mastered when using a self-inflating manual resuscitator is proper positioning and securing an airtight seal of a face mask.

2 Masks are constructed of black rubber or various combinations of transparent plastic and vinyl, which permits visual observation of the patient's mouth.

3 Face masks consist of three major parts:

   a The body

   b The seal

   c The connector

4 The *body* forms the main structural portion of the mask. Frequently it can be molded to better fit the patient's face.

5 The *seal* contacts the patient's face and prevents gas leaks between the face and mask. Mask seals may be inflatable air cushions or malleable material. Another type of seal is the rubber or plastic *flange,* which is a molded part of the mask body and is not inflatable.

6 The *connector* is the small opening in the body that allows the mask to be attached to the resuscitator or other system. Masks have two types of connectors: 22 mm outer diameter male, and 15 mm inner diameter female.

7 The secret to securing a proper seal with a face mask includes the following:

   a Selecting the proper mask size

   b Positioning the patient's head

   c Adjusting the seal

   d Fitting the mask to the face

   e Securing the mask in place

8 When selecting a face mask, a good rule is to select the

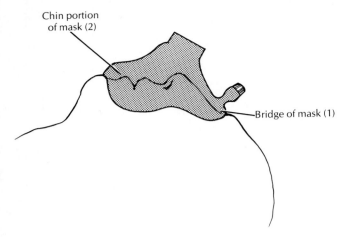

FIGURE 22-9 Proper placement of resuscitation unit mask over patient's face.

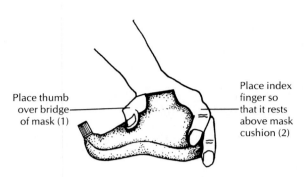

FIGURE 22-10 Proper hand positioning when holding resuscitator mask to patient's face.

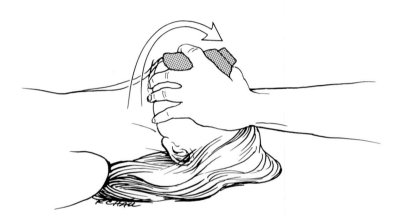

FIGURE 22-11 Proper placement of hands to hold resuscitator mask to patient's face and perform head-tilt maneuver.

smallest size that will provide a tight seal. This reduces dead space and is easier for the operator to hold in place. Masks are available in all sizes, from premature infants to large adults. Most masks can be shaped to fit most patients' faces. Patients' faces that create the *most difficulty* are those that are edematous, those that are burned or have other types of trauma, those that have beards, receding jaws, or flattened noses, or those that have nasogastric tubes in place.

9 Figs. 22-9, 22-10, and 22-11 show how a mask should be held with one hand. Detailed instructions that accompany the illustrations can be found in Procedure 22-3 at the end of this module.

10 The reader is encouraged to practice placing a face mask on a manikin, another person, and, if possible, a patient, according to Procedure 22-3.

13.0 USE OF OXYGEN-POWERED RESUSCITATORS—DEMAND VALVES

13.1 Oxygen-powered resuscitators—demand valves

1 A demand valve is a gas-powered mechanical resuscitator that operates in response to a patient's spontane-

ous breaths (assistor) or can be manually or automatically cycled if the patient is not breathing (controller).

2 Resuscitators are either *time cycled* or *pressure cycled*.

a A *time-cycled* device delivers a tidal breath for a preset length of time and cycles off.

b A *pressure-cycled* device delivers a tidal breath until a preset internal pressure is reached and then cycles off. In either case the patient may or may not have received an adequate tidal volume to ensure effective alveolar ventilation.

3 Oxygen-powered resuscitators should meet the following performance criteria*:

a Provide instantaneous flow rates of at least 100 L/min

b Have an inspiratory pressure safety release valve that opens at 50 cm H_2O

c Provide 100% O_2

d Operate satisfactorily under environmental conditions, including all temperature extremes found in North America

---

*According to the Aug. 1, 1980, supplement to JAMA.

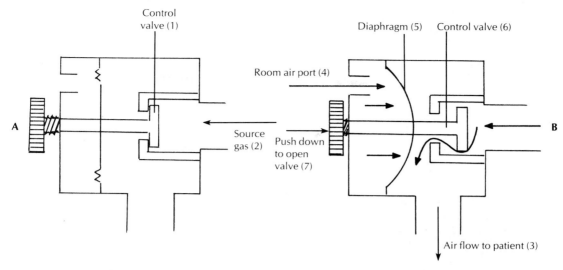

FIGURE 22-12 Demand valve. **A,** Closed position. **B,** Open position.

e Have a standard 15 mm/22 mm coupling for mask, endotracheal tube, esophageal airway, and tracheostomy tubes

f Have a rugged, breakage-resistant mechanical design that is compact and easy to hold

g Have a trigger (OFF/ON button) positioned so that both hands of the rescuer can remain on the mask to hold it in position while supporting and tilting the head and keeping the jaw elevated

4 Because most demand valves are similar, the Robertshaw valve is presented as an example. Many of the operational and theoretic characteristics of this unit can be applied to other types of demand valves. Fig. 22-12, *A* and *B,* illustrates the principle by which most demand valves operate.

a In Fig. 22-12, *A,* the demand valve is closed because the control valve *(1)* is resting on its seat, blocking supply gas *(2).*

b In Fig. 22-12, *B,* the valve is opened by the patient, who takes a spontaneous breath, causing the air to leave the area behind the diaphragm *(3).* This causes a reduced pressure gradient and the atmosphere enters a port *(4),* pushing the diaphragm *(5)* over in an attempt to equalize the pressure on the two sides of the diaphragm. As the diaphragm is pushed over, the valve is removed from its seat *(6)* and gas flows to the patient.

c When pressure is equalized again, the spring on the control button causes the diaphragm to move back to its original position, interrupting gas flow.

d If the patient is *not* breathing, an operator can open the valve by pushing in on the spring *(7),* which forces the valve off its seat, allowing gas to flow to the patient.

5 The Robertshaw valve (Fig. 22-13) is an oxygen-powered resuscitator cycled by the inspiratory efforts of a spontaneously breathing patient or by pressing a switch

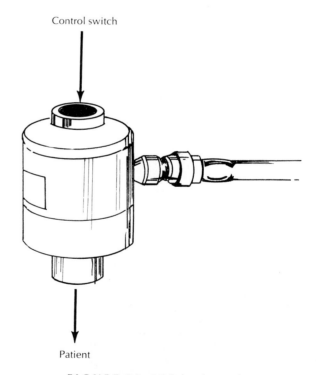

FIGURE 22-13 Robertshaw valve.

located on the back side of the valve (see *arrow*).

6 As is characteristic of demand valves, the flow from the valve increases in response to the patient's inspiratory demands (pressure gradient) until a maximum shutoff pressure of approximatley 40 mm Hg is reached.

7 If the patient is not breathing, the valve is cycled by the operator, who depresses the control button until the desired tidal volume is delivered or until the shutoff pressure is reached. CAUTION: When using these, the operator must observe the chest for ventilation and be

aware that the stomach can be inflated from the rapid gas flow and high airway pressure.

8 The Robertshaw valve has the following specifications:

a Supply pressure—40 to 90 psig (275 to 620 kPa).

b Flow—as required on demand, 0 to 160 L/min at 40 psig (275 kPa). For resuscitation, 160 L/min minimum at 40 psig (275 kPa). Shut off pressure, 40 mm Hg.

c Inlet fitting—standard diameter index safety system (DISS) $9/16$ to external thread. Special inlet connectors for mechanical resuscitators or piped O_2 systems are available at extra cost.

d Filter—65 micron sintered bronze (replaceable).

e Outlet—22 mm outside diameter × 15 mm inside diameter (fits standard medical masks, endotracheal catheters, and tracheotomy tubes).

f Finish—anodized aluminum and black polycarbonate.

g Duration—the useful duration of a system (how long the unit will operate on a given supply of gas) depends on many factors, such as breathing or resuscitation rate, mask fit, patient size, and cylinder capacity. Therefore the times below are only approximate. Obviously, duration is not a factor when using piped O_2 from a wall source. Duration times: breathing patient, 60 minutes*; nonbreathing patient, 15 minutes.

9 A typical method for operating a demand valve is included as Procedure 22-4 at the end of this module.

10 The reader is encouraged to observe and if possible operate a demand valve, because variations of the units are also used for intermittent mandatory ventilation in ventilators and continuous positive airway pressure systems.

14.0 MECHANICAL CARDIOPULMONARY RESUSCITATORS

14.1 Mechanical cardiopulmonary resuscitators

1 This device is also called the "thumper."

2 A well-trained team and coordinated effort are necessary when using any automatic chest compressor. These devices eliminate the operator fatigue that causes variation in cardiac output and provide simultaneous ventilation with high O_2 concentration; but although they do afford more regular and uninterrupted CPR, they do have limitations. They are as follows:

a Most are relatively heavy and difficult to move because of the necessary O_2 tanks and components.

b When transporting a patient, the plunger may frequently slip out of place if not carefully monitored.

c At the present time most models are available only for use on adults.

3 Compressor ventilators should be employed only with a cuffed endotracheal tube or esophageal airway or, if used with a mask, only by well-trained and experienced personnel.

*Based on 6 to 8 L/min.

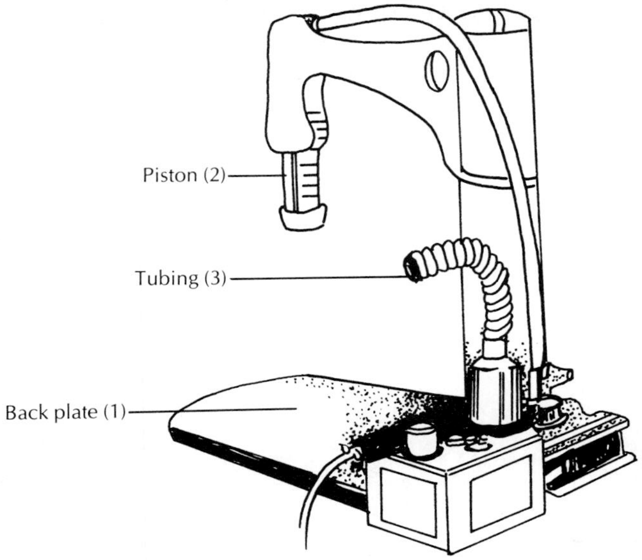

FIGURE 22-14 Mechanical chest compressor ("thumper").

Piston (2)
Tubing (3)
Back plate (1)

4 One commonly used automatic chest compressor is the HLR 50-90 machine. This device is strapped to the patient's chest and is less popular in the hospital setting than some other devices because of the difficulty in strapping it in place.

5 Another mechanical chest compressor is the Michigan Instruments, Inc., product, commonly known as the "thumper." This particular device has proved to be popular both in hospital and prehospital (emergency vehicle and on-site) settings.

6 An experienced health care provider can assemble and apply this device on a patient in under 1 minute's time, and an experienced team can apply the machinery with little or no interruption of external cardiac compression (see Fig. 22-14).

7 To apply the "thumper," its own back plate *(1)* is slipped under the patient and the arm unit is attached to the back plate with the piston *(2)* extending over the patient's chest. Quickly, the piston is placed at the midsternum area, locked in place, and then three switches are turned on; numbered 1, 2, and 3.

8 At this point the piston on the arm starts chest compression. Ventilations will occur automatically every 5 seconds, either through the mask attached to the machine, or through the tubing *(3)* that can be adapted to an endotracheal tube or esophageal obturator.

9 These machines, like any machine, must be handled, applied, and monitored properly by human hands in order to function efficiently and effectively. There are many contraindications for the use of mechanical chest compressors; however, in prolonged resuscitation they can prove to be irreplaceable if properly applied and used.

10 Adequate chest excursion with the use of mechanical chest compressors must be evaluated continuously; the same principles apply as in manual chest compression.

The rescuer must observe that the chest is compressed at a depth of 1½ to 2 inches.

11 The rescuer must note that the arm and piston of the chest compressor are positioned at the midsternum and that this position does not change with any movement of the patient.

12 Generally, mechanical chest compressors are found in the emergency department, where patients frequently undergo extensive resuscitation procedures, and on board emergency transport vehicles.

13 Some hospitals have elected to have a mechanical chest compressor available to travel with the code team in the event that they are needed for prolonged resuscitation.

14 For additional information on the thumper refer to supplement 22-3.

SUPPLEMENT 22-1 Checklist for cleaning/service protocol for Resusci-Anne

I Cleaning schedule for Resusci-Anne, following each class or after each 25 uses:

1 Replace lung bag.

2 Remove, wash, and decontaminate airway input tube.

3 Clean and decontaminate inside of mouth and connecting airway.

4 Clean and decontaminate skin of face.

II Cleaning procedures

_____ **1** Remove chest cavity.

_____ **2** Remove pressure plate and spring.

_____ **3** Remove head by turning it facedown and pulling it straight out.

_____ **4** Remove airway input tubing from neck.

_____ **5** Remove exhaust tubing.

_____ **6** Remove clear plastic airway intake and exhaust adapters; to remove adapter, pull straight up.

_____ **7** To remove chest plate, rotate lever on left side of plate to right and lift chest plate straight up.

_____ **8** Lift lung bag and remove it by pulling shortest of two white nozzles.

_____ **9** With bag out, check bottom plate for cracks and tears.

_____ **10** Spray external levels of ventilation and compression switch with silicone.

_____ **11** Inspect and spray "wrong hand indicator" located below compression switch.

_____ **12** Inspect and check battery output by removing blue cable from its receptacle and connecting it to ohm meter.
  • 12 to 15—good
  • Less than 12—battery needs replacing

_____ **13** Replace new bag by inserting thumb with bag into large hole. Keep point of bag toward head of manikin.

_____ **14** Clean all disassembled parts with scrub brush and with warm, soapy water. *Do not wash electric parts.*

_____ **15** Decontaminate disassembled parts by soaking them in Cidex according to manufacturer's specifications.

_____ **16** Clean and decontaminate inside of manikin's mouth and external skin of face with soapy water, then rinse and apply approved decontaminant according to manufacturer's specifications.

_____ **17** Reassemble manikin and test for operation; use the manual resuscitation unit to check chest rise.

_____ **18** Tag unit as cleaned and store it in its box.

SUPPLEMENT 22-2. Sample departmental procedure—initial steps to cardiopulmonary resuscitation

I Be familiar with location and use of equipment.

In a cardiac arrest situation, time is of the essence; immediate and correct action must be taken by whomever is present. It is important that this action be well organized. Therefore, before an arrest everyone should be familiar with the location and contents of the following:

1 Resuscitation kit (in clear plastic bag)
  a 1 Laerdal resuscitator with medium mask and reservoir or Puritan manual resuscitator (PMR) with medium mask
  b 1 Flowmeter with connecting tube
  c 1 All-purpose mask
  d 3 Airways (small, medium, large)
  (The pediatrics kit has additional airways and masks for infant and child and also a pediatric-size mask.)

2 Suction kit (in clear plastic bag)
  a 1 Regulator and bottle with connecting tube
  b 1 Extra connecting tube with plastic connector
  c 4 Sterile gloves
  d 4 14 Fr catheters
  e 3 Airways (small, medium, large)
  (The pediatric kit has additional airways—infant and child sizes; 10 French catheters are substituted for 14 French.)

3 Emergency O$_2$ kit (gray box)
  a 1 Flowmeter with nipple adapter
  b 3 Cannulas
  c 1 Connecting tube and connector
  d 1 All-purpose mask
  (The pediatric kit also has child-size all-purpose masks.)

II Be aware of the various types of arrests.

1 Respiratory. Patient is apneic.

2 Cardiac. Patient has no palpable pulse.

3 Combined. Patient is apneic and has no palpable pulse (cardiopulmonary arrest).

III Know ways in which one can determine type of arrest.

1 Respiratory. Feel gently for movement of air at site of patient's airway, mouth and nose, tracheostomy, or endotracheal tube, with palm of one's hand, while observing for chest or abdominal moment. If you feel none, patient has respiratory arrest. In case of doubt, assume that there are inadequate respirations.

2 Cardiac. Feel for a carotid or femoral pulse. If none is palpable, patient has cardiac arrest. In case of doubt, assume patient has cardiac arrest.

3 Combined. Combination of both respiratory and cardiac arrest.

IV Know action to be followed after determination of an arrest.

1 Observe time.

2 Observe patient's pupillary response. Pupils begin to dilate within 45 seconds of anoxia to the brain and are fully dilated in 120 seconds.

  a Pupils that are constricted and react to light indicate adequate oxygenation to brain.

  b Pupils that are dilated and react to light indicate decreased oxygenation to brain.

  c Pupils dilated and nonreactive to light indicate inadequate oxygenation to brain and death is imminent if immediate steps are not taken.

3 While doing No. 1 and No. 2 simultaneously, summon help by calling *Code Blue* followed by room number. *Do not leave patient.*

4 Begin cardiac and/or pulmonary resuscitation immediately (ABCs).

V Perform pulmonary resuscitation. Respiratory arrest: To properly oxygenate the blood, there must be a patent airway.

1 Make sure oropharynx is free of foreign material or secretions. Emergency suction kit is provided for this purpose. Negative pressure for aspiration can be controlled from 0 to 200 mm Hg by placing right-sided flag on regulated suction and turning front pressure control in clockwise direction for increasing negative pressure. Should more negative pressure be desired, right-sided flag can be rotated to line suction. This will provide −400 mm Hg pressure.

2 Hyperextend head maximally to establish an airway. This may relieve pharyngeal obstruction and improve airway to a degree that may even *permit* patient to breathe spontaneously. Hyperextension of head is accomplished as follows:

  a Place patient supine on flat surface.

  b Place one hand on chin and other on back of head.

  c Elevate chin and push top of head back simultaneously to extend neck.

3 Once airway has been established, it must be kept patent. Place an oral airway as follows:

  a Hyperextension of head is usually sufficient to open mouth.

  b Select properly sized airway (if too small, it could slip down to laryngopharynx).

  c Place airway in mouth so that rounded tip curves downward, making sure that tongue is not forced back but instead lies just under airway.

  d Insertion is complete when flared ends of airway come to rest on patient's lips.

  e If patient starts to gag, remove airway.

4 If spontaneous respiration is *not* restored by hyperextension, begin artificial respiration, mouth-to-mouth or mouth-to-tracheostomy; remember to seal nose and mouth, or use manual resuscitator. Give two slow, deep breaths every 1 to 1.5 seconds initially, then breathe:

  a 12 times per minute for an adult

  b 15 times per minute for children from 2 to 6 years of age.

  c 20 times per minute for an infant

5 Assess effectiveness of ventilation. Observe rise and fall of chest. If rise and fall of chest does not occur in response to ventilation, airway is not patent or air is entering stomach, increasing danger of vomiting and subsequent aspiration.

VI Perform cardiac resuscitation. In cardiac arrest, to circulate blood in absence of heart muscle activity, external cardiac massage must be done. External cardiac massage is varied in rate according to age of patient. Technique consists of 50% compression and 50% relaxation of pressure on lower half of patient's sternum. When external cardiac massage is done properly, circulation is 30% to 33% of normal.

VII Apply CPR to adults and children over 6 years of age as follows:

1 Place victim on firm surface, bed board, or floor.

2 Locate lower half of sternum.

  a Locate suprasternal notch and xiphoid process.

  b Find midpoint between these two "landmarks."

  c Lower half of sternum is portion immediately below that midpoint.

3 Give patient single thump to chest—lower half of sternum. If this is not sufficient to stimulate heartbeat, begin closed chest massage immediately. (NOTE: This is not currently recommended by AHA.)

  a Place heel of one hand in midline of body over lower half of sternum, avoiding xiphoid process.

  b Place heel of other hand over that of first.

  c Alternately compress and release sternum until femoral or carotid pulse can be felt. This usually is accomplished by compressing sternum 1½ to 2 inches. Maintain smooth, rhythmic motion without removing hands from sternum, keeping fingers off chest wall.

  d Closed chest massage is done at rate of 80 to 100/min for adult patient.

VIII Chest compression of children 2 to 6 years of age is as follows:

1 Place child on firm surface such as pedi-arrest board or tray.

2 Place heel of *one* hand on lower half of sternum.

  a Alternately compress and release sternum 1 to 1½ inches until carotid or femoral pulse is felt.

  b Closed chest massage is done at a rate of 80 to 100 min.

NOTE: CPR is continued until relief is available and should not be discontinued for longer than 15 sec. Individual doing compression does not stop for person who is ventilating patient. Ventilator must coordinate his or her activity with compression (i.e., lungs are ventilated at point when operator doing chest compression is in phase of relaxation [upstroke of compression cycle]).

IX Perform combined cardiopulmonary resuscitation for a heart and lung arrest.

  1 If there is one rescuer only
   a Establish airway.
   b Give patient *four* breaths initially.
   c Deliver *15* compressions.
   d Continue resuscitation by giving 2 breaths and then 15 compressions (2:15) alternately until help arrives.

  2 If there are two rescuers
   a Rescuer No. 1 breathes for patient (mouth-to-mouth or resuscitator):
    • *12 times per minute* for adult or child over 6 years (1 breath per 5 compressions)
    • *15 times per minute* for child 2 to 6 years of age
   b Rescuer No. 2 does closed chest massage:
    • *80 to 100 times per minute* for adult or child over 6 years of age
    • *80 to 100 times per minute* for child 2 to 6 years of age

The ABCs of resuscitation

I Airway care
  1 Remove pillow.
  2 Place patient on back.
  3 Clear mouth and nose of secretions.
  4 Hyperextend head maximally.
  5 Place oral airway. This will help keep airway patent.
  6 Always be sure airway is patent.

II Breathe for the patient
  1 Adult—Apply mouth-to-mouth, nose, or artificial airway ventilation. Give two slow, deep breaths, then ventilate 15 times per minute.
  2 Child (2 to 6 years)—Apply mouth-to-mouth, nose-and-mouth, or artificial ventilation. Give two slow, deep breaths, then ventilate 15 times/min.
  3 Bag and mask should be used when possible, making sure bag is supplied with O_2.
  4 Place mask as follows:
   a Narrow part is fitted on bridge of nose.
   b Flare out soft rubber around edges of mask.
   c Apply bottom of mask over mouth and onto face at level of jaw.
   d Secure mask in place with no air leaks.
    • Thumb and index finger secure mask to face.
    • Three fingers work to hyperextend jaw.
  5 Use oxygen if it is available.
   a Use mouth-to-mouth if O_2 is not available.
   b Manual resuscitation—Make sure O_2 connecting tubing is connected to inlet of bag. Place flowme-

ter in wall and place on flush flow. Resuscitator should be tested before inflating patient's lungs.
   c NOTE: Resuscitation must never be delayed by obtaining O_2 or setting up equipment.

III Circulation (compress the chest 1½ to 2 inches)
  1 Always give patient four good breaths before beginning compression or unoxygenated blood will be circulated. (Remember A-B-C must be in order.)
  2 Have a firm surface under patient's back and kneel to one side of patient so that your hands can be placed in center of chest.
  3 Feel for sternal notch and xiphoid process.
   a Eliminating the xiphoid process, divide the sternum in half, and place over the heel of one hand on lower half of sternum directly midline; place other hand on top of first hand.
   b Both hands work together as one unit; use upper part of body with elbows straight.
   c Compress sternum 1½ to 2 inches, until femoral or carotid pulse is felt. Remember 50% of time is compression and 50% is relaxation.
   d During relaxation phase do *not* remove heel of hand from sternum. This could result in improper placement.
  4 Individual doing compression stops and allows time for ventilation at end of each cycle of compression.

SUPPLEMENT 22-3. Cardiopulmonary resuscitator (Thumper)

I The need for mechanical heart-lung resuscitation

Perhaps the primary reason external cardiac compression, coupled with mouth-to-mouth ventilation, is the preferred technique for CPR is that as a first aid measure it can be performed on a patient without the need for any adjuncts or mechanical devices. Thus the rescuer, properly trained and experienced, can apply this lifesaving technique immediately and effectively, with the following assumptions:

  1 The rescuers are sufficiently strong and physically competent in proportion to the size of the patients that they can provide adequate levels of chest compression and ventilation.
  2 The rescuers, in the excitement of the emergency, can adequately recall the basic points of their training and have had sufficient experience to reduce these opints of training theory to actual practice.

In general it is possible to achieve adequate levels of training and experience to effectively carry out manual heart-lung resuscitation as the first phase of CPR. In most cases, however, where CPR is started, the final question of a successful resuscitation or a futile attempt will not and cannot be resolved for some time after the attempt is begun. In most cases the resuscitative techniques are merely supportive and will not result in the return of the normal cardiac function. The objective during this interim period, before definitive therapy can be brought to bear, is to maintain viability, particularly that of the central nervous system. Definitive therapy will in most cases require intracardiac or intravenous administration of drugs and, if the patient is in ventricular fibrillation, will nearly always require the use of electroshock therapy to restore normal heart rhythm. The clinical diagnosis of the cardiac arrhythmia, the administration of drugs, and the use of the defibrillator all require a significant amount of time. Moreover, it may very well be necessary to reestablish by artificial means the return of endogenous function; the time spent in bringing this all about will normally run from a minimum of 15 minutes to a maximum of, in many cases, several hours before the heart is either restarted or a decision can be reached that the attempt is indeed futile. During this time the manual technique becomes extremely strenuous and tiring and the effectiveness of technique suffers. Gone is the advantage of the manual technique, and its major disadvantages now begin to show themselves. Continued application requires team effort and the changing of personnel; rhythm and coordination suffer. Improper hand placement and control of force can very readily produce trauma. Inadequate ventilation in the stress of the manual technique can very well produce gastric insufflation with its risk of subsequent aspiration of vomitus; and unless mouth-to-mouth ventilation is diligently and properly performed, pulmonary atelectasis may develop with its attendant atrioventricular shunting.

A good mechanical device that, through proper organization and planning, can be readily available early after the onset of the cardiac emergency is the ideal answer for the developing inadequacies of the manual technique. In most cases, however, it serves the function of an improved "second-aid" device, in much the same way as an oxygen respirator takes over from the manual technique of artificial respiration. Once the mechanical device has been brought into play, it is now possible to specify and control what might be regarded as the important subtleties of the technique. For example, it has been experimentally found that chest compression should be held for a minimum of 50% of the total cycle. Rhythm should be constant and should be capable of being maintained for long periods of time. Force on chest should not vary, and it is desirable to initiate the force rather gradually and to release it rather suddenly. Optimum synchronization between chest compression cycling and ventilation cycling should be maintained. For example, it is desirable to start ventilation immediately at the end of systole, and conversely, systole should begin immediately at the end of the ventilation cycle. Adequate volume of ventilation gas should be made available at a constant safe pressure to completely and safely fill the lungs on each breathing cycle. Here again it is desirable to shape the input pressure wave so that full pressure will develop gradually at the start of the breathing cycle. All of these considerations are important in the optimization of the cardiopulmonary resuscitation technique, but such control cannot be realistically expected from the manual technique.

Other advantages of the mechanical technique over the manual are as follows:

1 Ventilation is with O_2-enriched air.
2 The mechanical technique has the ability to measure the true magnitude of sternal deflection.
3 It allows for the maintenance of a truly perpendicular direction on the sternum.
4 It allows for the maintenance of proper point-of-force application on the sternum.
5 The properly designed mechanical device eliminates the problem of mattress and spring deflection associated with manual technique.
6 The mechanical device is definitely labor saving and can eliminate at least one, or possibly two, personnel from the cardiac emergency team.

This is not to say that the mechanical device can ever completely replace manual techniques of CPR. These techniques will remain as the primary technique of first aid. However, it is definitely true that more adequate levels of CPR can be established by mechanical means and can be maintained for much longer periods of time.

II Description and operation

The "thumper" is a portable, nonelectrical, oxygen-powered, heart-lung resuscitator. It performs by pneumatic and mechanical means the optimized techniques of external cardiac compression and intermittent positive pressure breathing in a coordinated and synchronized manner.

The "thumper" operates from O_2 or air at 40 to 78 PSI (average adult consumption is 77 cubic feet an hour). If a high pressure tank O_2 is to be used, a regulator with quick disconnect fitting is available. The double E tank setup would last approximately 30 to 40 minutes at typical adult settings. The 40 to 78 PSI covers all hospital pipeline O_2 so that no regulator is necessary with this input.

III Applying the "thumper" to the patient

1 It has been determined that clinical death exists.
2 Two persons are present, knowledgeable in CPR.
3 Manual CPR has already been started.
4 First person will stop manual CPR and roll patient onto side (an alternative is merely to lift one shoulder).
5 Next, patient is rolled back onto backboard; manual CPR is continued by first person (time lost to patient should be less than 5 seconds).
6 Second person loosens constricting garments over chest and abdomen (constriction of abdomen during external cardiac compression can cause internal injury). Belts and clothing around neck and chest are removed or loosened.
7 Second person now hooks arm to base and main supply line to input on base. All action dials and switches are in OFF position, and ventilator dial reads zero and is in OFF position.
8 Next, swing arm is positioned on chest of patient during ventilation phase from person number one who is applying CPR. Since displacement is proper

criterion for setting force, marking rings on plunger are provided to facilitate this adjustment. Wide rings are 1½ inches apart; displacement of adult chest should be approximately space between two of these wide rings. Additional rings are provided at ½-inch intervals to aid in establishing smaller amounts of compression. After setting on chest has been accomplished, cardiac compression switch is turned on.

9 With first person continuing mouth-to-mouth breathing after every fifth chest compression, person No. 2 will now attach breathing hose to ventilator outlet.

10 With cardiac compressor operating at force on chest setting of at least 30 pounds, ventilation switch is turned on. Ventilation pressure is set to desired value (normally, 25 to 30 cm H_2O) by turning ventilation pressure control knob. (It is turned clockwise to increase pressure-read gauge during ventilation cycle.) The 25 to 30 cm H_2O pressure setting will safely and adequately ventilate most patients, both adult and pediatric. This setting may be utilized as constant, preset parameter but should be checked periodically. For unusual conditions of low compliance and/or high resistance, setting may be increased up to 50 cm H_2O.

11 Smaller end of breathing hose is connected either to standard male, 15 mm endotracheal tube fitting if patient is intubated or to face mask supplied. (If patient is to be ventilated by face mask, airway must be unrestricted and patency maintained by backward head extension. Leak around mask must be minimized.)

PROCEDURE 22-1

Procedure for assessing operation of a self-inflating manual resuscitator

No.	Steps in performing the procedure
	The practitioner will perform the following procedure for assessing operation of a self-inflating manual resuscitator.
1	Select manual resuscitator.
2	Remove it from its container.
3	Squeeze ventilator bag.
	3.1 Note rise and fall of nonrebreathing valve and air intake valve.
	3.2 Feel air leave outlet port of nonrebreathing valve.
4	Test resuscitator for leaks.
	4.1 Occlude outlet port of nonrebreathing valve and squeeze bag.
	4.2 If bag empties (slow or fast), there is a leak that must be corrected.
5	Disassemble manual resuscitator according to manufacturer's instructions and/or hospital procedure
	5.1 Remove major components.
	a Nonrebreathing valve
	b Ventilator bag
	c Oxygen reservoir (if present)
6	Disassemble each component.
	6.1 Arrange pieces so that they can be reassembled in reverse order and number.
	6.2 Name and number each part and give its function as it is disassembled.
7	Reassemble manual resuscitator.
	7.1 Use manufacturer's directions as unit is reassembled.
8	Squeeze bag and note movement of valves. Feel air leave outlet port of nonrebreathing valve.
9	Retest for leaks and correct as necessary.
10	Practice with test lung. Note ventilation volume; count breathing frequency.
11	Add supplemental O_2 and use manual resuscitator on test lung. Note changes in bag response time or in operational characteristics.

PROCEDURE 22-2

Emergency ventilation using a self-inflating manual resuscitator

No.	Steps in performing the procedure
1	The practitioner will use a self-inflating manual resuscitator with and without supplemental O_2 to provide ventilation to a patient. Gather necessary equipment. **1.1** Self-inflating bag **1.2** Mask or tracheal tube **1.3** Adapter **1.4** Oxygen flowmeter **1.5** Oxygen connecting tubing **1.6** Oral airway
2	Wash hands.
3	Assemble equipment.
4	Connect flowmeter to O_2 source, and turn to flush or 15L/min.
5	Clear airway, if necessary. **5.1** Hyperextend head. **5.2** Insert oral airway.
6	Seal mask over patient's mouth and nose, and secure with one hand.
7	Ventilate patient by intermittently squeezing bag. Look for chest wall excursion and correct as necessary. **7.1** Deliver adequate tidal volume. **7.2** Ventilate using proper frequency.
8	Continuously monitor patient for effective ventilation.
9	Check for incidental emesis and prevent aspiration.
10	Continue ventilation until relieved or until procedure is terminated.
11	Return all used equipment for decontamination.
12	Wash hands.
13	Discuss performance with a practitioner.
14	NOTE: If patient is intubated, learner is responsible primarily for delivering adequate tidal volume at adequate frequency. Care must be taken not to move or dislodge endotracheal tube.

PROCEDURE 22-3

Securing a face mask using a one-hand grip

No.	Steps in performing the procedure
1	The practitioner will use one hand to secure a face mask in place on a manikin, another student, then a patient, without leaks while operating a resuscitation bag with the other hand. Gather necessary equipment: **1.1** Self-inflating bag **1.2** Assorted sizes of masks **1.3** Assorted sizes of oral airways
2	Wash hands.
3	Place patient in supine position with shoulders slightly elevated. NOTE: Modified position must be used in cases of spinal injury (refer to Module Twenty).
4	Insert oral airway by correct technique (unnecessary for student practice).
5	With mask *detached* from resuscitator bag, place bridge (nose portion) of mask over bridge of patient's nose (see Fig. 22-9, *1*).
6	Place thumb of left hand over bridge of mask, above mask connector (see Fig. 22-10, *1*).
7	Place index finger opposite thumb below connector so that it rests just above mask cushion (see Fig. 22-10, *2*).
8	Position chin portion of mask over front of lower jaw, keeping mask in straight line (see Fig. 22-9, *2*).
9	Place three fingers (middle, ring, pinky) along ridge of mandible (see Fig. 22-11). **9.1** Secure mask by lifting jaw, causing face to be raised under mask, while simultaneously hyperextending head. **9.2** Adjust thumb and index finger to correct for any leaks. **9.3** Reposition head as necessary to improve airway.
10	Attach resuscitator bag to mask with free hand, and squeeze bag to deliver breath. NOTE: *In actual patient situation, resuscitator bag is not detached from mask during mask placement.*
11	Do not attempt to correct for air leaks by pressing down on mask. Proper technique is to rearrange fingers and hyperextend head while *lifting face into mask.*
12	Note rise and fall of patient's chest.
13	Readjust hand position as necessary to prevent leaks.
14	Continue ventilation until relieved or until procedure is terminated.
15	Return used equipment for decontamination.
16	Wash hands.

PROCEDURE 22-4

Operate a demand valve to assist and control ventilation*

No.	Steps in performing the procedure
	The practitioner will select and operate a demand valve with a mask as an assistor and a controller.
1	Wash hands.
2	Select equipment:
	2.1 Demand valve
	2.2 Pressure hose
	2.3 Assorted sizes of masks
	2.4 Assorted oral airways
3	Connect delivery hose to 40 to 90 PSI supply pressure source.
4	Depress control button and listen for flow of gas from outlet.
5	Release control button and note that gas flow ceases.
6	Attach appropriate size of mask to valve outlet.
7	Position patient in supine position. Insert oral airway.
8	Apply mask by hyperextending head and lifting patient's face into mask.
9	Hold mask in position with two hands.
10	If patient is not breathing, depress control button with a thumb until chest rises, then remove thumb. Note fall of chest. *Do not overinflate*
11	If patient is breathing, note valve's response to patient's inspiratory efforts.
12	Check and correct for air leaks and stomach inflation.
13	Continue ventilation until relieved or until procedure is terminated.
14	Turn off supply gas.
15	Remove demand valve and mask for decontamination.
16	Wash hands.

*Optional.

BIBLIOGRAPHY

Bond WW, Petersen NJ, and Favero MS: Viral hepatitis B: aspects of environmental control, Health Lab Sci 14:233, 1977.

Bond WW et al: Inactivation of hepatitis B virus by intermediate to high-level disinfectant chemicals, J Clin Microbial 18:535, 1983.

Centers for Disease Control: Acquired immune deficiency syndrome (AIDS): precautions for clinical and laboratory staffs, MMWR 31:577, 1982.

Centers for Disease Control: Prevention of acquired immune deficiency syndrome (AIDS): report of inter-agency recommendations, MMWR 32:101, 1983.

Eisenberg M, Bergnerb L, and Hallstrom A: Epidemiology of cardiac arrest and resuscitation in children, Ann Emerg Med 12:672, 1983.

Elling R and Politis J: An evaluation of emergency medical technicians' ability to use manual ventilation devices, Ann Emerg Med 12:765, 1983.

Favero MS: Sterilization, disinfection and antisepsis in the hospital. In Lenette EH et al, editors: Manual of clinical microbiology, ed 4, Washington, DC, 1985, American Society of Microbiology, 129.

Jude JR, Kouwenhoven WB, and Knickerbocker GB: Report of application of external cardiac massage on 118 patients, JAMA 178:1063, 1961.

McIntyre KM: Art of hospital cardiopulmonary resuscitation: liability risk of the layman. In Proceedings of the National Conference on the Medical/Legal Implications of Emergency Medical Care, Dallas, 1976, American Heart Association.

McIntyre KM and Hampton AG: Status of liability for out-of-hospital cardiopulmonary resuscitation (CPR), Circulation 54(suppl 2):224, 1976.

Melker R: Asynchronous and other alternative methods of ventilation during CPR, Ann Emerg Med 13(pt 2):758, 1984.

Melker R: Recommendations for ventilation during cardiopulmonary resuscitation. Time for change? Crit Care Med 13:882, 1985.

Safar P: The pathology of dying and reanimation. In Schwartz G et al, editors: Principles and practice of emergency medicine, ed 2, Philadelphia, 1985, WB Saunders Co.

Standards and guidelines for cardiopulmonary resuscitation (CPR) and emergency cardiac care, JAMA 255:2841, 1980.

Mechanical ventilation

11.3 Calculate dead space to tidal volume ratio (V_D/V_T).

12.1 Differentiate between volume-displacement spirometers, flow-activated spirometers, and heated-probe flowmeters.

12.2 Describe operation of the Wright respirometer to measure exhaled volumes.

13.1 Calculate dynamic compliance of patients.

13.2 Calculate static compliance of patients.

14.1 Explain how pneumotachometers measure gas flow.

14.2 Discuss how the system pressure manometer on a ventilator and pressure transducers are useful indicators of gas pressure.

14.3 Describe how ventilators monitor the patient's fraction of inspired concentration of oxygen (FIO_2).

14.4 Explain how and why it is important to monitor the temperature of a patient's inhaled gas.

14.5 Discuss other types of monitors that are being used with patients receiving ventilation.

15.1 Explain the operational features that are available with different types of volume ventilators.

16.1 Describe the various terms used to classify the Bennett MA-1 ventilator.

16.2 Point out the different parts of a Bennett MA-1 ventilator.

16.3 Locate and operate each of the Bennett MA-1 ventilator controls according to recommended procedures.

17.1 Differentiate between the different signals and systems comprising the Bennett MA = 1 ventilator monitoring system.

17.2 Operate the Bennett MA-1 ventilator according to simulated orders under simulated clinical conditions.

18.1 Explain the use of an air-oxygen blender used to deliver exact FIO_2 concentrations.

18.2 Explain the rationale for using intermittent mandatory ventilation (IMV) in lieu of more conventional ventilation methods.

18.3 Differentiate among the different types of IMV systems.

18.4 Give examples of how conventional ventilator breathing circuits can be modified for special functions (IMV, PEEP, etc.).

18.5 Assemble an IMV breathing circuit for use with the Bennett MA-1 ventilator.

18.6 Describe the general procedure for using IMV.

18.7 Describe the operation of the Bennett IMV demand valve.

18.8 Differentiate between the various controls and displays on the BEAR 2 ventilator.

19.1 Identify the steps involved in checking a ventilator for proper function.

19.2 Change ventilator breathing circuits according to recommended procedure.

20.1 Describe the setup and operation of the Emerson 3-PV, Emerson 3-MV, and Monaghan 225 ventilators according to recommended procedures.

21.1 Decontaminate ventilators according to departmental policy and recommended procedure.

22.1 Appreciate the changes that have evolved in the new generation of ventilators by discussing the primary differences between these units and previous modules.

22.2 Explain the operating principle or the Siemens Servo Ventilator (models 900 and 900B).

22.3 Differentiate between models 900B and 900C of the Siemens Servo ventilators.

22.4 Discuss features and performance specifications of the Bennett model 7200 microprocessor ventilator.

22.5 Point out the unique features and technical specifications of the Medishield Cpu 1 ventilator.

22.6 Discuss the features of the Hamilton Medical Veolar Ventilator and point out the major difference between it and other third-generation devices.

22.7 Differentiate between the Hamilton and Amadeus ventilators.

22.8 Appreciate the growth of neonatal technology.

22.9 Discuss the technical specifications of the Babybird 2 ventilator.

22.10 Discuss the technical specifications of the Sechrist model IV-100 B infant ventilator.

22.11 Discuss the technical specifications of the Bourns BEAR Cub Infant Ventilator.

22.12 Give a brief history of the development of high frequency ventilation.

22.13 Describe Bird's newest generation of volumetric diffusive ventilators (VDR) and differentiate between them and high frequency ventilation (HFV) concepts.

22.14 Discuss the use of VDR in clinical situations.

23.1 Define respiratory failure.

23.2 Point out the causes of respiratory failure.

23.3 Describe the clinical signs of respiratory failure.

23.4 Describe the treatment of respiratory failure.

23.5 Point out a treatment of respiratory failure.

24.1 Describe typical types of monitors and alarms used with ventilators.

24.2 Explain how a low pressure (disconnect) alarm works.

24.3 Point out and discuss desirable features of low pressure monitors/alarms.

1.0 MECHANICAL VENTILATION: BASIS INFORMATION
1.1 General need for mechanical ventilation

The concepts and skills presented in his module integrate the theory and applications covered in Modules Eight, Ten, Eleven, Twelve, Sixteen, and Twenty. For this reason it is recommended that the reader review these materials, since they are expanded and applied in this module.

1 The natural process of breathing results in a flow of air in and out of the lungs, which is called *ventilation*. In the healthy and nondrugged patient, ventilation occurs through work of the ventilatory muscles that cause the chest to expand and contract in a rhythmic fashion.

2 In patients who are critically ill because of disease, trauma, or drugs, breathing may become depressed, absent, or inefficient as a result of the energy required to cause breathing to occur. It is under these circumstances that alternate methods of providing ventilation are implemented.

These methods are called *artificial* ventilation. If ventilation is caused by a machine, it is referred to as *mechanical* ventilation.

3 The use of mechanical ventilators has gained widespread prominence as a life support modality. This is evidenced by the fact that as early as 1959, Mushing, et al. *(Automatic Ventilation of the Lungs),* described over 85 different brands of mechanical ventilators.

In this module we present 20 of the most popular ventilators used in the United States. These ventilators were chosen as examples of state-of-the-art practice and variations in theory of operation.

■ ■ ■

The following units of instruction continue where the discussion on expired air ventilation ended in Module Twenty-two. They provide the reader with the knowledge and skills necessary to assess a patient's ventilatory needs and subsequently select and implement continuous artificial ventilation for prolonged periods of time or until the patient's therapy is discontinued.

1.2 Causes of respiratory failure and indications for mechanical ventilation*

1 Initiation of mechanical ventilation is an interim life support measure that gives the physician an opportunity to medically correct or stabilize a patient's cardiopulmonary problem.

2 Providing mechanical ventilation to a patient does *not* cure the patient even though it may prolong life. Unfortunately, once mechanical ventilation has been started, a moral, legal, and professional question emerges; under what circumstances should it be terminated?

For this reason, the decision to begin mechanical ventilation is important because it involves a large

commitment of human and other resources that can become a long-term obligation by all involved. The reader may wish to talk to physicians regarding medical, philosophic, legal, or other considerations before a decision to administer mechanical ventilation is made.

3 The *medical indications* for mechanical ventilation should be based on a careful review of the pathophysiologic abnormalities presented by the patient. For this reason, mechanical ventilation, except under *extenuating circumstances,* should be initiated only by a physician's order. And first, questions concerning how the ventilator will improve the patient's chances for recovery should be explored.

a Another consideration is whether mechanical ventilation may worsen the patient's condition. For example, a patient with a large left-to-right shunt will not benefit from mechanical ventilation. It may instead decrease the cardiac output, increase the shunt, and therefore increase the patient's hypoxemia.

b Generally, mechanical ventilation is indicated to prevent patients from going into respiratory failure or to provide life support and stabilize patients who are already in respiratory failure.

4 There are many different criteria for identifying respiratory failure. One that is easy to remember is that of a *deteriorating* clinical picture combined with arterial blood gas values with an arterial oxygen tension (Pao_2) *less than 50 torr* and an arterial carbon dioxide tension ($Paco_2$) *greater than 50 torr* while the patient is breathing air. Exceptions to this criterion are based on whether the Pao_2 should be evaluated using room air or 100% oxygen. To avoid confusion, a Pao_2 of less than 50 torr using room air will be used in this unit as one of the indicators of respiratory failure.

5 Clinical manifestations of acute respiratory failure include the symptoms peculiar to the underlying pulmonary disease in addition to:
a Restlessness
b Confusion
c Tachycardia
d Diaphoresis
e Headache
f Central cyanosis
g Hypotension
h Tremors—asterixis
i Poor chest expansion
j Depressed ventilation
k Papilledema
l Unconsciousness
   • These conditions are almost directly related to the O_2 and CO_2 levels in the patient's arterial blood.

6 Diseases and conditions leading to respiratory failure can be grouped under three broad categories:
a Those that cause *impaired ventilation.*
b Those that *impair alveolar-capillary gas exchange.*
c Those that cause *ventilation-perfusion abnormalities and venous admixture.*

7 Impaired ventilation can be caused by diseases and

---

*Refer to Module Eight for a review of specific diseases and terminology used in this unit.

T A B L E 2 3 - 1 Restrictive defects

Decreased lung expansion	Limited thoracic excursion	Decreased diaphragmatic movement
Interstitial fibrosis	Chest surgery	Severe obesity
Pneumothorax	Flail chest	Abdominal surgery
Fibrothorax	Kyphoscoliosis	Peritonitis
Pleural effusion		

conditions leading to chronic airway obstruction, restrictive defects, neuromuscular defects, and central nervous system (CNS) depression or damage.

  a Diseases causing chronic airway obstruction include emphysema, chronic asthma, and chronic bronchitis.

  b Diseases causing restrictive defects such as decreased lung expansion, limited thoracic excursion, and decreased diaphragmatic movements are listed in Table 23-1.

  c Diseases causing neuromuscular defects include:
  • Myasthenia gravis
  • Guillain-Barré syndrome
  • Multiple sclerosis
  • Tetanus
  • Spinal injuries
  • Drugs and poisons
  • Poliomyelitis

  d CNS damage or depression can be caused by agents or conditions such as:
  • Anesthetics
  • Narcotics
  • Barbiturates
  • Tranquilizers
  • Head trauma

8 Impaired alveolar-capillary gas exchange can be caused by diseases such as:
  a Fibrosing alveolitis
  b Pneumoconiosis
  c Sarcoidosis
  d Pulmonary edema
  e Thromboemboli
  f Pneumonectomy
  g Tumor or other masses
  h Collagen diseases
  • For review, see Module Eight.

9 Ventilation-perfusion abnormalities and venous admixture can be caused by anatomic and physiologic shunts.
  a Anatomic shunts result in blood flowing from the right side of the heart to the left side without passing through the pulmonary vasculature.
  b Physiologic shunts can be caused by diseases such as:
  • Emphysema
  • Asthma
  • Chronic bronchitis
  • Bronchiolitis
  • Atelectasis
  • Thromboemboli
  • Respiratory distress syndrome
  • Pneumonia

1.3 Criteria for institution of mechanical ventilation

The criteria for beginning mechanical ventilation will vary from hospital to hospital. The following are representative of most criteria:

1 Decreasing level of consciousness
2 Vital capacity: less than 15 mg/kg
3 Pao_2: less than 70 torr with fraction of inspired concentration of oxygen (FIo_2) of 0.4
4 Alveolar to arterial diffusion of oxygen (A-aDo_2): greater than 400 torr with FIo_2 of 1.0
5 $Paco_2$: greater than 50 torr (in previously normocapnic patient)
6 Dead space tidal volume ratio (Vd/Vt): greater than 0.6
7 Inspiratory force: less than −25 cm H_2O

1.4 Preparing the patient for mechanical ventilation

1 Patients must be prepared *psychologically* and *physically* for mechanical ventilation. Lack of control of the breathing process, combined with inability of the intubated patient to speak, is very frightening to both patient and family. Too frequently in the rush to provide quality care, clinicians overlook the patient's needs as a *feeling* human being.

2 The conscious patient must be carefully informed of the purpose of the ventilator, how it will aid in recovery, and the limitations it will place on the individual's ability to talk, eat, move about, etc. The family or others who may be with the patient also should be informed of the process, its benefits, and possible complications.

3 The conscious patient should be gently coached in the best methods of breathing in conjunction with the ventilator and given other instructions on how to cough, move, acquire assistance, and go about other necessary daily tasks.

4 If possible, to gain the patient's confidence, it is probably desirable to ventilate the patient by hand before switching to the ventilator.

5 The patient who has been attached to the ventilator should not be left until stabilization has occurred and the individual's anxiety has diminished somewhat.
  NOTE: Ideally, patients on ventilators should be in a special care unit or have special duty personnel to monitor their progress to make any necessary adjustments in the ventilator's operation.

6 The patient should be placed in a supine position initially, conditions permitting. Patient movement should be carefully planned so that stress is *not* placed on the airway and the patient's attachment to the ventilator.
  a As previously stated, very small movements by the patient such as flexion of the head can cause the tracheal tube to move approximately 1.9 cm toward the carina.
  b Head extension can cause the tube to move approximately 1.9 cm away from the carina.
  c Lateral head rotation can cause the tube to move approximately 0.7 cm away from the carina.

7 Therefore once a patient has been positioned, *bilateral* breath sounds must be auscultated to determine that the tracheal tube has not been accidentally misplaced from a functional location in the trachea.

8 Patient comfort is an important consideration for the ventilator patient who spends hours, days, or even weeks in the same location. In these units patients can lose their contact with reality and themselves. When this occurs, their will to live diminishes, they frequently become uncooperative, and their personalities weaken.

The term most frequently used to describe this behavior is intensive care unit (ICU) stress or syndrome.

9 The most important service to the ventilated patient is a *caring* attitude, as demonstrated by frequent visits and special actions such as rearranging a pillow or positioning breathing tubes so they are not resting on a patient's chest. Not only are the visits necessary to maintain the ventilator and to aid in the patient's comfort but they help the patient's mental state.

10 Patient orientation is especially important and can be assisted by simple devices such as placing a calendar in the room or leaving the radio or television on in the room. Above all, the practitioner should treat ventilator patients not as a part of the machinery but as sensitive and frightened human beings.

1.5 The physician's order for respiratory care

1 The first step in determining a patient's ventilatory needs is to review the physician's order sheet. Standing or verbal orders should *not* be used for implementing mechanical ventilation except in emergency situations where no other option is available.

Resp. Setting										
Tidal Volume										
VT Press. Limit										
Resp. Rate										
Flow Rate										
FIO_2										
Sensivity IMV-ASS'T-CONT										

Resp. Setting		Changes	
Peep Or Expir. Resist			
Sigh Volume			
Sigh Press. Limit			
Sigh Rate			
Multi-Sigh			

	ACTUAL									OBSERVATION				WEANING						
DATE	Sys. Press.	Resp. Rate	Tidal Vol.	Flow Rate	Eff. Compl.	Temp.	FIO_2	IMV Rate/V_T	I:E Ratio	Patient Position (RS) (LS) (B)	Auscultation	Alarm Check	Circuit Change	Resp. Rate	Tidal Vol.	Minute Vol.	Vital Cap.	ABG's pH	ABG's $PaCO_2$	ABG's PaO_2	INITIAL
7 AM																					
8 AM																					
9 AM																					
10 AM																					
11 AM																					
12 N																					
1 PM																					
2 PM																					
3 PM																					
4 PM																					
5 PM																					
6 PM																					
7 PM																					
8 PM																					
9 PM																					
10 PM																					
11 PM																					
12 M																					
1 AM																					
2 AM																					
3 AM																					
4 AM																					
5 AM																					
6 AM																					

Diagnosis ____________

Orders by ____________

Date Started ____________

FIGURE 23-1 Typical form used to order and monitor continuous mechanical ventilation.

Continued.

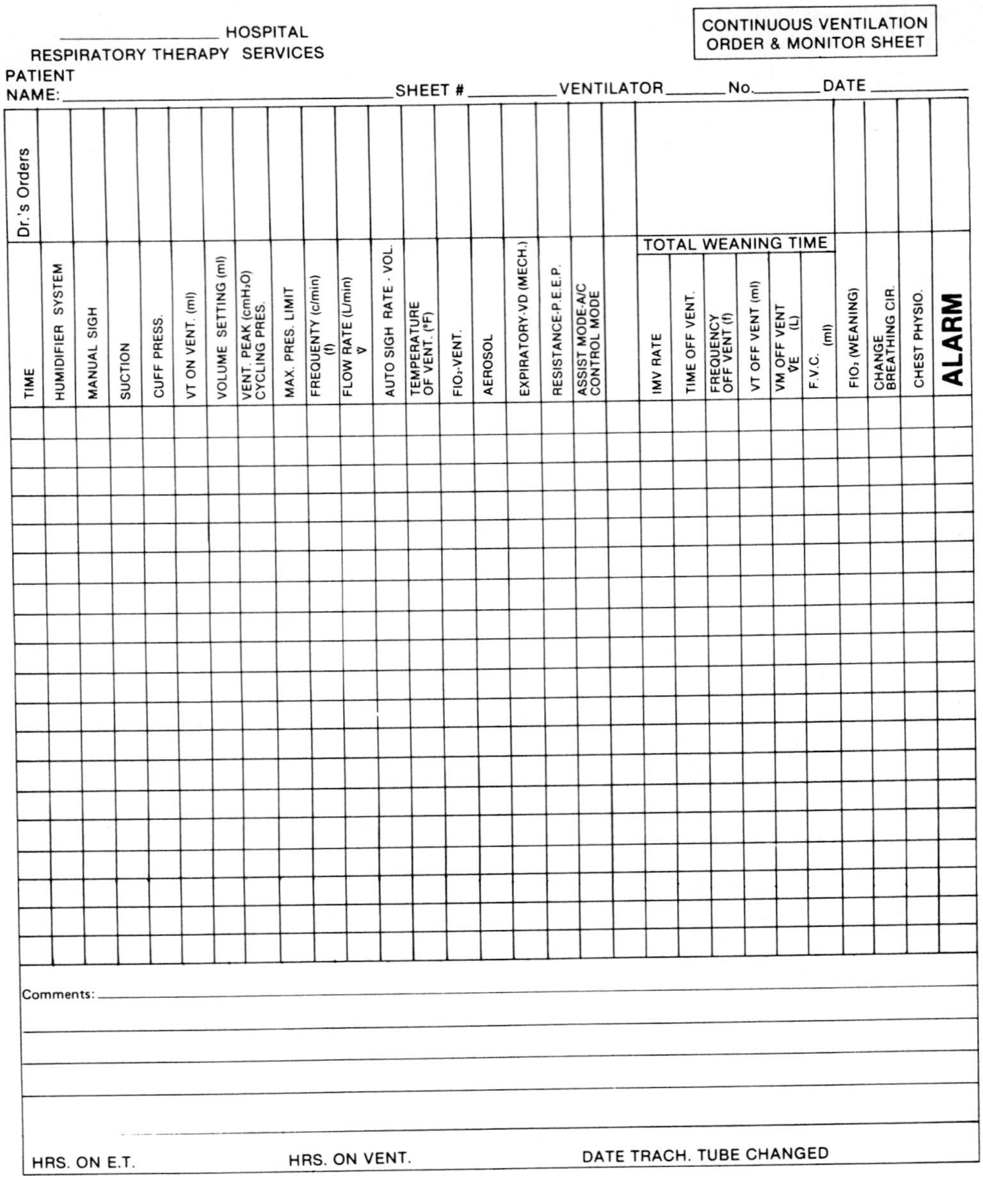

HOSPITAL
RESPIRATORY THERAPY SERVICES

CONTINUOUS VENTILATION
ORDER & MONITOR SHEET

PATIENT
NAME:_____   SHEET #_____   VENTILATOR_____ No._____ DATE_____

Column headers:
- Dr.'s Orders
- TIME
- HUMIDIFIER SYSTEM
- MANUAL SIGH
- SUCTION
- CUFF PRESS.
- VT ON VENT. (ml)
- VOLUME SETTING (ml)
- VENT. PEAK (cmH$_2$O) CYCLING PRES.
- MAX. PRES. LIMIT
- FREQUENCY (c/min) (f)
- FLOW RATE (L/min) V̇
- AUTO SIGH RATE · VOL.
- TEMPERATURE OF VENT. (°F)
- FIO$_2$ VENT.
- AEROSOL
- EXPIRATORY-VD (MECH.)
- RESISTANCE-P.E.E.P.
- ASSIST MODE-A/C CONTROL MODE
- TOTAL WEANING TIME
  - IMV RATE
  - TIME OFF VENT.
  - FREQUENCY OFF VENT (f)
  - VT OFF VENT (ml)
  - VM OFF VENT V̇E (L)
  - F.V.C. (ml)
- FIO$_2$ (WEANING)
- CHANGE BREATHING CIR
- CHEST PHYSIO.
- ALARM

Comments: _____

HRS. ON E.T. _____   HRS. ON VENT. _____   DATE TRACH. TUBE CHANGED _____

VENTILATOR MONITOR SHEET

FIGURE 23-1, cont'd Typical form used to order and monitor continuous mechanical ventilation.

A physician's order for continuous ventilation should provide the following information:

a Routine information
- The type of ventilator (i.e., volume constant or pressure)
- Cycling frequency (cycles per minute)
- Oxygen percentage (FIo$_2$)
- Maximum pressure limit (cm H$_2$O/torr)
- Inspiratory to expiratory (I:E) ratio
- Pao$_2$ and Paco$_2$ to be maintained.

b Special information
- Intermittent mandatory ventilation (IMV) rate (mechanical breaths per minute).
- Positive end expiratory pressure (PEEP) level (cm H$_2$O/torr)
- Sigh volume and frequency
- Expiratory retard
- Special drugs
- Weaning instructions including levels of pressure support

2 A typical form for *ordering* and *monitoring* continuous ventilation is presented in Fig. 23-1.

NOTE: This form is comprehensive and covers many variables that are not applicable to all hospitals.

3 *Before a patient is placed on a ventilator*, the following information regarding operation of the ventilator should be determined:

a Tidal volume (V$_T$) or minute volume (V$_M$)

b Cycling rate—frequency (f)

c FIo_2—percent oxygen

d PI maximum—inspiratory pressure limit

e I:E ratio—inspiratory to expiratory ratio

f $\dot{V}$—flow rate

Formulas for calculating these and other useful parameters for implementing and monitoring mechanical ventilation are presented in a subsequent unit.

2.0 MECHANICAL VENTILATION TERMINOLOGY
2.1 Terms and definitions

Many of the following terms and definitions are more completely defined in Module Eight.

1 Airway pressure release ventilation. A ventilator modality that briefly vents the patient's lungs to atmosphere at the end of each ventilator cycle.

2 Assisted ventilation. The ventilator assists the spontaneously breathing patient.

3 Compliance. Forces opposing expansion of a substance. (i.e., volume change per unit of force [pressure] applied) $C = V/P$ (see Module Eight). The greater the pressure (P) required to expand (increase the volume) of a substance (V), the lower the compliance.

4 Constant. A continuous action used to describe operation of a ventilator, regardless of internal and external influences (e.g., time, pressure, flow, or volume constant).

5 Controlled ventilation. The ventilator automatically maintains ventilation for the nonbreathing patient.

6 CDAP (constant distending airway pressure). Refers to a constantly elevated respiratory baseline pressure in relationship to the atmosphere and a resting lung volume. This term can be used in lieu of CPAP or PEEP although these two are most popular in the literature.

7 CPAP (continuous positive airway pressure). A method of generating PEEP. Frequently CPAP and PEEP are used interchangeably because they both cause the patient to have an elevated functional residual capacity (FRC).

8 CPPV (continuous positive pressure ventilation). Used to describe situations where PEEP is generated with a mechanical ventilator.

9 V_D (dead-space ventilation). The portion of inhaled gas that does *not* participate in gas exchange; a ratio of tidal volume (V_T to V_D) to calculated dead space. This is estimated to be approximately *1 ml per pound* of body weight in the adult patient.

10 Elastance. Force required to cause a substance that has been expanded to return to its resting state.

11 Fluidics. In respiratory care, the science of using air flows, rather than mechanical valves, to perform logical functions and deliver tidal volumes for artificial ventilation.

12 Gas compression. The amount of gas that is contained in a ventilator circuit or internal space as a result of the pressure generated to cause gas flow.

13 Generator. A device that creates a gas pressure, flow, or volume.

14 IDV (intermittent demand ventilation). A system that allows the patient to breathe spontaneously, using assisted ventilation until a predetermined time period has passed and a controlled mechanical breath is delivered.

15 Impedance. That which causes opposition. In physiology, factors causing airway impedances include primarily resistance and compliance.

16 IMV (intermittent mandatory ventilation). The spontaneously breathing patient is given a mechanical breath (mandatory) at predetermined intervals.

17 Inflation hold. The technique of inflating the lung and holding it inflated for a preset time by preventing exhalation from occurring. This maneuver theoretically increases gas diffusion and distribution throughout the lung.

18 IPPB (intermittent positive pressure breathing). In this situation a positive pressure breath is delivered to the patient's airway, resulting in inspiration. Exhalation occurs passively when the positive pressure is interrupted and the expanded chest deflates; hence intermittent *positive pressure* is generated. (See Module Seventeen.)

19 IPPV (intermittent or inspiratory positive pressure ventilation). This term differs from IPPB in that the patient is mechanically ventilated for longer periods.

20 Mandatory (minimum) minute ventilation. A method of *partial* ventilatory support using SIMV in which the ventilator ensures the delivery of a minimum preset minute volume by adjusting rate and/or the tidal volume.

21 One-way valve. A valve that allows gas to move only in one direction.

22 PEEP. An airway maneuver resulting in positive end expiratory pressure when used with a ventilator. PEEP is applied during the expiratory phase of the breathing cycle, preventing the patient from exhaling fully. This causes a positive pressure to be generated in the airway during both inspiration and exhalation resulting in an artificially increased functional residual capacity (FRC) (see page 684).

23 Pressure-limited, volume-variable ventilator. A device that ends inspiration when a *preset airway pressure* is reached. Volume may vary, dpending on the status of the patient's airway, gas flow rate, etc.

24 PSV (pressure support ventilation). A method of partial ventilatory support that is used to compensate for increased resistance to gas flow after a spontaneous inspiratory effort. A predetermined constant airway pressure is developed and maintained until the patient's flow decreases to a preset minimum value.

25 SIMV (synchronized intermittent mandatory ventilation). This approach is used by ventilator manufacturers to prevent a mandated breath from being delivered on top of a spontaneous breath (stacking controlled breaths). If "stacking" were to occur, lung volumes would be uncontrollably increased, causing excessive airway pressures and possible barotrauma.

26 Solenoid valve. An electromechanical valve that is

used in many mechanical ventilators to control and/or alter the pattern of the main flow of gas through the ventilator.

27 Surfactant. Lipoprotein substances that cover the air surface of alveolar units to prevent collapse as the volume is decreased during exhalation.

28 Valve. A device that controls or directs gas (or liquid) flow.

29 Ventilator breathing circuit. The external tubing, humidifier, water traps, and other devices that link the patient to the ventilator.

30 Volume-limited, pressure-variable ventilator. A device that ends inspiration after a preset lung volume has been delivered. Airway pressure as caused by the ventilator will automatically be increased or decreased as necessary to deliver the preset tidal volume.

3.0 DEVELOPMENT AND GROWTH OF MECHANICAL VENTILATION
Significant persons and events

1 Vesalius (1514-1564) described the effects of depriving animals of air. In 1542 he performed a tracheotomy on an animal and ventilated it by intermittently blowing through a reed. Additional historical events relative to artificial and mechanical ventilation can be found in Module Two.

2 Because of a polio epidemic in 1931, John Haven Emerson of Cambridge, Massachusetts, built a simplified version of the early negative pressure ventilators (iron lung).

3 During World War II, significant contributions were made to the whole area of oxygen and positive pressure breathing as a result of high altitude flying.

4 In the United States, manufacturers such as the Bennett Corporation designed the Bennett valve, which subsequently was modified for the delivery of IPPB and medications. (See Module Seventeen.)

5 In Sweden the polio epidemic of the 1950s caused the development of mechanical ventilators that could maintain a patient's ventilation for prolonged periods. Engström was foremost in this development.

6 During the late 1950s the Bird Corporation of Palm Springs, California, developed the first of a series of ventilators that would deliver IPPB and continuous mechanical ventilation. (See Module Seventeen.)

7 During the 1960s and 1970s, the manufacture and sale of mechanical ventilators became big business. The devices themselves became more sophisticated and, in the late 1970s, emphasis began to be placed on alarms and monitoring devices rather than on methods of delivering the positive pressure breath.

8 The late 1970s also saw the development of optional ventilator functions such as PEEP, IMV, and other variations of the basic positive pressure breath.

4.0 UNDERSTANDING HOW DIFFERENT POWER SOURCES ARE USED TO GENERATE A MECHANICAL BREATH AND HOW THEY ARE INTEGRATED INTO THE FOUR PHASES OF VENTILATOR PERFORMANCE.
4.1 Methods of generating mechanical breaths

1 The principles applied for creating an artificial breath are not complicated. During inspiration, gas flow occurs and a tidal volume is delivered as a result of a difference in pressure (gradient) between two points, such as a ventilator and the lungs.

2 Pressure gradients can be generated by many methods. These include:

a Squeezing (emptying) a compressible container (Figs. 23-2 and 23-3) that has an opening to the atmosphere. An example would be a bulb, bellows, or bag-type ventilator (resuscitator).

b Rapidly spinning vanes, such as fan blades in a turbine; these unidirectional blades (Fig. 23-4) push air from one point to another.

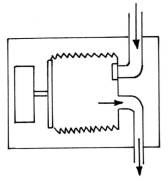

FIGURE 23-3 Creating a pressure gradient by compressing a bellows that has an opening to the atmosphere.

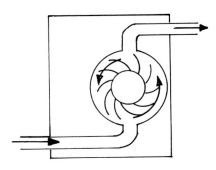

FIGURE 23-4 Pressure gradient is created by spinning blades that push air from one point to another.

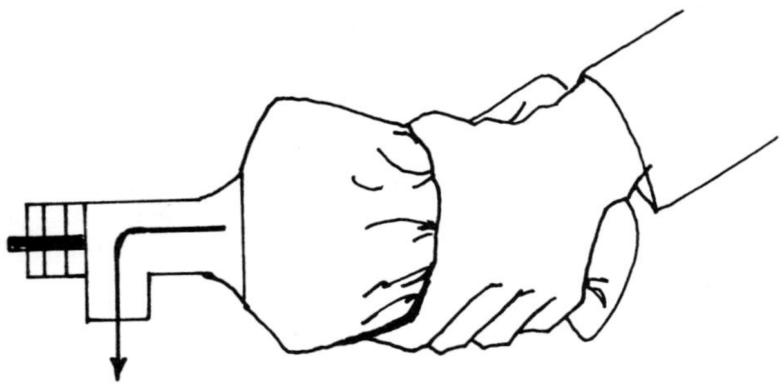

FIGURE 23-2 Creating a pressure gradient by manually squeezing ventilator bag.

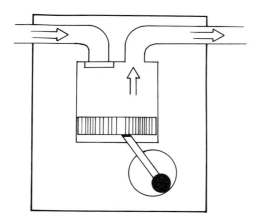

FIGURE 23-5 Pressure gradient created by piston pushing air from a cylinder.

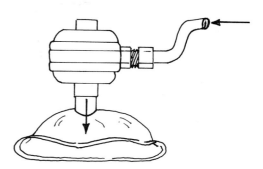

FIGURE 23-6 Pressure gradient created by gas being released from a high-pressure source.

c A rigid piston moves and causes air to leave a fixed-size cylinder (Fig. 23-5).

d The controlled release of gas (Fig. 23-6) from a high pressure source such as a cylinder or wall outlet.

e Fluidics—an application of the Coanda effect, where a continuous flow of gas is switched back and forth by other gas impulses to cause inspiration and expiration. A fluidic ventilator uses gas channels and gas impulses to generate patient volumes and control functions.

3 Mechanical ventilators were developed primarily for the purpose of relieving hospital personnel from having to manually ventilate patients for long periods.

4 The theoretic simplicity of artificially generating a tidal volume can be explained by the following illustrations.

a In Fig. 23-7, a continuous gas flow is allowed to escape from a high-pressure cylinder through a regulator *(1)*. The pressure of the gas escaping from this cylinder is the same as the internal pressure of the regulator attached to the cylinder, and the gas flow is greater than the patient's peak inspiratory demands.

b The gas leaves the cylinder and flows through a delivery hose *(2)* and a T piece *(3)* to the atmosphere.

c A rubber balloon representing the patient *(4)* is attached to the open port of the T piece. The other port is left open to the atmosphere *(5)*.

NOTE: The bag does *not* inflate because the flowing gas takes the path of least resistance—the atmosphere.

d When the open port is occluded by a finger or a valve *(6)*, the gas flowing from the regulator again takes the path of least resistance, causing the balloon to inflate. The balloon (simulating the patient's lungs) will continue to inflate *(7)* until the occluded port is opened or the pressure in the bag causes enough resistance to stop the flow of gas from the regulator or the bag ruptures. Gas flow will not cease until the pressure inside the bladder equals the pressure preset on the valve inside the regulator. (See Module Seven for a review of the operation of pressure regulating devices.)

Although this explanation may appear to be very simple, these steps can be easily related to the parts of a very sophisticated mechanical ventilator.

5 Using a Bird Mark 7 ventilator (Fig. 23-8, *A* and *B*) as an example, the cylinder can be compared to the power source that operates the Bird unit and ultimately delivers a tidal volume. In other devices the power source may be caused by electricity that moves a piston or turbine. The regulator functions as the main ventilator switch that starts or stops gas flow through the ventilator. In the Bird illustration, gas flow is started and stopped by the ceramic switch *(1)*. In the Bennett ventilator, it is the Bennett valve and in electronic ventilators, a solenoid valve (not shown).

a The delivery tubing can be compared to the more sophisticated patient breathing circuits *(2)*.

b The T piece stimulates the patient connector *(3)* that provides the attachment between the ventilator and patient.

c Finally the operator's finger or valve, which manually intermittently blocks and unblocks the exit port, represents the exhalation valve *(4)* that is opened *(5)* and closed to automatically cause inspiration and expiration to occur.

6 Conceptually, the simple T piece-type system can be applied to the most sophistocated ventilators if one remembers that for gas flow to occur (inspiration), a pressure difference must be created and a switching mechanism must intermittently interrupt this flow to allow exhalation to occur.

4.2 Four phases of mechanical ventilation

1 Mechanical ventilators generate and deliver gas to a patient's airway by causing a positive pressure difference to occur at the ventilator when *compared* to the patient's lungs. This pressure difference (gradient) causes gas to flow into the patient's lungs until the pressure in the patient's system and that of the ventilator equalize. If a high gas pressure is generated by the ventilator, a larger gradient will exist and a faster flow will occur unless it is controlled.

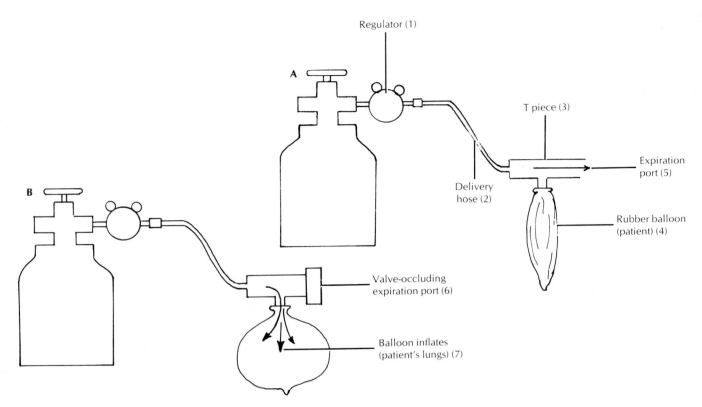

FIGURE 23-7 Simplified mechanical ventilator. **A,** Air leaves system when expiration port is open. **B,** Air inflates balloon (lungs) when expiration port is closed.

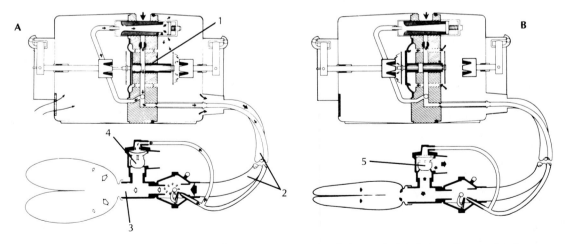

FIGURE 23-8 Basic principles of Mark 7 respirator. **A,** Inhalation. **B,** Exhalation. (Courtesy Medical Products Division/3M, St Paul, Minn.)

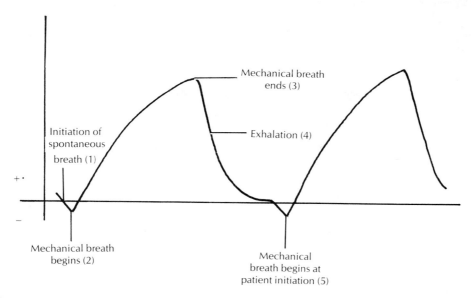

FIGURE 23-9 Typical pressure curve for pressure-cycled ventilator in assist mode attached to spontaneously breathing patient showing the phases of the mechanical breath.

2 The mechanical actions performed by the ventilator to provide artificial ventilation can be divided into *four* distinct phases:

  a Inspiration. The point at which a ventilator causes an exhalation valve in the patient's breathing circuit to close and allows a flow of gas to pressurize the patient's system.

  b Changeover from inspiration to expiration (cycling). The point at which the ventilator interrupts the main flow of gas to the patient's system and opens an exhalation valve, releasing pressure from the patient's system allowing the patient to exhale.

  c Expiration. Exhalation begins and continues from the point when the main ventilator flow is stopped (or interrupted) and the exhalation valve in the patient's breathing circuit is opened until the exhalation valve is once again closed.

  d Changeover from expiration to inspiration ("triggering") occurs whenever a ventilator switches from exhalation to inhalation. This can be automatic or by a spontaneous breathing effort. Either way, the point at which the exhalation valve is closed in the patient's breathing system and the ventilator's main flow begins is the changeover phase.

3 The various phases of a mechanical ventilation cycle can be seen and/or recorded by attaching the patient to a strip chart recorder or oscilloscope. Fig. 23-9 represents a typical pressure curve for a pressure-cycled ventilator attached to a spontaneously breathing patient. This pressure curve can be used as a means of visualizing the various phases of a mechanical breath. When using an x-y graph, pressure points above the baseline (marked *zero*) are positive (+) and, below the baseline, subambient (−).

  a At point *1* the patient has taken a spontaneous breath, causing the curve to *drop* below the baseline.

At this time the exhalation valve has closed but no gas is flowing from the ventilator. This conclusion is based on the continued downward movement of the pressure curve. At point 2 the exhalation valve is held closed and a mechanical breath has begun. This is represented by the fact that the pressure curve has started an upward movement. The time elapsed between point *1* and point *2* is the ventilator's *response time,* or the patient's triggering effort. This time delay between initial inspiratory effort and the beginning of ventilation is critical, because it represents patient work and wasted ventilatory volume, since muscles moved to generate a breath and breathing did not occur.

    The time delay factor can be adjusted in most ventilators by setting the *sensitivity control* to a more sensitive position.

  b Once begun, inspiration continues until the main flow of gas is interrupted *(3)*. At this time the exhalation valve opens and the patient begins to exhale passively, as represented by a downward movement of the curve.

  c Exhalation *(4)* is the point at which the curve starts downward and continues until the patient takes another breath *(5)*.

  d In the apneustic patient the pressure pattern would appear as represented by Fig. 23-10. The primary difference between Figs. 23-9 and 23-10 is shown in nos. *1* and *2*. In the controlled situation, the patient is not breathing and the pressure curve does *not* drop below the baseline because the ventilator is automatically cycled. In positive-to-positive phase ventilators, pressurization begins at the baseline *(6)* during the control mode of operation.

  e Exhalation is defined as the point at which flow is interrupted *(7)* and continues to the point where flow begins again *(8)*.

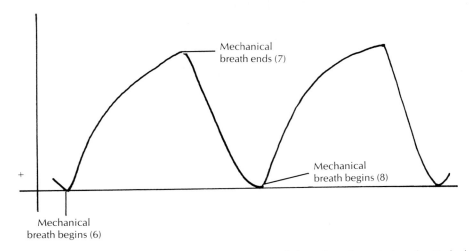

FIGURE 23-10 Typical pressure curve for pressure-cycled ventilator in control mode attached to apneustic patient.

5.0 CLASSIFYING VENTILATORS

5.1 Basic performance differences

1 Most simply defined, mechanical ventilators are devices that help patients breathe. They accomplish this by assisting the spontaneously but inadequately breathing patient to take a deeper breath or by automatically delivering a breath (controlled breathing) for the apneustic patient.

2 Therefore, by function and by definition, a ventilator can be called an *assistor* if it helps one who is already breathing and/or a *controller* if it assumes the breathing function.

When a ventilator is referred to as an assistor and/or a controller, the clinician immediately is able to identify two important operational features of the ventilator.

A verbal description of a ventilator's operational characteristics is referred to as "classification of the ventilator."

3 The following seven units present various methods for classifying ventilators. It is important that clinicians understand these methods so that they will be able to assess the functional operational characteristics of a ventilator based on its design specifications before it is purchased or before it is used on a patient.

4 Understanding classification also allows one to evaluate how a ventilator should perform on a patient and therfore assess whether the ventilator is operating properly under clinical conditions.

5 All mechanical devices can and will fail at some point as they reach and exceed their designed performance limits and as malfunctions occur. It is only through careful observation and applied knowledge of these ventilators by the operator that these potentially dangerous patient care situations can be prevented and/or corrected.

6 The specific method for classifying a ventilator varies according to the point of view of the person describing the ventilator. For this reason there are numerous classification methods that generally describe how the ventilator generates the tidal volume and the characteristics of gas flow that result in delivery of this volume to the patient, along with other performance characteristics.

The following classification terminology is general enough that it can be used to describe (classify) most of the ventilators available for patient use today.

5.2 Methods of classifying ventilators

Ventilators are classified according to:

1 Methods of generating tidal volume.

2 The mechanism for triggering from exhalation to inhalation.

3 The mechanism for cycling from inhalation to exhalation.

4 Assessment of the inspiratory and expiratory phases of the breathing cycle.

5 The mechanism by which the tidal volume is delivered to the patient.

6 Special functions it can perform.

5.3 Methods of generating tidal volume

During inspiration a ventilator may be classified as a *constant* or *nonconstant-flow generator* or a *constant* or *nonconstant-pressure generator*.

1 The pure *constant-flow generator* (CFG) is a ventilator type that produces and maintains a continuous rate of gas flow to the patient (liters per minute) during inspiration regardless of increasing impedances in the ventilator patient system distal to the ventilator.

   a To accomplish this, the ventilator must use an unlimited high pressure source (head) that will always be greater than any distal impedances to gas flow created by ventilator circuits and the patient's lung pathways.

   b To protect the patient against direct exposure to a high pressure source, the ventilator system incorporates a fixed-size orifice that causes the internal pres-

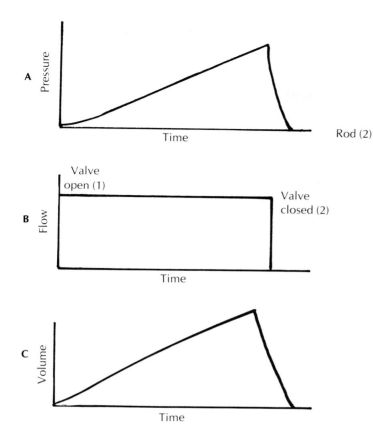

FIGURE 23-11 Graphs. **A,** Pressure. **B,** Flow. **C,** Volume pattern for a constant-flow generator.

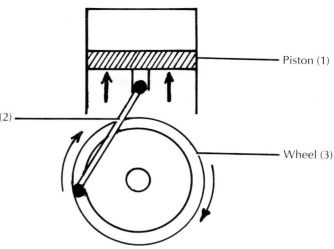

FIGURE 23-12 Piston of nonconstant flow generator.

sure to decrease as it crosses the orifice and enters the patient's breathing circuit.

c Even though the internal ventilator pressure is decreased on the distal side of the orifice, the potential pressure head on the proximal side of the orifice is such that a large pressure gradient is always present between the ventilator and the patient's airway. This pressure gradient, as long as it is maintained, results in a constant flow to the patient.

In Fig. 23-11, graphs *A* through *C* show a typical pressure, flow, and volume pattern for a CFG when plotted on an x-y axis.

• In graph A, a pressure is generated and constantly maintained to generate the high level of flow shown in graph B. Because this flow rate is constantly maintained throughout inspiration, a straight line is plotted on the flow graph. By subtracting the portion of the tracing related to the initial opening of the valve *(1)* and the venting of the valve causing exhalation *(2)*, one can easily see the square wave flow pattern that is characteristic of constant-flow generators.

d Volume ventilators such as the Bennett MA series and the Bourns BEAR series generate this type of flow pattern and therefore can be classified as constant-flow generators.

NOTE: It is important that the clinician understands that a constant-flow generator will deliver a constant flow—hence constant volume—only as long as the internal *driving pressure of the ventilator exceeds the distal impedances to gas flow.* When distal impedances equal or exceed the internal driving force of the ventilator, the constant-flow generator will cease to operate as such, and a desired tidal volume may not be delivered. As this point is reached, the flow pattern will become less of a square wave and resemble the peaked wave of a constant pressure generator. All ventilators have a maximum performance level at which point the ventilator ceases to operate as it was designed. Clinicians must be aware of a ventilator's limitations and performance characteristics under varied clinical conditions so that dangerous assumptions will not be made as to the ventilator's performance capabilities under changing clinical conditions.

2 A *nonconstant-flow generator* (NCFG) is a type of ventilator that delivers the same inspiratory flow pattern to the patient regardless of changing airway characteristics. The Emerson 3-PV and Engström ventilators are examples of NCFG.

a The consistency of this pattern is created because a piston powered by an electric motor is used to deliver a preset volume of air from a rigid cylinder (Fig. 23-12).

b Because the piston *(1)* is linked to a fixed rotating wheel by a rigid rod *(2)*, the flow pattern that is created is always the same as the piston moves up and down, causing inspiration and exhalation.

c The gas volume is varied by changing the distance that the piston travels within the cylinder to empty a preset volume.

d As the cam, which is attached to a wheel, rotates *(3)*, the piston movements are smaller at the beginning of inspiration and at the end of inspiration. This

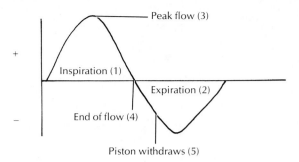

FIGURE 23-13 Sine wave–type flow pattern as generated by piston ventilator.

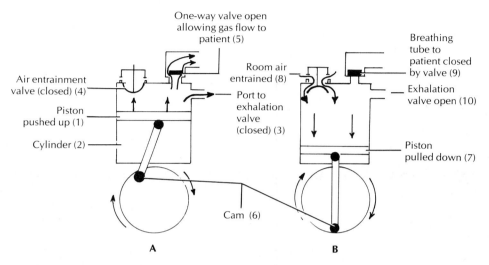

FIGURE 23-14 Basic design of a piston-type ventilator. **A,** Inspiration. **B,** Expiration.

causes a gradually increasing flow rate as the wheel continues to rotate through 90 degrees and a decreasing flow rate as it reaches the end of its compression stroke at 180 degrees. The greatest volume of air is moved as the wheel and cam pass through 90 degress of arc.

e This type of wheel rotation produces a sine wave–type flow pattern such as that illustrated in Fig. 23-13.

f In Fig. 23-13, inspiration is represented by the (+) sign and the gradually and decreasing one-half sine wave pattern above the baseline *(1)*. Exhalation is represented by the (−) sign and the one-half sine wave below the baseline *(2)*. The peak flow rate *(3)* is generated during inspiration as the piston in the ventilator reaches its point of greatest movement. Once peak flow has been delivered, the piston in the ventilator will continue to travel, but at a much shorter distance, causing a decaying flow-wave pattern that eventually reaches the baseline or zero as the piston reaches the end of its present stroke distance *(4)*.

g Exhalation occurs as the piston withdraws *(5)* to pull in fresh gas for another inspiration. This portion of

the waveform is not generally displayed by most texts because during the recovery period of the piston, the patient is exhaling and the breathing circuit is vented to the atmosphere. Fig. 23-14 represents a basic design for a piston-type ventilator such as the Emerson 3-PV.

h In this illustration, the patient's volume is determined by the distance the piston *(1)* moves upward in the cylinder *(2)*. The inspiratory flow rate is determined by the speed at which the piston moves upward so that the maximum volume that could be delivered by this ventilator is 2000 ml or a full stroke of the piston.

i As the piston starts upward, an increasing gas pressure in the cylinder causes gas to leave a port *(3)* to close the patient's exhalation valve located in the breathing circuit, to close the air entrainment valve *(4)*, and to open a one-way valve *(5)* allowing main gas to flow to the patient.

j As the wheel *(6)* continues to rotate, the piston is pulled downward *(7)*, causing room air to be entrained at the valve *(8)*. Simultaneously, the one-way valve *(9)* is seated to prevent a negative pressure from being pulled into the patient's airway by the descending piston, and the exhalation valve is opened *(10)*, allowing air to leave the patient's lungs. Inspiration begins again as the wheel continues to rotate, causing the piston to start upward.

k One of the theoretic *physiologic advantages* of this type of ventilator is that maximum flow occurs simultaneously with a maximum distending airway pressure. Also, inspiration does not end abruptly but decays as the descending side of the sine wave is generated. This exposes the airways to a slowly decreasing pressure and flow, which may increase gas distribution and delay small airway closure.

3 A *constant pressure generator* (CPG) is a type of ventilator that produces and maintains the same ventilator system pressure level throughout inspiration, regardless of changes in the patient's airway, (i.e., the *pressure is preset*). To accomplish this, the ventilator must use an unlimited source of pressure when compared to possible alveolar pressure so that a pressure gradient will exist and gas flow will occur.

a In a true CPG the ventilator pressure and internal resistance are usually low and approximate those in the patient's lungs at the end of an inspiration.

b The inspiratory flow rate begins high and gradually decreases during inspiration as the pressure gradient becomes less between the patient and the ventilator. In this type of device, flow can be interrupted by equalization of the pressure gradient between the ventilator and the patient or by time. In either case a predetermined volume may or may not have been delivered.

c Typical pressure, flow, and volume curves for a CPG, when plotted on an x-y axis, are presented in Fig. 23-15.

  • In *graph A* the ventilator produces a high initial flow rate *(1)*, which slows as the pressure gradient decreases within the lung during inspiration *(2)*.

  • In *graph B*, as the ventilator cycles ON, the high inspiratory flow rate results in an increasing airway pressure, which causes an increasing lung volume.

d IPPB devices, such as the Bird Mark 7 or Bennett valve-type ventilators, perform as CPG when they are operated *without air entrainment*.

4 A *nonconstant-pressure generator* (NCPG) is a ventilator that automatically changes the pressure of gas delivered to the patient's breathing circuit in response to changing airway conditions. In this type of ventilator the pressure patterns remain the same even though the airway pressure levels vary. This type of ventilator is rarely used today.

5.4 The mechanism for cycling from exhalation to inhalation

1 A general method of classifying a ventilator is to describe the mechanism by which inspiration is initiated.

2 A ventilator is an *assistor* if it triggers to inspiration (turns ON) in response to a patient's spontaneous inspiratory attempts and serves to augment the patient's spontaneous breathing.

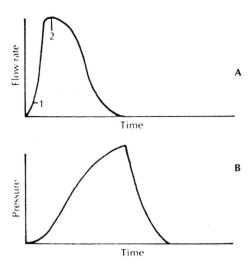

FIGURE 23-15 Typical pressure, flow, and volume curves for a CPG. **A,** Flow rate is initially high, but it slows as pressure builds up in the lung. **B,** High initial flow rate results in an increasing airway pressure and an increasing lung volume.

3 A *controller* is a ventilator that begins inspiration automatically and inflates the patient's lung regardless of the patient's efforts. This is usually accomplished by an electric or pneumatic timer that causes the ventilator to begin an inspiratory phase.

4 An *assistor-controller* is a ventilator that can respond to the patient's spontaneous breathing attempts and can also automatically assume the patient's ventilation should it deteriorate below an acceptable frequency or volume.

5 Most ventilators today have assist/control capabilities.

5.5 The mechanism for changing from inhalation to exhalation

The variables that can cause a ventilator to change from inhalation to exhalation (cycling or switchover) include *time, pressure,* and/or *volume.* One or more of these methods is incorporated by various types of ventilators.

1 *Time* is a constant that can be determined by the operator. In a time-cycled ventilator, inspiration is allowed to continue for a preset time interval. Exhalation begins when the inspiratory gas flow is blocked or stopped regardless of airway pressure or volume delivered. In a true time-cycled device, inspiration will end regardless of whether the ventilator is attached to the patient and regardless of the patient's lung characteristics.

a A time-cycled ventilator can function as a volume ventilator provided enough time is allowed for inspiration to occur and enough pressure is generated to cause a volume to be delivered. To accomplish this, time-cycled devices usually incorporate a high working pressure that will allow the ventilator to create an airway pressure gradient necessary to generate a gas flow, regardless of changing airway impedances. Examples of time-cycled ventilators are the Emerson 3-

PV volume ventilator and the Siemens Servo 900 series ventilators.

b It must be remembered that all ventilation occurs as a function of time. This time function results in calculation of a ratio between the time allowed for inspiration and that for exhalation and is known as the *I:E ratio*. This ratio is usually not allowed to become less than 1 to 1.5 except in special circumstances where *inverse* I:E ratios are established. More details on calculating I:E ratios are presented in a subsequent unit.

2 Switchover (cycling) caused by *pressure* describes a situation where inspiration continues until a preselected ventilator system pressure is reached, causing a valve at the ventilator to close, terminating inspiratory gas flow.

Ventilators that "cycle" because of pressure are also classified as *pressure-preset (limited)* and *volume-variable*. This is generally descriptive of their performances because the ventilator terminates inspiration in response to back pressure that is generated anywhere in the ventilator-patient system. Frequently a ventilator pressure cycles in response to "kinks" in the breathing circuit, mucus in the patient's airway, or deliberate or unintentional resistance of inspiration by the patient ("fighting the machine"). When early cycling occurs, the patient generally does *not* receive a desired tidal breath (volume). Hence the tidal volume may vary from breath to breath, depending on the changing impedances presented by the patient's breathing circuit or airway. However, in a pressure preset (cycled) ventilator gas flow will *not* cease, allowing exhalation to occur unless the preset pressure level is attained or it is manually or time cycled. For example, a leak anywhere in the system between the ventilator and the patient's lungs will cause the ventilator to remain in a continuous state of inspiration (gas flowing) until the leak situation is corrected.

3 Switchover resulting from *volume* is a situation where inspiration continues until a preselected volume of gas has been delivered into the patient's circuit. In a closed circuit, pressure will rise in direct proportion to the volume of gas delivered. In a true volume-cycled device, a preselected volume will be delivered regardless of the airway pressure needed to deliver the volume. Hence these ventilators are also classified as *volume-present (limited), pressure-variable devices*. As a precaution against excessive inflation pressure, pressure-limiting ("pop-off") valves are incorporated in most systems.

CAUTION: It is at this point when excess pressure is vented that the ventilator no longer functions as a volume-cycled device but as a pressure-cycled (limited) device. Consequently, the preselected tidal volume may or may not have been delivered. If this were allowed to continue, the patient would be hypoventilated and in danger of ventilatory insufficiency.

Clinically, there are few if any pure volume-cycled

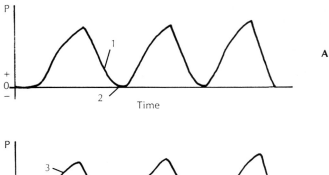
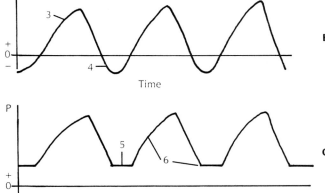

FIGURE 23-16 Graphs of expiratory pressure *(P)* patterns. **A,** Positive-to-ambient. **B,** Positive-to-negative. **C,** Positive-to-positive.

ventilators, because of the integration of pressure limits or time as alternate cycling mechanisms.

5.6 Classification according to expiratory phase

1 Exhalation begins when the ventilator and patient circuit are opened to ambient or held at some elevated predetermined expiratory baseline. Exhalation may be described as *passive, retarded, subambient,* or with *positive end expiratory pressure* (PEEP).

2 Ventilators incorporate one, or a combination, of the following expiratory patterns (Fig. 23-16):

a *Positive-to-ambient (A).* A positive pressure airway pressure *(1)* is released by venting it to the atmosphere. This type of exhalation normally is passive and unrestricted except for the minimum resistances offered by the flow of the exhaled gas through the breathing circuit and exhalation valve. During exhalation the patient's airway pressure is allowed to return to ambient *(2).*

b *Positive-to-negative (B).* A positive pressure during inspiration *(3)* is exposed to a subambient pressure gradient during exhalation *(4).* This type of pattern is not normally used during exhalation except in situations where the expiratory system is restricted by the small diameter of the tubing such as in neonatal-pediatric systems.

CAUTION: When using a positive-to-negative system, care must be taken *not* to allow the subambient pressure to be transmitted to the patient's airway. This situation can cause removal of oxygen and alveolar volumes, resulting in atelectasis, hypoxemia, and airway collapse.

c *Positive-to-positive (C).* A positive pressure during inspiration is released but maintained at a positive pressure level during exhalation *(5).* This pressure pattern shifts the baseline upward, causing the patient to breathe at an elevated baseline *(6)* called PEEP or CPAP.

5.7 Classification according to the internal system by which the tidal volume is delivered to the patient

1 Gas may be delivered to the patient by way of a direct connection with the ventilator's power source or indirectly from an intermediate chamber such as a bag or bellows.

2 A ventilator that delivers gas directly from its power generator (gas or piston) to the patient is a *single-circuit* device. Characteristically, this type of ventilator can generate greater pressure levels than a double-circuit system. Also, the wave patterns are different from those generated by a double-circuit device because of the cushioning effect caused by the bellows, bag, or other type of intermediate chamber as internal pressure is created in a double-circuit system.

3 A *double-circuit* ventilator delivers gas from its power source to empty a bag or bellows that delivers its contents to the patient. In this context a double-circuit device incorporates a "pneumatic hand" to compress a bellows, such as in the Bennett MA-1 or 2 ventilator, or to squeeze a bag such as in the Engström ventilator.

5.8 Classification according to special functions

Special ventilator functions include intermittent mandatory ventilation (IMV), synchronized intermittent mandatory ventilation (SIMV), continuous positive airway pressure (CPAP), positive end expiratory pressure (PEEP), and more recently with the new generation devices, pressure support ventilation, airway pressure release ventilation, and mandatory minute ventilation.

1 IMV describes a ventilator function that allows the patient to breathe spontaneously without assistance and, at predetermined intervals delivers a mechanical breath. The rationale for using this type of system is that it:

  a Allows the patient to adjust his or her own Pa_{CO_2}

  b Decreases the need for suppressant drugs

  c Facilitates transition from mechanical ventilation to spontaneous breathing (weaning)

  d Can be used with high and low levels of PEEP

  e Helps stabilize FI_{O_2}

  f Decreases the length of time of ventilator use by reducing psychologic dependence and helps patient maintain muscle tone of ventilatory muscles

  g Decreases O_2 consumption caused by the patient "fighting the ventilator."

    • Fig. 23-17 illustrates an IMV breathing pattern, showing the patient's spontaneous breath *(1),* followed by a periodic mechanical breath delivered by the ventilator *(2).* After this breath, the patient returns to spontaneous breathing *(3).* Technical de-

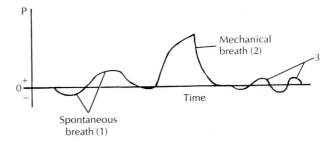

FIGURE 23-17 Graphic representation of IMV breathing pattern showing spontaneous and mechanical breaths.

tails on the use of IMV are presented in Unit 18.4.

2 As previously stated, SIMV, sometimes called intermittent demand ventilation (IDV), is a term describing another technique for applying IMV. In this method the delivery of the mechanical breath is synchronized with the patient's spontaneous breathing attempts. This prevents the possibility of "stacking a breath" (i.e., a mechanical breath delivered on top of a spontaneous inspiration).

3 CPAP may be used in conjunction with a mechanical ventilator or without it.

  a As previously explained, a CPAP system uses a high-pressure reservoir and a constant flow of gas that exceeds the patient's inspiratory peak flow demands.

  b With this system the patient breathes a constant elevated baseline pressure.

4 PEEP may be used in conjunction with assisted or controlled ventilation or with a spontaneously breathing patient. When used with a ventilator, an elevated baseline pressure level is established and positive pressure is delivered in addition to this level.

  a During exhalation (end of the mechanical breath) the airway pressure level returns or remains at the preset PEEP level until the next breath begins.

  b Spontaneous PEEP uses an open reservoir system with positive pressure held during the expiratory phase.

  c The difference between CPAP and PEEP is that the patient on PEEP must drop the airway pressure below baseline (ambient) to initiate gas flow. Thus with a PEEP system a patient must work harder to move a gas volume.

5 Discussion on pressure support ventilatory airway pressure release ventilation and mandatory minute ventilation is presented in Unit 22.1.

6.0 PARTS OF VENTILATORS AND HOW THEY FUNCTION

6.1 Parts of a ventilator system

Today there are many different types of ventilators produced by many manufacturers. Although the shapes, sizes, and features vary from one ventilator to the other, the

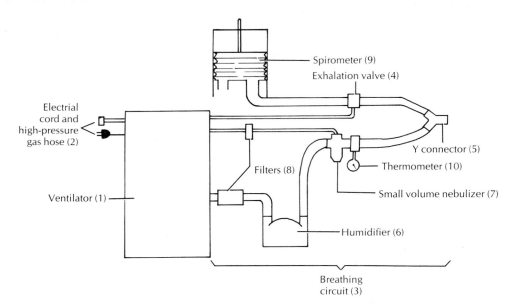

Spirometer (9)

Exhalation valve (4)

Electrial cord and high-pressure gas hose (2)

Y connector (5)

Thermometer (10)

Filters (8)

Small volume nebulizer (7)

Ventilator (1)

Humidifier (6)

Breathing circuit (3)

FIGURE 23-18 Typical ventilator system showing ventilator and breathing circuit.

overall ventilation systems remain essentially the same (Fig. 23-18).*

1 Ventilators are made up of two major systems:
   a The internal circuits, usually covered by a cabinet
   b The patient breathing circuit, consisting of a breathing tubes with exposed tubing and accessories such as humidifiers, water traps, gas filters, and nebulizers

2 The ventilator (see Fig. 23-18, *1*) is the apparatus that cycles ON and OFF to augment or provide a patient's ventilation.

3 The ventilator usually comes as a unit with an electrical power cord *(2)* (if it is electrically powered) and/or a high-pressure hose for connection to an external gas source.

4 A patient or *breathing circuit* refers to all the tubing and other accessories that attach the ventilator to the patient *(3).* The patient end of a breathing circuit usually contains an exhalation valve *(4),* which closes to the outside during inspiration and opens for exhalation, and a Y connector for attachment of the breathing circuit to the patient's airway *(5).*

5 Most breathing circuits also incorporate a humidifier *(6)* to humidify the relatively dry gas before it reaches the patient; a small volume nebulizer for the administration of medication *(7);* filters *(8)* to remove any gross contaminants from the inhaled gas; and a spirometer to monitor exhaled volumes *(9).*

6 Other ventilator features may include monitors for temperature *(10)* and IMV or PEEP assemblies (not shown).

*The reader is encouraged to locate each ventilator part as it is presented in the following text by referring to the figure and, if possible, to the actual ventilator.

6.2 Characteristics of breathing circuits

Patient breathing circuits are identified either as *standard* or *circle* systems and are constructed of *permanent* or *disposable* types of materials.

1 A *standard* breathing circuit (Fig. 23-19) refers to a tubing system that connects to the ventilator outlet at one end *(1)* and an exhalation valve *(2)* at the other. The distinguishing characteristic is that the patient inhales or exhales through the *same* tubing pathway. In the illustration, dotted arrows indicate gas flow during inspiration. Solid lines indicate exhalation. A standard breathing circuit has a larger *dead-space* volume than a circle system.
   a This arrangement causes the patient with each inspiration to rebreathe carbon dioxide that remains in the exhalation manifold and its attachments at the end of expiration. The volume of gas that occupies a space in the breathing circuit but does not make a useful contribution to alveolar ventilation is referred to as *mechanical dead space.*
   b In adults the dead-space volume may not be significant; however, in pediatric patients with small tidal volumes, this volume could cause the patient to be inadequately ventilated and oxygenated. (See Module Twenty-six.)
   c In Fig. 23-19 the dead-space volume is indicated by no. *3.* In this example the mechanical dead space would be approximately 100 ml or the volume of the patient connecting tubing and manifold *up to the point of the exhalation valve.*
   d Standard-type breathing circuits are used primarily for the administration of IPPB therapy with a mask or mouthpiece and for short-term mechanical ventilation (e.g., emergency room, recovery room).

2 A *circle* breathing circuit (Fig. 23-20) is a system that incorporates two tubes, one for inhalation *(1)* and the

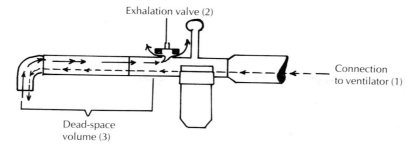

FIGURE 23-19 Standard breathing circuit.

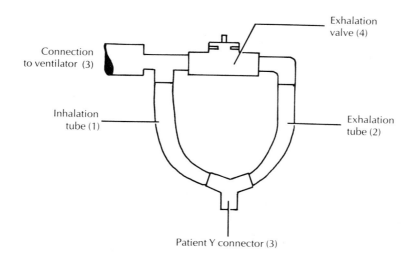

FIGURE 23-20 Circle breathing circuit.

other for exhalation *(2),* joined by a Y connector at the patient connection *(3).* Manufacturers market different models of the circle concept. However, most incorporate a two-tube system with an exhalation valve *(4)* to prevent rebreathing and a Y connector for patient attachment. Mechanical dead space is usually limited to the volume of the Y connector, a negligible amount.

Circle-type breathing circuits are used in situations requiring prolonged ventilation where a tracheal tube is in place and almost always for the ventilation of pediatric patients.

3 A *permanent-type* breathing circuit is one that can be decontaminated and reused numerous times. Permanent circuits are generally constructed of more durable materials than disposable circuits. For this reason they are more expensive and require repair because of the assembly and reassembly involved in the decontamination process.

4 *Disposable-type* circuits are very popular because they come already assembled and sterilized and can be discarded after patient use. This reduces the personnel time and facilities required for the decontamination proceess.

NOTE: Because disposables were not designed to be recycled as permanent items, they should not be reused. Once exposed to decontamination agents, they may fail

to function properly. Also, disposable tubing is much more difficult to properly clean and rinse.

6.3 Exhalation manifolds

1 The exhalation manifold (valve) is an integral part of any breathing circuit. Its function is to close the circuit from the atmosphere to allow pressurization of the system during a positive pressure breath and to open at the end of inspiration to allow exhalation to occur.

2 It is important to realize that *all* gas that is contained in the ventilator system, including internal tubing and patient's breathing circuit, as well as the patient's exhaled volumes, passes by this valve during exhalation.

3 Exhalation valves are integrated parts of a ventilator's main gas source. This linkage allows the exhalation valve to close just before the main breathing circuit is pressurized and to open simultaneously with the closing of the main flow valve.

4 Fig. 23-21 shows a simple exhalation valve arrangement using gas pressure to inflate a rubber balloon–type valve.

  a As the main valve in the ventilator *(1)* opens, a gas pressure is transmitted by means of a small bore-conducting tube to inflate the rubber balloon *(2)* (diaphragm). The inflated diaphragm covers the open port of the exhalation manifold *(3),* creating a seal

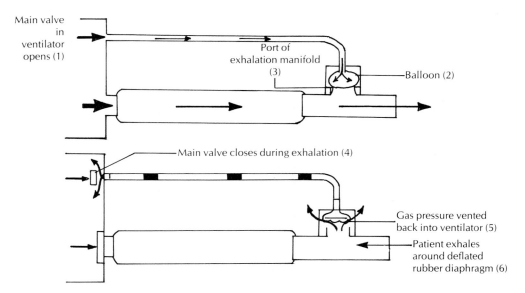

FIGURE 23-21 Simple exhalation valve arrangement using gas pressure to inflate a rubber balloon—type valve.

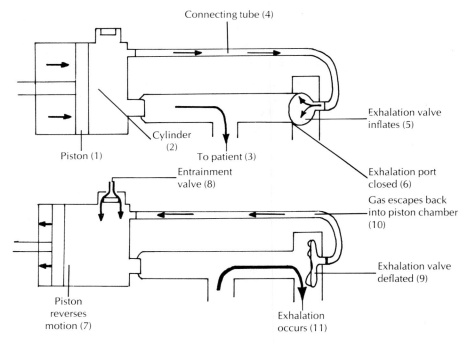

FIGURE 23-22 Exhalation valve arrangement in the Emerson 3-PV ventilator.

and preventing any pressure loss during the mechanical breath.

b During exhalation, the main valve closes, interrupting pressure to the exhalation diaphragm *(4)*. When this occurs, gas pressure that was holding the valve inflated is vented back into the ventilator *(5)*. The valve deflates and the patient is able to exhale around the deflated rubber diaphragm *(6)*.

c This cycle of inflating and deflating a rubber diaphragm is used by most ventilators for opening and closing the patient breathing circuit during inhalation and exhalation.

5 Fig. 23-22 represents another application of this system in a ventilator, such as the Emerson 3-PV, which generates gas flow by movement of a piston.

a During the inspiratory phase, the piston *(1)* moves forward to compress air in the cylinder *(2)*, causing it to move into the patient *(3)*.

b Simultaneously, as the piston begins its forward movement, pressurized gas travels down the connecting tube *(4)*, causing the exhalation valve *(5)* to inflate, closing the exhalation port *(6)*, and causing the positive pressure to enter the patient's lungs.

c Once the piston completes its forward motion, it reverses *(7)*, causing air to be drawn into the chamber by means of an entrainment valve *(8)* and to leave the inflated exhalation valve.

d The exhalation valve now is deflated *(9)* and opened to the atmosphere because the withdrawn piston causes gas within the hollow inflatable valve to escape back into the piston chamber by way of the connecting tube *(10)*, allowing exhalation to occur *(11)*.

6 The ventilator cycle, involving valve inflation and deflation, occurs simultaneously with the generation and interruption of the main gas flow at the ventilator, creating the inspiratory and expiratory phases of the mechanical breathing process.

7 In some ventilator systems, such as the Siemens Servo 990B and 900C, the exhalation valve is opened and closed electronically in conjunction with the opening and closing of a main *solenoid valve* at the ventilator. (See Module Seventeen for a discussion on electronic valves.) In others the exhalation valve may be adapted to perform special functions such as PEEP or gas collection for the monitoring of exhaled volumes. Special function exhalation valves are presented in the following unit.

8 A gas-collection manifold is a modified type of standard exhalation valve that channels all exhaled gases through a single port rather than allowing them to randomly disperse to the atmosphere (Fig. 23-23). This manifold is used when an attachment is needed to monitor exhaled volumes.

a In *A* the patient exhales past an exhalation valve *(1)* into the atmosphere *(2)*.

b In *B* the patient exhales past an exhalation valve *(3)* into a chamber that surrounds the valve, forcing ex-

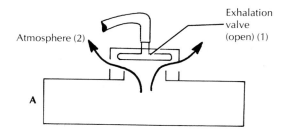

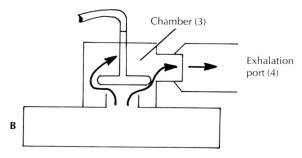

FIGURE 23-23 Exhalation past the exhalation valve of a breathing circuit into the atmosphere **A,** and a gas-collection manifold **B.**

haled gases to leave through a single port *(4)*. A spirometer or respirometer could be attached (at point *4*) to measure the patient's exhaled volume.

7.0 FLOW OF GAS THROUGH A BIRD (POSITIVE) Q CIRCLE AND A BENNETT MA-1 BREATHING CIRCLE

7.1 Breathing circuits for the Bird ventilator

1 The Bird Mark 7 ventilator incorporates either a standard-type breathing circuit for use with a mouthpiece and/or mask or a modified circle system. See Module Seventeen for use of the standard circuit with IPPB therapy.

2 The Bird Mark 7 ventilator also incorporates a modified type of circle system called a *positive Q circle* breathing system. This system can be used for prolonged ventilation with an intubated patient (Fig. 23-24).

a A ventilator *(1)* powered by gas at 45 to 55 psig delivers two gas flows to the patient's breathing circuit by way of two-channel connecting tube *(2 and 3)*.

b The large bore tubing *(3)* carries the main gas flow at respiratory pressures to a hollow block assembly *(4)*. The small bore tubing is known as the inspiratory power drive line and transports gas at a higher velocity and pressure to a T adapter *(5)*.

c One end of the T is inserted in the large volume nebulizer *(6)* and the other to a connecting tube *(7)* leading to the rear of the exhalation valve *(8)*.

d The main gas flow *(9)* continues through the block assembly, in and out of a 500 ml nebulizer for humidification *(6)*, to the inspiration side of the breathing circuit, and past a water trap *(10)*. At this point, any particulate moisture collecting in the tubing is removed before the gas travels to the Y connector *(11)* and the patient.

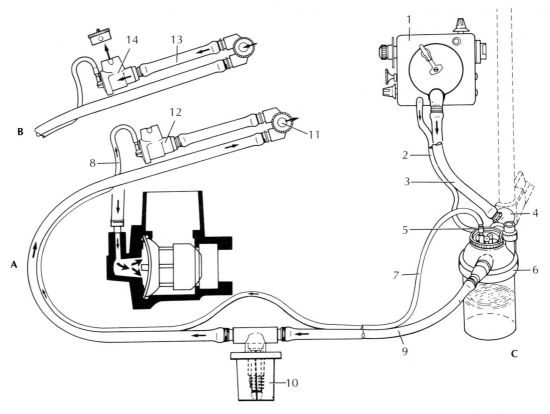

FIGURE 23-24 Bird Mark 7 and ten principles of positive phase Q circle system. **A,** Inhalation flow diagram. **B,** Exhalation flow diagram. **C,** Inline nebulizer. (Modified from a drawing by Medical Products Division/3M, St Paul, Minn.)

e Gas in the inspiratory drive line divides at the T to power the nebulizer and seat the exhalation valve *(12).*

f On exhalation, gas leaves the patient by way of the Y and the short expiratory limb of the breathing circuit *(13)* past the exhalation valve *(14),* completing a breathing circle.

3 Other assemblies will vary according to special functions, although all Bird circuits incorporate pneumatics (gas) to open and close valves.

Fig. 23-24 may be used to assemble a Bird Q circle according to Procedure 23-1.

7.2 Breathing circuit for the Bennett MA-1 ventilator

1 The Bennett MA-1 is a volume ventilator used primarily to provide prolonged continuous ventilation to intubated patients.

2 The MA-1 ventilator incorporates a circle-type breathing circuit designed for use with adults (Fig. 23-25).* This circuit incorporates a standard model cascade humidifier *(1),* an exhalation valve assembly (manifold) *(2)* with a thermometer *(3),* nebulizer *(4),* and inspira-

tory *(5)* and expiratory breathing tubes *(6).* These tubes connect the exhalation valve assembly to a patient Y connector *(7).* Also included in the breathing circuit are a bacteria filter *(8)* and a gas collection tube *(9)* that conducts exhaled gas to a water trap *(10),* then up a hollow pipe *(11)* to a monitoring spirometer *(12)* and, eventually, to the room.

3 The manner in which the exhalation valve operates in the MA-1 is very similar to that of the Bird Q circle in that gas pressure causes the valve to seat during inspiration. During exhalation, gas flow to the valve is interrupted, allowing it to deflate and the patient to exhale.

4 During inspiration (Fig. 23-26) a gas flow always 5 cm H_2O *greater* than the patient's system pressure leaves the MA-1 by way of a small port on the side of the cabinet *(1)* and travels to inflate a rubber diaphragm located on the side of the exhalation manifold *(2).*

a Simultaneously, the main gas flow *(solid arrows)* travels from the outlet port of the cascade humidifier *(3)* through the small volume nebulizer and to the patient by way of a Y piece *(4).*

b On exhalation, flow is stopped to the exhalation balloon and the valve opens, allowing gas to flow past the gas collection manifold *(dotted arrows)* to a collector tube *(5)* leading to the spirometer *(6)* by way of the water trap and hollow post.

---

*This circuit may be modified to add or delete accessories according to the needs of the patient. Pediatric tubing is available as an option. If possible, the reader is encouraged to point out each of the assemblies on an actual MA-1 ventilator as this unit is being studied.

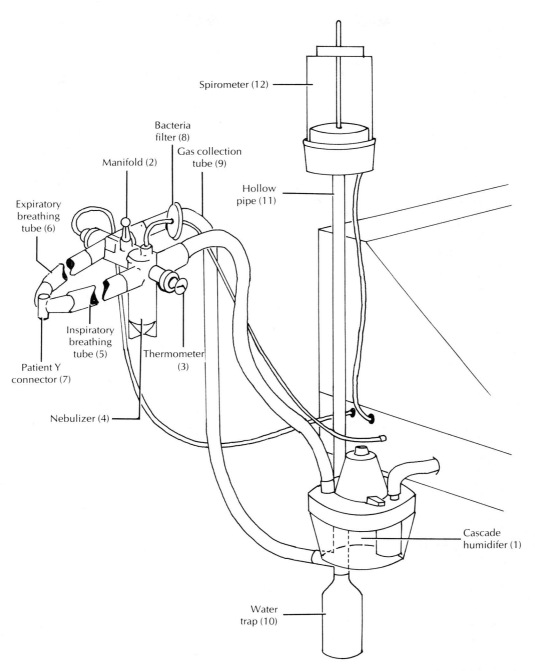

Spirometer (12)

Bacteria
filter (8)

Gas collection
tube (9)

Manifold (2)

Hollow
pipe (11)

Expiratory
breathing
tube (6)

Inspiratory
breathing
tube (5)

Thermometer
(3)

Patient Y
connector (7)

Nebulizer (4)

Cascade
humidifer (1)

Water
trap (10)

F I G U R E 2 3 - 2 5 Bennett MA-1 ventilator breathing circuit. (Courtesy Puritan-Bennett Corp, Carlsbad, Calif.)

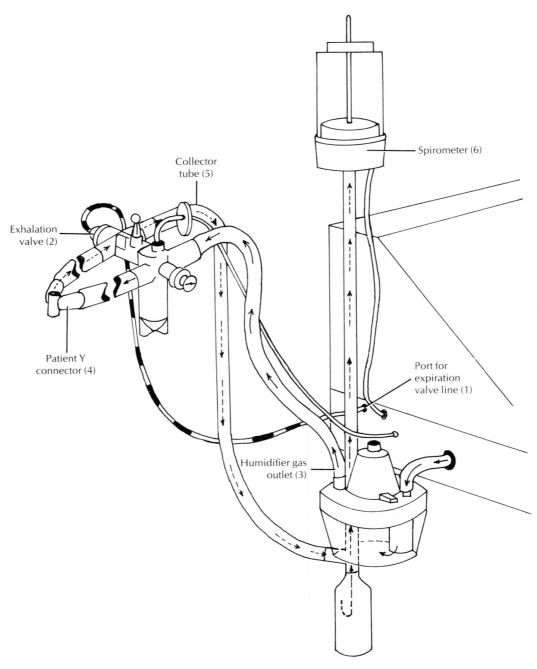

Exhalation valve (2)

Collector tube (5)

Spirometer (6)

Patient Y connector (4)

Port for expiration valve line (1)

Humidifier gas outlet (3)

FIGURE 23-26 Inspiration *(solid arrows)* and expiration *(broken arrows)* through Bennett MA-1 ventilator breathing circuit. (Courtesy Puritan-Bennett Corp, Carlsbad, Calif.)

7.3 Assembly and operation of a Bennett MA-1 ventilator

The steps involved in assembly of a ventilator will vary from one model to another. Thus it is important that the reader be able to follow a manufacturer's instruction manual and hospital procedure manual for assembly of a particular type of ventilator.

The Bennett MA-1 ventilator is used as an example of the type of instructions to follow in assembling a ventilator.

Procedure 23-2 (at the end of this module) provides instructions on connecting a Bennett MA-1 breathing circuit to a MA-1 ventilator and for operating a Bennett MA-1 ventilator.

7.4 Comparing the Bennett MA-1 to the Bennett MA-2 ventilator*

The *drive mechanisms* for the Bennett MA-1 and MA-2 ventilators are very similar. The primary difference between these ventilators are the following factory-installed features on the Bennett MA-2 ventilator. These features were not available on the MA-1 or were available only as add-on options.

1 *Continuous positive airway pressure* (CPAP). The ventilation cycling function can be locked out and the PEEP mechanism operated to provide demand CPAP with the patient breathing spontaneously.

2 *Demand valve.* A demand valve is integrated into the ventilator circuit that opens to provide gas flow to the patient whenever:

   a The patient continues to inhale at the end of a mechanical inspiration

   b Demand CPAP is used

   A primary consideration for use of this or any demand valve used in a ventilator circuit is sensitivity of the valve to open pressure and to peak flow rate.

   A valve that is not sensitive enough to a patient's inspiratory efforts will be slow in opening (prolonged response time). This causes the patient to perform additional work of breathing, resulting in a diminished tidal volume.

   The practitioner should also be aware that a demand valve by definition satisfies the patient's inspiratory demands by providing adequate gas flow, which for most adult patients is 120 to 150 L/min.

3 *Synchronized intermittent mandatory ventilation* (SIMV).[†] The benefit of this feature is that the machine does *not* deliver the mechanical breath on top of a spontaneous breath, which can cause excessive airway pressure and lung volume.

   a One problem that has been noted with this type of system is that the ventilator interprets negative pressure in the breathing circuit to be a spontaneous breath and does not deliver the preset mechanical breath.

   b Clinically, a patient with hiccups or other causes of negative airway pressure may cause a delay of ventilator cycling to the point that adequate alveolar ventilation is not provided. This is because the ventilator interprets the hiccup as a spontaneous breathing effort.

4 *Postive end expiratory pressure* (PEEP). The PEEP mechanism is built in and may be adjusted to pressures of 45 cm H_2O.

5 *Inspiratory hold.* An inspiratory hold for a period of up to 2 seconds can be adjusted to provide plateau holds.

6 *Humidification.* The ventilator is provided with a Bennett Servo II Cascade humidifier, which automatically adjusts preset water temperature based on feedback from a probe inserted at the patient's airway.

7 *Monitors measure:*

   • Respiratory rate. A digital presentation of the actual rate

   • Temperature. A digital readout of temperature

   • Oxygen concentration. A digital display of actual FIo_2

8 Alarms. The following are available to warn the practitioner of possible problem(s).

   a FIo_2. An alarm will sound if the FIo_2 exceeds or fails to meet preset concentration levels.

   b Low pressure alarm. This alarm sounds to inform the operator that the airway pressure during a mechanical breath did not exceed 10 cm H_2O above baseline pressure. It also sounds if the system pressure falls to 5 cm H_2O below baseline pressure for more than 1 second. This alarm is sometimes referred to as a tubing disconnect alarm.

7.5 Breathing circuit for the Emerson 3-PV volume ventilator*

1 The Emerson 3-PV volume ventilator, also known as the Post-OP ventilator, is a dependable controller. It can also be modified to be an assistor and IMV ventilator.

2 The breathing circuit on the 3-PV is located outside and inside the ventilator cabinet, with the humidifier enclosed behind a door.

3 Fig. 23-27 shows a complete tubing system for the 3-PV and is used to discuss the patient breathing circuit.[†] (Tubing sizes are not drawn exactly to scale.)

   a As the piston (1) starts upward in its chamber, a positive pressure is generated, which closes the gas inflow valve (2), forcing the gas to leave the piston chamber by means of a descending tube (3) and simultaneously closes a rubber diaphragm blocking open port in the exhalation valve (4). (Refer also to the magnified view, B.)

   b Descending gas opens a flutter valve (one-way) (5)

---

*The Bennett MA-2 ventilator is not shown.

[†]As described in previous modules, IMV is a function where the patient breathes spontaneously with preset mechanical breaths delivered to maintain a desired minimum respiratory rate.

---

*If possible, the reader is encouraged to have an Emerson ventilator available for reference while studying this unit.

[†]Fig. 23-27 can also be used as a diagram for putting together the assembled parts of an Emerson 3-PV breathing circuit.

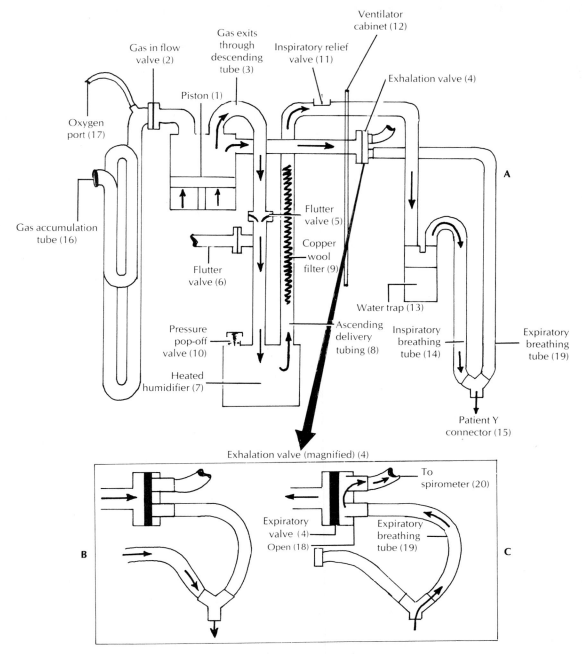

FIGURE 23-27A, Tubing system for the Emerson 3-PV ventilator and breathing circuit. **B,** Expanded view of exhalation valve during expiration. **C,** Inspiration. (Modified from a drawing by JH Emerson Co, Cambridge, Mass.)

and closes the flutter valve in the tube from the sigh generator *(6)*.

c The descending gas continues in and out of a heated humidifier ("hot pot") *(7)* into the ascending delivery tubing *(8)*, which carries gas at respiratory pressures toward the patient. En route to the patient, the gas travels through a copper wool filter *(9)* that reacts with oxygen to form copper oxide, which theoretically serves as a bacteria inhibitor. A maximum pressure limit can be adjusted by the "pop-off" valve located atop the humidifier *(10)*.

d The gas then enters an upper elbow and seats an inspiratory relief valve *(11)* as it passes out of the ventilator through the cabinet *(12)* at the outlet port.

e At this point the external portion of the inspiratory breathing circuit begins with a tube conducting the gas through a water trap *(13)*.

f Gas leaves the water trap and enters the inspiratory limb of the patient tubing *(14)* leading to a patient Y connector *(15)* and the patient.

g On exhalation, the piston reverses and moves downward, causing the gas entrainment valve *(2)* to open,

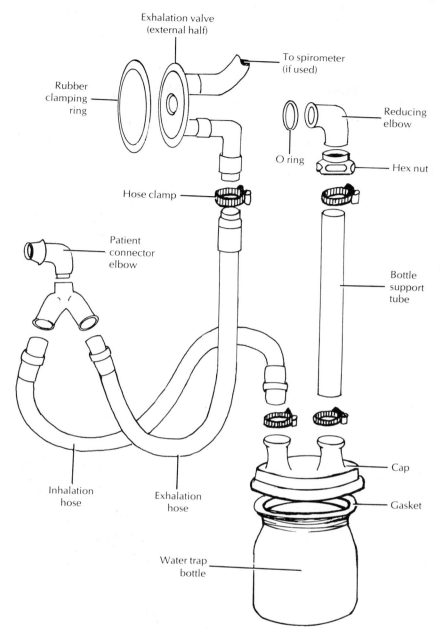

FIGURE 23-28 Expanded view of Emerson 3-PV ventilator external breathing circuit. (Modified from a drawing by JH Emerson Co, Cambridge, Mass.)

allowing room air that has entered a gas accumulation tube (trombone) *(16)* and oxygen, if it is flowing into the oxygen port *(17)*, to enter the piston chamber.

h Simultaneously, because there is no positive pressure being generated, the patient's exhalation forces the rubber diaphragm in the exhalation valve to move away from the port *(B, 18)*, allowing expiratory gas to travel out the expiratory side of the Y *(19)*, to pass the expiratory valve *(4)*, and to reach a spirometer *(20)*.

4 The inspiratory circuit of the 3-PV includes all the tubing and humidifier from the top of the piston chamber *(3)* to the patient's Y piece.

5 The mechanical dead-space volume of the circuit includes the Y piece *(15)*, the expiratory timer of the breathing circuit (not shown), the exhalation valve *(4)*, and tubing to the spirometer, if it is used in the system. Fig. 23-28 presents an expanded view of the external breathing circuit.

Procedure 23-4 serves as a guide to assembling an Emerson 3-PV external breathing circuit.

8.0 CONTINUOUS DISTENDING AIRWAY PRESSURE (CPAP, PEEP, sPEEP, AND EPAP)
8.1 Recording normal airway pressure

Before studying the use of continuous positive airway pressure (CPAP), it is helpful to review a graphic example

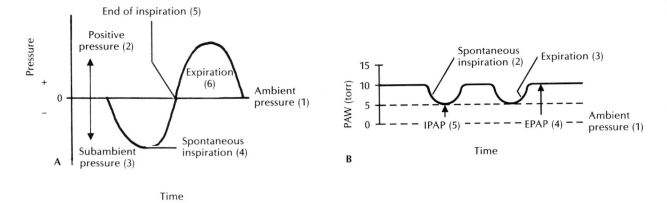

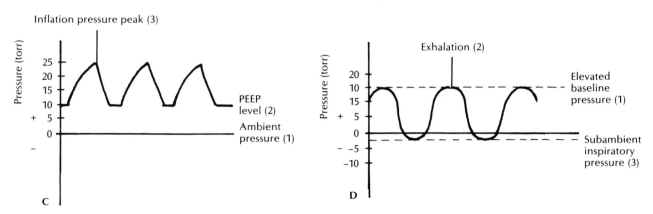

FIGURE 23-29 Pressure tracings of various ventilator pressure modes. **A,** Normal spontaneous breathing. **B,** CPAP. **C,** PEEP. **D,** Spontaneous PEEP.

of a normal pressure pattern for a spontaneously breathing patient.

1 CPAP, in the most general terms, refers to any situation that prevents the patient from exhaling completely before beginning another inspiration.

2 Physically, CPAP can be easily experienced by taking a deep breath, exhaling partially, and then taking another breath even though the chest feels partially filled.

3 As shown in Unit 4.2, airway pressure can be traced by monitoring the breathing cycle with an x-y recorder. Fig. 23-29 *(A)* represents a typical pressure tracing seen in monitoring the spontaneous breathing of a patient on an x-y recorder such as an oscilloscope, strip recorder, or chart paper.

  a Ambient pressure is presented as a baseline marked *zero (1)*.

  b Any upward movement *(2)* of the baseline or of a pressure-wave pattern from this original baseline represents a positive pressure when compared to ambient.

  c And downward *(3)* movement represents a subambient pressure when compared to ambient.

  d During a spontaneous breath, lowering of internal airway and lung pressures causes a corresponding drop in the pressure tracing below the baseline *(4)*.

  e As gas flows into the lungs from the atmosphere, the inspiratory pressure gradient becomes less and eventually equalizes with ambient as indicated by the pressure tracing returning to the baseline *(5)*.

  f During exhalation, pressure in the lungs and airway becomes greater than ambient, causing gas to leave the lungs to the atmosphere. This is represented by an upward, then gradually a downward, movement of the pressure tracing *(6)* as the expiratory flow rate begins high and tapers toward the end of exhalation.

  g At the end of exhalation, airway pressure once again equals ambient and gas flow ceases, causing the pressure tracing to return to the ambient baseline.

8.2 Recording continuous positive airway pressure as elevated baseline pressure

1 The terms and definitions describing the use of constant distending airway pressure (CDAP) have undergone almost constant change since Dr. Gregory and his colleagues originally described constant positive pressure breathing in the early 1970s.

2 Continuous positive airway pressure (CPAP) is a term used to describe the position of the inspiratory and expiratory pressure levels relative to ambient baseline. During CPAP, the *entire* breathing cycle must be performed at pressure levels above ambient (see Fig. 23-29, *B*).

a In illustration *B* the ambient baseline is indicated by the horizontal *x* axis marked *zero (1)*. Inspiration is indicated by 2 and exhalation by *3*.

b Note that spontaneous breathing is similar to illustration *A,* except that the complete breathing cycle occurs *above* the ambient baseline; in this example, +15 torr higher than ambient or a CPAP level of +15 torr *(4)*.

c During inspiration, the pressure pattern drops, but not to the baseline *(1)* so that inspiration begins not at ambient as in illustration *A* but at an elevated pressure base of +15 torr *(4)*.

d In reviewing the CPAP tracing, one can see that the breathing cycle can be subdivided into two distinct components: end positive airway pressure *(EPAP) (4)* and inspiratory positive airway pressure *(IPAP) (5)*.

e During inspiration, the degree to which the airway pressure drops toward ambient (i.e., the airway pressure at the maximum point of inspiration) is called IPAP. In this illustration, IPAP would be +5 torr *(5)*.

f EPAP describes the baseline at the end of exhalation *(4)*. EPAP in this illustration is +15 torr.

3 It may be useful to describe both IPAP and EPAP levels when charting CPAP because investigators have shown that alteration of either can influence the shunt and hence oxygenation.

8.3 Positive end expiratory pressure

1 Positive end expiratory pressure (PEEP) is a term describing a method whereby positive pressure is maintained on the airway of a patient *on a ventilator* during exhalation or during spontaneous breathing. (See Fig. 23-29 *C*.)

2 When PEEP is used with a mechanical ventilator, the pressure baseline is shifted upward from ambient *(1)* so that the inflation pressure caused by the mechanical breath begins at the PEEP level *(2)*, In this example the PEEP level would be 10 torr.

3 Inflation pressure caused by the mechanical breath becomes a *combination* of the PEEP pressure and the pressure required to deliver the tidal volume *(3)*. In this example, the ventilator system manometer would reflect an inflation pressure of 25 torr.

4 During inspiration and exhalation the baseline does *not* return to ambient, causing some to comment that this method should be called CPAP instead of PEEP. Obviously, a controversy exists in the field over expiratory elevated baseline nomenclature. In cases such as this, PEEP is used to describe any method of attaining an expiratory elevated baseline whenever the patient is attached to a ventilator.

5 CAUTION: The practitioner should be aware that high levels of PEEP combined with large tidal volumes can cause excessive airway pressures, leading to possible barotrauma, decrease in cardiac output, and other pressure-related complications. Instructions on the application of PEEP are presented in a subsequent unit.

8.4 Spontaneous positive end expiratory pressure

1 Spontaneous positive end expiratory pressure (sPEEP; also called EPAP) (see Fig. 23-29, *D*), describes a method of providing an elevated baseline *(1)* to a spontaneously breathing patient, using a mask or tracheal tube.

2 sPEEP is applied only during exhalation *(2)*, and the patient must be allowed to drop his or her airway pressure to ambient or slightly below ambient during a spontaneous inspiration *(3)*. sPEEP in this example would be 10 torr.

9.0 TYPES OF CONTINUOUS DISTENDING AIRWAY THERAPY (CPAP, PEEP, ETC.)
9.1 Methods of generating constant distending airway pressure (CDAP)

1 CPAP and PEEP are forms of constant distending airway pressure (CDAP) generated by limiting (restricting) exhalation so that a positive pressure effect is created as the patient exhales against the impedance. Inspiration begins before exhalation is completed so that the entire breathing cycle occurs above ambient pressures, except in sPEEP application.

2 The practitioner can simulate CDAP by performing a deep inspiration and using his or her hands to block exhalation after approximately one half of exhalation has occurred. Another inspiration is performed at this point, even though the lungs are only half empty. Continuous breathing at this elevated level will simulate the full feeling experienced in the chest by the patient breathing on a mechanically induced CPAP or PEEP system. Breathing too rapidly or exerting excessive expiratory force against the blocked airway may cause dizziness or changes in heart rate or pulse pressure. Similar symptoms may be experienced by the patient whose elevated baseline is not properly adjusted.

3 Constant distending airway pressure (either CPAP or PEEP) is generated by systems that cause exhaled gases to be directed:

a Into a tube that is submerged under water (Fig. 23-30).

b Against an exhalation diaphragm that is regulated by a spring (Fig. 23-31).

c In opposition to an exhaled gas flow (Fig. 23-32).

d Against a weighted exhalation diaphragm (Fig. 23-33).

4 The following explanations and illustrations focus primarily on the expiratory side of a breathing circuit.

Fig. 23-30 *(1)* represents a patient who is exhaling past an open gas collection–type exhalation valve *(2)* into a tube with one end attached to the expiratory port of the exhalation valve *(3)* and the other submerged under water *(4)*.

a To exhale the atmosphere, the patient must first generate enough positive pressure on exhalation to force (blow) water out of the submerged tube so the air can escape to the surface.

b The amount of PEEP or CPAP generated is equiva-

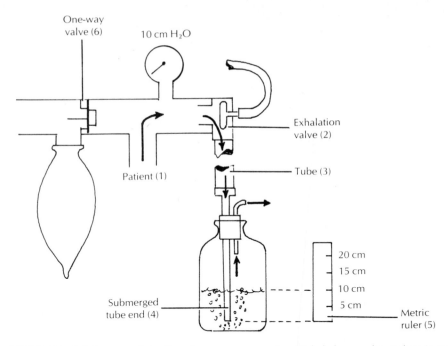

FIGURE 23-30 Constant distending airway pressure system. Exhaled gases directed against tube submerged under water.

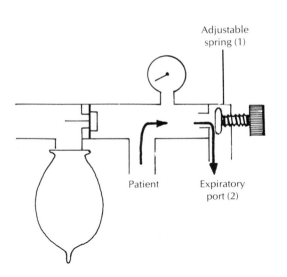

FIGURE 23-31 Constant distending airway pressure system. Exhaled gases directed against exhalation diaphragm regulated by spring.

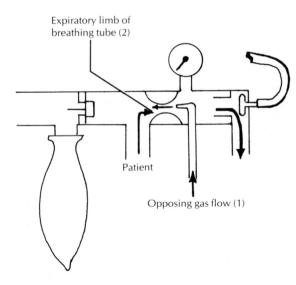

FIGURE 23-32 Constant distending airway pressure system (PEEP or CPAP). Exhaled gases directed against opposing gas flow.

lent to the distance, in centimeters, that the tube is submerged under the water.

   c In this model, the tube is submerged 10 cm, as measured by a metric ruler *(5)*.

   d This forces the patient to generate enough positive force on exhalation to displace the mass caused by 10 cm of water (i.e., generating 10 cm H_2O pressure CPAP or PEEP during exhalation with each breath).

   e The one-way valve *(6)* prevents the ambient pressure from being directed back into the ventilator breathing circuit.

   In Fig. 23-31 the principle is the same except the pa-

tient must now exhale against the force caused by an adjustable spring *(1)* that attempts to hold the valve closed during exhalation. The amount of expiratory positive pressure the patient must generate to overcome this resistance *(2)* and open the closed valve can be read directly from a pressure manometer inserted in the circuit as cm H_2O or torr.

5 Positive end expiratory pressure generated by an opposing gas flow is a concept incorporated in the Bird CPAP or PEEP system.

   a In Fig. 23-32 a gas flow *(1)* is directed against the expiratory gas as it enters the expiratory limb of the breathing circuit *(2)*.

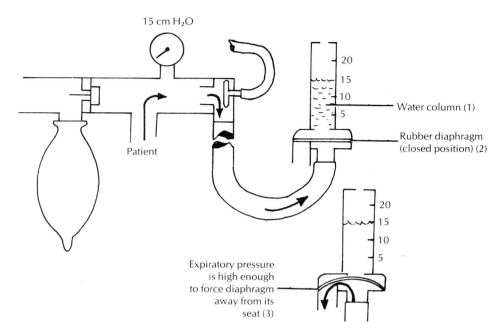

FIGURE 23-33 Constant distending airway pressure system. Exhaled gases directed against weighted exhalation diaphragm.

b The opposing gas flow causes a resistance to exhalation that the patient must overcome.

c The expiratory pressure generated to overcome the increased resistance results in a positive force that can be read on the system manometer as cm H$_2$O or torr.

d CPAP or PEEP levels can be increased or decreased by altering the opposing gas flow.

6 Fig. 23-33 represents a system that is a variation of the tube under water.

a The principle of operation is the same except that the weight of the water *(1)* is determined by its height in a column supported by a rubber diaphragm *(2)*.

b As the patient exhales, the diaphragm is held closed by the water until enough expiratory pressure is generated by the patient to force the diaphragm with its weight of water away from its seat *(3)*, allowing exhalation to occur.

c In this system the higher the water in the column, the greater the PEEP or CPAP in cm H$_2$O.

7 Valves used to generate PEEP or CPAP can be classified as either a *threshold-resistor* or *flow-resistor* valves.

Most ventilator systems use threshold-resistor valves because they allow expiratory pressure to remain relatively constant in the face of changing expiratory flows. This is not the case with flow-resistor valves where expiratory positive pressure varies directly with changing flow rates (i.e., the greater expiratory flow rate, the higher the levels of CPAP or PEEP).

a Examples of threshold-resistor valves include the Bird CPAP demand system and the Emerson water column PEEP valve.

b Examples of flow-resistor valves include the Sie-

mens ventilator PEEP valve and the Babybird outflow valve.

9.2 Using the Bennettt MA-1 ventilator PEEP attachment

1 The Bennett MA-1 PEEP attachment is available as an option to the standard MA-1 ventilator. The attachment is self-contained and easily mounted on the side of the ventilator cabinet accessory panel (Fig. 23-34).

NOTE: This type of PEEP system is used only as an example, since most ventilators for continuous care now have built-up PEEP and CPAP modalities.

2 The MA-1 generates PEEP by holding the exhalation valve in the patient manifold inflated so that the manifold is blocked, preventing the patient from exhaling to a zero baseline. This is similar in concept to the PEEP device shown in Fig. 23-31.

3 The pressure level at which the exhalation diaphragm is maintained is determined by rotating the knob on the PEEP device.

This can be demonstrated by removing the exhalation valve from the patient manifold, "dialing in" (adjusting) PEEP, and manually cycling the ventilator. Note that the diaphragm remains inflated at the end of inspiration. By removing the PEEP, the diaphragm deflates after inspiration has ended.

Procedures 23-5 and 23-6 may be used for providing PEEP on the MA-1 ventilator.

9.3 Criteria for applying and monitoring continuous expiratory elevated baselines

1 CPAP and/or PEEP-type maneuvers are used primarily in cases of *acute respiratory failure* (ARF). This condition is seen clinically with decreasing expiratory lung volume (functional residual capacity—FRC) early

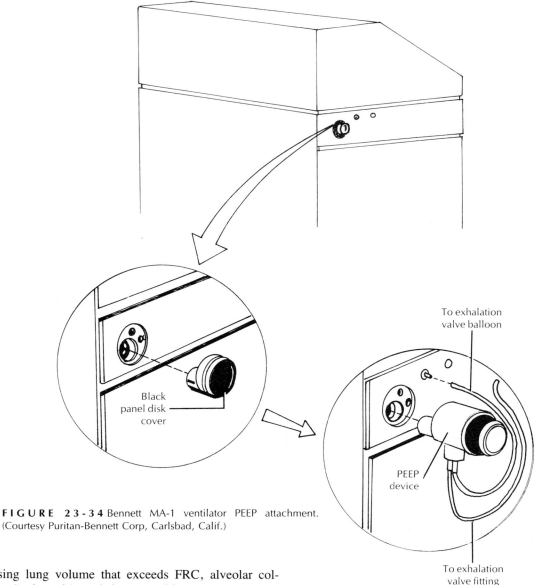

FIGURE 23-34 Bennett MA-1 ventilator PEEP attachment. (Courtesy Puritan-Bennett Corp, Carlsbad, Calif.)

closing lung volume that exceeds FRC, alveolar collapse (atelectasis), and shunt conditions causing hypoxemia.

2 FRC decreases with a patient's age, body size (obesity), and anatomic position (supine). It is also decreased by abdominal surgery, distension of the abdomen, and acute respiratory insufficiency.

3 The purpose of CPAP and PEEP is to *stabilize* the alveolus in a position of function (open) once the critical opening pressure has been achieved by hyperinflation.

4 CPAP/PEEP works on applying an *internal gas pressure* to hold the alveolus open. Physiologically, this causes the pressure within the alveolus to remain *higher* than the extra-alveolar pressure throughout inspiration and expiration. Once the alveolus has been opened (i.e., *critical opening pressure* has been reached), PEEP/CPAP keeps the alveolus from collapsing during exhalation, thereby preventing atelectasis and associated shunt conditions. This causes an increase in the expiratory lung volume (FRC) and reduces hypoxemia that is caused by a decreased FRC.

5 One goal of this therapy is to achieve a Pa_{O_2}/FI_{O_2} greater than 300 torr and a $\dot{Q}sp/\dot{Q}T$ (shunt) less than 0.15 while maintaining a normal cardiac output. Another is to maintain an arterial oxygen tension (Pa_{O_2}) of 50 to 60 mm Hg at nontoxic oxygen concentrations.

6 Elevated expiratory baseline pressure can be delivered by tracheal tube or by mask (face-mask PEEP). Either technique is functional, although better control of the pressure level (fewer leaks) and prevention of aspiration are best achieved with a tracheal tube system.

7 Ideally, patients on elevated expiratory baseline pressure therapy should be monitored for arterial/venous blood oxygen tensions, intrapulmonary shunt, and cardiac output by a *Swan-Ganz* catheter. (See Module 28, Unit 8.0.)

a The *purpose* of using a Swan-Ganz catheter (thermodilution type) is to:
• Monitor pulmonary artery pressure

- Measure pulmonary arterial occlusion pressure (wedge pressure)
- Measure cardiac output
- Provide an avenue for obtaining mixed venous blood samples for gas analysis

b Normal values during use of the Swan-Ganz technique are:
- Mean pulmonary artery pressure (MPA): 12 to 18 torr
- Pulmonary artery occlusion or wedge pressure (PAO): 4 to 10 torr
- Central venous or right atrial pressure (CVP): 3 to 12 torr

NOTE: In patients with compromised left ventricular function, postoperative stress, or postmyocardial infarction (MI), the desirable pressure ranges may be higher than normal values listed for a healthy individual. For example, an optimum PAO in a patient with cardiac involvement may be 13 to 17 torr, instead of 4 to 10 torr.

c During use of CPAP/PEEP therapy, the expiratory pressure level is gradually increased until the shunt is reduced to less than 0.15 and the pulmonary artery pressure (PAP) is less than 15 torr, with a functionally stable cardiac output. More details on determining PEEP levels follow.

8 Selecting the best method of providing CPAP/PEEP (i.e., maximum decrease in shunt, maximum Pao_2 for lowest FIo_2, and maximum cardiac output) is of prime consideration for the clinician.

For example, if spontaneous PEEP (sPEEP) is used, some patients, because of the increased work of breathing, may not tolerate airway levels greater than 10 cm H_2O pressure. In this case, CPAP or PEEP may prove more beneficial.

9 CPAP/PEEP therapy is started by establishing an initial elevated baseline pressure level of 5 cm H_2O and gradually increasing the baseline in 2 to 3 cm H_2O increments and waiting 20 to 40 minutes at each level until the desired physiologic effect is reached. Clinically, a reduced shunt level of less than 0.15, a functionally stable cardiac output, best dynamic compliance, and highest Pao_2 with lowest FIo_2 are considered indicators of appropriate PEEP or CPAP levels.

10 One of the most difficult clinical judgments is to decide appropriate ("optimum" or "best") PEEP or CPAP levels. If a Swan-Ganz catheter is in place, the patient's clinical picture can be compared to measured values for a more objective judgment.

a If a catheter is *not* used, "best" PEEP and CPAP levels must be *estimated* based on changing Pao_2, $Paco_2$, systemic blood pressure, and dynamic compliance.

b Clinical indications for evaluating "best" or "optimum" PEEP or CPAP (CDAP) levels are listed in Table 23-2.

TABLE 23-2 Clinical indicators of "best" or "optimum" levels of constant distending airway pressure (PEEP or CPAP)

Desirable criteria	Undesirable criteria
1 At a given FIo_2, Pao_2 increases as elevated baseline is incrementally applied. When possible, FIo_2 should be maintained at less than 0.6.	As "best" or "optimum" elevated baseline pressure is reached, Pao_2 will incrementally decrease.

NOTE: At elevated baseline levels greater than 15 cm H_2O, Pao_2 is *not* an adequate measure to determine cause and effect of PEEP and CPAP. This is because of elevated baseline greater than 15 cm H_2O, the lung function may be improved but the cardiac output may be reduced, causing a lower Pvo_2 in the shunted blood, which causes a further desaturation when mixed with arterialized blood.

2 As elevated baseline is applied, the dynamic compliance as determined by serial tidal volume and system pressure measurements will improve until "best" PEEP or CPAP levels are reached.	As "best" PEEP or CPAP levels are reached, the dynamic compliance will begin to decrease as elevated baseline is increased.

NOTE: A measurement of dynamic compliance can be used as an indicator of "best" elevated baseline levels because, as the patient's FRC approaches normal, the patient begins to breathe on a more favorable part of the compliance curve (i.e., greater expansion at lower inflation pressure).

3 As elevated baseline is applied, cardiac output will increase slightly if depressed or remain stable until "best" elevated baseline pressure is exceeded.	As "best" PEEP or CPAP levels are exceeded, cardiac output will begin to decrease as elevated baseline is incrementally increased.

NOTE: A Swan-Ganz thermodilution catheter is the best method of accurately measuring and tracking cardiac output. Patients who require greater than 25 cm H_2O elevated baseline pressure should be monitored with this technique because of possible hypotension as a result of decreased cardiac output of 15% or greater. If a Swan-Ganz catheter is unavailable, hypotension is considered severe if mean blood pressure is less than 60 torr. Mean blood pressure is calculated by the formula:

$$\text{Mean arterial pressure} = \frac{\text{Pulse pressure}}{3} + \text{Diastolic pressure}$$

Clinical experience has shown that undesirable effects of PEEP on cardiorespiratory values can be improved by increasing the patient's fluid load before and after each incremental increase in the PEEP level. This technique is still relatively new and should be used by the physician only if the patient has both Swan-Ganz and radial artery catheters. For more information on volume loading, refer to current journals and periodicals.

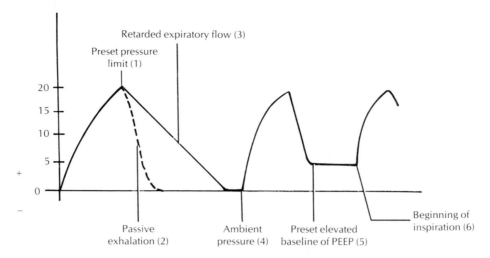

Preset pressure limit (1)

Retarded expiratory flow (3)

Passive exhalation (2)

Ambient pressure (4)

Preset elevated baseline of PEEP (5)

Beginning of inspiration (6)

FIGURE 23-35 Graphic comparison of pressure tracings caused by expiratory retard and PEEP.

9.4 Hazards of using constant distending airway pressure

1 The major hazards relatd to using continuous elevated baseline pressures are associated with conditions classified as barotrauma and cardiovascular depression.

2 Barotrauma is a general term describing extra-alveolar air (EAA). These conditions include:
   a Pneumothorax
   b Pneumomediastinum
   c Interstitial emphysema
   d Subcutaneous emphysema
   e Tracheal rupture
   f Peripheral airway rupture

3 These conditions are most frequently related to high levels of PEEP (greater than 20 cm H_2O). They also occur most frequently in patients with predisposed weaknened lungs (i.e., bullae or necrotizing pneumonia) or when PEEP is misused or malfunctions.

4 Excessive airway pressure may result in cardiovascular depression as a result of transmural pressure from the lungs that causes the great vessels of the heart to collapse, impeding venous return. This, combined with other influences, can cause decreased cardiac output with possible poor tissue perfusion, hypotension, and renal insufficiency.

5 Excessive PEEP levels can also cause a decrease in Pao_2 and compliance and an increase in volume of shunted blood flow per tidal volume of blood flow ($\dot{Q}s/\dot{Q}T$) and dead space tidal volume ratio (VD/VT).

6 As previously cited these parameters can be used as indicators for identification of best PEEP levels. For example, as lung function improves, the VD/VT ratio becomes lower (a value of less than 0.6 is clinically acceptable).

7 The detrimental cardiac effects caused by PEEP can be minimized or eliminated when PEEP is used in conjunction with IMV (see Unit 18.2).

9.5 Expiratory retard versus PEEP or CPAP

1 Many ventilators incorporate a mechanism for *lengthening* a patient's expiratory flow time.

2 The usual method is to *retard* or restrict a patient's expiratory flow rate by partially obstructing gas flow past the exhalation valve.

3 *Expiratory retard* is different from PEEP or CPAP in that even though expiratory flow is restricted, system pressure must return to *ambient* before each inspiration.

4 Fig. 23-35 compares a pressure tracing caused by expiratory retard to PEEP.
   a During a normal mechanical breath, a positive pressure is generated to a preset pressure limit *(1)*, causing the ventilator to cycle off, allowing a passive exhalation to occur *(2)*.
   b When expiratory flow is retarded, the time required for exhalation is extended as resistance to flow is generated throughout the expiratory phase. This is indicated by the more gradual slope of the expiratory pressure curve *(3)*. Note, however, that the patient's airway pressure *returns to ambient* before the next inspiration *(4)*.
   c If PEEP is used, expiratory pressure drops normally to a preset *elevated* baseline *(5)*, where it is maintained until the next inspiration *(6)*. A positive force is applied only at the end of the expiratory phase and not throughout exhalation as is true with retard. Also with PEEP, the patient's airway pressure does *not* return to baseline before each inspiration.

5 A simple method of causing expiratory retard is to place a cap with calibrated holes over the outflow part of the exhalation valve (Fig. 23-36). As the patient exhales, impedance to expiratory flow by the calibrated hole retards exhalation. The amount of resistance can be changed by selecting larger or smaller holes on the cap.

6 Another method used is to restrict the movement of the exhalation valve away from its seat by a spring, such as in the Bennett MA-1 ventilator.

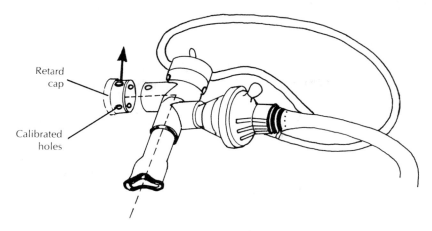

FIGURE 23-36 Expiratory retard is created by placing a cap with calibrated holes over the outflow port of the exhalation valve.

10.0 COMPUTING CLINICAL VARIABLES NECESSARY FOR OPERATION OF MECHANICAL VENTILATORS

10.1 Estimating required tidal volume and cycling rate

Before implementing mechanical ventilation, one should calculate an *estimated* required tidal volume (VT) for the patient.

1 An adult patient's *tidal volume can be estimated* by converting the patient's body weight from pounds to kilograms (divide by 2.2) and multiplying the body weight (kg) by 12 to 15 ml/kg. The ventilator cycling *rate (f)* for an adult patient also can be *estimated* at a rate of 10 to 15 breaths per minute.

2 The *formula* for estimating an initial tidal volume and cycling rate for a ventilator patient is:

$$V_T = 12 \text{ to } 15 \text{ ml/kg at a frequency of } 10 \text{ to } 15/\text{min}$$

EXAMPLE: Calculate an estimated tidal volume for a 170 pound patient:

a Step one: $170 \div 2.2 = 77$ kg
b Step two: $V_T = 12$ ml $\times 77$ kg $= 924$ ml

3 The *formula* for calculating actual breathing frequency is:

$$f = \frac{60}{T_I + T_E}$$

EXAMPLE: Calculate the breathing frequency of an inspiratory time of 2 sec and an expiratory time of 3 sec:

$$f = \frac{60}{2 + 3} = 12/\text{min}$$

4 Once the tidal volume has been calculated, one can easily compute the *minute volume* (V̇E) by multiplying the estimated tidal volume by the cycling frequency.

a The *formula* for computing a patient's minute volume is:

$$\dot{V}_E = V_T \times f$$

b Generally, patients who are ventilated at faster cycling rates require proportionately smaller tidal volume.

5 Minute volume measurements are probably more useful to the clinician, especially if the patient is assisting or on IMV. This is because the tidal volume may change from one breath to another, although the average tidal volume may be adequate when calculated for 1 min.

EXAMPLE: Using a tidal volume of 770 ml at 12 breaths per minute, the patient's *minute volume* would be:

$$770 \text{ ml} \times 12 = 9240 \text{ ml}$$

or

$$\dot{V}_E = \frac{9240 \text{ ml}}{1000 \text{ ml}} = 9.24 \text{ L}$$

6 It is important to note that the body weight formula for calculating a patient's tidal volume is an *estimate* used for determining only the *initial* value for setting the mechanical breath to be delivered by the ventilator. The adequacy of this calculation to provide necessary alveolar ventilation *must be confirmed* by an analysis of the patient's arterial blood gases.

7 It is important that an arterial blood gas sample be acquired before initiating ventilatory assistance and as a follow-up procedure. A comparison of these values will indicate necessary alterations in the patient's minute volume.

8 Another method of estimating a patient's ventilatory requirements is to use the *Radford nomogram* (Fig. 23-37). This nomogram was developed during the 1950 polio epidemic for predicting the ventilatory needs of people with primary healthy lungs; it compares the body weight, age, sex, and breathing frequency to arrive at a predicted tidal volume. For this reason the predicted values are low for patients with unhealthy lungs. This discrepancy can be adjusted by *adding approximately 50%* to the predicted lung volume if the patient has lung disease.

9 Other corrections for fever, daily activity, altitude, tracheal tube, metabolic acidosis, or mechanical dead space are compensated for by adding the values presented as corrections to the nomogram.

10 To use the nomogram, place a straight edge across the three vertical columns.

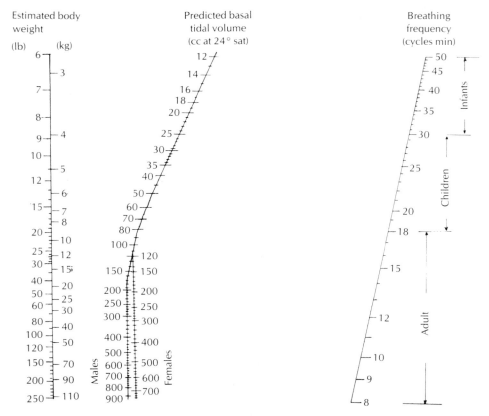

FIGURE 23-37 Radford nomogram used to estimate a patient's ventilatory requirements. (From Scanlan CL, Spearman C, and Sheldon R: Egan's fundamentals of respiratory therapy, ed 5, St Louis, 1990, The CV Mosby Co; modified from Radford EP Jr: Ventilation standards for use in artificial respiration, J Appl Physiol 7:451, 1955.)

a One end of the straight edge is placed at the line closest to the calculated body weight; the other edge is placed at the line indicating the measured or desired breathing frequency for adults, children, and infants.

b The predicted tidal volume is read on the center column at the point where the straight edge crosses the column.

c For example, a 170 pound male breathing at 10 breaths/min would require a predicted tidal volume of approximately 625 ml.

11 The patient with chronic obstructive pulmonary disease (COPD) requires an additional 313 ml, giving a total predicted tidal volume of 938 ml at sea level and normothermia. This value equals 12 ml/kg, which closely fits the body weight formula of 12 to 15 ml/kg estimated tidal volume.

10.2 Correcting the tidal volume to ventilatory needs

1 Once the patient has been placed on a ventilator, the tidal volume must be *adjusted* to provide the desired $Paco_2$ and pH, according to the physician's order. A rule of thumb is that 20% change in V_T equals approximately 4 to 6 mm change in $Paco_2$.

2 The respiratory component of this relationship depends on proper adjustment of the expired gas volume per minute ($\dot{V}_E$), which reflects alveolar ventilation ($\dot{V}_A$). When assessing the relationship between alveolar ventilation and $Paco_2$, one will find that the $Paco_2$ *decreases* as the alveolar ventilation is *increased*. This relationship, which extends to minute volume, can be used to predict a patient's corrected minute ventilation.

The *formula* for correcting a patient's minute volume is:

$$\text{New } \dot{V}_E = \frac{\text{Old } \dot{V}_E \text{ in liters } \times \text{ Patient's } Paco_2}{\text{Patient's normal } Paco_2}$$

and

$$\text{New } V_T = \frac{\text{New } \dot{V}_E}{f}$$

a EXAMPLE: A 55 kg woman with drug overdose is placed on a volume ventilator with a controlled rate of 10 breaths/min, an initial tidal volume of *660 ml*. ABGs after 20 minutes reveal the following values:
- $Paco_2$: 75 torr
- pH: 7.20
- HCO_3^-: 26 mEq/l

b These blood gases indicate that the patient is still in respiratory acidosis resulting from hypoventilation. This condition is acute because the HCO_3^- has not changed from normal. The most obvious action required is to increase the patient's minute volume from the initial value.

c To calculate the required new minute ventilation to compensate for the hypoventilation, apply the values to the first equation under 2.

• Old minute volume = 10 × 660 = 6600 ml or 6.6L

• New minute volume = $6.6 \times \dfrac{75}{40} = 12.4$ L

• The new tidal volume keeping the frequency constant = $\dfrac{\text{new } \dot{V}_E}{f}$

$$\frac{12.4}{10} = 1.24 \text{ L or } 1240 \text{ ml}$$

3 Certain clinical circumstances, such as the prevention of atelectasis or treatment of an already atelectatic lung, may require the maintenance of large tidal volumes combined with relatively high cycling rates. This combination can cause a hyperventilation state with resultant alkaline blood gases.

4 To correct for alkalosis, the physician can maintain normal respiratory rates and use *mechanical dead space* to cause the patient to rebreathe a small amount of exhaled carbon dioxide. Dead space is created by adding additional measured lengths of tubing to the expiratory side of the patient's breathing circuit.

This technique is effective in maintaining normal Pa_{CO_2} and pH, provided the mechanical dead-space volume (V_D) is accurately calculated by using the nomogram or by adding dead-space in 100 ml increments and confirming by blood gases.

10.3 Determining the ratio of inspiration to expiration (I:E)

1 A breathing cycle is composed of a total amount of time divided between inspiration and expiration.

2 Calculation of an I:E ratio is important because enough time must be allowed for inspiration to occur so that a desired tidal volume be delivered. Also, an appropriate length of time must be allowed for exhalation to occur to prevent air trapping and inadvertent PEEP situations. *Inadvertent PEEP is dangerous* and can lead to decreased cardiac output and other undesirable outcomes.

3 A general rule is that expiration time should be at least *1.5 times* the length of inspiration, and inspiration should not exceed *0.5 to 2 sec* in any mode. Most ventilators are set to alarm if the I:E ratio becomes equal to or less than 1:1.

4 The length of inspiration is determined by the inspiratory flow rate. This flow rate reflects the length of inspiration and refers to the volume change per unit of time, expressed as liters per second or per minute.

5 In adult patients, inspiratory flow rates of 40 to 60 L/minute are generally adequate unless the patient is breathing at abnormal frequencies (greater than 25/min).

6 Calculation of the I:E ratio is probably the most useful criterion for adjusting the inspiratory flow rate.

The formula for calculating an I:E ratio is:

$$\text{I:E ratio} = \frac{T_I}{T_E}$$

To calculate an I:E ratio, use the following steps:

a Observe and count number of breaths per minute.

b Divide total breaths per minute into 60 to compute total time of one breath.

c Observe and time the length of inspiration.

d Subtract inspiratory time from the total time to compute expiratory time of one breathing cycle.

e Substitute values into the formula. Divide the numerator (T_I) and denominator (T_E) by the numerator to obtain a fraction.

f Write the numerator of the fraction in front of the denominator instead of over it to obtain the desired I:E format.

7 EXAMPLE: Calculate the I:E ratio of a patient on a ventilator at a rate of 10/min using this method, according to the following steps:

a 10 breaths/min

b 60 ÷ 10 = 6 sec for each breath

c $T_I = 1.5$

d $T_E = 6 - 1.5$ or 4.5 sec

e $I:E = \dfrac{1.5}{4.5} = \dfrac{1}{3}$

f Ratio = 1:3

8 The length of inspiration (inspiratory time) is determined by the *inspiratory flow rate* and the cycling rate if a ventilator is in the control mode. Calculation of the inspiratory flow rate is important to ensure that enough time is allowed for inspiration to occur to reach a predetermined tidal volume.

9 In certain situations, one may need to calculate the length of inspiration and expiration, given a desired I:E ratio and ventilation frequency.

The formula for determining the length of inspiration when given a desired I:E ratio and frequency is:

$$T_I \text{ (sec)} = \frac{60/f \text{ (min)}}{I + E}$$

a EXAMPLE: Calculate the time allowable for inspiration, given a desired I:E ratio of 1:2 and a cycling frequency of 10/min.

b Solution:

• Calculate total time allowed for one breath:

$$\frac{60 \text{ sec}}{10} = 6 \text{ sec/breath}$$

• Substitute into the formula:

$$T_I = \frac{60/10}{1 + 2}$$

$$T_I = \frac{6}{3}$$

$$T_I = 2 \text{ sec}$$

10 Using the same desired I:E ratio and cycling frequency as cited, the *formula* for calculating length of expiration is as follows:

$$T_E = T_{(TDT)} - T_I$$
$$T_E = 6 - 2 = 4 \text{ sec}$$

Therefore I:E = 2 sec/4 sec.

11 Most ventilators provide a separate control for setting the flow rate. This control is usually calibrated in liters per minute (L/min), although some manufacturers use liters per second (L/sec).

The formula for converting liters per minute to liters per second is:

$$L/sec = \frac{L/min}{60}$$

EXAMPLE: Convert 40 L/min to L/sec:

$$L/sec = \frac{40}{60} = 0.67 \text{ L/sec}$$

The formula for converting liters per second to liters per minute is:

$$L/min = 60 \times L/sec$$

EXAMPLE: Convert 0.67 L/sec to L/min:

$$L/min = 60 \times 0.67 = 40 \text{ L/min}$$

12 When using a constant flow generator such as the Bennett MA-1 or Emerson volume ventilator, an unknown can be calculated, given the other two values:

The *formula* for calculating an unknown, given two other values is:

$$V_T = \dot{V} \times T_I$$

EXAMPLE: Calculate the tidal volume of patient on a Bennett MA-1 ventilator with an inspiratory flow rate of 40 L/min and an inspiratory time of 1.5 sec.

SOLUTION:

• Convert liters per minute to liters per second:

$$40 \text{ L/min} = 0.67 \text{ L/sec}$$

• Substitute known values into the formula:

$$V_T = 0.67 \text{ L/sec} \times 1.5 \text{ sec}$$
$$V_T = 0.67 \times 1.5 = 1.00 \text{ L} \times 1000, \text{ or } 1000 \text{ ml}$$

EXAMPLE: Calculate the predicted inspiratory flow rate for a patient on a Bennett MA-1 to deliver a 1000 ml tidal volume.

• Use the formula:

$$\dot{V} = \frac{V_T}{T_I}$$

• Convert milliliters to liters (1000 ml = 1.00 L)
• Substitute in the formula:

$$\dot{V} = \frac{1.00 \text{ L}}{1.5 \text{ sec}}$$

$$\dot{V} = 0.67 \text{ L/sec}$$

• Convert liters per second to liters per minute:
$$0.67 \times 60 = 40 \text{ L/min}$$

EXAMPLE: Using the formula:

$$T_I = \frac{V_T}{\dot{V}}$$

• Calculate the inspiratory time required to deliver a 1000 ml tidal volume at a flow rate of 40 L/min.

SOLUTION:

• Convert $\dot{V}$ from liters per minute to liters per second:

$$40 \text{ L/min} = 0.67 \text{ L/sec}$$

• Convert V_T from milliliters to liters:

$$1000 \text{ ml} = 1.00 \text{ L}$$

• Substitute in the formula:

$$T_I = \frac{V_T}{\dot{V}} = \frac{1.00}{1.5 \text{ sec}} = 0.67 \text{ L/sec}$$

• Convert liters per second to liters per minute:
$$0.67 \times 60 = 40 \text{ L/min}$$

10.4 Determining the peak inspiratory flow rate

Once an I:E ratio has been established by determining the length of time allowed for inspiration, an *inspiratory flow rate* can be determined.

1 The formula for calculating an inspiratory flow rate, given the time of inspiration is:

$$\dot{V} = \frac{V_T}{T_I}$$

where $\dot{V}$ = flow (ml/sec), V_T = tidal volume; T_I = length of inspiration.

EXAMPLE: Given an adult patient with a desired tidal volume of 800 ml, a frequency of 10, and inspiratory time of 1.5 sec, calculate the required inspiratory flow rate:

a Convert 800 ml to liters: 0.8 L.
b Substitute into the formula:

$$\dot{V} = \frac{0.8}{1.5} = 0.53 \times 60$$

c $\dot{V}$ = 31.9 or 32 L/min

2 Patients with obstructive disease usually require extended time for exhalation to occur. This can be expressed as a percent of the total breathing cycle.

The formula for calculating the percent of inspiratory time to the total breathing cycle

$$\text{Percent inspiratory time} = \frac{T_I}{T_I + T_E}$$

EXAMPLE: Calculate percent inspiratory time of a patient breathing at a rate of 12 breaths/min with 2 sec for inspiration and 3 sec for expiration:

SOLUTION:

a Substitute into the formula:

$$\% \text{T}_\text{I} = \frac{2}{2+3} = 0.4 \times 100$$

b $\% \text{T}_\text{I} = 40$

11.0 APPLYING MATHEMATICS TO ESTIMATE THE CAUSE OF HYPOXEMIA

Determining the cause of hypoxemia

1 The cause of hypoxemia can be estimated by calculating the alveolar to arterial oxygen tension ($P(A\text{-}1)o_2$) gradient.

2 Once the gradient has been determined, it can be used to assess whether the cause of hypoxemia results primarily from a volume of gas/flow of blood per unit of time ($\dot{V}/\dot{Q}$) *imbalance* or *hyperventilation.*

3 A $\dot{V}/\dot{Q}$ imbalance or physiologic shunt occurs when blood, which was not well oxygenated as it passed through the lungs, mixes with arterial blood.

4 A normal range for the $P(A\text{-}a)o_2$ is *less than 10 torr in room air* except in older patients where the range is increased to less than 30 torr. (See the following formulas.) The normal range with 100% oxygen is less than 100 torr.

5 The formula for predicting normal Pao_2 in patients breathing room air, based on their age and anatomic position, is:

Predicted Pao_2 if patient is seated: $Pao_2 = 104.2 -$
$(0.27 \times \text{Age})$

Predicted Pao_2 if patient is supine: $Pao_2 = 103.5 -$
$(0.42 \times \text{Age}) \pm 4$

6 If the Pao_2 is less than expected, the $P(A\text{-}a)o_2$ gradient for oxygen is increased because of shunting. This cannot be corrected by increasing the FIo_2.

7 $\dot{V}/\dot{Q}$ is also caused by an increase in $P(A\text{-}a)o_2$ gradient for oxygen. This can be corrected by increasing the FIo_2.

8 A rule of thumb formula for calculating the expected Pao_2 is:

Expected $Pao_2 = FIo_2 \times 5$ for FIo_2 less than 0.3

EXAMPLE: A patient breathing 60% oxygen (FIo_2 0.60) should have a Pao_2 of approximately 300 torr.

9 A useful clinical formula to calculate approximate $P(A\text{-}a)o_2$ is:

$$PAo_2 = PIo_2 - \frac{Paco_2}{0.8}$$

where PIo_2 = partial pressure of inspired oxygen and 0.8 is the estimated respiratory quotient, which remains stable under most clinical conditions.

EXAMPLE: Calculate the $P(A\text{-}a)o_2$ gradient for a patient breathing room air, yielding a measured Pao_2 of 50 torr and a $Paco_2$ of 40 torr.

a Convert FIo_2 of 21% to PIo_2

$$P_B - 47 \ (H_2O \text{ vapor}) \times 0.21 = 150 \text{ torr}$$

where P_B = barometric pressure

b Use the formula:

$$PAo_2 = 150 - \frac{40}{0.8} = 100 \text{ torr}$$

c Subtract: $100 - 50 = PA(A\text{-}a)o_2$ or 50 torr

$P(A\text{-}a)o_2 = Pao_2 \text{ (ideal)} - Pao_2 \text{ (determined by ABG)}$

where ABG = arterial blood gas

10 In *comparing calculated gradient to norms* for room air of 5 to 30 torr: a $P(A\text{-}a)o_2$ gradient greater than 30 torr indicates a $\dot{V}/\dot{Q}$ imbalance.

a The Pao_2 and $Paco_2$ are added. If the sum is less than 120 torr, the hypoxemia is a result of venous admixture, *not* hypoventilation.

EXAMPLE: A patient with the following:

$$Pao_2 = 50 \text{ torr}$$
$$Paco_2 = 45 \text{ torr}$$
$$\text{Gradient} = \overline{95} \text{ torr}$$

b The value confirms the hypoxemia is caused by a $\dot{V}/\dot{Q}$ imbalance rather than hypoventilation.

11.2 Calculation of percent shunt and required FIo₂

1 The shunt calculation is used to determine the *amount of shunt* that is occurring in a patient with a reduced Pao_2 when breathing 100% oxygen (normal 600 torr).

2 The following formula can be used to *approximate* the percent of shunt at sea level if the PaO_2 exceeds 200 torr on *100% oxygen.*

$$\% \text{ shunt} = (700 - Pao_2) \times 5\%$$

a EXAMPLE: Calculate the percent shunt in an adult patient breathing 100% oxygen at sea level for 20 minutes if the measured Pao_2 is 100 torr. Substitute in the formula:

$$\% \text{ shunt} = (700 - 100) \times 0.05$$
$$= 600 \times 0.5$$
$$= 30\% \text{ shunt}$$

b A *normal* physiologic shunt is 3% to 5%.

3 Laboratory findings have shown that the percent shunt is increased whenever a patient is given 100% oxygen. For this reason many clinicians believe that the administration of 100% oxygen may be harmful to the patient and should not be given even for a short time.

4 Table 23-3 can be used to calculate the percent shunt and/or the required FIo_2 for a desired Pao_2 at various oxygen percentages.

a To find a percent shunt value, enter the table with an FIo_2 figure, which represents the inspired oxygen concentration supplied to the patient, and with a Pao_2 figure, which represents the arterial oxygen tension of the patient. For instance, if the patient's FIo_2 is 0.95 (or 95%) and Pao_2 is 80 mm Hg, then the percent shunt value is 39. Or if the FIo_2 is 0.70 (or 70%) and the percent shunt value is 21, then the resulting Pao_2 would be 160 mm Hg.

TABLE 23-3 Determining percent shunt values: FIO_2 (1.00 = 100%)

	0.35	0.39	0.42	0.45	0.49	0.53	0.56	0.60	0.63	0.66	0.70	0.74	0.77	0.81	0.84	0.88	0.91	0.95	0.98	1.00
30	65	65	65	65	65	66	66	66	66	67	67	67	67	68	68	68	68	68	69	69
40	53	53	54	54	55	55	55	56	56	57	57	57	58	58	58	59	59	59	60	60
50	41	42	43	43	44	45	45	46	46	47	47	48	48	49	49	50	50	51	51	52
60	34	34	35	36	37	38	38	39	40	40	41	42	42	43	44	44	45	45	46	47
70	26	27	28	29	30	31	32	33	34	35	35	36	37	38	39	39	40	41	41	42
80	23	24	26	27	28	29	30	31	32	32	33	34	35	36	37	37	38	39	40	40
90	19	20	21	22	24	25	26	27	28	29	30	31	32	33	33	34	35	36	37	37
100	15	17	18	19	20	22	23	24	25	26	27	28	29	30	31	32	33	34	35	35
120	10	11	13	14	15	17	18	19	21	22	23	24	25	26	27	28	29	30	31	32
140	10	11	13	14	15	17	18	19	21	22	23	24	25	26	27	28	29	30	31	32
160	7	9	11	12	14	15	16	18	19	20	21	22	24	25	26	27	28	29	30	31
180	5	7	9	10	12	13	15	16	17	19	20	21	22	23	25	26	27	28	29	30
200	5	7	9	10	12	13	15	16	17	19	20	21	22	23	25	26	27	28	29	30
225			2	4	5	7	9	10	12	13	15	16	18	19	20	21	22	24	25	26
250			0	1	3	5	7	8	10	11	13	14	16	17	18	20	21	22	23	24
275				0	1	3	4	6	8	9	11	13	14	15	17	18	19	21	22	23
300					1	3	4	6	8	9	11	13	14	15	17	18	19	21	22	23
325							2	4	6	7	9	11	12	14	15	16	18	19	20	21
350								2	3	5	7	9	10	12	13	15	16	17	19	20
375									1	3	5	6	8	10	11	13	14	16	17	18
400											2	4	6	8	9	11	12	14	15	17

Modified from Division of Pulmonary Disease, Hahnemann Medical Center and Hospital, Philadelphia, Penn.

- Percent shunt is calculated from the following formula:

$$\text{Percent shunt} = \frac{(PAO_2 - PaO_2)\,.0031}{(A\text{-}VO_2) + (PAO_2 - PaO_2)\,.0031}$$

$$\text{and } PAO_2 = (FIO_2 \times 713) - (PaCO_2 \times 1.25)$$

- The shunt table is calculated with a hemoglobin of 15, an $A\text{-}VO_2$ difference of 4, and a pH of 7.5.

b For example, to determine the percent shunt if the patient's FIO_2 is *0.49* and the measured PaO_2 is *60 torr*:

- Locate the FIO_2 value across the top of the table.
- Follow the column of figures under the FIO_2 value until the PaO_2 value is located on the vertical axis of the outside column.
- The value representing the point where the FIO_2 and PaO_2 intersect is the percent shunt.
- In this example the percent shunt is *37*.

c EXAMPLE: Determine the required FIO_2 to raise the PaO_2 to 90 torr.

- Locate the desired PaO_2 on the outside vertical column (90).
- Follow the column horizontally across the page until the percent shunt is located (37%).
- At this point follow the column vertically and read the required FIO_2 at the top of the column (98).
- To achieve a PaO_2 of 90 torr with a 37% shunt, use an FIO_2 of 0.98.

11.3 Calculating wasted ventilation (VD/VT)

1 The determination of effective ventilation (alveolar ventilation) is critical for the adequate maintenance of a patient on a ventilator.

a Tidal volume (VT) equals dead space (VD) minute volume plus alveolar ventilation (VA).

b Alveolar ventilation equals expired volume (VE) minus physiologic dead-space ventilation per minute.

2 To ensure adequate alveolar ventilation and the efficiency of CO_2 removal, one must estimate the total dead space to the tidal volume. This value, expressed as the VD/VT ratio, is approximately 0.35 although it increases with age. Clinically, patients with VD/VT ratios of 0.6 or greater will usually require mechanical ventilation.

3 The $PaCO_2$ and the partial pressure of expired oxygen ($PECO_2$) are needed to calculate the VD/VT ratio.

a The formula for calculating the VD/VT of a patient *not* on a ventilator using the Enghoff modification of the Bohr equation is:

$$VD/VT = \frac{PaCO_2 - PECO_2}{PaCO_2}$$

b EXAMPLE: Determine the VD/VT of a patient on a ventilator with a measured $PaCO_2$ of 60 and a mean expired PCO_2 of 6%.

SOLUTION:

- Convert 6% expired CO_2 to torr (760×0.06) = 45.6 torr.
- Substitute values into the equation:

$$\frac{VD}{VT} = \frac{60 - 45.6}{60} = 0.24$$

4 Individually, dead space normally equals 20% to 40% of a measured tidal volume with anatomic dead space equal to approximately 1 ml/lb of body weight.

5 As long as the actual VD/VT is less than 0.7, an estimated ratio can be obtained by the formula:

$$\frac{VD}{VT} = \frac{\dot{V}E \text{ measured}}{\dot{V}E \text{ predicted}} \times \frac{PaCO_2 \text{ measured}}{PaCO_2 \text{ normal}} \times 0.33$$

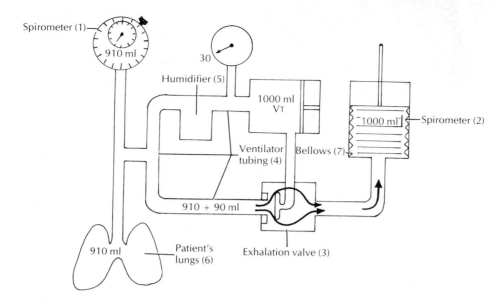

F I G U R E 2 3 - 3 8 Measurement of expiratory volume by two spirometers. One is placed by the patient's airway and the other after the exhalation valve.

where the predicted volume expired per minute ($\dot{V}E$) can be obtained from the Radford nomogram and the measured $\dot{V}E$ is obtained by a Wright respirometer placed after the exhalation valve on the ventilator. (See Unit 12.1.)

12.0 FLOW/VOLUME GAS MONITORS
12.1 Monitoring exhaled gas

1 The *general purpose of monitoring* is to guard against accidental trauma or death resulting from mechanical or human error by closely watching the patient's progress and ventilator status.

2 Today's ventilators are equipped with numerous types of devices to warn the practitioner of ventilator malfunctions. However, very few of these instruments are available to alert the practitioner of a failing patient until the patient's condition has radically changed. For this reason mechanical monitoring devices cannot and should not be used to replace respiratory care personnel in areas where a patient is being mechanically ventilated.

3 The measurements of exhaled tidal volume, airway pressure, FIO_2, and temperature are essential measurements to monitor when a patient is receiving continuous ventilation.

4 Exhaled tidal volume can be measured by several types of devices. One method is the *volume displacement spirometer*. This is a bellows device equipped with an alarm to indicate when the patient's exhaled volume is less than or exceeds a desired exhaled volume.

5 The accuracy of these devices can be greatly altered by the following circumstances:
  a Location of the spirometer in the circuit
  b Ventilator and tubing dead space
  c Mechanical drag because of inertia or friction of the bellows

d Gas volume expansion resulting from changes in temperature
  e Shunting of inspiratory gases into spirometer
  f Leaks in the expiratory circuit
  g Auxiliary gas flow from continuous flow nebulizers
  h Use of expiratory retard or PEEP

6 The accuracy of a gas volume reading to reflect the patient's exhaled volume will depend on the location of the spirometer in the breathing circuit. Ideally, a spirometer should be placed on the *expiratory side* of the breathing circuit and located as close as possible to the patient's airway connection. This is because the clinician is primarily interested in the exhaled gas volume that has entered and left the patient's lungs.

7 Fig. 23-38 shows two spirometers (*1* and *2*) located at different points on the expiratory side of the breathing circuit.
  a The location of one spirometer (*2*) is after the exhalation valve (*3*). This location is *not* desirable because the spirometer collects and measures *all the gas* contained in the ventilator system. This includes gas compressed within the ventilator tubing (*4*) and accessories such as the humidifier (*5*) during inspiration and the patient's exhaled volume (*6*).
  b The volume of gas compressed in the ventilator system is called *tubing compliance* or *compressed gas volume*. This gas has *not* passed into the patient's lungs and therefore has *not* contributed to the patient's ventilation. It is in essence a wasted gas volume. In Fig. 23-38 the compressed gas volume is equal to 90 ml.
  c Patients, especially infants with normally small tidal volumes, may be hypoventilated if this volume is measured by a spirometer (*2*) and used for the calculation of alveolar ventilation. For this reason the spirometer must be placed as close to the patient's

airway as possible *(1)*, so that it will record only the gas that leaves the patient's lungs *(6)*. In this example, the actual expired volume is 910 ml.

d If a spirometer is located after the exhalation valve *(3)*, corrections of the recorded volumes for gas compression, bellows drag, and temperature must be made. Bellows drag occurs as a result of the inertia of the bellows *(7)* to move from a fixed position and the resistance of the bellows to unfold and move against gravity.

8 The formula for correcting a tidal volume for gas compression is:

$$\text{Corrected V}_T = V_L - (P_S \times V_{CT})$$

where V_L = volume of gas leaving the lungs; P_S = system pressure; and V_{CT} = gas volume compression factor.

EXAMPLE: Compute the corrected tidal volume for a patient on a Bennett MA-1 ventilator receiving 1000 ml with a system pressure manometer reading 30 cm H_2O.

a NOTE: The Bennett MA-1 has a compression factor of 3 ml per cm/H_2O ventilator system pressure, using a nondisposable circuit.

b Calculate gas compression: $3 \times 30 = 90$ ml

c Complete equation:

$$V_T = 1000 \text{ ml} - 90 \text{ ml} = 910 \text{ ml corrected tidal volume}$$

9 To be completely accurate, a bellows also should be corrected for temperature changes because gas volume will increase or decrease as temperature of the gas rises or falls within the bellows. Clinically, this correction is not significant except when extremely small tidal volumes are used to ventilate the patient. Under these circumstances, a more sensitive type of spirometer should be used.

10 The volume of gas compressed within a ventilator will vary according to the ventilator. Fig. 23-39 is a gas compression nomogram that was developed using different ventilators in a laboratory.

a Using this nomogram to estimate the volume of gas compressed, the practitioner selects the system pressure indicated on the ventilator manometer along the vertical axis and lays a straight edge to horizontally cross the ventilator compression line. The amount of compressed gas volume is read by drawing a vertical line from the intersect of the straight edge to the volume line across the bottom of the graph.

b For example, the Emerson Post-Op ventilator has a gas compression volume of 125 ml at 30 cm H_2O cycling pressure. Most manufacturers provide gas compression figures with the ventilator.

11 Volume displacement (collection) spirometers are usually large and require permanent mounting to the ventilator. Because of their size and performance characteristics, these devices usually are not as accurate in recording exhaled volumes as are flow-activated spirometers.

a Examples of flow-activated spirometers include the *Wright Respirometer* and the *Boehringer turbine (rotary) counter spirometer*. These devices use a turbine or vane assembly that is rotated by exhaled tidal volume flow directed through the meter. The number of rotations are counted and shown on the meter as volume. Spirometers that incorporate rotating vanes or turbines to measure volume are also known as *turbinometers*.

b The accuracy of these devices is affected by:
- Maximum and minimum gas flows that are *not* within the design limits of the meter
- Location of the meter in the ventilator circuit
- Moisture content of the exhaled gas
- Contamination by environmental exposure to dust and by respiratory tract expectorates

12 Typical volume measuring devices include:

a Wright Peak Flow Meter. Measures single breath flow up to 1000 L/min.

b Wright Respirometer (a different device from *a*). Uses a spinning vane to measure flows that are recorded as volume. It is capable of measuring cumulative volumes up to a total of 100 L.

c Boehringer rotary counter spirometer. Uses a spinning turbine to measure flows that are recorded as volume. The advantage of this system over the Wright respirometer is that the counter is *not* exposed to the patient's gases, and the turbine, which is exposed, can be separated for sterilization. This system prevents cross-contamination and allows a turbine to remain with each patient. The intended volume-flow range is 2000 ml tidal volume in 1 sec expiratory time, up to a forced vital capacity in healthy adults.

d Dräger Volumeter. Larger than the Wright Respirometer and measures air flow in both directions. Cumulative gas volume to 5 L.

e Bennett respiratory ventilation meter. Similar to Dräger in that it responds to flow in both directions. Cumulative up to 5 L gas volume. Effectiveness is limited by moisture.

f Parkinson and Courin dry displacement gas meter. Larger than the devices already listed, but accuracy

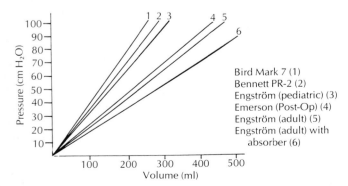

FIGURE 23-39 Gas compression nomogram for different ventilators.

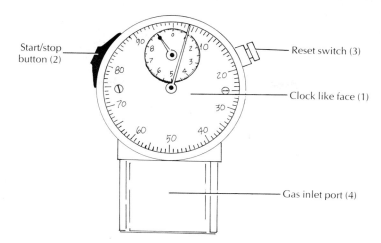

Start/stop button (2)

Reset switch (3)

Clock like face (1)

Gas inlet port (4)

FIGURE 23-40 Components of Wright Respirometer. (Modified from operating instructions, Wright Respirometer, Harris Calorific, Cleveland, Ohio.)

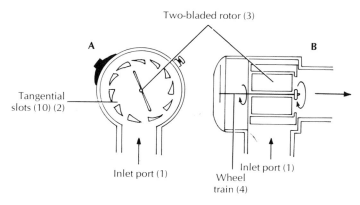

Two-bladed rotor (3)

A   B

Tangential slots (10) (2)

Inlet port (1)

Inlet port (1)
Wheel train (4)

FIGURE 23-41 Internal structures of Wright Respirometer. **A,** Frontal view. **B,** Side view. (Modified from operating instructions, Wright Respirometer, Harris Calorific, Cleveland, Ohio.)

and toughness have prompted their use in some ventilators (i.e., Emerson and Engström).

g Heated probe flowmeter. Reflects the rate of cooling of a heated probe by a passing gas stream. The change in temperature is reflected as increased current energy flow, which is proportional to a tidal volume change. Some tidal volume electrical monitoring devices use this method of relating gas flow to tidal volume.

13 Useful observations when using spirometers to measure exhaled volumes include the following.

  a Spirometers should be placed as close to the endotracheal tube as possible.

  b Exhaled tidal volume measures on the expiratory limb of the circuit should be considered only an estimate of what the patient actually received.

  c Spirometers should be routinely serviced and checked for accuracy.

  d Spirometers are potential agents for spreading infection and should be used with one-way valves and frequently decontaminated.

  e Possible situations causing the spirometer to fail or to show an erroneous reading should be noted.

12.2 The Wright Respirometer

1 The Wright Respirometer (Fig. 23-40) was invented by B. M. Wright, MD, of the Medical Research Council at the Pneumoconiosis Research Unit of Cardiff, England, to measure the respiratory volume of coal miners while at work underground. This device represents a broad class of spirometers known as *turbinometers*, which record gas volume through the measurement of gas flow.

2 Because of its small size and light weight, this unit is easily portable and may be carried by the practitioner to measure changing ventilatory volumes at the patient's bedside. It must be noted that because of its size and sensitive clocklike mechanism, this unit must *not* be dropped or bumped. Mistreatment of any type may result in a nonoperational unit or, even more *dangerous* to the patient, an inaccurate instrument.

3 Fig. 23-40 shows a view of the Wright Respirometer with the clocklike dial face *(1)*, a start-stop button *(2)*, a reset switch *(3)*, and the gas inlet port *(4)*.

4 Fig. 23-41 is a diagram of the Wright showing the various internal structures.

  a Gas is directed into the inlet port *(1)*, where it passes

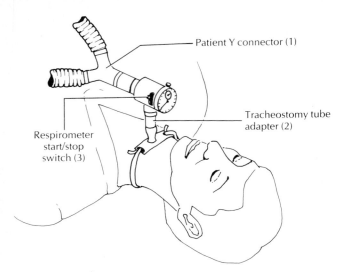

FIGURE 23-42 Wright Respirometer being used to measure exhaled volume of a ventilator patient with a tracheostomy. (Modified from operating instructions, Wright Respirometer, Harris Calorific, Cleveland, Ohio.)

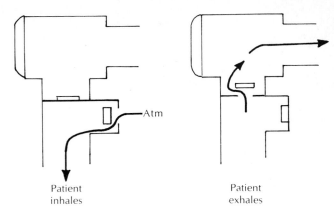

FIGURE 23-43 Wright Respirometer and one-way valve arrangement to measure exhaled volumes directly from patient. (Modified from operating instructions, Wright Respirometer, Harris Calorific, Cleveland, Ohio.)

through 10 tangential slots *(2)* in a cylindric ring and out the outlet port.

b Gas passing through the instrument causes a flat two-bladed rotor to spin *(3)*, which in turn drives a wheel train attached to the hands of the dial *(4)*.

c Movement of the hands around the dial of the meter indicates cumulative gas volumes that are actually a measure of gas flow through the instrument.

5 The Wright Respirometer is simple to operate and can be adapted to fit into most ventilator circuits. As with other monitoring devices, the Wright Respirometer should be placed on the expiratory side of the breathing circuit as close as possible to the patient.

6 Fig. 23-42 shows the Wright Respirometer being used to measure exhaled volumes in a circle system *(1)*.

a In this arrangement the Wright is turned OFF so that the inspiratory gases pass through the respirometer and enter the patient by way of a tracheostomy tube *(2)*.

b On exhalation, the Wright is switched ON *(3)*, and the volume is recorded by the hands moving around the dial.

c NOTE: The Wright Respirometer, used in this manner, is contaminated by the patient's exhaled gas and should *not* be used with another patient until it has been cleaned. It must not be left in the circuit because of possible damage from humidity.

7 When the Wright Respirometer is attached directly to the patient (not used with a ventilator), it is recommended that a low-resistance multifunction one-way valve be placed between the patient and the instrument to prevent possible cross-infection of the patient from use of the instrument on previous patients (Fig. 23-43).

8 Operational ranges and calculations for the Wright Respirometer are as follows:

a Flows

- Minimum 2 L/min
- Maximum 300 L/min

b Graduations on the small dial face
- 100 small-dial graduations
- Each small-dial graduation = 0.01 L

c Graduations on the large dial face
- 100 large-dial graduations
- Each large-dial graduation = 1 L

d Temperature maximum 140° C (284° F)

e Differential pressure between inside and outside = 6 cm Hg (1.2 PSI)

f Resistance to flow = 2 cm H_2O at 100 L/min

g Accuracy ± 2% at 6L/min flow

h NOTE: This instrument measures flow only in *one* direction and should not be exposed to flows, temperatures, or pressures beyond design limits.

9 Situations to avoid when using the Wright Respirometer include the followng.

a Do not reset the dials when the meter is ON. The vanes are very sensitive and are easily broken if they are reset in one direction while they are moving in the other.

b Do not expose the meter to peak flow rates in excess of design capabilities. This will warp the vanes and require expensive repair.

c Do not drop the unit or allow it to strike hard surfaces.

d Because of possible damage from humidity, do not leave the unit in a ventilator circuit.

e Do not submerge the unit in solutions while cleaning.

13.0 SOLVING MATHEMATICAL PROBLEMS RELATED TO CALCULATION OF PULMONARY COMPLIANCE
13.1 Calculation of dynamic compliance

1 The bedside measurement of compliance during mechanical ventilation allows the practitioner to estimate the stiffness of the lungs and chest to inflation. Because this measurement is obtained during air flow conditions, it is called *dynamic* or *effective* compliance (C_{dyn}).

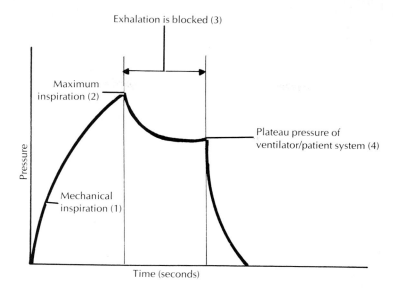

FIGURE 23-44 Graphic representation of a ventilator pressure pattern with an inflation hold.

2 Dynamic compliance is calculated by the following formula:

$$C_{dyn} = \frac{V_T \text{ (corrected)}}{PIP - PEEP}$$

where V_T corrected = (V_T − compressed gas volume); PIP (peak inspiratory pressure) = maximum pressure observed on the ventilator pressure manometer at the end of inspiration, and PEEP = positive end expiratory pressure.

3 EXAMPLE: Calculate dynamic compliance of a patient on a Bennett MA-1 ventilator that delivers a tidal volume of 800 ml with an indicated peak manometer pressure of 20 cm H_2O and zero PEEP.

a Correct the tidal volume for compressed gas volume. This value is provided by the manufacturers; in the MA-1, 3 ml/cm H_2O pressure is indicated. In this example, 20 × 3 = 60 ml. Subtract the compressed volume from the measured tidal volume.

$$800 \text{ ml} - 60 \text{ ml} = 740 \text{ ml (corrected)}$$

b Substitute in the formula:

$$C_{dyn} = \frac{740 \text{ ml}}{20} \text{ or } \frac{0.74 \text{ L}}{20} =$$

$$0.03 \text{ L/cm } H_2O \text{ or } 30 \text{ ml/cm } H_2O$$

c Compare compliance to normal; a normal *static* compliance for the total respiratory system is *0.1 L/cm H_2O*.

d A *decrease* in the dynamic compliance figure indicates an increase *in the stiffness* of the lungs/chest. This occurs in conditions causing increased airway resistance such as asthma and in resistant tissue such as pulmonary fibrosis.

e Clinically, serial measurements of dynamic compliance are useful indicators for detecting airway changes that increase impedance to air flow. Mucous plugs and linked ventilator tubing can both cause *de-*

creases in compliance. Sudden increases in compliance may indicate the presence of a tension pneumothorax, which would not be desirable and must be treated as a medical emergency.

13.2 Calculation of static compliance

1 Compliance measured under zero gas flow conditions at any lung volume is known as *static* compliance (C_{st}). In a clinical situation static compliance determinations can be made if the patient is on a ventilator that can be adjusted to deliver an *inflation hold* at the end of inspiration.

NOTE: Some authorities believe that static compliance, not dynamic compliance, is the best indicator of optimum PEEP.

2 The zero gas flow condition represents true alveolar pressure. This allows differentiation between that portion of the inspiratory pressure caused by airway resistance and lung compliance.

3 An inflation hold is created by the ventilator that results in closing the expiratory limb of the breathing tube for a brief time after inspiration has ended (inspiratory pause).

4 Fig. 23-44 graphically represents a ventilator pressure pattern with an inflation hold.

a No. *1* represents a mechanical inspiration that ends at maximum inspiration *(2)*. Exhalation is blocked for a brief pause *(3)*, which causes the pressure in the ventilatory system, the airway, and the alveoli to equalize.

b This equalization is represented by a decay of the peak pressure to a plateau level *(4)*.

c This pressure is read from the ventilator system manometer as the plateau pressure, and it is used in calculating static compliance. The difference between inflation pressure and plateau pressure represents the pressure difference caused by air-flow resistance of the patient and ventilator system.

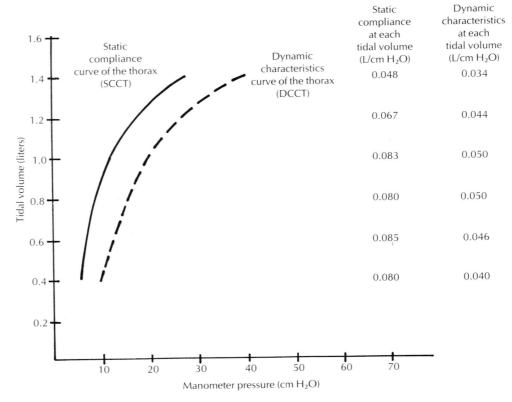

Static compliance at each tidal volume (L/cm H_2O)	Dynamic characteristics at each tidal volume (L/cm H_2O)
0.048	0.034
0.067	0.044
0.083	0.050
0.080	0.050
0.085	0.046
0.080	0.040

FIGURE 23-45 Static and dynamic compliance curves and values of the thorax.

5 The equation for calculating static compliance is:

$$C_{st} = \frac{V_T \text{ (corrected)}}{PC}$$

where PC = compliance caused by pressure.

6 Fig. 23-45 illustrates a static compliance curve of the thorax (SCCT).

a The continuous curve on the left represents an SCCT. The dashed curve on the right represents a dynamic characteristic curve of the thorax (DCCT). The static compliance of the thorax of each tidal volume is calculated by dividing the tidal volume by the "plateau" pressure at that tidal volume.

b A shift to the right of the SCCT occurs with lung disease that increases lung recoil. The dynamic characteristics of the thorax at each tidal volume is calculated as in no. 5 by dividing the exhaled tidal volume by the peak pressure at end inspiration. A shift to the right of the DCCT occurs with diseases associated with increased airway resistance such as bronchospasm or mucous plugging.

7 EXAMPLE: Calculate the static compliance of a patient on a Bennett MA-1 ventilator that delivers a tidal volume of 800 ml at an inspiratory pressure of 20 cm H_2O. The observed plateau pressure is 15 cm H_2O.

a Convert tidal volume of 800 ml to a corrected figure using a ventilator compliance factor that equals 3 ml/cm H_2O:

$$800 \text{ ml} - 60 \text{ ml} = 740 \text{ ml or } 0.74$$

b Substitute in the formula:

$$C_{st} = \frac{0.74 \text{ L}}{15 \text{ cm } H_2O} = 0.049 \text{ L/cm } H_2O \text{ or } 49 \text{ ml/cm } H_2O$$

c Compare compliance value to norm and to dynamic compliance.

Procedure 23-7 can be used to evaluate a patient's need for mechanical ventilation.

14.0 CONCEPTS FOR MEASURING GAS FLOW, GAS PRESSURE, FIO_2, AND PATIENT TEMPERATURE
14.1 Using pneumotachometers to measure flow

Gas flow can be measured electronically by a device known as a *pneumotachometer*. (See also Module 24, Unit 3.5.)

1 Pneumotachometers measure flows by using one of three principles. The *first* principle is based on a pressure drop across a resistance. A drop in pressure occurs whenever flow leaves a pressure source. This pressure drop is a linear function of flow and therefore can be measured by using a differential pressure transducer.

a Fig. 23-46 illustrates linear flow resistance meters or pneumotachometers using specially designed flow-resistive elements.

b The Silverman, Wittenberg, and Lilly pneumotachometers *(A)* use a fine wire mesh screen *(1)* as a resistance unit. Gas flow is introduced at one end of the hollow tubelike unit *(2)* and exists at the other

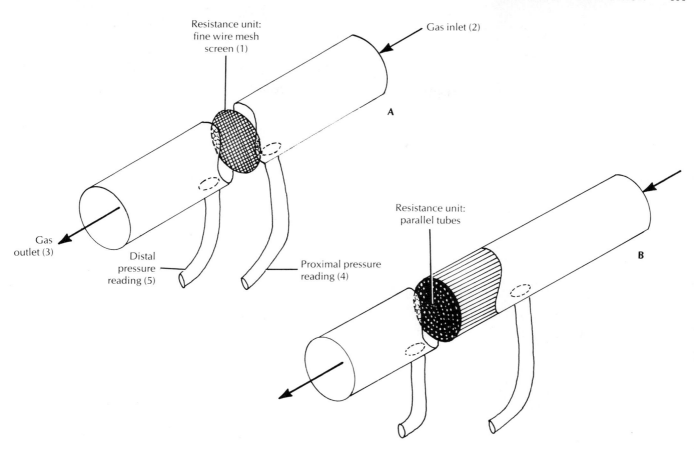

FIGURE 23-46 A, Silverman pneumotachometer. **B,** Fleisch pneumotachometer.

end *(3)*. As the gas reaches the proximal side of the screen, a pressure reading is taken *(4)*. A second reading is taken on the distal side of the screen *(5)*.

• The pressure drop that occurs as a result of the gas crossing the resistor is measured by the pressure transducer and reported as flow.

• The greatest problem with the screen-type unit is increased resistance because of humidity condensate. For this reason most units require a *heated* screen for continuous in-line flow measures.

c The Fleisch Pneumotach is a *second* type of pneumotachometer *(B)*. It uses the same principle of comparing pressure drop across a resistor for flow determination.

• The *difference* between these two types of units is that *type B* incorporates concentric tubes, parallel plates, or a large bundle of parallel tubes as a resistance unit.

• An initial pressure is monitored as the gas enters the round, tubelike pneumotachometer unit. After the gas has traveled the length of the unit, a second pressure reading is taken. The pressure difference is measured by a differential pressure transducer and reported as flow.

3 The BEAR flow transducer is a relatively new and *third* type of flow and volume monitor in which tidal volume delivery is determined by a *vortex* flow sensor that contains an ultrasonic transducer and a sensor.

a Vortices are waves that may be generated in a fluid stream. In the BEAR flow sensor, the vortices are caused by air tumbling over a strut or rod placed in the airstream. As the air passing over the strut moves down the flow tube, the air continues to vibrate from side to side inside the flow tube the way a flag waves in the wind.

b The faster the airstream flows past the strut, the faster the airstream vibrates in the tube. The tube-strut combination in the BEAR sensor is designed to generate one beat, or vortex, each time 1 ml of gas passes the strut.

c The waving motion of the airstream is detected by an ultrasonic beam. An electronically powered crystal transducer transmits an ultrasonic sound wave across the flow stream. The vibrating airstream intermittently changes the ultrasonic beam strength. A second crystal receives the ultrasonic beam and converts the variations or counts into an electronic signal directly proportional to flow. An electronic circuit processes the vortex-modulated signal and computes the tidal volume. The vortex concept is not substantially affected by gas stream composition, temperature, or humidity.

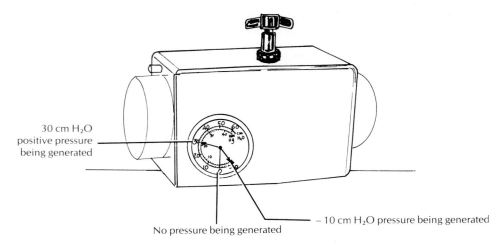

30 cm H_2O positive pressure being generated

No pressure being generated

− 10 cm H_2O pressure being generated

FIGURE 23-47 Pressure manometer on face of Bird Mark-7 ventilator.

14.2 Monitoring pressure (Fig. 23-47)

1 The pressure manometer located on the panel of a ventilator can be a valuable indicator of changes that may be occurring in a patient-ventilator breathing system, much the same as a speedometer indicates a car's forward movement. This manometer usually is calibrated in cm H_2O and mm Hg and shows positive (+) and negative (−) pressures being generated.

2 It is important to emphasize that this pressure does *not* necessarily reflect the patient's airway pressure (P_{aw}). This is so because of the pressure drop that occurs as gas passes through the numerous mechanical passages and anatomic structures on its way to the alveoli.

3 Alveolar distending pressure is ultimately determined by the source pressure generated by the ventilator, the characteristics of gas flow, the gas volume, and the length of time the pressure is held in the airway.

4 Thus the pressure recorded by the ventilator pressure manometer is a reflection of gas pressure in the ventilator and breathing circuit (i.e., system pressure), and not the lung units themselves. Except in cases of inspiratory hold, airway pressure is usually greater than alveolar pressure.

5 For this reason, in volume ventilators the *pressure manometer* can be used to reflect changes in airway impedance rather than as an absolute measure of airway pressure.

6 In volume ventilators the tidal volume, rate, and sometimes the flow are set by the operator. Once these variables are set, the pressure required to deliver the present volume will automatically vary to provide the pressure gradient necessary to deliver the preset tidal volume. Therefore changes in the pressure manometer are probably caused by airway changes.

7 For example, the manometer will show a pressure increase from an initial reading if water collects in the breathing tube, if mucus obstructs the trachea, if the tracheal tube becomes accidentally misplaced, or if the patient's compliance decreases, even though the volume remains approximately the same.

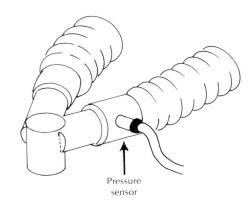

Pressure sensor

FIGURE 23-48 Desired location of a pressure sensor in the patient breathing circuit: close to the patient.

8 A general rule is that an *increasing system pressure* from a previous reading means increasing airway or breathing circuit impedance, providing the tidal volume, flow, and rate are not altered.

9 The manometer also reflects *decreased pressure readings* if a leak occurs in the system, if the patient has a tension pneumothorax (early stage), if a mucous plug moves from obstructing a major bronchus, or if compliance increases. In this example the tidal volume, flow, and rate remain the same but the system pressure decreases.

10 A negative deflection of the pressure manometer can be used to indicate the inspiratory effort exerted by the patient who is in the assist mode or receiving intermittent mandatory ventilation (IMV).

11 With elevated baseline pressure, the manometer is used to indicate PEEP or CPAP levels or plateau pressure for monitoring static compliance. A working manometer that does not return to zero at the end of exhalation indicates PEEP either prescribed or inadvertent. As previously noted, *inadvertent* PEEP indicates air trapping, which, if uncorrected, can cause cardiovascular complications and/or barotrauma.

12 The pressure manometer also shows the point at which pressure is released or vented from the system. This

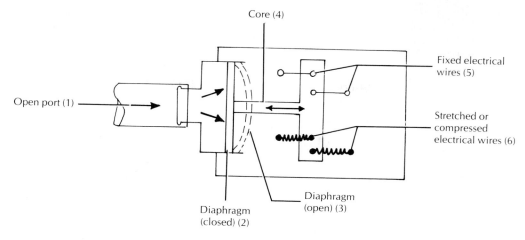

FIGURE 23-49 Strain gauge used to measure pressure.

situation occurs whenever the system pressure reaches the maximum safety pressure normally set at the factory, the maximum working pressure, or the pressure limit set by the operator.

13 The most accurate clinical reflection of airway pressure is to place a pressure-sensing probe as close as possible to the patient-ventilator airway connection.

14 Fig. 23-48 illustrates where a manufacturer has located a pressure sensor in the breathing circuit. An important consideration is that the pressure tap for attaching the transducer tube should be located *as close as possible* to the patient connection.

15 Pressure sensing probes usually are attached to devices called *bidirectional differential pressure transducers,* which are a part of a system consisting of an electronic amplifier and a meter or indicator. Pressure transducers measure strain or displacement of a sensor caused by internal force generated by gas pressure. Both types measure pressure.

16 A *strain gauge* consists of a single pressure-sensing element diaphragm enclosed in a hermetically sealed chamber (Fig. 23-49).

 a An open port *(1)* allows tubing to conduct the pressure to be measured to a diaphragm *(2).*

 b The diaphragm moves in response to the pressure in the test chamber *(3).*

 c As the diaphragm moves, it moves a core *(4)* that has one pair of electrical wires that are fixed *(5)* and another pair *(6)* that are stretched or compressed.

 d When a wire is stretched or compressed, it undergoes a change in resistance. These wires are carrying an electrical charge that is balanced by a wheatstone bridge circuit. (See Module Thirteen.)

 e The voltage charge that occurs across the bridge is proportional to the change in the wire resistance as the wires to the core are stretched or compressed. The unbalanced bridge reflects the voltage change on a strip recorder or oscilloscope as a pressure signal.

17 Other types of transducers are available depending on a particular need, such as measuring arterial blood pressure.

14.3 Monitoring fraction of inspired concentration of oxygen (FIo$_2$)* (See also Module 28, Critical Care Cardiorespiratory Monitoring.)

1 Most modern ventilators that are used for continuous ventilation incorporate monitors that keep track of the oxygen percentage of the inspired air (FIo$_2$) and initiate an alarm if a preset oxygen level is *not* maintained. These alarms usually incorporate *visual* and *audible* signals.

2 If a ventilator uses an oxygen analyzer–type monitor, the probe should be located on the *inspiratory side* of the patient's breathing circuit. Also, it should be located in the system so that the gas sample monitored reflects any *supplemental* oxygen that may be added to the main gas volume by small volume nebulizers or other devices that will be powered by oxygen (i.e., distal to the point where the supplemental oxygen is added).

3 In Fig. 23-50 the oxygen percentage of the main gas flow leaving the ventilator is 40% (FIo$_2$ 0.4) *(1).* At point 2 a side-arm nebulizer powered by 100% oxygen *(3)* is used to deliver an aerosolized medication to the main gas flow. This results in an increased oxygen percentage to the patient *(4)* when compared to the sample taken at the ventilator. Therefore the FIo$_2$ of patient gas equals the FIo$_2$ of the main gas flow plus any supplemental oxygen. The actual amount of oxygen increase depends on the flow rate and the percent of the oxygen added to the total volume.

4 When placing a remote oxygen sensor into the patient-ventilator breathing circuit, care must be taken not to allow a gas leak in the system. If the sensor is left in the circuit for continuous monitoring, it should be pro-

---

*For a review of details on the theory and operation of various oxygen monitors, see Module Thirteen.

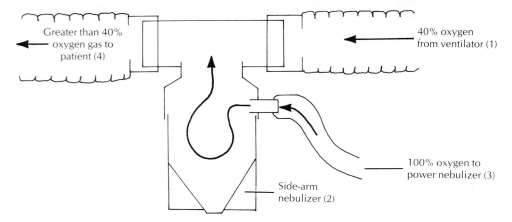

FIGURE 23-50 Enlarged view of nebulizer in patient breathing circuit. Supplemental oxygen is added to main gas source when nebulizer is powered by 100% oxygen.

tected against or not affected by elevated humidity levels.

5 Once an effective FI_{O_2} level has been established and confirmed by arterial blood gas sampling, routine FI_{O_2} readings should be taken and recorded on the patient-ventilator monitoring sheet according to departmental procedure.

6 NOTE: Although many ventilators use oxygen analysis–type monitors, some do *not*. In these units FI_{O_2} is calculated mechanically or pneumatically by the use of an air-oxygen mixer or blender (see Unit 18.1) and requires specific gas pressures (approximately 50 pSIG) to operate properly. What these ventilator oxygen monitors indicate is whether sufficient gas pressure is entering the system to allow the blender to operate properly. Analysis of the delivered gas of an external oxygen analyzer is very important to verify the operation of the ventilator's blender.

Procedure 23-8 can be used to monitor a patient receiving continuous mechanical ventiltion.

14.4 Measuring the temperature of patient gas

1 The introduction of heated humidity to ventilator circuits requires accurate determinations of gas temperature at the patient's airway. Heated gases above 37° C can cause tissue irritation and even severe airway burns unless the temperature is known and controlled. As in measuring airway pressure, the thermometer should be located in the inspiratory circuit as close as possible to the patient's airway.

2 A thermometer placed elsewhere in the circuit would *not* accurately reflect the temperature of the gas entering the airway. This is because of the changes in temperature resulting from environmental cooling of the gas as it passes through the tubing, changes in tidal volume and peak flow, and the influence of any supplemental or entrained gases.

3 Fig. 23-51 shows the location of a mechanical ther-

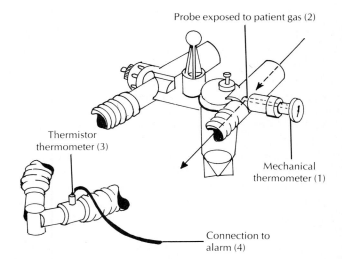

FIGURE 23-51 Location of a mechanical thermometer and thermistor temperature sensor in a Bennett ventilator breathing circuit. (Courtesy Puritan-Bennett Corp, Carlsbad, Calif.)

mometer and an electronic temperature sensor as they are used in a Bennett ventilator breathing circuit.

a A *mechanical* (bimetallic) thermometer *(1)* is placed in the inspiratory side of the breathing circuit. An adapter allows a temperature probe to be exposed to patient gas in the breathing circuit *(2)*.

b The bimetallic mechanical thermometer monitors temperature in response to the expansion and contraction of a metal filament exposed to changing airway temperatures. These devices normally are not very accurate for measuring air temperature. For this reason the accuracy of the thermometer should be confirmed by comparing it with a more accurate instrument.

c *Thermistor* (electronic) thermometers *(3)* are semiconductors made from metallic oxides. The resistance of the thermistor to the passage of an electrical current decreases as the temperature being monitored rises. This type of thermometer is usually very stable and accurate and has a very rapid response time. These characteristics make this thermometer useful for monitoring the temperature of respiratory gases. Several ventilator companies use thermistor-type thermometers combined with a meter to allow the operator to read the temperature using light-emitting diodes (LED) on the panel of the ventilator.

d These electronic sensors are usually connected to an audible and visual alarm *(4)* that activates when temperatures greater than preset are reached.

4 Some humidifiers can be preprogrammed so that the temperature of the ventilator gas at the patient's airway is monitored by a thermistor and is fed back by means of an electrical connection to cause the heater in the humidifier to cycle OFF and ON. This automatic cycling maintains a constant gas temperature to the patient. These humidifiers are said to be *servo-controlled* because a desired temperature at a distant point serves to operate (control) the heating element back at the humidifier.

5 Another type of thermometer that may be used is the *resistance-wire* thermometer. This device operates on the principle that the resistance of certain type wires increases as their temperature increases. This change in resistance is usually linked to a balanced wheatstone bridge-type circuit, which displays the imbalance caused by changing temperature as a temperature readout.

NOTE: The wires in these devices can become very hot and therefore should *not* be used in an explosive atmosphere.

14.5 Other monitoring considerations

1 Current technology has improved such devices as CO_2 analyzers to measure CO_2 concentration in exhaled volumes (PE_{CO_2}) and correlate this to arterial carbon dioxide tention (Pa_{CO_2}) levels. Transcutaneous arterial oxygen ($tcPa_{O_2}$) analyzers are available, permitting continuous monitoring (without repetitive arterial sticks) of oxygen levels in the patient.

2 In the well-perfused patient, tcP_{O_2} readings have correlated closely with direct in vivo Pa_{O_2} readings.

3 The development of more noninvasive devices for monitoring, as well as application of computers to continuously monitor the patient, is a probability. Computer technology will enable the monitoring of trends in the patient's condition, alerting the practitioner in time to make adjustments to prevent major problems. However, computers cannot replace the conscientious and competent practitioner.

15.0 VARIOUS FEATURES OF VOLUME VENTILATORS
15.1 Available options

1 Again, most volume ventilators are powered by one of four sources:
a Compressor

b Blower (turbine)
c Piston
d Compressed gas

2 The power sources serve to inflate the lungs directly (single-circuit system) or indirectly by emptying a bag or a bellows (double-circuit system).

3 Other than the noted differences in the methods of generating the tidal volume, most volume ventilators offer various combinations of operational features such as:
a Respiratory rate
b Inspiratory time
c I:E ratio
d Expiratory time
e Total cycle time
f Minute ventilation
g Continuous flow
h Inspiratory pressure
i Inspiratory pressure limit
j Inflation hold
k Oxygen concentration
l Tidal volume
m Continuous positive airway pressure (CPAP)
n Positive end expiratory pressure (PEEP)
o Expiratory resistance
p Expiratory retard
q Inspiratory flow
r Sigh
s Intermittent mandatory ventilation (IMV)
t Control-assist
u Assist
v Control
w Square wave
x Tapered wave
y Sine wave
z Humidity

4 All of these operational variables can be confusing to clinicians who are not familiar with a particular ventilator or do not frequently use it in different clinical situations.

5 Integration of the power source with time, flow, and other features causes the ventilator to perform in a certain way (i.e., as a constant pressure generator, constant flow generator, nonconstant flow [sine wave] generator).

6 This unit and subsequent units present *examples* of ventilators that are powered by one of four methods and incorporate various combinations of operational options.

16.0 CONTROLS OF THE BENNETT MA-1 VENTILATOR
16.1 Classification of the Bennett MA-1 ventilator

1 Classification. The Bennett MA-1 ventilator is an electrically powered, volume-cycled, double-circuit, constant-flow generator that can be operated as an *assistor,* a *controller,* or an *assist-controller.*

Even though this unit has been available since the early 1970s, it is still the ventilator of choice in many hospitals.

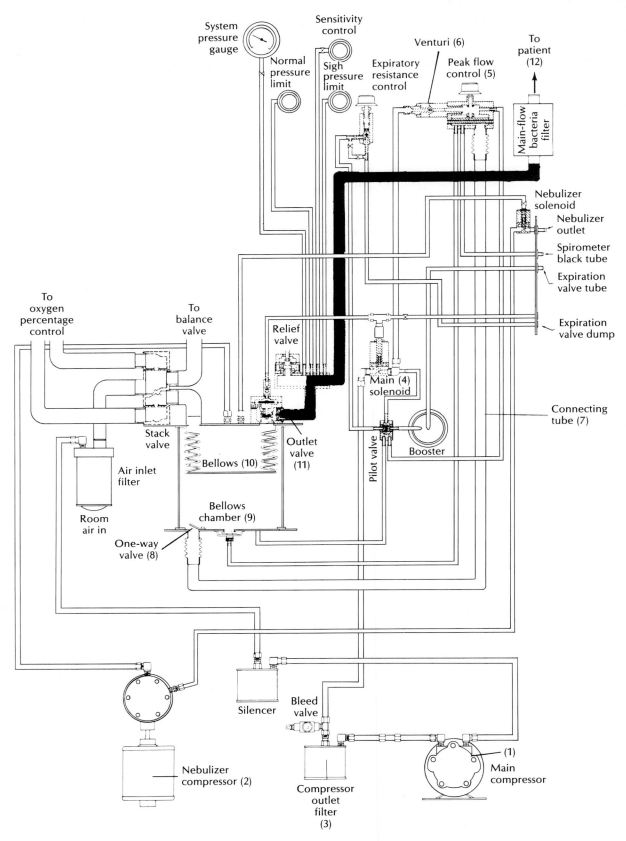

F I G U R E 2 3 - 5 2 Bennett MA-1 ventilator showing two electrical air compressors. (Modified from functional diagram for Bennett MA-1 ventilator. Courtesy Puritan-Bennett Corp, Carlsbad, Calif.)

a Special features that are available as options include PEEP, IMV, and a servo-controlled humidifier.

b The Bennett MA-1 ventilator also can be pressure-cycled, causing it to perform as a pressure-limited device.

c The following is an explanation of the Bennett MA-1 ventilator classification terminology.

NOTE: The principles detailed in this explanation *can be applied to other ventilators* that have similar structural and performance characteristics.

2 Electrically powered

a The Bennett MA-1 ventilator has two air compressors that are powered by electricity (Fig. 23-52).

b The main compressor is a Bell and Gossett 0.5 HP, 115-volt, AC, 60 cycle, single phase, rotary motor, which is capable of delivering a maximum tidal volume of 2200 ml at a peak flow of 100 L/min.

c The second compressor is much smaller and is used to generate a gas flow of 6 to 8 L/min to operate a small volume nebulizer located at the breathing manifold.

d The ventilator also has an oxygen inlet with a high-pressure hose attached to the rear panel (Fig. 23-53, *1*). This hose is connected directly to a 50-PSI oxygen source by means of an adapter if an FIO_2 greater than room air is desired.

e NOTE: The ventilator will *not* operate unless the electrical cord on the rear panel *(2)* is plugged into a 115-volt, AC, 60-cycle outlet and the OFF-ON switch is activated, even though oxygen may be flowing through the high-pressure hose.

3 Volume-cycled system

a The Bennett MA-1 ventilator is said to be a volume-cycled ventilator because a desired tidal volume can be preset by rotating the *normal volume control* on the front panel of the ventilator.

b Tidal volume is adjusted in 100 ml increments to a maximum of 2200 ml.

c When the ventilator is operational, inspiratory pressure will increase automatically to provide power necessary to deliver the preset tidal volume, provided a pressure limit is *not* reached.

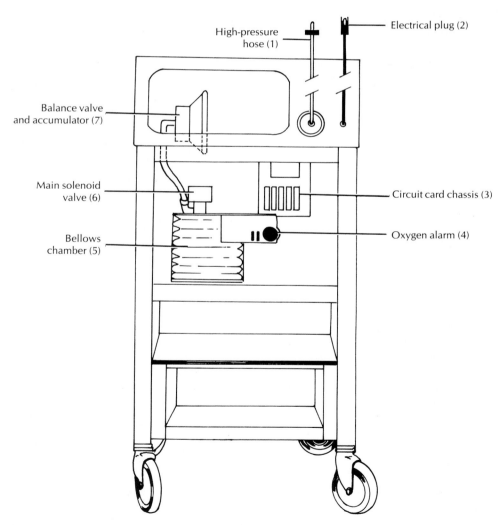

FIGURE 23-53 Internal components of Bennett MA-1 ventilator as seen from back after removal of back panel. (Courtesy Puritan-Bennett Corp, Carlsbad, Calif.)

d If a *pressure limit* ("pop-off" pressure) is reached, the inspiratory pressure will be vented to the outside, even though the desired tidal volume may not have been achieved.

e At this point, the ventilator does *not* function as a volume-cycled ventilator but as a pressure-cycled device.

f A "pop-off" pressure limit can be established by adjusting the *normal pressure limit control* on the face of the ventilator panel.

g CAUTION: If this pressure limit is set too low, the ability of the ventilator to function as a volume-cycled device may be severely restricted, since airway impedance increases and the patient may *not* receive a desired tidal volume.

4 Double-circuit system

a The Bennett MA-1 ventilator incorporates *two independent gas* systems, which interact with each other to generate the patient's tidal volume.

b In Fig. 23-52, gas flow (inspiratory phase) generated by the *main compressor (1)* passes through an *outlet filter (3)* and proceeds upward through a *main solenoid (4)* to the peak flow control *(5)*.

c As gas enters the peak flow control assembly, it is directed through a Venturi *(6)*. At this point, entrainment of room air is used as necessary to supplement (increase) the gas flow rate from approximately 30 L/min before the Venturi to as much as 100 L/min after air entrainment. The exact flow rate is adjusted from a minimum to 100 L/min by adjusting the *peak flow control* on the panel of the ventilator.

d The adjusted peak flow proceeds down a connecting tube *(7)* to open a one-way valve *(8)* and enter the bottom of the bellows chamber *(9)*.

e At this point, the positive pressure created in the chamber forces the bellows *(10)* upward, causing its gas contents (the preset tidal volume) to pass through an outlet valve *(11)* and enter a main tube that carries the tidal volume (dark line) to the patient *(12)*.

To reiterate, the Bennett-MA-1 ventilator is a double-circuit system, because one system conducts gas from the compressor to the bellows and the second system conducts patient gas from inside the bellows to the patient.

NOTE: Although unlikely, if a hole were to occur in the bellows *(10)*, the ventilator would function as a single-circuit device with gas moving directly from the compressor through the hole to the patient's lungs. This is not desirable and could cause excessive airway pressure and inaccurate FIO_2.

5 Constant-flow generator

a The Bennett MA-1 ventilator performs as a constant-flow generator at system pressures less than 40 cm H_2O gauge.

b Because of the low internal driving force of the bellows, the gas flow decreases as impedance to gas flow increases. This causes the characteristic square flow wave of a constant flow generator to taper like

that of a constant pressure generator. (See Unit 5.2.)

c When the ventilator begins to function like a constant pressure ventilator, preset volumes may *not* be delivered.

d If this situation develops, either the impedance to flow must be reduced or the ventilator should be changed to one that generates more power.

e The Bennett MA-1 ventilator flow rate is set by the operator by adjusting the *peak flow control*.

6 Assistor functions

a The Bennett MA-1 ventilator will trigger ON in response to a patient's spontaneous inspiratory efforts, provided the solenoid valve is set to be sensitive enough to detect the decrease in system pressure caused by spontaneous breathing.

b The ability of the ventilator to detect a patient's spontaneous inspiratory efforts is called *sensitivity*. The degree of sensitivity can be set by adjusting the *sensitivity control* on the panel of the ventilator.

c The more sensitive a ventilator is, the faster it will detect and respond to spontaneous breathing.

d NOTE: If the ventilator is made *too* sensitive, it will self-cycle. This uncontrolled cycling, referred to as "chattering," is not desirable in that it can lead to ineffective ventilation and hypoventilation of the patient.

7 Controller functions

a The Bennett MA-1 will automatically cycle to ventilate the apneic patient at rates adjustable from *6* to *60* times per minute.

b Rates are set by adjusting the "rate in cycles per minute" control on the panel of the ventilator.

c A special rate card is provided by the manufacturer to modify the ventilator for IMV rates of less than 6/min (if it was not already set up to do so).

8 Assist-control mode

a The Bennett MA-1 can be set to function as an assistor-controller by adjusting the *rate control* to cycle the ventilator at a preset frequency.

b This automatic cycling rate will occur should the patient fail to breathe at a rate equal to or greater than the preset cycling minimum.

16.2 Identification of the parts of a Bennett MA-1 ventilator*

1 The major components of the Bennett MA-1 (Fig. 23-54) are the *cabinet,* consisting of a control panel *(1)* covered with a lid (not shown), a storage compartment accessed by a swing-down door on the front of the ventilator (not shown), a humidifier *(2),* and a spirometer *(3)* mounted on the left side of the ventilator, with a breathing circuit for connecting the ventilator to the patient *(4)*.

A high-pressure hose for attachment to a supplemen-

---

*If possible, it is recommended that the reader have an assembled Bennett MA-1 ventilator with a rubber test lung, the manufacturer's instruction manual, and the departmental procedures manual available for reference before beginning this unit.

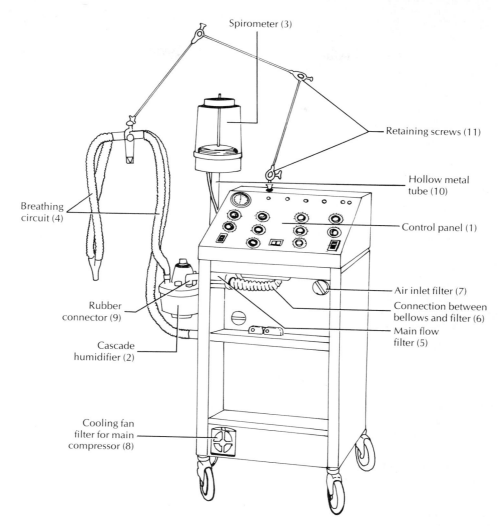

Spirometer (3)

Retaining screws (11)

Breathing circuit (4)

Hollow metal tube (10)

Control panel (1)

Rubber connector (9)

Air inlet filter (7)

Connection between bellows and filter (6)

Main flow filter (5)

Cascade humidifier (2)

Cooling fan filter for main compressor (8)

FIGURE 23-54 Major components of the Bennett MA-1 ventilator. (Courtesy Puritan-Bennett Corp, Carlsbad, Calif.)

tal oxygen source and an electrical power cord are located on the rear of the cabinet.

The operator proceeds as follows.

a Attach the rubber test lung to the patient Y adapter.

b Uncoil the power cord from the rear of the ventilator and insert it into a 115-volt, 60-cycle outlet.

c Before operating the MA-1, locate the following assemblies. Open the front cabinet door and identify:
  • Main flow filter inside of front cabinet *(5)*
  • Corrugated tubing connecting gas from the bellows to the main flow filter *(6)*
  • Air inlet fiber *(7)*
  • Cooling fan filter for main compressor *(8)*.

d On the left side of the cabinet, locate the rubber-angled connector leading from the machine outlet to the inlet port of the cascade humidifier *(9)*. This tube conducts gas from the main flow filter into the cascade.

e Trace the inspiratory limb of the patient's breathing circuit, which carries gas from the outlet port of the cascade humidifier to the inlet side of the patient manifold.

f Follow the white small-bore nebulizer tubing (not shown) from the white connector on the top of the nebulizer to the white connector on the side of the ventilator cabinet. Note the small nebulizer bacteria filter that is inserted in-line in front of the nebulizer inlet. This tube conducts gas from the nebulizer compressor to the nebulizer only if the nebulizer is turned on.

g Trace the large collector tube from the expiratory side of the manifold outlet to the inlet pole of the water trap adapter.

This tube conducts exhaled gas to the spirometer by way of the large chrome hollow tube *(10)* that connects the exit port of the water trap adapter to the bottom of the spirometer.

h Follow the small bore black tube leading from the bottom of the spirometer base (not shown) to the spirometer port located on the left side of the ventilator cabinet. This tube conducts air from the ventilator during inspiration to open the poppet valve in the spirometer, allowing the bellows to empty and descend.

i Adjust the supporting arms by loosening the black retaining screws *(11)*, and position the patient manifold so that it can be easily reached.

j Note the two flex tubing-type breathing tubes that connect from the patient Y adapter to the inspiratory and expiratory ports of the patient manifold. These tubes form the distal parts of the patient's breathing circuit and connect the patient by means of a Y adapter to the ventilator.

k Trace the small bore tube leading from the exhalation valve to the chrome fitting marked "exhalation valve" on the side of the cabinet (not shown). This tube conducts air from the ventilator during inspiration to seal the exhalation valve so that a positive pressure can be generated in the system. During exhalation, this tube allows gas in the valve to travel back to the machine and vent, causing the exhalation valve to deflate. This allows the patient to exhale.

2 If the back panel of the MA-1 chassis is removed (see Fig. 23-53), the internal workings can be studied. It is helpful to understand the placement and use of the following:

a Circuit card chassis *(3)*. Holds several printed circuit cards that are responsible for various preprogrammed functions and controls.

b Oxygen alarm *(4)*. A monitor to detect reduced operating pressure from a 50-PSIG source or the lack of it.

c Bellows chamber assembly *(5)*. The main compression source of the double-circuit system.

d Main solenoid valve *(6)*. Controls excursion of the bellows that regulates volume delivered to the patient.

e Balance valve and accumulator *(7)*. Accumulates oxygen and delivers to the air-mixing valve.
CAUTION: Disconnect the ventilator from any electrical source before removing the back panel.

16.3 Identification and function of the controls of a Bennett MA-1 ventilator

1 The control panel of the MA-1 ventilator is conveniently arranged into a left and right grouping of controls.

2 The controls comprising the left-hand grouping, with the exception of the oxygen percentage controls, are those that are used for general operation of the ventilator. The right-hand control grouping consists of special function controls.

3 If a ventilator is available before studying the function of each control, prepare the ventilator for operation by following these steps.

a Attach a complete breathing circuit.

b Attach a test lung to the patient Y adapter.

c Plug the black power cord located on the rear panel of the ventilator into a 115-volt, 60-cycle circuit.

d Depress the power switch located in the left-hand corner of the control panel to ON.

4 If a ventilator is not available, refer to the Bennett MA-1 control panel (Fig. 23-55) for study.

A *Basic controls*

1 The *pressure manometer* and light indicators are horizontally arranged in a row across the top of the panel. These are used to monitor the patient and the ventilator functions.

2 The *sensitivity control* is used to adjust the ventilator to respond to the patient's spontaneous breathing attempts. The range of inspiratory effort required to trigger the machine ON can be adjusted from -10 cm H_2O gauge to -0.1 cm H_2O gauge pressure and to an oversensitive (self-cycling) level. The greater the sensitivity, the easier it is for a spontaneously breathing patient to trigger the ventilator ON.

3 The *peak flow control* establishes the maximum flow (liters per minute) to the patient during inspiration. This control is adjustable from 15 to 100 L/min. Adjustment of this control combined with the cycling frequency establishes the *length* of the inspiratory phase and the I:E ratio for a given tidal volume. A normal peak flow range for most adults, using a 12 to 15 ml/kg tidal volume and an I:E ratio of 1:2 or less, is 40 to 50 L/min.

4 The *power switch* turns the electrical functions of the machine OFF and ON. This is the master switch that must be activated before the ventilator will perform any electrical function.

5 The *normal pressure limit control* allows the operator to set maximum inspiratory pressure limits from 20 to 60 cm H_2O as monitored by the system pressure manometer. Maximum pressure limits are critical in determining the ventilator's ability to deliver a predetermined tidal volume under conditions of increasing airway impedances.

a NOTE: When the normal pressure limit is reached, the ventilator will vent its system pressure to the atmosphere. This action ends the inspiratory cycle *regardless of whether or not a desired preset tidal volume was delivered* by the ventilator. At this point the ventilator may or may not be functioning as a volume ventilator depending on whether the preset volume was delivered before the normal pressure limit is met.

b The normal pressure limit control should be set approximately *10 cm H_2O pressure greater than the system pressure* required to deliver the desired tidal volume or at a level to prevent pressure trauma to patients with known lung structural weakness such as blebs.

c A ventilator *that is venting* because operation within the normal pressure limit may indicate:
- The pressure limit initial setup is set too low for the desired tidal volume.
- Increases in system and/or airway impedances. This includes increases in resistance resulting from a kinked breathing circuit, mucus in the tracheal tube, bronchospasm, or decreases in pulmonary compliance.

d For these reasons, the system pressure manometer and the normal pressure limit can be clinically useful for

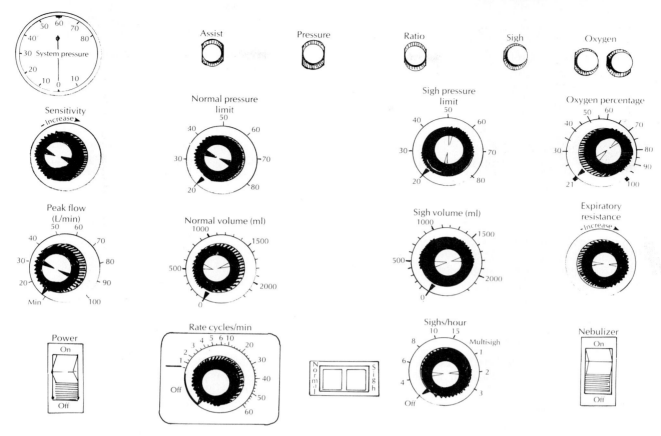

FIGURE 23-55 Bennett MA-1 control panel. (Modified from Bennett MA-1 control panel. (Courtesy Puritan-Bennett Corp, Carlsbad, Calif.)

monitoring *changes* in the ventilator-patient systems.

6 *Normal volume.* The normal volume control allows the operator to set a desired tidal volume (in milliliters) to be delivered by the ventilator. This volume is calibrated between 0 and 2200 ml and is reflected on a spirometer if the spirometer is located distal to the exhalation valve. It is important that the operator realizes that the tidal volume delivered by the ventilator and measured by the spirometer is *not* the volume that participates in alveolar ventilation. The alveolar volume is less than the delivered volume because of gas compression in various ventilator tubes and accessories such as the humidifier (ventilator dead space and tubing compliance).

7 *Rate—cycles per minute.* The frequency control establishes the number of respirations per minute when the ventilator is operated in the control or assist-control mode.

a If the ventilator is operated as a pure assistor, the rate control should be OFF. Frequency is calibrated between 6 and 60 cycles per minute in the standard MA-1 model. Frequencies less than 6 cycles/min for IMV can be obtained by changing the rate card, although most new models already have this modification.

NOTE: As a safety function, in clinical use it may be desirable to set a control rate at a value less than the spontaneous breathing rate.

b When establishing the cycling frequency, the practitioner must consider norms from a particular age-group, and desired I:E ratio, the tidal volume, and the peak flow. All of these must be adjusted to accommodate a particular cycling frequency, since time of inspiration and exhalation constitutes a single cycling frequency. Clinically, a respiratory rate is established for a 1-minute time frame.

8 *Sigh pressure limit.* This is the first control that constitutes the special function controls of the ventilator (right side of the control board). The sigh pressure limit functions the same way as the normal pressure limit control except that it controls the maximum system pressure delivered during a sigh breath.

a The sigh function is an artificial way of providing periodic lung hyperinflations larger than that of a normal tidal volume. It is theoretically used to prevent patchy microatelectasis that may occur with constant volume ventilation.

NOTE: The effectiveness of routine "sighing" is considered controversial by many physicians and it is included as a function control on most ventilators today.

b The sigh pressure limit is adjustable between 20 and 80 cm H_2O pressure. It is normally set at 5 to 10 cm H_2O higher than the normal pressure limit. It is believed that artificial sighs may not be indicated if an initial tidal volume is established on the basis of 12 to 15 ml/kg of the patient's body weight.

9 *Sigh volume.* This control sets the volume of gas that is to be delivered (in milliliters) during the artificial sigh up to a maximum of 2000 ml. This volume is normally set at twice the normal tidal volume being delivered to the patient; however, all special functions of the ventilator should be prescribed by the physician.

10 *Sighs per hour.* This control regulates the number of sighs that are to be delivered per hour. It can be adjusted to deliver 2 to 15 sighs/hour. This means that at 2 sighs/hour the ventilator will deliver one sigh every 30 minutes and, at 15 sighs/hour, one sigh every 4 minutes. A normal range is one sigh every 15 minutes.

a In addition, a function lever located on the control will allow the operator to program the ventilator to deliver 1, 2, or 3 sighs sequentially.

b For example, if the control were set to deliver 4 sighs/hour and the function lever were set on 2, the patient would receive 2 sighs in sequence every 15 minutes.

11 *Oxygen percentage.* This control establishes the oxygen percentage of the patient's inspired air (FIo_2). It is calibrated and can be set between the range of 21% and 100% oxygen.

a It is important for the operator to be aware that on the MA-1 oxygen-air mixing occurs as the result of a Venturi that entrains oxygen from an accumulator (reservoir). This oxygen mixes with air that is pulled into the bellows during its descent following an inspiration (ascent). If the control is set at 100% oxygen, no room air is entrained, and a bellows fills with gas drawn entirely from the accumulator.

b Air-oxygen mixing is based on a *proportion theory,* which is used with air-oxygen blenders. The critical consideration is that the oxygen accumulator must be connected to an oxygen source by means of the high-pressure hose and not some other gas such as compressed air.

c NOTE: If such a mistake were to occur, the oxygen alarm would *not* be activated because it monitors physical pressure (cm H_2O) by the gas in the accumulator. It does *not* test the air in the accumulator for the actual presence or absence of oxygen molecules (i.e., a patient could be receiving compressed air even though the oxygen control is set at 100%).

12 *Expiratory resistance.* This control is used to *retard* exhalation by holding the exhalation valve inflated (closed) at the end of a mechanical inspiration. If the control is adjusted to "full increase," the exhalation valve will momentarily completely block exhalation. This technique is used to create an inspiratory plateau for measuring static compliance.

a Partial adjustment of the control only partially holds the expiratory valve closed, resulting in expiratory retard. The effects of expiratory resistance can be observed on the system pressure manometer by noting a delayed return of the indicator to zero at the end of inspiration.

b NOTE: When using expiratory retard the cycling frequency must be adjusted to allow the patient a *complete exhalation* (i.e., the pressure indicator returns to zero before beginning a subsequent inspiration). Failure to allow adequate time for a complete exhalation will result in the creation of an inadvertent PEEP condition.

13 *Nebulizer control.* The nebulizer OFF and ON switch controls the small compressor used to provide gas at 8 to 10 PSI to power a small volume medication nebulizer located at the breathing manifold. When this compressor is ON, gas is pulled from the bellows volume by the compressor to power the nebulizer. This approach is clinically important, because no additional gas volume is added to the preset tidal volume by the nebulizer flow.

14 *Manual switch.* Two push-button controls allow the operator to manually initiate a normal or a sigh mechanical breath. This control is used to cycle the ventilator during a check before putting the ventilator on a patient and in clinical situations where manual control of the patient is desired. Depressing this control will *override* any previous frequency control setting as long as the button is pushed. Care must be taken when manually cycling the ventilator to allow time for a complete exhalation before manually starting another inspiration.

■ ■ ■

The following performance checks are presented as examples of how the various controls on the Bennett MA-1 ventilator should perform when tested under specified conditions.

To actually perform these checks the reader will need to have an MA-1 ventilator available.

If a ventilator is *not* available, the following information will be useful as an overview of how each control generally effects operation of the ventilator in test and clinical situations.

B *Sensitivity control orientation and performance check*

1 If a ventilator is available, it should be adjusted in the following manner.

a Lift the lid covering the control panel on the front of the ventilator.

b Turn power switch ON.

c Set peak flow to 40 cm H_2O.

d Set normal volume to 500 cm H_2O.

e Set normal and sigh pressure limits to 80 cm H_2O.

f Set sensitivity to full left (OFF).

g Set rate to OFF.

2 Operate the sensitivity control.

a Rotate knob full right until unit self-cycles (chatters); this is too sensitive and is not used clinically.

b Note that the amber assist light at top left of the control panel flashes with each cycle.

c Rotate the knob *full left* (unit should cycle OFF).

d Grasp the rubber test lung in one hand.

e Squeeze and release the test lung until -20 cm H_2O pressure is indicated on the system pressure manometer located on the panel.

f The ventilator should *not* cycle ON at this point, indicating an assist "lockout." This is used to prevent a patient from assisting during mechanical ventilation.

g Rotate the knob three quarters turn from a full OFF position.

h Squeeze and release the test lung.

i Note that at least -9 cm H_2O pressure should be generated before the unit triggers ON.

j Also note that the assist light illustrates and remains ON for approximately half a second.

k Continue to rotate the knob in one-half turn increments, creating negative pressure by squeezing and releasing the test lung at each step.

l The subambient pressure required to trigger the unit ON, according to the manometer, should be lower after each rotation.

m Continue this adjustment activity until approximately -0.25 cm H_2O is required to trigger the ventilator ON. This is the *maximum* sensitivity level that can be set before the ventilator self-cycles.

n Rotate the knob counterclockwise until it is once again in the OFF position.

o Remove the test lung and occlude the opening on the patient Y with your hand.

p Continue to block the Y with your hand, and adjust sensitivity until the ventilator self-cycles.

q Now rotate the sensitivity control until the ventilator cycles OFF and remains off.

This method can be used to quickly adjust the maximum sensitivity limit for a patient with a weakened inspiratory force for whom assisted ventilation is prescribed.

If this method is used in a "real patient" situation, to prevent contamination of the patient Y adapter, use a sterile object such as the inside of a sterile wrapper (instead of your hand) to block the Y.

C *Peak flow control orientation and performance check*

1 If a ventilator is available:

a Turn power switch ON.

b Set normal volume at 2200 L/min.

c Clamp the black small bore tubing on base of spirometer.

d Remove test lung and connect a Wright Respirometer to the patient outlet side of the Y adapter.

e Set rate OFF.

f Turn nebulizer switch OFF.

2 To operate the peak flow control:

a Adjust peak flow control to each of the following values and manually cycle the unit:

Control set	Flow
Minimum	14 to 17 L/min (Wright)
20	18 to 22 L/min
40	36 to 44 L/min
50	45 to 54 L/min
70	63 to 75 L/min
100	91 to 107 L/min

b Note that peak flow limits increase as the control is rotated clockwise.

c Remove Wright Respirometer, and attach a test lung unit to the patient's Y piece.

d Set the peak flow control to minimum, and manually cycle the ventilator.

e Time the length of inspiration.

f Set the peak flow control to 40 L/min, and manually cycle the unit.

g Time the length of inspiration.

h Set the peak flow control to 100 L/min, and manually cycle the unit.

i Time the length of inspiration.

j Note that the length of inspiration decreases as the peak flow is incrementally increased.

k Leave peak flow control set at 100 L/min, and reduce normal volume control to 1100 ml.

l Unclamp small black tube on base of spirometer.

m Cycle the unit manually.

n Time the length of inspiration.

o Observe that the length of inspiration can be controlled by altering peak flow and/or desired volume.

p Leave normal volume control at 1100 ml.

q Set peak flow control to 20 cm H_2O.

r Set rate to 30 cycles per minute.

s Note tidal volume recorded by the spirometer.

t Time the length of inspiration to length of expiration (determine I:E ratio).

u Observe that the length of inspiration can be controlled by the relationship between the:
- Peak flow rate
- Desired tidal volume
- Cycling frequency

v Also observe that if the ratio warning indicator flashes, the I:E ratio is in fact less than 1:1.

w Gradually increase the peak flow rate until the ratio light remains OFF, indicating an I:E ratio of at least 1:1.

x Practice adjusting flow rate, volume, and cycling frequency until you understand the relationship that exists between the three variables in establishing the I:E ratio.

D *Normal pressure limit control orientation, and performance check*

1 If a ventilator is available:

a Turn power switch ON.

b Set normal volume at 2200 ml.

c Set sigh volume at 2200 ml.

d Set peak flow at minimum setting.

e Turn nebulizer switch OFF.

f Turn rate control OFF.

2 To operate the normal pressure limit control:

a Set normal pressure limit at 20 cm H_2O.

b Block patient outlet Y adapter.

c Cycle the unit manually, and note pressure reading on system pressure manometer.
- System pressure reading should correspond to preset pressure limit ± 3 cm H_2O.

d Increase the normal pressure limit incrementally to 80 cm H_2O, and note system pressure manometer for corresponding readings.

e Observe that the pressure indicator light flashes and an audible signal is sounded each time the pressure limit is reached.

f Attach a test lung to the patient outlet port of the Y adapter.

g Set the normal volume at 1000 ml.

h Set the peak flow at 40 L/min.

i Record the volume indicated on the spirometer.

j Change normal pressure limit from 80 to 20 cm H_2O.

k Record exhaled volume on spirometer.

l Note system pressure manometer reading.

m Observe that the pressure warning light flashes ON and the audible alarm sounds, indicating that the preset pressure is being reached and vented.

n Slowly increase the normal pressure limit control until the alarms cease.

o Record volume measured by the spirometer. This is the airway pressure required to deliver the preset volume at a preset flow rate.

p Partially obstruct the test lung, and observe the alarms and loss of volume recorded by the spirometer.

q Increase the normal pressure limit by 10 cm H_2O, and observe airway pressure and alarm function.

r Set normal pressure limit to 30 cm H_2O.

s Reduce normal volume until alarms are no longer activated.

t This is the maximum volume that can be delivered by the ventilator, given this pressure limit restraint. At this point, the MA-1 ceases to function as a volume-cycled device and becomes a pressure-cycled device.

u Systematically change volume, flow rate, and normal pressure limit, and measure the effect on exhaled volume until you are familiar with the interaction that occurs between adjustment of these controls and the patient's tidal volume.

v Remember that the pressure control can be used to warn the operator of increases in a patient's airway impedance because of secretions, decreases in compliance, kinked tubes, etc.

w NOTE: Many ventilators incorporate a gas compression factor that should be subtracted from the measured tidal volume to correct for ventilator dead space. To more accurately measure a patient's alveolar volume, the operator should place the spirometer as close as possible to the patient's airway.

x CAUTION: The preset tidal volume may *not* be delivered if:
- The normal pressure limit is reached and the system pressure is vented.
- Airway pressure exceeds 40 cm H_2O because of lung impedances. At this level the ventilator will begin to function as a constant pressure generator rather than a constant flow generator.
- A leak occurs in the patient and/or ventilator system.
- A blockage occurs in the patient and/or ventilator system.

E *Normal volume control orientation and performance check*

1 If a ventilator is available:
a Turn power switch ON.
b Attach a test lung to patient Y adapter.

2 To operate the normal volume control:
a The volume control is electrically powered by the no. 3 circuit card and a bellows potentiometer.
b Set normal volume at 200 ml.
c Set peak flow at 20 L/min.
d Set normal pressure limit at 80 cm H_2O.
e Cycle the unit manually, and note a spirometer reading of 250 ml (± 10).
f Observe system pressure on pressure manometer.
g Set normal volume at 500 ml.
h Set peak flow at 40 cm H_2O.
i Cycle the ventilator manually.
j Time the length of inspiration.
k Check spirometer reading for 545 ml.
l Observe system pressure on pressure manometer.
m Set normal volume at 2000 ml.
n Set peak flow at 90.
o Manually cycle the unit.
p Time the length of inspiration.
q Check spirometer reading for 1955 to 2105 ml.
r Observe system pressure on pressure manometer.
s Note the relationship that exists between increasing volumes, increasing system pressure, flow rate, and inspiratory time.
t With the ventilator set as in *m* and *n,* manually twist the rubber test lung, simulting partial restriction.
u Cycle the unit manually and observe:
- Volume on the spirometer
- Length of inspiration
- System pressure

F *Rate in cycles per minute control orientation and performance check*

1 If a ventilator is available:
a Follow steps *1* and *2* outlined in the sensitivity exercise (see *B* on p. 710).
b Remove the test lung from the patient Y tube, leaving the patient outlet open to the room.

2 To operate the rate control, which is electrically powered by the no. 1 circuit card and a potentiometer:
a Set the peak flow control at 100 L/min.
b Set the normal volume control at 0.
c Set sensitivity control to OFF (counterclockwise).
d Set sighs per hour to OFF.
e Set rate control to 6 cycles/min.

3 Measure the time between cycles (approximately 10 sec).

4 Set the rate control at 60 cycles/min.

5 Measure the time between cycles; approximately 1 sec.

6 Set the rate control at 30, and measure the time between cycles (approximately 2 sec).

7 Set the rate control at 15, and measure the time between cycles (approximately 6 sec).

8 Attach the test lung to the open port of the patient Y adapter.

9 Set the normal volume at 800 ml.

10 Set the peak flow at 40 L/min.

11 Set the control at 12 cycles/min.

12 Note the expired tidal volume on the spirometer.

13 Increase the rate to 60 cycles/min.

14 Note the expired volume on the spirometer.

G *Sigh pressure limit control orientation and performance check*

1 If a ventilator is available:

  a Turn power switch ON.

  b Set normal volume at 1000 ml.

  c Set sigh volume at 2200 ml.

  d Set peak flow at minimum setting.

  e Turn nebulizer OFF.

  f Turn rate control OFF.

2 To operate the sigh pressure limit control:

  a Set normal pressure limit at 30.

  b Set sigh pressure at minimum.

  c Block the patient outlet port of Y adapter.

  d Cycle the sigh mechanism manually, and observe what happens by noting exhaled volume recorded on spirometer.

  e Attach a test lung to the patient Y adapter.

  f Increase the sigh pressure limit incrementally, cycle the unit, and observe system pressure readings and exhaled volumes.

  g Note that the sigh-pressure limit and normal-pressure limit both function to pressure-limit the ventilator.

H *Sigh volume control orientation and performance check*

This control operates in the same way as the normal volume control except that it establishes the inflation volume that will be delivered during a mechanical sigh.

I *Sighs per hour orientation and performance check*

1 If a ventilator is available:

  a Turn power switch ON.

  b Set normal volume at 100 ml.

  c Set peak flow at 40 cm H_2O.

  d Set normal pressure limit at 30 cm H_2O.

  e Set sigh volume at 1500 ml.

  f Set sigh pressure limit at 40 cm H_2O.

  g Set rate at 12 cycles/min.

2 To operate the sigh rate control:

  a Attach a test lung to the patient Y adapter.

  b Set the sighs per hour to 15.

  c A single sigh should occur in 4 min.

  d Note system pressure and exhaled volume.

  e Set multisigh lever to 3.

  f Wait 4 min, and observe ventilator function.

  g The ventilator should deliver three sequential sighs.

J *Oxygen percentage control orientation and performance check*

1 If a ventilator is available:

  a Remove the smoke-colored transparent view panel on the rear of the ventilator cabinet and the blue rear-cabinet panel.

  b Connect the high-pressure hose (see Fig. 23-53, *1*) to a 50 PSI oxygen source.

  c Identify the circuit card chassis and cards *(3)*. *Do not touch.*

  d Identify the oxygen alarm *(4)*.

  e Identify the bellows *(5)*.

  f Identify the main solenoid valve *(6)*.

  g Identify the accumulator *(7)*.

  h Set normal and sigh rate controls OFF.

  i Set expiratory resistance control OFF.

  j Set normal pressure limit at 80 cm H_2O.

  k Set peak flow at 100 L/min.

  l Set normal volume at 2000 ml.

  m Set oxygen percentage at 21%.

  n Turn nebulizer OFF.

  o Set sensitivity OFF.

2 To operate the oxygen percentage control:

  a While watching the oxygen accumulator, turn the power ON.

    • Because the oxygen percentage selector is set on 21%, the accumulator should *not* fill.

  b Set the oxygen percentage at 80%.

    • The accumulator should fill, the oxygen warning indicator on the panel should light, and a buzzer should sound.

    • As the accumulator fills, both signals should cease.

  c Disconnect the oxygen supply hose from the 50 PSI gas source.

  d Cycle the ventilator manually, and observe the accumulator and bellows. It should empty as oxygen is drawn from it to fill the descending bellows.

  e Change the oxygen adapter on the end of the supply hose to an air adapter.

  f Connect the hose to a PSI-compressed air source.

  g Note the accumulator as it fills with compressed air.

  h Note that the alarm lights do not signal the fact that the patient is *not* receiving 80% oxygen.

  i CAUTION: Change the air adapter on the supply hose back to an oxygen adapter.

  j Connect the oxygen hose to a 50 PSI gas supply.

  k Set normal volume at 2200 ml.

  l Set peak flow at 100 L/min.

  m Set oxygen percentage at 100%.

  n Attach a test lung to the patient Y connector.

  o Cycle the ventilator manually, and note the volume recorded by the spirometer.

  p Conclude the check by replacing the cabinet panel on the rear of the ventilator.

K *Expiratory resistance control orientation and performance check*

1 If a ventilator is available:
   a Attach a test lung to the patient Y adapter.
   b Set rate at 10 cycles/min.
   c Set peak flow at 60 L/min.
   d Switch unit ON.
   e Adjust volume until spirometer reads 800 ml.
2 To operate the expiratory resistance control:
   a Set expiratory resistance control to full ON (clockwise).
   b Cycle the ventilator manually.
   c Note inspiratory pressure on system manometer.
   d Observe delay in exhalation, and note inspiratory plateau as indicated by the pressure indicator reaching a peak and slowly decaying and holding at a lesser pressure level.
   e Observe and record the exhaled volume on the spirometer.
   f Set the rate control to 12 cycles/min.
   g Decrease the expiratory resistance incrementally by rotating the control counterclockwise.
   h Time the length of expiration, and note that pressure on the manometer returns to zero before each inspiration.
   i Increase the rate to 30 cycles/min.
   j Observe that a stacking of breaths occurs in that the ventilator does not allow time for exhalation to occur before each inspiration. This is *dangerous* and will lead to elevated baselines and high levels of inadvertent PEEP.

17.0 OPERATING AND MONITORING THE BENNETT MA-1 VENTILATOR.

17.1 The Bennett-MA-1 ventilator monitoring system

One of the outstanding features of any modern day ventilator is its capabilities to monitor the patient. The Bennett MA-1 ventilator uses indicator lights and/or audible alarms (each with the following functions) to inform the operator of the patient/ventilator status (see Fig. 23-55).

1 *Assist light.* An amber light that flashes on each time a spontaneous breath is generated or if the sensitivity control is "overset," causing the machine to self-cycle.
2 *Pressure light.* A red light that flashes (combined with a buzzing alarm) when a preset pressure is reached ("pop-off" or vent pressure). It indicates that lung pressure is lower than the system pressure and that there is increased impedance in either the tubing system or the patient's airway. The cause of increased impedance should be immediately located and corrected (e.g., suctioning the patient, unkinking tubing).
3 *Ratio light.* A red light appears when the I:E ratio becomes less than 1:1. Once the ventilator has been initially set up, this is usually caused by reduced compliance and increased resistance. Usually the undesirable I:E ratio can be corrected by:
   a Clearing the patient's airway
   b Increasing the flow rate
   c Decreasing the cycling rate
   d Decreasing the tidal volume
4 *Sigh light.* A white light flashes on each time the patient is sighed by machine control or manually.
5 *Oxygen light.* A green light appears when the high-pressure hose has been attached to an external gas source of at least 40 PSI, regardless of the composition of the gas. A red light appears and a high-pitched alarm sounds when the desired oxygen inlet pressure is *not* being delivered. This may mean a low source pressure or a leak in the system.
6 *Spirometer alarm.* A shrill whistlelike sound is heard if the desired tidal volume is not being reached and will continue until the problem is corrected or the alarm is shut off. It is usually indicative of a disconnect or a gas leak in the tubing system. Usually the problem can be quickly corrected by checking the patient/ventilator system, beginning with the patient and working backward toward the ventilator.

NOTE: Bennett ventilators sold before 1981 were equipped with Bennett SA-1 or SA-2 monitoring spirometers and spirometer alarms. These devices under certain conditions of flow, volume, and rate would *not* alarm if the expiration diaphragm tube became disconnected and/or the exhalation diaphragm became damaged and nonfunctional. When this situation occurs, it was possible for the spirometer to alternately fill and empty in *reverse* order, simulating ventilation even though the patient was receiving little or no ventilation. In 1981 the Puritan-Bennett Corporation replaced the models SA-1 and SA-2 spirometers on new ventilators with an SA-3 model that does alarm to indicate that preset tidal volumes are not being exhaled and/or there is inadequate positive pressure being generated. This alarm properly indicates a leak in the system and/or an inoperative exhalation valve.

In 1985 a letter was mailed to hospitals indicating that the model SA-2 spirometer was obsolete and would no longer be serviced by the Puritan-Bennett Company. In today's environment of intensified litigation it is important to note that whenever a ventilator or its breathing circuit is modified in the field from the factory model, it may cause the ventilator and its monitoring and alarm functions to fail or perform inaccurately.

7 *Cascade humidifier.* This device provides a continuous source of warm, moist gas to the patient. The thermostat control on top of the cascade electrical unit can be adjusted to provide temperature ranges between room temperature and 50° C (120° F). A thermometer or electric thermistor is inserted into the breathing tube circuit to monitor the gas temperature before it enters the airway. The type of cascade alarm depends on the MA-1 model; several are available.

17.2 Operating the Bennett MA-1 ventilator

The following procedures at the end of this module serve as guides.

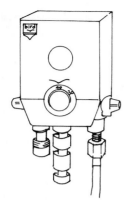

FIGURE 23-56 Bird Oxygen Blender. (Courtesy Medical Products Division/3M, St Paul, Minn.)

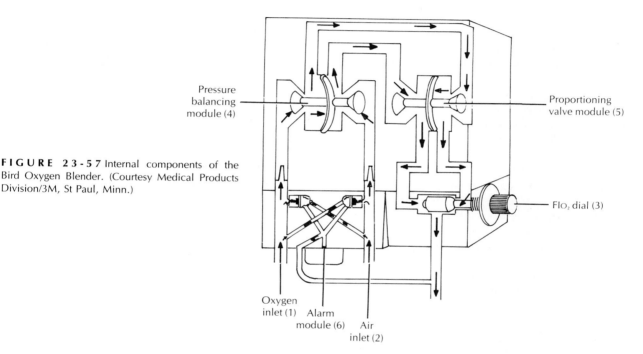

Pressure balancing module (4)

Proportioning valve module (5)

FIGURE 23-57 Internal components of the Bird Oxygen Blender. (Courtesy Medical Products Division/3M, St Paul, Minn.)

FIo₂ dial (3)

Oxygen inlet (1)   Alarm module (6)   Air inlet (2)

1 Procedure 23-9 can be used to estimate and deliver a patient's ventilator requirements with a volume ventilator.

2 Procedure 23-10 can be used to set up a volume ventilator.

3 Procedure 23-11 can be used to monitor a patient on continuous ventilation.

18.0 INDICATIONS FOR AND METHODS OF APPLYING INTERMITTENT MANDATORY VENTILATION (IMV)

18.1 Air-oxygen blenders

1 It is important that the clinician have the means of providing *precise oxygen* concentrations to a patient. In the past a lack of technology forced respiratory care personnel to attempt to mix gases at the bedside or to use expensive premixed gases in cylinders. Currently, most ventilators incorporate their own systems for delivering exact oxygen concentrations to the patient.

2 Each manufacturer has its own method of delivering precise levels of oxygen and air, although most use

some type of oxygen-air mixing valve. Although these valves have different names such as Bennett Air-Oxygen Mixer or Bird Oxygen Blender, they function similarly. The *Bird Oxygen Blender* is used here as an example of a typical air-oxygen mixing valve (Fig. 23-56).

3 The Bird Blender allows the operator to dial a precise oxygen concentration. Once selected, this oxygen concentration will not change regardless of changes in the ventilator settings or fluctuations in supply gas pressures. This is a result of the mixing occurring before the gas enters the ventilator.

4 Like most blenders, the Bird unit is easy to operate and can be used to supply precise concentrations of gas to a ventilator, T adapter, or continuous positive airway pressure (CPAP) system. The accuracy of this blender system is ±3% of the predialed oxygen percentage.

5 The Bird Oxygen Blender (Fig. 23-57) uses two *independent* sources of oxygen *(1)* and air *(2)*, from either a pipeline system or cylinders, for operation of the blender.

6 The desired inspired oxygen (FIO₂) is set by turning a dial on the front of the blender (3).

7 Internally, the blender is made up of three separate modules:

a The pressure balancing module (4), which compensates (balances) for any differences in the inlet pressures between the oxygen and air so that oxygen and air enter the second chamber at the same pressure levels.

b The proportioning valve module (5), where oxygen and air mix to the desired FIO₂ as set on the control dial.

c The alarm module (6), which sounds an audible tone if the inlet pressures (1 and 2) differ more than 20 PSI.

8 If a gas source were to fail or to become 20 PSI less than the other source, the gas with the highest pressure would bypass the blender, sound the alarm, and continue operation of the ventilator.

CAUTION: When this occurs, the patient will be receiving 100% oxygen or compressed air, depending on which gas source failed. This must be corrected immediately so that the patient will receive the prescribed FIO₂.

9 The mixed gas leaves the bottom of the blender at approximately 2 PSI less than the inlet pressure or 48 PSI.

10 The mixed gas can be used to power any device requiring approximately 50 PSI to operate (e.g., resuscitators, ventilators, flowmeters, or nebulizers).

18.2 Use of intermittent mandatory ventilation (IMV)

1 IMV is the periodic delivery of a mechanically induced positive pressure breath to a spontaneously breathing patient.

2 Graphically, an IMV breathing pattern would present a tracing of the patient's spontaneous breaths, followed by a periodic mechanical breath delivered by the ventilator. After this breath, the patient returns to spontaneous breathing.

3 IMV was initially used in surgery by anesthesiologists who would occasionally squeeze the anesthesia bag to hyperinflate the lungs of a spontaneously breathing patient.

4 In 1971 Kirby et al., in *Anesthesia/Analgesia*, described IMV used in conjunction with a "new pediatric ventilator." IMV was successfully used to treat infants with idiopathic respiratory distress syndrome and as an option for weaning patients from mechanical ventilation.

5 Benefits of this technique were recognized and applied to children and adults. These include:

a Allowing the patient to adjust his or her own arterial carbon dioxide tension (PaCO₂)

b Decreasing the use of suppressant drugs

c Facilitating transition from mechanical ventilation to spontaneous breathing (weaning)

d Placing fewer demands on the staff during the wean-

ing process than required using the traditional method

e Decreasing the length of ventilatory time by reducing the patient's psychologic dependency for the ventilator and helping the patient maintain muscle tone of ventilatory muscles

f Helping stabilize FIO₂

g Decreasing O₂ consumption and CO₂ production by the patient, which are caused by "fighting the ventilator"

h Allowing use with high and low levels of PEEP

i Giving the physician another option to the use of assisted or controlled ventilation

6 The patient can adjust PaCO₂ by establishing his or her own rate and depth of ventilation during the period of spontaneous breathing. The intermittently delivered mechanical breath serves to hyperinflate the lung, prevent atelectasis, and facilitate CO₂ elimination in much the same way as the physiologic or mechanical sigh.

7 IMV decreases the need for suppressant drugs because it allows breathing at the patient's own rate. Spontaneous breathing occurs by means of low resistance one-way valves from either the atmosphere, a reservoir bag, or a demand valve while the patient is still attached to the ventilator. This differs from the more traditional methods of practice in which the hyperpneic or tachypneic patient is sedated to depress abnormal ventilatory rate. Once the patient's spontaneous breathing is depressed, controlled ventilation could be effectively used without the patient's breathing in opposition to ("fighting") the ventilator.

8 IMV facilitates the weaning process because the patient never becomes completely dependent on mechanical ventilation. IMV forces the spontaneously breathing patient to continue to participate in his or her own breathing process except during the mandated mechanical breath. With IMV the weaning process actually begins from the moment the patient is placed on the ventilator. With the traditional method of ventilation, weaning does not occur until the end of the mechanical ventilation process, which may have involved days, weeks, or even months.

9 Traditional weaning methods usually required the patient to be "off" and "on" the ventilator until the individual could tolerate longer periods off the ventilator and could maintain ABGs on room air or oxygen. This procedure is time-consuming and requires a great deal of attention by the staff.

10 *Traditional criteria* for weaning attempts varied from one physician to the other, although the criteria that follow represent a collection of the more popular parameters for weaning.

a PaO₂ greater than 80 torr with FIO₂ 0.6 or less

b Alveolar-to-arterial diffusion of oxygen (A-aDO₂) less than 300 to 350 torr with FIO₂ of 1.0

c PaCO₂ less than 55 torr

d Vital capacity (VC) greater than 10 to 15 ml/kg

e Forced expiratory volume at 1 second (FEV₁) greater than 10 ml/kg

f Inspiratory force greater than -20 to -30 cm H_2O pressure

g Dead space/tidal volume ratio (V_D/V_T) less than 0.55 to 0.6

h V_T 3 to 4 ml/lb ideal body weight

i V_T at 50% at predicted volume after ventilator is removed

j Respiratory rate 12 to 15 per minute

NOTE: These values are also useful as indicators for *intubation* and *ventilation* in the deteriorating patient, as well as indicators for weaning the patient from mechanical ventilation.

11 IMV eliminates the need for gathering elaborate weaning values, because in most cases the patient who can maintain acceptable ABG values at an IMV rate of *one or less per minute* with a tracheal tube in place will probably remain stable with similar values after termination of ventilation and extubation.

12 During the period of complete assisted or controlled mechanical ventilation, the patient usually develops a psychologic dependency for the ventilator and panics at the thought of being weaned. In addition, these patients lose muscle tone because of inactivity and a dependency on the ventilator to actively inflate their chests. IMV helps the patient maintain muscle tone of ventilatory muscles because they must be actively used during the periods of spontaneous breathing. These periods normally exceed those devoted to the mandated breaths delivered by the ventilator.

13 The FIO_2 can be stabilized by IMV because it reduces the possibility of respiratory alkalosis resulting from aggressive mechanical ventilation. Respiratory alkalosis, when superimposed on the patient with acute respiratory failure, can cause:

a A decrease in cardiac output

b A decrease in cerebral blood flow

c An increase in airway resistance

d A decrease in pulmonary compliance

e An increase in oxygen consumption

14 Any of these conditions can hinder O_2 delivery uptake and use, which subsequently increases cellular hypoxia. These changing conditions also make it more difficult for the physician to select and maintain FIO_2 levels that will render a desired PaO_2 or mixed venous oxygen tension $P\bar{v}O_2$.

15 IMV reduces the tendency of a patient to resist the ventilator, which uses energy and increases O_2 consumption. Experience has shown that the patient quickly learns to synchronize with the ventilator during the periods of mechanical ventilation. Manufacturers, however, have developed *cycling integrators* called synchronized IMV *(SIMV)* that prevent the ventilator from delivering a mechanical breath if the patient has already begun a spontaneous breath.

16 IMV can be effectively used in conjunction with constant distending airway pressure such as PEEP. Experience has demonstrated that patients may respond more favorably to PEEP/IMV with less cardiovascular involvement than is used with conventional mechanical ventilation methods. This is attributed to the fact that the patient's *mean intrapleural pressure* is less with IMV than at the same level with conventional mechanical ventilation. With IMV there are fewer positive pressure inflations that decrease venous return and more spontaneous breaths that cause the intrapleural pressure to decrease and facilitate venous return, hence cardiac output. It has also been shown that less barotrauma occurs with high levels of PEEP (greater than 15 cm H_2O) used with IMV as compared to conventional ventilation.

17 IMV gives the physician still another option to assisted and controlled ventilation than is offered by more traditional ventilators. Assisted ventilation requires that the patient create an inspiratory effort sufficient enough to trigger the ventilator to inspiration. This necessitates that the ventilator sensitivity and response time be adjusted so that the ventilator delivers a mechanical breath with minimum effort and without wasted movement of the patient's ventilatory muscles. With IMV, assisted ventilation is not necessary provided the patient is breathing and provided the mandated ventilation is adjusted to maintain adequate alveolar ventilation.

18.3 Types of IMV systems

There are basically *three types* of IMV systems. These systems attach to the inspiratory side of the ventilator breathing circuit and incorporate one-way valves to cause all gas to flow only into the inspiratory side of the breathing circuit during inspiration. During spontaneous breathing the patient receives gas from a reservoir source located to the proximal side of the one-way valve. This reservoir may be ambient, a pressurized anesthesia bag, or a demand valve.

1 An *ambient* reservoir IMV system (Fig. 23-58) allows the patient to breathe spontaneously from a humidified gas source flowing continuously from a nebulizer *(1)* at the same FIO_2 as the ventilator *(2)*. During the mandated breath, a one-way valve *(3)* prevents positive pressure loss back through the nebulizer. This type of system cannot be used with continuous distending airway pressure (CDAP), but it does allow monitoring of exhaled volumes with a spirometer *(4)*.

2 The *pressure* reservoir IMV system (Fig. 23-59) incorporates a large 3 to 5 L anesthesia bag attached to the one-way valve for a gas source. This bag is attached to a one-way valve installed proximal to a humidifier. (This system is explained in detail in Unit 18.5)

3 The *demand* valve–type IMV system uses a demand regulator (valve) in place of an anesthesia bag or other continuous flow systems. The principles of operation for a demand valve are presented in Module Twenty-two (demand valve resuscitators). A possible problem when using a demand valve is that the triggering mechanism may not respond to the patient's inspiratory demands so that the valve will not turn on, or it may re-

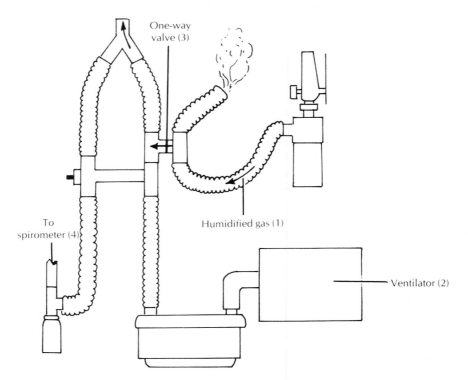

FIGURE 23-58 Ambient reservoir IMV system.

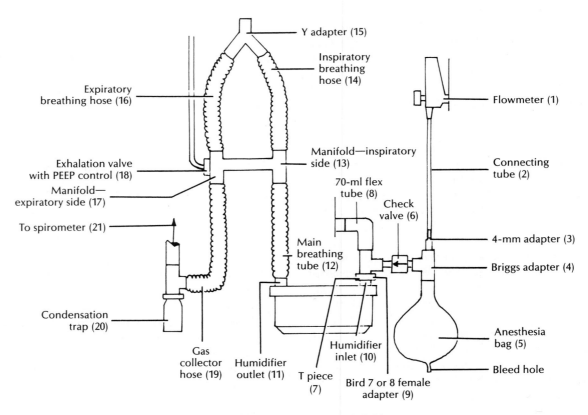

FIGURE 23-59 Pressure reservoir IMV system.

spond too slowly, causing the patient to increase the work of breathing.

4 Some ventilators using a demand-type IMV system are the Bennett MA-2, BEAR 1 and 2, and Emerson IMV. Models such as the Bennett MA-1 and Emerson Post-Op ventilators can be modified by adding a demand regulator to the unit.

18.4 Modifying conventional breathing circuits for special functions

Ventilators today are very flexible, allowing the clinician to vary the ventilator's performance according to special needs of the patient. These needs are based on an assessment of what physiologic components are abnormal and can be stabilized or temporarily adjusted by modifying the ventilator's performance.

NOTE: Most ventilators have built-in CPAP, PEEP, and IMV functions.

Those ventilators that do not have these modalities may be modified as follows.

1 It is important to realize that a ventilator does *not* correct the physiologic problem; it serves only to stabilize the patient and maintain life support until the patient's condition can be medically corrected.

2 Two particular ventilator functions that require special breathing circuits are *positive end expiratory pressure* (PEEP) and *intermittent mandatory ventilation* (IMV) (discussed in Unit 8.2).

3 In review, *IMV,* intermittent demand ventilation *(IDV),* and *SIMV* are techniques that use the delivery of periodic mechanical breaths to a spontaneously breathing patient. To accomplish this, the ventilator is set to cycle at low frequencies (1 to 3 breaths/min), and a special breathing circuit must be used to allow the patient to breathe spontaneously. IMV circuits can be easily assembled from existing breathing circuits by incorporating one-way valves, a 3 to 5 L anesthesia bag, an oxygen-air blender, and some tubing.

4 Fig. 23-60, *A,* illustrates a typical IMV setup, including an oxygen-air blender *(1)* that delivers a *constant* flow of gas at a predetermined FIo_2 to a reservoir bag *(2)* and the IMV circuit to the point of the one-way valve *(3).* As the patient takes a breath *(4),* the pressure is decreased in the breathing circuit, causing gas to flow *(5)* through the one-way valve to the patient. This flow will continue with the patient drawing gas from the reservoir bag *(2)* until spontaneous inspiration ends. The ventilator *(6)* has been adjusted *not* to respond to the patient's inspiratory efforts and remains OFF.

5 As inspiration ends, expiration begins (Fig. 23-60, *B),* with the patient exhaling *(7)* to close the one-way valve *(3)* that stops gas flow from the reservoir bag. The ventilator *(6)* is still cycled OFF and the patient is forced to exhale against a fixed resistance on the expiratory limb of the breathing circuit, which causes 10 torr of continuous positive airway pressure (CPAP) to be generated *(8).*

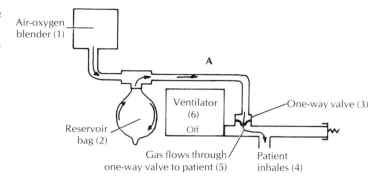

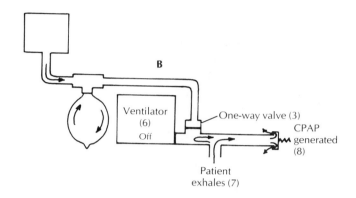

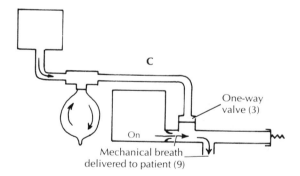

FIGURE 23-60 Typical IMV setup. **A,** Spontaneous inspiration. Patient draws gas from reservoir bag. Ventilator remains off. **B,** Expiration against a fixed resistance to create 10 mm Hg CPAP. **C,** Positive pressure breath delivered by ventilator at predetermined intervals.

6 Fig. 23-60, *C,* illustrates the ventilator, which has been set at a slower cycling rate than the patient is breathing, cycling ON, causing a mechanical breath to be delivered to the patient *(9).* As the positive pressure breath is delivered, the one-way valve *(3)* is forced closed, preventing pressure from escaping into the reservoir bag. Simultaneously, the patient receives a preset tidal volume and the ventilator cycles OFF. This breath is subsequently exhaled against the fixed resistance, causing PEEP to occur, since the patient is not allowed to exhale to ambient before the resistance valve closes.

7 With the ventilator OFF once again, the patient reverts

to a spontaneous breathing mode incorporating the IMV system described in Fig. 23-60, *A*.

8 If a ventilator is not equipped for delivering IMV at the factory, there are many commercial systems available. These usually incorporate a *demand valve* to provide the patient with a constant gas source instead of a reservoir bag. Otherwise these systems theoretically function the same as the simple anesthesia bag system previously described.

18.5 IMV circuit for the Bennett MA-1 ventilator

1 Fig. 23-59 shows an IMV assembly for a Bennett MA-1 ventilator using standard adapters and a 3 L anesthesia bag. The components of this system include:

  a An air-oxygen blender with flowmeter to provide consistent FIO_2 *(1)*

  b A connecting tube to conduct gas from the blender to a standard endotracheal adapter *(2)*

  c A standard size 4 mm entotracheal tube adapter to fit into one side of a Bird T piece *(3)*

  d A Bird T piece or Briggs adapter *(4)*

  e A 3 or 5 L anesthesia bag with bleed hole to serve as an inspiratory reservoir *(5)* NOTE: If bleed hole is not provided, the monitoring spirometer will not operate properly.

  f A flapper check valve (one-way valve) to control gas flow from the reservoir only during inspiration *(6)*

  g A T piece (same as *4*) with one end inserted into a 70 ml flex tube *(7)*

  h A 70 ml flex tube with the other end attached to outlet of ventilator *(8)*

  i A Bird 7 or 8 female adapter *(9)* inserted between T piece *(7)* and inlet port of cascade humidifier *(10)*

  j Outlet port of cascade humidifier *(11)*

  k Main breathing tube *(12)*

  l Inspiratory side of Bennett manifold *(13)*

  m Inspiratory breathing hose *(14)*

  n Y adapter and patient connector *(15)*

  o Expiratory breathing hose *(16)*

  p Expiratory side of Bennett manifold *(17)*

  q Exhalation valve with PEEP control *(18)*

  r Gas collector hose *(19)*

  s Condensation trap *(20)*

  t Monitoring spirometer post to spirometer *(21)*

2 This same type of circuit can be used with other ventilators, although different size adapters may be required to attach the circuit to the ventilator and to the exhalation valve. Other ventilators may or may not have built-in PEEP capabilities. If not, a special PEEP circuit can be attached to the exhalation valve.

18.6 General procedure for using IMV

1 The *indications* for the use of IMV are the same as those for mechanical ventilation except that the patient must be breathing spontaneously at the same rate and tidal volume. Otherwise, the patient would require controlled mechanical ventilation.

2 If the patient is breathing spontaneously, mechanical breaths can be programmed to occur at any time during the patient's spontaneous breathing cycle.

3 The *primary consideration* is to establish a controlled rate and tidal volume by the ventilator that will ensure the patient of acceptable ABG values. Patients who require ventilatory rates greater than 10/min have virtually the same needs as those requiring controlled ventilation.

4 The general procedure for using IMV follows.

  a Draw and analyze an arterial blood gas (ABG) sample.

  b Attach the spontaneously breathing patient to the ventilator.

  c Use PEEP as required to maintain Pao_2.

  d Draw another ABG to confirm best ventilator settings.

  e Reduce ventilatory cycling rate incrementally to establish desirable IMV rate by allowing the patient to breathe spontaneously.

  f Redraw ABG.

  g Adjust ventilator rate, tidal volume, and/or FIO_2 as necessary to continue stable ABG.

  h Allow adequate time for the patient to stabilize at each new level of IMV (6 to 24 hours) before moving to a lower IMV rate.

5 CAUTION: It is difficult to accurately measure the exhaled volumes of patients who are on IMV (with or without CPAP or PEEP) because of the continuous gas flow from the PEEP valve or from the IMV circuit that does not participate in alveolar gas exchange.

6 Some modern ventilators have monitors that allow the operator to obtain a direct readout of only exhaled volumes. Unfortunately, not all ventilators have such monitors, and some method is required for identifying exhaled gas volumes from constant gas flows. Fig. 23-61 shows one type of isolation valve that can be used with IMV, PEEP, or CPAP for measuring exhaled volumes without being influenced by other gas flows. In this example, a Bard-Parker disposable-type exhalation manifold is used in conjunction with a Bird one-way check valve.

  a Fig. 23-61, *A*, illustrates that, during spontaneous breathing, the patient opens a low-resistance one-way valve *(1)*, causing gas to flow through from IMV system through the central inner channel of the exhalation manifold *(2)*, to a tracheal tube adapter *(3)*. During spontaneous inspiration, the exhalation valve fills to cover the exhalation port *(4)* to prevent entrainment of room air.

  b During exhalation (see Fig. 23-61, *B*), the one-way valve *(6)* is closed by the pressure of the exhaled gases. The exhalation valve *(7)* is then forced away from the exhalation port, allowing the exhaled gases to flow around the valve from the inner channel of the exhalation manifold into an outer channel *(8)* leading to the gas collection port and the spirometer *(9)*.

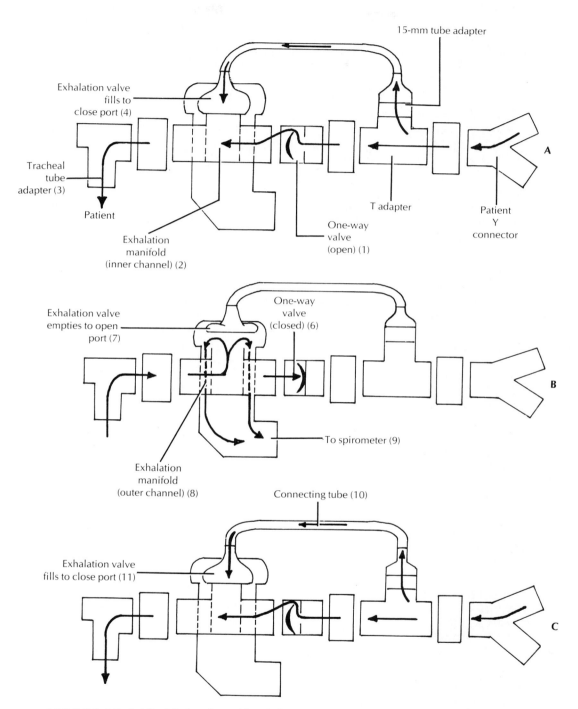

15-mm tube adapter

Exhalation valve
fills to
close port (4)

Tracheal
tube
adapter (3)

Patient

Exhalation
manifold
(inner channel) (2)

One-way
valve
(open) (1)

T adapter

Patient
Y
connector

A

One-way
valve
(closed) (6)

Exhalation valve
empties to open
port (7)

To spirometer (9)

Exhalation
manifold
(outer channel) (8)

B

Connecting tube (10)

Exhalation valve
fills to close port (11)

C

F I G U R E   2 3 - 6 1 Bard-Parker disposable exhalation manifold used with Bird one-way check valve during spontaneous inspiration **A,** expiration, **B,** and mechanical inspiration **C.**

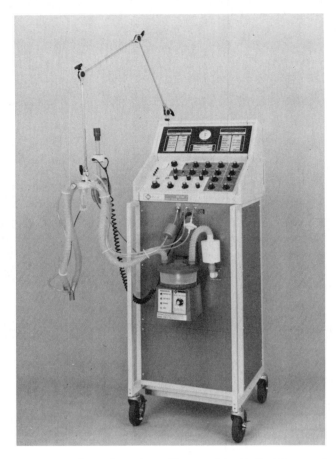

FIGURE 23-62 BEAR 2 mechanical ventilator. (Courtesy Bear Medical Systems, Inc, Riverside, Calif.)

c During a mechanical breath (Fig. 23-61, *C*), the rising positive pressure in the breathing circuit is transmitted by means of a connecting tube *(10)* to inflate the mushroom valve *(11)* and prevent the loss of the mechanical tidal volume. Other components of the valve function as in Fig. 23-61, *A*.

d During exhalation the positive pressure ends and gas leaves the exhalation valve *(7)*, allowing the patient to exhale (see Fig. 23-61, *B*).

Procedure 23-12 can be used to assemble and provide IMV with a Bennett IMV demand valve.

18.7 The Bennett IMV demand valve

1 Both the Puritan-Bennett and Emerson Corporations offer an optional IMV demand regulator to modify ventilators for IMV and continuous elevated baseline systems. The Bennett demand regulator is used here as an example of a typical unit.

2 When used only as a demand regulator, it is mounted on the side of the MA-1 ventilator by removing the round black disk from its place on the mounting plate and inserting the regulator into the open port.

3 The regulator requires a *separate gas source* from the MA-1 and can be powered by air, oxygen, or a mixture of air and oxygen.

4 The IMV regulator can also be used to generate continuous elevated baseline pressures from 0 to 15 cm H_2O.

5 Once the IMV regulator is attached, the patient can open the valve with an inspiratory effort of -2 cm H_2O, and inspiratory flow rates can be adjusted by turning the control located on top of the regulator.

18.8 BEAR 1 and 2 ventilators

1 The BEAR (models 1 and 2) ventilators are electronically controlled, pneumatically powered, time, pressure, or volume-cycled ventilators.

2 They provide control, assist/control SIMV, and CPAP modes. Because both are so similar, only the BEAR 2 ventilator is discussed here (Fig. 23-62).

3 The boxed material explains the BEAR 2 control panel, which is shown in Fig. 23-63.

4 In addition to a comprehensive control panel, the BEAR 2 ventilator offers 29 different display signals and alarms to help the clinician maintain the ventilator and the patient (Fig. 23-64 and the boxed material).

5 The outstanding characteristics of the BEAR 2 ventilator are:

a SIMV. Once an IMV rate is established, the machine monitors the patient's spontaneous breaths. If the patient has received an assisted breath, the ma-

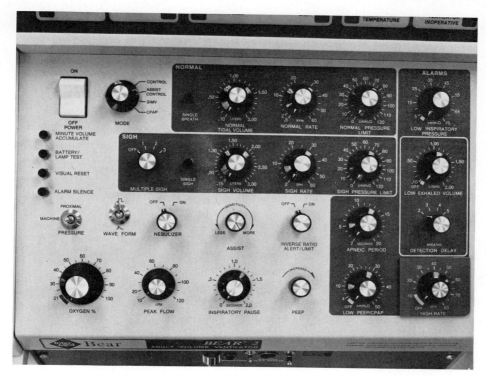

FIGURE 23-63 BEAR 2 control panel. (Courtesy Bear Medical Systems, Inc, Riverside, Calif.)

Control panel (see Fig. 23-63)

1 Power on/off. Controls electrical power to the ventilator.

2 Mode control. Selection of mode of operation.

3 Normal single breath. Manual breath; operable 350 msec after the end of exhalation. Operates in all modes.

4 Tidal volume. 100-2000 ml. When tidal volume is delivered, inspiration ends. (Exhaled tidal volume and minute volume are displayed.)

5 Normal rate. 0.5-60 BPM. (Rate display indicates the sum of the machine and patient breaths.)

6 Normal pressure limit. 0-120 cm H_2O. When the selected pressure is reached, inspiration ends and terminates volume delivery. (Audiovisual alert [*pressure limit*] on display panel shows that pressure limit was reached.)

7 Multiple sigh. Number of sighs to be delivered in succession at preset intervals (*control* and *assist-control* modes only.)

8 Single sigh. Manual sigh; operable 350 msec after the end of exhalation when *Multiple sigh* is set at 1, 2, or 3 position.

9 Sigh volume. 150-3000 ml. When sigh volume is delivered, sigh breath ends.

10 Sigh rate. 2-60 sighs/hour (*control* and *assist-control* modes only).

11 Sigh pressure limit. 0-120 cm H_2O. When the selected sigh pressure is reached, inspiration ends and terminates volume delivery. (Audiovisual alert-[*pressure limit*]-on display panel shows that pressure limit was reached.)

12 Minute volume accumulate. Tidal volume accumulates for 1 min, displays for second minute, and then automatically returns to tidal volume. (*Minute volume accumulate* indicator blinks during accumulation and remains lit during the display of minute volume.)

13 Battery/lamp test. Activates all digital and LED displays, as well as testing the battery-powered, power-loss sensing circuit.

14 Visual reset. All activated visual alarm/alert indicators remain on, until the *visual reset* button is pushed.

15 Alarm silence. Allows silencing of all audible alarms except the *Vent inoperative* alarm. The alarm system will reset automatically in 60 sec or can be reset manually by depressing the *alarm silence* pushbutton (display panel light shows *alarm silence* on).

16 Proximal pressure switch. *Proximal* position: pressure measured at patient Y; *Machine* position: pressure measured upstream of the mainflow bacteria filter (Read on *Proximal airway pressure* gauge).

17 Waveform. Controls flow pattern delivered during positive pressure breaths.

18 Nebulizer. Allows intermittent administration of medication during positive pressure breaths (14 PSIG at 11 L/min). Does not alter oxygen concentration of tidal volume (display panel light shows *nebulizer* on).

19 Assist-sensitivity. Adjustable from *less* (−5 cm H_2O) to *more* (−1 cm H_2O). Senses patient effort in *assist-control* and SIMV modes to deliver synchronized positive pressure breaths (display light shows inspiratory source).

20 Inverse ratio alert/limit—Off. Allows *inverse I:E ratio* (visual alert only; display panel light indicates *inverse ratio* is off). On: Prevents inverse ratio; 1:1 ratio terminates inspiration (audiovisual alert).

21 Oxygen % −21%-100% oxygen (+3%). Connect to 30-100 PSIG oxygen source for concentrations higher than 21%. Audiovisual alert on display panel shows oxygen source pressure less than 30 PSIG with *oxygen %* control setting higher than 21%.

22 Peak flow. 10-120 L/min. Controls initial flow rate during positive pressure breaths; no effect on spontaneous flow.

23 Inspiratory pause. 0-2.0 sec. Delays the beginning of exhalation.

24 PEEP—0-50 cm H_2O. Leak compensated in all modes except *control* (effective leak compensation is the available flow less the patient demand, as long as PEEP exceeds 1 cm H_2O to keep the demand valve open).

NOTE: *Assist* sensitivity may be compromised if excessive leak compensation is required.

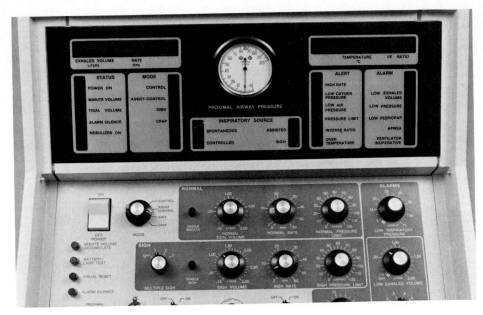

F I G U R E 2 3 - 6 4 BEAR 2 display signals and alarms. (Courtesy Bear Medical Systems, Inc, Riverside, Calif.)

Display signals and alarms (see Fig. 23-64)

1 Digital display of **exhaled volume** on a breath-to-breath basis or *minute volume*.

2 Digital display of the number of **breaths per minute.** Shows the average breath rate, based on the total spontaneous and machine breaths in the last 20 sec and continuously updates every second.

3 Displays level of pressure at the proximal airway from −10 to 120 cm H_2O. Machine (system) pressure may also be read on the **proximal airway pressure gauge** by moving the *proximal pressure* toggle switch to the left or to the right.

4 Displays the gas temperature at the patient Y.

5 Digital display of inspiratory time to expiratory time ratio, breath-to-breath in the **control** and **assist-control** modes. A flashing display indicates greater than a 1:9.9 machine *I:E ratio*.

6 **Power on.** The machine is plugged into an operating AC power outlet and the *power* switch is "on".

7 **Minute volume.** The *exhaled volume* is being accumulated for 1 minute (flashing LED indicator), or the minute volume is displayed (continuously illuminated LED indicator).

8 **Tidal volume.** The *exhaled volume* displays the breath-to-breath *tidal volume*.

9 **Alarm silence.** Audible alarm silenced for 60 sec (except for *vent inoperative*).

10 **Nebulizer on.** Nebulizer is on during mechanical inspiration cycle.

11 **Control.** Ventilator set in *control* mode.

12 **Assist-control.** Ventilator set in *assist-control* mode.

13 **SIMV.** Ventilator set in SIMV mode.

14 **CPAP.** Ventilator set in CPAP mode.

15 **Spontaneous.** Patient breath, unassisted (SIMV, CPAP modes).

16 **Controlled.** Ventilator-initiated positive pressure breath (*control, assist-control, SIMV* modes).

17 **Assisted.** Patient-initiated positive pressure breath (*assist-control,* SIMV modes).

18 **Sigh.** Sigh breath delivered (automatic: *control, assist-control;* single: all modes).

19 **High rate.** The total spontaneous and machine-delivered breaths exceeded the *high rate* control setting.

20 **Low oxygen pressure.** Oxygen inlet pressure less than 30 PSI and *oxygen %* control set above 21%.

21 **Low air pressure.** Internal air compressor presssure and external air pressure less than 9.5 PSI.

22 **Pressure limit.** Machine pressure has reached preset level and terminated inspiration (exhaled volume may be less than selected tidal volume).

23 **Inverse ratio.** Inspiratory time interval exceeds expiratory time, I:E ratio less than 1:1. If the *inverse ratio alert/limit* control is *on* and the ventilator is in *control* mode, the ventilator will terminate inspiration and provide an audible and visual alarm when a 1:1 I:E ratio is reached.

24 **Overtemperature.** Inspired gas temperature exceeds 41° C, or the electrical connection of the temperature probe inadvertently is disconnected, or the temperature probe is defective.

25 **Low exhaled volume.** Exhaled volume has not exceeded level set on *low exhaled volume* alarm for the number of consecutive breaths selected with the *detection delay* control. Disconnect of clamshell from flow tube will cause alarm on next breath.

26 **Low pressure.** Inspiratory pressure has not exceeded level set on the *low inspiratory pressure* alarm, or the expiratory pressure has not dropped below the level set on the *low inspiratory pressure* alarm.

27 **Low PEEP/CPAP.** PEEP/CPAP pressure is less than that set on the PEEP/CPAP control.

28 **Apnea.** The number of seconds selected on the *apneic period* control has elapsed since the beginning of the last breath (spontaneous or mechanical).

29 **Ventilator inoperative.** Indicates total air pressure source or AC power failure, or certain internal electronics failure.

CPAP, Continuous positive airway pressure; LED, light-emitting diodes; PEEP, positive and expiratory pressure; SIMV, Synchronized intermittent mandatory ventilation.

chine will not deliver another breath until adequate time has passed for exhalation to occur. This approach prevents breath stacking leading to increased airway pressure and possible barotrauma.

b A comprehensive alarm package that enables the clinician to easily and quickly assess the patient and ventilator for alarm functions.

19.0 DEMONSTRATING ABILITY TO CHANGE VENTILATOR CIRCUITS AND TO IDENTIFY VENTILATION MALFUNCTION
19.1 Testing a ventilator for proper function

1 The steps involved in checking a ventilator for proper function will vary according to the ventilator involved and hospital procedure. In most hospitals the ventilator is decontaminated, serviced, and tested after each patient. A completely assembled ventilator is used when the final checkout is performed.

2 A complete assembly generally includes:
a Attachment of patient breathing circuit
b Attachment of humidifier
c Attachment of spirometer and/or other accessories

3 Checking a ventilator for proper operation should include a systematic testing of all components, using a typical operational *checklist* to ensure that steps are not missed.
a Check for presence and proper attachment of patient breathing circuit and accessories such as a humidifier.
b Check for presence and proper attachment of all patient gas filters.
c Visually inspect unit for cleanliness and any signs of damage.
d Move all controls and check for smooth operation.
e Ensure that the needle pointer on the system pressure manometer is at zero or according to manufacturer's specifications.
f Ensure that the thermometer is accurate: ± 2° F.
g Inspect the power cord for any signs of wear or exposed wires.
h Plug the power cord into a proper electrical outlet making sure the unit is grounded and does not spark.
i If a separate humidifier is used, plug in the power cord and check for operation of the heating element.
j Turn on the power switch and check for operation of the main compressor.
k If present, turn on the nebulizer power switch and check for operation of the nebulizer compressor.
l Pressure-check the ventilator for any gas leaks.
- Set volume to maximum.
- Set flow rate to maximum.
- Set pressure limits to maximum.
- Obstruct the patient Y adapter.
- Cycle the ventilator manually and note system pressure, expansion of breathing tubes, any sounds of leaks, and operation of pressure alarm.
m Check operation of pressure relief valves and pres-

sure alarms by obstructing patient Y piece and cycling the unit at various pressure limits.
n Attach a respirometer to the exhaust side of the patient manifold.
o Set a range of tidal volumes, and note that measured volume is within 150 ml of the preset volume.
p Set an automatic cycling rate and time it for accuracy.
q Check operation of any special controls such as IMV or PEEP.
r Measure the oxygen percentage (±2% of what is set).
s Check all alarms and monitors for visual/audible operation.
t Label the ventilator as having been checked before storage.

4 It is also a good practive to *perform a final check* when removing a ventilator from storage and at the bedside before attaching the ventilator to the patient. This *bedside check* includes:
a A visual check for filters
b A visual check of tubing and accessories
c A proper level of solutions in the humidifier
d Operation of the compressor
e Delivery of a flow rate/volume
f Pressure check for leaks
g Operation of pressure relief valves and exhalation valve
h Operation of alarms/monitors
i Operation of rate control
j Operation of any special controls such as IMV, PEEP, or CPAP

19.2 Changing a ventilator circuit

1 The bedside service of an operating ventilator is an important function of respiratory care personnel.
2 It is necessary that, during this service, the patient continue to receive ventilatory volume levels, rate, and FIO_2 as close as possible to that which was being delivered by the ventilator.
3 It is also important that the circuit change and other services be performed as quickly and as proficiently as possible to minimize the time that the patient is off the ventilator. Adequate time, however, must be taken to test the new circuit to ensure that it is attached and operating properly before reconnecting the patient.
NOTE: Even though a patient may be ventilated manually during a circuit change, any interruption in PEEP and/or CPAP can result in drastic drops in Pao_2 that may take up to 20 minutes to regain.
4 The specific steps involved in changing a ventilator circuit will vary according to the ventilator, although certain general principles should be followed. Procedure 23-13 can be used for a general procedure for changing a ventilator circuit.
5 Procedure 23-14 can be used to identify and correct ventilator malfunction.

20.0 COMPARISON OF VOLUME VENTILATORS: THE EMERSON 3-PV, EMERSON 3-MV, AND MONOGHAN 225

20.1 Applying concepts and principles to set up and operate volume ventilators according to hospital policy and accepted procedures

The previous units of instruction were devoted to developing *generic* concepts and specific skills for using mechanical ventilation. These concepts and skills can be applied to the operation of most ventilators, even though the Bennett MA-1 ventilator is used as an example in this module. What follows is a comparison of the general procedures for setting up the Emerson 3-PV, Emerson 3-MV, and Monaghan 225 volume ventilators. Compare and contrast these procedures with the previously described procedure for setting up the Bennett MA-1.

A *General procedure for operation of the Emerson 3-PV Post-Op ventilator*

1 Characteristics

  a A constant volume, pressure-variable ventilator, it can operate with assisted or controlled ventilation of the patient. Preset volumes can be delivered without concern for changes in lung compliance.

  b Maximum pressure settings are based on lung compliance.

  c A modified kettle is incorporated in the system to achieve adequate humidification of the inspired air. By use of a hot plate, the kettle is heated to about 50° C (120° F). Supplementary gases can be delivered through a hose in the rear of the ventilator.

    NOTE: Another type of humidifier, such as a cascade, may be substituted for the kettle humidifier.

2 Equipment assembly

  a Attach tubing to the reducing elbow of inspiratory outlet and tighten with screw clamp provided. Remaining end attaches to condensation trap bottle.

    Inspiratory tubing is attached to the condensation trap jar provided and tightened with screw clamp provided.

    Both inspiratory and expiratory tubing are attached to a Y piece with a 15 mm elbow on the inspriatory side.

  b Next, secure expiratory tubing to the exhalation valve assembly and tighten with screw clamp provided.

  c Next, attach tubing to the exhalation port elbow. The remaining end of the tubing is attached to the spirometer.

3 Controls of ventilator

  a Pressure gauge. System pressure designated in centimeters of water. Maximum pressure can be set by turning knob located on the safety valve on the kettle.

  b Volume scale measures preset volume.

  c Volume. The tidal volume is adjusted by means of a handwheel located on front of the ventilator. The scale shows the desired stroke volume. It should be

remembered that the actual delivered amount will be less than the stroke volume delivered because of loss through compression of dead space air.

  d Gas dilution. Room air is normally delivered; however, supplemental oxygen may be added. Remember to always monitor inline oxygen concentrations. Given two values:

    • Oxygen percentage desired

    • Minute ventilation in liters based on manufacturer's setting of ventilator, you can calculate the amount of oxygen in liters per minute required.

EXAMPLE:

$$\frac{(\% \, O_2 - 21 \times \text{Minute ventilation})}{79} =$$

Liters per minute of oxygen

To deliver an O_2 concentration of 50% with a minute ventilation of 5 L, how many liters per minute of oxygen must you supply?

$$\frac{(50 - 21) \times 5}{79} = \frac{29 \times 5}{79} = \frac{145}{79} = 1.835 \text{ or } 2 \text{ L/min } O_2$$

  e Inspiratory and exiratory time controls. Adjustable separately from 12 to 70 rpm.

  f Trim screw. This is located between inspiratory and expiratory adjustments. When operation is on abnormal line voltage, this adjustment permits speed compensation.

  g Pump switch. Activates motor.

  h Humidity switch. Thermostatically controls temperature.

  i Fuse light. Warning that, when lighted, it must be changed.

  j Moisture kettle. Delivers humidification to patient.

  k Assist attachment. Switch for use as an assistor or controller.

  l Deep breathing or sigh. A blower device that is activated periodically to provide hyperinflation for a few breaths. Time adjustments between sighs and can be set. A manual sigh phase is also available.

  m Spirometer. The spirometer unit is mounted above the ventilator. Gas exhaled with each breath through the exhalation port advances the spirometer needle, which in turn indicates approximate volumes.

  n As with all ventilator patients receiving oxygen, continuous in-line O_2 monitor should always be used.

4 Patient initiation

  a Connect power cord to alternating current.

  b Fill humidifier with warm water to the appropriate level.

  c Turn the heater switch to high.

  d Initiate ventilator through pump switch.

  e Adjust the tidal volume by turning the handwheel in front of ventilator.

  f Set maximum pressures required.

  g To set respiratory rate, adjust both inspiratory and expiratory controls.

h Add additional concentrations of oxygen to rear of unit if necessary.

i Set sigh volume and time.

j Select mode: assist or controller.

k Based on model, set ventilator alarm.

B *General procedure for operation of the Emerson 3-MV (IMV) ventilator*

This Emerson model is basically the same as the 3-PV model in design and characteristics except for its special functions. It is operated by the following procedures.

1 Attach the power cord, properly grounded, to an alternating current 115-volt, 60 Hz electric outlet.

2 Put warm water in the humidifier kettle until its level is near the top. Turn on the main power switch, and adjust the humidifier control (maximum if a patient is about to use the ventilator).

3 Put water in the PEEP exhalation valve to the desired level. (During filling, lift the elbow on top of the transparent tube. A squeeze-bulb with extension is convenient for adding or removing water.)

4 Adjust to the desired stroke volume by turning the crank (high on the right side of the ventilator) while observing the tidal volume indicator on the panel. (A somewhat smaller volume will actually be delivered to the patient's lungs because there is a small loss from compression of dead-space air.)

5 The ventilator uses compressed air or oxygen; both are normally blended by a mixing valve to the proportion that has been prescribed. This source should be set up and adjusted. The mixture flowing from the mixing valve goes into two reservoir bags. The right-hand bag supplies the patient's spontaneous respirations. The left-hand bag collects gas for the intermittent mandatory breaths.

6 Turn on the pump and adjust the frequency of mandatory breaths, using the digital switch to the left of the pressure gauge. (The time displayed is for a total cycle.) At the beginning of treatment, the mandatory breaths may be set at the rate of the patient's spontaneous respiration (as in ordinary controlled ventilation). The interval between breaths is then gradually increased as the patient's condition improves. Eventually, mandatory breaths are spaced so far apart that the patient scarcely relies on them at all, and weaning is completed.

7 After connecting the patient to the ventilator, recheck all adjustments that have been made previously:

a The flow of (mixed) gas into the right-hand reservoir bag should not distend the bag excessively but should be enough to supply all spontaneous breathing and, at the same time, maintain any level of PEEP that has been selected.

b The flow to the left-hand bag should be adequate for the mandatory breaths.

c Check the PEEP level as shown on the system pressure gauge. (This reading will be slightly greater than the height of the water column in the transpar-

ent tube because a charging line from the piston adds about 3 cm of pressure to keep the valve closed during inspiration.)

d Check the temperature of the gas being delivered to the patient and adjust the humidifier control accordingly. Higher settings will be needed for higher minute volumes, and the humidifier will need repeated attention. Ideally, there should be a thermometer in the Y piece as a guide to the humidifier setting.

e Check the proportions of the oxygen-air mixture going to the patient.

f Check the adequacy of the patient's total ventilation by observation of spontaneous breathing efforts and by periodic analysis of blood gases.

8 The alarm (No. 3MV-1) may be used normally if mandatory breaths are fairly frequent—at least 4/min. If mandatory breaths are less frequent than 4/min, the alarm will respond properly only to a Pneumotube (3MV-G8).

a Stretch the Pneumotube lightly around the patient's chest, fastening it with the Velcro straps. The tension should be just enough so that the corrugated tube (in front) will expand with each inspiration. The air moved in this way can activate the alarm, and a moisture barrier is not required.

b Adjust the alarm sensitivity to *A* and allow it to warm up for at least 1 min. With the ventilator running and the patient connected, turn the sensitivity knob slowly clockwise until a "beep" signal is heard. Back it off counterclockwise until no signal is heard. When the adjustment is turned to its extreme clockwise position, the alarm is most insensitive: it will become quiet only in response to very strong breathing (high pressures and/or rates). When the adjustment is far counterclockwise (and yet at a point where the signal is still given), it is highly sensitive and will become quiet in response to small inpulses (low pressures and/or rates). An adjustment between these extremes should be selected.

c Recheck sensitivity after the machine has been on for half an hour. If patient compliance changes, the alarm must be reset.

d CAUTION: Do not place excessive reliance on the alarm. If properly adjusted, it will signal emergencies of several kinds (such as electric current failure), but other emergencies may not trigger it. A patient using a ventilator should be attended at all times.

9 O_2 Check Oxygen Analyzer (No. 3MV-OA). Turn the calibration knob to bring the needle to 21% and allow a minute for the reading to stabilize in room air. The dial will now display the oxygen percentage and the mixed gas as it flows to the humidifier, with the sensor in line. (For detailed specifications and instructions, see Form No. 3MV-OA-I that accompanies the O_2 Check Unit.)

10 After use, remove Y piece, elbow hoses, and associated parts for sterilization. Ethylene oxide sterilization with adequate aeration is recommended. In prolonged use of the ventilator, it is desirable to change (and re-sterilize) these parts every 24 hours or more often because they tend to pick up contamination from the patient.

11 The delivery tubing (up from the humidifier) is packed with copper wool. This serves as a coarse filter, it increases the surface area from which moisture is added to the airstream, and it has active bactericidal properties. The copper's protective action is greatest when it is clean and bright. Occasional washing in mild acetic acid or the like— and subsequent rinsing—is recommended. In any case, the copper wool should be replaced when it begins to get thin and fragile. (A new piece can be drawn into the tube readily by a string tied to one end.)

12 At various points in the breathing circuit, mushroom valves direct flow in a specific direction. If piping is ever disconnected, note carefully the position of these valves so they can be replaced correctly (when the piping is rejoined securely).

C *General procedure for operation of the Monaghan 225 ventilator*

The Monaghan fluidic ventilator offers a method for providing mechanical ventilatory support for patients who are unable to provide adequate support for themselves.

The MRI version of the 225/SIMV ventilator has no electronic components and virtually no ferrous materials that would interfere with the diagnostic imaging (Fig. 23-65, *A* and *B*).

 1 *Equipment:*
  a Monaghan 225
  b Humidifier with heating element
  c Arm support
  d Standard ventilator circuitry (disposable or nondisposable)
  e 24 inch large-bore tubing
  f Thermometer
  g Thermometer plug
  h 500-PSI line and O_2 adapter
 2 *Assembly*
  a Slide the Cascade humidifier up over the heater assembly. Turn the two knobs, wide end toward the heater untile they click into place.
  b Attach the 24 inch large-bore tubing from the bacteria filter to the port on the Cascade-labeled inlet.
  c Place ventilator tubing through arm support.
   • Take one tube, connect it to the Cascade labeled "outlet"; the other end of this tube connects to the nebulizer side of the manifold.
   • Take the other tube that is the same size as the one that you just placed on the machine and connect this tube from the exhalation port on the manifold to the Monaghan 225 transducer if it is to be used.
   • Attach the remaining tubing with the patient Y connector onto the remaining side of the ventilator manifold.

   • Connect nebulizer line and exhalation line to appropriate place on the Monaghan 225 labeled "nebulizer" and "exhalation."
 3 *Cleaning*
  a Remove and discard all disposable tubing.
  b Remove Cascade.
  c All removable parts are to be chemically decontaminated in a solution such as gluteraldehyde or pasteurized with the exception of the following parts:
   • Thermometer (wiped with alcohol only).
   • Transducer (can be cleaned by gently swishing through mild detergent solution followed by swishing through water).
 4 *Testing and calibration*
  a Assemble unit, and make connection to 50 PSI source.
  b Attach test lung to patient connection.
  c Test and set controls:
   • Assist-control (A-C) sensitivity
   • Volume at 600 cc (try various volumes)
   • Rate of 12 cycles/min
   • Test pressure limit and set below test resistance.
  d Correct all leaks.
  e Using white adhesive tape, initial and date time of check.
 5 *Connection for patient use*
  a Add water to Cascade; plug in heating element, and adjust Cascade temperature control to approach 37° C in inspiratory line.
  b Connect 500 PSI tubing to 50 PSI source.
  c Retest controls.
  d Set A-C by dialing the sensitivity knob clockwise until oscillation begins: dial back until oscillation ceases.
  e Inform patient of therapy.
  f Connect patient: check for exhaled volume with Wright Respirometer or Monaghan 225 digital spirometer; auscultate lungs.
  g Set pressure limit 10 cm H_2O above peak pressure.
  h Check all controls.
   • Set peak flow to at least match patient's flow rate and promote laminar flow.
   • Check volumes for accuracy.
   • If PEEP is instituted, adjust sensitivity as necessary to ensure ventilator response with a negative deflection of 1 cm H_2O.
   • Monitor as prescribed on flow sheets.

21.0 CONCEPTS AND PRINCIPLES OF MICROORGANISM CONTROL
21.1 Ventilator decontamination

The general principles for the control of microorganisms, prevention of cross-infection, and decontamination are presented in Module Nine. These principles apply to the use and culturing of all equipment that comes into contact with patients.

It is critical that ventilators be properly decontaminated and closely monitored to ensure their continued asepsis be-

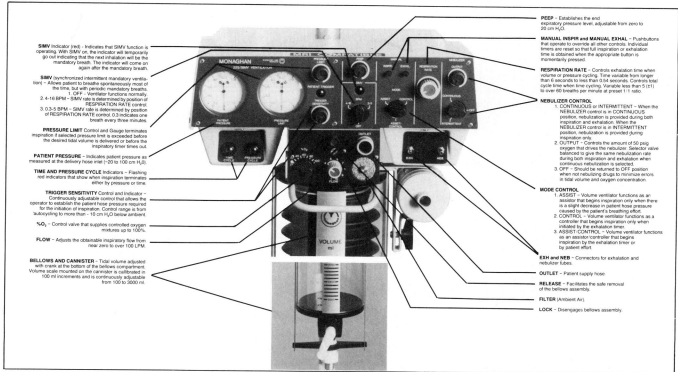

A

B

SIMV Indicator (red) - Indicates that SIMV function is operating. With SIMV on, the indicator will temporarily go out indicating that the next inhalation will be the mandatory breath. The indicator will come on again after the mandatory breath.

SIMV (synchronized intermittent mandatory ventilation) – Allows patient to breathe spontaneously most of the time, but with periodic mandatory breaths.
  1. OFF - Ventilator functions normally.
  2. 4-16 BPM – SIMV rate is determined by position of RESPIRATION RATE control.
  3. 0.3-5 BPM – SIMV rate is determined by position of RESPIRATION RATE control. 0.3 indicates one breath every three minutes.

PRESSURE LIMIT Control and Gauge terminates inspiration if selected pressure limit is exceeded before the desired tidal volume is delivered or before the inspiratory timer times out.

PATIENT PRESSURE – Indicates patient pressure as measured at the delivery hose inlet (−20 to 100 cm H_2O).

TIME AND PRESSURE CYCLE Indicators – Flashing red indicators that show when inspiration terminates either by pressure or time.

TRIGGER SENSITIVITY Control and Indicator – Continuously adjustable control that allows the operator to establish the patient hose pressure required for the initiation of inspiration. Control range is from autocycling to more than − 10 cm H_2O below ambient.

%O_2 – Control valve that supplies controlled oxygen mixtures up to 100%.

FLOW – Adjusts the obtainable inspiratory flow from near zero to over 100 LPM.

BELLOWS AND CANNISTER – Tidal volume adjusted with crank at the bottom of the bellows compartment. Volume scale mounted on the cannister is callibrated in 100 ml increments and is continuously adjustable from 100 to 3000 ml.

PEEP – Establishes the end expiratory pressure level, adjustable from zero to 20 cm H_2O.

MANUAL INSPIR and MANUAL EXHAL – Pushbuttons that operate to override all other controls. Individual timers are reset so that full inspiration or exhalation time is obtained when the appropriate button is momentarily pressed.

RESPIRATION RATE – Controls exhalation time when volume or pressure cycling. Time variable from longer than 6 seconds to less than 0.54 seconds. Controls total cycle time when time cycling. Variable less than 5 (±1) to over 60 breaths per minute at preset 1/1 ratio.

NEBULIZER CONTROL
  1. CONTINUOUS or INTERMITTENT – When the NEBULIZER control is in CONTINUOUS position, nebulization is provided during both inspiration and exhalation. When the NEBULIZER control is in INTERMITTENT position, nebulization is provided during inspiration only.
  2. OUTPUT – Controls the amount of 50 psig oxygen that drives the nebulizer. Selector valve balanced to give the same nebulization rate during both inspiration and exhalation when continuous nebulization is selected.
  3. OFF – Should be returned to OFF position when not nebulizing drugs to minimize errors in tidal volume and oxygen concentration.

MODE CONTROL
  1. ASSIST – Volume ventilator functions as an assistor that begins inspiration only when there is a slight decrease in patient hose pressure caused by the patient's breathing effort.
  2. CONTROL – Volume ventilator functions as a controller that begins inspiration only when initiated by the exhalation timer.
  3. ASSIST/CONTROL – Volume ventilator functions as an assistor/controller that begins inspiration by the exhalation timer or by patient effort.

EXH and NEB – Connectors for exhalation and nebulizer tubes.

OUTLET – Patient supply hose.

RELEASE – Facilitates the safe removal of the bellows assembly.

FILTER (Ambient Air).

LOCK – Disengages bellows assembly.

FIGURE 23-65 A, Full-view of Monaghan 225/SIMV MRI ventilator. **B,** Monaghan MRI version of 225/SIMV ventilator control panel. (From Monaghan Medical Corp, Plattsburg, New York.)

cause they provide a direct route into the patient's unprotected airway.

Micro air filters are useful in helping to prevent the spread of bacteria and in filtering particles 1 to 5 µg from the gas source to the patient.

The use of disposable breathing circuits has helped to reduce the incidence of cross-infection by contaminated tubing and poor sterilization technique. It is important that respiratory care personnel adhere to department policy regarding the cleansing of ventilators and their accessories. If such a policy is not available, the general guidelines that follow may be useful in establishing a decontamination procedure.

A *Cleaning, disinfection, decontamination, and sterilization of respiratory therapy equipment*

1 *Purpose:* to prevent the spread of infection by way of respiratory therapy equipment, either directly or through cross-contamination.

2 *General information:*

a A continuing bacteriologic monitoring program is the only assurance that current cleaning and disinfection procedures are effective.

b The continuing use of disposable equipment is a major step in reducing cross-infection, since the possible contagion is eliminated as the circuits are changed. Costs in cleaning, packaging, and time are greatly reduced.

c For safety, anyone cleaning equipment should wear a plastic apron and rubber gloves. Report any skin reaction to the department head immediately.

3 *Respiratory therapy equipment:* The purpose of cleaning equipment is twofold. Initially, the practitioner should be interested in freeing the equipment surface of all organic material or soil. This exposed surface will now be exposed to the sterilizing agent used. It is most important to examine the equipment while it is being cleaned, observing that broken or damaged parts are replaced. Minute parts should be closely inspected.

B *General decontamination procedure*

1 Disassemble, scrub with detergent, and rinse all parts that have come into direct contact with the patient. Do *not* disassemble electrical parts or parts of the ventilator unless so instructed by the manufacturer or hospital policy.

2 Prepare ventilator for gas sterilization or decontamination according to manufacturer's instructions.

3 Immerse disassembled parts in liquid decontamination agent as directed by the agent manufacturer.

4 Remove disassembled parts after appropriate exposure time, and rinse thoroughly with sterile, distilled water.

5 Reassemble all parts using appropriate aseptic technique.

6 Package assembled parts, label as to date of decontamination, and store in designated area.

7 Aerate ventilator after exposure to ethylene oxide to remove any residual gas.

8 Store ventilator in designated area.

C *Service procedure*

The following procedure is recommended to help prevent infection of the patient once the ventilator is in operation.

1 Always use a decontaminated ventilator and breathing circuit for each new patient. Do not rotate attachments between patients.

2 Change the breathing circuit and accessories every 8 hours.

3 Use sterile, distilled water in the humidifier.

4 Drain any condensate that collects in the breathing tube into a container. Do not empty condensate back into the humidifier.

5 When changing a used breathing circuit, place dirty equipment into a closed container to transport back to the department to be disposed of or decontaminated.

6 Wipe the external surface of the ventilator with an aseptic agent.

7 Remove any used items from the room for decontamination.

22.0 SUPPLEMENTAL MATERIALS ON MECHANICAL VENTILATION

22.1 New generation ventilators

The use of microprocessors to control ventilator function has resulted in a new third generation of ventilators.

These units produce and deliver tidal volumes in the same manner as their predecessors except for high-frequency devices.

1 The primary differences are in the ways in which function modes are set and monitored.

2 Some new third generation ventilators use an electronic central processing unit (CPU) to automatically scan the ventilator's circuits for proper function and to monitor the unit's ability to meet preset clinical parameters.

3 Any variations from factory performance specifications and/or preset clinical parameters activate warning systems at the bedside and even at remote stations.

4 With these devices the need for *ventilator checks* by personnel is diminished. However, the need for patient rounds is not diminished and may in fact become more frequent as the new and sophisticated technology gives the practitioner many more options for controlling a patient's ventilation. Some of these options are listed below.

5 Pressure support ventilation (PSV)

a Pressure support ventilation describes a procedure that was introduced in the mid-1980s as a means of complementing the ventilatory efforts of a spontaneously breathing patient.

b This technique requires a ventilator that has a pressure support feature and a patient that is capable of triggering his or her own ventilator breath.

c Simply described, once inspiration is triggered by the patient, the ventilator immediately adjusts gas flow rates to provide preset inspiratory support pressure. This preset PSV level is maintained throughout the inspiratory phase.

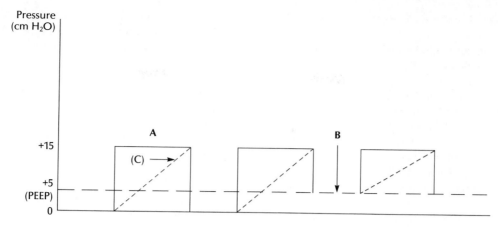

FIGURE 23-66 A, Schematic representation of airway pressure measured at the proximal airway of a spontaneously breath's patient on a mechanical ventilator with PSV. **B,** +5cm H_2O PEEP. **C,** *Dotted line* represents waveform by conventional ventilation without PSV.

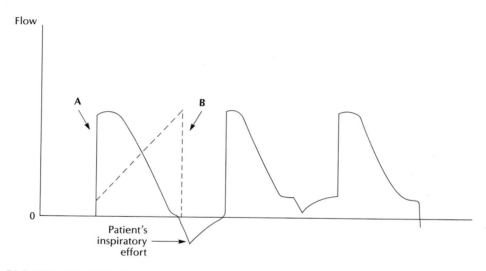

FIGURE 23-67 A, Schematic representation of inspiratory flow rates generated to initiate and maintain PSV throughout the inspiratory cycle. **B,** *Dotted line* represents accelerating flow pattern by conventional ventilator without PSV.

d Fig. 23-66 (*A*) shows the preset PSV level of 15 cm H_2O. In addition, a +5 cm H_2O PEEP is added (*B*). The dotted line (*C*) represents the waveform generated by a conventional IPPB device.

e Fig. 23-67 shows the flow rates delivered by the ventilator to initiate and maintain the preset level of PSV throughout the inspiratory phase.

Also note how rapidly the ventilator responds to the patient's spontaneous effort to initiate inspiration.

f PSV levels can vary between 1 and 100 cm H_2O pressure depending on the ventilator model.

g With PSV the inspiratory phase is terminated when a certain minimum inspiratory flow rate is reached or whenever an excessive airway pressure is monitored. For example, on the Servo 900C ventilator, inspiration ends when the flow decreases to 25% of the peak flow generated for the inspiratory phase or the inspiratory pressure rises to +3 cm H_2O above the preset inspiratory pressure.

h PSV differs from the traditional assisted ventilator mode using IPPB in that:
- With the beginning of inspiration, an accelerated inspiratory flow rate is delivered by the ventilator so that the PSV level is immediately reached.
- As inspiration continues, flow rates are automatically adjusted to maintain a constant preset pressure level throughout inspiration.
- With conventional IPPB or controlled mechanical ventilation, airway pressure levels gradually increase during inspiration, reaching peak pressure just before the end of the inspiratory cycle. During inspiration, airway pressure fluctuates up and down as the patency of the airway and compliance and resistance change.

i Physiologic rationale for PSV includes:
(1) Interacts with mechanoreceptors (pressure receptors) located in the lungs and chest wall to enable the patient to establish a more physiologic venti-

latory control over rate, tidal volume, and flow rate.

 (2) Causes the patient to actively participate in his or her own ventilation. PSV enables the patient to maintain control over ventilation and to use his or her own muscles without the undesired stress or fatigue that may occur with unassisted and controlled work of breathing.

j PSV used with intermittent mandatory ventilation combines the benefits of having the patient breathe on his or her own with the added assurance that a minimum level of minute ventilation can be mandated by the ventilator.

k Clinically PSV may be most useful in patients that are being weaned and in situations where it is desirable for the patient to assist in ventilation without the added fatigue that accompanies the work of breathing.

l PSV *alone* probably should not be used on patients with an unstable ventilatory drive, excessive secretions, bronchospasm, frequently changing airway resistance and compliance, and severely weakened physical condition.

m Further research is necessary to document the clinical application of PSV. It remains a controversial procedure.

6 Airway pressure release ventilation (APRV)

 a The purpose of APRV is to allow a patient's lungs being maintained by CPAP to briefly *vent to ambient* at the end of a ventilatory cycle and then rapidly reinflate to regenerate the elevated baseline with the subsequent inspiration.*

 b The physiologic advantage of this modality is that with CPAP the higher unrestricted gas flow allows for unrestricted spontaneous ventilation and a very brief interruption of elevated airway pressure to *facilitate* venous return and *eliminate* CO_2.

 c An important consideration is that with APRV peak airway pressure (Paw) never exceeds the CPAP level, which should result in fewer incidents of barotrauma than occur with conventional ventilation.

7 Mandatory (minimum) minute ventilation (MMV)

 a Mandatory minute ventilation is a relatively new modality that enables the ventilator to automatically adjust a patient's IMV rate or level of pressure support to maintain a preset minute volume.

 b The purpose of MMV is to decrease the weaning time for a ventilation patient. Examples of patients in whom MMV may be useful include drug overdose and postoperative respiratory depression.

 c It is important to note that MVV does *not* substitute for mandated breaths in situations where apnea may occur.

■ ■ ■

Although there are numerous devices that could qualify,

the following ventilators are examples of a new generation of devices that undoubtedly will become even more automated as the blending of microprocessors with ventilators is more fully accepted as a safe and dependable method of controlling a ventilator's function and monitoring patients. Although these devices are different brands, they incorporate the following similar operational features. (See also Module Thirty.)

8 Similarities of third generation ventilators

 a A CPU ventilator control.

 b Electromechanical valves to control and adjust waveforms for gas flow.

 c Numerous ventilatory modalities including pressure support ventilation.

 d Extensive monitoring and alarm packages.

22.2 Siemens Servo Ventilators

1 The Siemens Servo Ventilators (900, 900B, and 900C) are among the first to use electronic feedback loops with an integrator unit to deliver a guaranteed tidal volume.

2 Even though a microprocessor is not used with these ventilators, the control of input gas flow based on output delivery with automatic adjustment to meet a preset volume places these ventilators on the leading edge of the transition to a computer-controlled device.

3 The primary difference is that the microprocessor-controlled ventilators use preprogrammed software to direct the functional logic of the ventilator.

4 The Siemens 900B and 900C Ventilators are time-cycled, pneumatically powered, and electronically controlled.

5 They can be operated as an assistor, a controller, or assistor/controller.

6 Special functions include synchronized intermittent mandatory ventilation (SIMV), continuous positive airway pressure (CPAP), and positive end expiratory pressure (PEEP).

7 The principle of operation for all of the models is the same although some differences exist in the features offered by the more modern model C ventilator.

8 The pneumatic power system of the Servo Ventilator is unique in that it incorporates mechanical forced generated by spring tension (Fig. 23-68, *1*) to compress (empty) a gas-filled bellows *(2)*.

9 As the bellows *(2)* is compressed (moved up), gas flows out past an electronically controlled inspiratory valve *(3)* at a constant flow rate.

 This flow rate is ensured by the constant spring tension against the bellows and by the opening and closing of the electronic inspiratory valve.

10 Both the 900B and C ventilators incorporate electromechanical scissors (chopper) valves that open and close in response to electrical signals. These valves control tidal volume, flow rates, flow pattern, inspiratory time, expiratory time, and expiratory pressure on the 900C. (Figs. 23-68 and 23-69).

11 Fig. 23-29, *A* and *B*), illustrates a scissors valve in the

*Stock CM and Downs JB: Airway pressure release ventilation: a new approach to ventilatory support during acute lung injury July 1987, Respir Care 32:7.

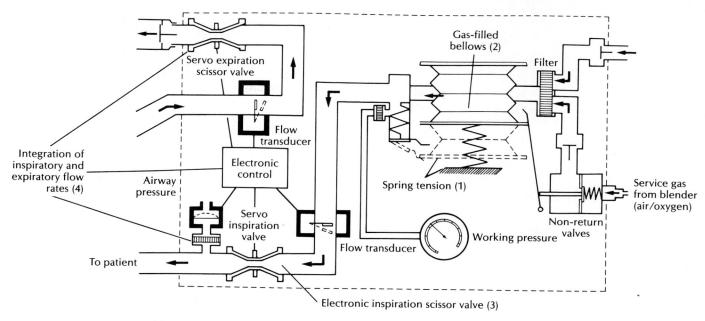

FIGURE 23-68 Functional flow diagram for Siemens Servo Ventilator. (Modified from diagram courtesy Siemens Corp, Union, N.J.)

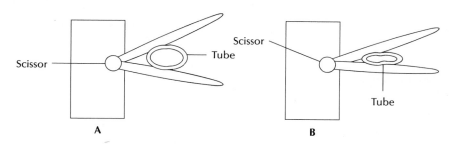

FIGURE 23-69 A, Scissor valve open allowing gas flow. **B,** Scissor valve closed pinching the tube and interrupting gas flow. Electromechanical valve can be partially or completely opened or closed during a cycle to limit gas flow and establish ventilatory waveforms.

opened and closed position.

12 These inspiratory and expiratory valves are electrically opened and closed for a given period of time to allow the tidal volume to be delivered to the patient.

13 During mechanical inspiration the expiratory valve closes and the inspiratory valve opens and vice versa.

14 Both valves respond to a preset signal for time, flow rate flow patterns, and tidal volume.

15 A motor on the inspiratory valve constantly corrects the valve opening to obtain preset values.

16 The use of a spring-driven bellows between the service gas and the patient makes the ventilator a double circuit system and causes it to perform as a constant flow generator.

17 This classification is appropriate because the force of the spring against the bellows plate creates a constant force, hence gas flow throughout the inspiratory cycle. This performance classification remains valid as long as the working pressure exceeds airway resistance and other opposition to gas flow.

18 The combination of feedback electronics integrated into the inspiratory and expiratory gas circuits enables the ventilator to continuously electronically monitor, compare, and adjust inspiratory gas flow rates. These flow rates are adjusted as needed to deliver the preset minute volume *(4)*.

19 If resistance to gas flow increases inspiration, causing expiratory flow to be reduced, the ventilator's integrated electronic control system automatically increases inspiratory flow rates to produce the tidal volume necessary to achieve a preset minute ventilator ($V_T \times f$).

In other words, gas flow rate from the ventilator is increased or decreased ("servoed") as needed to deliver the preset minute volume, giving the ventilator its name.

A *Ventilator controls*

Since the Siemens 900B and 900C ventilators are very similar, the 900B is discussed first, followed by an explanation of changes made on the 900C. For the reader to acquire a better understanding of the relationship of the con-

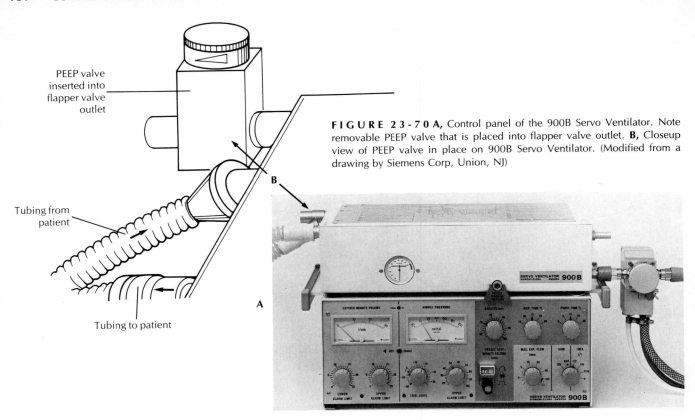

PEEP valve
inserted into
flapper valve
outlet

Tubing from
patient

Tubing to patient

FIGURE 23-70 A, Control panel of the 900B Servo Ventilator. Note removable PEEP valve that is placed into flapper valve outlet. **B,** Closeup view of PEEP valve in place on 900B Servo Ventilator. (Modified from a drawing by Siemens Corp, Union, NJ)

trols and their locations on the control panel, the following explanations are coordinated with Fig. 23-70, *A* and *B*.

1 *Preset working pressure.* Used to set the maximum pressure available to empty the bellows to deliver gas to the patient (adjustable to 100 PSIG).

2 *Preset inspiratory minute volume.* Used to establish the desired minute volume to be delivered to the patient. It can be adjusted from 0.5 L/min to 25 L/min for neonatal or adult ventilation.

3 *Breaths per minute* (BPM). Used to set the cycling frequency (adjustable from 6 to 60 BPM).

4 *Inspiratory time percentage.* Used to adjust the length of inspiration, which varies with the preset cycling frequency (adjustable time between 15% and 50% of the breathing cycle). This control adjusts the peak flow rate as a function of time.

5 *Pause time percentage.* Used to set the end expiratory pause as a percentage of the respiratory cycle. This pause occurs at the end of an inspiration but before the beginning of an exhalation (adjustable 0% and 30%). During this pause the lungs remain inflated, causing a plateau pressure waveform.

6 *Flow pattern selector switch* (Fig. 23-71). This switch can be used to select either a square wave *(A),* accelerating flow wave *(B),* or decelerating flow wave *(C).*

7 *Maximum expiratory flow.* Used to create expiratory retard. When activated, this control prolongs the length of exhalation by causing the patient to exhale against a preselected resistance (see Fig. 23-71, *D*).

8 *Sigh function.* Used to preset periodic sighs, which are

delivered when the sigh system is activated and following every 100 breaths.

NOTE: This function is activated by the same knob as the IMV control.

9 *Intermittent mandatory ventilation (IMV).* Used to set the rate at which a machine-delivered breath is delivered to the patient. In the intervals between each machine-delivered breath, the patient breathes spontaneously without ventilator support.

NOTE: The 900B delivers IMV in a manner synchronized with patient effort. If the patient has already begun a spontaneous breath when it is time for the machine breath, the machine cycle is delayed until it no longer conflicts with the patient's spontaneous breathing efforts.

10 *Continuous positive airway pressure/positive end expiratory pressure (CPAP/PEEP).* An external (spring-loaded PEEP) valve must be attached to the expiratory outlet (flap valve) of the ventilator to generate desired PEEP or CPAP levels (Fig. 23-70, *B*)

Two valves are available: 0 to 20 cm H$_2$O and 0 to 50 cm H$_2$O.

The resulting pressure is then read on the airway pressure manometer.

11 *Trig level.* This knob is used to adjust the sensitivity of the ventilator when it is operated in the assisted or IMV mode. It determines the sensitivity level (patient effort) that will be required to open the inspiratory valve to deliver a mechanically assisted or spontaneous IMV breath. It is usually set at 2 to 3 cm below the baseline working pressure.

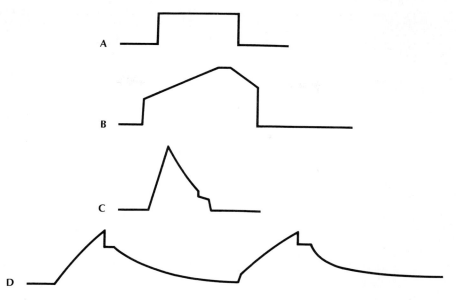

FIGURE 23-71 A through **D,** Siemens 900B and C flow waveforms. (Courtesy Siemens Corp, Union, N.J.)

12 *Oxygen percentage.* There is no specific control for setting a desired inspired oxygen (FIo$_2$) level. Desired O$_2$ concentration is adjusted on an air-oxygen blender that is attached to the lower inlet of the source gas inlet connection.

13 *Humidification.* The Siemens does not provide a humidifier. Humidity may be provided by a Cascade-type unit or other acceptable humidification system.

B *Monitors and alarms*

The Servo has monitors available to show expired minute volume and airway pressure. An optional monitor is available to provide end tidal CO$_2$ values.

C *Alarms*

1 The ventilator has visual and audible alarms to indicate high or low minute volumes in variance with preset values. These alarms are useful to detect hyperventilation, patient disconnects, cuff leaks, or high airway pressure because of kinked tubing, etc.

2 Specifications for the Siemens Servo 900B Ventilator are presented in Table 23-4.

22.3 The Siemens Servo Ventilator 900C

1 The 900C is an updated model of the 900B ventilator.

2 The operating principle is the same as that for the 900B ventilator.

3 The following features have been added to the 900C ventilator (Fig. 23-72) that were not available on the 900B model:

a Working pressure. Increased to 120 cm H$_2$O.

b Pressure support. A new mode has been added to give pressure support during spontaneous breathing in the synchronized intermittent mandatory ventilation (SIMV) mode. Once a preset pressure level has been set, it is maintained throughout the inspiratory

TABLE 23-4 Specifications for Siemens Servo Ventilator 900B

Minute volume	0.5 to more than 25 L/min
Rate	6 to 60 BPM on assist-control mode or 6 to 60 BPM divided by 2, 5, or 10 on IMV
Inspiration percent	15%, 20%, 25%, 33%, or 50% of set ventilatory cycle time established by rate control
Pause time percent	0.5%, 10%, 20%, or 30% of set ventilatory cycle time established by rate control
Sensitivity (patient triggering)	Variable from −20 to +45 cm H$_2$O pressure
Pressure limit	Adjustable up to 100 cm H$_2$O pressure
Working pressure (driving force)	Adjustable up to 100 cm H$_2$O pressure
Flow pattern switch	Square wave or sine wave
Sigh system	One sigh every 100 breaths at double tidal volume or off
Displays	
Pressure meter	−20 to 100 cm H$_2$O
Expired minute volume meter	0 to 30 L/min
Alarms	
High and low minute volume	Audio and visual
High pressure limit	Audio and visual
2-min alarm silence	Automatically reset
Electric power disconnect	Approximately 1 min audio signal

Courtesy Siemens-Elema Ventilator Systems, Elk Grove Village, Ill.

cycle. The advantage to this system is that it helps the patient to overcome tubing and other circuit resistance during spontaneous breaths.

c Respiratory rate. Adjustable between 0.5 and 120 BPM compared to a maximum of 60 BPM on the 900B.

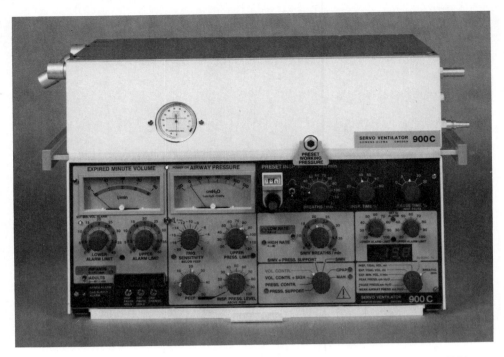

F I G U R E   2 3 - 7 2 Siemens Servo Ventilator 900C. (Courtesy Siemens Corp, Union, N.J.)

d Pressure control. The ventilator may be operated as a pressure-cycled unit by setting the mode control to "Press. Contr." and adjusting inspiratory pressure control to the desired pressure level.

e Minute volume. Increased from 25 to 30 L/min to 40 L/min.

f Inspiratory time percent. Increased from a maximum of 50% to 67% and 80%, enabling reverse I:E ratios to be delivered.

g Triggering levels. Triggering level (sensitivity) can be set at a level below the preset positive end expiratory pressure (PEEP) level.

As PEEP is changed, the triggering level is automatically compensated to maintain the same degree of inspiratory triggering effort.

h PEEP. PEEP capability is built into the unit and can be electronically adjusted from 0 to 50 cm H$_2$O.

i Monitors. Direct in-line monitoring of FIo$_2$ inspired and expired tidal volume, breaths per minute, expired minute volume, peak pause, and mean airway pressure is available by turning a selector knob.

j Alarms. A selection switch allows for expired volume alarms based on an adult or infant scale.

k Fresh gas. A flush button is available to allow injection of a completely fresh concentration of gas into the patient.

NOTE: Performance specifications for the Siemens 900C Ventilator are the same as those for the 900B model except for the changes noted in this section.

22.4 The Bennett 7200 Series Microprocessor Ventilator (Fig. 23-73)

1 The Bennett 7200 Series unit is an electrically powered, pneumatically driven, microprocessor-controlled

volume ventilator. It can be used for pediatric patients and adults but not neonates.

2 It functions primarily as a constant flow generator delivering the characteristic inspiratory square wave flow pattern (Fig. 23-74).

3 In addition, the operator may select either a *descending ramp waveform* or a *sine wave* (Fig. 23-73, *B* and *C*).

4 The ventilator offers four operational modes: controlled mechanical ventilation (CMV), synchronized intermittent mandatory ventilation (SIMV), continuous positive airway pressure (CPAP) and SIMV with pressure support (optional).

5 During CMV the ventilator functions as an assistor or a controller. As a controller the tidal volume may be machine initiated or manually cycled by the operator.

6 During SIMV, breaths may be manually (operator) generated, machine initiated, or triggered by the spontaneously breathing patient.

7 If pressure supported SIMV is used, flow accelerates to the preset pressure supported level whenever airway pressure is dropped by the spontaneously breathing patient to the sensitivity level of the triggering flow.

8 Once the preset pressure support level is reached, inspiratory flow rate is automatically adjusted to maintain this pressure level throughout inspiration.

9 Inspiration ends whenever the flow rate decreases to 5 L/min or when airway pressure reaches 1.5 cm H$_2$O above the preset pressure support level.

10 During CPAP, breaths are primarily generated by the spontaneous breathing efforts of the patient. The exception is a manually cycled breath by the operator.

11 Regardless of the mode of operation, all normal inspiratory gas flows are generated from pressurized air and oxygen. The source for these gases may be a wall

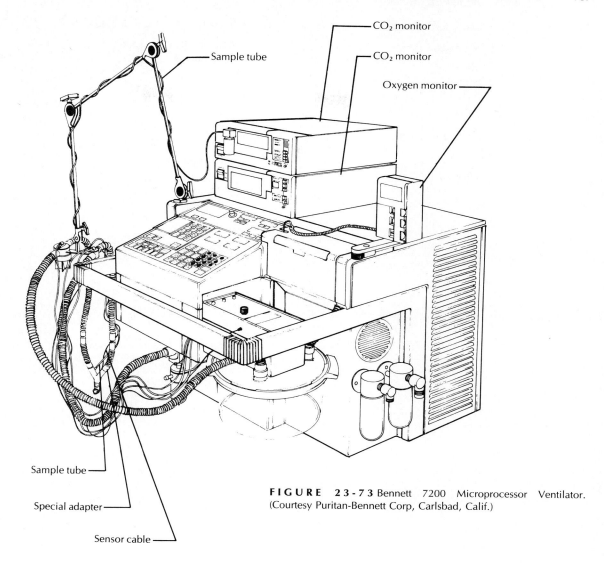

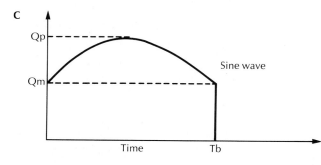

FIGURE 23-73 Bennett 7200 Microprocessor Ventilator. (Courtesy Puritan-Bennett Corp, Carlsbad, Calif.)

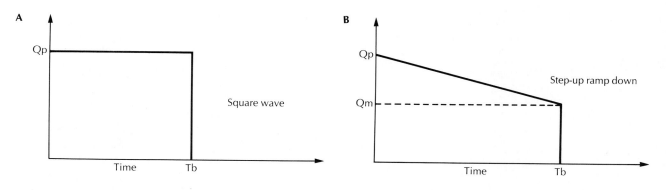

FIGURE 23-74 A through **C,** Flow patterns for Bennett 7200 Microprocessor Ventilator. (Courtesy Puritan-Bennett Corp, Carlsbad, Calif.)

TABLE 23-5 Technical data and specifications for the model 7200 microprocessor ventilator

1 PHYSICAL CHARACTERISTICS

Dimensions

Ventilator module	Height: 41.9 cm (16.5 in) Depth: 56.5 cm (22.5 in) Width: 55.9 cm (22.0 in)
Ventilator module with compressor pedestal	Height: 102 cm (40.0 in) Depth: 64.8 cm (25.5 in) Width: 55.9 cm (22.0 in)

Assembly weight

Ventilator module	50.8 kg (112 lb)
Ventilator module with pedestal	95.3 kg (210 lb)
Ventilator module with compressor pedestal	114 kg (250 lb)
Pedestal	44.5 kg (98.0 lb)
Compressor pedestal	62.6 kg (138 lb)

Shipping weight (approximate)

Ventilator module	79.4 kg (175 lb)
Ventilator module with pedestal*	
Ventilator module with compressor pedestal	172 kg (380 lb)
Pedestal	72.6 kg (160 lb)
Compressor pedestal	90.8 kg (200 lb)

2 ENVIRONMENTAL REQUIREMENTS

Altitude

Operating	3048 m (10,000 ft)
Storage/shipping	15.240 m (50,000 ft)

Environmental temperature

Operating	16° to 41° C (60° to 105° F)
Storage	−34° to 71° C (−30° to 160° F)

Relative humidity

Operating	0% to 90% noncondensing
Storage	0% to 100% noncondensing
Clearances for air circulation	Minimum of 15 cm (6.0 in) on all vertical sides

Storage requirements

Less than 200 days	None
More than 200 days	Replace batteries (2) before returning to use

3 ELECTRICAL SPECIFICATIONS

Model	Voltage (AC)	Amperes (rms)†	Frequency (Hz)
Ventilator module	115 ± 10%	2.8	60 ± 5%
	100 ± 10%	‡	60 ± 5%
	100 ± 10%	3.4	50 ± 3%
	220 ± 10%	‡	50 ± 3%
	240 ± 10%	1.6	50 ± 3%
Compressor pedestal	115 ± 10%	4.7	60 ± 5%
	100 ± 10%	‡	60 ± 5%
	100 ± 10%	6.4	50 ± 3%
	220 ± 10%	‡	50 ± 3%
	240 ± 10%	2.6	50 ± 3%

Leakage current: ventilator module with compressor pedestal	Less than 100 µg amperes at 115 V
Power cord	125 (240) V AC hospital grade, UL and CSA approved, 305 cm (10.0 ft)
Internal batteries (2)	Lead acid, 2.1 V DC typical, General Electric, sealed X-cell, 5 ampere-hour rating

4 PNEUMATIC SPECIFICATIONS

Source pressure

Oxygen (DISS 9/16-18), medical grade, dry	241 to 689 kilopascal (35 to 100 PSIG)
Air (DISS 3/4-16), medical grade, dry	241 to 689 kilopascal (35 to 100 PSIG)
Source flow: air and oxygen	190 L/min, minimum at 35 PSIG

5 VENTILATOR DATA

Gas inlet protection:

Filtering capability, air and oxygen	Particle size 0.3 µg with 99.8% efficiency
Water filter	Not intended to remove water vapor from gas. Use dry gas only.

Operator-selected parameters

Tidal volume	0.10 to 2.50 L
Respiratory rate	0.5 to 70 BPM
Peak inspiratory flow, maximum	10 to 120 L/min, operator selected 180 L/min, during spontaneous breathing
Sensitivity, inspiratory	0.5 to 20 cm H_2O below PEEP
O_2%	21% to 100%
Plateau	0.0 to 2.0 seconds
PEEP/CPAP pressure	0 to 45 cm H_2O

Operator-selected alarm thresholds

High-pressure limit	10 to 120 cm H_2O
Low inspiratory pressure	3 to 99 cm H_2O
Low PEEP/CPAP pressure	0 to 45 cm H_2O
Low exhaled tidal volume	0.00 to 2.50 L
Low exhaled minute volume	0.00 to 60.0 L
High respiratory rate	0 to 70 BPM

Operator-selected modes

CMV	
SIMV	Selects modes of ventilation
CPAP	
§	(Reserved for future enhancements)

Inspiratory flow waveforms

Square	
Descending ramp	Selects waveform for mandatory breaths
Sine	

Operator-selected submodes:

100% O_2 suction	Switches O_2% to 100 for 2 min
Manual inspiration	Commands the delivery of one mandatory breath
Manual sigh	Commands the delivery of one mandatory sigh breath (1.5 × Tidal volume)
Automatic sigh	One sigh breath every 100 breaths
Nebulizer	Activates nebulizer for 30 min

Operator-selected alarm control keys

Alarm silence	Silences audible alarm for 2 min
Alarm reset	Resets ventilator to prealarm state of alert

Alarm indicators

High-pressure limit	Airway pressure* exceeds alarm threshold

Courtesy Puritan-Bennett Corp, Carlsbad, Calif.

*The ventilator module and pedestal will be shipped separately.

†Power consumption and amperage assume the connection of a Cascade II or equivalent humidifier.

‡Values not specified at this printing.

§Airway pressure is measured at the patient Y.

Continued.

TABLE 23-5 Technical data and specifications for the model 7200 microprocessor ventilator—cont'd

5 VENTILATOR DATA—CONT'D

Low exhaled tidal volume	Tidal volume is below alarm threshold	Breath-type indicator lights (automatic)	
Low pressure O_2 inlet	Supply O_2 pressure is below 35 PSIG	Assist	
Low inspiratory pressure	Airway pressure during delivery of a mandatory breath is below alarm threshold	Spontaneous Sigh Plateau	Illuminates during appropriate breath or breath cycle
Low exhaled minute volume	Minute volume is below alarm threshold	Mean airway pressure Peak airway pressure PEEP/CPAP pressure	In cm H_2O: three digit display (maximum of two digits to the right of the decimal)
Low pressure air inlet	Supply air pressure is below 35 PSIG	Plateau pressure Respiratory rate	In breaths per minute: three digit display (maximum of one digit to the right of the decimal)
Low PEEP/CPAP pressure	Airway pressure is below alarm threshold		
High respiratory rate	Actual respiratory rate exceeds alarm threshold		
Low battery	Less than 1 hr reserve power for audible alarm	I:E ratio	Two digit display (maximum of one digit to the right of the decimal)
Apnea	No breath detected for 20 sec	Tidal volume	In liters: three digit display (maximum of two digits to the right of the decimal)
I:E	Actual value greater than 1:1	Minute volume	
Exhalation valve leak	Gas flow past the exhalation flow. Sensor during breath delivery is 50 ml or 10% of delivered volume, whichever is greater	Spontaneous minute volume Safety modes of operation Apnea ventilation Backup ventilator Disconnect ventilation	Temporary ventilatory support with factory preset parameters
Power disconnect alarm	AC power to the ventilator is interrupted	Safety valve open	Patient breaths room air unassisted by ventilator
Alarm summary display Ventilator inoperative (red) Alarm (red) Caution (yellow) Backup ventilator (red) Safety valve open (red) Normal (blue)	Illuminates to indicate ventilator status	Self-diagnostics Power-on-self test (POST) Extended self-test (EST)	Automatic after power on (10 sec duration) Operator-selected (2-3 min duration)
Operator-selected or monitored parameters		Ongoing checks	Automatic, continuous during ventilator operation
Airway pressure	Continuous display, breath-by-breath	I:E ratio check	Automatic, with parameter changes
Exhaled volume	Continuous display, breath-by-breath	Lamp test Output signals Remote nurse's call Analog signals for pressure and flow	Operator selected For remote indication of alarm For display of parameters on separate recording device

piping system or, in the case of air, an internal compressor (optional).

12 The operating pressure for the ventilator is 35 to 100 PSIG for both air and oxygen, resulting in a flow rate of 190 L/min unrestricted flow.

13 The peak inspiratory flow rate during CMV is 120 L/min and 180 L/min during spontaneous breathing.

14 Tidal volumes may be adjusted from 0.10 to 2.50 L at rates of 0.5 to 70 BPM and maximum pressure limits of 120 cm H_2O.

15 Both CPAP and positive end expiratory pressure (PEEP) are created by restricting deflation of the exhalation balloon that covers the exhalation port of the patient breathing circuit.

These elevated baseline pressures are adjusted by turning a knob from 0 to 45 cm H_2O.

16 Technical data and specifications for the model 7200 microprocessor ventilator are presented in Table 23-5, which points out this model's many control, monitoring, and safety features.

17 Mechanically, it is similar to other ventilators in that the tidal volume and variations to the pressure and flow patterns are available on other units.

18 The uniqueness of this device is the electronic memory and control of ventilator functions by the microprocessor.

For example, gas flow through the ventilator is controlled by the coordinated operation of seven different solenoids (electromechanical valves).

Once the operator has set the waveform, tidal volume, respiratory rate, peak inspiratory flow, plateau, and oxygen concentration, the microprocessor automatically regulates the opening and closing of the *proportional solenoid valves* to deliver the specified tidal volume. The microprocessor then continuously monitors gas flow during subsequent breaths and converts it to a measurement at body temperature, ambient pressure, saturated with water (BTPS), with 100% humidity. This flow is then compared to actual flow, and adjustments are automatically made as needed to provide the preselected tidal volume.

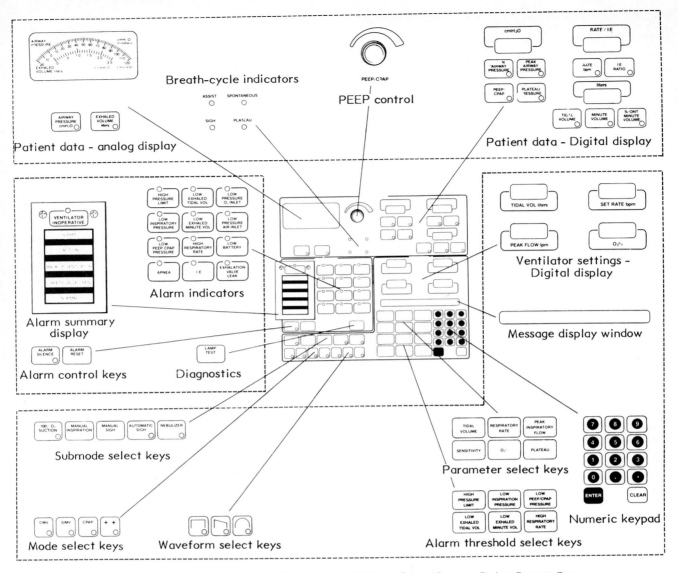

FIGURE 23-75 Control panel of the Bennett 7200 ventilator. (Courtesy Puritan-Bennett Corp, Carlsbad, Calif.)

19 Other functions controlled by the microprocessor include:
  a The entire pneumatic system that, through the proportional solenoid valves, mixes and shapes inspired gases
  b The correction circuit that converts delivered gases to BTPS (discussed in no. *15*)
  c Memory storage of operational data
  d Monitoring alarm and digital and message display systems
20 An example of the safety feature incorporated into this unit includes the microprocessor self-testing systems that automatically search for any operational problems and activate relevant corrective or safety overrides. These systems are called Power-on self-test (POST), extended self-test (EST), Lamp test ongoing checks, I:E ratio check, and nebulizer flow check. Both POST and EST should be used to determine whether the ventilator is operational.

If a major problem is detected, the ventilator automatically switches to a standby mode until the difficulty is overcome.

The extensive options offered by this ventilator are presented in Fig. 23-75, which shows the control panel.

It is beyond the scope of this work to discuss further details about this ventilator. Additional information can be obtained by contacting the manufacturer.

22.5 The Ohmeda CPU1 ventilator (Figs. 23-76, 23-77, 23-78) and Advent ventilator (Fig. 23-79).

1 The Ohmeda CPU1 ventilator (distributed in the United States by Ohio Medical Products*) is another example of a ventilator that is microprocessor controlled.
2 The CPU1 is powered by air and oxygen from an external blender connected to 50 PSIG gas sources. The

*Ohmeda, A Division of The BOC Group, Inc, Madison, Wis.

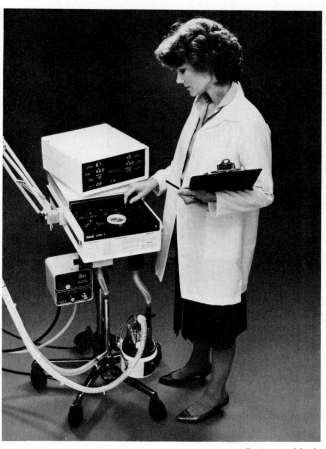

A

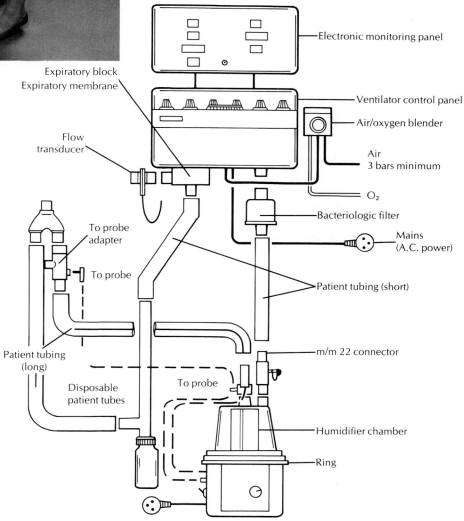

FIGURE 23-76 A, Medishield CPU1 ventilator showing accessories and tubing hook-up. **B,** Detailed listing of major external components of Medishield CPU1 ventilator. (Courtesy Ohmeda, A Division of The BOC Group, Inc, Madison, Wis.)

B

Electronic monitoring panel

Expiratory block
Expiratory membrane

Ventilator control panel

Air/oxygen blender

Flow transducer

Air
3 bars minimum

O_2

Bacteriologic filter

To probe adapter

Mains
(A.C. power)

To probe

Patient tubing (short)

Patient tubing (long)

m/m 22 connector

Disposable patient tubes

To probe

Humidifier chamber

Ring

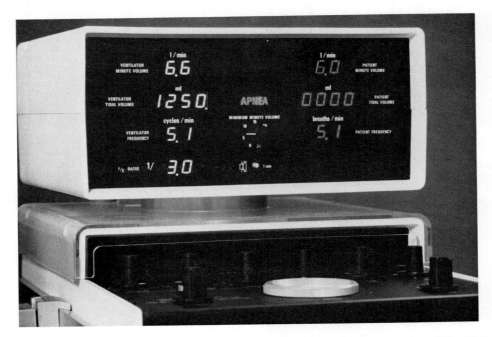

F I G U R E 2 3 - 7 7 CPU1 electronic monitoring panel. (Courtesy Ohmeda, A Division of The BOC Group, Inc, Madison, Wis.)

ventilator can be operated as an assistor or controller and has built-in continuous positive airway pressure (CPAP), positive end expiratory pressure (PEEP), intermittent mandatory ventilation (IMV), and synchronized intermittent mandatory ventilation (SIMV) capabilities.

3 The unique pneumatic control system enables the patient to breath spontaneously from a demand valve in all ventilator modes. As a controller, the ventilator functions as a time-cycled, constant flow generator or as a pressure cycle unit. As a constant flow generator, it produces a characteristic square wave inspiratory flow pattern.

4 The pneumatic functions of the ventilator are controlled by six solenoids operated by the microprocessor.

5 This logic enables the ventilator to compare exhaled gases to a preset minute volume and to automatically adjust the cycling frequency to provide the preset (mandated) minute ventilation.

6 Basically the functions of the microprocessor are:
To receive signals from the command circuit, the expiratory flow transducers, the inspiratory flow detector, and the airway pressure limit detector and to generate the respiratory cycle in response to this information. In addition, the microprocessor controls all monitoring and alarm functions.

7 As a safety feature it conducts internal status checks on itself and the pneumatic system to detect any problems and to warn the operator.

8 The simplicity of assembly, operation, and service of this ventilator, combined with sophisticated, but functional alarms, makes this a good example of one of the new generation products that uses a microprocessor to make the operator's job easier and the patient safer.

9 Figs. 23-77 and 23-78 show the CPU1 control panel and electronic monitoring module.

Note the relatively small number of controls and monitoring readouts because of microprocessor control. This approach is functional and practical and reduces confusion caused by more complicated panels.

The ventilator is housed in two cases mounted one above the other. The upper case contains the microprocessor and associated electronics together with a cooling fan and provides the digital display of ventilation parameters together with alarm displays. The control for setting the minimum minute volume threshold is also contained on this front panel, together with the alarm mute button. At the rear of this case are the cooling fan air intake with its protective filter, an elapsed time meter and the main ON/OFF switch. The lower case contains the pneumatic components together with their associated switching solenoids and controls. Situated at the rear of this case are a system pressure gauge, calibration potentiometers, battery test button, and option selector switches. At the underside of the case are the supply gas input hose, a socket for the power supply to the humidifier, patient gas outlet, and expiratory block. There is also a tubing nipple to provide driving gas to power a nebulizer.

a The box on the opposite page presents performance specifications for the CPU1.

b Additional details on this unit can be obtained by contacting the distributor.

10 Currently the Ohmeda Advent TM ventilator is in the process of being introduced. This ventilator will incorporate the best features of the CPU1 ventilator plus new features not included on the CPU1 (Fig. 23-79).

11 Features and specifications of the new Ohmeda Advent ventilator are presented in the box on p. 744.

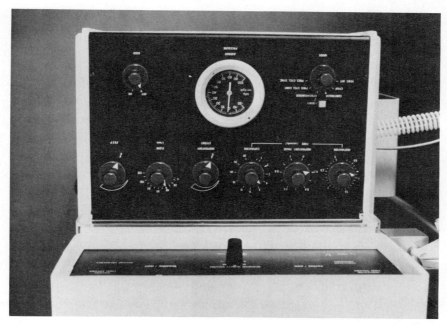

FIGURE 23-78 Looking down at top of CPU1 control panel. (Courtesy Ohmeda, A Division of The BOC Group, Inc, Madison, Wis.)

Performance specifications for the CPU1 ventilator

MODES OF OPERATION

- Spontaneous respiration with continuous positive airway pressure (CPAP)
- Controlled ventilation with adjustable I:E ratio and plateau
- Assisted ventilation with constant tidal volume
- Intermittent mandatory ventilation (IMV)
- Synchronized intermittent mandatory ventilation (SIMV)
- Pressure cycled with imposed expiratory time
- Pressure cycled assistance with patient triggering
- Programmed mandatory minute volume (MMV)

SUPPLY

O_2 and air at 300-600 kilopascals (KPa) (O_2 + N_2O optional) 100-240 V-50 or 60 Hz

CONTROLS

- Mode selection switch
- Inspiration time (T_I) 0.3-3.0 sec
- Inspiratory pause time (T_P) (plateau) 0-1.0 sec
- Expiration time (T_E) 0.6-30 sec
- Inspiratory flow (3-120 L/min
- Inspiratory effort 0-10 cm H_2O
- PEEP 0-30 cm H_2O
- Sigh (manual or every 100 breaths)
- Aiway pressure 5-100 cm H_2O (when pressure cycled mode selected)
- Mandatory minute volume (when MMV mode selected)
- Inspired O_2 mixture (FIo_2) 21% to 100%
- Temperature of humidified gas delivered to patient

CALCULATED DISPLAY (DERIVED FROM CONTROL SETTINGS)

- Frequency 0.5-66 cycles/min
- I:E ratio 1:0.2-1:99
- Tidal volume 20-6000 ml
- Minute volume 1-50 L/min

MONITORED DISPLAYS (MEASURED)

- Frequency 0.1-99 c/min
- Tidal volume 25-6000 ml
- Minute volume 0.1-99 L/min

ALARMS

- Apnea (includes patient disconnect)
- Minimum volume 0-30 L/min
- Maximum airway pressure 5-100 cm H_2O
- Comprehensive alarms for machine/patient circuit faults (see text)

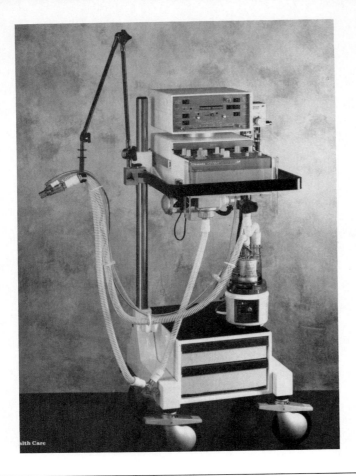

FIGURE 23-79 Ohmeda Advent ventilator. (Courtesy Ohmeda, Columbia, Md.)

Specifications for Ohmeda Advent ventilator

The Ohmeda Advent ventilator combines advanced concepts of user and patient friendliness into one highly flexible package capable of ventilating a full range of adult and pediatric patients.

The ventilator incorporates low work-of-breathing by:

- Proximal airway pressure sensing
- Very short response time to patient effort
- High flow capability
- Low resistance expiratory valve

Pressure support is available to augment spontaneous tidal volumes.

The "message window" concept enhances user friendliness. It provides one place to look for all alarm messages and monitoring information, including such enhanced diagnostic data as:

- Mean airway pressure
- Spontaneous inspiratory flow rate
- Percent spontaneous minute volume
- Auto PEEP level

The Advent ventilator provides all of the below modes plus pressure support and room for future expandibility:

- CPAP
- SIMV
- Mandatory minute volume (MMV)
- Assist/control
- Pressure control (with assist)

CONTROLS

- Modes: Assist-control, SIMV, MMV, CPAP, pressure control (with assist)
- Tidal volume: 70-2000 ml
- Minute volume: 1-85 L/min
- Compliance compensation: on monitor
- Machine rate: 0.5-85 breaths/min
- Sensitivity: −0.5-−10 hPa (cm H_2O)
- Peak flow: 10-150 L/min
- Waveforms: square and decelerating
- Airway pressure: −20-120 hPa (cm H_2O)
- PEEP: Off-30 hPA (cm H_2O)
- Pressure support: Off-30 hPa (cm H_2O) above PEEP level
- Inspiratory pause: 0-1 sec
- Inspiratory time (in pressure control with assist): 0.3-4 sec
- Sigh rate: 1 each 100 breaths
- Sigh volume: Vt × 1.5
- Manual sigh: yes
- Manual breath: yes
- Expiratory hold: yes
- Nebulization program: yes (internal/external even during spontaneous ventilation)

Patient monitoring: minimum and maximum airway pressure, disconnection, apnea, minimum minute volume, low spontaneous Vt, high respiratory rate.

- I/E limit: yes
- Apnea delay: 30 sec or 45 sec with backup ventilation
- Machine monitoring: Program, gas, mains supply, expiratory valve leak

INPUTS

- Electrical: 100, 120, 127, 220, 240 volts 50 or 60 Hz
- Pneumatic: 350 ± 70 kPa (52 ± 10 PSIG)

OUTPUTS

- Remote humidifier supply
- Remote synchronization signal for 2 Advents: optional
- Remote alarm: optional
- RS 232 communication: optional
- Monitor: available

Dimensions of the ventilator on the trolley:

- D: 690 mm (27 in)
- W: 620 mm (24.4 in)
- H: 1600 mm (62.9 in)
- Weight of the ventilator without accessory: 27 kg (59.5 lb)
- Weight of the ventilator with accessories on trolley: 80 kg (176.3 lb)

22.6 Hamilton medical veolar ventilator (Fig. 23-80)

1 The Hamilton Veolar ventilator is still another example of a new or third generation–type device.

2 Like the Bennett 7200 series, the Siemens Servo 900 series and the BEAR 5, it uses electromechanical valves (solenoids) to provide various ventilation modes, flow patterns, and monitoring and alarm options.

3 It primarily differs from the Bennett and Siemens Servo ventilators in that it offers an option called minimum minute volume with pressure support.

4 The minimum minute ventilation mode on the Veolar ventilator enables the ventilator to monitor the patient's exhaled ventilation and to supplement the patient's efforts with varying levels of pressure support. This pressure support is automatically adjusted until the patient's spontaneous minute volume meets or exceeds a preset minimum level.

5 The BEAR 5 ventilator offers a similar type of mandatory minute volume mode called augmented mandatory minute ventilation (AMV). AMV can be used with or without pressure support and with assisted or mandated ventilation modes.

6 Specifications for the Hamilton Veolar ventilator are included in the box below.

Specifications for Hamilton Veolar ventilator

CONTROLS

- Modes — Assist/control, SIMV, spontaneous, minimum minute ventilation, pressure control ventilation—with or without spontaneous breathing and pressure support
- Special functions — Single breath, reservoir tank flush, medication nebulizer
- CMV frequency — 5-60 breaths/min
- SIMV frequency — 0.5-30 breaths/min
- Tidal volume — 20-2000 ml
- I:E ratio — 1:9 to 4:1
- Plateau/pause — 0-8 sec
- Peak flow — to 180 L/min (indirectly adjusted)
- Flow patterns — Sine, square, decelerating, accelerating, and 50% decelerating, 50% accelerating modified sine
- Sensitivity — Off or 1-15 cm H_2O below baseline; response time <100 msec
- Peak pressure — 110 cm H_2O
- PEEP/CPAP — 0-50 cm H_2O
- Pressure support — 0-50 cm H_2O
- Oxygen — 21%-100%
- MMV range — 1-25 L/min
- Alarm loudness — 60-68 dBA
- Pressure control — Up to 99 CM H_2O

PATIENT-MONITORED INFORMATION

- Patient expiratory time and I:E ratio
- Respiratory frequency: total and spontaneous*
- Tidal volume: inspired and expired (at airway)
- Expired minute volume*
- Pressure: maximum, mean, PEEP and on-line
- Static lung-thorax compliance*
- Airflow resistance: inspiratory* and expiratory*
- Inspired oxygen concentration
- Inspiratory flow, mandatory and spontaneous

*Trended over 15 min and 2 hr

ALARMS

Operator adjustable alarms
- High respiratory frequency — 10-70 breaths/min
- High pressure — 10-110 cm H_2O
- Low minute volume — 0.2-50 L/min
- High minute volume — 0.2-50 L/min
- Low oxygen concentration — 18% to 103%
- High oxygen concentration — 18% to 103%

Nonadjustable alarm
- Apnea — 15 sec
- Fail to cycle — 20 sec
- Disconnection — 2 breaths
- Tidal volume mismatch — 3 breaths
- Flow out of range — >180 L/min
- Oxygen/air supply pressure — <29 PSI (2 bar)

Set trigger; turn flowsensor; power supply; dysfunction

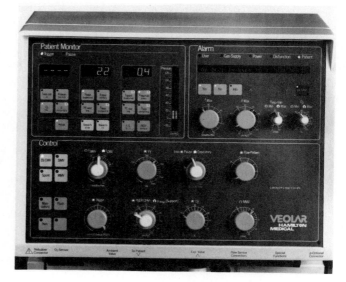

FIGURE 23-80 Hamilton Medical Veolar ventilator for pediatric and adult patients. (Courtesy Hamilton Medical, Reno, Nev.)

Courtesy Hamilton Medical, Inc, Reno, Nev.

Specifications for Hamilton Amadeus adult/pediatric ventilator

CONTROLS

- Modes   (S)CMV (ASSIST/CONTROL), SIMV, SPONT
- Special functions   Calibration: oxygen, flow, tightness test, O_2flush
- CMV frequency   5-120 BPM
- SIMV frequency   0.5-60 BPM
- Tidal volume   20-2000 ml
- I:E ratio (% cycle time)   1:9-4:1
- Pause   0-8 sec
- Peak flow   to 180 L/min (indirectly adjusted)
- Flow patterns   Two patterns user selectable
- Sensitivity   off of 1-10 cm H_2O below baseline; response time <100 msec
- Peak pressure   110 cm H_2O
- PEEP/CPAP   0-50 cm H_2O
- Pressure support (p_{insp})   0-100 cm H_2O
- Oxygen   21% to 100%
- Alarm loudness   65 dBA

PATIENT MONITORED INFORMATION

- Rate
- Expired tidal volume at airway
- Expired minute volume
- Pressure: maximum, PEEP, on-line
- Static lung-thorax compliance
- Inspiratory airway resistance
- Inspired oxygen concentration
- Inspiratory peak flow

ALARMS

Operator adjustable alarms
- High rate   20-130 BPM
- High pressure   10-110 cm H_2O
- Low exp. minute volume   0.2-50 L/min
- High exp. minute volume   0.2-50 L/min
- Oxygen limits ± 5%   16%-105% O_2 or off

Nonadjustable alarms
- High pressure
- Disconnection   2 breaths
- Apnea   15 sec
- Exp. minute volume
- Oxygen concentration
- High rate
- Power
- Gas supply   <2 bar (29 PSI)
- Inoperative
- User alarms: Flow out of range   >180 L/min
            Set trigger
            Flow sensor

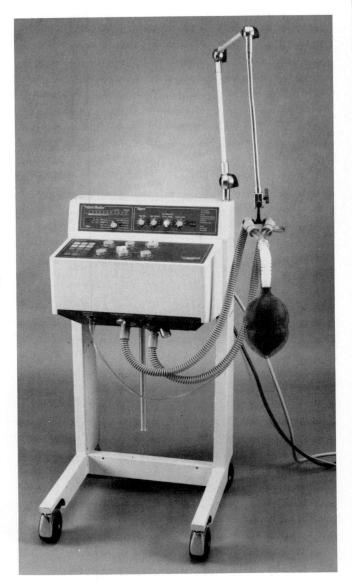

FIGURE 23-81 Hamilton Amadeus intensive care ventilator for pediatric and adult patients. (Courtesy Hamilton Medical, Reno, Nev.)

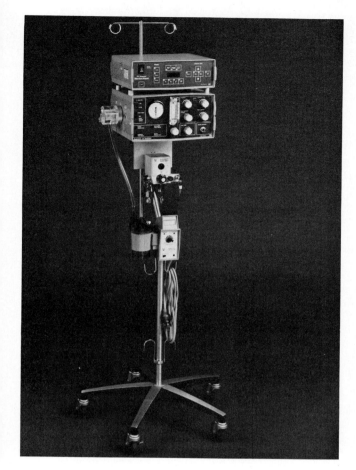

FIGURE 23-82 Babybird 2A ventilator. (Courtesy Medical Products Division/3M, St Paul, Minn.)

22.7 Hamilton Amadeus adult/pediatric ventilator

1 The Amadeus was designed for use in intensive care (Fig. 23-81) on pediatric and adult patients.
2 It was introduced in December, 1988, as an advanced model to the Veolar ventilator presented in Unit 22.6. Specifications for the Amadeus ventilator are presented in the box on p. 746.

22.8 Neonatal ventilators

The development of neonatology as a medical specialty has resulted in the availability of a complete new technology designed specifically for neonates.

In addition to the ventilators already mentioned for use with adults and neonates, the ventilators discussed in the following units are used exclusively for newborn infants.

Each ventilator and its performance specifications are presented so that the reader can compare the technical similarities and differences in these units.

22.9 Babybird 2 ventilator (Fig. 23-82)

The Babybird 2A ventilator is an electronically controlled, pneumatically powered, time-cycled, and pressure limited continuous flow ventilator with controlled mechanical ventilation (CMV), intermittent mandatory ventilation (IMV), and continuous positive airway pressure (CPAP) capabilities. Like its predecessor, the Babybird, its princi-

---

Specifications for Babybird 2A ventilator (model 8900A)

An electronically controlled, pneumatically powered, time-cycled and pressure limited continuous flow ventilator that provides three basic support modes to ventilate critically ill babies: CMV (controlled mechanical ventilation), IMV (intermittent mandatory ventilation), and CPAP (continuous positive airway pressure).

DIMENSIONS
- H: 7½ in
- W: 12¾ in
- D: 11¾ in

WEIGHT
- 15 lb (6.8 kg)

POWER REQUIREMENTS
- Ventilator — 115 V/60 Hz or 220 V/50 Hz
- Current leakage — Less than 100 microamperes
- Circuit breaker (fused) — 1 amp

PARAMETERS REGULATED
- Inspiratory time — 0.1-2.5 sec
- Expiratory time — 0.2-30 sec
- Cycling frequency — OFF to 2-150/BPM
- Peak inspiratory pressure — 0-80 cm H_2O ± 10% at 10 L/min
- Flow — 3 to 30 L/min ± 10%
- Patient overpressure — 15 cm H_2O to 80 cm H_2O ± 10%
- Elevated baseline: PEEP/ CPAP — 0-30 cm H_2O % 10 L/min
- Source gas pressure
  - Oxygen — 45-55 PSIG (clean and dry)
  - Air — 45-55 PSIG (clean and dry)
- Inspiratory time limit — 4.25 sec

ALARMS
- Source pressure low
- Incompatible timer setting
- Power failure, electrical
- Inspiratory time
- Babybird 2A ventilator gas consumption for pneumatics

VISUAL AND AUDIBLE
- Factor preset at 38 + 2 PSIG
- Factory preset at 0.2 sec expiratory time
- Loss of 115 V/60 Hz or 220 V/50 Hz
- Factory preset at 4.25 sec 16 L/min

Bird Products/3M, 3M Center 225-55, St. Paul, MN 55144.

---

ples of operation are consistent with IMV. In this mode the operator must select mandatory machine breaths that will assume physiologic arterial blood gas levels. Both inspiratory and expiratory time are adjustable, giving the operator a wide range of breathing frequencies and I:E ratios.

The primary difference between the Babybird and the newer model Babybird 2A ventilator is the extensive electronic monitoring/alarm package and the calibrated controls for faster, more accurate operation by inexperienced or unfamiliar operators.

More details on the performance of the Babybird 2A ventilator are presented in the box above.

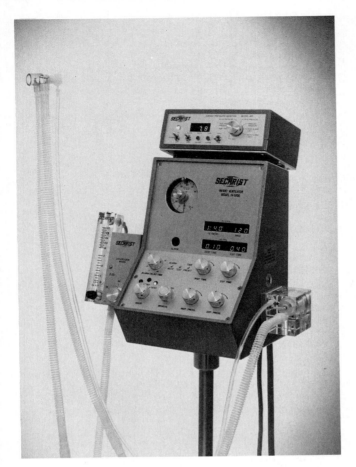

FIGURE 23-83 Sechrist infant ventilator model IV-100B. (Courtesy Sechrist Industries, Inc, Medical Products Division, Anaheim, Calif.)

22.10 Sechrist model IV-100B ventilator (Fig. 23-83)

The Sechrist ventilator is a time-cycled, pressure limited, pneumatically powered, fluidic and electronically controlled ventilator with CMV, IMV, and CPAP capabilities. It incorporates a microprocessor to open and close a solenoid valve that supplies inspiratory gases.

Like most time-cycled units, both inspiratory and expiratory times can be independently controlled, producing rates to 200 breaths/min with standard and review I:E ratios.

The microprocessor, in conjunction with opening and closing of the exhalation valve, gives the ventilator waveform modification capabilities of either a square wave or modified sine wave. The model 600 Airway Pressure Monitor may be added as an option to graphically display the patient's spontaneous breathing along with the ventilator pressure waveform.

This feature enables the operator to more easily synchronize the ventilator to the patient and to establish the correct flow rate to minimize the patient's work of breathing.

Additional details on the performance of the Sechrist ventilator are provided in the box above.

Performance specifications of the Sechrist model IV-100B ventilator*

- Recommended applications: neonate, pediatric ventilation
- Flow: 0 to 32 L/min, flush 40 L/min, FIo$_2$: 21-1.00
- Mode: OFF, CPAP, VENT
- Inspiratory time: 0.10-2.90 sec
- Expiratory time: 0.20-60.0 sec
- I:E ratio: 14.5:1-1:600 (readout 1:0.1-1:99)
- Rate: 1-200 BPM
- Expiratory pressure: −2-15 cm H$_2$O
- Inspiratory pressure: 7-70 cm H$_2$O
- Manual breath: yes
- Alarm: independent from microprocessor; low airway pressure, leaks, patient disconnect, fail to cycle, source gas failure, power failure (battery backup), apnea, and prolonged inspiration
- Alarm delay time: 3-60 sec
- Alarm mute: 25 sec ± 5 sec
- Safety pressure pop-off: yes (adjustable)
- Indicators: Inspiratory time, expiratory time, I:E ratio, mode selection, alarm, and alarm set point
- Manual test: checks microprocessor function, displays, alarm function
- Safety auto lock-out circuit: Yes, inspiratory phase terminated at 4 sec even if microprocessor fails
- Microprocessor self-test: yes
- Timing preset: Yes
- Dimensions: H: 13 in (33.02 cm)
  W: 14 in (35.56 cm)
  D: 9 in (23.00 cm)
- Weight: Model IV-100 B-F
  Net   16 lb (7.13 kg)
  Shipping 41 lb (18.6 kg)
    Model IV-100B-M
  Net   22 lb (10.00 kg)
  Shipping 46 lb (20.90 kg)
- Power requirements: 117 VAC 50/60 Hz, circuit breaker protected, 3-wire SJT power control provided, hospital-grade plug, current leakage less than 20 microamps when tested per UL 544
- Overseas voltage requirements available

Courtesy Sechrist Industries, Inc, Anaheim, Calif.
*Specifications are subject to change.

22.11 Bourns BEAR Cub Infant Ventilator BP 2001 (Fig. 23-84)

The Bourns BEAR Cub Ventilator BP 2001 is an updated version of the BEAR BP-200 Ventilator. It is a time-cycled, pressure-limited controller with CPAP, PEEP, CMV, and IMV modes.

It offers continuous gas flows of 3 to 30 L/min and cycling frequencies from 1 to 150 breaths/min with inspiratory times of 0.1 to 3.0 sec.

The monitoring and alarm system is extensive, offering digital displays and audible signals for 19 different parameters. All controls are calibrated and clearly labeled, making it an easy ventilator to operate.

Other details regarding its performance capabilities are presented in Table 23-6.

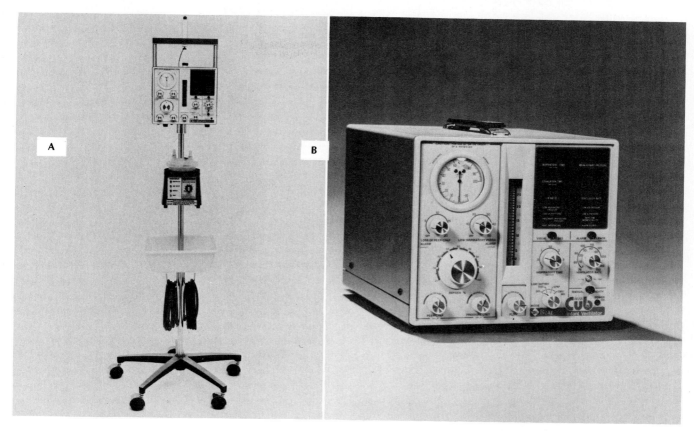

FIGURE 23-84 A, Bourns BEAR Cub Infant Ventilator BP 2001 showing stand humidifier and accessory tray. **B,** Closeup of BP 2001 showing control panel with control knobs, flowmeter, and manometer. (Courtesy Bear Medical Systems, Inc, Riverside, Calif.)

22.12 High-frequency ventilation

High-frequency ventilation (HFV) is still an evolving technology that has been used primarily in rigidly controlled laboratory and clinical studies. Its specific clinical applications are still to be defined and documented.

High-frequency mechanical ventilation refers to the use of mechanical ventilators that can deliver cycling rates greater than 60 breaths/min.

A History

The documented history of HFV can be traced back to 1949, when James L. Whittenberger, MD, worked with panting dogs.

As early as 1954, Virginia Apgar, MD, and Richard Day, MD, tried high-frequency ventilation on newborns with atelectasis.

In the early 1970s the Swedes experimented with reverse I:E ratios for the ventilation of neonates.

More recently Kim Bland, MD, et al., reported a 92% survival rate with the use of HFV on neonates with respiratory distress syndrome (RDS).

In 1980 and 1981 Forrest Bird, MD, expanded the concept of HFV to include intermittent percussive ventilation with monopulsing and counterpulsing intrapulmonary percussion on adults and neonates. This approach not only provides alveolar ventilation but it also causes internal percussion to the airway to promote clearance of secretions.

B Terms/definitions

Some terms and definitions that are currently used to describe HFV and its application include:

1 Wave: complete respiratory cycle
2 Amplitude: size of the wave (force)
3 Frequency: number of waves passing a given point in 1 sec
4 HFPPV/HFV: high-frequency positive pressure ventilation
5 cps: cycles per second (rate)
   Hz: Hertz, cycling frequency (one wave/sec)

C HFV described

1 High-frequency ventilation is a generic term describing the operational performance of ventilators that deliver *rapid* respirator rates at *small* tidal volumes.
2 The exact cycling rates that qualify a device as a high-frequency ventilator are still undecided. The Food and Drug Administration (FDA) has established *150 breaths per minute* (BPM) to qualify a ventilator's performance as high frequency.

TABLE 23-6 Performance characteristics and specifications of the BEAR Cub model BP 2001 ventilator

VENTILATOR

Controls

Mode	OFF, battery/lamp test, CPAP, CMV/IMV
Manual breath pushbutton	Permits delivery of a single breath in the CPAP mode only
Rate	1-150 BPM (dual scale 1-75 and 76-150)
BPM range toggle switch	Selects either 1-75 or 76-150 BMP range
Inspiratory time	0.1-3.0 sec
Pressure limit	0-72 cm H_2O
PEEP/CPAP	−2-20 cm H_2O
Flow	3-30 L/min
Oxygen percentage	21%-100%
Low inspiratory pressure alarm	OFF: 50 cm H_2O
Loss of PEEP/CPAP alarm	OFF: 20 cm H_2O
Alarm loudness	Adjustable, minimum to maximum (65-75 dB)
Alarm silence pushbutton	30 sec
Visual reset pushbutton	Clears visual alarms and alerts

Indicators

Power ON	Indicates electrical power to the ventilator has been turned on
Alarm	Low inspiratory pressure loss of PEEP/CPAP
	Prolonged inspiratory pressure ventilator inoperative
Alert	Low oxygen pressure
	Low air pressure
	Rate/time incompatibility
	Alarm silence

Displays

Inspiratory time (digital)	0-9.99 sec*
Exhalation time (digital)	0-99.9 sec*
I:E ratio (digital)	1:0.0-1.99*
Ventilator rate (digital)	0-199 BPM*
Mean airway pressure (digital)	0-99 cm H_2O*
Flow (flowmeter)	3-30 L/min
Proximal airway pressure (gauge)	−10 to 100 cm H_2O
Air and O_2 inlet pressure (gauges)	0-100 PSIG (0-7 kg/cm^2) or
	0-160 PSIG (0-11 kg/cm^2)
Elapsed time (meter)	0-99, 999.9 hr

Remote monitor

Proximal airway pressure	
Analog output jack	BNC type connector, 10 mv/cm H_2O scale, 0-100 cm H_2O range

Preset values

Minimum exhalation time	0.25 sec
Maximum working pressure	87 cm H_2O (measured at the "To Humidifier" outlet)

Alarms, alerts, and subambient pressure relief valve

Low inspiratory pressure	Audible and visual alarm
Loss of PEEP/CPAP	Audible and visual alarm
Prolonged inspiratory pressure	Audible and visual alarm
Ventilator inoperative	Audible and visual alarm, includes:
	Fail to cycle
	Electrical power failure/disconnect
	High/low inspiratory time
	Panel control malfunction
	Prolonged solenoid ON time
	Timing circuit failure
Low air pressure	Audible and visual alert
Low O_2 pressure	Audible and visual alert
Excessive inverse I:E ratio	Audible and visual alert
Rate/time incompatibility	Visual alert
Alarm silence	Visual alert
Subambient pressure relief valve	Allows the patient to breathe room air provided he can overcome the resistance of the patient circuit and −2.0 cm H_2O for the subambient pressure relief valve should a total gas failure occur

Inputs

Electrical inputs	117 VAC, 60 Hz, less than 50 watts. Foreign models available—specify voltage and frequency.
	3 conductor 18 AWG SJT power cord
	0.5 amp circuit breaker
	Current leakage less than 100 microamperes

Courtesy Bear Medical Systems, Inc, Riverside, Calif.

*Indicates potential range of display, limited by minimum/maximum ventilator parameters.

Continued.

TABLE 23-6 Performance characteristics and specifications of the BEAR Cub model BP 2001 ventilator—cont'd

Inputs—cont'd

Pneumatic inputs	30-75 PSIG air (2-5 kg/cm$_2$) and 30-75 psig O$_2$ (2-5 kg/cm^2) at 46 L/min
	DISS connections (male thread)

Miscellaneous

9 VDC output jacks	Two 9 VDC, 200 ma each or 400 ma total, 3-pin female connector. Protected by a ½ A, 250 V fuse.

Physical dimensions, weights, and shipping information

Ventilator dimensions	10 high × 10 in wide × 14 in long (25.4 cm × 25.4 cm × 35.6 cm)
Overall dimensions	52 high × 27" wide × 26 in long (132 cm × 68.6 cm × 66 cm)
Ventilator weight	27 lb (12.3 kg)
Shipping weight, ventilator	30 lb (13.6 kg)
Accessories weight	24 lb (10.9 kg)
Shipping weight accessories	26 lb (11.8 kg)
Net weight of complete system	51 lb (23.2 kg)
Net shipping weight of complete system	56 lb (25.5 kg)

HUMIDIFIER, INFANT, BEAR MEDICAL LS460

Control module

Power requirements	117 VAC, 60 Hz
	Foreign models available—specify voltage and frequency
Input power	107 watts
Current leakage	20 ua max (ventilator mounted)
	30 ua max (table, slide, pole mounted)
Power cord (table, slide, pole mounted)	3 wire, 18 gauge, SJT, light gray, 10 foot, with hospital grade plug
Fuse rating	1.25 amp, fast blow
Water temperature range	75° F (24° C) to 170° F (77° C)
Warmup time	10-30 min
Air temperature regulation	±2° F at steady state conditions
Inoperative indicator	Occurs within 8 sec of a heater or control module malfunction
Indicators (visual)	WAIT (white)
	NORMAL (green)
	ADD WATER (amber)
	INOPERATIVE (red)
Overall dimensions	7 in × 7 in × 7 in (17.8 cm × 17.8 cm × 17.8 cm)
Weight	6 lb (2.7 kg)

Infant humidifier cover and jar assembly

Reservoir capacity	180 ml at FULL line
	60 ml at ADD line
Usable volume	120 ml
Compliance	0.12 ml/cm H$_2$O at FULL line
	0.25 ml/cm H$_2$O at ADD line
Flow resistance	0.1 cm H$_2$O/1/sec at FULL line
(at 30 L/min [0.5 L/sec])	Negligible at ADD line
Overall dimensions	5½ in × 3½ in (14.0 cm × 8.9 cm)
Weight	¾ lb (0.34 kg)

Control module and infant humidifier cover and jar assembly

Overall dimensions	7 in × 7 in × 10½ in (17.8 cm × 17.8 cm × 26.7 cm)
Weight	6¾ lb (3.04 kg)

360 DEGREE ALARM LIGHT (OPTIONAL)

Electrical inputs	9 VDC, 150 ma, provided by 9 VDC output jack on rear of ventilator
Visibility	20 feet minimum
Bulb rating	T 3¼, bayonet base, 14 V industry #1815
Overall dimensions	5 in × .87 in × .87 in (12.7 cm × 2.2 cm × 2.2 cm)
Weight	5 oz (0.14 kg)
Shipping weight	1 lb (0.45 kg)

ACCESSORY MOUNTING RAIL ASSEMBLY (OPTIONAL)

Mounting clamps	Compatible with Fairfield or Eastern type
Maximum accessory weight	Rail is not designed to support greater than 10 lb
Maximum accessory size	Rail is not designed to support items that extend more than 12 in above the ventilator cover or extend beyond the sides of the ventilator cover.
Overall dimensions	Rail, 11 in × 1⅛ in (27.9 cm × 2.8 cm)
Weight	1.5 lb (0.68 kg)
Shipping weight	2 lb (0.91 kg)

Specifications for the P-7 scanner monitor/alarm models 9000 and 9900C

An electrically powered, microprocessor-controlled monitor with touch sensitive control panel. Automatic and/or adjustable alarm limits for peak inspiratory pressure (PIP), mean airway pressure ($P\overline{aw}$) and PEEP/CPAP levels allow flexible application.

POWER REQUIREMENTS
- Model 9900 — 115 V; 50/60 Hz (±10%)
- Model 9900C — 220 V; 50/60 Hz (±10%)

Circuit breaker (fused):
- Model 9900 — ¼ amp (slow-blow)
- Model 9900C — ⅛ amp (slow-blow)
- Current leakage — Less than 25 microamperes

WEIGHT
- 8 lb (3.6 kg)

PARAMETERS MEASURED AND DISPLAYED / **LIMITS**
- Peak airway pressure (PIP) — 2 to 150 cm H_2O ± 2.1% of full scale
- Mean airway pressure ($P\overline{aw}$) — 1-100 cm H_2O ± 1.7% of full scale
- Positive end expiratory pressure (PEEP) — 0-100 cm H_2O ± 2.1% of full scale
- Continuous positive airway pressure (CPAP) — 0-100 cm H_2O
- Inspiratory time (T_I) — 0.1-30 sec ± 1.5% of full scale
- Expiratory time (T_E) — 0.1-60 sec ± 0.6% of full scale
- Ventilator frequency (f) — 1-20 BPM ± 1.7% of full scale
- — 21-200 BPM ± 0.7% of full scale
- — 201-900 BPM ± 0.9% of full scale
- I:E ratio (I:E) — 0.1 to 300

ALARMS
- Disconnect alarm — T_I + T_E + 25% (T_I + T_E) + 2 sec set latest AUTOSET
- Automatic alarm limits — The AUTOSET switch sets pressure alarm limits 20% above their latest reading for high limit and 20% below for low limit, rounded to nearest digit. Disconnect (no activity) timer is set at the latest T_I + T_E + 25% (T_I + T_E + 2 sec)
- Automatic power-up sequence — The monitor analyzes the waveform until the first PIP event following 30 sec is reached, then computes for $P\overline{aw}$ and performs an internal autoset to set alarm limits
- Adjustable sensitivity — Pressure swing that monitor must detect to register a ventilation cycle
- Parameter alarms (high/low) — Distinct audible and visual alarms—automatic or adjustable, self-canceling when alarm condition ceases, but alarmed parameter is placed on HOLD
- Temporary alarm mute — 60 sec
- Battery failure — Test sequence will read failure if output voltage from the 9-volt battery falls below 6.8 volts
- Power failure alarm — Activated whenever power is lost when the ON-OFF switch is ON
- Chart recorder output — 0-4 volts, DC; 100 cm H_2O = 2.5 volts
- Sampling rate — 1.2 msec (833/sec) for each parameter except mean airway pressure, which is sampled every 4.8 msec

Bird Products/3M, 3M Center 225-55, St. Paul, MN 55144.

3 Forrest Bird, in an article published in the 1980 summer issue of the *Flying Physician*, used the following definitions for describing ventilator cycling rates.

Low frequency diffusion ventilation (LFV):	0-120cpm—1-2 Hz
Medium frequency diffusion ventilation (MFV):	120-360cpm—2-6 Hz
Very high frequency diffusion ventilation (VHFV):	360-900cpm—6-15Hz
Ultra high frequency diffusion ventilation (UHFV):	900(+)cpm—15 Hz

Although there is disagreement as to which cycling rates constitute a high-frequency ventilator; there is general acceptance of the fact that HFV is primarily generated by one of three methods discussed next.

D *High-frequency positive pressure ventilation (HFPPV)*

HFPPV describes a ventilator that cycles in the range of *60 to 150* BPM and has adjustable I:E ratios. The delivered tidal volume approximates the dead space of the patient to prevent CO_2 buildup, and inspiration is *active* followed by a *passive* exhalation. A conventional ventilator can be modified to function as this type of device.

E *High-frequency jet ventilation (HFJV)*

1 A high-frequency jet ventilation is a custom-designed device that delivers small tidal volumes of *3* to *6* ml/kg at *60* to *900* BPM. As with the HFPPV, inspiration is *active*, followed by a *passive* exhalation.

2 HFJV is based on the principle of a source gas delivered to a rapidly cycling electromechanical valve called a solenoid. When the valve is open, gas streams through a narrow cannula, which is placed inside a tracheal tube. As gas exits the cannula opening (jet), it is accelerated and entrains supplemental gas before entering the trachea (Fig. 23-85).

3 In this mechanism, inspiratory gas travels through the

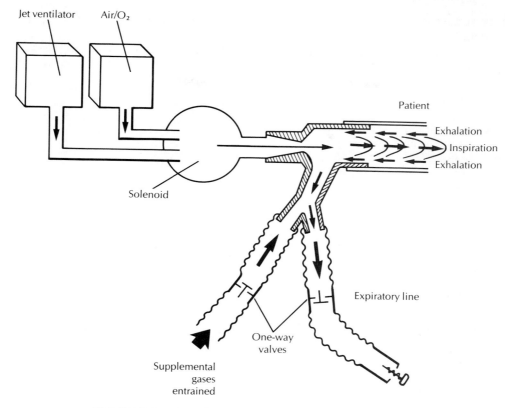

FIGURE 23-85 Schematic representation of high-frequency jet ventilator.

center of the tube while exhalation occurs simultaneously along the walls of the tubes (see coaxial flow in Figs. 23-85 and 23-86).

4 A stated advantage of this type of device is the fact that adequate ventilation may be achieved in patients with major airway complications with relatively *low peak inspiratory pressure*. This technique may offer an alternative to situations where, with conventional ventilation, high peak airway pressures interfere with cardiac output.

F High-frequency oscillation (HFO)

High-frequency pulse generators provide the greatest range of cycling frequencies. These devices are capable of delivering rates at 3000 to 4000 BPM. Tidal volumes are small, and oscillation occurs during both *inspiration* and *exhalation*. Oscillation is created by a rapidly vibrating radio-type speaker, a rubber diaphragm, or a rapidly cycling piston.

G Dynamics of gas flow

An exact explanation for the dynamics of gas flow during HFV has not been formulated. The following theories are postulated:

1 Augmented diffusion or enhanced diffusivity. HFJV causes turbulence that excites proximal molecules, which in turn excite distal molecules until diffusion gradients are satisfied throughout the lung.

2 Coaxial flow. With HFV, gas flow is laminar and bidirectional. In coaxial flow, inspiration occurs through

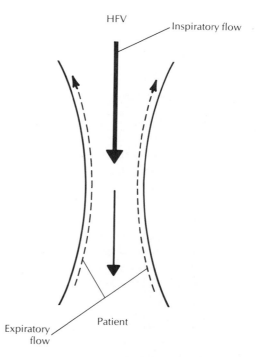

FIGURE 23-86 Coaxial flow. Inspiration occurs through center of tube while exhalation occurs along the walls of the tube in opposite direction.

the center of the airway while simultaneous exhalation (CO_2) is leaving the lung along the walls of the airway (Fig. 23-86).

H *Benefits of HFV*

Noted benefits of HFV include:
1 Reduced barotrauma
2 Reduced interference with intracranial pressure
3 Reduced interference with cardiovascular pressure
4 Prevention of aspiration during CPR with expiratory rates greater than 66% of the total cycle and cycling rates greater than 60 BPM
5 Increased ventilation in noncompliant lung with bronchopulmonary fistula
6 More uniform ventilation in cases with obstructed airways

I *Disadvantages of HFV*

1 Inadvertent PEEP and CO_2 retention at cycling rates greater than 200 BPM
2 Retards mucocilliary transport
3 Poor humidification systems
4 A lack of understanding of HFV

J *Future of HFV*

1 It is still too early to determine exact indications and contraindications for HFV. Human and animal studies are still under way at selective medical centers, and data are being gathered and compared.
2 The technology is new and problems such as poor humidification and medication administration by means of aerosols still must be resolved. In general, clinical data have shown that in certain patients HFV does work better than other methods of ventilation. Perhaps HFV can be compared to the use of CPAP, PEEP, and IMV just a few years ago.
3 Clearly, it is an interesting technology that should be developed and used when indicated, such as when more conventional ventilatory methods do not achieve the desired results.

22.13 Examples of high-frequency ventilators

State of the art high-frequency ventilation is still evolving as data are gathered in laboratories and from clinical trials.
1 As previously cited, in 1979 Forrest Bird developed still another approach to known high-frequency techniques. Bird's system incorporated a ventilator that would provide oscillation at frequencies to 1200/min (20 Hz) with adjustable I:E ratios of 3:1 to 1:3.
2 The primary difference between Bird's ventilator and others was that it integrated high-frequency oscillation with bulk gas movement. This allowed the operator to schedule intermittent percussion rather than a constant use of either bulk gas movement or oscillation.

These early ventilator systems have been modified and improved based on data on neonatal and adult pa-

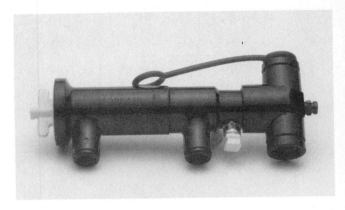

FIGURE 23-87 Bird Phasitron. (Courtesy Bird Airlodge, Sand Point, Idaho.)

tients obtained from clinical trials in the United States and abroad.
3 The key to Bird's newest generation of volumetric diffusive respirators (VDR) is a matrix device called a Phasitron (Fig. 23-87).
4 The Phasitron (Fig. 23-88, *A* and *B*) provides a phsyiologic/mechanical interface for volumetric diffusive respiration. The unique sliding Venturi provides for respiratory gas injection during inspiration *(A)* and physiologic pulmonary outflow during exhalation *(B)*.
5 The synchronous gas delivery and exhalation features of the Phasitron enhance the high-frequency delivery of subtidal volumes with minimum inadvertent gas trapping at the end of exhalation.
6 This feature reduces the risk for barotrauma, which is a potential problem with some high-frequency devices.
7 The monojet (single) jet system used by the Phasitron enables the VDR unit to be simply and easily programmed for many different functions because all gas enters and exits through a single Venturi orifice.
8 Bird's new generation of intrapulmonary diffusive ventilators (IPV) and volumetric diffusive respirators (VDR) has been expanded to include more than 10 different models. These models offer the operator a wide selection of cabinet shapes and sizes, ventilatory patterns, operational modes, and monitoring and alarm options.

A *IPV units*

1 Functionally and physiologically the Bird IPV units were designed to replace the more traditional IPPB machine for the delivery of volume-assisted aerosol therapy.
2 The primary difference is the manner (rate and pattern) in which the tidal volume is delivered combined with internal airway percussion.
3 Percussive ventilation may be more effective in providing alveolar ventilation at lower mean airway pressure and increasing bronchial airway clearance through internal percussion.

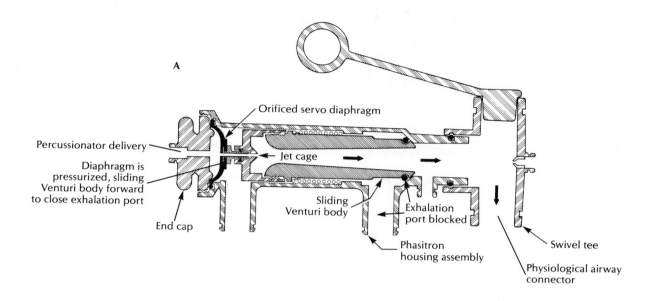

A

Orificed servo diaphragm

Percussionator delivery

Jet cage

Diaphragm is
pressurized, sliding
Venturi body forward
to close exhalation port

Sliding
Venturi body

Exhalation
port blocked

End cap

Phasitron
housing assembly

Swivel tee

Physiological airway
connector

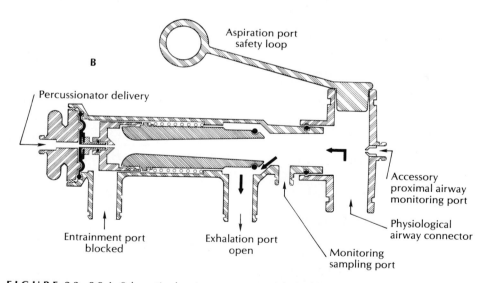

B

Aspiration port
safety loop

Percussionator delivery

Accessory
proximal airway
monitoring port

Physiological
airway connector

Entrainment port
blocked

Exhalation port
open

Monitoring
sampling port

FIGURE 23-88 A, Schematic showing cross-section of Bird Phasitron pressurized (closed) to provide inspiration. **B,** Schematic showing cross-section of Bird Phasitron unpressurized (open) allowing exhalation. (Courtesy Bird Airlodge, Sand Point, Idaho.)

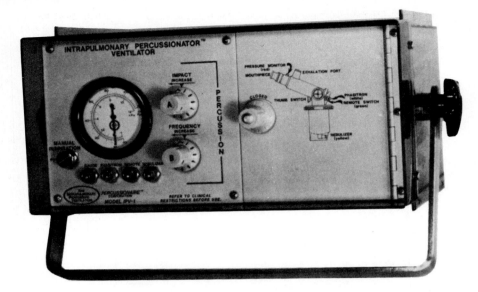

FIGURE 23-89 Control panel of Percussionaire Basic Intrapulmonary Percussionator. (Courtesy Percussionaire Corp, Sand Point, Idaho.)

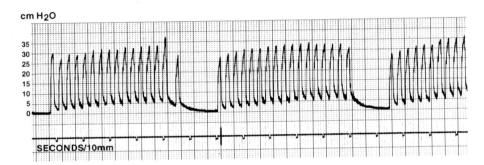

FIGURE 23-90 Typical IVP pressure waveform measured at proximal physiologic airway. (Courtesy Percussionaire Corp, Sand Point, Idaho.)

B *VDR ventilators*

1 The VDR units were designed to supplement and/or replace traditional volume ventilators.
2 The primary differences in the VDR units are the cycling rates, delivery of effective alveolar ventilation at lower mean airway pressure, and the option of superimposing percussive frequencies over conventional sinusoidal waveforms.
3 These options provide the clinician with still another alternative for adjusting ABGs and bronchial hygiene.
4 Rather than attempt to explain each model the following units are presented as examples of the Bird IPV/VDR series.

C *IPV-1 percussion (Fig. 23-89)*

1 The primary institutional IPV-1 percussionator was built to replace the traditional IPPB machine. (Note the simplicity of the control panel.)
2 With this unit the operator need only adjust percussive impact and frequency until an ideal breathing rate and volume are obtained.
3 Note also that individual breaths (tidal volume) are dif-

ferent for each patient although rates of 100 to 120 BPM at 20 to 25 ml are most commonly selected for adult patients.

4 A typical waveform for the Percussionaire Basic Intrapulmonary Percussionator is shown in Fig. 23-90. In this example it can be seen that the ventilator is delivering approximately 2 breaths/sec at an average cycling pressure of 30 to 35 H_2O. After approximately every 10 sec, a pause occurs. During these pauses airway pressure returns to baseline and the patient has an opportunity to expectorate any raised secretions.

D *Generic VDR-3 respirator (Fig. 23-91)*

The generic VDR-3 respirator is a transitional conventional IMV ventilator that enables the operator to use traditional IMV/CPAP modes with the option of using a VDR/IPV percussion program.

E *VDR-II sinusoidal percussionator (Fig. 23-92)*

1 The VDR-II Sinusoidal Percussionator incorporates intrapulmonary percussion with conventional methods for critical care.

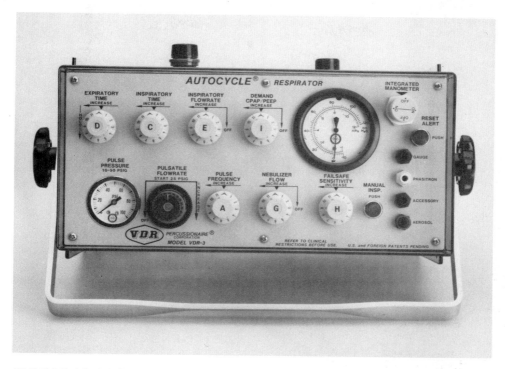

FIGURE 23-91 Generic VDR-3 conventional time-cycled IMV ventillator with independent, selectable, oscillatory VDR programming. (Courtesy Percussionaire Corp, Sand Point, Idaho.)

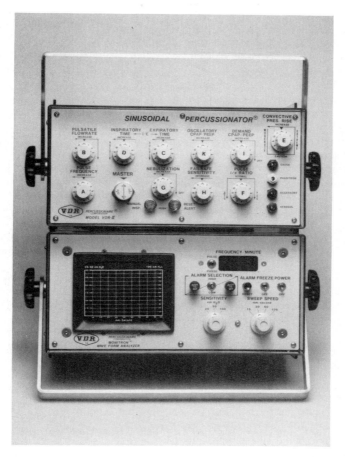

FIGURE 23-92 VDR-II Sinusoidal Percussionator combined with the Monitron unit. (Courtesy Percussionaire Corp, Sand Point, Idaho.)

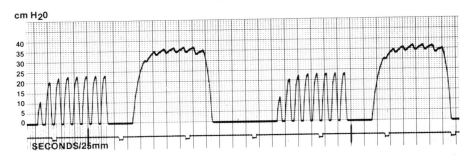

FIGURE 23-93 Waveform for the Volumetric Diffusive Ventilator.

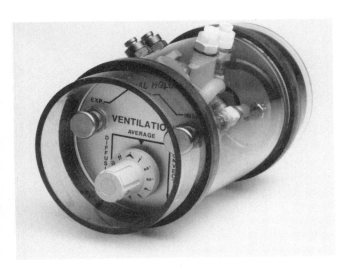

FIGURE 23-94 TXP military transporter respirator. Military transporter respirator is an acute care, time-cycled respirator for both civilian and military applications. (Courtesy Percussionaire Corp, Sand Point, Idaho.)

2 The Monitron monitoring and alarm unit enables the operator to visually observe airway pressure tracing of waveforms and serves as a disconnect alarm.

3 Fig. 23-93 shows a waveform for the Volumetric Diffusive Ventilator. Note that the patient is ventilated using a combination of high-frequency oscillations followed by a conventional controlled mechanical breath. With this ventilator, the most commonly used breathing frequencies are 200 to 400 BPM for adults and 400 to 600 BPM for neonates.

F *TXP military transporter respirator (Fig. 23-94)*

1 A small, rugged cannister-shaped respirator that was developed for prehospital and inhospital transport and resuscitation.

2 A single-knob control allows the operator to select conventional or diffusive ventilation.

3 Conventional ventilation can be adjusted from 6 to 80 BPM and diffusive ventilation from 6 to 375 BPM.

G *The IPV therapy breathing circuit (Fig. 23-95)*

1 This assembly can be used on all the IPV percussionator devices but not on the VDR or TXP units.

2 The breathing circuit attaches to the Phasitron unit to complete the connection to the patient.

H *The VDR intensive care breathing circuit Fig. 23-96*

Fig. 23-96 shows the VDR intensive care breathing circuit that can be used on all VDR and TXP devices, as well as the IPV-2 percussionator. This circuit is color coded to match outlet connections on the ventilation cabinet for easy assembly and incorporates half-turn connectors to prevent accidental disconnects.

22.14 Clinical trials

The case histories presented in this unit* were documented by Carl J. Bodenstein, MD, during his service in the neonatal facilities advanced by Welzie M. Allen, MD, and Hrair Garabedian, MD. These case histories provide examples of how volumetric diffusive respiration (VDR) may be used in neonatal management.

It must be understood that high-frequency ventilation is an experimental technique to be used only in research protocols. Thus these cases may help the clinician develop additional research protocols for human experimentation with, of course, research committee approval.

A *Clinical monitoring requirements in volumetric diffusive respiration (VDR)*

Although neonatal monitoring provisions will vary greatly from one facility to another, there are certain cardinal requirements as neonatology makes the transition from the role of survival into a more defining scientific body. As a result of mandated therapeutic means, the future impetus must be that of minimizing "handicap." Advanced monitoring and therapeutic devices will play a major role in the reduction of therapeutic "side effect."

Conventional cardiopulmonary management in the majority of neonatal pathologic conditions involves only limited invasive monitoring, namely the umbilical artery cath-

---

*Reprinted and modified with permission of F.M. Bird, MD. The following abbreviations are used: *UAC*, umbilical artery catheter; *UVC*, umbilical venous catheter; *CVP*, central venous pressure; *PIE*, pulmonary interstitial emphysema; *BPD*, bronchopulmonary dysplasia; *RLF*, retrolental fibroplasia; *CBG*, capillary blood gas; *HMD*, hyaline membrane disease; *MAP*, maximum airway pressure; *PIP*, peak inflation pressure; *SEM*, systolic ejection murmur; *RVH*, right ventricular hypertrophy; *BP*, blood pressure; *ABP*, arterial blood pressure; *HR*, heart rate; *PPHT*, persistent pulmonary hypertension; *RUL*, right upper lobe; *NS*, normal saline; *SVN*, small volume nebulizer; *EGA*, extrauterine gestational age; *PA*, pulmonary artery; *IRB*, investigative research board.

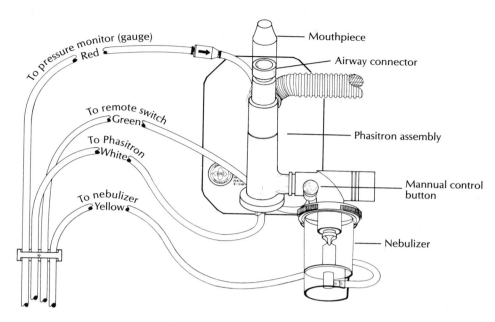

FIGURE 23-95 IPV therapy breath circuit. (Courtesy Percussionaire Corp, Sand Point, Idaho.)

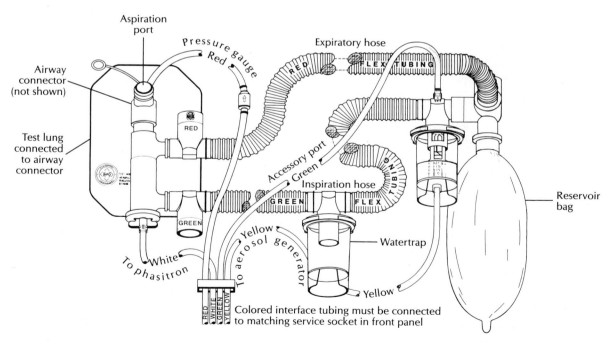

FIGURE 23-96 VDR fail-safe intensive care breathing circuit can be used on all VDR and TXP devices and the IPV-2 percussionator. (Courtesy Percussionaire Corp, Sand Point, Idaho.)

eter. Current technologic advances in transcutaneous oxygen and CO_2 monitoring and in noninvasive blood pressure monitoring systems may, at times, circumvent the need for arterial catheterization. Neonatal VDR, especially when used as a result of failure of conventional therapy, demands extended clinical monitoring capabilities for optimum management. Continuous heart rate, arterial blood pressure, $tcPO_2$, and temperature monitoring are mandatory. Central venous pressure measurement by way of an umbilical venous catheter or other suitably placed central line will aid in management and become an absolute requirement in the most difficult cases encountered. Continuous waveform display of both arterial and central venous pressures can provide vital information regarding cardiac response to VDR programming, as well as to changes in thoracic compliance. The latter may be augmented by the continuous measurement of transesophageal pressure. Additionally, although still in its infancy in many neonatal centers, placement of a multilumen Swan-Ganz catheter for measurement of pulmonary artery pressure and even thermal dilution cardiac output determination may add significant information toward the management of the most recalcitrant neonates with persistent pulmonary hypertension.

The key to an "aggressive" invasive monitoring approach is the anticipation of monitoring requirements and the mobilization of appropriate instrumentation before a critical state is reached. Risks inherent to instrumentation must always be carefully weighed against the benefits of augmented cardiorespiratory management.

B *Functional analysis through case history presentation*

The following case histories reflect a learning curve associated with the rescue of (twelfth hour) neonates under investigative protocols. Failing neonatal patients were removed from traditional cardiopulmonary management and placed on Bird-conceived volumetric diffusive respiration (VDR). The reader must remember these were patients of last resort and the clinicians were on absolutely new ground with little documented resource to draw on. Competent opinion would imply that several of these patients were initially maintained beyond previous therapeutic limits; that is, clinical reversal occurred with overwhelming deficits and repeated insults as attempts to get back on familiar ground were made.

The format for each case presentation is the same. Patient and practitioners are obscured by the substitution of alpha codes. The absolute numbers and facts are not altered in any way.

Following each case presentation is a discussion relative to what was learned from each clinical course and suggestions relative to how improvement could be endangered.

Case presentations encompass a wide spectrum of premature and term babies with multiple reasons for clinical intervention. Following the case histories, a general summary is presented.

Finally, a detailed expansion of neonatal VDR program-

ming is set forth and discussed. A specific program generally associated with each case history is interrelated.

1 *Neonatal VDR case presentation: baby boy (A)—Carl J. Bodenstein, MD.*

Baby boy *(A)* is a 1275 g, 30-week (estimated) gestational age white male neonate, born to a 20-year-old G2, P1, Rh-negative (well) white woman without prenatal care who presented completely effaced and dilated in breech position. Delivery was by cesarean section for premature breech. Apgar scores were 8 at 1 minute and 7 at 5 minutes with rapid onset of severe respiratory compromise requiring intubation at 4 minutes of age. First arterial blood gas (ABG) on conventional ventilation with 22/3 equaled manometer pressure 22 cm H_2O with a PEEP of 3 cm H_2O, IMV 40, IT 0.6, FIO_2 0.95 showed pH 7.26 PcO_2 45, PO_2 67, BE -5.8. Initial chest x-ray (CXR) demonstrated a near "white out" with subtle pulmonary interstitial emphysema (PIE) already present. Physical examination was remarkable only for the 30-week gestational age. Initial CBC demonstrated Hb 14.5, hct 42.7, WBC 11,000 without left shift. Umbilical catheters were inserted with UAC at L4 and UVC in right atrium. Initial arterial blood pressures were 45/20 with CVP of 3. Blood and endotracheal cultures were obtained (subsequently negative), and antibiotic therapy was begun.

Status remained stable with weaning of ventilatory parameters to 21/3 and FIO_2 0.58 until 17 hours of age when a right tension pneumothorax occurred; this was initially well-relieved by a 12 Fr thoracotomy tube insertion. Subsequent CXRs demonstrated worsening bilateral PIE with a continued right pneumothorax, despite a vigorously bubbling chest tube, necessitating the placement of a second right chest tube. Pancuronium (Parulon) was administered at this point. Ventilatory parameters required an increase to 32/4, IMV 100, IT 0.3, FIO_2 1.0 to maintain acceptable ABGs. At 42 hours of age, a left pnumothorax occurred. This was initially controlled by a 12 Fr thoracotomy tube insertion but later required a second tube to maintain relief. Despite a continuous rapid bubbling from both chest tubes, the left pneumothorax reaccumulated and thoracotomy tube location was changed with good relief. By this time PIE and pneumatocele formation were severe, ventilatory parameters had been subsequently weaned to 25/4, IMV 60, FIO_2 remained at 1.0, and it was elected to begin a trial of Bird volumetric diffusive respiration (VDR) (Fig. 23-97).

Immediately before switchover, ABGs on the Babybird ventilator with 22/4, IMV 55, FIO_2, 1.0 were pH 7.29, PcO_2 41, PO_2 60, BE -5.6. The initial VDR program was set up with an FIO_2 of 1.0, a frequency of 580/min, with a 1:1 I:E ratio and a continuous oscillation with a mean oscillatory pressure of 14 and a rise of 10. Fifteen minutes into the VDR program, ABGs demonstrated pH 7.35, PcO_2 35, PO_2 95, BE -4.1. After 1 hour into the VDR program, ABGs demonstrated

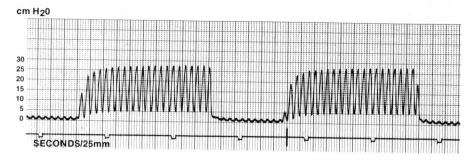

F I G U R E 2 3 - 9 7 Classical percussive neonatal VDR waveform program. (Courtesy Percussionaire Corp, Sand Point, Idaho, and Hewlett-Packard.)

pH 7.33, P_{CO_2} 39, P_{O_2} 198, BE −4.5. After 6 hours into the VDR program, CXRs demonstrated liittle change; however, FI_{O_2} had been weaned down to 0.5 with mean airway pressures reduced to 7 with the left air leak significantly decreased. Six-hour ABGs were pH 7.42, P_{CO_2} 34, P_{O_2} 77, BE −1.1. Additionally, a marked diuresis had ensued with vital signs remaining stable. After 24 hours into the VDR program, air leaks had abated and CXRs were somewhat improved; however, severe PIE changes remained. After approximately 30 hours into the VDR program, schedules were FI_{O_2} 0.57, frequency 560/min, with a 1:1 I:E ratio, mean airway pressure 11.5 with a rise of 10. ABGs at 30 hours were pH 7.45, P_{CO_2} 33, P_{O_2} 55, BE +2.0.

With a stable patient, the better part of valor was judged to go back to the conventional Babybird ventilator. Therefore, after 30 hours into the VDR program, the patient was switched back to conventional ventilation on the Babybird ventilator. The Babybird was set up with FI_{O_2} 0.57, pressures 14/5, IMV 60, IT 0.5. After 2 hours into the conventional program, the ABGs were not remarkably changed; however, the left pneumothorax had reaccumulated and the FI_{O_2} had been increased to 1.0. Noting the unexpected deterioration, the patient was transferred back to the VDR program.

At 36 hours back into the VDR program, large volumes of secretions and plugs were suctionable from the airway. Over the next 6 hours, FI_{O_2} was weaned down to 0.78, an oscillatory frequency of 600/min, with a 1:1.5 I:E ratio; mean airway pressure was 10. ABGs demonstrated pH 7.45, P_{CO_2} 40, P_{O_2} 83, BE +4.4. At this time the patient was allowed to recover from Pavulon. The patient remained stable with little change in CXRs. A metabolic alkalosis was present with diuresis continuing. At 72 hours into the VDR program, a marked impedance to cardiac output was noticed. This required constant volume pushes to maintain a CVP of 6 to 9, plus the initiation of dopamine therapy.

A short trial of conventional therapy was attempted: FI_{O_2} 1.0, pressure 25/4, IMV 50, IT 0.5. Oxygenation was extremely poor and VDR was reinstated. VDR parameters were FI_{O_2} 1.0, frequency 600/min, with a 1:1

I:E ratio, mean oscillatory airway pressure 12 to 13 with a rise of 10. A 0.8 sec oscillatory interruption interval was scheduled 20 times per min. During the switchover, bilateral air leaks had reaccumulated, and after the insertion of dual 16 Fr thoracotomy tubes, good resolutions were obtained. Over the next 24 hours, FI_{O_2} was weaned down to 0.86, with air leaks abating. CXRs demonstrated little change.

After 7 consecutive days of VDR, a midnight insecurity caused a brief return to conventional ventilation resulting in the reestablishment of air leaks. After VDR was reinstated, the air leaks rapidly arrested. Subsequent CXRs demonstrated massive hyperinflation of the right lung with a notable decrease in PIE on the left side.

After the next 10-day run of VDR, both chest tubes were removed. Shortly thereafter, while hand bagging during breathing circuit exchange, a tension pneumothorax occurred on the right side.

NOTE: Hand baggng pressure was limited to 15 cm H_2O. A right thoracotomy tube was reinstalled. VDR programming was FI_{O_2} 1.0, frequency 480 with a 1:1 I:E ratio, mean airway pressure 11 with a rise of 10. Oscillatory interruption intervals were established at 0.8 sec at a rate of 24 times/min. Over the next 24 hours, a marked weaning was established with parameters set at FI_{O_2} 0.32, frequency 440 with a 1:1 I:E ratio; mean airway pressure was reduced to 7. CXRs underwent startling changes, with a return to a complete "white out" status followed by a rapid clearing.

At this time, the patient was 21 days old with 18 of these spent on VDR programming. The patient was breathing spontaneously through a program of 420 cycles per minute with a mean oscillatory pressure of 8. Interruption intervals were as previously programmed

Two days later, conventional ventilation was reestablished. The patient's status deteriorated with CXRs revealing a return to a "white out." Although ABGs initially improved, subsequent CXRs revealed PIE on the left side at 2 hours and bilateral pneumothorax at 4 hours. A left thoracotomy tube was reinstalled. Subsequently, VDR was reinstated, and air leaks resolved rapidly, allowing the removal of the thoracotomy tube 24 hours later. FIO_2 was weaned back down to 0.30, with major improvement in CXRs. VDR parameters at this time were a frequency of 540 and a mean airway pressure of 7 with a rise of 10. The interruption interval was 1 second 30 times each minute. The patient was now 28 days old, being extremely alert and active. Serialized cranial ultrasounds and EEG findings were normal for gestational age. Continuous drip nasoduodenal tube feedings were started, the patient having been previously maintained on hyperalimentation with Aminosyn and Intralipid.

After 27 days of VDR, final weaning was commenced. The VDR program was changed to FIO_2 0.3, frequency of 560 with a mean airway pressure of 6. Two days later, oscillatory CPAP was terminated with conventional demand CPAP established. The patient was successfully extubated 7 days later at 42 days of age. Despite continued CXR findings of perihilar infiltrates, the patient was weaned in 5 days to room air and demonstrated no clinical stigma or bronchopulmonary dysplasia. Feedings by nipple/gavage were instituted and the patient's neurologic status appeared normal. The patient was discharged home at 67 days of age weighing 5 pounds, 1 ounce (2996 g). Resting respiratory rate was 25 without retractions, and feedings were well tolerated without tachypnea or cyanosis. Final CXR before discharge demonstrated continued perihilar changes with minimal BPD displayed peripherally. Serial retinal examination showed grade II active phase RLF, arrested and resolving. Neurodevelopmental status at 6 months is normal.

a Discussions baby boy (A):

With a new device having unknown characteristics being used on a critically ill patient without qualified clinical backup, combined with days of 24-hour surveillance away from home, the tendency was to wean back to conventional ventilation as early as possible. This would be a natural human tendency. Without operational manuals or previous mechanical or clinical experience, functioning under an investigative protocol, with associated potential legal complications, the clinicians were under extreme personal duress to complete the VDR programming and return to known conventional management.

b Suggestions and possibilities:

Set up a VDR apparatus in or near the nursery on a test lung before clinical intervention is anticipated. Schedule on a time-available basis hands-on familiarization by all attending. Teach the logic and programming of VDR schedules. Evaluate attending for comprehension.

Once committed, a patient successfully programmed on VDR may not always be safely returned to conventional ventilation; therefore, a logical weaning schedule must be considered.

Volumetric diffusive respiration in this case was able to minimize barotrauma while maintaining acceptable ABGs, allowing reversal of trauma initialized by conventional ventilatory means.

The importance of a well-seasoned professional clinical team is illustrated.

With familiarization resulting from hands-on experience, the VDR device, like the Babybird, becomes a routine clinical management tool with advanced potential to meet extended clinical pathophysiology. Each clinical course better prepares the attending for the next procedure.

The importance of an aggressive, constant, vital parameter clinical monitoring setup, including CVP, is demonstrated.

Possibly an initial advanced critical care station can be organized in each nursery to allow normal clinical progression from pure survival techniques to protocols that minimize potential residual effects.

The less compliant the breathing circuit, the greater the opportunity for barotrauma as demonstrated with a compression bag device and/or conventional ventilation. The VDR phasitron provides pneumatic clutching at the proximal airway without breathing circuit compliance.

Respiratory management must be considered as effective cardiopulmonary management. Tendencies toward a metabolic acidosis, tachycardia, and decrease in renal output all must be in part controlled with an effective VDR program.

2 *Neonatal VDR case presentation: baby boy (B)—Carl J. Bodenstein, MD.*

Baby boy *(B)* is a 3600 g, 36-week estimated gestational age white male neonate born to a 24-year-old G3, P2, A-positive (well) white woman with unremarkable pregnancy, delivered by repeat cesarean section. Agpar scores were 4 at 1 minute and 8 at 5 minutes with suctioning, stimulation, and mask CPAP given for resuscitation. The patient was placed at 0.60 FIO_2 hood in which initial CBG showed pH 7.28, Pco_2 47, Po_2 46, BE -4.3. Initial CXR showed mixed pattern of retained fetal fluid superimposed on mild HMD. A UAC was placed at T7 and UVC in right atrial CVP position. ABGs showed pH 7.24, Pco_2 57, Po_2 58, BE -2.9. The patient was intubated with 3.5 ET, and bloody fluid was aspirated from the airway. CXR was now consistent with moderate HMD. Initial ventilator settings were 20/4, IMV 38, IT 0.6 (1:2) and FIO_2 0.98. ABGs showed pH 7.38, Pco_2 37, Po_2, 278, BE -1.7. Initial CBC showed Hb 15.8, hct 50.5 WBC 16.5 without left shift. Blood culture was obtained (subsequently negative), and antibiotic therapy was begun. Physical examination was remarkable only for 36 weeks gestation. Admission diagnosis was unexpected HMD with possible blood aspiration.

In the first 36 hours of life, ventilatory parameters requires an increase to 40/5, IMV 80, FIO_2 1.0 with CXR showing good aeration without initial pulmonary interstitial emphysema (PIE), followed by the later

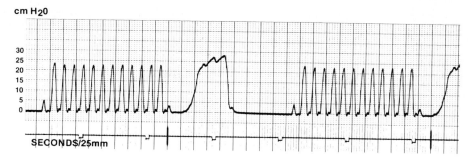

FIGURE 23-98 Classical waveform with a positive I:E ratio. (Courtesy Percussionaire Corp, Sand Point, Idaho, and Hewlett-Packard.)

demonstration of moderate pneumomediastinum. The patient subsequently required maintenance of P_{CO_2} below 30 to maintain adequate oxygenation, and echocardiographic systolic time intervals demonstrated pulmonary hypertension. The patient was paralyzed with Pavulon, started on dopamine at 12.5 µg/kg/min, and Priscoline at 4 mg/kg/hr. Response was minimal. Over the next 24 hours there was progression of the pneumomediastinum, and on day three of life, a tension pneumoperitoneum occurred. A 14-gauge catheter was placed on the peritoneal cavity with good resolution of the pneumoperitoneum; however, the pneumomediastinum has progressed significantly. Ventilatory parameters were increased to the maximum of 53/7, IMV 120, MAP 26, FI_{O_2} 1.0 to maintain acceptable blood gas parameters while cardiac output was being significantly impeded. Later, a left pneumothorax occurred with initial chest tube placement ineffective. Subsequently a 16 Fr chest tube was inserted after a mediastinal stripping was performed. CXRs showed resolution of the pneumothorax and some improvement in the degree of loculation of the pneumomediastinum.

At this time, ventilatory parameters were 49/7, IMV 120, IT 0.2, FI_{O_2} 1.0, and MAP 22. Urine output was minimum, and the patient was 350 g above birth weight, with a BUN of 17, creatinine at 1.1.

At 3½ days of age, the patient was established on volumetric diffusive respiration (Fig. 23-98). Initial program was frequency 500, 34/5, 1:1.5 I:E, and a conventional breath with a peak pressure of 30 delivered 15 times per minute. IT was 0.4 and expiratory time was 0.6 seconds. MAP was 20. A conventional breath was required, as chest observation during initial oscillatory pause programming demonstrated no significant chest deflation. The lungs were severely stinted with PIE. Initial blood gases on VDR showed pH 7.46, P_{CO_2} 34, P_{O_2} 57, BE +2.2. Over the next 30 min, oscillatory amplitude was increased to 44/12 with conventional breaths programmed 20 times per minute with a peak pressure of 45. MAp was 31. Resultant ABGs showed pH 7.36, P_{CO_2} 37, Pa_{O_2} 52, BE −2.7. CXR at this time showed some resolution of pneumomediastinum. The chest tube was now inactive, as was the peritoneal catheter. Mean arterial blood pressure

was 8 points lower than measurements before initiation of VDR. Various manipulations of oscillatory frequency were next tried, with changes documented by blood gases taken 5 minutes apart:

a freq. 460, 43/12, MAP 31. Conventional PIP 46 15/min: pH 7.37, P_{CO_2} 37, P_{O_2} 48, BE −2.7.

b freq. 400, 43/12, MAP 21. Pauses without tidal delivery: pH 7.36, P_{CO_2} 41, P_{O_2} 41, BE −1.2.

c freq. 600, 48/4, MAP 18. Conventional PIP 52 20/min: pH 7.41, P_{CO_2} 41, P_{O_2} 71, BE +2.4.

Three hours into VDR on the last settings, CXR showed significant resolution of pneumomediastinum. ABGs obtained at this time showed pH 7.51, P_{CO_2} 30, P_{O_2} 159, BE +2.8. Amplitude of both oscillations and conventional breath were lowered to 48/4, freq. 600 and 43/4 at 20/min, with subsequent ABGs of pH 7.50, P_{CO_2} 31, Pa_{O_2} 101, BE +2.8. ABG was now 81/54, CVP 4, and diuresis had ensued. CXR 16 hours into VDR was remarkably improved, and the abdominal catheter was removed. The patient continued to required moderate respiratory alkalosis to maintain oxygenation, and no ventilatory weaning was tolerated.

Forty hours into the VDR procedure, CXR showed return of PIE on the left side. An attempt to wean conventional breath amplitude and frequency was met by decompensation with pH 7.19, P_{CO_2} 68, P_{O_2} 40, BE −3. Subsequently, the patient was reestablished on pulsatile settings of freq. 600, 47/7, conventional breath 35/6, and later 35/2, 20/min. ABGs showed 7.49, P_{CO_2} 32, P_{O_2} 162, BE + 2.0. Blood pressure was 96/57, CVP 4. The left thoracotomy tube had reactivated, air had reaccumulated in the abdomen, and a 14 Fr peritoneal catheter was reinserted.

The patient was allowed to recover from curare at this point with hopes that spontaneous tidal volume ventilation on oscillation with pause programming would be safer than conventional tidal programming. Oscillations were maintained at freq. 600, 46/5, MAP 25, FI_{O_2} 100 with pauses of 1.6 sec. ABGs showed a pH of 7.50, P_{CO_2} 33, Pa_{O_2} 136, BE + 3.9. Stability over the next 20 hours allowed FI_{O_2} to be weaned to 0.89. CXR showed improvement in PIE, and the peritoneal catheter was again removed. Oscillatory settings were weaned to 37/5.

At 5 days of age, the patient received hyperalimentation with Aminosyn and Intralipid. Vital signs remained stable, the patient had recovered from paralysis well, and had diuresed to within 60 g of birth weight. Twenty four hours later, severe PIE had reaccumulated, and it was decided that weaning of oscillatory pressures was sential despite pulmonary hypertension, which, if present, now appeared fixed and unresponsive. Priscoline was subsequently withdrawn, although the patient was reparalyzed, and oscillatory pressures weaned slowly from freq. 540, 45/4, MAP 23.5 to 26.7, down to a MAP of 18. CXR showed good resolution of PIE, and the question of BPD changes arose. ABGs showed pH 7.37, Pco_2 44, Po_2 130, BE + 1.2 on an FIo_2 of 90%. Thoracotomy tube continued to demonstrate active air leak (although minimum); however, the left tension pneumothorax recurred when the tube occluded with serous fluid, and the chest tube was changed with good resolution. At this time, marked dependent flank edema was treated with a 6 hr albumin/Lasix dosing for 24 hours. Diuresis of 400 g ensued. FIo_2 had been weaned to 0.50, and oscillatory parameters of freq. 560, 28/10, MAP 13.8, with resultant ABGs of pH 7.41, Pco_2 45, Po_2 72, BE + 4.0. CXR showed improvement in PIE, although haziness persisted. FIo_2 was slowly weaned over the next 48 hours to 30, and the patient was then allowed to recover from paralysis. Oscillatory parameters were freq. 540, 22/5, MAP 10 with pauses every 20/min. The chest tube was removed, and CXR was consistent with residual BPD changes.

After 13 days of VDR, the patient was placed on oscillatory CPAP of freq. 540, 10/4, MAP 6.5. However, ABGs showed CO_2 retention to 62, and programmed pauses were reinstituted at 16/5, MAP 6.3, freq. 420 with CO_2 returning to the 40s. CXRs remained unchanged. Oscillatory CPAP was reinstituted successfully successfully 2 days later and maintained for 48 hours, after which a conventional CPAP of 4 was used at an FIo_2 of 0.30. The patient was started on Decadron for 24 hours before successful extubation at 22 days of age.

Several days later, a grade III/VI SEM was audible, and repeat echocardiography failed to demonstrate a significant pathologic condition. Cardiac catheterization was performed, with FIo_2 needs increasing to 0.60 and ECG demonstrating marked RVH. Catheterization revealed pulmonary valvular stenosis. The patient was started on routine Lanoxin, Lasic therapy, and hypercaloric formula. He was weaned down to an FIo_2 of 0.25, requiring occasional bavage feedings. CXR at 35 days of age continued to show moderate BPD changes and right ventricular enlargement. Neurologic status was normal was were EEG, BAER, and eye examination. Weight gain was subsequently well established over the next 30 days. The patient was discharged at 76 days weighing 4620 g. Neurodevelopmental status at 6 months is normal. RVH on the basis of pulmonic stenosis remains prominent and surgery was anticipated. Over the subsequent months improvement was marked and repeat catheterization failed to demonstrate significant pulmonary valvular pressure gradient. Minimal residual BPD is present. The patient continues to thrive.

a Discussions baby boy *(B):*

The demonstrated rush to get back to what was considered safe ground in baby boy *(A)* was overcome. The major quest was to find a compatible program that would best serve to stabilize the patient. The importance of reducing sustained dissecting pressure in the presence of latent or active intrapulmonary air leaks is well documented. The critical balance between diffusive and convective waveforms was well presented. The maintenance of both Pao_2 and $Paco_2$ was independently governed by control over diffusive and convective functions. Subsequent cases have demonstrated the effectiveness of a "stepladder" (step and backstep) VDR programming. This type of ventilatory pattern may provide for the enhancement of both diffusive and convective parameters with a minimum component of dissecting pressure rise for a given tidal exchange.

b Suggestions and possibilites:

A clear understanding of waveform generation will facilitate the ability to select a balance between critical parameters.

The use of a waveform analyzer to determine clinical programming is not only an excellent teaching tool but also is a must in overall clinical management.

Organization of physical hardware is a key to long-term management.

The flow sheet recording of all vital and respiratory parameters is a key to a rapid means of projecting logically based therapeutic maneuvers.

Control over airway caliber is greatly influenced by the correct aerosol generation. Although a thermal system to heat aerosol is not projected as a means of controlling body temperature, it does reduce possible thermal reflex response to cold within the upper physiologic airways. By installing a humidified thermal element downstream of the aerosol generator, proximal airway delivery temperatures of 30° to 33° C can be maintained.

NOTE: This must be in conformance with the Bird-conceived percussive breathing circuit.

CAUTION: Resultant insensible water gains must be anticipated in fluid and electrolyte management.

3 *Neonatal VDR case presentation: baby boy (C)—Carl J. Bodenstein, MD.*

Baby boy *(C)* is an outborn +4040 g, 43-week estimated gestational age white male neonate, born to a 31-year-old G3, P2, A+ obese but otherwise well white woman, by emergency cesarean section for fetal distress with thick meconium present. Apgar scores were 3 and 4 at 1 and 5 minutes respectively, the baby being succm H2O

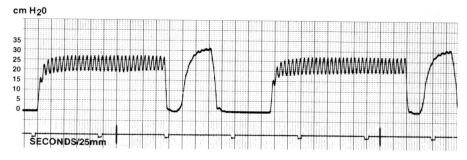

F I G U R E   2 3 - 9 9 Classical diffusive-connective VDR waveform. (Courtesy Percussionaire Corp, Sand Point, Idaho, and Hewlett-Packard.)

tioned and given blow by oxygen. Initial ABG showed pH 7.05, Pco_2 37, BE -15.0 in hood FIo_2 0.50. Initial CXR showed right pneumothorax and pneumomediastinum, as well as severe changes of meconium aspiration. The patient was intubated and transported on conventional ventilator settings of 30/0, IMV 80, FIo_2 1.0, with ABGs showing pH 7.43, Pco_2 33, Po_2 124, BE-1.3 on arrival at the neonatal center.

Ventilatory parameters were rapidly weaned down to 25/0, IMV 50, FIo_2 1.0. CXR showed severe meconium aspiration; however, air leaks had spontaneously resolved. Physical examination on admission was positive only for postmaturity. ABPs were 71/54, CVP 2, HR 130. Ampicillin and gentamicin were initiated after blood cultures (subsequently negative) were obtained. Within 8 hours of admission, ventilation was weaned to 18/2, IMV 20, FIo_2 1.0; however, CXRs revealed a large pneumomediastinum. oxygenation gradually worsened over the next 24 hours and CXRs showed little change. Pulmonary hypertension was documented by echocardiographic systolic time intervals and trial of hyperventilation was undertaken. The patient was given Pavulon and started on dopamine. ABGs before Priscoline trial were pH 7.54, Pco_2 26, Po_2 38, BE $+1.0$, Priscoline resulted in no response whatsoever. After several hours of severe hypoxia, it was elected to enter into a volumetric diffusive respiration ventilatory protocol (Fig. 23-99).

ABGs just before VDR showed pH 7.52, Pco_2 26, Po_2 41, BE -0.5 on 33/0, IMV 80, FIo_2 1.0. VDR was initiated at freq. 540, 32/8, MAP 17. Initial ABGs showed pH 7.36, Pco_2 35, Po_2 35, BE -5.0. When pauses were then added, Pco_2 rose to the 50s so frequency was lowered to 480 and a conventional breath 30/2 followed by a pause 20 times per minute was established with resultant ABGs of pH 7.133, Pco_2 42, Po_2 66, BE -3.2 one hour after start on VDR. Over the next 3 hours, oxygenation improved dramatically and conventional breath amplitude was weaned to 20/2, ABGs showing pH 7.48 to 7.60, Pco_2 22 to 29, Po_2 105 to 230, BE $+1.0$ to 4.0. Vital signs were stable at BP 80/60, CVP 0-2, HR 160 to 180.

CXR obtained 6 hours after initiation of VDR was markedly improved. Over the next 24 hours, oscillatory

parameters were weaned to 24/5, freq. 480 MAP 13, FIo_2 0.95 with resultant ABGs of pH 7.56 to 7.64, Pco_2 17 to 24, Po_2 97 to 139, BE 0.5 to $+3.0$. CXRs showed little change. The patient was maintained on Priscoline, 2 mg/kg/hr; dopamine, 10 μg/kg/min; and Pavulon, as well as hypocarbic alkalosis with all Po_2 greater than 100 for treatment of PPHT. By 48 hours into the VDR protocol, the conventional breath was omitted and a 1.4 sec pause, 10/min was programmed. Settings at this time were freq. 600, 23/2, MAP 9, FIo_2 0.9, and ABGs pH 7.56, Pco_2 25, Po_2 112, BE $+1.5$. Subsequent attempts to wean oscillatory amplitudes were met by marked decreases in oxygenation and required a return to an FIo_2 of 1.0 whenever Pco_2 was greater than 30, with a pH of less than 7.46. CXRs continued to show little change.

After 48 hours "locked in" at freq. 480, 36-40/6, MAP 15-17, FIo_2 0.88 to 0.95, with programmed pauses, oxygenation improved, allowing weaning of FIo_2 to 0.70, ABGs remaining pH 7.50 to 7.57, Pco_2 17 to 21, Po_2 120 to 156, BE -2.2 to -5.4. CXR showed better aeration but little other change. Twenty four hours later, however, lung fields were massively overexpanded. During this time, BP remained 90s/60s, CVP 0 to 2, HR 125 to 140. ABGs were unchanged with FIo_2 weaned to 0.54.

After 10 days of VDR, the patient was brought up from Pavulon with oscillator settings of 24/5, freq. 480, MAP 14, FIo_2 0.40 with a programmed pause as previously established. CXR showed good improvement. Dopamine was withdrawn and Priscoline was tapered over the next 24 hours. CXR now showed a RUL collapse. ET aspirate subsequently grew *Pseudomonas* species that was later reported by the manufacturer as a contaminant of our NS for suction vials. RUL atelectasis persisted over the next 6 days despite vigorous PT, aerosol SVNs, and antibiotic therapy. Despite this, oscillatory amplitudes were gradually weaned to freq. 480, 13/7, MAP 8, FIo_2 0.30.

After 13 days of VDR, oscillatory CPAP was begun, and the patient was extubated 1 day later with weaning to room air over the next 5 days. CXR continued to show some patchy RUL infiltrates and perihilar bilateral infiltrates. Feedings were begun and progressed slowly with gavage required for 1 week.

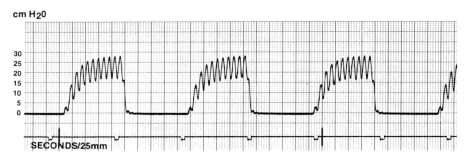

FIGURE 23-100 Classical VDR ascending (step and backstep) waveform. (Courtesy Hewlett-Packard and Percussionaire Corp, Sand Point, Idaho.)

The patient was discharged at 34 days of age, weighing 3970 g, with respiratory function and neurologic examination normal for his age. Additionally, EEG and CT scans were within normal limits. Neurodevelopmental status at 6 months is normal.

a Discussions baby boy (C):

After reviewing baby boys (A and B), baby boy (C) appears to be without major challenge. This is far from the truth. Each patient presented parallel but in many ways different challenges. Probably the most significant factor was the expanded clinical base of understanding. The original suspicions toward the once alien device were replaced with ever-increasing confidence in both device and clinical protocols. With expanded qualification of attending personnel, coverage was being distributed on a more uniform basis. Overall analysis was becoming more critical, with the desire to search for more effective VDR programming without fear of losing clinical ground already gained. With a greater trust in the device, the protocol, and each other, communications between attending exponentially improved. The ability to provide the severe respiratory alkalosis required for PPHT without induced barotrauma was demonstrated.

b Suggestions and possibilities:

The more involved each individual member of the attending team becomes, the more effective the total coverage.

Initial time spent in understanding reflects in earlier and more effective patient stabilization.

The application of a CRT presenting proximal airway waveform provides a most logical approach toward programming and the teaching of waveform analysis.

Oscillatory CPAP may be considerably more effective in maintaining PaO_2, when compared to static demand CPAP.

Each member of the clinical programming team must be highly proficient in waveform selection (on a clinical basis) as well as in control logic.

4 *Neonatal VDR case presentation: baby girl (D)—Carl J Bodenstein, MD.*

Baby girl *D* is a 2900 g, 38-week EGA, born to a G6, P4, AB 1 white woman. Pregnancy was complicated by polyhydramnios, and at elective induction and artifical rupture of membranes, significant late decelerations were seen with maternal vaginal bleeding. These events were followed by an emergency cesarean section. Apgar scores were 1 and 6 while initial ABGs on 40% FIO_2 showed a pH of 7.17, CO_2 of 88, and a PO_2 of 39. The patient was intubated and placed on 100% FIO_2, then bagged with pressures approximating 23 to 25 with a rate of approximately 60. Blood cultures were obtained (subsequently negative), and ampicillin and gentamicin were begun. Initial CXR demonstrated an extremely high right diaphragm with a small bilateral thoracic dimension. Liver was well palpable 4 cm below the right midcostal margin. Transport was performed on a conventional ventilator, 27 pressure, 80 rate, 1:1 I:E. Blood gases on institutional arrival demonstrated a pH of 7.32, PCO_2 of 46, PO_2 of 38, and base deficit of 2.0. Ventilation was established with 27/4, subsequently increased to 32 and then to 38 cm H_2O.

Blood gases showed a pH of 7.45, PCO_2 of 30, PO_2 of 57, with a BE of -1.3. PEEP was subsequently removed with a delivery pressure of 38/0, rate of 60, 1:1 I:E with ABGs pH 7.52, PCO_2 of 25, PO_2 of 75, and a BE of -0.3.

Physical examination was significant only for small thoracic size. Additional significant history obtained from the family was that of a previous sibling that had died at 6 hours of age of a bilateral pneumothorax, approximately 1 year before delivery of this infant. Assessment on admission was pulmonary hypertension with possible pulmonary hypoplasia on the basis of asphyxiating thoracic dystrophy of a Lejeune autosomal dominant basis.

Blood pressure at the time of admission was 75/40 with an HR of 140. Subsequently oxygenation became extremely poor and decreased (despite CO_2 kept well in the low 30s with a moderate respiratory alkalosis) to a PaO_2 of 18.

It was elected at this time that a VDR trial (Fig. 23-100) be performed and additionally a Swan-Ganz catheter be placed. Ventilation before transfer to a Baby-bird ventilator was 50/0, IMV 60, FIo_2 100%. The VDR Percussionator was programmed with an ascending waveform (step and backstep) ventilation. Parameters were 64/5, mean airway 24, frequency 680/min, stepladder segments repetitively programmed at a rate of 40/min. Step and backstep were of equal duration. Initial blood gases showed pH of 7.33, Pco_2 of 36, and Po_2 of 32. Blood gases 15 min later demonstrated a pH of 7.43, with Pco_2 of 30 and Po_2 of 28. A Swan-Ganz catheter was inserted at this time. Immediately after insertion, ABGs demonstrated a pH of 7.56, Pco_2 of 30, Po_2 of 28, and a BE of + 6.3. Initial pulmonary artery pressures (PAP) showed a mean of 42 with a systemic mean of 52. A Priscoline push was administered per Swan-Ganz catheter resulting in blood gases revealing a pH of 7.48, Pco_2 of 35, and a Po_2 of 21. Subsequently, the stepladder interval was lengthened and the repetitive rate decreased to 34/min. Using a 2:1 ratio of step to backstep, ABGs then demonstrated a pH of 7.54, Pco_2 of 27, and a Po_2 of 39. CXR obtained after placement of the Swan-Ganz catheter showed the PA line in the main pulmonary artery. A right pulmonary effusion was now demonstrated. The effusion was relieved with a 20-gauge angiocath with removal of 14 ml of straw-colored fluid. After initial drainage, a 12 Fr catheter was inserted laterally and posteriorly for chronic drainage of the pleural effusion.

Laboratory studies indicated the effusion was a transudate, and the cause was believed to have resulted from right heart failure.

Oxygenation remained extremely poor over a significant time interval, representative of severe hypoxia with a Po_2 of 30 or less, despite the maintenance of Pco_2 in the 30 to 40 range with an associated respiratory alkalosis. As a result of the inability of the VDR protocol to provide oxygenation, a transfer back to conventional ventilation was made. Shortly after transfer back to conventional ventilation, the patient died with an increasing respiratory and metabolic acidosis. Postmortem examination demonstrated bilateral pulmonary hypoplasia. The pulmonary architecture was well preserved without evidence of PIE. Severe acute hepatic congestion and cerebral edema with a marked venous congestion were noted. In addition to the recognized right pleural effusion, a left pleural effusion containing 20 ml of fluid was found. The presumptive diagnosis of Lejeune's asphyxiating thoracic dystrophy is in concert with the previous sibling's respiratory death.

a Discussions baby girl *(D)*:

The lack of barotrauma documented at autopsy, despite pulmonary hypoplasia and the use of an ascending waveform (step and backstep) programming, was impressive in this case. This would suggest that the backstep breakup of an ascending pressure gradient may serve to break up hoop stress sufficiently to minimize tendencies toward the pneumatic dissection of pulmonary airway.

A consistent team approach and decision-making process made this case, despite an inevitable fatal outcome, a rewarding experience for all attending, including nurses, respiratory therapists, and physicians alike.

b Suggestions and possibilities:

The ascending VDR (step and backstep) waveform may well present a clinical program that should be further investigated. Possibly, an ascending waveform providing for a maximum convective exchange with a minimum of sustained hoop stress within the pulmonary airways is the most logical primary VDR program.

5 *Neonatal VDR case presentation: baby boy (E)—Carl J. Bodenstein, MD.*

Baby boy *(E)* is a 1900 g, 4 pound 3 ounce, 31-week EGA white male neonate born to a 31-year-old G4, P2, B-positive white woman by repeat cesarean section caused by premature labor unabatable with tocolytics. Apgar scores were 7 at 1 minute, 8 at 5 minutes, and the baby was initially placed in 0.60 FIo_2 with ABGs of pH 7.21, Pco_2 46, Po_2 125, BE −9.5. The initial CXR was near white out, compatible with severe HMD. ABGs at 1 hour of age demonstrated a pH of 7.15, Pco_2 of 54, Po_2 of 77, and a BE −11.0. The patient was intubated with a 3.0 Fr endotracheal tube. Ventilatory parameters of 22/4, IMV 40, FIo_2 0.5 demonstrated a pH of 7.33, Pco_2 of 38, Po_2 of 215, and a BE of −5.1. A UAC had been inserted to L3 level and a UVC was placed to the right atrial position for CVP monitoring. Blood cultures (subsequently negative) were obtained, with ampicillin and gentamicin started. Over the next 4 hours, FIo_2 was weaned to 0.4 with other parameters unchanged. CXR demonstrated some clearing with early PIE changes. Over the next 24 hours, ventilatory parameters were weaned to 20/4, IMV 40, and an FIo_2 of 0.5. All ABGs showed pH 7.30 to 7.35, Pco_2 32 to 41, and Po_2 50 to 80. CXR at 36 hours of age demonstrated moderate bilateral PIE. A right tension pneumothorax occurred 4 hours later and was well relieved with a 12 Fr thoracotomy tube insertion. Ventilatory parameters required an increase to 23/2, IMV 40, and an FIo_2 0.8 over the next 8 hours. Pavulon was administered. ABGs demonstrated pH 7.25. to 7.30, Pco_2 44 to 48, po_2 76 to 90 with BEs of −5 to −7.5. Weight at this time was down 15 g from birth with a declining urine output. BP was 65/4, CVP 1, HR 150s. Serialized cranial ultrasounds were within normal limits. With vigorous and accelerating right air leaks and increasing ventilatory parameters, a trial of volumetric diffusive respiration was started at 52 hours of age (Fig. 23-101).

The VDR-1 Percussionator was initially programmed at 38/7, MAP 17.2, freq. 760, FIo_2 0.72 with as oscillatory interruption interval at an oscillatory baseline 38 times per minute (oscillatory IMV) with a step to backstep I:E ratio of 1:1.5. First ABGs showed pH 7.22, Pco_2 48, Po_2 87, with a BE of −8.0.

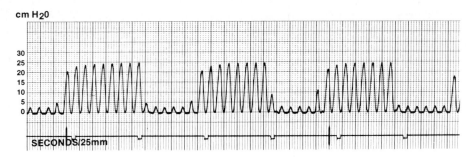

FIGURE 23-101 Classical intrapulmonary percussive ventilation with an accented baseline oscillatory CPAP. (Courtesy Percussionaire Corp, Sand Point, Idaho, and Hewlett-Packard.)

VDR parameters were reprogrammed to 38/7, oscillatory IMV 40, 1:1 I:E ratio causing a rise in CVP from 5 to 8. Second ABGs revealed pH 7.19, Pco$_2$ 59, Po$_2$ 74, with a BE of -7.0. Reprogramming for additional convective exchange resulted in a frequency decrease to 600/min, IMV of 30, 42/4, 1:1 I:E with new blood gases demonstrating a pH of 7.23, Pco$_2$ of 47, Po$_2$ of 82 with a BE of -8.0. Finally, 10 min after increasing convective component, ABGs revealed a pH of 7.27, Pco$_2$ 41, Po$_2$ 91 with a BE of -7.5, the CVP remained between 8 and 9, with ABP 66/42 and HR in the 150s. Over the next 3 hours, Pco$_2$ declined to 31, pH 7.36, and Po$_2$ around 80. CXR demonstrated some decrease in PIE findings.

In an impatient attempt to increase Pao$_2$ (still at an FIo$_2$ of 0.72) the diffusive frequency was increased to 720/min, causing oscillatory pressures to rise to 57/12. (NOTE: Amplitude and/or I:E [E] should have been used to decrease FRC after frequency increase.) After reprogramming, Pco$_2$ declined into the 20s, pH rose to 7.45, FIo$_2$ weanable to 0.7 at the expense of AM chest plates revealing a reaccumulation of air on the right requiring a tube for resolution. Insertion of a 12 Fr thoracotomy tube brought about resolution. A diuresis of 120 g had occurred since initiating the VDR program. With a rapid weaning of ventilatory programming to 57/12, 47/10, 42/8, 37/4, 33/0 with a frequency of 730/min, an FIo$_2$ of 0.7, and an IMV of 36, ABGs demonstrated a Pco$_2$ of 43 and Po$_2$ of 82. With an overshoot during weaning, the patient was reprogrammed over the next 2 hours for elevations in Pco$_2$ requiring an increase in oscillatory delivery pressures back up to 42/0, which provided Pco$_2$ of from 43 to 51. From this point positive reprogramming was started with a frequency of 600, then down to 540/min, 36/3, IMV 36, 1:1 I:E wtih a subsequent weaning of FIo$_2$ from 0.7 to 0.49. Peak inspiratory pressures of from 36 down to 32 were maintained over the next 10 hours. CXRs at this time demonstrated clearer lung fields with PIE less prominent. Weaning was continued with reprogramming to a freq. of 440, 35/5/, IMV 36, 1:1 I:E whereupon FIo$_2$ was weaned to 0.36. At this time one chest tube was removed and the patient was allowed to recover from paralysis. Returning spontaneous ventilatory activity was slow, demonstrating rhythmic and nondistressed breathing through the previously established VDR program. After 36 hours of VDR, oscillatory CPAP was initiated. ABGs were then pH 7.30 to 7.37, Pco$_2$ 41 to 51, Po$_2$ 70 to 92 on an FIo$_2$ of 0.40, decreasing to 0.32. A favorable diuresis had continued, with the patient now 230 g below birth weight. Hyperalimentation with aminosyn and scant lipids were begun. CXR was significantly clearer and PIE changes were absent. The patient was extubated after 12 hours of CPAP. Six hours later in the prone position, during a vigorous crying session, the right pneumothorax reaccumulated. This was easily relieved by the existing chest tube when the patient was rotated into the supine position. Positional change did not resolve decompensation with a pronounced tachypnea, and the patient was placed back on oscillatory CPAP with an FIo$_2$ of 0.60. Weaning from this point was rapid with extubation following in 24 hours. Weaning to room air was accomplished within the next 24 hours with removal of the chest tube. CXRs continued to show some increased perihilar markings. The patient was started on nipple feedings, which progressed slowly but well. He was discharged at 22 days of life with a weight of 1960 g (4 pounds, 5 ounces). Neurologic examination is normal for age and opthalmologic examination is within normal limits.

a Discussions baby boy (*E*):

Earlier VDR intervention may markedly shorten duration of therapeutic process.

Program change must be closely monitored to negate potential miscalculation. Parameter alteration must be performed singly with blood gas determination before reprogramming. Each programming change must reflect lag and effect as verified by positive documentation.

Patience remains a virtue. Establish a single logic for weaning with strict adherence unless blood gas parameters dictate otherwise. Do not enter into a circle of confusion; confirm, then act. All members of the team must be totally familiar with the weaning schedule and acceleration because communication gaps are human and must be guarded against.

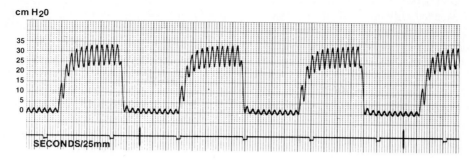

F I G U R E   2 3 - 1 0 2 Classical ascending waveform (step and backstep) with pronounced convective waveform. (Courtesy Hewlett-Packard and Percussionaire Corp, Sand Point, Idaho.)

CAUTION: Avoid overheparinization resulting from the use of heparinized flush solutions when numerous blood gases are obtained over a short period of time.

b Suggestions and possibilities:

When stroke volume delivery frequency is increased, both inspiratory and expiratory time intervals are decreased proportionately; however, a disproportionate increase in functional residual capacity (FRC) occurs because the passive expiratory flow interval is reduced. By reducing expiratory flow time, the delivered stroke volume progression is unable to backflow to the original FRC. With an increased FRC, peak delivery pressures will be increased by delivering against lower compliance within the airways, increasing tendencies toward pneumatic dissection. Therefore, when oscillatory frequency is increased, either concomitantly decrease delivery amplitude or extend the (E) component of the oscillatory I:E ratio to decrease or maintain FRC.

The asecending waveform continues to demonstrate clinical efficacy.

6 *Neonatal VDR case presentation: baby boy (F)—Carl J. Bodenstein, MD.*

Baby boy *(F)* is a 3005 g birthweight 36 week LGA outborn neonate born to a 29-year-old G2, P1, A-positive white woman with premature rupture of membranes. Subsequent labor was augmented with Pitocin, accompanied by late decelerations, and Pitocin was discontinued. Delivery was by way of vaginal vertex, Apgar scores were 7 and 9, but respiratory distress was present from birth. The patient was initially placed in a hood with an FIo_2 of 0.4; however, apnea intervened at 2 hours of age requiring intubation and mechanical ventilation. An umbilical artery catheter was introduced. Blood cultures were obtained (subsequently negative) with antibiotics started. Transport was on conventional ventilation with 32/5, IMV 60, I:E 1:1, FIo_2 1.0. Initial ABGs showed pH of 7.29 to 7.31, Pco_2 of 43 to 45 and Po_2 of 26 to 47. CXRs were consistent with moderate HMD. Physical examination was positive only for an IDM-looking LGA 36-week neonate with respiratory distress. UVC was placed for

CVP monitoring *(5)*, and cardiac echo was performed to rule out cyanotic heart disease (negative). Systolic timing intervals were consistent with pulmonary hypertension. Ventilatory parameters were 40/4, IMV 60, I:E 1:1, FIo_2 1.0. ABGs were pH 7.31, Pco_2 39, Po_2 45, with a BE of −5.1. Ventilatory parameters were then increased to 42/4; following ABGs were pH 7.12, Pco_2 60, Po_2 81 with a BE of −10. Over the next 10 hours, CO_2 and pH corrected; however, all Po_2 were less than 50. CXR remained consistent with severe HMD. With increasing inability to provide adequate ventilation, despite Pavulon, an increase in IMV to 80, and a PIP of 46, it was elected to initiate a trial of volumetric diffusive respiration (Fig. 23-102).

Before transfer to a VDR program, ventilatory parameters were 46/2, IMV 60, I:E 1:1, FIo_2 1.0. ABGs were a pH of 7.62, Pco_2 of 27, Po_2 of 79, with a BE of −8.3. VDR was initiated with an ascending waveform (step and backstep) with 43/5 with a repetitive stepladder of 30. Initial frequency was 990/min, which was subsequently lowered to 800/min; step to backstep ratio was 1:1. First post-VDR blood gases demonstrated a pH of 7.51, Pco_2 of 32, Po_2 of 98, with a BE of +3.8. Following blood gases ranged to pH 7.61 with Pco_2 of 29, Po_2 of 146 and a BE of +8.7. Within 2 hours of VDR initiation FIo_2 was weaned to 0.8. Soon therafter ventilatory parameters were weaned to 28/3, IMV 30, frequency 800 with following ABGs all having Po_2 above 100 with respiratory alkalosis of pH 7.45 and Pco_2 of 30 to 35. Hypocapnia and hyperoxia were maintained in the face of persistent pulmonary hypertension. Dopamine 10 µg/kg/min, was started. After about 12 hours into VDR ventilation, the PIP required was increased to 33 with an associated increase in FIo_2 to 0.96. Following blood gases revealed a pH of 7.59, Pco_2 of 30, Po_2 of 136, and a BE of +8.6. A marked diuresis had ensued while blood pressure was maintained at a mean of 10 points above pre-VDR levels. CVPs were maintained from 3 to 6. CXRs remained consistent with severe hyaline membrane disease. On day 3 of life, the patient was started on hyperalimentation, and lipid was withheld due to lung findings. CXR now demonstrated significant clearing. After 36 hours into the VDR program, the patient had been weaned to

26/4, IMV 30, frequency 800/min, and an FIo_2 of 0.8. Subsequently, oxygenation again became labile, and required pressures were increased to 39/3. The stepladder rate had been weaned to 20 in the intervening time frame. Blood gases demonstrated a respiratory alkalosis with Po_2 greater than 100 and BE of from +3 to +5. The baby had diuresed significantly and now was 180 g below birth weight. Active weaning was initiated, and over the next 24 hours, ventilatory parameters had been reduced to 23/3, IMV 24, FIo_2 to 0.3. Dopamine and Pavulon were withdrawn. After a 4-day run on VDR, with nearly clear CXRs, the patient was started on a course of oscillatory CPAP at 4 cm H_2O. Following blood gases were a pH of 7.40, Pco_2 of 36, Po_2 of 92, with a BE of 0 to −3. After 5 days of VDR, the patient was extubated to 30% hood at 6 days of age. Subsequently, the patient was weaned to room air within 24 hours; feedings were then commenced and progressed very well. The patient was discharged at 10 days of age with a weight of 3060 g. Neurologic examination was normal.

a Discussions baby boy *(F):*

Rapid weaning of oscillatory peak inspiratory pressures (PIP) may be accompanied by the later onset of CO_2 retention to a greater degree than would be expected with conventional ventilation. The cause of this commonly observed phenomena may be the slow "derecruitment" of functional alveolar units.

As experience is gained by the neonatal management team, the VDR protocols have become increasingly predictable. It would appear that the earlier the initiation of VDR, the less stormy the therapeutic regime.

b Suggestions and possibilites:

The greatest value of the Bird-conceived VDR concept beyond survival may remain with minimizing residual effects resulting from mandated therapeutic means.

C *Case history summarization*

Six of the initial anecdotal neonates out of the first ten patients studied under volumetric diffusive respiration (VDR) by the Spokane group have been presented under "real life" conditions. The other three survivors were parallel to cases presented. The other neonate that died had nonreversible pathologic conditions: severe birth asphyxia (pH 6.83), with massive meconium aspiration and pulmonary hypertension (pulmonary artery pressure to 110/80). Hopefully, the lessons learned have been elucidated sufficiently to enable following clinicians a clearer understanding of the overall management capabilities and limitations of Bird-conceived VDR protocols.

The learning curve experienced by each clinical team embarking into VDR will vary widely, based on the clinical settings encountered. However, as demonstrated in the preceding cases, key points can be drawn together to form a logical approach toward VDR programming, initiation, maintenance, and successful weaning. Many of these points have already been enumerated in the discussions of each case.

A general review of the clinical experience provided by Dr. Bodenstein and his colleagues follows:

1 Ten cases, all failing conventional procedures, were treated by VDR device. There were eight survivors, all with no, or minimal, residual effects. The restricted IRB (FDA device exemption) protocol mandates the application of criteria associated with advanced potentially terminal disease in patient selection. Therefore, by denying early application of VDR in this patient population, optimal clinical protocol is compromised. Clinical judgment, when maximal survival with minimal residual is the goal, should not be hampered by "absolute" criteria or protocol.

2 The VDR program with minimal barotrauma-inducing component, namely an interrupted oscillatory pattern with regular return to baseline, may be attempted in most cases. Clinical experience regarding "thoracic excursion" will dictate whether augmented convective ventilatory component is required. Reaffirmation by blood gas determinations is paramount. Augmented convective component may be accomplished by the:

a Reduction of oscillatory frequency range providing larger stroke volume (viable range in neonatal factoring in both diffusive and convective component appears to be 350 to 800 cpm).

b Expansion of the I:E (E) component of the oscilltory cycle.

c Programming of more frequent returns to baseline (viable range appears to be 20 to 45 min).

d Introduction of convective ventilatory component by convectional breath programming (probably the most barotrauma inducing component).

e Augmentation of both diffusive and convective component by the use of the step and backstep waveform program with repetitive rates of 20 to 45 min.

3 Intermittent return to baseline appears essential to the maintenance of adequate cardiac output and venous return. Impedance of cardiac output is frequent in the smaller infants maintained on VDR. Augmented preload and pressor therapy may be useful adjuncts to an *appropriately adjusted VDR program.* Unstable neonates cannot overcome the adverse effects of inappropriate programming.

4 Weaning may be logically accomplished by the serial lowering of the inspiratory pressures, then the prolongation of the baseline pause interval *without provoking a major change in the successful VDR program.*

23.0 IDENTIFICATION AND TREATMENT OF RESPIRATORY FAILURE
23.1 Respiratory failure

Because it requires volumes to cover the topic of respiratory failure, this unit focuses only on the use of mechanical ventilation in respiratory failure.

1 *Definition*. There is no clear-cut definition that identifies respiratory failure. Instead, there are generally agreed on conditions that usually are present together or individually when a patient is diagnosd as being in respiratory failure. These conditions include:

a Acute dyspnea

b Pa_{O_2} less than 50 mm Hg with the patient on room air

c Pa_{CO_2} greater than 50 mm Hg

d A pH less than 7.35

2 There are two primary types of acute respiratory failure (ARF).

a Type I. Patients with hypoxemia, and eucapnia or hypocapnia. These patients usually have acute lung injury such as adult respiratory distress syndrome (ARDS).

b Type II. Patients with hypoxemia and hypercapnia. These patients primarily have chronic obstructive pulmonary disease or central causes of hypoventilation.

23.2 Causes of respiratory failure

The causes of respiratory failure can be traced to conditions that affect the following:

1 Brain. Drug overdose, trauma, poliomyelitis, etc.

2 Spinal cord. Guillian-Barré syndrome, trauma, etc.

3 Neuromuscular system. Myasthenia gravis, tetanus, neuromuscular blocking antibiotics, etc.

4 Thorax and pleura. Massive obesity, trauma, pneumothorax, pleural effusion, etc.

5 Upper airway. Tracheal obstruction, sleep apnea, epiglottis, laryngotracheitis, etc.

6 Cardiovascular system. Pulmonary embolism, cardiogenic pulmonary edema, etc.

7 Lower airway and alveoli. Aspiration, sepsis, bronchiolitis, chronic obstructive pulmonary disease, atelectasis, bronchiectasis, etc.

23.3 Clinical signs of respiratory failure

The primary clinical signs of respiratory failure are similar to those that accompany hypoxemia. They include:

1 Tachycardia

2 Tachypnea

3 Mild hypertension

4 Peripheral vasoconstriction

5 Mental confusion (later)

6 Bradycardia (later)

7 Cyanosis (later)

23.4 Treatment of respiratory failure

Treatment of respiratory failure consists primarily of correcting the hypoxemia and/or hypercapnia without causing additional complications as a result of oxygen toxicity and/or barotrauma associated with mechanical lung inflation.

When mechanical ventilation is used to treat respiratory failure, two major goals are pursued: (1) alveolar ventilation must be maintained and (2) hypoxemia must be corrected.

Once a patient has been placed on mechanical ventilation, arterial blood gas (ABG) must be measured to determine effectiveness of the ventilator to provide alveolar ventilation. This measurement should be drawn approximately 30 min after the patient has been placed on mechanical ventilation.

To assess change the ABG values should be compared to preventilator measurements.

A Pa_{O_2} level of 50 to 60 mm Hg is considered acceptable with a Pa_{CO_2} of 40 to 50 mm Hg and a pH of 7.35 to 7.50. NOTE: Some patients normally exist with abnormally high Pa_{CO_2} values.

If changes are required in the ventilation values expected, the following simple equation may be used to determine new ventilatory parameters.

$$\text{Desired respiratory rate} = \text{Prior rate} \times \frac{\text{Prior } Pa_{CO_2}}{\text{Desired } Pa_{CO_2}}$$

If supplemental oxygen is required, the lowest possible FI_{O_2} to attain a Pa_{O_2} of 50 to 60 mm Hg should be used. An FI_{O_2} greater than 0.5 for prolonged periods (greater than 12 hours) can cause oxygen toxicity.

If an FI_{O_2} of 0.5 does not result in an adequate Pa_{O_2}, one should consider the use of continuous elevated baseline pressure: continuous positive airway pressure (CPAP) or positive end expiratory pressure (PEEP).

One way of assessing the effectiveness of oxygen therapy is to determine the arterial (a)/alveolar (a) oxygen gradient.

A useful abbreviated formula is:

$$PA_{O_2} = PI_{O_2} - \frac{Pa_{CO_2}}{R}$$

where PI_{O_2} = Barometric pressure (PB) minus water vapor pressure or (PB − 47) and R = Respiratory quotient assumed to be 0.8.

Once the PA_{O_2} is determined, the a/A gradient can be calculated by:

$$\text{a/A gradient} = \frac{Pa_{O_2}}{PA_{O_2}}$$

A normal a/A ratio is greater than 0.75.

Given this ratio the new Pa_{O_2} that will result from a change in the FI_{O_2} can be predicted by using the following equation:

$$\frac{\text{Prior } Pa_{O_2}}{\text{Prior } PA_{O_2}} = \frac{\text{New } Pa_{O_2}}{\text{New } PA_{O_2}}$$

24.0 VENTILATOR MONITORS AND ALARMS
24.1 Typical monitors and alarms

1 Most modern ventilators have built-in monitoring and alarm systems that assess whether or not the ventilator is operating properly and if the patient is responding according to preset (desired) results.

2 Module 28 includes a more comprehensive presentation of the parameters and clinical application of critical care cardiorespiratory monitoring, and Module 30 addresses applications of computer technology to ventilators and patient assessment.

3 Typical monitoring and alarm systems on ventilators include:

Monitoring function	Reason for alarm
Source pressure (air/oxygen) or power	Drop in inlet pressure caused by cylinder depletion or wall piped service or loss of electrical power.
Failure to cycle	Electrical failure or ventilator failure.
Stand by (ventilation)	Ventilator "on" but not delivering breaths for a set time period such as 60 sec.
High-system pressure	Breathing system pressure exceeds preset level and is being dumped or inspiration is being terminated.
Low-system pressure	Breathing system pressure has not been reached or has dropped below a preset level during inspiration such as occurs with a patient disconnect.
Low PEEP/CPAP	PEEP or CPAP levels are less than that preset by the control.
Low exhalation volume	Exhaled tidal volume or minute volume is less than that selected for the patient.
Apnea	Failure of the patient to breath spontaneously, or of ventilator to deliver a breath in a preset time period.
I:E ratio	Ventilator fails to maintain preset I:E ratio or ratio becomes less than 1:1
Oxygen percent	Failure of ventilator to deliver preset FIo2.
Temperature	Temperature of gas delivered to patient is not within the range preset on the humidifier.

4 For details regarding the characteristics and performance of monitors and alarms for specific ventilators the reader is referred to factory operating manuals.

24.2 Low-pressure (disconnect) monitors and alarms

1 A low-pressure monitor and alarm is a safety device that should be used whenever a patient is attached to a ventilator or closed breathing circuit.

2 For this reason it is presented here as an example of a typical monitor and alarm system. The purpose of a low-pressure monitor and alarm is to advise the practitioner if a desired positive pressure or gas flow rate is *not* reached or has dropped below a preset level in the patient's breathing circuit during inspiration, be it mechanically or patient generated.

3 Monitoring of positive pressure in the patient breathing circuit during the inspiratory phase of the ventilator is important because this pressure indicates the driving force available to generate the patient's tidal volume.

4 NOTE: It is equally important to measure the patient's exhaled volume because a desired positive pressure may be indicated in the breathing circuit even though the patient has not received an adequate tidal volume.

5 Low-pressure monitoring alarms may be built into the ventilator at the factory or purchased as free-standing units.

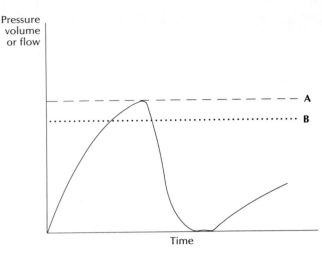

FIGURE 23-103 A, Ventilator inspiratory waveform showing preset desired pressure volume or flow-rate point (no alarm) versus, B, preset alarm point, usually set at 10% to 20% below desired performance with 10- to 12-second delay.

6 Alarms that monitor low pressure and high pressure operate similarly with the primary difference being the alarm points.

7 High-pressure alarms signal if a pressure exceeds a preset limit during inspiration.

8 Low pressure alarms signal if a preset minimum pressure or flow is *not* reached within a set interval of time.

9 Free-standing monitoring alarm units usually incorporate both the monitoring and alarm function into a single cabinet.

10 The free-standing device may be attached to a patient's breathing circuit at the Y piece with a connecting tube or at the exhalation valve manifold.

11 Once in place, the operator sets a minimum pressure or flow rate that must be reached in a preset period of time or the alarm will sound (Fig. 23-103).

In other words, the alarm is always armed. If the preset or flow rate is delivered within the preset time period, the alarm is automatically reset so that it does not activate.

12 If for some reason the preset pressure or flow rate is not reached within the preset time period no. 2, a pressure-sensing flow-sensing switch in the unit completes a circuit to establish the alarm function. Most units incorporate both a visual and audible signal that has battery backup power.

24.3 Desirable features of low-pressure monitor alarm

a AC and DC power source.

b Key operated OFF/ON switch.

c Manually adjustable control for desired variables such as pressure, flow, volume, and time.

d Manual reset control.

e Audible and visual alarm with audible silence option.

f Adjustable sensitivity.

g Responds to disconnected or inoperative exhalation valve.

PROCEDURE 23-1

Connecting a Bird (positive) Q circle to a Bird Mark 7 ventilator

No.	Steps in performing the procedure
	The practitioner will connect assembled parts of a Bird (positive) Q circle to a Bird Mark 7 ventilator. (See Fig. 23-24 for illustration.)
1	Insert patient Y adapter *(11)* into the longest and shortest lengths of large channel tubing forming the inspiratory and expiratory breathing tubes.
2	Insert other end of short breathing tube into open port of exhalation valve *(12)*, and attach the small channel inspiratory drive line to the exhalation valve fitting *(8)*.
3	Insert water trap *(10)* between long and short piece of large channel tubing.
4	Attach large channel tube to the outlet port of the 500 ml nebulizer *(6)*.
5	Connect the end of the small channel inspiration drive line to the main channel of a T adapter *(5)*.
6	Attach the chrome nebulizer block assembly *(4)* to the mounting post, and secure it with the retaining screw.
7	Insert the inlet port of the 500 ml nebulizer into the block assembly.
8	Attach one end of the shortest length of large bore tubing *(3)* to the chrome tubing connector atop the block assembly *(4)*.
9	Attach the end of the large channel breathing tube to the outlet port of the ventilator.
10	Attach the remaining end of the inspiration drive line to the small chrome connector located beside the outlet port of the ventilator *(2)*.
11	Check the circuit for operation and leaks.
12	Correct any malfunctions.

PROCEDURE 23-2

Connecting a Bennett MA-1 breathing circuit to a Bennett MA-1 ventilator

No.	Steps in performing the procedure
	The practitioner will connect assembled parts of a Bennett MA-1 breathing circuit to each other and to a Bennett MA-1 ventilator. This assembly assumes that the ventilator is not brand new, has already been prepared for use with assembled hardware, etc. (See Fig. 23-25 for illustration.)
1	Position support arm to receive manifold by loosening all black retaining screws.
2	Loosen retaining screw and insert knob of manifold *(2)*.
3	Position manifold so that large openings face the ventilator.
4	Tighten retaining screw holding the manifold in this position.
5	Insert nebulizer bacteria filter *(8)* with small bore tube to white connector extending from top of small volume nebulizer *(4)*.
6	Attach one end of large bore corrugated tubing to humidifier outlet.
7	Attach other end of large bore tubing to manifold inlet (large opening beside small volume nebulizer with thermometer port).
8	Connect white small bore nebulizer tube to the open port of the bacteria filter and to white connector on the side of the ventilator to the right of the spirometer post.
9	Attach one end of the large bore spirometer collector tube *(9)* with large adapter to manifold outlet.
10	Connect water trap jar into white collector tube T adapter *(10)*.
11	Connect water trap to bottom of spirometer post.
12	Attach other end of large bore collector tube to the water trap inlet.
13	Connect one end of small bore clear expiration valve tube to tapered translucent adapter of exhalation manifold.
14	Connect other end of expiratory valve tube to the aluminum connector on the side of the ventilator to the left of the spirometer post.
15	Fit small bore tubes into the white retainer rings along the large bore tubes.
16	Install thermometer probe into port on inspiratory side of nebulizer (toward the patient) *(3)*.
17	Connect one end of each of the two smaller bore corrugated tubes to the patient side of the exhalation manifold *(5 and 6)*.
18	Connect other end of tubes to the patient Y adapter *(7)*.
19	Check the circuit for function and leaks.
20	Correct any malfunctions.

PROCEDURE 23-3

Assembly/operation of the Bennett MA-1 ventilator

No.	Steps in performing the procedure	No.	Steps in performing the procedure
	The practitioner will attach patient breathing circuit, humidifier, and other accessories to completely assembled Bennett MA-1 ventilator and operate it in the clinical setting.	10	Press the power control ON.
1		11	Set sensitivity adjustment at lock-out position by turning fully counterclockwise. Set up as controller.
1	Select a decontaminated ventilator from storage.		
2	Gather necessary accessories:	12	Set normal volume control to secure the desired tidal volume (spirometer volume minus 3 ml/cm H$_2$O uncorrected tubing compliance correction). Normal tidal volume between 600 to 1000 ml (cc) for most average size adults.
	22.1 Breathing circuit		
	2.2 Humidifier		
	2.3 Spirometer		
3	Wash hands.	13	Set maximum flow adjustment control to secure desired I:E ratio. If ratio is less than 1:1 (if inspiration time is longer than expiration), the ratio warning light will turn ON.
4	Connect component parts to the ventilator. NOTE: All parts used in assembly must be sterile.		
	4.1 Fit the black tube to the black connector underneath the spirometer base and to the black spirometer connector on the unit.	14	Set normal pressure limit for the maximum pressure deemed safe. It can also be set for a pressure 10 cm H$_2$O higher than the observed peak system pressure, so that a relatively small increase in resistance or decrease in compliance will activate limit and the alarms. Visible and audible alarm will sound.
	4.2 Fit the humidifier cover to the heater assembly. Lock the two retainer knobs to secure.		
	4.3 Open the cabinet door on front of the unit. Fit the main flow bacteria filter through the hole at upper left corner of unit (observe flow direction indicated on the filter). Secure the filter with clamp and nut.	15	Set rate control as prescribed by physician (normal rate between 10 to 14/min for adults).
		16	Observe temperature of thermometer on manifold after humidifier has had time to warm up. If temperature is inadequate, adjust thermostat control on top of humidifier until desired temperature is reached.
	4.4. Fit the angled connector to the filter outlet and to the humidifier inlet port as labeled on the top of the humidifier.		
	4.5 Fit the right-angled tube to filter inlet and to the humidifier outlet port as labeled.	17	Set sigh pressure limit to the maximum pressure that is deemed safe, keeping in mind that this presure may be reached only during the periodic sigh inspiration.
	4.6 Attach the manifold assembly to the support arm with the large openings facing the ventilator.		
	4.7 Fit the small nebulizer bacteria filter to the white jet connector on the patient manifold; observe the arrow indicating flow direction on filter.	18	Set sigh volume control for the estimated desired volume. Normal sigh volume is from 1½ to 2 times the tidal volume.
		19	Set sighs per hour control to desired frequency. Normal settings is 15/hour. NOTE: Patient may be sighed manually by pressing manual sigh button.
	4.8 Connect large bore corrugated main tube to the humidifier outlet and to the manifold inlet facing the ventilator		
	4.9 Fit the small bore white nebulizer tube to the nebulizer manifold outlet facing the ventilator and to the spirometer vial adapter on the bottom of the chrome spirometer post.	20	Optional: Set expiratory resistance control by turning the control clockwise and observing the effects on the system pressure gauge until the desired plateau is reached.
			CAUTION: This control should not be used without the physician's conset.
	4.11 Fit the clear small bore expiration valve tube to the translucent expiration diaphragm attached to the cap located on the side of the manifold, and to the silver expiration valve connector on the side of the ventilator. Fit the expiration valve tube into the retainer tabs on the collector tube.	21	Attach angled Y adapter at end of breathing tube to either tracheotomy tube or endotracheal tube adapter.
		22	Inflate cuff on tracheal tube as necessary to ensure a closed system.
		23	Be sure that angled Y connector and adjacent tubings do *not* place stress on patient's tube.
	4.12 Fit one end of two shorter corrugated tubes to the two open connectors on manifold. Join the other end of the tubes with a Y adapter.	24	If nebulized medication is desired, add medication to nebulizer cup on manifold. Press nebulizer switch to ON position.
	4.13 Cover the Y with a clean cover to prevent contamination during transport.	25	Fill out ventilator check sheet.
5	Fill the humidifier with sterile distilled water only (do not use normal saline).	26	Check ventilator hourly or according to hospital procedure.
6	Transport assembled ventilator to patient area.		**26.1** Drain any water in tubes.
7	Place a NO SMOKING sign on door of patient's room and on ventilator.		
8	Start therapy. Insert and tape electrical plug into electrical outlet.		
9	If oxygen enrichment is desired, connect the oxygen hose on the rear of the cabinet to a 50 PSI oxygen source (limits are 40 to 75 PSI).		

Continued.

PROCEDURE 23-3

Assembly/operation of the Bennett MA-1 ventilator—cont'd

No.	Steps in performing the procedure
	26.2 Fill cascade humidifier as necessary (for least interruption to patient ventilation, remove the tube from the humidifier outlet and the connector from the main flow bacteria filter outlet; then connect the tube to the filter).
	CAUTION: Do not leave patient system disconnected from humidifier for extended period of time. The patient will be receiving unhumidified gas, which will result in pulmonary irritation.
	26.3 Make notes on ventilator check sheet.
27	Change all ventilator tubing and the cascade humidifier daily to prevent bacterial growth and patient contamination.
28	Start therapy as an assistor.
29	Turn sensitivity control clockwise to allow patient triggering. The more the control is advanced, the more sensitive the unit becomes.
30	Before making connection to patient, turn control until the assist lamp lights and the unit self-cycles; then back off until lamp does not light (approximately -0.5 to 1 cmH$_2$O should be indicated on the manometer).
31	Avoid increasing sensitivity to a point where the unit self-cycles. This setting may not be readily distinguishable from patient assist and may promote too fast a rate and too short an expiration.
32	For the patient who is breathing erratically or who may stop breathing, set the rate control slightly lower than the normal rate. With this, if the patient does not initiate inspiration by his or her own effort, the rate control will take over that function (assist/control).
	CAUTION: A minimal assist/control rate becomes unsatisfactory if the patient ceases to trigger inspiration for any extended period, as evidence by no signal from the assist indicator lamp. Volume or rate, or both, must then be increased, since the assist-control mode has passed into a full control mode.
33	Observe the system pressure gauge, and adjust the maximum flow control so that the gauge shows a positive pressure during early inspiration.
	NOTE: Patients who are initiating their own inspiration may require a higher inspiraory flow than the completely passive patient.
34	Chart the procedure and complete ventilator/patient checks, using appropriate departmental forms.

PROCEDURE 23-4

Connecting an Emerson breathing circuit to an Emerson 3-PV volume ventilator

No.	Steps in performing the procedure
	The practitioner will connect assembled parts of an Emerson 3-PV breathing circuit to an Emerson 3-PV volume ventilator. (See Figs. 23-27 and 23-28 for illustrations.)
1	Attach clear bottle support tube to reducing elbow.
2	Tighten clear tube to elbow with hose clamp.
3	Attach other end of clear tube to inlet of water trap and tighten clamp over tube.
4	Connect one end of long corrugated tube (inspiratory tube) to outlet port of water trap (13) and secure with screw clamp.
5	Insert other end of inspiratory tube (14) over one side of patient Y adapter (15) with pushing/twisting motion. Check for tight fit.
6	Insert one end of other long corrugated breathing tube (exhalation tube) (19) over elbow from exhalation valve, and secure with clamp.
7	Insert other end of expiratory tube firmly over other side of patient Y adapter with pushing and twisting motion. Check for fit.
8	Insert elbow in exhalation port (4), and connect corrugated tube to spirometer inlet (if used).
9	Check circuit for function and tightness.

PROCEDURE 23-5

Attaching the Bennett PEEP attachment

No.	Steps in performing the procedure
	The practitioner will attach and test the operation of the Bennett PEEP attachment to an assembled MA-1 ventilator.
1	Disconnect the small transparent expiration valve tube from the aluminum expiration valve connector protruding from the mounting plate on the side of the ventilator.
2	Pull the black disk cover from the mounting plate, exposing an open port.
3	Plug the PEEP attachment into the open port.
4	Attach the clear small bore tubing from either connector on the bottom of the attachment to the aluminum connector protruding from the mounting plate on the side of the MA-1.
5	Fit the end of the small clear exhalation valve tube leading from the cap of the exhalation valve to the other connector on the bottom of the PEEP attachment.
6	Set controls on the MA-1 as follows: 6.1 Set PEEP control at OFF. 6.2 Set peak flow at MAX. 6.3 Set normal pressure limit at MAX. 6.4 Set normal volume at 1500 ml. 6.5 Set expiratory resistance at OFF. 6.6 Set rate control at OFF.
7	Connect a rubber test lung to the patient Y adapter.
8	Turn power switch ON.
9	Manually cycle unit and check that system pressure manometer drops to zero at end of exhalation (no PEEP).
10	Set expiratory retard control full clockwise (right), and manually cycle the unit.
11	Observe spirometer for smooth slow filling, indicating expiratory retard.
12	Verify that pressure drops to zero at end of exhalation.
13	Turn PEEP control full right and cycle the unit.
14	System pressure mmanometer should indicate 9 to 14 cm H_2O pressure at the end of exhalation.
15	Turn expiratory resistance control full left and manually cycle the unit. System pressure gauge should read $\pm$ 2 cm H_2O pressure of previous reading.
16	Incrementally rotate PEEP control counterclockwise, and check for changing PEEP levels on the system manometer.
17	Return PEEP to zero and manually cycle unit.
18	Note that system manometer returns to zero at the end of exhalation indicating no PEEP.
19	Turn power OFF.

PROCEDURE 23-6

Using Bennett MA-1 ventilator to generate PEEP

No.	Steps in performing the procedure
	The practitioner will use a fully assembled MA-1 ventilator to deliver PEEP according to physician's orders.
1	Take fully assembled MA-1 to bedside.
2	Wash hands.
3	Explain procedure to simulated patient, especially the sensation of breathing against PEEP.
4	Plug ventilator to power source.
5	Turn power switch ON.
6	Set prescribed volume limit (15 ml/kg body weight).
7	Set normal pressure limit.
8	Set peak flow.
9	Set frequency to achieve desired minute volume.
10	Set FIo_2 to 0.6.
11	Set rate control to 10/min for adults.
12	Set other controls OFF.
13	Draw arterial blood gas (use simulation arm if possible).
14	Calculate volume of shunted blood per tidal volume of blood flow ($\dot{Q}s/\dot{Q}T$ less than 0.15).
15	Attach simulated patient to ventilator.
16	Measure static compliance.
17	Wait 15 minutes; draw another ABG.
18	Check Pao_2, which should be at least 50 to 55 torr but not greater than 70 torr.
19	Recheck static compliance.
20	If Pao_2 is greater than 70 torr, decrease FIo_2 to achieve a Pao_2 of 70 torr.
21	If Pao_2 is less than 50 torr, add 2 to 3 cm PEEP until desired results are obtained (assume Pao_2 less than 50 torr).
22	Wait 15 minutes, then recheck ABG.
23	Calculate increase in Pao_2 and static compliance.
24	Increase PEEP by 2 to 3 torr increments as required to reach Pao_2 of 50 torr. Wait 15 minutes at each step for ABG and compliance measurement (assume PEEP of 15 cm H_2O is necessary).
25	If Pao_2 does *not* increase, go to high levels of PEEP greater than 15 torr (raise PEEP to 25 cm H_2O).
26	Carefully observe cardiac output, mixed venous oxygen tension ($P\bar{v}o_2$), Pao_2, compliance, and any signs of tension pneumothorax or barotrauma (note distension of test lung).
27	Maintain patient at stable FIo_2 and PEEP level for 12 to 24 hours.
28	Carefully reduce FIo_2 and/or PEEP by 2 to 3 cm H_2O increments by checking desired parameters and allowing 6 to 24 hours at each step.
29	Reduce FIo_2 to lowest possible level and PEEP to 2 cm H_2O to maintain stable values.
30	Remove patient from PEEP and maintain on low flow oxygen if necessary until room will maintain stable Pao_2.
31	Chart patient's progress as required.

PROCEDURE 23-7

Evaluating need for mechanical ventilation

No.	Steps in performing the procedure
1	The practitioner will assess a patient's need for mechanical ventilation using the criteria listed below. NOTE: This task is a diagnostic determination that should be left to the physician, except in emergency situations or according to prearranged standing orders by the physician. Assess the patient generally for: **1.1** Respiratory activity (present, absent, effective, ineffective) **1.2** Work of breathing **1.3** Color **1.4** Vital signs **1.5** Level of consciousness **1.6** Anxiety level **1.7** Compliance
2	Measure clinical parameters with ventilation indicated for the following: **2.1** Respiratory rate is more than 35. **2.2** Vital capacity is less than 10 to 15 ml/kg. **2.3** Arterial to alveolar oxygen dead space gradient (a-AD$_{O_2}$) is more than 400 torr on 100% O_2. **2.4** Dead space to tidal volume ratio V_D/V_T is more than 60%. **2.5** Pa$_{CO_2}$ is more than 60 torr.
3	Gather and assess the patient's history and events relevant to the current situation.
4	Discuss the need for ventilation and procedure with patient and family as appropriate.
5	If ventilation is necessary, arrange for: **5.1** Tracheal intubation **5.2** Proper type of ventilator **5.3** Suction equipment **5.4** Support staff **5.5** Monitors

PROCEDURE 23-8

Monitoring oxygen percentage on a mechanical ventilator

No.	Steps in performing the procedure
	The practitioner will operate the Critikon Oxygen multipurpose Differential analyzer* to measure Fl$_{O_2}$ on a patient being mechanically ventilated.
1	Collect Critikon and appropriate adapters.
2	Check accuracy of analyzer in room air environment.
3	Check accuracy of analyzer in 100% oxygen environment.
4	Change membrane cartridge if necessary.
5	Change batteries if necessary.
6	Clean silver anode if necessary.
7	Wash hands.
8	Use analyzer in upright position to measure Fl$_{O_2}$ of gas in the inspiratory side of the ventilator circle. Allow to stabilize.
9	Accurately read the oxygen percentage on the dial.
10	Wash hands.
11	Chart results.

*Or similar brand.

PROCEDURE 23-9

Estimating ventilation requirements

No.	Steps in performing the procedure
	The practitioner will estimate the patient's ventilatory requirements for continuous mechanical ventilation using a volume ventilator.
1	Determine body weight of patient (ml/kg).
2	Select mode of ventilation based on patient's condition (assist-control).
3	Estimate a functional breathing rate (adult, child, infant).
4	Set tidal volume in ml/kg.
5	Set inspiratory flow rate; initially 40 to 50 L/min.
6	Set FIo_2, initially 0.21.
7	Set cycling frequency (adult, child, infant).
8	Connect ventilator to patient during exhalation phase.
9	Count respiratory rate.
10	Measure exhaled tidal volume.
11	Readjust inspiratory flow rate for desired I:E ratio.
12	Draw ABG after 15 min or according to procedure.
13	Readjust tidal volume and respiratory rate to achieve desired ABG values.
14	Readjust FIo_2 as required.
15	Use PEEP if indicated (according to procedure).
16	Redraw ABG in 15 min, according to procedure.
17	Make adjustments to tidal volume and rate, FIo_2, and PEEP as appropriate until desired level ABG is reached.
18	Keep physician informed of all values/changes according to procedure.

PROCEDURE 23-10

Setting up a volume ventilator

No.	Steps in performing the procedure
	The practitioner will set up a volume ventilator.
1	Confirm physician's orders.
2	Select ventilator to meet patient's needs:
	2.1 Volume
	2.2 Frequency
	2.3 IMV, CPAP, PEEP
	2.4 FIo_2
3	Collect support items:
	3.1 Gas source or hose adapter
	3.2 Respirometer or spirometer
	3.3 Oxygen monitor
	3.4 Sterile, distilled water
	3.5 Patient breathing circuit
4	Wash hands.
5	Assemble and test ventilator before bringing it to the patient area.
6	Introduce yourself.
7	Identify patient by ID band.
8	Discuss procedure with patient and family, if appropriate.
9	Reassure patient.
10	Estimate patient's needs and set ventilator for:
	10.1 Tidal volume
	10.2 Flow rate
	10.3 Frequency
	10.4 I:E ratio
	10.5 PEEP or CPAP
	10.6 IMV
	10.7 FIo_2
11	Connect patient to ventilator.
12	Check for chest expansion and listen for bilateral breath sounds.
13	Listen for proper exhaust sounds.
14	Listen for gas leaks.
15	Use respirometer to measure minute volume.
16	Chart ventilation values.
17	Recheck patient in 15 to 20 min and adjust ventilator as necessary.

PROCEDURE 23-11

Monitoring the patient on continuous ventilation

No.	Steps in performing the procedure
1	The practitioner will monitor a patient for adequate ventilation according to the following steps. Use visual/audible signs.
	1.1 Visually assess patient and ventilator.
	1.2 Visually evaluate chest expansion, level of physical activity, facial expression, use of ventilatory muscles.
	1.3 Visually check alarms/monitors.
	1.4 Listen for audible alarms, unusual sounds made by the ventilator, and patient noises.
2	Measure/record ventilation values using ventilator/patient monitoring form.
3	Check operation of humidifier, and record temperature.
4	Empty condensate or other solution from tubing and water traps.
5	Use suction on the patient as necessary.
6	Evaluate vital signs and monitors.
7	Assess arterial blood gases compared to ventilation tidal volume, rate, PEEP, and FI_{O_2} as appropriate.
8	Make corrections according to hospital procedure.
9	Handle emergencies by responding appropriately to the situation and assessing life support function.

PROCEDURE 23-12

Using a pressure reservoir for intermittent mandatory ventilation (IMV)

No.	Steps in performing the procedure
1	The practitioner will assemble and operate a pressurized reservoir system for IMV with a Bennett MA-1 ventilator on a test lung and on a patient. Collect necessary equipment:
	1.1 Assembled MA-1 ventilator
	1.2 Oxygen blender
	1.3 Connecting tubing
	1.4 IMV equipment
2	Wash hands.
3	Assemble IMV setup according to Fig. 23-59.
	3.1 Attach one-way valve to T piece with direction of flow toward inspiratory circuit.
	3.2 Connect T tube to proximal end of one-way valve.
	3.3 Attach 5 L anesthesia bag to T tube on proximal end of the one-way valve.
4	Explain procedure to patient.
5	Draw ABG for baseline data.
6	Attach IMV valve to inspiratory side of ventilator circuit proximal to humidifier.
7	Verify valve operation and no leaks by occluding patient Y and cycling ventilator.
8	Adjust ventilator to prescribed rate, which will allow patient to breathe spontaneously.
9	Observe spontaneous rate and depth of breathing and valve function.
10	Be sure bag does not collapse between ventilator cycles.
11	Set cycling frequency so that control rate ensures adequate ABG.
12	After 20 to 30 min, draw ABG.
13	Adjust ventilator rate and/or tidal volume to correct for best ABG.
14	Chart results.
15	Continue to monitor patient, and incrementally adjust control rate as spontaneous breathing and ABG become adequate.

PROCEDURE 23-13

Changing ventilator breathing circuits

No.	Steps in performing the procedure
1	The practitioner will change the patient's breathing circuit on various types of volume ventilators according to the following steps. Collect necessary equipment: **1.1** Sterile breathing circuit **1.2** Humidifier **1.3** Sterile, distilled water for humidifier **1.4** Manual resuscitator with necessary adapters **1.5** Flowmeter with connecting tube **1.6** Sterile gloves **1.7** Plastic bag
2	Wash hands.
3	Assemble components of sterile breathing circuit outside patient area.
4	Fill humidifier with sterile, distilled water.
5	Obtain assistance.
6	Carry preassembled circuit into patient area.
7	Explain procedure to patient.
8	Have assistant set up manual resuscitator at bedside with appropriate FI_{O_2}.
9	Turn to OFF ventilator alarms and ventilator.
10	Put on sterile gloves.
11	Disconnect patient from ventilator.
12	Have assistant manually ventilate patient by matching as closely as possible the tidal volume, oxygen percentage, and rate delivered by the ventilator.
13	Remove used ventilator circuit, empty humidifier, and immediately place it in a plastic bag.
14	Remove and place gloves in the bag.
15	Place new circuit on ventilator.
16	Turn ventilator to ON.
17	Pressure check new circuit for gross gas leaks, and check function by occluding patient Y piece on circuit with a sterile object and manually cycling the ventilator.
18	Connect ventilator to patient during expiratory phase.
19	Observe patient for chest expansion.
20	Auscultate the chest for bilateral breath sounds.
21	Turn to ON all alarms/monitors.
22	Measure ventilatory values and compare to prechange values.
23	Correct any noted discrepancies.
24	Dispose of contaminated ventilator circuit (if disposable), or process contaminated permanent equipment according to hospital procedure.
25	Complete any required records.

PROCEDURE 23-14

Identifying/correcting ventilator malfunction

No.	Steps in performing the procedure
1	The practitioner will recognize and take appropriate action to correct any malfunction of a ventilator used for continuous ventilation. Ensure that a manual resuscitator is readily available to each ventilator in service.
2	Recognize that a malfunction is occurring by: **2.1** Change in patient's level of consciousness, color, breathing activity **2.2** Unusual sounds by patient **2.3** Absence of sounds or unusual sounds by ventilator **2.4** Changes in system pressure manometer **2.5** Ventilator tubing expansion
3	Disconnect the patient and provide manual ventilation.
4	Manually ventilate patient, duplicating as close as possible ventilator settings.
5	Reassure/comfort the patient.
6	Report the situation and ask for assistance.
7	With patient disconnected, check the appropriate ventilator alarm. **7.1** Check all hose/adapter connections. **7.2** Check humidifier seal. **7.3** Check source gas. **7.4** Check electrical connection. **7.5** Check IMV valve and PEEP valve, if appropriate.
8	Attach a test lung and confirm complete ventilator function.
9	Replace ventilator, if appropriate.
10	Reconnect the patient to the ventilator.
11	Explain the problem to the patient and/or visitors, as appropriate.
12	Chart activity according to procedure.

BIBLIOGRAPHY

Banaszak EF et al: Home ventilator care, Respir Care 26:1262, 1981.

Bone RC: Complications of mechanical ventilation and positive end-expiratory pressure, Respir Care 27:402, 1982.

Bone RC: Monitoring patients in acute respiratory failure, Respir Care 27:700, 1982.

Bone RC: Mechanical trauma in acute respiratory failure, Respir Care 28:618, 1983.

Bone RC: The adult respiratory distress syndrome: treatment in the next decade, Respir Care 29:249, 1984.

Boros SJ: Principles of ventilator care. In Thibeault DW and Gregory GA, editors: Neonatal pulmonary care, ed 2, Reading Mass, 1986, Addison-Wesley Publishing Co Inc.

Boysen PG: Respiratory considerations in the postoperative period. In Civetta JM, Taylor RW, and Kirby RR, editors: Critical care, Philadelphia, 1988, JB Lippincott.

Branson RD, Hurst JM, and DeHaven, CB: Synchronous independent lung ventilation in the treatment of unilateral pulmonary contusion: a report of two cases, Respir Care 29:361, 1984.

Breivik H et al: High frequency and conventional positive-pressure ventilation do not decrease cardiac output in acute cardiac tamponade in dogs, Respir Care 28:291, 1983.

Burton GG and Hodgkin JE, editors: Respiratory care—a guide to clinical practice, ed 2, Philadelphia, 1984, JB Lippincott Co.

Carlon GC: Monitoring in respiratory failure, based on pathophysiologic considerations, Respir Care 27:696, 1982.

Chatburn RL, Lough M, and Primiano FP Jr: Modification of a ventilator pressure monitoring circuit to permit display of mean airway pressure, Respir Care 27:276, 1982.

Chatburn RL, McClellan LD, and Lough MD: A new patient-circuit adaptor for use with high frequency jet ventilators, Respir Care 28:1291, 1983.

Cooper KR and Morrow CF: Pulmonary complications associated with head injury, Respir Care 29:263, 1984.

Demers RR, Pratter MR, and Irwin RS: Use of the concept of ventilator compliance in the determination of static total compliance, Respir Care 26:644, 1981.

Downs JB: Ventilatory patterns and modes of ventilation in acute respiratory failure, Respir Care 28:586, 1983.

Ershousky P and Krieger B: Changes in breathing pattern during pressure support ventilation, Respir Care, 32:1011, 1987.

Gallagher TJ: Acute respiratory failure: rationale of therapy, Respir Care 27:1527, 1982.

George RB and Richard RR: Sudden development of cyanosis and markedly decreased compliance during mechanical ventilation, Respir Care 27:79, 1982.

Gilmartin M and Make B: Home care of the ventilator-dependent person, Respir Care 28:1490, 1983.

Guilfoile TD: High frequency ventilation in the management of persistent fetal circulation of the newborn, Respir Care 27:174, 1982.

Halevy A et al: Long term evaluation of patients following the adult respiratory distress syndrome, Respir Care 29:132, 1984.

Heebink DM: The high frequency ventilation saga, Respir Care 26:991, 1981.

Heebink DM: The critical care frontier, Respir Care 28:207, 1983.

Henry WC, West GA, and Wilson RS: An evaluation of a gas collection valve for use in metabolic measurements in high flow CPAP systems, Respir Care 27:282, 1982.

Holtackers TR, Loosbrock LM, and Gracey DR: The use of the chest cuirass in respiratory failure of neurologic origin, Respir Care 27:271, 1982.

Hudson LD: Evaluation of the patient with acute respiratory failure, Respir Care 28:542, 1983.

Irwin RS and Demers RR: Mechanical ventilation. In Rippe JM et al, editors: Intensive care medicine, Boston, 1985, Little Brown & Co.

Kacmarek RM: The role of pressure support ventilation in reducing work of breathing, Respir Care 33:99, 1988.

Kinasewitz GT: Use of end-tidal capnography during mechanical ventilation, Respir Care 27:169, 1982.

Kirby RR, Smith RA, and Desautels DA: Mechanical ventilation, New York, 1985, Churchill Livingston Inc.

Lewis RM: Automatic increases in mean airway pressuring during mechanical ventilation, Respir Care 27:675, 1982.

MacIntyre NR: Pressure support ventilation: effects on ventilatory reflexes and ventilatory-muscle workloads, Respir Care 32:6, 1987.

Mathewson HS and Gish GB: New volume ventilators (editorial), Respir Care 27:553, 1982.

Maxwell C: Monitoring maximal expiratory PCO_2, Respir Care 27:734.

McGough EK, Banner MJ, and Boysen PG: Pressure support ventilation and intermittent positive pressure ventilation in acute lung injury, Chest 94(suppl):25, 1988.

McPherson SP and Spearman CB: Respiratory therapy equipment, ed 4, St Louis, 1990, The CV Mosby Co.

Murray JF: Pathophysiology of acute respiratory failure, Respir Care 28:531, 1983.

Mushin WW et al: Automatic ventilation of the lungs, ed 3, Oxford, England, 1980, Blackwell Scientific Publications Inc.

Op't-Holt TB et al: Comparison of changes in airway pressure during continuous positive airway pressure (CPAP) between demand valve and continuous flow devices, Respir Care 27:1200, 1982.

Osgood CF et al: Hemodynamic monitoring in respiratory care, Respir Care 29:25, 1984.

Pearce L, Lilly K, and Baigelman W: Effects of positive end-expiratory pressure (PEEP) on intracranial pressure, Respir Care 26:754, 1981.

Pierson DJ: Persistent bronchopleural air leak during mechanical ventilation: a review, Respir Care 27:408, 1982.

Pierson DJ: Indications for mechanical ventilation in acute respiratory failure Respir Care 28:570, 1983.

Pierson DJ: Weaning from mechanical ventilation in acute respiratory failure, Respir Care 28:646, 1983.

Pierson D, Capps JS, and Hudson JD: Maximum ventilatory capabilities of four current-generation mechanical ventilators, Respir Care 31(11):1054, 1986.

Pratter M, Demers RR, and Irwin RS: Adult respiratory distress syndrome: an inadequately stressed feature of Legionnaires' disease, Respir Care 26:875, 1981.

Puckett JD, Smith JD, and Smith RB: Synchronized versus nonsynchronized IMV and high frequency ventilation for IMV, Respir Care 27:289, 1982.

Sivak ED, Cordasco EM, and Gipson WT: Pulmonary mechanical ventilation at home: a reasonable and less expensive alternative, Respir Care 28:42, 1983.

Sjostrand UH et al: IPPV, HFPPV/PEEP in dogs with acute cardiac tamponade, Respir Care 28:767, 1983.

Sjostrand UH, Smith RB, and Babinski MF: An experimental comparison of high frequency ventilation (HFPPV and HFJV) in open ventilator systems, Respir Care 28:761, 1983.

Smith JD: Application of mechanical ventilation in acute respiratory failure, Respir Care 28:579, 1983.

Spearman CB, Sheldon RL, and Egan DF: Egan's fundamentals of respiratory therapy, ed 5, St Louis, 1990, The CV Mosby Co.

Pulmonary function

6.15 State the importance of instantaneous flow as a screening device for small airway disease.

6.16 Estimate various flow rates from a representative tracing of flow to volume.

6.17 Point out the various flow volume loops for:
a A normal test.
b A patient mildly obstructed.
c A patient severely obstructed.
d A patient with reduced MID and terminal flow rates.
e A patient mildly restricted.

6.18 Given flow volume loops, point out and explain various parameters that can be calculated from the tracings.

6.19 Explain advantages to flow-volume loop studies compared with flow-time.

6.20 Define specifics of maximum voluntary ventilation.

6.21 Outline the procedure involved in calculation of maximum voluntary ventilation.

6.22 Describe the usefulness of the maximum voluntary ventilation test.

6.23 List problems with the maximum voluntary ventilation test.

7.1 Identify the relationship of ATPS, BTPS, and STPD to pulmonary function testing.

7.2 Identify and use Boyle's, Charles', Dalton's and Gay-Lussac's laws in temperature conversion.

7.3 Describe the effect of temperature on water vapor pressure.

7.4 Convert ATPS to BTPS and STPD.

8.1 Identify tests of gas exchange.

8.2 Outline a test for dead space.

8.3 Identify factors of diffusion of a single-breath test.

8.4 Identify factors of a steady-state diffusion test.

9.1 Explain how the results of spirometry reflect impairment in patients with and without obstructive or restrictive defects.

9.2 Describe general trends in interpretation of test results of lung mechanics.

9.3 Explain the results of positive tests of small airway function.

9.4 Explain how the results of gas distribution tests reflect lung volume in healthy and unhealthy patients.

9.5 Differentiate overall trends between restrictive and obstructive diseases.

9.6 Differentiate between chest wall restriction and parenchymal restriction.

10.1 Explain how deep inspirations involved in spirometry may elicit bronchoconstriction.

10.2 Identify hazards of heart overstimulation when testing for bronchodilator effect.

10.3 Identify hazards associated with patient conditions of dyspnea or equipment contamination.

11.1 Describe the importance of patient cooperation in testing procedures.

11.2 Apply techniques designed to encourage patient effort—adequate instruction, coaxing, and coaching in spirometry.

11.3 Describe the need for accuracy in pulmonary function testing interpretation.

11.4 Distinguish between test values that are effort-dependent and those that are not effort-dependent.

12.1 Describe the relationship of respiratory mechanics and work of breathing to pulmonary function testing.

12.2 Identify information needed to correlate pulmonary function results to disease processes.

12.3 Discuss the value of routine pulmonary function tests.

12.4 Briefly describe the role of computers in pulmonary function testing.

13.1 through **13.4** Using examples given, interpret the pulmonary function tests for patients 2 through 5.

14.1 through **14.6** Using flow-volume loop patterns shown in Figs. 24-28 to 24-34, determine the type and location of the airway obstruction.

1.1 DEFINITIONS, USES, AND CONTRAINDICATIONS OF PULMONARY FUNCTION TESTING

1.1 Definition of pulmonary function

1 Pulmonary function is a general term describing a broad area of testing to assess a patient's ability to effectively ventilate his or her lungs.

2 The tests primarily involve having patients perform certain inspiratory and expiratory maneuvers to measure lung volumes and capacities, flow rates, diffusion capacities and distribution of ventilation.

3 Results of these tests provide essential information about the impact of disease on pulmonary function, and are of particular benefit in assessing the extent of a respiratory disability. These studies are also used to evaluate surgical risk, and to detect, early on, pulmonary disease.

4 There are many different types of pulmonary function equipment that range from simple mechanical devices to very complex electronic computerized units.

1.2 Pulmonary function and surgery

1 Spirometry screening is of great benefit in determining a patient's baseline normals before surgery so that evaluation of the patient's status after surgery will be more accurate.

2 Thoracic surgery, particularly abdominal surgery, may result in a decrease of 50% to 75% of the vital capacity on the first day after surgery.

3 In the preoperative evaluation, vital capacity, maximum expiratory flow rate, and maximum voluntary ventilation are some of the best tests to indicate surgical risks.

4 Complications can be predicted as highly probable in patients with maximum expiratory flow rates (MEFR) under 200 liters/minute (L/min), maximum voluntary ventilation (MVV) less than 50% of predicted, or a vital capacity (VC) below 1 L.

5 Other relative contraindications to surgery would be an increased residual volume (RV)/total lung capacity (TLC) ratio above 50% or a diffusing capacity below 50% of predicted.

1.3 Pulmonary function and evaluation of bronchial hygiene

1 Many disease conditions and situations that involve change of lung air flow dynamics (like postoperative atelectasis and acute bronchial asthma) are treated by the use of chest physical therapy and bronchodilator drugs or techniques.

2 To accurately assess the benefit of airway hygiene techniques, pulmonary function testing (especially forced VC improvement in overall volume or time-flow improvement) may be used.

1.4 Spirometry in initial screening and disability

1 The shape of a spirometer tracing, as well as the flow rates calculated from it, are useful in categorizing the dysfunction and in estimating the amount of disability.

2 The screening tests of pulmonary function and the slightly more advanced tests of functional residual capacity (FRC) and diffusion can assist in differentiating between physiologic problems and in identifying and locating the problems as specific to the airways, alveoli, vascular bed, or combined areas.

3 Pulmonary function results can indicate whether or not patients have abnormalities with air flow, VC, and expiratory flow. These problems may be termed *obstructive*. Those problems with decreased lung volumes may be termed *restrictive* abnormalities.

4 Once an abnormality has been determined, its effects can be determined by more specific function tests.

5 Evaluation of disability may involve a number of factors including results and comparisons of VC, MVV, MEFR, and exercise testing.

6 In evaluating disability, dyspnea (subjective shortness of breath) is a prime consideration. Exercise testing, various comparisons of MVV, and forced VC are related to electrocardiogram (ECG), heart rate, and blood gas values. These indexes and values and the shape of a flow-volume loop (which is discusssed later) are the most important for differentiating true disability from malingering and psychosomatic concerns.

7 In grading dyspnea, flow rates (especially peak expira-

tory flow rates below 200 L/min) are an important evaluation.

8 The air velocity index and dyspnea index can be used to indicate probable dyspnea.

a Air velocity index $= \dfrac{(\% \text{ predicted MVV})}{(\% \text{ predicted VC})}$

b Dyspnea index $= \dfrac{(\text{Minute volume})}{\text{MVV}}$

1.5 Determination of flow compliance in the pulmonary system

1 Flow rates serve to measure obstruction in airways, but they must be related to the volume at which they are measured.

2 Expiratory air flow depends on recoil and airway diameter, so maximum flows will occur at highest lung volumes where recoil force is highest and airways are larger. Reduced flows indicate a disease process reducing lung recoil or airway diameter; both are characteristic of obstructive conditions.

3 Conditions that have already produced symptoms of an obstructive or restrictive impairment are relatively easy to identify with simple spirometry (forced vital capacity [FCC], forced expiratory volume [FEV], maximum voluntary ventilation [MVV]) and correlate with blood gas results, distribution of ventilation, and physical assessment.

4 The more difficult conditions to test are those in which impairment is probable but not easily detected or those patients that may be asymptomatic. This is the situation with early obstruction and small airway diseases that may lead to obstruction.

5 To detect disease in small airways (those less than 2 mm in diameter), the measurements of flow and resistance need to be performed at low lung volumes. Some specialized tests are known, but the significance of small airway disease and its relation to chronic obstruction are still being researched. The effectiveness of determining early airway disease is a subject of professional controversy.

6 Tests of small airway function include a measurement of frequency dependence of compliance that takes a measure of compliance (change in volume/change in pressure cm H_2O) and the fact that measurements of this value do not change in healthy subjects with changes in respiratory rate but do change in patients with obstruction in large or small airways. Only in patients with normal spirometry results does this test help to detect small airway obstruction.

7 Other tests of small airway dysfunction use conventional testing equipment modified for special purposes. Calculation of flow can be made from a spirogram such as the forced expiratory flow (FEF) 25% to 75% calculation or volume of isoflow by using helium to create a flow-volume loop over a patient's normal loop. A closing volume determination is made by using inhaled oxygen and measuring the dilution of nitrogen on a nitrogen meter while the patient exhales at a slow but steady flow rate. NOTE: A similiar test measures distribution of ventilation and uses a similar technique but does not control flow rate. It is called the single breath nitrogen test.

1.6 Contraindications to pulmonary function testing

1 A patient with poor coordination or lack of ability would contraindicate pulmonary function testing. Patients with severe dyspnea, the very old, the very young, and those who (for whatever reason) cannot follow specific instructions make poor candidates for pulmonary function testing.

2 Patients with severe asthma may have adverse reactions to some of the bronchodilating agents used in testing and would require modifications. It may be necessary to omit post-bronchodilator testing if the patient is having bronchospasm.

3 Patients with certain illnesses would require modifications to testing, if they are able to be tested at all. Patients with aneurysms, hernias, pulmonary emboli, or arrhythmias may not be candidates as a result of the stress involved in testing. Patients with contagious diseases like tuberculosis also may not be candidates.

2.0 ABBREVIATIONS, DEFINITIONS, AND DIAGNOSTIC VALUE OF PULMONARY FUNCTION TESTING*

2.1 Lung volumes and capacities

1 The lung volumes can be divided into four basic sections for study purposes.

 a *Tidal volume* (TV or V_T). The volume of gas inspired or expired during normal respiration.

 b *Residual volume* (RV). The volume of gas remaining in the lungs after a maximum expiration.

 c *Inspiratory reserve volume* (IRV). The maximum volume that can be inspired after a normal inspiration.

 d *Expiratory reserve volume* (ERV). The maximum volume that can be exhaled after a normal expiration.

2 There are also four lung capacities. Each capacity is composed of two or more primary volumes.

 a *Functional residual capacity* (FRC). The total amount of volume in the lungs after a normal expiration; consists of ERV plus RV.

 b *Inspiratory capacity* (IC). The maximum amount of gas that can be inspired after a *normal* expiration; consists of V_T plus IRV.

 c *Vital capacity* (VC). The maximum amount of gas that can be exhaled after maximum inspiration; consists of TV plus IRV plus ERV.

 d *Total lung capacity* (TLC). The total amount of gas in the lung at maximum inspiration includes TV plus IRV plus ERV plus RV.

3 Some authorities also include closing volume and closing capacity in discussions of lung volume (Fig. 24-1). However, these are not considered "primary" and are discussed in the units on special testing procedures and small airway disease.

2.2 Abbreviations of pulmonary function testing results

1 FVC. Forced vital capacity; vital capacity with maximum forced expiratory effort.

2 FIVC. Forced inspiratory vital capacity.

3 FEV_T. Forced expiratory volume, timed; (e.g., FEV_1 equals forced expiratory volume in 1 second).

4 $FEV_T/FVC\%$. Forced expiratory volume (timed) to forced vital capacity ratio as a percentage.

5 FEF_X. Forced expiratory flow related to some part of the FVC curve (X).

6 FEF 75%. Forced expiratory flow at the point when 75% of FVC is exhaled.

7 FEF 25% to 75%. Mean forced expiratory flow during the middle half of FVC (formerly MMEFR).

8 PEFR. Peak expiratory flow rate.

9 MVV. Maximum voluntary ventilation (formerly MBC); estimated from $FEV_1 \times 34$ for males; $FEV_1 \times 40$ for females.

10 R_{aw}. Airways resistance.

11 D_X. Diffusing capacity of the lung.

12 C_{st}. Static compliance of the lung.

13 C_{dyn}. Dynamic compliance of the lung.

14 AVI. Air velocity index, percent predicted MVV/percent predicted VC.

15 DI. Dyspnea index. Percent MVV predicted from

$$\frac{\text{Minute volume}}{\text{MVV}}$$

2.3 Types of evaluation testing to assist in diagnosis of pulmonary disorders

1 *Physical assessment* uses history and physical examination procedures to arrive at a preliminary diagnosis before other tests are initiated.

2 *Pulmonary pathology* relies on the results of biopsy or bronchoscopic examinations.

3 *Radiology* uses radiation, particularly lung x-ray films (roentgenography), to identify specific areas of the lung that may be diseased.

4 *Laboratory and blood examinations,* including arterial blood gas analysis, electrolytes, hemoglobin, etc., help confirm other findings, particularly pulmonary function results.

5 *Physiology and mechanical testing* involves the use of various testing devices to determine the patient variance from established normal values, (i.e., pulmonary function testing).

2.4 Limitations of pulmonary function tests

1 Pulmonary function testing is limited by the skill of the practitioner performing and calculating the results of the test and by the equipment used to perform the test.

2 Many sophisticated types of pulmonary function tests

---

*The interested reader is encouraged to contact the American Thoracic Society and the American College of Chest Physicians for publications related to pulmonary function testing.

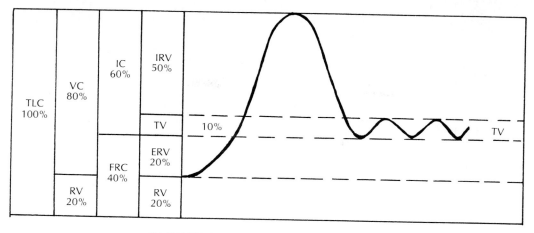

FIGURE 24-1 Lung volumes and capacities.

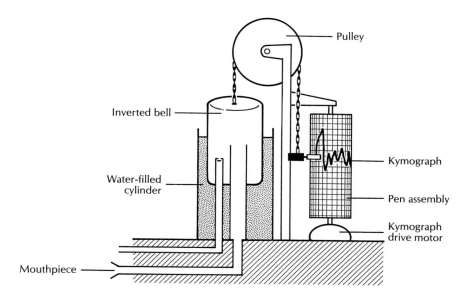

FIGURE 24-2 Water-seal spirometer.

for airway resistance and compliance changes yield results that are inconclusive at the present time. Future research and development may justify their clinical usefulness. The potential usefulness of pulmonary function tests in clinical practice was addressed by a 1978 statement issued jointly by the American Thoracic Society and the American College of Chest Physicians. This statement supported the use of pulmonary function testing as a means for identifying lung disease and as a mechanism for assessing the value of a particular treatment.

3.0 PULMONARY FUNCTION EQUIPMENT

Many pulmonary function measurements are made with a device called a *spirometer*. There are several different kinds of spirometers available today. They are primarily used to measure lung volumes and capacities, and air flow rates.

3.1 Water-sealed spirometers (Fig. 24-2).

A water-sealed spirometer consists of a thin-walled, lightweight cylindrical bell suspended in a container of water with the closed end up and the open end below the surface. The bell is suspended by a chain and pulley mechanisms that connects to a pen for recording the bell movements on graph paper mounted on a rotating drum called a kymograph. As the patient inhales air from the bell, it moves the bell downward, causing the pen to rise proportionately. Gases exhaled into the bell cause the reverse to occur. As the pen rises and falls, a tracing is made of the respiratory efforts on graph paper.

To prevent the accumulation of exhaled carbon dioxide in the breathing circuit, a cannister filled with carbon dioxide crystals is placed on the expiratory port within the spirometer. To prevent rebreathing the same air,

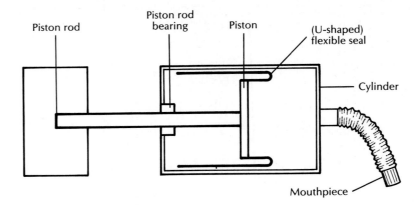

FIGURE 24-3 Dry rolling-seal spirometer.

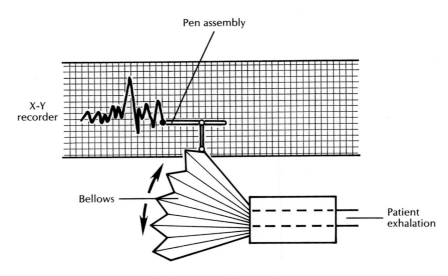

FIGURE 24-4 Wedge spirometer.

one-way valves are placed in the circuit. A stopcock on the side of the spirometer permits the entry of additional fresh air to the bell.

Water-seal spirometers are commonly used to measure:
Lung volumes and capacities
Diffusion capacities (D_{LCO})
Flow measurements (FVC, $FEV_{1,3}$, FEF, MVV)

3.2 Dry rolling-seal spirometer (Fig. 24-3).

The dry rolling-seal spirometer is similar to the water-seal spirometer. Gas from the patient enters a cylinder and displaces a piston that is sealed into the cylinder by a rolling diaphragm-like seal. An electric potentiometer detects the piston's movements and provides an electric signal for recording the data on a graph or scope. The dry rolling-seal spirometer is suitable for performing the same tests as the water-seal spirometer.

3.3 Wedge spirometer (Fig. 24-4).

The wedge spirometer incorporates the use of an expandable bellows to collect exhaled volumes, and a graph is used to display volume and time. As a volume of gas enters the spirometer, the bellows expands, moving upward. The amount of this movement is recorded by a pen on a graph calibrated in volume (liters). A motor moves the pen horizontally at a certain rate so that time measurement may be made. The wedge spirometer is usually used to measure vital capacity, timed vital capacities, flow rates and maximum voluntary ventilation.

3.4 Flow sensing devices

Flow sensing devices such as the Wright Respirometer and pneumotachs function by measuring the volume of air passing through them as a function of time.

1 Wright respirometer (Fig. 24-5). The Wright

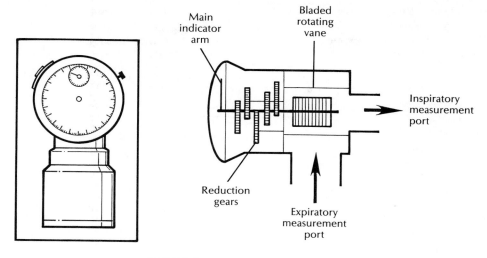

FIGURE 24-5 Wright Respirometer.

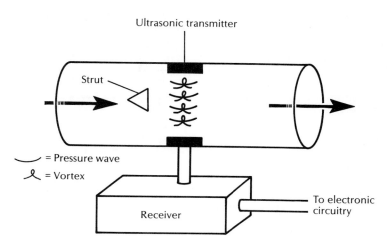

FIGURE 24-6 Pressure drop pneumotach.

Respirometer is a small hand-held device that is commonly used at the bedside to measure tidal volume, minute volume and vital capacity. As gas flows through this device, it spins, rotating vanes. Through a series of gears the vane movement is indicated on a dial calibrated in liters. For more details on the Wright Respirometer refer to Module 23, Unit 12.0.

3.5 Pneumotachs

1 Pneumotachs. A pneumotach is a flow-sensing device that integrates flow signals to obtain a volume measurement. These devices utilize various physical principles to measure air flow. There are three common types of pneumotachs.

a Pressure-drop pneumotach (Fig. 24-6). This pneumotach consists of a tube with an element inside to offer resistance to air flow. When air flowing through the tube meets this resistance, its flow is impeded to some degree and pressure drops. This drop in pressure is measured by a sensitive pressure transducer that converts it into an electronic signal.

b Temperature-drop pneumotach (Fig. 24-7). This pneumotach, also called the hot wire flowmeter, utilizes King's law to measure flow and volume.
King's law:
"The velocity of gas flow over a heated element is proportional to the convective heat loss from the element."

c Ultrasonic flow pneumotach (Fig. 24-8). This pneumotach is a tube with struts placed inside to cause turbulence in the flow of gas. This turbulence creates waves (vortices) within the flow. At the same time an electronic transmitter sends ultrasonic sound waves vertically through the tube to a receiver. The turbulent flow waves hit the ultrasonic sound waves and change them. These changes in the ultrasonic sound waves, picked up by the receiver, are proportional to the flow of gas and are shown as liters per minute or second.

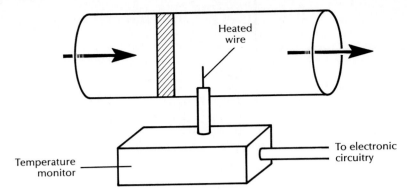

FIGURE 24-7 Temperature drop pneumotach.

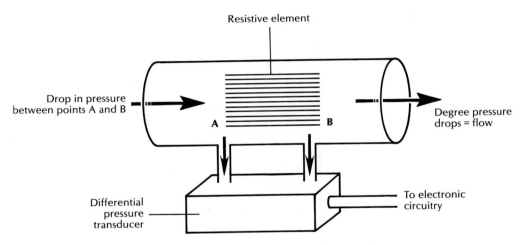

FIGURE 24-8 Ultrasonic flow pneumotach.

3.6 Body box

1 Body plethysmography (Fig. 24-9). The body plethysmography, also called a body box, is a large airtight box, much like a telephone booth, in which the subject sits. There are several types of body boxes but the most common are the variable pressure and the variable volume. With the variable pressure box the subject breathes air from within the box, and with the variable volume box, the subject breathes air through a mouthpiece-airway system that leads outside the box. Airway pressure changes and box pressure and volume changes are measured. From these measurements lung volumes can be derived by using Boyle's law:

$$P_1 V_1 = P_2 V_2$$

2 The body box is especially useful in the measurement of functional residual capacity and residual volume.

4.0 DIAGNOSTIC TESTS OF LUNG FUNCTION
4.1 Clinical types of diagnostic tests

1 The five general areas of pulmonary function testing follow.

a Spirometry, which measures pulmonary mechanics, volumes, and flows
b Tests to evaluate gas distribution
c Tests to evaluate gas diffusion across the alveolar-capillary membrane
d Exercise testing
e Blood gas analysis, which tests the effects of physiologic lung changes on the homeostasis of gas exchange by the tissues

2 Respiratory care uses pulmonary studies to measure mechanical ability, efficiency, and abnormalities; especially as applied to the pulmonary system when stressed.

4.2 Spirometry

1 Evaluation of ventilatory function can be very useful in determining a patient's ability to maintain adequate gas exchange without undue work of breathing. It can predict a patient's probable postoperative pulmonary status or ability to be weaned from mechanical ventilation.

2 Bedside ventilatory tests must be easily performed by

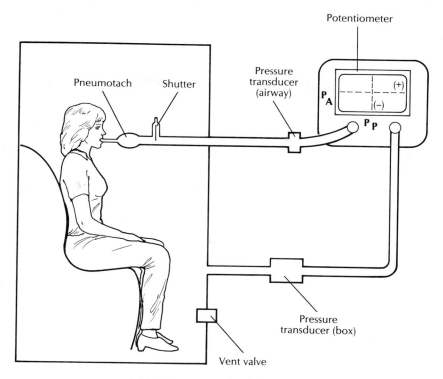

FIGURE 24-9 Body plethysmograph.

the patient and practitioner. They should distinguish between normal and abnormal results with portable equipment.

3 Bedside spirometry objectives are to identify a patient's ability to cough and increase ventilation. This is best measured by a forced vital capacity and the volumes calculated from it.

4 Spirometry is used to detect deviations in volumes and flow rates from normal so that a physician can determine if an obstructive or restrictive impairment exists.

5 Tests of pulmonary mechanics can distinguish overt restrictive impairments from obstructive ones and thereby determine if changes involve the airways or the lungs themselves.

6 Spirometry is the basic device used to evaluate the effects of bronchodilators on airway flow and on lung volumes.

4.3 Tests to evaluate gas distribution

1 Single-breath nitrogen distribution (SBN_2), helium wash-in, and nitrogen wash-out tests measure changes in ventilation distribution of the lung as measure functional residual capacity in the helium-wash-in and nitrogen wash-out test.

2 This information identifies lung regions with long time constants seen in airway narrowing and bullae forma-

tion. NOTE: Measurement of dead space to tidal volume aids in the diagnosis of pulmonary vascular occlusion.

4.4 Tests to evaluate gas diffusion

1 Tests of diffusion measure the amount of functional capillary bed that is in contact with functional alveoli.

2 Any factor that acts to deter diffusion or increase thickness of the membrane between the alveolus and the blood will result in a lower-than-predicted amount of carbon monoxide being transferred.

3 Carbon monoxide diffusion is limited by diffusion and not perfusion amount because carbon monoxide combines with hemoglobin so readily.

4.5 Exercise (stress) testing

1 Exercise testing is useful in distinguishing impairment of cardiac origin and pulmonary origin. With exercise malingering is more easily detected.

2 Exercise testing may help evaluate fitness for certain types of work or sports.

3 Exercise testing evaluates the effects and modifications in therapeutic and rehabilitation programs.

4 Cardiac output, maximum oxygen uptake, and oxygen consumption are all part of exercise testing.

5 One of the simplest stress tests is the maximum voluntary ventilation (MVV) test. It may be desirable to use this for preoperative evaluation.

4.6 Arterial blood gas (ABG) analysis*

1 ABG testing evaluates the hydrogen ion concentration in blood, which is the determinant of blood acidity. This acidity is very important to the red blood cell (RBC) when determining the amount of oxygen it will carry (oxyhemoglobin dissociation curve) (Module Eight, Unit 11.1).

2 ABG tests will assist in determining how much oxygen is being carried to the tissues and will also assist in determining the effectiveness of ventilation by analyzing the partial pressure of carbon dioxide (P_{CO_2}).

5.0 NORMAL VALUES OF PULMONARY MECHANICS, LUNG VOLUMES, VENTILATION, GAS DISTRIBUTION, AND GAS DIFFUSION

5.1 Factors involved in computing pulmonary function testing normals

1 Predicted values are a necessity in calculating pulmonary functions. Most normal values have been taken from research data collected in testing centers and military services over many years and are based on results of "healthy individuals." Abnormalities are therefore "relative" in nature and deviations of under 20% of predicted are not considered important. Patterns of deviation from normal, especially in more than one test, are suggestive of an abnormality.

2 Certain information must be known about personal data and the patient's history to evaluate results based on published "normals." Most results have nomograms that can be used to predict normals based on age, sex, and height.

3 To determine normals for spirometric values, one must know the patient's sex, height, and age. To determine maximum voluntary ventilation normals, one must calculate surface area based on weight and age. Values for peak expiratory flow rates require the use of body surface area or height. Many of the other tests have been established normal based on one normal or values based on age.

5.2 Computing predicted vital capacity and maximum voluntary ventilation

1 Predicted vital capacity (VC) can be determined by using charts of predicted values based on height and age.

2 Formulas corresponding to the predicted value charts are:

a For male patients VC = [27.6 − (0.112 × Age)] × Height (cm)

b For female patients VC = [21.8 − (0.101 × Age)] × Height (cm)

c Alternate formulas are available in many texts, but all allow the 20% deviation factor from the figure calculated.

3 Predicted maximum voluntary ventilation (MVV) values may also be figured from nomograms based on body surface area. Normal values for an adult male approach 170 to 180 L/min; up to 30% deviation is allowed.

4 An indirect determination of MVV can be based on the FEV_1 result times 30 to 40, but its use is quite limited since it requires values taken under conditions of stress.

5.3 Normal spirometric values

1 Normal computation of volumes may be taken from a VC tracing. Either a slow or fast tracing should normally yield the same volumes, although flow rates will differ. A fast, or forced, VC will yield results useful for disease interpretation (see Fig. 24-10).

2 Normal lung volumes are determined as a percentage from the total lung capacity after determining VC and functional residual capacity (FRC).

a FRC value—"resting lung level"—40% total lung capacity (TLC).

b VC value—70% to 80% of TLC.

c Reserve volume (RV) value—25% to 30% of TLC: this increases with age as a result of a loss of lung elasticity.

d Inspiratory capacity (IC) value—about 60% of TLC.

3 The reader is encouraged to compute normal values based on Fig. 24-1 and use of the vital capacity formula to figure normal values for a 150 lb. male, 5 feet tall, and 25 years old.*

a VC = _____ml

b TV = _____ml

c ERV = _____ml

d IRV = _____ml

e IC = _____ml

f FRC = _____ml

g TLC = _____ml

5.4 Forced expiratory volume calculated as a basis of forced vital capacity

1 Forced expiratory volumes (FEV) are flow rate calculations based on a forced vital capacity (FVC) and normally expressed as a percent of FVC (see Fig. 24-10).

2 These timed VCs may be based on volume expired in 1 second (FEV_1), ½ second ($FEV_{0.5}$), 3 seconds (FEV_3), or as a percentage of the total from a starting point in the middle of the curve (FEF 25%-75%) or at the end of the curve (FEV 0.75-85).

5.5 Values of FEV

1 The most common values are FEV_1 or FEV_3.

2 Normal formulas to calculate them are as follows.

a $FEV_1\% = \dfrac{FEV_1}{FVC} \times 100$ (normally = 75% to 83%)

b $FEV_3\% = \dfrac{FEV_3}{FVC} \times 100$ (normally = 95% to 100%)

---

*Review the units on arterial blood gases in Module Eight.

*a, VC = 4800 ml; b, TV = 500 ml; c, ERV = 1200 ml; d, IRV = 3000 ml; e, IC = 3600 ml; f, FRC = 2400 ml; g, TLC = 6000 ml.

5.6 Normals for ventilatory function and breathing mechanics

1 Maximal voluntary ventilation (MVV) = greater than 170 L/min.
  a MVV = $FEV_1 \times 34$ (males).
  b MVV = $FEV_1 \times 40$ (females).
2 FEV_1 = 83%.
3 FEV_3 = 97%.
4 Peak expiratory flow rate (PEFR) = greater than 600 L/min.
5 FEF 25% to 75% = 4.7 L/sec.
6 FEF 200 to 1200 = 6 L/sec.
7 Compliance of lungs and thoracic cage (C_{LT}) = 0.1 L/cm H_2O.
8 Compliance of lungs (C_L) = 0.2 L/cm H_2O.
9 Airway resistance (R_{aw}) = 1.6 cm H_2O/L/sec.
10 Diffusing capacity of lung for carbon monoxide (D_{LCO}) = 25 ml/min/mm Hg.
11 Diffusing capacity of lung for oxygen (D_{LO_2}) = 31 ml/min/mm Hg.
12 Single-breath nitrogen distribution = less than 1.5% N_2.
13 Seven-minute nitrogen emptying = less than 2.5% N_2.
14 RV/TLC ratio = less than 20% (young); less than 50% (elderly).
15 Closing volume = less than 10% on patients under 50 years of age; 10% to 40% on patients over 50 years of age.
16 Changing nitrogen (ΔN_2) = less than 2%.

6.0 LUNG VOLUME TESTS, VENTILATION TESTS, AND PULMONARY MECHANICS TESTS

6.1 Tidal volume (TV).

1 TV is the gas inhaled or exhaled during normal resting ventilation.
2 To measure TV, the patient breathes normally into a spirometer.
3 This should be done for 1 minute, so as to obtain an average volume. No two TV are the same. (Fig. 24-11 shows a typical spirometer tracing.)
4 To attain the average TV

$$TV = \frac{\text{Minute volume } (V_M}{\text{Respiratory rate } (f)}$$

5 V_M. The total amount of volume either inhaled or exhaled over 1 minute.
6 Respiratory rate (f). The total number of breaths taken over 1 minute.

6.2 Vital capacity (VC)

1 VC is equal to expiratory reserve volume (ERV) plus inspiratory reserve volume (IRV) plus tidal volume (TV) *or* inspiratory capacity (IC) plus ERV.
2 To measure VC, the patient inspires maximally and then exhales completely into a spirometer. There is no time limit on how long it takes the patient to exhale completely. (See Fig. 24-12 for a typical tracing.)
3 The normal values of VC are computed as follows.
  a For male patients VC = [27.6 = (0.112 × age)] × height (cm).
  b For female patients VC = [21.8 − (0.101 × age)] × height (cm).
  NOTE: the VC may vary up to 20% from the predicted normals in healthy individuals.
4 A decrease in VC can be caused by a decrease in compliance as a result of bronchogenic carcinoma, pneumonia, atelectasis, etc.
5 VC is normally 70% to 80% of the TLC.

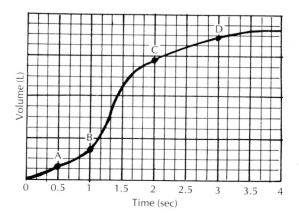

FIGURE 24-10 Forced expiratory volume (FEV).

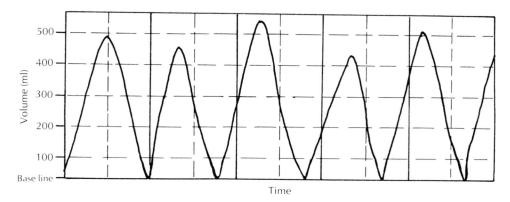

FIGURE 24-11 Measurement of tidal volume (TV).

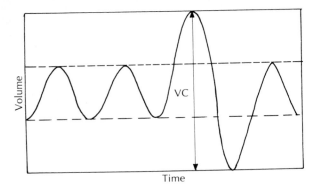

FIGURE 24-12 Vital capacity (VC) spirogram.

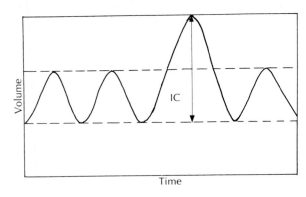

FIGURE 24-13 Inspiratory capacity (IC) spirogram.

6.3 Forced vital capacity (FVC)

1 FVC is the amount of air that can be exhaled forcefully after a maximum inspiration.

2 To measure the FVC, the patient inspires maximally and exhales completely as quickly as possible into a spirometer. (Fig. 24-12 shows a typical tracing.)

3 The FVC normally equals the VC in volume.

4 The FVC is measured over a period of time to determine how fast a patient can expire his/her VC.

5 The longer it takes for a patient to expire his/her entire VC, the more obstruction is likely in the airways, thus, a decreased FVC.

6 From the FVC, a number of other calculations can be made: $FEV_{0.5}$, FEV_1, FEV_3, $FEV_1\%$, $FEV_2\%$, and $FEV_3\%$ (see Fig. 24-10, *A-D*).

7 $FEV_{0.5}$, FEV_1, FEV_2, and FEV_3 can be read directly off the graph.

8 $FEV_1\% = \dfrac{FEV_1}{FVC} \times 100$ (normally 75% to 83%)

9 $FEV_2\% = \dfrac{FEV_2}{FVC} \times 100$ (normally 85% to 90%)

10 $FEV_3\% = \dfrac{FEV_3}{FVC} \times 100$ (normally 95% to 100%)

6.4 Inspiratory capacity (IC)

1 The IC is equal to the IRV plus the TV.

2 To measure the IC, the patient breathes normally for three to four breaths then inhales maximally.

3 The measurement on the spirogram is the point from resting expiration to maximum inspiration. (Fig. 24-13 shows a sample tracing.)

4 The IC normally is approximately 74% of the VC and 60% of TLC.

6.5 Expiratory reserve volume (ERV)

1 The ERV is the amount of gas that can be exhaled after a normal exhalation, ERV is equal to VC minus IC.

2 To measure the ERV, the patient breathes normally for three to four breaths and then, on the practitioner's signal, exhales completely. (Fig. 24-14 shows a sample tracing.)

3 The ERV is approximately 25% of the VC.

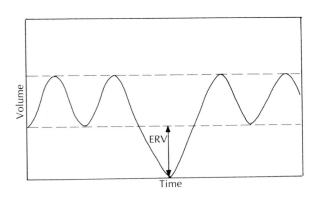

FIGURE 24-14 Expiratory reserve volume (ERV) spirogram.

4 The validity of the ERV determination is not of diagnostic value.

5 Fig. 24-15 summarizes lung volumes and capacities for the adult.

6.6 Theory of helium wash-in test

1 Functional residual capacity (FRC) and residual volume (RV) cannot be calculated from spirometric tracings because the FRC and RV are the volume of air left in the lung at the resting point following exhalation.

2 Various techniques have been developed to use or analyze a gas not consumed in normal gas exchange to help *indirectly* measure FRC and RV.

3 If the patient rebreathes from a closed spirometer or bag system that contains a known volume of air and small known concentration of an insoluble gas (helium), the helium is diluted by the air in the lungs and this amount of dilution can be measured.

4 The fall in concentration of helium is then a function of the ratio of lung volume to the volume of the closed circuit system.

5 A helium analyzer (catharometer) measures the helium concentration, and volume changes are recorded on a plotter or kymograph.

6 Knowing these volumes and concentrations, a simple dilutional equation can be used to calculate the lung

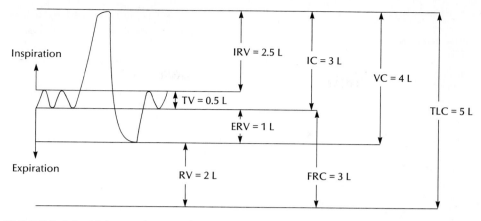

F I G U R E 2 4 - 1 5 Lung volumes and capacities for the adult. (Modified from Current Reviews in Respiratory Therapy—function: a practical approach, lesson 8, vol 2, p 9, 1980.)

volume after gas equilibration between the lung and spirometer.

6.7 Circuitry in the helium wash-in test

1 A closed circuit is required.
2 The amount of helium is small, and to estimate and correct for oxygen consumption, oxygen must be added to keep the system volume constant.
3 Soda-lime must be in the circuit to absorb exhaled carbon dioxide.
4 A one-way valve and unidirectional blower are used to assure gas mixing and flow by the helium analyzer.
5 An integrator pen should be used to allow calculation of the minute volume, tidal volume, and respiratory rate.
6 The reader is encouraged to visit a hospital pulmonary function laboratory to obtain more details about a specific system.

6.8 Calculations in the helium functional residual capacity test

1 Calculations for dead space of the rebreathing system must be made to subtract from the final volume to get a true FRC. (See the boxed material.)
2 A record must be made of initial and final helium concentration.
3 Calculations for functional residual capacity vary from system to system but must correct for dead space and switching error (patient into closed system) see Boxes *A* and *B* for examples of how to correct for dead space and for error in switching patient into a closed system).

6.9 Theory of nitrogen wash-out test

1 The nitrogen wash-out test for FRC has high precision and measurement of intrapulmonary mixing by determining the amount of gas washed out of the lung.
2 This test requires modifications of a special valve and no switching error in turning the patient into the system at exactly the FRC level.

Sample spirometer system dead space calculation and FRC test

CALCULATING DEAD SPACE USING A PULMONET*

1 Zero helium meter.
2 Admit 200 ml of helium to system and read helium concentration; if off scale, add sufficient air until able to read helium concentration (should be 80 or above).
3 Before reading this initial helium concentration, (He_I). wait about a minute
4 Add 3 to 5 L of air, wait a minute or so, and read final helium concentration (He_F).
5 Calculate dead space of spirometer system:

$$\text{Dead space} = \frac{\text{Volume air added} \times He_F}{He_I - He_F}$$

FUNCTIONAL RESIDUAL CAPACITY (FRC)

1 Zero helium meter.
2 Add about 240 ml He − 300.
3 Add air so that the total volume of spirometer system will be 8.5 L (if dead space is 5 L, add 3 L of air, etc.)
4 Read initial helium concentration (He_I).
5 Turn O_2 supply to ON and set O_2 flomweter at about 300 ml. Do not switch into spirometer.
6 Have subject breathe on mouthpiece open to room air.
7 Start kymograph of spirometer at slow speed.
8 Switch subject into spirometer at end-expiration and turn O_2 flow into spirometer.
9 Record He concentration every 30 seconds and stop test after concentration has remained steady for *1 minute* or after test has been run for 5 minutes.
10. Make adjustments in added O_2 to keep breathing record.

Gould Inc., Medical Products Division, 805 Liberty Lane, Dayton, OH 45449.
*This equipment is used only as an example. The reader is encouraged to investigate the many computerized systems that are avaiable today for FRC measurement.

A: Functional residual capacity (FRC) calculations

Vol_{DS} = Volume of dead space
He_I = Helium initial reading
He_F = Helium final reading
Volume × Concentration = Volume × Concentration
$Vol_{DS} × He_I = (Vol_{DS} + 4 L) He_F$
$Vol_{DS} × He_I = Vol_{DS} He_F + 4 He_F$
$Vol_{DS} (He_I − He_F) = 4 He_F$

$$Vol_{DS} = \frac{4 He_F}{He_I − He_F}$$

If Vol_{DS} = 5.3 L, then addition to 3.2 L would give a total volume system of 8.5 L at beginning at FRC test.
Volume × Concentration − Volume × Concentration
$8.5 × He_I = (8.5 + FRC) He_F$
$8.5 He_I = 8.5 He_F + FRC He_F$
$8.5 (He_I − He_F) = FRC He_F$

$$FRC = \frac{8.5 × (He_I − He_F)}{He} ± \text{Switching error} × \text{temperature}$$
correction factor − 0.0 with
0.0 standing for mouth piece
dead space

Switching error
a Subtract volume
b Subract volume
c Add volume

B: Functional residual capacity (FRC) calculations

He_I = 9.85
He_F = 6.40
Temperature = 25° C

$$Vol_{DS} = \frac{He\ added}{He_I} = \frac{590\ ml}{9.85\%} = 5990\ volume$$

Vol_{DS} = Dead space + Amount He added

Then: $FRC = Vol_{DS} × \dfrac{He_I − He_F}{He_F}$

$$= 5990 × \frac{9.85 − 6.40}{6.40} = 3228\ cc\ uncorrected$$

Then correct for:
1 Absorption of He (or 100 ml)
2 Temperature
3 Switching effort (if any)

3 Calculations involve special consideration of the following.
  a Bag volume (bag with room air)
  b Bag nitrogen concentration
  c Alveolar nitrogen
  d Correction for the small amounts of switching error
  e Correction for nitrogen excreted from the tissues
  f Correction for valve and mouthpiece dead space
4 The patient is switched onto a collection bag for expired gases when he is at the FRC level (end of tidal volume). The unknown FRC volume represents 80% of FRC (air is 79% to 80% nitrogen).
5 Knowing the volume exhaled and the amount of nitrogen at the end of exhalation, the volume of nitrogen in the lung can be calculated from what it was at the beginning of the test. This would represent 80% of starting FRC.
6 The exhaled nitrogen concentration should be displayed on a plotter. The plotted graph should show an exponential decay and be rounded at the top. Spiked tops may indicate obstructive disease (Fig. 24-16).
7 Note that the concentration of nitrogen should be below 2% (nitrogen index) by the end of a 7-minute period.
8 Calculations necessary to calculate FRC are as follows:
  a $FRC = \dfrac{Bag\ nitrogen\ \% × Bag\ volume}{80\ (N_2\ concentration) − Alveolar\ N_2}$
  b Note that the calculation above is uncorrected for dead space, switching error, and true alveolar nitrogen. A sample test is given below (uncorrected).

Minute volume = 2 L/min
Length of test = 5 mm
Final N_2 concentration = 40%

$$FRC\ (uncorrected) = \frac{TV × 0.4\ (N_2\%)}{0.79} = \frac{10 × 4}{0.79} = \frac{4\ L/min}{79} = 5.1\ L$$

  c Calculation of alveolar nitrogen is needed only on water-seal spirometers filled with air.

6.10 Single-breath dilution tests

1 Single-breath tests of dilution really end up being used as tests of distribution of ventilation. They cannot be used to measure FRC.
2 Single-breath tests are only of the open-circuit type (nitrogen) because helium tests require a closed circuit and rebreathing techniques. (See Fig. 24-16, A through C.)
  a In the single-breath test, the patient exhales fully and inhales fully a single breath of oxygen.
  b The subject exhales slowly and completely. A nitrogen meter measures the concentration and plots N_2 concentration against expired volume.
  c Exhalation will show how oxygen was distributed by dilution of the nitrogen. The change between 750 ml to 1250 ml should vary less than 2% in normal lungs.
3 The single-breath oxygen test is quite similar to tests for closing volume (detecting small airway disease), with the major difference being that the patient holds a slow and steady flow during expiration and the entire cycle is recorded.

6.11 FRC determinations by a body box (plethysmography)*

1 The gas analysis methods of determining FRC are very dependent on the patency of patient airways. If good

---

*See Ruppel G: Manual of pulmonary function testing, St Louis, 1983, The CV Mosby Co.

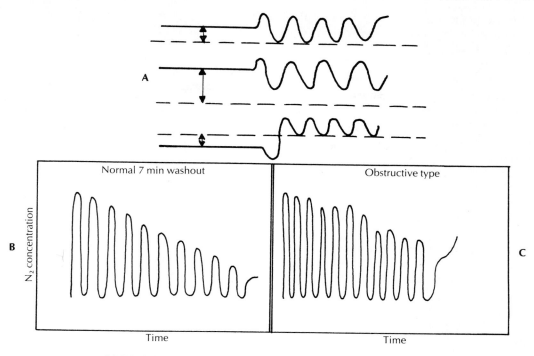

FIGURE 24-16 Nitrogen wash-out tests. Normal vs. obstructive.

gas communication is not sufficient, mixing time for helium may be high or the nitrogen emptying rate may be low. This may result in underestimating FRC, reserve volume (RV), and total lung capacity (TLC) calculations.

2 Use of the body box method of calculation gives much more accurate calculations, even in obstructed patients with air trapping. The body box method has recently been shown to overestimate lung volumes in some patients.

3 The body box is usually a variable pressure device, although variable volume types are available.

4 Although the procedure varies, the specifics of it include knowledge of the following:
   a Mouth pressure factors
   b Box factor (cc/cm)
   c Scope readings of tangents of slope
   d Constant: $Pk = (Bp - 47) \times 1.36$*

$$FRC = \frac{Pk \times Box\ factor}{Tan + FRC \times Mouth\ factor}$$

6.12 Concept of average flow

1 Note the technique of forced expiratory flow 25% to 75% (FEF 25%-75%) calculation shown below.
   a Take the total vital capacity (VC) (read off the graph) and divide by four.

b Measure up from the bottom of the curve and number as determined in Fig. 24.10 *A* and mark. Repeat coming down from the top of the curve.

2 Note that this concept is one of an average flow over the middle half of the expiratory cycle taken as a slope of the middle two lines of four dividing the vital capacity volume into four equal parts. This concept is best presented as an observed demonstration.

6.13 Calculations of FEF 25% to 75% and FEF 200 to 1200

1 Also called mid-maximal expiratory flowrate, the FEF 25% to 75% is a measure of change in volume (vertical) over time (base).

2 Maximum expiratory flow (FEF 25% to 75%) is the first abnormal parameter to appear in early chronic obstructive pulmonary disease (obstructive spirometry).

3 Calculation of the time of FEF 25% to 75% in seconds is called midexpiratory time (MET). Normal is 0.5 second.

4 Another calculation, but more slanted to large airway dysfunction detection is the FEF 200 to 1200 (MMF). The FEF 200 to 1200 uses similar calculations as the FEF 25% to 75%, but measures flow over the specific VC volume from 200 to 1200 ml and discards the first 200 ml expired.

6.14 Average flow compared with instantaneous flow

1 Average flow calculations are based on volume-to-time consideration over the slope of a line between two volume time points.

2 Instantaneous flow is used in recorders using pneumo-

---

*Pk, Constant; Bp, barometric pressure.

tachographs or electronic integration (x-y recorder plotter) that plots points of actual flow, which can be compared to time or volume.

3 In the usual setting, an x-y plotter recorder is used to trace flow vertically and volume horizontally.

4 The normal shape of an expiratory curve is an exponential delay function with most of the flow occurring at the highest lung volumes. Flow progressively decreases as elastic recoil pressures equalize to transpulmonary pressures.

6.15 Instantaneous flow as a screening device

1 The analysis of flow generated against volume expired measures lung volumes and lung mechanics simultaneously.

2 The extent of obstruction or restriction may be easily visualized. In addition, calculations of variations in the curve shape from the exponential function-type indicate air trapping or low volumes.

3 Since flow is related to volume and not just time, the curve should be reproducible each time of a patient is truly using maximum effort.

4 Detection of reduced flows at small volumes would give better indication of small airway dysfunction than would a volume-time spirogram.

6.16 Estimating various flow rates and volumes (Fig. 24-17)

1 Note that all the volume obtainable by spirometry may be read on the horizontal axis.

2 To be accurate in calculations, the graph paper must be calibrated to the machine or else the calibrations must be stated or indicated on paper.

3 Basically, the technique for having a patient perform a flow-volume loop is the same as a forced vital capacity during spirometry measurement.

4 The additional executions of a maximum inhalation after a maximum expiration creates the lower inspiratory portion of a flow-volume loop.

5 Each loop should have an identical shape; if not, one should suspect patient malingering or equipment error.

6.17 Flow volume loops for various conditions

1 Examples of flow volume loops for various disease states are presented as Figs. 24-18 through 24-27 listed below:

24-18 *A*. Example of FEV, using standard spirographic tracing

24-18 *B*. Normal test showing flow volume loops

24-19. Patient airway mildly obstructed

24-20. Patient airway severely obstructed

24-21. Reduce MID and terminal flow rates

24-22. Patient mildly restricted

2 In studying each of the above tests, note changes in shape of the inspiratory and expiratory positions of the loop from normal with each disease evaluated.

3 As the obstruction or restriction is increased or decreased the inspiratory and expiratory positions of the

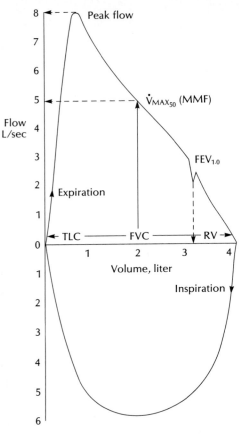

FIGURE 24-17 Normal flow-volume loop showing various components for calculation. (Modified from Current Reviews in Respiratory Therapy, 2:9, 1980.)

loop change by moving closer or further from a perpendicular axis.

6.18 Examples of flow volume loops with calculations

1 Figure 24-23 *A* and *B* shows how the FEV, which was depressed (*A*), returns to normal after bronchodilator therapy is given (*B*).

2 Additional examples of different parameters that can be calculated from various flow volume loops are presented as Figs. 24-24 through 24-26.

3 Fig. 24-27 summarizes normal, obstructive and restrictive flow volume loops by superimposing curves.

6.19 Advantages of flow-volume loops

1 Plotting two patient variables (flow and volume) against each other allows for standardization toward normal for patients of large size or very small volume outflow. This is especially true where an overestimate or masking of disease processes occurs with volume-to-time calculations.

2 Flow-volume loops aid in early obstructive disease detection. Modifications with the use of a helium study of a flow-volume loop superimposed over a flow-volume loop taken with room air (process of isoflow) may aid

Text continued on p. 808.

MALE   AGE: 27 yrs   HT: 65 in, 165 cm   WT: 135 lbs, 61 kg   BSA: 1.67

All Values BTPS	Predicted	Measured	% Predicted
FVC (L)	4.423	5.006	113
FEV_1 (L)	3.764	4.376	116
FEV_3 (L)	4.202	5.006	119
FEV_1/FVC (%)	75	87	116
FEV_3/FVC (%)	95	100	105
MMEF 25%-75% (L/sec)	5.513	5.179	94
PEFR (L/sec)	8.937	11.222	126
FEF 75% (L/sec)	8.036	8.921	111
FEF 50% (L/sec)	5.791	6.867	119
FEF 25% (L/sec)	3.217	2.761	86

COMMENTS: Normal test

FEV_1 example from
standard spirogram

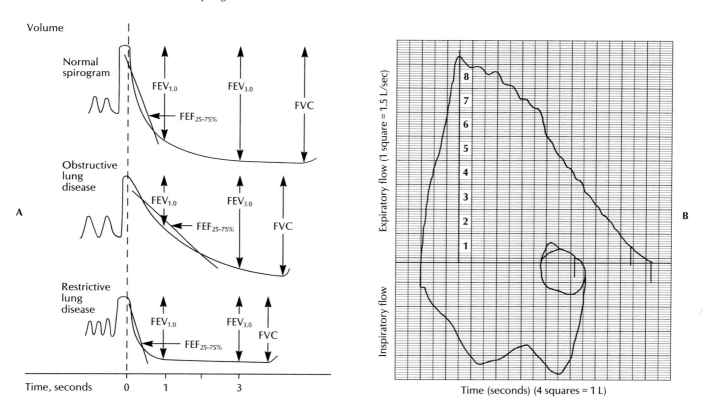

FIGURE 24-18 A, FEV, example from standard spirogram. **B,** Flow-volume loop—normal test.

MALE   AGE: 59 yrs   HT: 72 in, 182 cm   WT: 188 lbs, 85 kg   BSA: 2.07

All Values BTPS	Predicted	Measured	% Predicted
FVC (L)	4.572	4.591	100
FEV_1 (L)	3.526	2.549	72*
FEV_3 (L)	4.343	3.762	87
FEV_1/FVC (%)	75	55	73*
FEV_3/FVC (%)	95	81	85
MMEF 25%-75% (L/sec)	4.749	1.187	25*
PEFR (L/sec)	9.177	7.965	87
FEF 75% (L/sec)	8.026	3.292	41
FEF 50% (L/sec)	5.254	1.451	28
FEF 25% (L/sec)	2.157	.460	21

*Most significant.

COMMENTS: PT. Mildly obstructed.

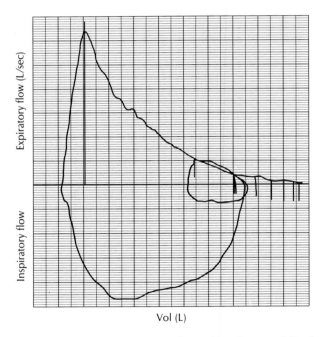

F I G U R E   2 4 - 1 9 Standard spirogram. Flow-volume loop—mildly obstructed.

MALE   AGE: 81 yrs   HT: 63 in, 160 cm   WT: 130 lbs, 59 kg   BSA: 1.61

All Values BTPS	Predicted	Measured	% Predicted
FVC (L)	2.423	2.318	96
FEV$_1$ (L)	2.064	1.028	50*
FEV$_3$ (L)	2.302	1.704	74
FEV$_1$/FVC (%)	75	44	59*
FEV$_3$/FVC (%)	95	73	77
MMEF 25%-75% (L/sec)	3.395	.432	13*
PEFR (L/sec)	7.353	3.504	48*
FEF 75% (L/sec)	6.776	1.026	15*
FEF 50% (L/sec)	3.987	.495	12*
FEF 25% (L/sec)	.931	.106	11*

*Most significant.

COMMENTS: PT. Severely obstructed.

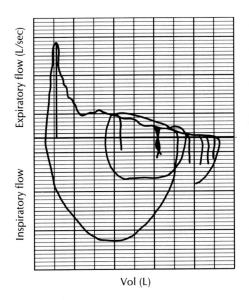

FIGURE 24-20 Standard spirogram. Flow-volume loop—severely obstructed.

FEMALE   AGE: 52 yrs   HT: 67 in, 170 cm   WT: 174 lbs, 79 kg   BSA: 1.90

All Values BTPS	Predicted	Measured	% Predicted
FVC (L)	3.548	3.271	92
FEV$_1$ (L)	2.375	2.426	102*
FEV$_3$ (L)	3.371	3.056	91
FEV$_1$/FVC (%)	75	74	99
FEV$_3$/FVC (%)	95	93	98
MMEF 25%-75% (L/sec)	3.927	2.002	51
PEFR (L/sec)	6.293	8.213	131
FEF 75% (L/sec)	5.782	6.230	108
FEF 50% (L/sec)	4.384	2.973	68*
FEF 25% (L/sec)	1.937	.743	38*

*Most significant.

COMMENTS: Reduced mid and terminal flow rates.

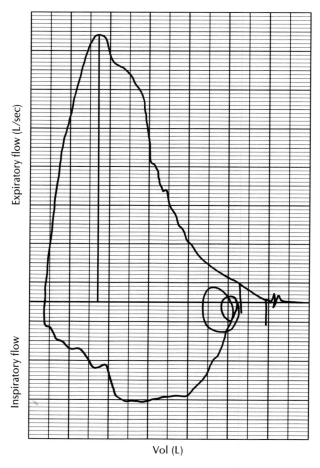

F I G U R E 2 4 - 2 1 Standard spirogram. Flow-volume loop—reduced mid and terminal flow rates.

FEMALE   AGE: 30 yrs   HT: 65 in, 165 cm   WT: 101 lbs, 45 kg   BSA: 1.48

All Values BTPS	Predicted	Measured	% Predicted
FVC (L)	3.680	2.610	71*
FEV_1 (L)	2.747	2.395	87
FEV_3 (L)	3.496	2.610	75
FEV_1/FVC (%)	75	91	121*
FEV_3/FVC (%)	95	100	105
MMEF 25%-75% (L/sec)	4.511	2.700	60
PEFR (L/sec)	6.507	7.257	112
FEF 75% (L/sec)	6.062	7.257	120
FEF 50% (L/sec)	4.766	3.150	66
FEF 25% (L/sec)	2.661	1.593	60

*Most significant.

COMMENTS: Mildly restricted.

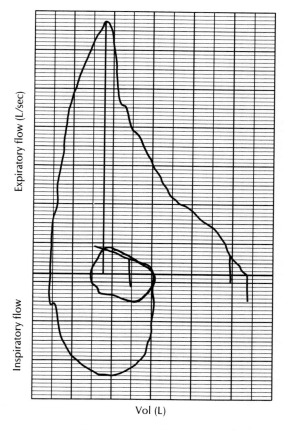

FIGURE 24-22 Standard spirogram. Flow-volume loop—mildly restricted.

COMMENTS:

Lung volumes: The vital capacity is normal. The total lung capacity and the residual volume are also normal. There is no evidence of any significant air trapping. Inspired air is evenly distributed.

Mechanics: The FEV_1 is at the lower limits of normal. The peak expiratory flow rate is normal. The mid and terminal expiratory flow rates are slightly reduced. Airway resistance is in the upper limits of normal.

Diffusing capacity: Diffusing capacity is normal through steady state and single breath methods of analysis.

Arterial blood gases: ABGs show mild hypoxemia, with the PO_2 80 mm. There is a mild respiratory alkalosis present. The hemoglobin in 14.4, and the carbon monoxide saturation is normal at 1.3%.

INTERPRETATION:

These studies show a very mild obstructive pattern, with complete reversibility following bronchodilator spray. These studies are consistent with, and classical of branchial asthma.

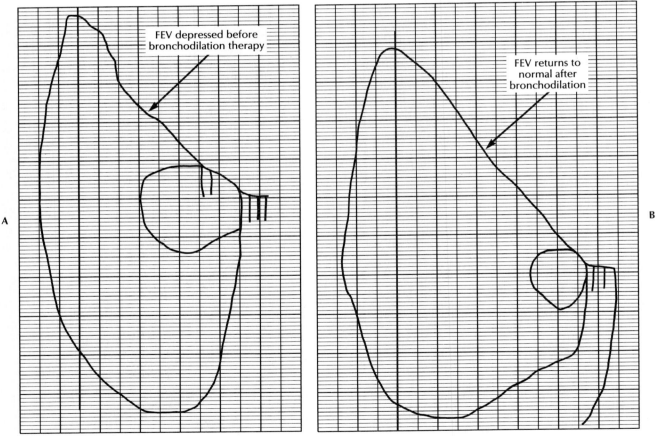

FIGURE 24-23 A, Flow-volume loop. FEV depressed before bronchodilation therapy. **B,** FEB returned to normal after bronchodilation.

1.) FEV = *3.30* L

2.) FEV 1.0 = *1.91* L

3.) VC^1 = *58%*

4.) PEFR (L/sec) = *5.7*

5.) FEF 25% (L/sec) = *4.5*

6.) FEF 50% (L/sec) = *2.0*

7.) FEF 75% (L/sec) = *0.5*

8.) Point A on the above trace represents the TLC.

9.) Point B on the above trace represents the RV.

10.) The segment AC on the above trace represents the IC capacity.

Calibrations:

1.) L Liter = 30 mm for volume

2.) 1 L/sec = 15 mm for flow

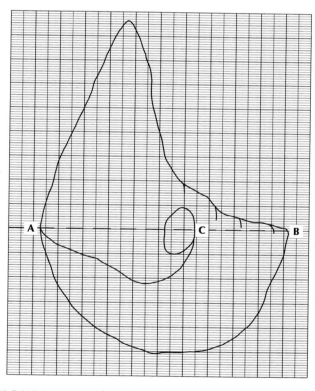

F I G U R E   2 4 - 2 4 Flow-volume loop showing various calculations.

1.) FVC = *4.18* L

2.) FEV 1.0 = *3.60* L

3.) VC$_1$ = *86%*

4.) PEFR (L/sec) = *7.9*

5.) FEF 25% (L/sec) = 6.4 (L/sec)

6.) FEF 50% (L/sec) = 6.2 (L/sec)

7.) FEF 75% (L/sec) = 3.5 (L/sec)

8.) Point A on the above trace represents the TLC.

9.) Point B on the above trace represents the RV.

10.) The segment AC on the above trace represents the IRV.

Calibrations:

1.) 1 Liter = 20 mm for volume

2.) 1 L/sec = 10 mm for flow

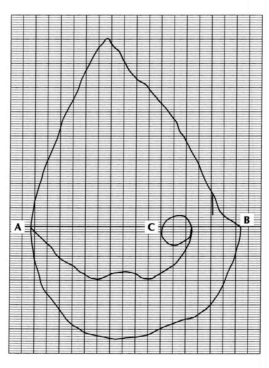

FIGURE 24-25 Flow-volume loop showing various calculations.

1.) FVC = *4.25* L

2.) FEV 1.0 = *3.27* L

3.) VC_1 = *77%*

4.) PEFR = *8.7* L/sec

5.) FEF 25% = *7.7* L/sec

6.) FEF 50% = *4.1* L/sec

7.) FEF 75% = *1.5* L/sec

8.) Point A on the above trace represents the TLC.

9.) The segment AB represents the IRV.

10.) The segment CD represents ERV.

11.) The segment AC represents the patient's IC.

12.) The segment AD represents the patient's FVC.

Calibrations:

1.) 1 Liter = 20 mm for volume

2.) 1 L/sec = 10 mm for flow

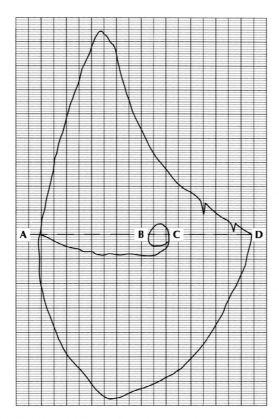

F I G U R E   2 4 - 2 6 Flow-volume loop showing various calculations.

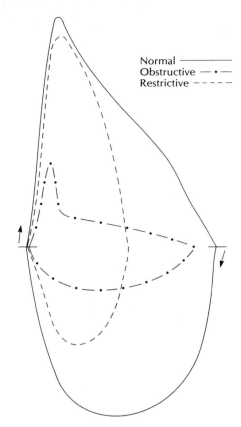

Normal ————
Obstructive — • —
Restrictive - - - - -

FIGURE 24-27 Normal, obstructive, and restrictive flow-volume loops. (Modified from Current Reviews in Respiratory Therapy 2:8, 1980.)

even further in detecting disease before it becomes clinically evident.

3 It is almost impossible for the malingering patient to regulate flows so as to have a reproducible tracing on a second attempt. Maximum efforts, however, will superimpose and should have the same overall shape. This can aid in evaluation of patient performance.

4 Five cases that will enable the reader to apply his/her understanding of flow-volume loops are presented as Unit 12.0 at the end of this Module.

6.20 Maximum voluntary ventilation

1 The maximum voluntary ventilation (MVV) test is the maximum volume of gas moved into and out of the lungs in a voluntary effort for a given number of seconds. It is expressed as liters per minute (L/min).

2 It differs from other tests by three specifics.
   a It involves both inspiratory and expiratory phases of ventilation.
   b It requires sustained maximum effort by the patient.
   c It requires good neuromuscular coordination.

3 The MVV is a dynamic test for overall lung function. It is really a miniature stress test and as such, it may not detect subtle physiologic changes but measures ventilatory reserve.

4 As a single-breath maneuver, the peak expiratory flow rate (PEFR) would be the counterpart of the MVV.

6.21 Procedures involved in the MVV test

1 The patient, in the standing position, ventilates maximally. The patient is instructed to breathe as rapidly and as deeply as possible for 15 seconds into and out of the apparatus.

2 Set a correct speed to allow calculation (160 mm/min with a Collins water-seal spirometer).

3 Calculation of MVV involves use of the integrator pen in water-sealed spirometers or direct integration for other units.

4 MVV may also be calculated by measuring the distance between the inspiratory-expiratory volume directly for a 15-second interval and multiplying the result by four (for 1 minute).

6.22 Usefulness of MVV testing

1 It is an overall function test, measuring the patient's ability to exchange air.

2 It may be used to identify air trapping.

3 MVV testing may be used to evaluate bronchodilator response if the FVC is nonspecific in results.

4 It may evaluate air trapping by the air velocity index (AVI) or dyspnea by the dyspnea index (DI):

$$AVI = \frac{(\% \text{ Predicted MVV})}{(\% \text{ Precited VC})} \qquad DI = \frac{\text{Minute volume}}{MVV}$$

6.23 Problems with MVV

1 MVV tests are greatly affected by nonpulmonary factors, such as muscular weakness, obesity, arthritis, or pain.

2 A MVV test may be overly strenuous to a compromised patient.

3 A MVV test may be normal in patients with pulmonary restriction.

4 To check for air-trapping, the air velocity index may need to be recalculated.

7.0 RELATIONSHIPS OF ATPS, BTPS, AND STPD
7.1 Correction from ATPS to BTPS to STPD

1 Even though the water-seal spriometer has been replaced in most hospitals by electronic devices, the concept of correcting a gas volume for temperature change is still important.

2 The condition under which air is collected in a spirometer is termed ATPS (ambient temperature and pressure, saturated with water vapor).

3 The condition under which gas volumes should be reported is BTPS (body temperature [37° C] and pressure, saturated). Volumes will be larger as a result of gas expansion at higher body temperature.

4 If a report on oxygen consumption is to be made, a different conversion is required to a smaller volume represented as STPD (standard temperature [0° C] and pressure [760 torr], dry [free of water vapor pressure]).

7.2 Gas laws and volume determination

1 Conversion of volumes from room temperature involves principles based on the understanding of what happens to a gas when it is exposed to different temperatures, pressures, and amounts of water vapor.

2 These conversions are based on the knowledge of Boyle's, Charles', Dalton's, and Gay-Lussac's laws, as well as the general knowledge that increased kinetic energy will expand a gas if the temperature is increased and if volume is available.

3 The gas laws are all derived from the ideal gas law:

$$\text{Pressure} \times \text{Volume} = nR \text{ temperature}$$

This expresses the relationship of pressure, volume, and absolute temperature if mass (n) and a constant (R) are used.

4 Charles' law gives the basis for temperature conversion and the need for the use of the absolute temperature scale for conversion. This is a result of the determination that, ideally, a gas will change $\frac{1}{273}$ of its total volume for every change in temperature of 1° C.

5 A combination of the empirical gas laws and the ideal gas law is given in the general gas law:

$$\frac{P_1 V_1}{T_1} = \frac{P_2 V_2}{T_2}$$

Where P equals atmospheric pressure and T equals temperature in degrees absolute (degrees C + 273). Pressure should be measured from a standard mercury barometer in the room and temperature from a thermometer on the spirometric device itself.

6 As a result of different coefficients of expansion between scales and the mercury barometer level, substract 2.5 mm Hg from the barometric pressure if room temperature is close to 24° C; otherwise use the correction provided with the barometer.

7.3 Temperature and water vapor pressure

1 According to Dalton's law of partial pressures, gases exert their effects and pressures according to their concentration in a gas mixture.

2 Water vapor is an exception to the principle of Dalton's law because the properties of a vapor are different from a gas and rely basically on temperature. A vapor exerts a pressure in a mixture based on its temperature.

3 A basic conversion in gas volumes collected by spirometry is necessary due to this vapor effect. Air collected over water or in a bellows is slightly contracted, so conversion from ATPS to BTPS involves initial subtraction of a greater water vapor pressure from atmospheric pressure. It also involves a correction by multiplications of a greater factor in room temperature to body temperature.

4 The total volume is usually about *8% higher* when all conversions from ATPS to BTPS are made.

TABLE 24-1 Correction factors for converting gas volumes to BTPS

Factor to convert volume to 37° C saturated*	When gas temperature is (C°)	Factor to convert volume to 37° C saturated	When gas temperature is (C°)
1.102	20	1.051	29
1.096	21	1.045	30
1.091	22	1.039	31
1.085	23	1.032	32
1.080	24	1.026	33
1.075	25	1.020	34
1.068	26	1.014	35
1.063	27	1.007	36
1.057	28	1.000	37

American Lung Association, Chronic obstructive pulmonary disease, ed 5, 1977, The Association.
*These factors have been calculated for barometric pressure of 760 mm Hg. Multiple observed gas volume by BTPS factor. It is unnecessary to correct for small deviations from standard barometric pressure at or near sea level.

7.4 Equations and conversions: ATPS to BTPS or STPD

1 Corrections must first be made for water vapor pressure with the following formula.

$$\frac{P_B}{P_B} - \frac{P_{H_2O}}{P_{H_2O}} \text{ at } 37° \text{ C}$$

2 Since the temperature of gas in the body is greater than in the spirometer, the volume must be increased by the factor:

$$\frac{273 + 37° \text{ C}}{273 + t \text{ (spirometer)}}$$

for absolute scale. See Table 24-1.

3 Combining the conversions gives the following formula:

$$\text{Volume}_{BTPS} = \text{Volume}_{ATP} \times \frac{273 + 37}{273 + T} \times \frac{P_B - P_{H_2O}}{P_B - 47}$$

4 For conversions from ambient to STPD, using the following formula:

$$\text{Volume}_{STPD} = \text{Volume}_{ATP} \times \frac{273}{273 + T} \times \frac{P_B - P_{H_2O}}{760 \text{ (dry)}}$$

5 Study the following example.
  a Volume equals 4.0 L at a temperature of 25° C and barometric pressure of 750 mm Hg.
  b Consulting Table 24-1 gives the factor figured from combining conversion factors—P_{H_2O} at 25° C = 24 mm Hg.
  c $\text{Volume}_{BTPS} = 4.0 \times \frac{(273 + 37)}{(273 + 25)} \times \frac{(750 - 24)}{(750 - 47)}$
  d $V_{BTPS} = 4.3 \text{ L}$

TESTS OF GAS EXCHANGE
8.1 Tests of gas exchange

1 Tests of gas exchange include procedures involved in blood gas determinations as well as a means of identifying changes in shunting, ventilation dead space, and gas exchange ratio differences.

2 Diffusing capacity tests are a pulmonary laboratory procedure used to measure transfer capacity of a highly soluble gas (carbon monoxide) across the alveolar capillary membranes in the lung.

3 Diffusion blocks or ventilation-perfusion abnormalities may show lower diffusion capacity results.

8.2 Tests for dead space

1 Testing for dead space involves calculation of the amount of physiologic dead space increase (anatomical and alveolar as a result of atelectasis or ventilation-perfusion imbalances.

2 The system is set with a one-way valve to a large Douglas bag collector.

3 Exhaled gas is collected for 3 minutes. At midpoint during the collection an arterial blood gas is drawn.

4 Calculations involve the standard Bohr equation, modified to:

a $$Vol_{DS}/TV = \frac{PaCO_2 - PeCO_2}{PaCO_2}$$

b Example: Pa = 40 mm Hg, mixed expired CO_2 = 30 mm Hg

$$Vol_{DS}/TV = \frac{40 - 30}{40} = \frac{10}{40} = 0.25$$

$$0.25 \times 100 = 25\% \text{ of TV}$$

8.3 Single-breath diffusion tests

1 The diffusing capacity test is one of the most sensitive indicators of dysfunction within the lung parenchyma and connective tissues.

2 In some conditions such as sarcoidosis, the diffusing capacity test may be the earliest indicator of abnormality. The diffusing capacity test will indicate an abnormality before chest x-ray examinations, volume studies, and blood gases are affected.

3 The gas used in diffusing capacity is carbon monoxide (CO), which has some 210 times the affinity for hemoglobin than does oxygen.

4 In the single-breath test, a patient inhales a specially-mixed gas containing less than .05% carbon monoxide, 10% helium, and 21% oxygen with the remainder composed of nitrogen.

a Helium and nitrogen meters are calibrated and readied for use.

b The patient rebreathes into the system, being turned into the system at the RV level.

c After a 10-second breath hold, the patient is switched into a spirometer.

5 Calculations must be made of alveolar carbon monoxide, alveolar volume, and D_{LCO}.

$$D_{LCO} = \frac{(V_A)\,(60)}{P_B - 47)\,T} \times \text{Log} \frac{FaCO_{11}}{FeCO_{12}}$$

Where

V_A = Alveolar volume (STPD)

60 = Correction from seconds to minutes

P_B = Barometric pressure

47 = Water vapor pressure (P_{H_2O})

T = Breath hold interval (in seconds)

Log = Natural logarithm

$FaCO_{11}$ = Fraction of CO in alveolar gas before diffusion

$FaCO_{12}$ = Fraction of CO in alveolar gas at the end of diffusion

8.4 Steady-state diffusion tests

1 Although it is not as popular as the single-breath test, the steady-state test is just as valid for testing diffusion.

2 Equipment for this test includes a collection bag and CO meter.

3 End-tidal CO measurements are analyzed and computed.

9.0 TYPES OF LUNG DISEASE

9.1 Spirometric results and impairment

1 Vital capacity (VC) may be lower than usual in patients with restriction or obstruction to airflow.

2 With restrictive disorders, reduced VC is the result of a reduced total lung capacity (TLC).

3 In obstructive disorders, VC is low because of increased residual volume (RV).

4 If TLC is increased, the lungs are probably abnormally distended. This *may* be abnormal, as in asthma or emphysema, or may indicate normal conditions resulting from aging (RV/TLC = about 50%). Hyperinflation by itself signifies no disease in particular.

5 Lower than normal volumes may indicate disease or inadequate effort.

9.2 General trends to interpret lung mechanics tests

1 Data obtained from lung mechanics tests (spirometry, MVV) cannot override results from the history and other assessment techniques.

2 Any function test can indicate disease only in relation to how it alters function, not its anatomic relationships.

3 The following relationships will show how the interpretation of lung mechanics tests gives an initial indication of obstructive or restrictive conditions. These indications must then be confirmed or denied by further tests (Table 24-2).

9.3 Results of tests for small airways function

1 Small airways are those defined as less than 2 mm in diameter (bronchioles).

2 Normally, small airways contribute little, if any, to airway resistance. This is the "silent zone" containing most of the lung's reserve. It is suspected of being the area that is first involved in obstructive disorders.

3 Only sophisticated types of tests can measure changes in volume and obstruction caused in small airways. Most techniques involve easily performed procedures, but require expensive equipment for calculations that are well beyond the limits of spirometry.

T A B L E   2 4 - 2 Interpretation of lung mechanics tests

PFT	Obstruction	Restriction
FVC	Decreased	Decreased
IC	Decreased or normal	Decreased
ERV	Decreased or normal	Decreased
TV	Increased	Normal or slightly decreased
RV	Increased	Decreased
RV/TLC	Increased	Decreased
FEV_1	Decreased	Normal (FEV_1/VC)
MEFR	Decreased	Normal
MVV	Decreased	Decreased
FEF 25% to 75%	Decreased	Normal

T A B L E   2 4 - 3 Gas distribution results (ΔN_2)

Single-breath oxygen test	Nitrogen wash-out test	Example
Increased N_2	Increased N_2	Asthma (acute attack); emphysema
Increased N_2	Normal	Bronchitis
Normal	Increased N_2	Bullous disease
Increased N_2	Normal	Cardiac asthma
Normal	Normal	Restrictive diseases

T A B L E   2 4 - 4 General trends for tests of obstruction and restriction

Test	Obstruction	Restriction
Volumes: IC	Decreased	Decreased
ERV	Decreased	Decreased
TV	Increased	Normal
RV	Increased	Decreased
TLC	Increased or normal	Decreased
Flows: FVC and FEV_1	Decreased	Decreased or normal
MEFR	Decreased	Normal
MVV	Decreased	Decreased
Diffusion	Decreased	Decreased
Resistance	Increased	Normal
ΔN_2	Increased (>2%)	Normal
Frequency dependent	Positive	Negative
Compliance	Increased or normal	Decreased
Closing volume	Increased (10% VC)	Normal
Volume of isoflow	Increased	Normal
Vol_{DS}/TV	Increased	Normal
Shunt ($\dot{Q}S/\dot{Q}T$)	Increased	Increased

4 Tests of small airway disease include:
  a FEF 25% to 75% determination from the spirogram
  b Flow-volume loop slope observations
  c Closing volume studies
5 Although *4a* and *4b* are relatively effective in identifying small airways disease, the most effective are:
  a Closing volume
  b Volume of isoflow
  c Frequency dependence of compliance
6 Closing volume determination is made from a single breath oxygen expiration test. It is modified so that the patient's expired flow is steady and constant throughout expiration.
  a It is based on the fact that the weight of the lung makes pleural pressure less in effect and alveolar volume smaller at lung bases than at the apices.
  b As a result, gas is preferentially deferred to the apices. Theoretically, lung airways should close off (air trapping) in lower (basal) airways earlier than at the top.
  c A nitrogen analyzer measuring this effect in a single-breath oxygen test should show an increase in nitrogen concentration at the end of the curve plotted by this test.
7 Volume of isoflow is used along with interpretation of flow-volume loop analysis for early airway closure as evidenced by a change in the shape of the loop. Volume of isoflow tests use helium to produce a flow-volume test graph that is placed over the normal air flow volume. The helium gas is much more diffusible than room air through obstructed airways, so it should show higher volume.
8 Frequency dependence of compliance is the optimum test for measuring presence of air trapping in the small airways. It is a difficult test to perform, however, requiring patient stress and discomfort as well as requiring pressure measurement by a balloon inserted into the esophagus. Dynamic compliance measurements will decrease (less volume per pressure change) in patients with airway disease.

9.4 Results of gas distribution tests

1 The single-breath oxygen test and the 7-minute nitrogen wash-out (functional residual capacity) tests are most often used to indicate maldistribution of ventilation.
2 Comparisons of these tests show that the single-breath test, besides being modified for closing volume determination, may give a change in nitrogen concentration (ΔN_2) result at the earliest stages of airway narrowing. The ΔN_2 calculated from the 7-minute wash-out (FRC) test may best identify bullous disease (Table 24-3).

9.5 Overall trends between obstructive and restrictive diseases

1 It should be noted that obstructive diseases, in general, affect airway flow diffusion and air trapping.
2 Restrictive conditions cause a reduction in overall volumes and diffusion.
3 General trends for most tests for restriction and obstruction are summarized in Table 24-4.

9.6 Chest wall restriction compared with parenchymal restriction

1 Consult the list in Table 24-5 for differences in test results in parenchymal restriction (e.g., atelectasis) from the chest wall type of restriction (e.g., kyphoscoliosis).

TABLE 24-5 Differences in parenchymal and chest wall restriction

Test	Parenchymal restriction	Chest wall restriction
Lung volumes	Decreased	Decreased
Vital capacity	Decreased	Decreased
FEV_1	Normal	Normal
FEF 25%-75%	Normal	Normal
MVV	Normal to decreased	Normal to decreased
DLCO	Decreased	Decreased
C_{st} C_{dyn}	Decreased	Decreased
R_{aw}	Normal	Normal
Closing volume	Increased	Variable

10.0 POTENTIAL HAZARDS ASSOCIATED WITH PULMONARY FUNCTION TESTING

10.1 Pulmonary function testing hazards with the asthma patient

1 Deep breathing required in spirometry and in the MVV test may be hazardous to a patient with irritable airways.

2 Because of the possibility of hypoxia and cardiac arrhythmias caused by exertion and bronchospasm, pulmonary function testing may have to be limited to testing bronchodilator response.

10.2 Hazards of bronchodilators

1 In testing for the effect of bronchodilators, the history and medication record of the patient is of prime importance.

2 It must be determined if the patient is having difficulty getting a satisfactory effect from his bronchidilator. Many of these drugs may have adverse effects on the heart, especially if tolerance develops and the patient takes increasing dosages to obtain the desired relief.

10.3 Hazards with certain patient conditions

1 Contagious lung diseases present particular problems if pulmonary functions are to be done, especially if limited equipment and supplies are available. It is advisable to postpone testing until the disease condition has run its course or has been brought under control.

2 Certain conditions contraindicate pulmonary function testing as a result of the stress on the patient. These are:
   a Pulmonary emboli
   b Aneurysms
   c Severe cardiac conditions
   Testing may be allowed if certain modifications are made.

11.0 IMPORTANCE OF PATIENT COOPERATION DURING PULMONARY FUNCTION TESTING

11.1 Important of patient cooperation

1 Almost all of the spirometric tests for pulmonary function are effort-dependent and still rely on patient cooperation with the procedure for results.

2 The importance of giving the patient a total explanation of the procedure cannot be overstated. Patient apprehension and lack of understanding may affect vital signs as well as cooperation and, therefore, affect test results.

11.2 Techniques to encourage effort

1 Adequate instruction is the first step in ensuring good effort in testing.

2 A strong voice and "cheerleading" abilities, especially when giving VC, peak flow, and MVV tests are not only advisable but mandatory. Loudly encouraging the patient with "more, more," or "go, go" is a standard part of the procedure.

11.3 Accuracy needed in interpretation

1 Interpretation of pulmonary function results must be put into perspective with the patient's history and blood gas determination for validity.

2 Since most pulmonary function screening devices are very effort-dependent, wrong interpretation based on less-than-maximum responses could be detrimental to the patient, financially and psychologically.

11.4 Lists of effort-dependent tests

1 Effort-dependent
   a VC
   b Flow rate tests
   c MVV
   d Frequency dependence of compliance
   e Gas dilution
   f FRC studies (FVC at end)
   g Flow-volume loops
   h Volume of isoflow

2 Not maximum-effort-dependent
   a Closing volume
   b Diffusing capacity

12.0 RELATIONSHIPS OF RESPIRATORY MECHANICS AND WORK OF BREATHING TO PULMONARY FUNCTION TESTING

12.1 Respiratory mechanics and work of breathing

1 Some advanced physiologic testing is used to determine oxygen consumption ($\dot{V}O_2$) and respiratory quotient ($\dot{V}O_2/\dot{V}E_{CO_2}$), which can be used to calculate a patient's metabolic status and amount of increase in ventilatory work.

2 Testing results for compliance can be determined by pressure-volume measurements in normal breathing. In mechanical ventilation, an estimation of this can be made by comparing pressures needed to ventilate to volumes inspired. Decreased compliance mechanisms increase the work of breathing as a result of changes in the FRC resting level of the lung.

12.2 Information needed to correlate pulmonary function test results to disease processes

1 Pulmonary function studies alone cannot diagnose a disease, nor the extent to which it impairs lung physiology.

2 Correlating blood gas studies with pulmonary function results gives a much better determination of the extent of the suggested damage to real disability.

3 Information on patient history and a current x-ray lung analysis can be most helpful in making a differential diagnosis. Inspiratory and expiratory differences may give another clue to the extent of air trapping or residual volume increases in obstructive conditions. Chest wall restrictive processes limiting inspiration may also be revealed.

12.3 Values of routine pulmonary function tests

Routine pulmonary function tests are useful in distinguishing causes of dyspnea, establishing potential surgical risk, possibly detecting early pulmonary diseases, testing the effects of bronchodilator therapy, and measuring the degree of pulmonary impairment.

12.4 Tests are calculated and analyzed by computers and by trained personnel.

1 The 1980s is undoubtedly the decade in which computers gained eminence in applications to clinical medicine and in the pulmonary function laboratory.

In 1982, the American Association for Respiratory Care dedicated a special issue to *"Computers in Pulmonary Medicine."* This issue pointed out the growth of computers since World War II and how they can be used in the pulmonary laboratory for quality control, storage and quick retrieval of data, and analyzing pulmonary function studies.

Computers undoubtedly will continue to grow in popularity because they are fast, accurate, and require less work in calculating results than did the mechanical methods.

In ending this module the authors would like to point out that even though computers can be of great assistance in the laboratory and at the bedside, they cannot replace the eye, intellect, and feelings of the trained observer who must interact with the patient to obtain maximum performance.

This module has focused on standard traditional pulmonary function techniques for the purpose of giving the reader the background necessary to appreciate and understand the basics of pulmonary function testing with or without computer interface.

2 It is important for the reader to appreciate that pulmonary function has grown as a separate profession.

3 On July 11, 1987, The National Board for Respiratory Care Inc., (NBRC) administered its first Registry Examination for Advanced Pulmonary Function Technologists (RPFT).

4 A total of 276 candidates sat for this first examination with over 57% passing. For more information about the RPFT examinations, the reader may contact the NBRC, 8310 Nieman Rd., Lenexa, Kansas, 66214.

13.0 INTERPRETATION OF PULMONARY FUNCTION TESTS (SPIROMETRY, LUNG VOLUMES, AND TRANSFER FACTOR):

Units 13.0 and 14.0 are presented as examples of patients where pulmonary function testing enabled the practitioner to better assess their pulmonary status. The reader is encouraged to apply his/her own knowledge and skills at assessing these patients by following the procedure as presented below. Answers to the problems are presented as Unit 13.9.

13.1 Purpose

1 To understand general principles in interpretation of pulmonary function tests.

2 To estimate physiological defects associated with impaired pulmonary function.

13.2 Procedure

1 Review the module and if necessary study other texts to become familiar with evaluation of ventilatory studies.

2 Use the following sample guide to systematically make commitments regarding spirometry, response to bronchodilators, residual volume, total lung capacity, and transfer factor.

3 Interpret the type of lung disease associated with the abnormality.

4 Interpret blood gases. (Normal values will vary depending on altitude.)

5 If previous studies are available, compare results with previous evaluation.

6 Suggest other tests that might more accurately define the physiological defect.

13.3 Sample guide for pulmonary function

This guide can be used to evaluate spirometry, lung volumes, transfer factor, and arterial blood gases. Interpretations of PFT/ABG can easily be computerized from this type of evaluation form.

1 Normal ventilatory studies.

2 Normal spirometry.

3 Spirometry demonstrates:

a Borderline obstructive defect (FEV_1/FVC 70% to 75%; MMF)

b Mild obstructive defect (FEV_1/FVC 65% to 70%)

c Moderate obstructive defect ($FEV_1/FVC < 65\%$; $FEV_1 > 1.5$ L)

d Moderately severe obstructive defect ($FEV_1 < 1.5$ L; > 0.75 L)

e Marked obstructive defect ($FEV_1 < 0.75$ L)

f Borderline reduction in vital capacity (FVC 75% to 80%)

g Mildly reduced vital capacity (FVC 60% to 75%)

h Moderately reduced vital capacity (FVD 50% to 60%)

i Markedly reduced vital capacity (FVC < 50%)

4 No change after single inhalation of bronchodilator (<10%).

5 Slight improvement after single inhalation of bronchodilator (10% to 20%).

6 Moderate improvement after single inhalation of bronchodilator (20% to 50%).

7 Marked improvement after single inhalation of bronchodilator (>50%).

8 Residual volume:

  a Normal (80% to 120%)

  b Decreased (<80%)

  c Slightly increased (120% to 150%)

  d Moderately increased (150% to 200%)

  e Markedly increased (>200%)

9 Total lung capacity:

  a Normal (80% to 120%)

  b Slightly decreased (70% to 80%)

  c Moderately decreased (55% to 70%)

  d Markedly decreased (<55%)

  e Slightly increased (120% to 140%)

  f Moderately increased (140% to 160%)

  g Markedly increased (>160%)

10 Transfer factor (diffusing capacity):

  a Within normal limits

  b Decreased

11 Abnormalities suggest:

  a Early obstructive pulmonary disease

  b Mild obstructive pulmonary disease

  c Mild, somewhat reversible obstructive pulmonary disease

  d Mild, highly reversible obstructive pulmonary disease

  e Moderate obstructive pulmonary disease

  f Moderate, somewhat reversible obstructive pulmonary disease

  g Moderate, highly reversible obstructive pulmonary disease

  h Moderately severe obstructive pulmonary disease

  i Moderately severe, somewhat reversible obstructive pulmonary disease

  j Moderately severe, highly reversible obstructive pulmonary disease

  k Severe obstructive pulmonary disease

  l Severe, somewhat reversible obstructive pulmonary disease

  m Severe, highly reversible obstructive pulmonary disease

  n With probable emphysematous component

  o With significant emphysematous component

  p With predominate emphysematous component

  q Mild restrictive pulmonary disease

  r Moderate restrictive pulmonary disease

  s Severe restrictive pulmonary disease

  t With borderline defect in transfer factor (diffusion)

  u With mild defect in transfer factor (diffusion)

  v With moderate defect in transfer factor (diffusion)

  w With severe defect in transfer factor (diffusion)

12 Arterial blood gases

  a Are normal

  b Demonstrate mild hypoxemia

  c Demonstrate moderate hypoxemia

  d Demonstrate severe hypoxema ($Po_2 < 50$)

	Age 20	Age 45	Age 70
(Po_2 = 65 to 80	62 to 75	60 to 70)
(Po_2 = 50 to 65	50 to 62	50 to 60)

13 No change from previous study.

14 Slight improvement from previous study.

15 Moderate improvement from previous study.

16 Marked improvement from previous study.

17 Slight deterioration from previous study.

TABLE 24-6 Patient one*

Interpret the following tests

Age 16   Height 62 in   Weight 90 lb

	PREDICTED	MEASURED	% PRED
SPIROMETRY			
Forced vital cap (FVC)	3.51 L	1.60 L	FVC 46 %
Forced exp vol in L/sec (FEV_1)	2.92 L	1.48 L	$\frac{FEV_1}{FVC}$ 93 %
Max mid-exp flow rate (MMF, $FEF_{0.25-0.75}$)	3.86 L/sec	2.46 L/sec	

LUNG VOLUME (HELIUM)		% PRED	PREDICTED
Insp cap (IC)	0.90 L		
Exp res vol	0.60 L		
Func resid cap (FRC)	1.21 L		
Resid vol (RV)	0.61 L	71 %	0.86 L
Tot lung cap (TLC)	2.11 L	52 %	4.09 L
RV/TLC	29 %		21 %

TRANSFER FACTOR ($D_{L_{CO}}$)

	Resting		
Single breath	11.4	$\frac{cc\ CO}{min}$ mm Hg	
			PREDICTED
Steady state		$\frac{cc\ CO}{min}$ mm Hg	Mean 26.5 Range 16.5 to 36.5

INTERPRETATION:

Spirometry demonstrates markedly reduced vital capacity.
Residual volume decreased.
Total lung capacity markedly decreased.
Transfer factor (diffusing capacity) decreased.
Abnormalities suggest severe restrictive pulmonary disease with moderate defect in transfer factor (diffusion).

COMMENT:

These pulmonary functions are typical for a patient with severe interstitial lung disease (eg, sarcoidosis, scleroderma, and interstitial fibrosis).

*Reprinted with permission, courtesy of AARC, Daedalus Enterprises, Dallas, Tex.

18 Moderate deterioration from previous study.

19 Marked deterioration from previous study.

20 Suggest lung volume study to further evaluate restrictive spirometric defect.

21 Suggest transport factor (diffusion) study.

NOTE: The following tables list tests run on five patients. The interpretation section has been completed on patient no. 1 in Table 24-6. Interpretation for patients 2 through 5 are to be done by the reader. Complete interpretations of the tests are given after each table.

TABLE 24-7 Patient two*

Interpret the following tests

Age 74   Height 62 in   Weight 196 lb

	PREDICTED	MEASURED	% PRED
SPIROMETRY			
Forced vital capacity (FVC)	2.47 L	2.33 L	FVC 94 %
Forced exp vol in L/sec (FEV$_1$)	2.00 L	1.64 L	$\frac{FEV_1}{FVC}$ 70 %
Max Mid-exp flow rate (MMF, FEF$_{0.25-0.75}$)	2.11 L/sec	1.03 L/sec	

LUNG VOLUME (HELIUM)	PREDICTED VOL		
Insp cap (IC)	2.03 L		
Exp res vol (ERV)	0.42 L		
Func resid cap (FRC)	2.82 L	% PRED	PREDICTED
Resid vol (RV)	2.40 L	133 %	1.80 L
Tot lung Cap (TLC)	4.85 L	111 %	4.38 L
RV/TLC	49 %		41 %

TRANSFER FACTOR (D$_{L_{CO}}$)

Resting

	cc CO	PREDICTED
Single breath 13.8	min	
	mm Hg	Mean 15.8
	cc CO	Range 5.8 to 25.8

INTERPRETATION:

(Write response here) _____

_____

_____

_____

*Reprinted with permisssion, courtesy of AARC, Daedalus Enterprises, Dallas, Tex.

Interpretations and comments for patients two through five

Patient two

1 Interpretation:

a Spirometry demonstrates mild obstructive defect.

b Residual volume slightly increased.

c Total lung capacity normal.

d Transfer factor (diffusing capacity) within normal limits.

e Abnormalities suggest mild obstructive pulmonary disease.

2 Comment:

a These pulmonary function values are typical for an asymptomatic person who has smoked cigarettes for years.

TABLE 24-8 Patient three*

Interpret the following tests

Age 34   Height 66 in   Weight 216 lb

	PREDICTED	MEASURED	% PRED
SPIROMETRY			
Forced vital capacity (FVC)	3.77 L	1.06 L	FEV 28%
Forced exp vol in L/sec (FEV$_1$)	3.12 L	0.93 L	$\frac{FEV_1}{FVC}$ 88 %
Max mid-exp flow rate (MMF, FEF$_{0.25-0.75}$)	3.52 L/sec	1.08 L/sec	

LUNG VOLUME (HELIUM)			
Insp cap (IC)	1.18 L		
Exp res vol (ERV)	0.45 L		
Func resid cap (FRC)	2.24 L	% PRED	PREDICTED
Resid vol (RV)	1.79 L	102 %	1.76 L
Tot lung cap (TLC)	3.42 L	64 %	5.38 L
RV/TLC	52 %		33 %

INTERPRETATION:

(Write response here) _____

_____

_____

_____

_____

*Reprinted with permission, courtesy of AARC, Daedalus Enterprises, Dallas, Tex.

Patient three

1 Interpretation:

a Spirometry demonstrates severely reduced vital capacity.

b Residual volume normal.

c Total lung capacity moderately decreased.

d Abnormalities suggest moderate restrictive pulmonary disease.

2 Comment:

a The pulmonary function values are typical for a patient with severe interstitial lung disease.

b Possibly some of the reduction in vital capacity results from obesity. A diffusion capacity (transfer factor) test might help to further define the physiologic defect.

TABLE 24-9 Patient four*

Interpret the following tests			
Age 59 Height 70 in Weight 154 lb			
	PREDICTED	MEASURED	% PRED
SPIROMETRY			
Forced vital capacity (FVC)	4.39 L	3.56 L	FVC 81 %
Forced exp vol in L/sec (FEV₁)	3.28 L	2.87 L	$\frac{FEV_1}{FVC}$ 81 %
Max mid-exp flow rate (MMF, FEF₀.₂₅₋₀.₇₅)	3.09 L/sec	2.51 L/sec	

LUNG VOLUME (HELIUM)			
Insp cap (IC)	3.30 L		
Exp res vol (ERV)	0.70 L		
Func resid cap (FRC)	2.92 L	% PRED	PREDICTED
Resid vol (RV)	1.81 L	123 %	2.22 L
Tot lung cap (TLC)	6.54 L	95 %	6.22 L
RV/TLC	28 %		36 %

TRANSFER FACTOR (D$_{L_{CO}}$)

	Resting		
Single breath 18.5	cc CO min mm Hg	PREDICTED	
Steady state	cc CO min mm Hg	Mean 21.0 Range 11.0 to 31.0	

INTERPRETATION:

(Write response here) _____

_____

_____

_____

*Reprinted with permission, courtesy of AARC, Daedalus Enterprises, Dallas, Tex.

Patient four

1 Interpretation:
   a Normal ventilatory studies.
   b Transfer factor (diffusing capacity) within normal limits.
2 Comment:
   a Although these pulmonary function values are within the range of normal, other pulmonary function studies such as tests of small airway disease or exercise tests might define a defect.

TABLE 24-10 Patient five*

Interpret the following tests			
Age 57 Height 72 in Weight 165 lb			
	PREDICTED	MEASURED	% PRED
SPIROMETRY			
Forced vital capacity (FVC)	4.68 L	2.44 L	FVC 52 %
Forced exp vol in L/sec (FEV₁)	3.52 L	0.70 L	$\frac{FEV_1}{FVC}$ 29 %
Max mid-exp flow rate (MMF, FEF₀.₂₅₋₀.₇₅)	3.43 L/sec	0.23 L/sec	

LUNG VOLUME (HELIUM)			
Insp cap (IC)	1.70 L		
Exp res vol (ERV)	1.45 L		
Func resid cap (FRC)	5.97 L	% PRED	PREDICTED
Resid vol (RV)	4.52 L	217 %	2.08 L
Tot lung cap (TLC)	7.67 L	113 %	6.76 L
RV/TLC	58.9 %		31 %

TRANSFER FACTOR (D$_{L_{CO}}$)

	Resting	PREDICTED
Single breath 7.2	cc CO min mm HG cc CO	Mean 21.5 Range 11.5 to 31.5

INTERPRETATION:

(Write response here) _____

_____

_____

_____

*Reprinted with permission, courtesy of AARC, Daedalus Enterprises, Dallas, Tex.

Patient five

1 Interpretation:
   a Spirometry demonstrates marked obstructive defect.
   b Spirometry demonstrates moderately reduced vital capacity.
   c Residual volume markedly increased.
   d Total lung capacity normal.
   e Transfer factor (diffusing capacity) decreased.
   f Abnormalities suggest severe obstructive pulmonary disease, probably with emphysematous component.
2 Comment:
   a These pulmonary function values are typical for a patient with severe chronic obstructive lung disease secondary to emphysema. The transfer factor is usually decreased with emphysema but not bronchitis with the same spirometric defect.

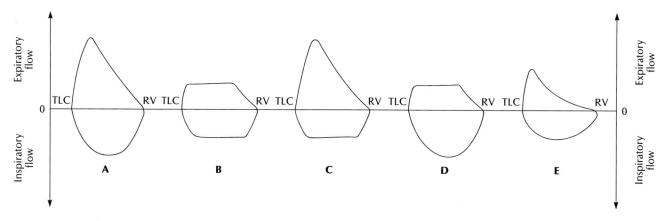

FIGURE 24-28 A to **E,** examples of the various flow-volume loop patterns. For each patient presented in the text, select the flow-volume loop pattern that most closely characterizes the type of obstruction. (Reprinted with permission, courtesy of AARC, Daedalus Enterprises, Dallas, Tex.)

14.0 USE OF FLOW-VOLUME LOOP PATTERNS TO DETERMINE THE TYPE AND LOCATION OF AIRWAY OBSTRUCTION

14.1 Purpose of and instructions to this exercise

1 The flow-volume loop (F-V loop) is a test of ventilatory function in which airflow is plotted against volume during a maximal forced expiratory vital capacity followed by a maximal inspiratory effort.

2 Various obstructive abnormalities of the airways produce characteristic patterns. These patterns are of diagnostic value in describing the type and location of various obstructions.

3 In the following cases, case histories of patients are shown and the reader will complete the statements that follow each case.

4 Each flow-volume loop may be selected once, more than once, or not at all.

5 Answers are presented following each case.

Patient one

1 A 59-year-old black woman with a 13-year history of a goiter controlled with thyroid medications.

2 The patient stopped taking the medications because of enlarged lymph nodes and a stiff jaw.

3 The goiter became larger and the patient began complaining of dyspnea on exertion.

4 Resting arterial blood gases were normal.

5 The pulmonary function test showed airway obstruction resulting from an enlarged goiter.

  a From Fig. 24-28 select the pattern resembling this patient's type of obstruction.

    Answer: Fig. 24-28, *B* resembles this patient's F-V curve.

    • A goiter will usually result in a fixed upper airway obstruction by compression of the trachea. Thus the airway diameter at the site of obstruction will not change with inspiration or expiration.

    • A constant flow seen as a plateau in the effort-de-

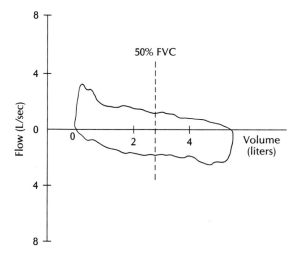

FIGURE 24-29 Flow-volume loop obtained from patient 1 characterizing a fixed upper airway obstruction. (Reprinted with permission, courtesy of AARC, Daedalus Enterprises, Dallas, Tex.)

pendent portion of the expiratory curve will be present, with no change in the effort-independent portion.

    • A plateau will also be observed on the inspiratory part of the curve, because both inspiration and expiration are affected.

  b Give the mid-FVC ratio of expiratory to inspiratory flow in this type of obstruction.

    Answer: A mid-FVC ratio of around 1 (within normal limits) is typical. The patient's actual curve appears in Fig. 24-29.

Patient two

1 A 32-year-old white man was admitted for precholecystectomy evaluation.

2 Spirometry and arterial blood gases are within normal limits. He denied any respiratory problems.

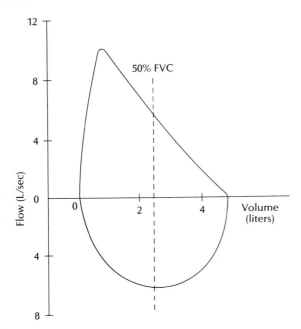

FIGURE 24-30 Normal flow-volume loop from patient 2. (Reprinted with permission, courtesy of AARC, Daedalus Enterprises, Dallas, Tex.)

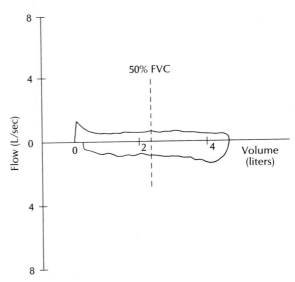

FIGURE 24-31 This flow-volume loop from patient 3 shows severe fixed upper airway obstruction (trachea stenosis). (Reprinted with permission, courtesy of AARC, Daedalus Enterprises, Tex.)

   a From Fig. 24-28 select the F-V loop that best resembles his pulmonary status.
   Answer: Fig. 24-28, *A* resembles this patient's F-V loop.
   • His F-V loop is normal.
3 The portion of the expiratory curve near total lung capacity (TLC) is effort-dependent and contains the flow rate termed "peak flow."
4 The portion of the expiratory curve near residual volume (RV) is independent of effort, with the flow limited by dynamic compression of the small airways.
   a Give the ratio of expiratory flow to inspiratory flow at the mid-FVC.
   Answer: At mid-FVC, the ratio in normal subjects is about 0.9. This patient's actual F-V loop appears in Fig. 24-30.

Patient three
1 A 23-year-old man suffered head injuries and required a tracheostomy with assisted ventilation for 2 weeks.
2 Several weeks following the removal of the cuffed tracheostomy tube he complained of symptoms from severe tracheal stenosis at the subglottic level.
   a From Fig. 24-28 select the F-V loop best depicting this patient's obstruction.
   Answer: Tracheal stenosis is usually a fixed obstruction, resulting in an F-V loop resembling that of Fig. 24-28, *B,* with the characteristics described for patient 1.
   • Fig. 24-31 shows this patient's F-V loop, showing the severity of his flow limitation of all lung volumes.

   b Give the ratio of the mid-FVC flows.
   Answer: The mid-FVC ratio is approximately 1.0. This patient underwent resection of the stenosis, with an end-to-end anastomosis resulting in restoration of normal flow rates (Fig. 24-32).

Patient four
1 A 51-year-old white man is evaluated for shortness of breath.
2 He has had dyspnea for 2 years.
3 Resting arterial blood gases show moderate hypoxemia.
4 He had increased sputum production for 2 months.
5 Spirometry shows obstructive lung disease.
   a From Fig. 24-28 select the F-V loop best resembling his actual loop.
   Answer: Chronic obstructive lung disease is characterized by Fig. 24-29, *E.*
   • The shape of the expiratory curve is mostly abnormal in the effort-independent part near RV, indicating greater dynamic compression of the diseased small airways. Thus we obtain a characteristic curvilinear shape. Give the normal mid-FVC ratio for this type of obstruction.
   Answer: The inspiratory curve is less affected, if at all, resulting in a mid-FVC ratio of less than 0.5. This patient's F-V loop is shown in Fig. 24-33.

Patient five
1 A 26-year-old man had dyspnea and noisy breathing on exertion for 3 years.

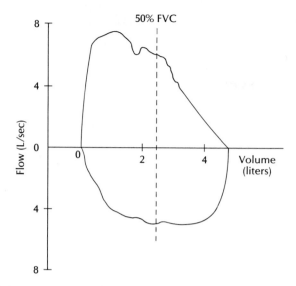

FIGURE 24-32 Flow-volume loop from patient 3 several weeks after corrective surgery. Notice the tremendous improvement in flow rate from that in Figure 24-31. (Reprinted with permission, courtesy of AARC, Daedalus Enterprises, Dallas, Tex.)

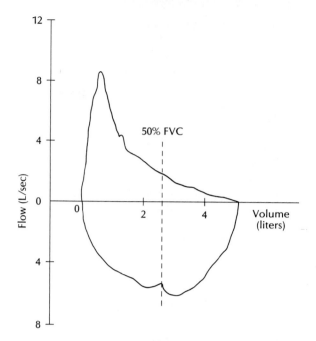

FIGURE 24-33 Flow-volume loop from patient 4. It is a common pattern seen in chronic obstructive pulmonary disease. (Reprinted with permission, courtesy of AARC, Daedalus Enterprises, Dallas, Tex.)

2 Two years earlier he had abnormal pulmonary function tests and had been put on oral bronchodilators and steroids.

3 He was re-examined and was found to have generalized expiratory stridor.

4 Flow-volume loops (Fig. 24-34) showed a variable intrathoracic obstruction that was confirmed by tracheal biopsy to be a grade 2 squamous cell carcinoma. From Fig. 24-28 select the F-V loop that resembles his expected F-V loop.

Answer: A variable intrathoracic upper airway obstruction results in an F-V loop resembling that in Fig. 24-28, *D*.

• In a variable obstruction, the location of the lesion is important.

• In a variable intrathoracic obstruction, the extraluminal pressure will be equivalent to intrapleural pressure or negative to intraluminal pressure during inspiration that favors dilatation of the airways.

• During expiration, extraluminal pressure is positive relative to intraluminal pressure, and narrowing of the airway occurs, which increases the obstruction.

• A plateau indicating constant flow will be seen during expiration on the F-V loop, while the inspiratory limb will be normal or near normal. Give the mid-FVC ratio usually obtained from this type of obstruction.

Answer: The mid-FVC ratio will be very low, resembling that of chronic obstructive lung disease.

• Here the shape is very important in the separation of the two.

• Fig. 24-28, *C* is an F-V loop produced by a variable extrathoracic upper airway obstruction.

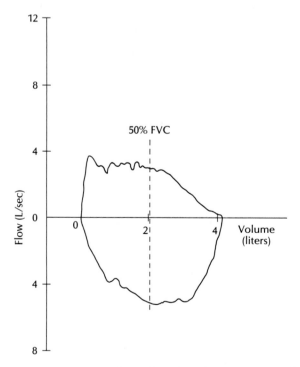

FIGURE 24-34 This flow-volume loop from patient 5 is characteristic of a variable intrathoracic upper airway obstruction. (Reprinted with permission, courtesy of AARC, Daedalus Enterprises, Dallas, Tex.)

- In this type of obstruction, the pressure inside the airway is markedly negative compared with the atmospheric pressure around the airway during forced inspiration that narrows the airways.
- During forced expiration, the pressure inside the airway is more positive than the atmospheric pressure around the airway; thus dilatation of the airway occurs. Consequently, in a variable extrathoracic obstruction, the obstruction becomes greater on inspiration and less on expiration, giving a mid-FVC ratio greater than one.
- Vocal cord paralysis is the usual cause of this form of upper airway obstruction, whereas tumors make up the majority of the variable intrathoracic upper airway obstructions.

BIBLIOGRAPHY

Altose MD: The physiological basis of pulmonary function testing, Ciba Clin Symp 31:139, 1979.

American Thoracic Society: Snowbird workshop on standardization of spirometry, Am Rev Respir Dis 119:813, 1979.

Bergman NA: New tests of pulmonary function: physiological basis and interpretations, Anesthesiology 44:220, 1976.

Burton GG, Gee GN, and Hodgkin JE, editors: Respiratory care: a guide to clinical practice, Philadelphia, 1977, JB Lippincott Co.

Cherniack RM: Pulmonary function testing, Philadelphia, 1977, WB Saunders Co.

Cherniack RM: Pitfalls in pulmonary function testing, Respir Care 28:434, 1983.

Conkle RG: Bedside spirometry, Curr Rev Respir Ther 3:2, 1980.

Crapo RO: Clinical applications of pulmonary function data, AART Convention Lecture Series, American Scientific Products, 1982.

Gardner RM et al: Computerized decision-making in the pulmonary function laboratory, Respir Care 27:799, 1982.

George RB: Bedside pulmonary function testing in the ICU, AART Convention Lecture Series, American Scientific Products, 1983.

Gibbs PS: Preoperative evaluation of the patient with lung disease, Curr Rev Respir Ther 6:1, 1983.

Hankinson JL: Quality control in the pulmonary function laboratory, Respir Care 27:830, 1982.

Knudson RJ et al: Changes in the normal maximal expiratory flow-volume curve with growth and aging, Am Rev Respir Dis 127:725, 1983.

Larson JK: Computer-assisted spirometry, Respir Care 27:839, 1982.

McPherson SP: Respiratory therapy equipment, ed 4, St Louis, 1990, The CV Mosby Co.

Milledge JS and Nunn JF: Criteria of fitness for anesthesia in patients with chronic obstructive lung disease, Br Med J 3:670, 1975.

Pilbeam SP: The physiologic basis for exercise testing, AART Convention Lecture Series, American Scientific Products, 1983.

Ruppel G: Manual of pulmonary function testing, St Louis, 1982, The CV Mosby Co.

Spearman CB, Sheldon RL, and Egan DF: Egan's fundamentals of respiratory therapy, ed 5, St Louis, 1990, The CV Mosby Co.

LEARNING OBJECTIVES

On completion of this module the reader will be able to:

1.1 Describe the social and economic impact of chronic pulmonary disease.

1.2 Explain the need for outpatient and home care programs.

1.3 Discuss the economic savings to the patient by well-designed outpatient and home care programs.

2.1 Explain the psychologic impact of chronic pulmonary disease.

2.2 Describe how patients with chronic pulmonary disease may view themselves.

2.3 Describe how the family of the chronic pulmonary disease patient may view the patient.

2.4 Explain how counseling for the patient and family can help with adjustment.

2.5 Define rehabilitation and list the goals of rehabilitation.

3.1 Identify pathophysiology associated with pulmonary diseases.

4.1 Identify disorders that may warrant a pulmonary rehabilitation program.

5.1 Describe the signs of pulmonary deterioration.

6.1 Explain special problems associated with the pediatric patient.

6.2 Explain special problems associated with the elderly patient.

7.1 Identify components that make home care and rehabilitation a specialty.

8.1 Outline a plan to care for the patient with chronic pulmonary disease in the hospital setting.

8.2 Outline a plan to care for the patient with chronic pulmonary disease in the outpatient clinic setting.

8.3 Outline a plan to care for the patient with chronic pulmonary disease in the home setting.

9.1 Explain the need for a multidisciplinary health care team to care for the home patient.

10.1 Construct a home care plan with the patient's physician.

11.1 Explain the need for education as a part of the home care plan.

12.1 Explain the concept of motivation with regard to the patient and family following a home care plan.

13.1 Identify causes of pulmonary emergencies in the home and describe a plan to be used in the event of an emergency.

14.1 Identify professional and community services required by the home patient.

Pulmonary rehabilitation and home care

14.2 Describe the role of the coordinator of patient services.

15.1 Identify sources on abuse of pulmonary rehabilitation, outpatient care, and home care programs.

15.2 Discuss the overall impact of the January 1, 1989 Medicare Catastrophic Health Insurance on health care.

1.0 SOCIAL AND ECONOMIC IMPACT OF CHRONIC PULMONARY DISEASE

1.1 Social and economic impact

1 Chronic lung disease, especially chronic obstructive pulmonary disease (COPD), represents one of the greatest health problems in the United States.
   a According to statistics reported by the American Lung Association in their booklet, *Lung Disease Changes Everything*, crippling lung disability is the cause of death for over 40,000 Americans annually, with 250,000 new cases reported each year.
   b Currently, approximately 15,000,000 persons suffer from some form of chronic obstructive pulmonary disease.
   c This booklet points out that "many of these patients do not receive proper medical care because the outpatient treatment is not carried by insurance. Also, the number of professionals to treat these lung patients is inadequate."

2 It has been estimated that almost 26 million work hours are lost as a result of the *disability* of chronic pulmonary disease each year.

3 In addition, over 18,000 individuals are added each year to Social Security disability rolls as a result of chronic pulmonary disease.

4 Of the individuals having chronic disease, some 150,000 to 250,000 are receiving long-term home care. These patients are diagnosed primarily as having pulmonary emphysema, chronic bronchitis, or asthma.

5 It is almost impossible to estimate the hospital costs, Medicare and Medicaid disability payments, and insurance reimbursements that are paid out as a result of the care required to treat pulmonary disease.

1.2 The need for outpatient and home care programs

1 In the hospitals, respiratory patients are seen by a well-trained staff of doctors, respiratory therapists, nurses, physical therapists, laboratory personnel, and dietitians, all of whom combine their skills to ensure the patient of a medically controlled environment.

2 Once released from the hospital, the respiratory patient is frequently sent home to surroundings that are *not* controlled and to people who are *not* informed of the special needs of the patient. This results is a vicious cycle of admission, release, and readmission into the hospital with acute episodes.

3 The recurring cycle of readmission and release from the hospital is expensive and psychologically demoralizing to the patient and his family.

4 Without some form of treatment intervention, this cycle usually continues until the patient dies as a result of an overwhelming infection and/or respiratory failure and cardiac arrest.

5 Where adequate outpatient clinic services and home care programs exist, it is possible with the cooperation of the patient and family to break this cycle and to improve not only the patient's survival rate but sometimes dramatically improve his or her quality of living.

1.3 Economic savings to the patient by well-designed outpatient and home care programs

1 Whether the patient will be able to maintain his or her treatment at home or will need to rely on the hospital outpatient service will depend on the *degree* of disability suffered by the patient.

2 With hospital costs rising annually, it is obvious that individuals with chronic illnesses are going to have to seek out methods of treatment other than hospitalization.

3 Many individuals who are ambulatory and/or not acutely ill would benefit from outpatient and home care programs.

4 It is not necessary to quote hospital room costs and the price of patient care to point out that it is much less expensive being treated at home than at the hospital.

5 In some situations, even the seriously disabled patient may benefit from proper home care in conjunction with periodic visits to the hospitals' outpatient clinic.

6 Under the Prospective Payment System of 1983, hospitals have moved toward shifting as much diagnostics and treatments as possible to outpatient and home care programs.

7 Actually, studies have shown that by supporting outpatient facilities and home care programs patients with chronic pulmonary disease go to the hospital less and that the visits are shorter, thereby saving money and reducing operating costs for the hospital. For example:

a Over 75% of one study group of pulmonary patients spent over 850 days in the hospital before home care. This amounted to about one admission per patient per year, with an average of about 16 days of hospitalization per admission.

b After home care, only about 40% of those patients had hospitalizations, with a total of only about 470 hospital days for that study group. This adds up to an average of approximately 6 admissions per patient per year, with an average of about 13 days per admission.

c By analyzing the costs for the total study population, the study showed an expense outlay of almost $130,000.00 before home care.

d After home care, the total cost of respiratory therapy, nursing, and equipment was approximately $98,000.00, or a savings of $32,000.00.

2.0 PSYCHOLOGIC IMPACT OF CHRONIC PULMONARY DISEASE ON THE PATIENT AND FAMILY

2.1 Psychologic impact

1 We are all subject to the beliefs of the culture in which we live. Our *reactions* to disease are influenced by our *beliefs* concerning sickness; in the United States it is generally believed that illness is to be avoided at all costs. In fact, happiness is sometimes defined as the absence of sickness, (e.g., the phrase, "at least we have our health."

2 Our culture is primarily depicted as:
a Youth-oriented
b Independent
c "On-the-go"
d "Live-for-today"

3 Compare this with a patient who is primarily:
a Old, or at least past middle age
b Dependent and getting more so
c Going nowhere
d Alive today and maybe not tomorrow because of a constantly impending chronic lung disease that can quickly become acute and terminal

4 From the above, it is relatively easy to understand the psychologic stress placed on the chronically ill patient. In an activity-oriented society, acceptance of life-long illness does not come easily, and resignation to the inevitable comes slowly, if at all: "at least he went out fighting," "he never gave up," etc. We as a people do not seem to have the ability to accept the fact that not all of life's problems have a solution via industry, medicine, or science.

2.2 How patients with chronic pulmonary disease may view themselves

1 In Module Five it was learned that in accepting death (or undergoing grief) an individual usually goes through distinct stages of
a Denial
b Anger and shock
c Bargaining

d Depression and grief

e Acceptance

2 When accepting the loss of a loved one, the loss of a limb, or the loss of one's health, it is quite understandable that an individual will move through the same stages.

3 A patient who has been growing slowly aware of his or her symptoms of shortness of breath may put off a visit to the doctor, avoiding the confirmation of illness.

4 However, once the diagnosis of chronic illness is confirmed, the patient must, for his or her own psychologic health, begin the work of acceptance.

5 How far a patient will work toward acceptance depends on:

a Cultural view of illness

b Previous life-style

c Ability to work through problems

d Level of psychologic health

e Availability of family help

f Availability of professional help

6 As discussed in Unit 2.1, the patient who has led an active life may feel "washed out," "over the hill," and/or "better off dead."

7 On the other end of the scale, there is the patient who will strive to "make the best of it" until the very end.

2.3 How the patient's family may be affected and how they may view the patient

1 The reactions of the patient's family are going to depend on many independent variables based on social, cultural, and economic factors.

2 It is possible that the patient's family may view the patient as a pulmonary cripple, pitiful, a burden, a horror, or some other negative image.

3 Help for the family will depend on the emotional and physical capabilities of the family members, their attitudes, their knowing what to do for the patient, and their willingness to deal with the added responsibility.

4 The fact is, for the rest of the patient's life, his or her family will have to make some adjustments in their life-style as a result of the patient's illness.

2.4 Counseling for the patient and the family

1 It is important that patients receive help with handling the stress of their disease. Help in the form of counseling is also of great benefit to the family and may take the form of talking to a therapist, nurse, or physician.

2 Counseling may involve the services of a minister, rehabilitation counselor, or mental health professional and may be done with the patient, the patient's family, the patient and the family, or a group of patients. Counseling help is usually available free of cost or nearly so, from local rehabilitation agencies, outpatient clinics, and various public service organizations.

2.5 Rehabilitation and goals of rehabilitation

1 Patients with chronic pulmonary disease are hospitalized more than is necessary overall. There are many reasons for this, some of which are included below.

a There is overdependence on the physician by the patient and his family.

b The patient and family are not helped to assume their share of responsibility for his or her care.

c Usually, if the patient gets a respiratory infection or is very short of breath, either the patient or the family calls the doctor.

d There are inadequate services and personnel available to care for the patient on an outpatient or at home basis.

e Patients do not have the financial resources to provide appropriate care at home nor are public funds or services available.

2 It is important that the patient be encouraged toward self-help and self-reliance.

a With training and support, patients get to know their disease better and learn ways to deal with it successfully without having to call the doctor as often.

b With increased understanding comes an improved outlook. The patient will do exercises more regularly, take medicine more regularly, be on the watch for a change in symptoms, be better equipped to deal with bouts of shortness of breath, and feel more like the master of the disease, rather than the other way around.

3 Like the patient, many physicians tend to use the hospital for the treatment of patients with chronic pulmonary disease more than is necessary. The hospital is especially overused for *evaluation* of the patient's condition. After initial evaluation in the local hospital (particularly if in a small town), if the patient does not improve significantly, the patient is often referred to a larger (and frequently more expensive) medical center.

4 The reevaluation seldom uncovers anything new, but the patient and famiily usually *feel* like something was done. Since little can be done to cure chronic pulmonary disease, it is important that patients be *taught* to live and function with their disease.

5 The following definition was adopted by the *Committee on Pulmonary Rehabilitation of the American College of Chest Physicians* in 1974: "Pulmonary rehabilitation may be defined as an art of medical practice wherein an individually-tailored multi-disciplinary program is formulated that, through accurate diagnosis, therapy, emotional support, and education, stabilizes or reverses both the physio- and psychopathology of pulmonary diseases and attempts to return the patient to the highest possible functional capacity allowed by his pulmonary handicap and overall life situation." Please note that the word *cure* is not mentioned in this definition.

6 Rehabilitation should work toward the following goals.

a Helping the patient to be independent

b Facilitating the patient's acceptance by others

c Improving the patient's ability to cope with disease and its limitations

d Attaining the *patient's* goals toward living

7 The patient must be taught to use "graded" goal attainment and to keep goals realistic with respect to the degree of the disability.

a Small goals are easier to achieve, and each successful attainment builds self-confidence.

b Chaining several small steps together or "grading" the task to be achieved helps accomplish larger goals that would otherwise be unattainable, and therefore, frustrating for the patient (Fig. 25-1).

c Goals must reflect what the *patient* feels is important. Respiratory care practitioners must overcome the temptation to give advice based on their own value system and needs.

d The length of time for completion, (i.e., 1 week, 1 month, etc.) should come from the patient.

e The parts (steps) of each goal should come from the patient, so that the steps can be set that are to be achieved by the end of 1 day, 1 week, 1 month, etc.

f The patient should have a copy of the Goal Attainment Chart, which may have as many goals as are realistic and in whatever time frame is considered realistic.

g As each step is checked off, it provides a visual record with which the patient can see progress, thus providing encouragement and positive feedback.

h It is almost impossible to fail to get positive attainment with this system because the schedule and time periods may be adjusted at any time once a realistic goal is chosen.

3.0 PATHOPHYSIOLOGY ASSOCIATED WITH PULMONARY DISEASES

3.1 Pathophysiology

1 *Respiratory failure* is a pathophysiologic condition in which the lungs are unable to meet the *metabolic* demands of the body.

a *Ventilatory failure* is a condition in which the lungs are unable to meet the metabolic demands of the body as far as carbon dioxide homeostasis is concerned.

• The characteristics of ventilatory failure are inadequate alveolar ventilation and a $Paco_2$ above 50 mm Hg; it may be acute or chronic.

• The causes of ventilatory failure are cardiopulmonary disease, central nervous system (CNS) depression, neurologic disease, musculoskeletal disease, hepatorenal disease, or fatigue.

b *Ventilatory insufficiency* is the presence of alveolar hyperventilation.

• The characteristic of ventilatory insufficiency is a $Paco_2$ of greater than 30-50 mm Hg; it may be acute or chronic.

• The causes of ventilatory insufficiency are hypoxemia, a response to metabolic acidosis, or a CNS response.

2 The following is a comparison of ventilatory failure, ventilatory insufficiency, and normal findings.

a Ventilatory failure is defined as a $Paco_2$ greater than 50 mm Hg.

b Normal $Paco_2$ is 30 to 50 mm Hg.

c Ventilatory insufficiency is a $Paco_2$ greater than 30-50 mm Hg.

3 Obstructive pulmonary disease

a An obstructive pulmonary disease is one in which there is a disproportionate reduction in expiratory flow, reflected in a low forced expiratory volume (1 second)/vital capacity (FEV_1/FC) ratio (less than 70%).

b The characteristics of obstructive disorders are upper airway obstruction, lower airway obstruction, lower or diffuse airway obstruction, reversible or irreversible airway obstruction, and increased airway resistance.

c Most common causes of obstructive disorders are bronchospasm, mucous plugging, tumor stenosis, or a lack of airway patency as a result of bronchospasm.

4 Restrictive pulmonary disorders

a A restrictive disorder is one that demonstrates reduced VC, but usually a normal FEV_1/VC ratio (greater than 70%).

b The characteristics of a restrictive disorder relate to extrapulmonary disorders, lung or pleural disorders, interstitial disorders, and decreased distensibility (compliance) of the thoracic cage.

c Causes of restrictive disorders are neuromuscular

Goals to be attained	First week	Second week	Third week	Fourth week
Walk to back yard without assistance	Walk to bedroom door and back ✔ Done	Walk to end of hallway and back ✔ Done	Walk to back door and back ___ Done	Walk to back yard and back ___ Done
Dress self without assistance	Put on shorts and undershirt ✔ Done	Put on shirts and trousers ___ Done	Put on socks and shoes ___ Done	Put on sweater or coat ___ Done

FIGURE 25-1 Goal attainment chart.

diseases, chest wall abnormalities, pleural diseases, or parenchymal lung diseases.

5 The following is a comparison of the obstructive and the restrictive disorders and normal findings:

   a *Normal.* VC is normal; FEV_1 is normal; $FEV_1/VC \times 100$ = greater than 70%.

   b *Restrictive.* VC is reduced; FEV_1 is normal or slightly reduced; $FEV_1/VC \times 100$ = greater than 70%.

   c *Obstructive.* VC is normal or slightly reduced; FEV_1 is reduced; $FEV_1/VC \times 100$ = less than 70%.

6 Functional abnormalities associated with normal spirometry

   a Functional abnormalities are those physiologic alterations that occur without dysfunction being indicated in spirometric studies.

   b This means that there is a diffusing capacity abnormality caused by either an alveolar-capillary block or anemia.

   c It could also mean that there is a blood gas disturbance caused by anatomic vascular abnormalities, small localized pulmonary abnormalities, a dysfunction of ventilatory drive, a maldistribution of inspired gas as a result of the presence of bullae or small airway dysfunction.

4.0 THE PULMONARY REHABILITATION PROGRAM
4.1 Disorders that may warrant pulmonary rehabilitation

1 *Neuromuscular diseases* are those that result in the impairment of consciousness and/or involuntary alteration of muscular movements. The characteristics of a neuromuscular disease are changed or reduced level of consciousness, increased weakness of muscles, changed or increased secretions, and changed or reduced lung function measurements.

   a *Myasthenia gravis.* A sporadic disease characterized by fluctuating muscular weakness, with a predilection for cranial muscles; characteristically improved by administration of cholinergic drugs.

   b *Guillain-Barré syndrome.* A polyradiculoneuritis with symmetric, ascending motor weakness and distal sensory impairment.

   c *Muscular dystrophy.* A disorder that affects motor neurons and peripheral nerves; primarily hereditary myopathies characterized by progressive weakness.

   d *Poliomyelitis.* An acute viral infection in which only a small percentage of those infected develop clinical signs—fever, headache, stiff neck and back, and sometimes flaccid paralysis of various muscle groups.

   e *Botulism.* An acute intoxication manifested by neuromuscular disturbances after ingesting food containing a toxin excreted by *Clostridium botulinum.*

   f *Tetanus.* An acute infectious disease characterized by intermittent tonic spasms of voluntary muscles and convulsions.

   g *Drug induced.* Following ingestion of toxic substances or overdose of other substances.

   h *Amyotrophic lateral sclerosis.* A disease of unknown etiology, characterized by motor neuron degeneration in the spinal cord, medulla, and motor cortex.

2 Chest wall abnormalities are those caused by alterations in the shape and/or stability of the chest wall.

   a Causes of chest wall instability are simple rib fractures, flail chest, and post-thoracotomy conditions of the chest.

   b Examples of chest wall deformities are:
   • *Kyphoscoliosis.* An angulation of the thoracic spine, both laterally and postero-anteriorly.
   • *Ankylosing spondylitis.* A vertebral joint immobilization and ossification of paravertebral ligaments.
   • *Pectus excavatum.* A congenital malformation of the chest wall characterized by a pronounced funnel-shaped depression, with its apex over the lower end of the sternum.

3 Disorders of the ventilatory drive function result from a variety of stimuli that may stimulate or depress the drive.

   a *Stimulation symptoms* are as follows.
   • CNS symptoms (dizziness, loss of consciousness)
   • Peripheral symptoms (numbness, coldness, etc.)
   • Muscular symptoms (spasms, tremors, etc.)
   • Respiratory symptoms (shortness of breath, excessive yawning, etc.)
   • Cardiac symptoms (palpitations, tachycardia, etc.)
   • Gastrointestinal symptoms (dryness of mouth, bloating, dysphagia, etc.)
   • Psychologic (anxiety, insomnia, etc.)
   • Fatigue
   • Hypocapnia

   b *Depression symptoms* are as follows.
   • Hypercapnia (hypoventilation)
   • Hypoxemia (decreased Pao_2, tachycardia, etc.)
   • Vital capacity less than 1 L
   • Acidosis
   • Abnormal CO_2 response curve

   c Disorders of the ventilatory drive function may be caused by the following.
   • *Drug intoxication* caused by interactions of different drugs, anaphylactic reaction of patient to drugs, and interaction of drugs and pre-existing respiratory insufficiency
   • *CNS effects* brought on by infections, tumors, vascular diseases, and trauma

   d Primary alveolar hypoventilation is a ventilatory drive disorder when ventilatory function and gas diffusion tests are normal, but the level of resting ventilation is decreased, resulting in hypoxemia and hypercapnia. Examples are:
   • *Pickwickian syndrome.* Gross obesity and chronic hypoventilation associated with somnolence, erythrocytosis, and hypoxemia.
   • *Non-obese hypoventilation syndrome.* Hypoventilation resulting in hypoxemia and hypercapnia, in the absence of obesity.
   • *Intermittent upper airway obstruction.* Occurs dur-

ing sleep and is sometimes misdiagnosed as pick-wickian syndrome.

   e Oxygen-induced hypoventilation. In severely hypoxic patients, in whom hypoxia is the respiratory stimulus, oxygen decreases respiration and thereby increases carbon dioxide retention, with resultant respiratory acidosis, coma, or death.

4 Pneumoconioses are diseases that cause changes in the lung as a result of the inhalation of dusts. (See also Module Eight.)

   a *Silicosis.* Caused by the inhalation of free crystalline silica or silicon dioxide as from underground mining, foundry work, pottery manufacture, and sand blasting. Pulmonary complications include a slowing of phagocytosis and clogging of the lymphatic system, which causes connective tissue damage and resultant fibrosis formation. Cavitation of lung tissue may occur as well as lung restriction and/or lung obstruction, hypoxemia, and early heart trouble.

   b *Asbestosis.* Physical and chemical irritation, as from making clutch facings, brake linings, roofing, insulation, etc. Pulmonary complications include a nonnodular type of fibrosis with shortness of breath, lung restriction, and early heart trouble. Bronchial carcinoma has been shown to result from asbestos as well as another rare form of cancer called mesothelioma.

   c *Coal worker's disease* ("black lung"). Similar to silicosis, but different as a result of pigmentation of the lung tissue.

   d Other pneumoconioses are byssinosis (cotton worker's lung or "brown lung"), farmer's lung, mushroom picker's lung, bagassosis, berylliosis, maple bark disease, and bird fancier's lung.

5 Effects of air pollution

   a Air pollution is a national problem resulting from industrial, automobile, and tobacco emissions (which form carbon monoxide, hydrocarbons, heavy metals, various toxins), the products of reaction (ozone, various chemical irritants), and materials of natural origin (allergens, dusts, etc.).

   b Complications from air pollution include general irritation and temporarily paralyzed cilia, a decreased resistance to disease and antigen formation, increased resistance to air flow, increased obstruction to air flow, and increased carcinogenesis.

6 Chronic obstructive pulmonary disease is a disease state with the following definitions (see Module Eight).

   a Loss of alveolar walls, mucous gland hyperplasia, mucosal inflammation with abnormal amounts of mucus

   b Persistent airway obstruction of uncertain etiology

   c Clinical state of dyspnea on exertion with objective evidence of reduced air flow, not explained by specific or infiltrative lung or heart disease

7 Types of chronic obstructive pulmonary diseases are listed here.

   a *Emphysema.* A state of the lungs in which the air spaces distal to the terminal bronchioles are abnormally increased in size, including destruction of the alveolar walls and recession of adjacent capillaries.

   b *Chronic bronchitis.* Chronic cough with excessive production of sputum, which is not due to known specific causes and which persists for more than 3 months of the year for 2 or more years.

   c *Bronchiectasis.* A permanent abnormal dilation and distortion of the bronchi, bronchioles, or both; usually accompanied by thick, purulent sputum production.

   d *Asthma.* Recurrent generalized airway obstruction which, in the early stages, is paroxysmal and reversible by medication and is accompanied by eosinophilia of the blood and sputum.

   e *Cystic fibrosis.* An inherited disease resulting from an autosomal recessive disorder involving the exocrine glands of the body, complicated by bronchiectasis, hemoptysis, pneumothorax, and atelectasis.

8 Another condition that may require rehabilitation is the *adult respiratory distress syndrome.* This is an acute lung injury resulting from several diverse insults, all of which produce a similar pathophysiology and clinical picture.

5.0 PULMONARY DETERIORATION
5.1 Signs of pulmonary deterioration

1 The greatest single problem encountered in the treatment of the pulmonary patient at home is a lack of awareness or denial that anything is wrong. This is an unfortunate situation and may be avoided through patient and family education. Cardinal signs of pulmonary deterioration are outlined in the boxed material that follows.

2 The signs of pulmonary deterioration listed in the boxed material may be subtle or obvious. They may occur singly or together. The patient and the practitioner must be aware of what conditions are normal for this patient. For example, a cough is *not* normal, and implies irritation of the tracheobronchial tree. Changes in the patient's coughing pattern or severity may indicate a change in the patient's condition.

3 The presence or absence of sputum is another indicator. Like the cough, it is not normal for a patient to expectorate sputum in any significant amount or to suddenly stop raising secretions.

   a It is normal for any person to unconsciously swallow mucus that moves to the pharynx from the bronchioles and nasal areas.

   b Changes in the volume of sputum raised over a 24-hour period and/or changes in the consistency, color, or odor can be significant, especially as related to the control of infection and maintenance of tracheobronchial hygiene.

4 The quantity of sputum produced varies greatly and depends on factors such as body hydration and the ratio between expectorated and swallowed mucus.

5 Sputum collection and analysis is an important component of any pulmonary assessment protocol. To be meaningful, the following steps should be observed in the collection and evaluation of sputum.

  a The patient should be educated as to the need for sputum collection and the importance of following proper collection procedures.

  b Good oral hygiene should be maintained to prevent contamination of the collection by microbes in the mouth.

  c The patient should only collect sputum samples that have been produced by a deep cough.

6 Visually, a sputum sample can be identified as mucoid, purulent, or mucopurulent.

  a Mucoid refers to sputum that is clean, transparent-to-light, and has air bubbles.

  b Purulent sputum is yellow or green with solids and is opaque to light.

  c Sputum that is both mucoid and purulent is identified as mucopurulent.

7 Episodic or constant chest pain can be pleuritic or anginal in origin.

  a Pleuritic pain is usually acute in onset and directly associated with a patient's breathing and coughing maneuvers. It is usually worsened during inspiration over specific areas of the lung, and may follow an infection, fever, or common cold.

  b Anginal pain differs in that it is normally induced by exertion and relieved by rest and/or nitroglycerin. An electrocardiogram (ECG) may or may not show changes during these isolated instances. Any cardiac pain should be handled as an emergency unless the condition is controlled by the physician.

8 Other clinical signs frequently encountered in the chronic pulmonary patient are extreme fatigue, unusual drowsiness (with or without headache), dizzy spells, and insomnia. These symptoms most frequently reflect hypercapnia and hypoxemia when associated with the patient's hallucinations of circling objects and bright multicolored lights.

Signs of pulmonary deterioration

  1 Cough
  2 Increase or decrease in volume of sputum
  3 Increase in consistency of sputum
  4 Change in color of sputum
  5 Increased levels and frequency of dyspnea or shortness of breath
  6 Episodic or constant chest pain
  7 Intermittent fever
  8 Ankle edema
  9 Extreme fatigue or unusual drowsiness
  10 Morning headaches, dizzy spells, loss of libido
  11 Orthopnea necessitating elevation of head
  12 Decreased levels of mental awareness and/or elevated combativeness
  13 Slurring of speech, somnolence, or insomnia

6.0 CARE OF PEDIATRIC AND ELDERLY PATIENTS
6.1 Special problems associated with the pediatric patient

1 The most obvious difference in working with the pediatric patient is size. However, it is crucial that one recognizes that *children cannot be treated as small adults*.

2 General anatomic differences between children and adults are that children have:

  a A smaller rib cage
  b More horizontal positioning of the ribs
  c Smaller airways
  d Smaller nasal passages
  e A higher diaphragm
  f Greater airway instability
  g A proportionately larger tongue
  h More anterior vocal cords
  i Smaller larynx and cricoid ring

3 Diseases of the pediatric patient differ somewhat from the adult. Typical childhood pulmonary diseases are respiratory distress syndrome, croup, asthma, bronchiolitis, bronchitis, and cystic fibrosis.

4 Another difference between adult and pediatric patients is in the type of equipment used. This equipment will need to be modified to accommodate the pediatric patient's ability and inclination to cooperate.

  a Tents are used to administer oxygen and mist. Cannulas, catheters, and masks are not tolerated well by children.

  b Aerosol therapy is the primary means of delivering medication; children do not normally tolerate and/or are unable to coordinate intermittent positive pressure breathing.

  c Mists or fogs are very popular in pediatric therapy and are delivered by vaporizers, compressor-powered nebulizers, or heated nebulizers.

  NOTE: High mist therapies must be used with caution, as premature infants may be seriously overloaded with fluid as a result of water added to their systems by nebulizers. Weighing the infant daily helps keep a record of its fluid intake.

5 Therapy undertaken with infants and children will differ from that with adults. For example, medication dosages are usually much smaller and are given for shorter periods of time for children. In order to gain a child's cooperation, most therapy initially is disguised as a game or something fun and interesting, and generally requires carefully controlled patience. It is necessary when working with infants and children to be acutely aware of the attitudes, feelings, and needs of the patient's parents as well as those of the child.

6 Pulmonary function testing of children is especially different from adults because of:

  a Different volumes and capacities
  b Flow rates
  c Different normals
  d Games and exercises necessary to encourage cooperation

6.2 Special problems associated with the elderly patient

For a more complete presentation of the elderly see Modules 24 and 29.

1 Problems associated with the elderly, or *geriatric*, patient are usually much different than those associated with the younger patient. These problems result from the normal changes of aging, in addition to the problems and disability brought on by chronic disease.

2 *Normal* changes of aging include:
  a Changes in skin structure and elasticity
  b Loss of high-frequency hearing ranges
  c Reduced smell and taste
  d Structural changes in bone, reduction in calcium, increasing brittleness
  e Hardening of ligaments that reduces range of motion
  f Thickening and/or hardening of arteries and vessels
  g Loss of muscle tone
  h Slowed reaction time
  i Reduced glandular secretions
  j Reduced digestion and appetite
  k Loss of some heart efficiency
  l Loss of some lung efficiency
  m Diminished ability and/or desire to follow directions

3 Normal changes in the aging lung include increased emphysema due to structural deterioration, reduced arterial oxygen tension, less efficient vascular networks, and less efficient protective functions.
  NOTE: *Senile emphysema* may be almost symptom-free compared with the COPD form of emphysema.

4 As a result of factors such as emotional, financial, or family problems and cognitive and affective changes brought on by stroke, cerebral ischemia, and personality changes, the following may affect the patient's ability to participate in home care.
  a Attitude
  b Willingness to work
  c Mental status, involving
    • Capability
    • Memory
    • Understanding
    • Personal responsibility
    • Depression
  d Physical ability to match the patient's mental willingness

5 In the event of difficulty resulting from any of the above, it may be necessary to make use of patient or family counseling, family training in care of the patient, and follow-up programs to encourage and assist the family.

7.0 COMPONENTS THAT MAKE HOME CARE AND REHABILITATION A SPECIALTY

7.1 Home care and rehabilitation as a specialty

1 Providing care to the outpatient and to the home care patient is a unique problem that should be handled as a specialty.

2 It requires a team of health care professionals that are specially educated and trained as to the needs of the chronic pulmonary disease patient. (See also Unit 9.1 in this module.)

3 Philosophically, a home care or outpatient program must consider the following assumptions.
  a The home care or outpatient has different needs and concerns from the hospitalized patient.
  b The home care or outpatient does not receive the expert attention of the hospitalized patient.
  c The home care or outpatient may have a precipitating disease that goes unnoticed until an emergency arises.

8.0 HOW TO PLAN CARE FOR THE PULMONARY DISEASE PATIENT IN THE HOSPITAL, OUTPATIENT, AND HOME SETTING

8.1 Caring for the chronic pulmonary disease patient in the hospital setting

1 The objectives of respiratory therapy in the treatment of chronic obstructive pulmonary disease (COPD) and other chronic pulmonary diseases are to control and alleviate, as much as possible, the symptoms of respiratory impairment and disability and to teach the patient how to achieve optimum ability to carry out daily activities of living.

2 Care in the hospital consists of two phases—the *acute phase* and the *stable phase*.

3 In the first phase, acute care in the hospital begins with an evaluation to determine the patient's current condition, current treatment, and causitive factors that might have contributed to his respiratory disease and admission complaint.

4 The initial in-hospital evaluation will help the respiratory practitioner make appropriate recommendations to the patient's physician and to the respiratory care health team. It will also provide information that will be of use in making out the home care or outpatient care plan (Fig. 25-2).
  NOTE: This evaluation form is meant to serve as an example only. In practice each hospital usually provides its own forms. The use of this form is to serve as an adjunct to the physician and *in no way* should be used in lieu of the physician's history and physical or to prescribe therapy without a physician's order.

5 The respiratory practitioner should also ascertain the patient's present physical and psychologic condition by interview, so as to make appropriate recommendations to the patient's physician and to the respiratory care health team. Factors to be considered are the patient's smoking habits, weight, diet, and physical activity (Fig. 25-3).
  NOTE: This information form is meant to serve as an example only. The use of this form is to serve as an adjunct to the physician and *in no way* should be used in lieu of the physician's notes or to prescribe therapy without a physician's order.

6 The respiratory care practitioner should also identify specific problems the patient has that may require treat-

Name _____ Patient no. _____

Room no. _____ Attending physician _____

Patient's age_____ Sex _____ Previous admission: Yes   No

Date of evaluation _____ 19_____ Diagnosis _____

_____

HISTORY (Include medical, emotional, occupational factors, smoking)

_____

_____

_____

_____

_____

_____

_____

_____

_____

_____

Current symptoms: Sputum amount_____ Color_____ Frequency _____

Cough: _____ When _____ Pain during cough: Yes_____ No

Chest pain: Yes_____ No _____ Nitroglycerin: Yes _____ No _____

If yes to nitroglycerin, how often _____

Elimination:_____

Special limitations_____

_____

Other factors:_____

_____

_____

_____

Continued.

FIGURE 25-2 Respiratory patient evaluation form.

GENERAL ADMISSION INFORMATION   FOR DISCHARGE PROGRAM

Smoking:_____   _____

Environment:_____   _____

Antibiotics:_____   _____

Fluid intake:_____   _____

MEDICATIONS:_____   _____

Bronchodilators_____   _____

_____   _____

Expectorants_____   _____

Steroids_____   _____

Digitalis_____   _____

Diuretics_____   _____

Other_____   _____

RESPIRATORY THERAPY:

Nebulizer_____   _____

Oxygen_____   _____

Humidity_____   _____

IPPB_____   _____

PHYSICAL THERAPY:

Breathing training_____   _____

Exercise training_____   _____

Respiratory hygiene_____   _____

OCCUPATIONAL THERAPY:

_____   _____

_____   _____

_____   _____

FIGURE 25-2, cont'd Respiratory patient evaluation form.

NUTRITION: _____

_____

_____

SOCIAL SERVICE:

Financial _____   _____

Personal needs_____   _____

Family needs _____   _____

PATIENT/FAMILY EDUCATION:

_____   _____

_____   _____

_____   _____

_____   _____

COMMENTS:

_____   _____

_____   _____

_____   _____

_____   _____

_____   _____

FIGURE 25-2, cont'd Respiratory patient evaluation form.

Name _____ Patient no. _____

Room no. _____ Sex _____   Previous admission: Yes   No

Date of this admission _____ , 19 Diagnosis _____

Interviewed by _____ Date of interview _____ , 19

GENERAL INFORMATION:

1. What name do you prefer to be called?

2. Does anyone else in your family have health problems?

3. How much do you smoke per day?   Pipe?   Cigar, etc.?

4. How many years have you smoked?   Pack/years:

5. If stopped, how long?

6. Does anyone else in your family smoke?

7. How many chest colds do you have per year?

8. How long do they last?

9. What do you do about them?

ENVIRONMENT:

1. Where do you live?   house?   apartment?

2. With whom do you live?

3. Will someone be able to care for you at home?

4. Do you live near a factory?   freeway?   open field?

5. Does your home get very dusty?

6. Do you have carpets?

7. Do you have air conditioning?   attic fan?   window fan?

8. Do you have pets?

9. Do you use a tub or shower?

10. Does steam from the shower bother you?

FIGURE 25-3 Respiratory patient interview form.

OCCUPATION/ACTIVITY:

1. What is your occupation?

2. Describe your work conditions.

3. What are your hobbies?   woodworking, gardening, mechanics, etc.

4. Who does your housework?

5. Do you use a vacuum or broom?

6. What tasks are you not able to do?

HABITS:

1. What are your usual meal times?

2. Do you eat snacks?   When?

3. What is your heaviest meal?

4. Describe a typical heavy meal.

5. How much fluid do you drink per day?   What kind?

6. Do you use alcohol?   How much?

ELIMINATION:

1. Do you have problems with constipation/diarrhea?

2. What do you use to treat elimination problems?

3. Any trouble while in hospital?

4. Are bowel movements daily or other?

5. Any difficulty voiding?   Frequency?

SLEEP/REST:

1. Are you usually well rested?

2. Do you sleep throughout the night?

3. If you awaken, why?

4. What helps you get back to sleep?

Continued.

FIGURE 25-3, cont'd Respiratory patient interview form.

5. Do you use sleeping medications?

6. Do you use wool blankets?

7. Do you use feather pillows?   How many?

8. Do you ever have to sit up to sleep?

EMOTIONAL/SPIRITUAL:

1. Do you have a religious preference?

2. Do you attend services regularly?

3. Have you had any recent emotional upsets? (Information may have to come from family)

4. What were they? (deaths, loss, family troubles)

5. What do you do when you get very upset?

PERCEPTION/KNOWLEDGE OF ILLNESS:

1. Could you tell me what you know about your illness?

   (Interviewer check)

   Very informed_____ Moderately informed_____ Barely informed_____

   No knowledge whatsoever_____

2. Who told you about your illness?

3. What things do you do that help with your breathing?

4. When do you see your doctor?

5. Do you have pain at home?

6. What relieves it?

7. Does your family understand your illness?

8. What have you told them about it?

FIGURE 25-3, cont'd Respiratory patient interview form.

INTERVIEWER OBSERVATIONS   (Check all that apply):

1. Did patient seem   _____

    Relaxed   _____

    Nervous   _____

    Frightened   _____

    Angry   _____

    Hostile   _____

2. Did the patient's nonverbal cues agree with his/her voice and behaviors?

3. Did patient appear

    Depressed   _____

    Incoherent   _____

    Irrational   _____

    Inconsistent   _____

INTERVIEWER COMMENTS:

_____

_____

_____

_____

_____

_____

_____

_____

_____

_____

_____

_____

FIGURE 25-3, cont'd Respiratory patient interview form.

ment. This is accomplished through a *problem list*.

7 The problem list should include, but not be limited to, the following.

   a Frequency of re-infections

   b Retained secretions

   c Bronchospasm

   d Hypoxemia

   e Hypercapnea

   f Respiratory center depression

   g Physical impairments affecting depression

8 The patient's *care plan* will be developed for the most part from the problem list. Proper management of the patient's airway and treatment of hypoxia and carbon dioxide retention are of primary importance to the respiratory care practitioner. Other respiratory therapy procedures that may be included are:

   a Inhalation of an appropriate bronchodilator via intermittent positive pressure breathing (IPPB) or air compressor

   b Chest auscultation, to include the type of sound heard, the pitch of sounds, and the breathing phase in which sounds are heard

   c Arterial blood sampling and analysis

   d Oropharyngeal and tracheal suctioning

   e Humidification therapy

   f Oxygen therapy

   g Sputum induction

   h Pulmonary drainage

   i Breathing exercises

9 *Ongoing evaluation* to determine effectiveness of care will include arterial blood gas analysis, pulmonary function testing and/or exercise tolerance testing, chest radiography, and sputum collection and analysis.

10 After reaching a *stable phase* in their illness, the patient is ready for the education component of his or her respiratory program. The *chief objective* of this program is to transfer responsibility from the respiratory health care team to the patient. To accomplish this objective, the respiratory care practitioner should:

   a Obtain an outpatient-home care history to ascertain and evaluate past home programs, if any (Fig. 25-4).

   b Instruct the patient in the use, maintenance, and cleaning procedures for home respiratory equipment.

   c Instruct and evaluate understanding and competence in the use of respiratory drugs.

   d Aid in teaching group classes for patients and their families in the aspects of COPD and in home care.

11 *Exercises* are considered necessary in teaching patients to deal effectively with their illness. A recommended grading of the exercises follows.

   a First week: 30 minutes a day exercise, scattered throughout the day in 5-minute sessions, not to exceed 5 minutes in any 1 hour.

   b Next 4 weeks: 45 minutes a day exercise, in sessions of 10 minutes, not to exceed more than 10 minutes in any 1 hour. Part of this time should be spent in postural drainage and in walking, if walking can be done without shortness of breath by this time.

   c After 4 weeks: 45 to 60 minutes daily, mainly in walking and in postural drainage.

These times are recommended only when the patient's health and physician permit their implementation.

12 *Exercise 1*. Efficient breathing, while sitting forward (Fig. 25-5). The following can be used as a sample patient teaching guide.

   a Sit on an armless chair with both feet flat on the floor, or if your legs are not quite long enough, put a stack of magazines under your feet.

   b Lean forward. Place your left elbow on your left thigh near the knee, and your right elbow on your right thigh near the knee. Try to keep your knees fairly close together, but if you are overweight, just keep the legs comfortably separated.

   c Rest your chin gently on your hands.

   d Now pucker your lips and slowly blow out the "stale air" steadily as you count silently: "1-2-3-4." Now, breathe in fresh air steadily *through your nose* while you silently count: "1-2."

   e Blowing out time should equal 4 counts or 4 seconds. Breathing in time should equal 2 counts or 2 seconds.

   f It is important that you master this exercise because it is very helpful in the following ways.

   • It helps get over attacks of breathlessness.

   • It can help prevent attacks of breathlessness.

   • It helps clear phlegm out of the throat when first getting out of bed or at any other time.

   • It can usually prevent an unwanted coughing spell or stop a coughing spell that seems out of control.

   • It can usually help overcome wheezing spells.

   g Follow one breath with another. If you take 10 complete breaths, you will have practiced for 1 minute. Practice for 1 minute every hour for the first 2 weeks, then do it every morning and night, and whenever you need help with breathlessness or coughing.

13 *Exercise 2*. Efficient breathing while sitting forward.

   a This exercise will help you "see" your breathing. Cut a 4 inch square from the newspaper and draw a bull's eye in the center.

   b Sit on an armless chair with both feet flat on the floor, or if your legs are not quite long enough, put a stack of magazines under your feet.

   c Lean forward with your elbows in the basic position (Exercise 1). Rest your chin in your left hand.

   d Grasp the paper square between your right thumb and index finger at the corner of the square (Fig. 25-6, *A* and *B*).

   e Hold the paper so that the bull's eye is not less than 1 inch from your lips and not more than 2 inches away from your lips.

   f Pucker your lips and blow out the "stale" air steadily toward the bull's eye as you count silently: "1-2-3-4," (Fig. 25-6, *A).*

   g Check to *see* that you are breathing properly by watching the paper being blown away from your lips

EQUIPMENT:

1. Does patient have respiratory equipment at home?

2. What type of equipment?

3. What medication is patient using?

    How often?

4. What frequency did physician prescribe?

5. How long has patient had equipment?

6. Where was it purchased?

7. Did patient receive training?

8. What therapy is patient receiving in hospital?

9. Will patient need equipment for discharge?

    What type?

    Vendor?

HUMIDITY:

1. Is patient getting any form of humidity at home?

    How?

    How often?

2. Does the patient have a preference for cool or warm mist?

3. What type of humidity is the patient getting in the hospital?

4. Does patient need training in this area?

5. Will patient need humidity equipment for discharge?

    What type?

    Vendor?

Continued.

FIGURE 25-4 Outpatient home care evaluation form.

OXYGEN:

1. Does patient have oxygen at home?

   What type of set-up?

   How often?

   Liter flow?

2. Is patient receiving oxygen in the hospital?

   How often?

   Liter flow?

3. Does patient need training in this area?

4. What are most recent arterial blood gases?

5. Do ABG results meet criteria for supplemental oxygen at home?

   How often?

   Liter flow?

6. What type set-up to be used at home?

   Vendor?

CLEANING:

1. Has patient been instructed to clean equipment at home?

   Method?

   How often?

2. Does patient need training in this area?

3. Will equipment be brought in for cleaning, sterilization, and repair during this admission?

FAMILY SUPPORT:

1. Does patient live with family or alone?

2. Is there someone trained to assist patient?

3. Is there anybody willing to learn?

FIGURE 25-4, cont'd Outpatient home care evaluation form.

INSURANCE:

1. What type of coverage is available to patient?

2. Will coverage assist in rental or purchase of equipment?

3. Does patient need the services of financial aid department or social services in this area?

SPIROMETRY:

1. Will patient have pulmonary testing?

2. Results:

COMMENTS:

_____

_____

_____

_____

_____

_____

_____

DISCHARGE CHECK LIST:

——   Evaluation completed

——   Patient has received physician's prescription

——   Patient has received training for home program

——   Patient has written instructions

——   Vendor has been supplied with necessary prescriptions

——   Blood gas/spirometry results copy for vendor (if insurance requires)

——   Patient knows how to contact respiratory rehabilitation person

——   Patient knows how to contact vendor

——   Discharge summary completed

F I G U R E   2 5 - 4 ,   c o n t'd Outpatient home care evaluation form.

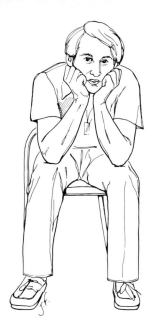

FIGURE 25-5 Efficient breathing while sitting forward—exercise 1.

and *held* there while you count for 4 seconds. As you breathe in, the paper should return toward your lips.

   h Practice with the paper square for ten breaths or one minute several times a day until proper breathing becomes natural.

14 *Exercise 3.* Efficient breathing while sitting forward.

   a This exercise will help you "feel" your breathing.

   b Sit on an armless chair, as in Exercises 1 and 2. Lean forward. Place your right elbow on your right thigh, near the knee. Rest your chin on your right hand.

   c *Firmly* place your left palm between your breastbone and your navel so that as you breathe you can feel the movement of that area (Fig. 25-7).

   d Pucker your lips and blow "stale" air out steadily while you count silently: "1-2-3-4." Now breathe in steadily *through your nose* while you count silently: "1-2."

   e Each time you blow air out, you should be able to *feel* your stomach being pulled back toward your backbone all the time that you are forcing the air out of your lungs.

   f Each time you breathe in, you should be able to feel you stomach being *pushed* out against your palm

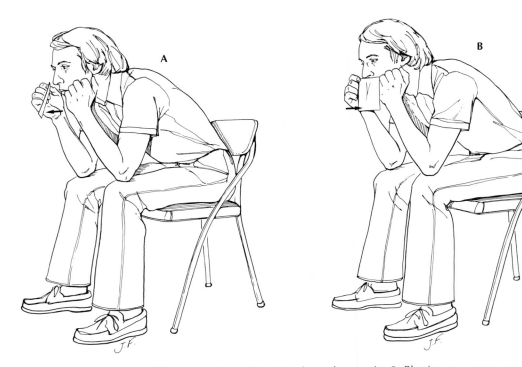

FIGURE 25-6 Efficient breathing while sitting forward—exercise 2. Blowing on a paper square, **A,** Exhalation and **B,** inhalation.

constantly as you are breathing in the fresh air.

g Practice breathing by feeling your stomach for ten breaths, or 1 minute, several times a day until you can train your brain and the muscles of your chest and stomach to stop breathing inefficiently and start breathing as you should.

15 As you build your strength and endurance after leaving the hospital, the exercises may be altered to fit your new skills and stronger breathing.

a Move from the leaning position to a straight sitting position (Fig. 25-8, *A* and *B*).

b Or, you may place both hands on your stomach (Fig. 25-9).

c Move to the standing position (Fig. 25-10, *A* and *B*).

16 *Exercise 4.* Walking with your breathing (not shown).

a As you have learned to breathe properly, you must now learn to coordinate your breathing with activity.

b Before starting to practice walking, stand with your hands just above your hips so that you can feel your stomach move in and out as your breathe. Counting silently: "1-2-3-4," blow out the "stale" air through pursed lips and feel your stomach contract. Now breathe in, counting silently: "1-2," while your stomach expands, pulling in fresh air.

c Once you have mastered breathing in rhythm, you

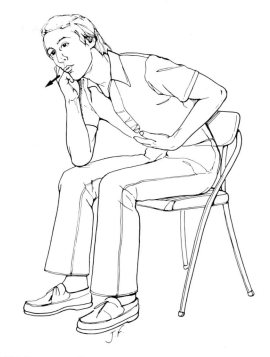

F I G U R E 2 5 - 7 Efficient breathing while sitting forward—exercise 3.

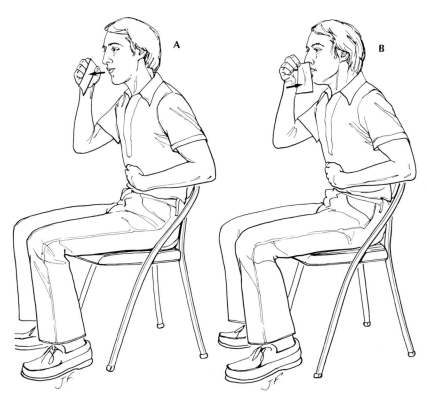

F I G U R E 2 5 - 8 Efficient breathing while sitting straight—position 1. **A,** Exhalation and **B,** inhalation.

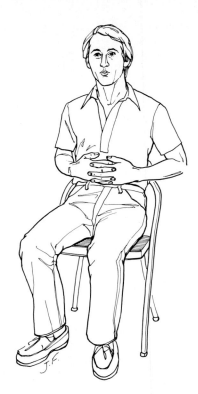

FIGURE 25-9 Efficient breathing while sitting straight—position 2.

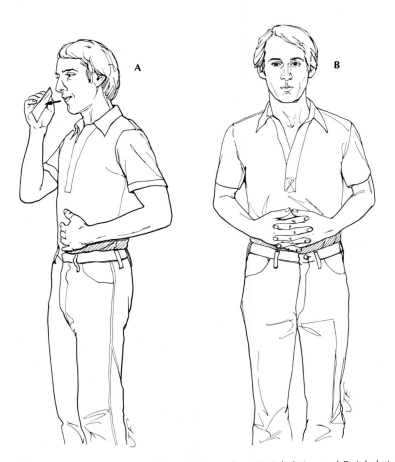

FIGURE 25-10 Efficient breathing while standing. **A,** Exhalation and **B,** inhalation.

are ready to step forward on the very first count when you breathe out.

d While you breathe *out:*
- Count "a" silently as you step forward with your *left* foot.
- Count "2" silently as you step forward with your *right* foot.
- Count "3" silently as you step forward with your *left* foot.
- Count "4" silently as you step forward with your *right* foot.

e While you breathe in:
- Count "1" silently as you step forward with your *left* foot.
- Count "2" silently as you step forward with your *right* foot.

f You have now taken 6 forward steps in one complete breath. Now stop walking. Check your breathing. By contracting your stomach muscles, you push the "stale" air out through puckered lips, "1-2-3-4." Now you expand your stomach, pulling in fresh air through your nose,"1-2."

g If you walk for 1 minute with your breathing exercise, you will have taken 60 steps. If you can do this exercise without getting short of breath and your physician agrees, gradually build up your walks as you are able. Walk gradually, and only on the level, in your house.

h As you are able, you can move outdoors and finally with *short steps* up *gentle slopes;* the steeper the slope, the shorter the step.

i Walking is not only necessary for getting about, but it is also excellent exercise. If walking is to be pleasant and useful, it must be done *faithfully every day* you are physically able to do so.

j Walking in place can be substituted in bad weather or if there are too many hills in your area. The amount of energy put into this exercise can be changed by the distance each foot is taken off of the floor with each "step." The rate of stepping, however, should not change appreciably.

17 *Exercise 5.* Walking up steps with your breathing (Fig. 25-11, *A* through *E*).

a This is one of the most difficult exercises a person with breathing problems can undertake, but if you have been walking faithfully and using your pursed-lip breathing and stomach muscles, it should be just another "step" for you to master.

NOTE:
- *Do not* attempt this exercise without your physician's approval.
- *Do not* walk up any steps without a handrail to hold on to.

b Stand at the bottom of the steps, one hand on the handrail and the other at your side, just above your hip, with fingers to the front and thumb at the back.

c Now for three breaths (3 × 6), check your breathing and counting as if you were going to walk in place (mark time) *(A).*

d Begin to walk up the steps—while you breathe *out*
- Count "1" silently, placing *left* foot on first step *(B).*
- Count "2" silently, placing *right* foot beside left *(C).*
- Count "3" silently, placing *right* foot on second step *(D).*
- Count "4" silently, plaing *left* foot beside right *(E).*

e While you breathe *in,* count "1-2" silently as you *rest* on the second step.

f Check your breathing. As you breathe out and count silently "1-2-3-4," you should feel your stomach contract, pushing out the stale air. As you breathe in, counting silently "1-2," expand your stomach muscles to pull in the fresh air.

g With one full breath, you are now on the second step. Do not go any higher on your first day. It will be easier to practice on the same first two steps than to go any higher.

h If your physician permits, practice on the first two steps several times a day.

i Remember, *breathe every breath correctly*. You must not allow yourself to go up fast enough nor far enough to get short of breath.

j If you do get short of breath, it may indicate that the next time you practice this exercise, you should take only *one* step for each full breath, then rest for one or two breaths.

k If you get short of breath and feel uncomfortable, turn around and sit down on the step and use *Exercise 1* in order to get back your breath.

l It would be wise to have someone stand by to help you until you feel confident with this exercise.

m Remember, *never try to exceed your ability*. Take your time. Muscles take time to strengthen and you will not be able to go any faster than it takes your muscles to condition themselves to these new challenges.

18 Keep in mind that the exercises described above are in easy-to-understand, everyday language. Make sure the patient receives instructions in a manner that he/she can easily grasp. There are many other exercises to use with the chronic pulmonary disease patient, most of which are forms of "games" to teach pursed-lip breathing (which many patients learn unconsciously) and diaphragmatic breathing. Some are listed below:

a Blowing out candles
b Blowing ping pong balls about on a table
c Blowing through a straw into a glass of water
d Breathing with hands on stomach (diaphragm)
e Lying down with a heavy book on the stomach and breathing so that the book rises and falls
f Twisting a large towel around the stomach and pulling on the ends during exhalation to "squeeze" the air out

19 Basically, however, the most important point that patients must understand, regardless of the teaching

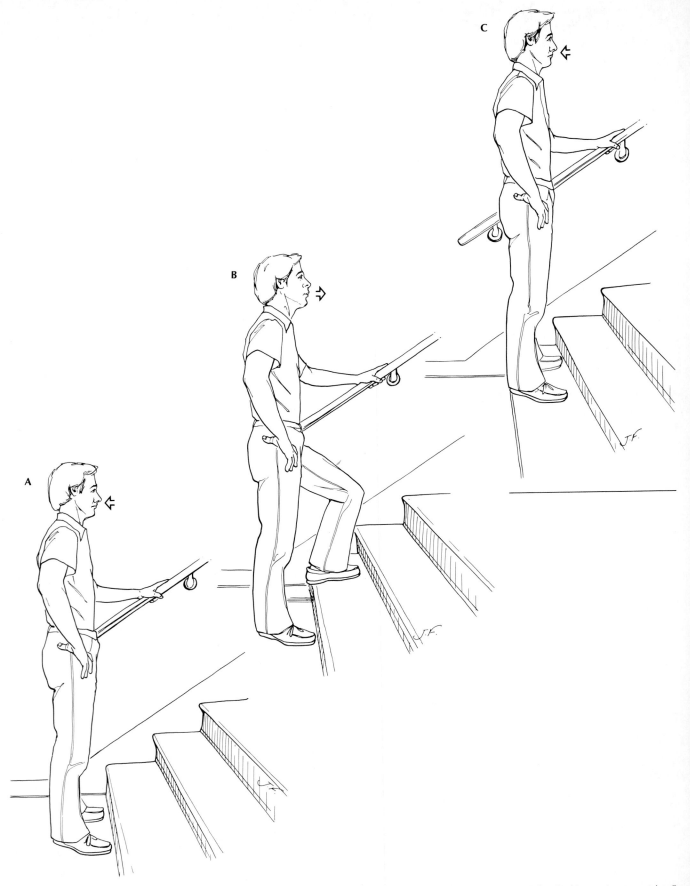

F I G U R E   2 5 - 1 1 A through **E,** Efficient breathing while climbing stairs—exercise 5.

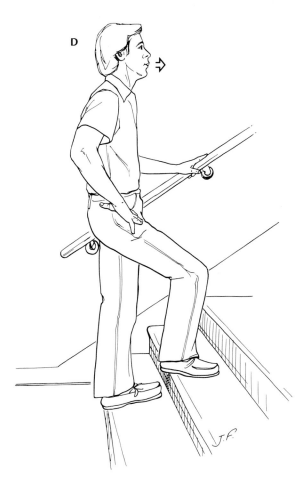

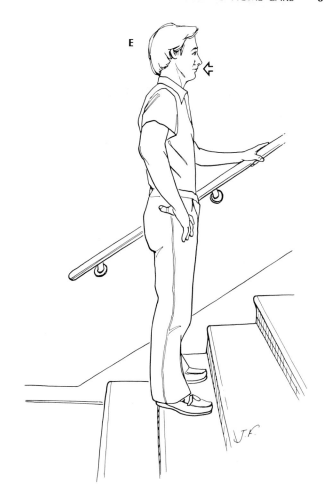

method used, is that their disease is one in which the lungs do not empty rapidly during exhalation. All techniques should help to maintain patent airways and to prevent air trapping.

a Humidity (refer to Module Eleven)

b Aerosol (refer to Module Twelve)

c Medication (refer to Module Fifteen)

d Pulmonary drainage (refer to Module Nineteen)

e Airway management (refer to Module Twenty)

20 Basic breathing exercises that are also considered useful are included here.

a Bilateral chest compression (Fig. 25-12, *A* and *B*).

• Exhale while you place your palms flat over the lower ribs and upper abdomen. Keep shoulders down, elbows straight out, and hands rigid. Blow your stale air slowly through pursed lips while contracting your abdominal muscles, and applying firm pressure with your fingers and palms. Maintain the pressure until the lungs have emptied.

• Now release some of the pressure being applied by your hands and inhale by expanding your abdomen, pulling in fresh air through your *nose*. Keep your hands and arms in position, *B*, and feel your chest expand against the pressure being applied by your hands.

b Diaphragmatic breathing (Fig. 25-13, *A* and *B*).

• Lie flat on a hard surface, rest left hand across chest, place right hand on abdomen. Inhale air through your *nose,* letting your abdomen expand against the pressure of your hand, *A*.

• Exhale *slowly* through pursed lips by contracting your abdominal muscles, *B,* and assisting exhalation by pressing down on your hand. This exercise also may be performed while standing with your back flat against a wall.

c Diaphragmatic breathing with bent knees (Fig. 25-14, *A* and *B*).

• Exercise as in *B,* bending the knees, causing abdominal contents to push the diaphragm upward.

d Diaphragmatic breathing with bent knees and forced exhalation (Fig. 25-15, *A* and *B*).

• Lie flat on a hard surface. Raise knees and inhale through your nose until you feel that your chest is fully expanded.

• Now lift your feet from the floor and exhale *slowly* through pursed lips while pulling your bent legs (hugging them) as close to your chest as possible with your arms until exhalation is completed, *B*.

e Diaphragmatic breathing against a weighted resistance (Fig. 25-16).

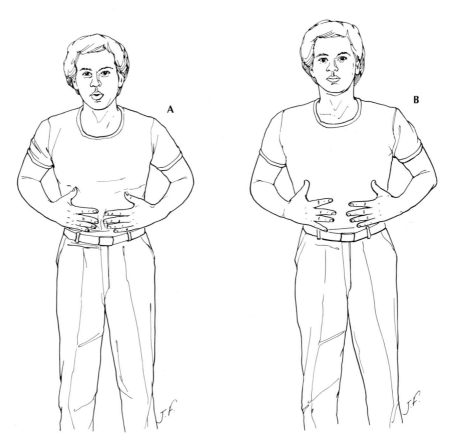

FIGURE 25-12 Bilateral chest compression exercise. **A,** Exhalation and **B,** inhalation.

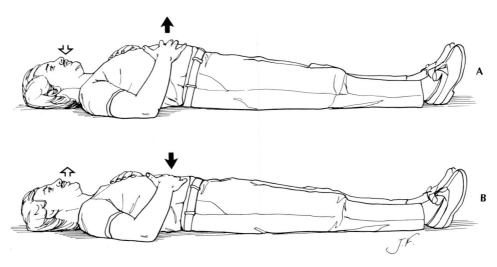

FIGURE 25-13 Diaphragmatic breathing—position 1. Lying flat with hands on chest and stomach. **A,** Inhalation and **B,** exhalation.

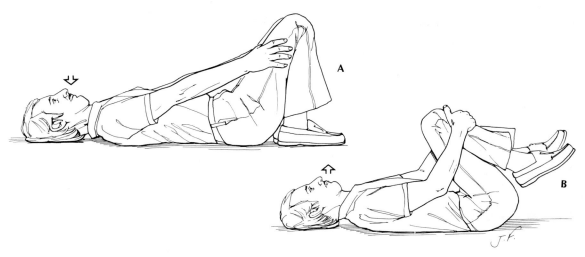

FIGURE 25-14 Diaphragmatic breathing—position 2. Knees bent, feet flat with hands on chest and stomach. **A,** Inhalation and **B,** exhalation.

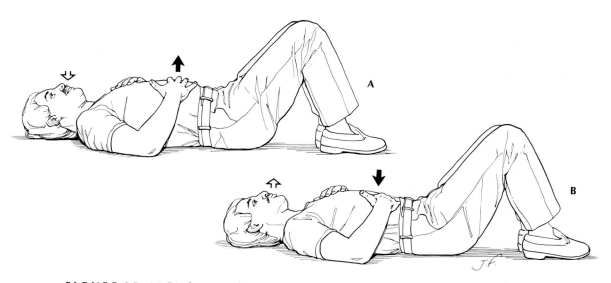

FIGURE 25-15 Diaphragmatic breathing—position 3. Knees bent with hands holding knees. **A,** Inhalation and **B,** exhalation.

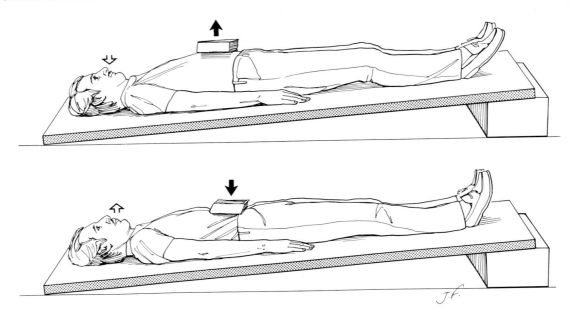

FIGURE 25-16 Diaphragmatic breathing—position 4. Lying flat with feet elevated and 5 pound object placed on abdomen.

- Lie on a flat surface with your feet elevated at least 14 inches (as in your drainage exercises). Place a 5-pound object on your abdomen (e.g., hot water bottle, dictionary, bag filled with sand, etc.).
- Breathe in deeply through your *nose,* while feeling and observing your chest and abdomen rising against the resistance of the weight.
- Breathe out *slowly* through pursed lips, allowing the weight to assist in exhalating by pressing down during exhalation.
- Your physician may want to increase the weight gradually as you get stronger.

f Resting position 1 (Fig. 25-17).
- This is helpful in reducing shortness of breath.
- Place your elbows *up* on pillows that have been placed on a table or desk.
- Use a pursed-lip position to breathe out slowly.
- *Always* use your abdominal muscles to breathe.

g Resting position 2 (Fig. 25-18).
- This is helpful in reducing shortness of breath.
- Place your elbows *up* on a wall, counter, or some other object about chest high.
- Use a pursed-lip position to breathe out slowly.
- *Always* use your abdominal muscles to breathe.

h Resting position 3 (Fig. 25-19).
- This is helpful in reducing shortness of breath.
- Sit on armless chair with your feet flat on the floor, or if your feet do not quite reach the floor, place them on a stack of magazines.
- Put your elbows on your thighs near the knees.
- Rest your chin on your hands.
- Use a pursed-lip position to breathe out slowly.
- *Always* use your abodminal muscles to breathe.

21 The next most important thing is knowing the *general health measures* that all patients should follow. These are listed below.

a Avoid *irritation* to the respiratory tract. Irritation can be caused by:
- Cigarettes, pipes, cigars (personally and from others)
- Smoke of any kind (burning trash, barbecuing, cooking, hobbies that rely on woodburners or soldering irons)
- Dust (use the vacuum frequently, filter heaters and air conditioners, avoid yard work in dry weather, avoid open windows and window or attic fans that pull in outside air, avoid using a broom)
- Allergies (learn to avoid exposure to agents such as feathers, animals, medicines, or foods that may cause a reaction)

b Practice good dietary habits.
- A diet should be well balanced to maintain energy, but not so much as to gain weight and compromise breathing ability through obesity.
- Very spicy, greasy, or hot foods should be avoided, as well as iced drinks and frozen foods (ice cream, etc.).
- Foods that cause gas should be avoided, since they may cause distention of the abdomen and compromise breathing ability.
- Meals should be moderate in amount. Large meals will cause bloating and may compromise breathing ability. If necessary, space four to six small meals over the day.

c Liquids are very important and most patients should drink *at least* six to eight glasses of water for hydra-

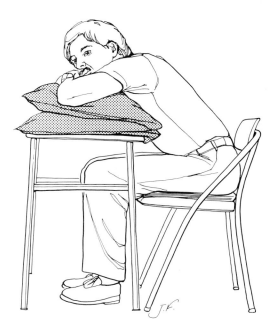

FIGURE 25-17 Resting—position 1. Sitting while leaning on elbows that have been placed on a table or desk.

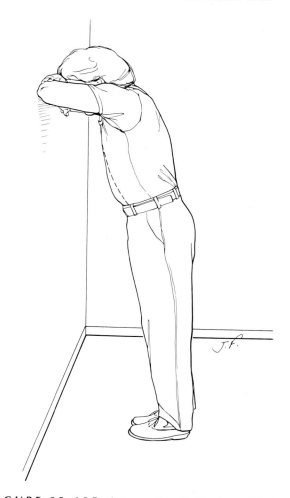

FIGURE 25-18 Resting—position 2. Standing while leaning on elbows that have been placed on a wall or chest-high object.

tion. NOTE: This must be approved by the physician in the event of cor pulmonale or renal problems.

d Temperature and humidity should be controlled as much as possible. Maintain room temperatures at approximately 66° F to 72° F and relative humidity greater than 70%. Patients should avoid extremes; for example, leaving a warm house and going out in winter weather without something over the mouth and nose.

e Changes in altitude can be very uncomfortable. Patients should avoid flying in unpressurized aircraft, and avoid for the most part, altitudes below 500 feet and above 5000 feet.

f Constipation should be avoided. Straining at stool may bring on shortness of breath, and a full bowel may press against the diaphragm and compromsie breathing ability.

g Patients should avoid exercise or exertion to the point of fatigue. Muscular exertion must be counterbalanced by appropriate rest.

h Changes in climate, unless there is a specific emotional reason or one resulting from problems in altitude, are not usually necessary. Many patients place far too much faith in the old concept of "moving to a better climate." Most patients are far better off learning to live in their accustomed climate where they have family, friends, traditions, etc., and other psychosocial advantages.

i Illnesses such as "flu" and colds must be avoided because they seriously compromise a patient's weakened breathing ability and reduce resistance. The patient should try to avoid crowded areas during "flu" season, get "flu" shots from his or her physician or

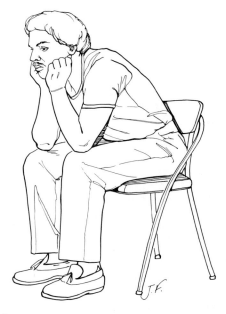

FIGURE 25-19 Resting—position 3. Sitting while leaning on hands.

health department, and avoid contact with friends and family who are sick. If a respiratory infection does occur, seek professional help *at once*.

j Be aware of the signs of pulmonary deterioration presented in the boxed material of Unit 5.1 in this module.

k Avoid over-the-counter drugs that promise "fast relief." The patient's physician will prescribe whatever is necessary, safe, and *effective*.

22 The last measure that all technicians, therapists, and rehabilitation workers must realize is that the *patient's attitude* about his or her illness is the single most important indicator of a patient's ability to do well.

a All the exercises, medications, and oxygen in the world are no good to a patient who will not use them.

b All the rehabilitation that money can buy will not help a patient who will not quit smoking.

c One must consider the *psychosocial aspects* of the patient and his or her family. Refer to what has already been studied concerning the role of the sick person in our society.

d Most rehabilitation workers will learn that the majority of patients will master breathing exercises and drainage positions readily. The bulk of their work will be to keep the patients active, interested, and enthusiastic about "staying alive."

e It is crucial that the patient be allowed to work toward and achieve his or her own goals and not the "goals" of a 25-year-old rehabilitation worker who tries to second-guess what the patient wants to be able to do. For example, the patient may want only to be able to walk to the patio and feed birds to be happy. Trying to convince this patient of how great it would be to walk to the corner drugstore to buy a newspaper is counterproductive and can produce frustration and all the negative effects that follow.

23 Oxygen therapy in conjunction with this module is an important point, especially while the patient is in the hospital.

24 The need for supplemental oxygen at home will differ from patient to patient and will depend on the activities undertaken. Oxygen is always ordered and prescribed by a physician.*

8.2 Caring for the chronic pulmonary disease patient in the outpatient setting

1 The philosophy of outpatient treatment should be to continue the work begun in the hospital.

2 Unfortunately, in many hospitals patients who have recovered from their acute insult are sent home only to get sick again through the same ignorance of care that put them in the hospital in the first place.

3 Obviously, with patients being sent home to an unhealthy physical and emotional environment and with treatment discontinued, the benefits derived from the

*Use of oxygen in the home will be discussed in more detail in Unit 8.3.

hospital can be completely and rapidly undone.

4 Outpatient programs may take on different forms. They may be connected directly to the hospital or a part of a social affairs agency, (e.g., the American Lung Association). Programs may be operated by a group of physicians, by a private business concern, or by an educational facility.

5 Outpatient programs may use different formats, such as (a) the quick, drop in, "puffing parlor," (b) an informal "come-in-when-you-need-us" operation, (3) a rigid, scheduled appointment program, or (4) those programs based on a "seminar" or learning experience, lasting perhaps all day.

6 However, most programs designed for outpatients contain general features such as those listed here.

a The patient comes into the facility, meaning that the patient must be either ambulatory or have someone bring him or her in for visits.

b Most programs feature at least treatment, training, education, and pulmonary function testing.

c The better programs offer additional services, such as:
  • Arterial blood gas analysis
  • Social programs, club meetings, speakers, etc.
  • Counseling and guidance
  • Classes in maintenance of equipment
  • Outreach facilities, such as "meals-on-wheels," home visits, etc.
  • Follow-up and referral services

7 A well-designed respiratory care outpatient facility should have the following personnel and offer the following services.

a Proper personnel, (i.e., a medical director, program supervisor, therapist, technician, and others) as necessary and depending on the size of the unit

b Oxygen and compressed air for equipment and transport

c Nebulizers

d Lung inflation devices

e Suctioning equipment

f Medications in stock

g Tilt table for pulmonary drainage

h Treadmill for graded exercise

i Stair steps

j Bicycle

k Pulmonary function devices (spirometers, flow rate devices, etc.)

l Separate cleaning and decontamination area

m Clean storage area

n Audio-visual area and/or equipment

o Stand-by ECG monitor, defibrillator, and resuscitation supplies

8 The facility should be located so that patients will *not* have to walk any great distance or climb any stairs.

9 The objectives of an outpatient facility should be to:

a Deliver therapy as ordered by a physician, and help the patient maintain patent airways.

b Provide educational opportunities for the patient and

family that deal with various aspects and treatment of the illness.

c Help the patient achieve personal goals on a long-term basis through physical conditioning and improved tolerance to activities.

d Aid the patient and family to cope with chronic illness through counseling and outreach services.

10 Specific details on therapy are found in earlier modules and will be not repeated here. However, the sample program below points out some of the details of a well-designed approach to a 1-day outpatient plan.

a Morning session—information gathering
- Pulse, blood pressure, temperature, and respiratory rate are taken
- Discussion of the home care program
- Review of medical history
- Pulmonary function test

b Morning session—therapy and exercise
- Aerosol/humidity with breathing exercises
- IPPB or other lung expansion maneuvers (if indicated) followed by postural drainage, chest percussion, and coughing exercises on the tilt table
- Exercise on treadmill/bicycle/stairs (with oxygen if indicated)

c Morning session—education
- Review of key points in home care (or talks by dietitians, social workers, counselors, etc.)

d Lunch
- If possible, with outpatient staff and other outpatients
- Social interaction encouragement

e Afternoon session—training and retraining
- Breathing patterns
- Diaphragmatic breathing

f Afternoon session—therapy and exercise
- Aerosol/humidity with breathing exercises
- IPPB or other lung expansion maneuvers (if indicated) followed by postural drainage, chest percussion, and coughing exercises on the tilt table
- Exercise on treadmill/bicycle/stairs (with oxygen if indicated)

g Afternoon session—education and evaluation of day
- Review of equipment upkeep and cleaning
- Question and answer period with medical director
- Review of day's activities and evaluation

11 The sample program above could be attended on whatever schedule was appropriate for each patient. For example, the patient could come in every Monday, Wednesday, and Friday for the first 2 weeks after discharge; then, every Monday and Thursday for 2 weeks, then, finally, once a week continuously.

12 Patients who cannot stay the entire day because of job responsibilities could come in for 1 exercise period several times a week and attend educational sessions in the evening.

13 Social activities are very rewarding and give patients needed contact with others. They are also a means to encourage peer support in a manner similar to the suc-

cessful Alcoholics Anonymous concept. Examples would be dinners or picnics together, group tours and outings to various entertainments, and group discussion and/or counseling sessions. A daily phone call service where members of the "club" can call others to inquire as to their progress or simply to chat has been very rewarding in some communities.

14 There are two distinct parts to evaluating the patient's progress—that which can be measured and that which cannot be measured.

a *Measurable indicators* include:
- Physical examination
- Auscultation
- Chest x-ray examinations
- Gas analysis of arterial blood
- Electrocardiogram
- Baseline ventilatory function (FEV_1 or FEF 25%-75%) and lung volumes
- Exercise performance measures of maximum oxygen uptake

b Indicators for which there are *no reliable measures* include:
- The patient's report on his progress
- The family's report on the patient's progress
- The patient's self-image
- The patient's outward affect

15 It should be noted that many patients seem "happy," "well-adjusted," and "full-of-life," even though their measurable indicators show a worsening of their disease. Although the term is overused, "mind over matter" accurately describes how many patients react to their chronic pulmonary disease. Some patients, on the other hand, react with anxiety, depression, and compulsive somatic concern over the smallest symptoms and soon resign themselves to the role of "pulmonary cripple."

16 Evaluation and follow-up should be scheduled in intervals, such as initial evaluation, 2 weeks, 6 weeks, 3 months, 6 months, 1 year, and 2 years after discharge from the hospital phase.

17 Each evaluation and follow-up should include the following:

a Review of medication

b Review of medical history

c Physical examination

d A measure of forced expiratory volume timed to forced vital capacity ($FEV_1/FVC\%$), FEV_1 volume, and maximum voluntary ventilation (MVV)

e A review of the patient's home care program by a member of the home care team who has appraised the patient's home situation and skill in self-treatment

f A report or questionnaire to be filled in by the patient that includes:
- Questions relating to psychologic adjustment
- Questions relating to social and family adjustment
- Space for patients to comment on personal reactions

- Space for patients to describe tolerance to activity and exercise

8.3 Caring for the chronic pulmonary disease patient in the home setting

1 Many patients who are cared for primarily in the home setting are also treated as outpatients.
2 Caring for the patient in the home setting has certain *advantages*.
 a The patient feels more comfortable in his or her own surroundings and in actively participating in his or her own rehabilitation.
 b The patient does not have to leave the house, go out in adverse weather, or expend energy traveling to an outpatient facility.
 c The patient's family is nearby to help out when needed.
 d Home care is less expensive.
3 Caring for the patient in his or her home has noted *disadvantages*.
 a Trained personnel are difficult to locate, and assistance is intermittent.
 b The patient's use of medication is not closely monitored.
 c The patient does not have the specially designed equipment of the outpatient facility, (i.e., tilt table, treadmill, etc.).
 d Because there is less need to "get up and get out," there is also a greater tendency to stay in pajamas and robe and neglect hair care and shaving, etc. This may adversely affect psychosocial aspects.
 e Care and cleaning of equipment may be neglected.
 f The patient's baseline state of health may not be properly assessed and followed.
 g It is too easy for the patient to lapse back into old habits without contact with others, especially others who share the same problems.
4 Although home care programs have some undesirable characteristics, many patients do very well treating themselves and manage to stay active and productive. In some cases, the patient's *attitude* helps to defeat the effects of the disease. A home care plan (see Unit 10.1) should be designed with the knowledge of the patient's background, stage of disease, medication needs, and exercise tolerance. See Fig. 25-2 for a sample form that will help design a home care plan after a patient is discharged from the hospital.
5 Since the home care patient is not being seen regularly by professional personnel, it is necessary that some type of contact, either telephone or personal, be arranged. (Refer to Unit 9.1 for a discussion of the health care team.)
6 Visits should be scheduled so that the patient's care can be evaluated, usually with the help of a *form*. Each visit should include:
 a Patient's vital signs and overall assessment
 b Review of therapy
 c Review of oxygen usage
 d Simple spirometry
 e Instruction as necessary
 f Equipment check
 g Equipment cleaning procedure check
7 The completed forms are necessary for program record keeping, patient follow-up, a means for reporting to the attending physician, and information for third party reimbursement.
8 Oxygen plays a large part in many home care patients' daily routine. Studies have shown that oxygen can reduce the need for hospitalization and improve survival by controlling or reducing the effects of COPD, pulmonary hypertension, secondary polycythemia, and cor pulmonale.
9 Oxygen can also miprove physical endurance and exercise tolerance. However, patients with a diagnosis of COPD and associated severe hypoxemia (a PO_2 of less than 55 mm Hg on room air), who also exhibit cor pulmonale, secondary polycythemia, or exercise limitation (which is responsive to oxygen administration) are the only *indicated* individuals to benefit from oxygen therapy. In the absence of the above complications, the home administration of oxygen will *probably not* be of any real value.
10 The home administration of oxygen requires the consideration of both ease of administration and reasonable expense to the patient. The two most commonly prescribed methods are the:
 a Nasal cannula. One of the simplest and least expensive methods; usually run at 1 or 2 L/min; generally comfortable and well-tolerated.
 b Mask. Regardless of type, is not usually practical because of the large amount of oxygen flow necessary. Even controlled-percentage masks (entrainment-type) use too many liters per minute to be economical. Masks are generally less well-tolerated than the nasal cannula. (See also Module Ten.)
11 The next consideration is the oxygen source.
 a The most practical method for the ambulatory patient is the *liquid reservoir system;* for example, the "Linde Walker" and storage system (see Module Seven). This allows complete walking freedom, is relatively inexpensive, is simple to operate and maintain, and can be used for leaving the home (portable unit) or as a stationary base. It also requires very little storage space.
 b The *oxygen cylinder* has always been popular but has several disadvantages. Tanks are generally heavy, except for the small ones with very few cubic feet of gas in them, which need to be changed frequently.
 - Changing tanks requires skills that some older or very sick patients could not perform. Refilling small tanks from a larger one is not practical or safe.
 - Small tanks are very difficult to move around with.
 - Depending on usage, cylinders may be the *least expensive* means of supplying oxygen to the home patient at this time.

c Oxygen concentrators and enrichers have grown in popularity and are rapidly replacing other methods of providing oxygen to the home patient.

d These units usually use a *molecular sieve,* which selectively removes the nitrogen, carbon dioxide, carbon monoxide, and other gases from the room air and leaves an enriched oxygen supply.

- This supply is about the size of a large suitcase and is primarily used for a stationary supply. The actual cost of the oxygen it produces (filters) is nothing, although rental fees, maintainence costs, and increased electric bills *may be more expensive* than using other oxygen sources.
- Oxygen percentages from 22% to 90% can be produced with flow rates inversely proportional to the concentration produced. For example, a 22% concentration could be produced in flows greater than 3.5 L/min, where a 90% concentration would only be produced at around 1 L/min.

e Other sources of oxygen exist but are generally impractical as a result of high cost, unavailability, and lack of volume to last for any extended period of time. These include the solid chemical cannisters that cannot be shut off once activated; the aerosol-type cans with attached masks; and the very small cylinders (similar to those used to power pellet rifles) that can be hidden in canes, walking sticks, etc.

12 Whether or not a home patient should receive oxygen therapy should be determined by rigid standards based on both clinical and laboratory data. The *average* Pao_2 agreed upon by most physicians as reasonable and desirable for COPD patients is approximately 60 mm Hg. However, this figure is subject to much discussion among rehabilitation experts.

9.0 A MULTIDISCIPLINARY HEALTH CARE APPROACH FOR THE HOME CARE PATIENT
9.1 The need for the health team approach in the care of the home patient

1 As mentioned earlier, professional visits to the home care patient will be limited, primarily because of the inability of one person to spend as much time with one patient as is sometimes necessary.

2 The solution is in using different people from different professional areas. There are two reasons for this. First, it supplies the number of visits necessary for good home care, and second, since no one person can be expert in everything, most major areas of skills are represented.

3 The following professions can be used in serving as part of the home care health team for patients with pulmonary disease. After each *profession* is a list of its special talents.

a *Respiratory care*
- Assists in delivering therapy
- Helps set up equipment and maintain it
- Delivers inhalation medications
- Performs simple spirometry

- Instructs and informs the patient
- Assesses the patient's pulmonary and general health
- Reports to the physician

b *Nursing*
- Assists in physical evaluation
- Instructs and informs the patient
- Delivers and instructs in the use of medication
- Instructs patient's family in bedside care

c *Physical therapy*
- Assists in breathing exercises
- Assists in postural drainage
- Assists in exercise program
- Instructs and informs the patient

d *Occupational therapy*
- Performs evaluation of activities for daily living
- Helps adapt home environment for patient's needs
- Assists in physical training
- Instructs and informs the patient

e *Electrocardiology*
- Performs ECG tests
- Performs bicycle or treadmill ergometry (done only in laboratory)

f *Dietetics*
- Assists in proper diet
- Helps with simplified food preparation
- Instructs and informs the patient

g *Social work/counseling*
- Helps patient deal with personal problems
- Evaluates home situation
- Provides assistance in obtaining financial help, insurance coverage, etc.
- Provides information about available community resources
- Provides psychologic support to patient and family

10.0 THE HOME CARE PLAN
10.1 Constructing a home care plan with the help of the patient's physician

1 The reader is encouraged to take the time to actually develop a patient care plan for a simulated patient in a home care situation. This exercise will help the reader develop a broader perspective as to scope of activities involved with home care. (Information from the form presented in Fig. 25-2 may be useful in designing a health care plan.)

This care plan is a simulation only and should *not* be used to care for an actual patient unless it is modified to meet the specific needs of the patient. Procedure 25-1 may be used as a procedure for constructing a health care plan for the home patient.

2 A care plan may be designed according to the following list of major areas of concern for the patient.

a *Environment*
- Add humidifier and/or special filter to central heat/air conditioning system
- Eliminate irritants to respiratory tract
- Stop smoking

b *Prevent complications*
- Get flu shot
- Avoid crowds
- Be aware of condition

c *Airway maintenance*
- As prescribed, aerosol therapy with 1 ml iso-etharine in 3 ml of normal saline, delivered with a compressed air nebulizer, four times a day
- Postural drainage to follow aerosol treatment

d *Exercises*
- Breathing exercises three times a day: on arising, early afternoon, and before bedtime
- At least one daily walk of at least 10 minutes duration with 1 L of oxygen

e *Basic health care*
- Diet as prepared by hospital dietitian
- Six to eight glasses of water daily
- Medication as ordered by physician

f *Sterilization of respiratory equipment*
- Wash in hot soapy water, rinse in hot water
- Soak in a mixture of ½ cup of white vinegar to 4 cups water for 20 minutes
- Run this vinegar solution through spinning-disk nebulizers for at least 20 minutes, or soak small pieces in this solution for at least 20 minutes

g *Outpatient check-up*
- Report to rehabilitation unit 2 days a week for the first month
- After first month report to rehabilitation unit 1 day a week from then on

11.0 EDUCATION AS A PART OF THE HOME CARE PLAN
11.1 The need for education as part of the home care plan

1 Education is regarded as the cornerstone of management of all chronic diseases. The long-proved model of patient education is the diabetic who is taught many difficult concepts, including self-administration of intradermal injections. COPD patients can also learn what is necessary for the maintenance of their illness.

2 Patients must be part of their own treatment team. Education should be directed toward *prevention* and *avoidance*. The avoidance of smoking, respiratory irritants, other's infections, and of situations causing breathlessness.

3 Education must be tailored to the needs of patients and to their ability to understand and carry out the instructions. Aids to teaching may include:

a Charts
b Diagrams
c Booklets
d Filmstrips and tapes
e Movies
f Demonstrations using manikins
g Demonstrations using the patient

12.0 UNDERSTANDING THE CONCEPT OF MOTIVATION WITH REGARD TO THE PATIENT AND FAMILY FOLLOWING A HOME CARE PLAN
12.1 Motivating the patient and family to follow a home care plan

1 Unfortunately, what motivates John may have little or no effect on Mary. There is no set of rules, games, or exercises to increase motivation. However, the respiratory care practitioner may be able to improve motivation by understanding what motivation is. Other than what we see externally in a patient, we should also be concerned with how a patient feels about particular things or situations and how he or she experiences the world. Mr. Smith, for instance, may feel angry and act angry, yet he may also feel so without making his anger apparent to others.

2 How, then, can we determine what another person's *subjective* experiences are—the way they feel on the inside?

a First of all, we cannot take part in this private experience. All we see is Mr. Smith's overt behavior. And although by watching Mr. Smith's behavior and the situation we may *infer* that he feels angry, we must recognize that our statement about his subjective state is *only* an inference rather than a direct observation.

b Frequently, our inferences are based on someone's non-verbal cues: a tensing of jaw muscles, a tapping of the toe, drumming of fingertips.

c In other instances, we "guess" how the other person must feel based on how we would feel in the same situation.

d Regardless of our method, we must be constantly aware that making statements about another's experience is always a matter of inference.

e Individuals also differ in their ability and readiness to make inferences about another's experiences. For example, two technicians at a rehabilitation facility see Mr. Smith throw a box of tissues across the room.
- Technician A says, "Mr. Smith just threw a box of tissues."
- Technician B says, "Mr. Smith feels frustrated."

f Technician A passes over any interpretation and simply describes the overt behavior. Technician B infers that Mr. Smith is angry and that the anger is the result of *felt* frustration. Actually, both points of view are necessary in the understanding of patient motivation and personality.

3 In 1937, the psychologist, Gordon W. Allport, said that:

Personality is something and does something. It is not synonymous with behavior or activity; least of all is it merely the impression that this activity makes on others. It is what lies behind specific acts and within the individual. The systems that constitute personality are in every sense determining tendencies, and when aroused by suitable stimuli, provoke those adjustive and expressed acts by which the personality comes to be known.

4 In other words, to cause an outward reaction, an individual requires a stimulus. So, to get a patient to *respond* with a desired behavior (motivation or desire to take his therapy), we must supply the required stimulus (whatever it will take).

5 *"Why"* is the important concept. *Why* does Mr. Smith stay angry with his wife? *Why* does he refuse his oxygen, although he admits he feels better with it? *Why* does he get depressed at particular times of day? The emphasis in such questions is on the motivation underlying the observed behavior.

6 Motivation to take home care can also be defined as "will to live," since the patient is usually well aware that carrying out home care will improve his or her quality of life. There are no concrete methods for getting a patient to "want to get better." Certain individuals do show a certain knack for motivating others, but studies are contradictory about what special quality these people possess.

7 For the rest of us, we should ask ourselves, "What is this person willing to live for?" It may be any one of the following list of emotional stimuli.
  a The love of a family member
  b A favorite pet
  c The ability to work in the garden
  d The ability to do their own shopping
  e Getting together with cherished friends
  f *Anything* where the patient says that all the work of exercise and therapy is worth having or doing it

8 Obviously, the patient is not always going to be able to answer the question of what will "turn him or her on" simply because he or she has probably never connected the lack of will to live to the loss of anything except difficulty in breathing.

9 *Inducing* motivation is not the skill of an amateur. It rests in the hands of the counselor, clergyman, or social worker. However, all health workers can be alert to obvious problems that affect a patient's life and can be effective and patient listeners.

10 The simple emotional bond between the patient and the practitioner who seems to *genuinely* care about the patient's treatment may be all it takes to assist the patient to "re-enter" life.

11 Topics included in a typical patient education program:
  a Whom to contact for help. Key people and service agencies.
  b Anatomy and physiology of lung disease. A simplified approach to the heart and lung.
  c Pathology and pharmacology. A layperson's presentation of lung disease; how it works and how it can be treated, including the benefits and dangers of drugs.
  d Individual therapeutic modalities. A detailed instruction for the patient involving use of his or her own medications, equipment, and procedures, including cleaning and care of the equipment.
  e Exercises for daily living. An exercise program to

teach the patients to care for themselves, walk, and otherwise achieve maximum use of their own lung function.
  f Stress relaxation exercise. A program to help the patient and family to recognize and to cope with stress.
  g Environmental hygiene. Instruction to help the patient and family to recognize, avoid, and/or correct unhealthy physical and environmental situations.
  h Dietary planning. Instruction to help the patient and family to understand what to eat, how to prepare it, and when to eat.
  i Self-assessment. When and who to call for help. Instruction to help the patient and family to recognize situations that require professional assistance.

13.0 CAUSES OF PULMONARY EMERGENCIES IN THE HOME
13.1 Identify the causes of pulmonary emergencies in the home and a plan to deal with them

1 The patient with chronic pulmonary disease and his or her family must be thoroughly educated as to what constitutes an emergency and what to do should an emergency arise.

2 The boxed material that follows lists some of the primary causes of emergencies in the home. Although this list is not totally inclusive, it does point out those areas that are most frequently reported in the literature.

3 Dust and mold collecting on air conditioning filters, vents, and in refrigerator drip trays are frequently overlooked as sources of bronchial irritation.
  a Aerosols from hairsprays and other pressurized containers present a more obvious source of irritation and must be avoided.
  b Heavy aftershaves and perfumes should be used in very small quantities.

4 Exacerbation of a pulmonary infection will usually result in increased production and retention of secretions and can usually be controlled with prescribed medications by the patient's physician. Secretions must be

---

Causes of pulmonary emergencies in the home

1 Bronchial irritants from dust, smoke, and other inhalants
2 Production and retention of excessive secretions
3 Exacerbation of pulmonary infections
4 Misuse of drugs, e.g., bronchodilators, expectorants, etc.
5 Physical strain resulting from excessive exercise
6 Equipment malfunction
7 Improper diet, e.g., too little or too much food
8 Dehydration leading to inspissated mucous plugs and infection
9 Misuse of respiratory care equipment including excessive oxygen concentrations and overdependence on intermittent positive pressure breathing (IPPB)
10 Accidents resulting from falls
11 Emotional stress resulting from psychosocial factors

controlled by hydration and by removal to prevent possible increased levels of carbon dioxide and hypoxemia.

5 Another source of pulmonary emergency can be attributed to the *misuse* of respiratory care equipment and drugs. The misuse and overuse of IPPB and oxygen is well known. Abuse of equipment and drugs is generally caused by a lack of understanding by the patient as to the benefits of IPPB or oxygen. Drugs, such as oxygen, bronchodilators, and even aspirin are frequently misused by patients who seek relief from perpetual discomfort. All of these drugs are potentially harmful and must be prescribed. For example, 1 person per 1000 can have a toxic reaction to aspirin, a drug considered "safe" for almost everyone.

6 Emotional stress (espcially anxiety and "panics") experienced by the uninformed patient and his or her family frequently causes undue upset and complications associated with mental and physical fatigue.

7 Reporting the emergency and seeking qualified assistance is just as important as recognizing the problem.

8 Since the family is the first responder to most emergencies in the home, the family members (and close friends) must be taught *cardiopulmonary resuscitation,* as well as other first aid techniques. They must be able to recognize and correct situations leading to airway obstruction, as well as the method of contacting local rescue agencies. The best precaution is to form an emergency plan; and if an emergency occurs, to follow that plan.

14.0 UTILIZING PROFESSIONAL AND COMMUNITY RESOURCES IN CARE OF THE HOME PATIENT
14.1 Professional and community services required by the home patient

1 Chronic lung disease imposes a serious mental and physical strain on the patient and family. In 1975, the American Lung Association published the results of a study conducted by a combined task force of the Association and their medical wing, the American Thoracic Society.

2 This report delineated thirty-six services that would be needed by most chronic lung patients who have been released from the hospital. These services listed by the task force fall into six major categories.

3 Follow-up data on the patient is essential because it is the link that monitors the patient's progress and provides the information necessary for the physician to make informed decisions about the patient's care plan.

4 Education should involve as many of the patient's contacts as possible and should be offered on a formal basis according to a schedule.

5 Respiratory care should be of the highest quality within realistic economic considerations. It should also be carefully monitored by a team who understands respiratory care and total patient assessment.

6 Keep in mind that, regardless of attempts at economy, the home patient usually has financial difficulties as a result of continuous ongoing care. Family income is usually limited and, traditionally, external support is from third party payers and other sources (Blue Cross-Blue Shield, Medicare, Medicaid, CHAMPUS, etc.).

14.2 The coordinator of patient services

1 The services required by chronic lung patients are many and complex. To be useful, the services must be readily and easily available.

2 One way of helping patients to avail themselves of these services is through the use of a patient services coordinator.

3 The coordinator should be located in a central location and physicians informed of the process for using the coordinator's services.

4 The primary function of the coordinator is to work with the physician to arrange the team care of the home patient.

5 This coordination involves everything from visits from the respiratory therapy personnel to transportation of the patient to the physician for a check-up.

15.0 SUPPLEMENTAL MATERIAL ON REHABILITATION
15.1 Abuse of pulmonary rehabilitation, outpatient care, and home care programs

1 The American Association for Respiratory Care (AARC) has adopted the following three important standards regarding the quality of care, ethical practice, and fraud in respiratory home care programs.

a *Standards for Respiratory Therapy Home Care* (adopted July 27, 1979). Four standards of a quality home care program (services) are described along with discussions of each standard.

b *Ethical Performance of Respiratory Home Care* (adopted April 15, 1982). Conflict of interest is discussed, along with possible disciplinary actions by the AARC.

c *Statement of Principles on Fraud and Abuse in Home Care* (adopted April 14, 1983). Situations constituting fraudulent and abusive practive are defined according to the AARC and Medicare/Medicaid Act—Fraud and Abuse Amendments of 1977 (PL 95-142). The reader who is interested in home care is encouraged to acquire all of the above standards and to be knowledgeable of all federal laws governing this practice. Violations of these laws can result in a large fine and imprisonment. Standards may be acquired by contacting the American Association for Respiratory Care, 11030 Ables Lane Dallas, Texas 75229.

15.2 Medicare Catastrophic Health Insurance

1 Beginning January 1, 1989, the federal government expanded Medicare coverage to protect the elderly and disabled patient against catastrophic health care costs.

2 Benefits are mandated by the Medicare Catastrophic Act of 1988 (PO 100-360).

TABLE 25-1 Summary of Catastrophic Medicare benefits

Service	Year begins	Patient pays	Medicare pays	Restrictions on costs, length of stay, number of readmits
Hospitalization	1989	Single annual deductible, $564	100% remaining bill after deductible	None
Skilled nursing facility	1989	50% for first 8 days	50% for first 8 days, then 100%	150 days
Home health care	1990	None	100%	6 days/wk with medication of 7 days needed 38 days of care

3 This new law limits the amount that Medicare beneficiaries must pay for hospitalization, physician visits, medical supplies, and outpatient drugs covered by Medicare.

4 It also increases access to and fees to pay for home health care, skilled nursing facilities, hospitals, respite care, and breast cancer screening.

5 Examples of expanded coverages are presented in Table 25-1 below.

6 The economic impact of this new law on the various states can be considerable. Even though it is based on a matching formula with the federal government, it is estimated that it may cost the states' Medicaid programs $33 billion over the next four years. This added expense will undoubtably be passed through to the taxpayers.

7 The short- and long-range implications of expanded health care benefits for an estimated 32 million Medicare beneficaries on respiratory care and other allied health personnel is staggering.

8 As is pointed out in Module Twenty-nine, by the year 2050, one out of every three individuals in our society will be 55 years old or older. The 65+-year-old age group will comprise about 25% of the total U.S. population. During this time, the 75+-year-old group will be approximately the same size as the 65+ year age group is in 1989.

9 Clearly the need for qualified allied health personnel to care for the elderly can become a health care emergency unless it is addressed immediately. The Bureau of Labor Statistics predicts that the number of health care workers is expected to increase by 26% by 1995, but this increase still will not meet the expanding demands.

10 These professionals must be educated to deliver care in the hospital and alternative care settings such as nursing homes, skilled nursing facilities, outpatient care facilities, and in the home.

11 For more details regarding Medicare and other third party payers and services to the elderly, contact local insurance carriers and/or home health agencies.

PROCEDURE 25-1

Constructing a health care plan for the home patient

No.	Steps in performing the procedure
	The practitioner will follow these steps in constructing a health care plan for the home patient.
1	Choose an appropriate patient.
2	Contact and explain assignment to patient's attending physician.
3	Receive permission to design plan from physician.
4	Outline therapy:
	4.1 Aerosol and/or IPPB
	4.2 Postural drainage
	4.3 Breathing exercises
	4.4 Oxygen
	4.5 Medications
5	Outline program for control of infection (decontamination).
6	Outline basic health care.
7	Outline visitation program by health care team.
8	Schedule outpatient visits (if necessary and if outpatient unit is available).
9	Obtain approval from patient's physician regarding your plan. (NOTE: It is understood that the physician may *not* want to send the patient home on such a plan, but that he or she simply grant approval about the planning.)

BIBLIOGRAPHY

Boroch M: Diversification—beating new paths in respiratory care, AARC Times 10:8, 1986.

Bunch D: RT involvement in home care—what does the future hold? AARC Times 7:11, 1983.

Bunch D: RTs at home, alternative site opportunities increase, AARC Times 9:11, 1985.

American Association for Respiratory Therapy, Standards for respiratory therapy home care, an official statement, Respir Care 24:1080, 1979.

Balk R, Bone RC: Classification of acute respiratory failure, Med Clin North Am 67:551, 1983.

Beckett J: Katie Beckett—The little girl who caught the country's eye, AARTimes 9(6):41, 1985.

Bone RC: Treatment of respiratory failure due to advanced chronic obstructive lung disease, Arch Intern Med 140:1018, 1980.

Bone RC: Acute respiratory failure and chronic obstructive lung disease: recent advances, Med Clin North Am 65:563, 1981.

Bunch D: Rt involvement in home care: what does the future hold? AARTimes 7:24, 1983.

Bunch D: Pennsylvania SNFAs expanded services. AARTimes 9(7):21, 1985.

Cotton RD: Hospital conditions of participation: a guide for the respiratory care practitioner, AARTimes 11:1, 1987.

Garrett SS and Giese MA: Between therapist and patient, the language of caring, Respir Ther 11(5):51, 1981.

Hopp JW and Gerken CM: Making an educational diagnosis to improve patient education, Respir Care 28:1456, 1983.

Libby DM et al: Acute respiratory failure in scoliosis or kyphosis, Am J Med 73:532, 1982.

Malkus BL: Respiratory care at home, Am J Nurs 76:1789, 1976.

McDonald GJ: A home care program for patietns with chronic lung disease, Nurs Clin North Am 16:259, 1981.

MacDonell RJ Jr: Suggestions for establishment of pulmonary rehabilitation programs, Respir Care 26:966, 1981.

Pitty TL: Home oxygen therapy for COPD: practical aspects, Postgrad Med 69:102, 1981.

Porte P: Legislation and respiratory rehabilitation, Respir Care 28:1498, 1983.

Porte P: Wading through the rules, AARTimes 8(11):23, 1984.

Weimer MP: Home respiratory therapy for patients with chronic obstructive pulmonary disease, Respir Care 28:1484, 1983.

Neonatal and pediatric respiratory care

1.0 PRINCIPLES OF NEONATAL, PEDIATRIC, AND ADULT RESPIRATORY CARE

1.1 Physiologic considerations

1 In beginning the study of pediatric respiratory care, the reader must be aware that newborns and children are not just adults on a small scale. Neonates, infants, and older children have specific problems related to their ages and general problems not seen in adult patients.

2 The relationship of age to disease is sometimes related to anatomic factors.

a The infant's larynx is higher and softer than the adult's, and it is prone to spasm. This may lead to respiratory and/or cardiac arrest.

b Small airways, which do not have full cartilaginous support, are prone to collapse. They also become obstructed easily because of small lumen size.

c The ribs are not fully calcified, making the chest wall soft and pliable.

d Changes resulting from growth and development are considerations in the decision of therapeutic and supportive measures used in the treatment of pediatric patients.

3 An adult with chronic lung disease is usually treated with supportive measures, the goal being to make the patient as comfortable and functional as possible until death inevitably occurs. A pediatric patient with chronic lung disease (e.g., bronchopulmonary dysplasia) is also treated with supportive measures, but the goal is to keep the patient as comfortable and functional as possible until the lungs develop further and to hope the disease process diminishes with growth.

4 The development of other systems has an influence on the respiratory system.

a The upper digestive tract may have not matured functionally or anatomically, causing repeated aspiration and respiratory problems.

b Immunologic reaction to various infections may not be fully developed. Placental transfer of antibodies protects against certain bacteria and viral infections but not against others. The antibody that protects against enteric organisms is not transferred across the placenta, and infants are especially susceptible to this type of infection.

5 Just as important as recognizing the difference between adult and pediatric respiratory care is the fact that most principles and facts of adult respiratory care apply or can be applied to pediatric respiratory care.

6 Even though goals for pediatric patients with chronic lung disease may differ, most young patients have excessively thick mucous production leading to obstruction. Like their adult counterparts, they breathe functionally by hypoxic drive.

7 To help in the study of pediatric respiratory care, the reader must remember:

a Growth and development are especially important factors to diagnosis, treatment, and recovery from pediatric pulmonary diseases.

b There are disease processes generally limited to pediatrics that must be treated with special considerations to age-group.

c Pediatrics requires a special relationship with the patient and the parents for successful treatment.

d Precision and careful measurements are a necessity. Pediatric patients will require more precise observation, therapy, and evaluation than adults.

e Most adult principles and facts apply to pediatric respiratory care, usually differing only in technique and with special consideration for development, age, and size of the patient.

8 The majority of specialists in all branches of pediatric medicine received their initial training in adult medicine.

2.0 THE PSYCHOLOGY OF PEDIATRIC CARE
2.1 Psychologic considerations for neonates and their parents

1 In pediatrics, health care professionals learn quickly that patient care not only involves care of the child but care of the *parents* as well. Understanding and supporting the parents and child are basic principles of pediatric care.

2 The bonding between mother and child, enhanced by seeing, touching, holding, and feeding, was previously disrupted when the child had to be placed in the intensive care nursery.

3 The importance of maternal bonding is now being emphasized, and personnel in intensive care nurseries are encouraging early and frequent visits between relatives and the sick infant.

4 Parents usually feel frustration and guilt when they learn their new baby is ill or has congenital abnormalities. The visions of their "beautiful baby" are shattered, and parents will require strong psychologic support.

5 Even very sick infants on ventilators and with numerous tubes can be seen and touched by parents and relatives after proper hand washing and gowning.

a If parents are not allowed to see their sick or deformed infant, regardless of severity, they often imagine the condition to be far worse than it actually is.

b Parents have expressed a prolonged feeling of emptiness and grief when they are not allowed to see their infant, even if the child is dying or dead.

c If the parents never saw the infant, they cannot fully express their grief for what seems to them a nonexistent baby. This creates a prolonged mourning period for the parents.

2.2 Psychologic considerations for children and their parents

1 The hospital is a frightening experience for most people, and children are no exception. Respiratory problems usually produce even more fear and anxiety. Children in this emotional state require warmth and assurance. Wtih children (as with adults) cooperation of the patient leads to the best therapeutic results.

2 Cooperation is best accomplished by a friendly, patient, understanding person, who, with a firm voice, explains and directs therapy.

3 Honesty with children is also important. Children who are told "It won't hurt at all" before an arterial puncture do not have to be very old to figure out afterward that they were not told the truth. A more honest, direct approach would be, "When I stick you, it will hurt. But if you hold still, maybe we can get the blood with one stick. If you jerk and move around, we will probably have to stick you more than once, and it will just hurt more." By saying this, the child knows:

a What is about to happen.

b The procedure is painful (being prepared helps).

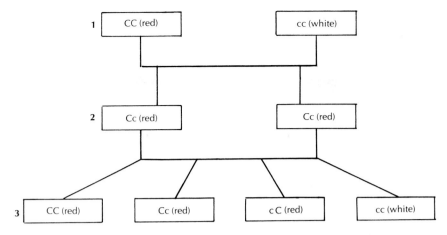

F I G U R E 2 6 - 1 Combinations of gene alleles that can be passed down through three generations.

c What behavior is expected for the procedure.

d It will be beneficial to all, including himself or herself, if he or she cooperates.

Honesty and firmness are often of some help, even with the most uncooperative children.

2.3 Psychologic considerations for chronic illness

1 Parents often express shock, disbelief, grief, and guilt when they are told their child has a chronic illness.

2 It is important to allow parents to express their feelings about the situation and to provide honest answers, support, and understanding.

3 Understanding of chronic illness prepares parents to make rational decisions when helping make care plans, along with the child (if possible) and the rest of the medical team.

4 Participating in the planning of care for the child is important because it encourages a close relationship with the child and helps parents overcome the initial shock, disbelief, and guilt.

3.0 ROLE OF GENETICS IN NORMAL AND ABNORMAL DEVELOPMENT

3.1 Introduction to basic genetic theory

1 Genes are the basic hereditary structures that carry the code for organismal development.

2 There is genetic influence in virtually all disease processes, which plays an unnoticeable part in some illnesses and which underlies the total etiology in others.

3 *Genes* are composed of *deoxyribonucleic acid* (DNA) molecules, which have the ability to reproduce. DNA also influences the *ribonucleic acid* (RNA) composition sequence, which will influence the function of cells.

4 *Chromosomes* are rod-shaped structures in cell nuclei that carry several thousand genes. Humans normally have 46 chromosomes (23 pairs) in each cell. Twenty-two (22) pairs of chromosomes are normally identical, and these are known as *autosomes. Sex chromosomes* comprise the remaining single pair.

5 Sex chromosomes determine an individual's sex. Females normally have two X chromosomes for the twenty-third pair, whereas a male will normally have an X and a Y chromosome for the twenty-third pair.

6 Since the X and Y chromosomes are not identical, they are called heterologous. The autosomes, being identical, are referred to as being homologous.

7 Chromosomal arrangement of genes consists of a specific number at a specific location. Since each cell has pairs of chromosomes, it logically follows that each will have pairs of genes. These genes at the same chromosomal location can exist in different forms called alleles, which determine alternative characters in inheritance.

8 A specific gene may have many alleles, but a person has only two alleles for each gene. Each parent contributes one allele to form the pair.

9 The Austrian biologist Gregor Mendel's classic work with flowers is an example of alleles. He worked with the gene for flower color, which had two alleles of the gene—one producing red flowers and one producing white flowers (Fig. 26-1).

10 The first generation, CC, is the homozygote for red color flower, cc is the homozygote for white color flower. C is a dominant allele, c is a recessive allele *(1)*.

11 The second generation consists of two heterozygote offspring. Since the dominant allele is present, both plants are red *(2)*.

12 The third generation has two homozygotes and two heterozygotes *(3)*.

a If the homozygote has dominant alleles, flowers will be red.

b In the heterozygote alleles, the dominant alleles will be expressed, and flowers will be red.

c In the homozygote, where there are two recessive genes, the recessive alleles in pair will produce white flowers.

13 A person with similar alleles is referred to as a homozygote. A person with different alleles is referred to as a heterozygote.

14 If an effect is expressed with only a single gene present, it is called a dominant gene (or allele). If an

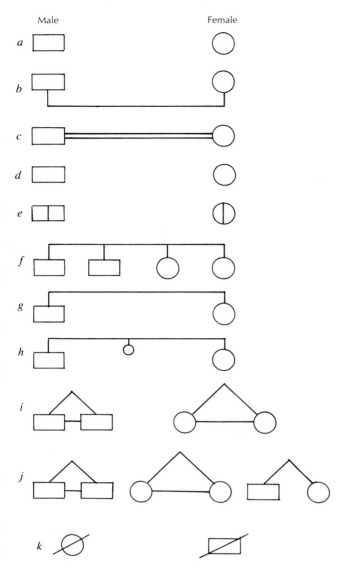

Male   Female

a

b

c

d

e

f

g

h

i

j

k

FIGURE 26-2 Family pedigree.

Siblings (or sibs), the brothers and sisters *(f)*

The same information represented in a shorter form *(g)*

An abortion or a miscarriage represented by the small circle *(h)*

Identical (monozygote) twins *(i)*

Nonidentical (dizygotic) or fraternal twins: male, female, one male, one female *(j)*

Deceased *(k)*

3.2 Genetic disorders

1 Because they are most easily understood, mendelian or single-gene disorders have been the ones most thoroughly studied. These disorders exist in four types:

a Autosomal dominant

b Autosomal recessive

c X-linked recessive

d X-linked dominant

2 X-linked refers to the gene or its effect being located on the X chromosome (sex chromosome). In other words, some disorders are passed primarily by the sex chromosome, such as baldness in men.

3 *Cystic fibrosis* (CF) is a mendelian recessive disorder. The patient who has the disease is a homozygote, whereas nonaffected parents are heterozygotes. There is no present method to determine the outcome of future pregnancies. Each pregnancy carries the same chance of an infant affected by CF, regardless of the number of affected and nonaffected siblings of previous births (Fig. 26-3).

a A family with four children would include:

• The heterozygote parents (not affected)

• The sib who is a homozygote (is affected, has CF)

• The sib who does not carry the gene (not affected)

• The two sibs who are heterozygotes (not affected, but they carry the gene)

b The affected sib mates with a noncarrier of the gene. The offspring will carry the gene, but are not affected.

c The unaffected sib who carries the gene has union with a noncarrier. One half of the offspring will carry the gene, but not be affected. One half will not carry the gene nor be affected.

As can be seen from Fig. 26-3, the heterozygote carriers outnumber the homozygote-affected individuals. The normal siblings of CF heterozygote parents have a two-out-of-three chance of being carriers. Interfamily mating quadruples the risk of having an affected child; the more carriers who intermarry, the greater the risk of producing children with the disease.

4 The four types of single-gene disorders have more than 1500 known conditions associated with them. Since single-gene disorders are more easily studied, the probability of affected offsprings can be predicted.

5 Autosomal dominant disorders carry a 50% chance of reappearance, without regard for sex, for each individual pregnancy. If the affected individual has a negative family pedigree (a new appearance), the chance of reappearance in the offsprings is zero, but one half of the offspring risk being dominant carriers.

effect is expressed only in the presence of an identical pair of genes, it is called a recessive gene (or allele).

15 In a heterozygote, the dominant allele will express itself over the recessive allele. Recessive alleles express themselves when a homozygote possesses a pair of recessive alleles.

16 The primary method of genetic observation in humans is the construction of a family tree or *pedigree*. This will show family traits and their order of appearance (Fig. 26-2). These symbols will help the reader understand basic genetic charts.

17 The labels for the pedigree symbols that appear in Fig. 26-2 are as follows:

Normal male and normal female *(a)*

Normal mating *(b)*

Mating by related persons *(c)*

Individuals affected by the disease or trait *(d)*

Heterozygote individuals *(e)*

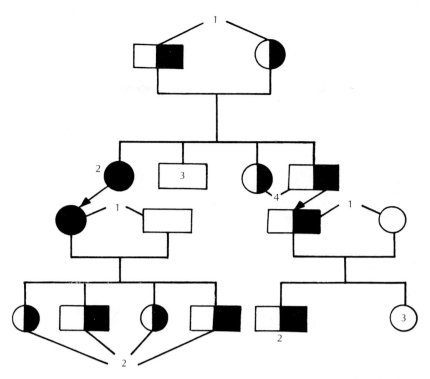

FIGURE 26-3 Genetic origination of cystic fibrosis. *1*, Noncarrier; *2*, unaffected offspring who carry the gene; *3*, offspring who are neither affected nor carry the gene; *4*, affected offspring.

6 Autosomal recessive disorders carry a 25% chance of reappearance with each individual pregnancy. Interfamily mating increases this risk.

7 X-linked (sex-linked) recessive disorders do not affect female siblings of the heterozygous females. One half of all male siblings carry the risk of being affected.

8 X-linked dominant disorders in affected females carry a 50% chance, regardless of sex, of reappearance. In an affected male with the disorder, all female siblings and no male siblings carry a chance of reappearance.

9 Some of the more notable single-gene disorders are albinism, hemophilia, sickle cell anemia, phenylketonuria, Huntington's chorea, and Tay-Sachs disease.

10 Other heredity-related disorders are the *multiple-gene* disorders.

11 Appearance of the disorder in a sibling with normal parents and no previous occurrence in the family tree carries a one-out-of-20 chance of another sibling being affected. Actually, the normal risk for any parent is about one out of 20 for this type of disorder to appear and offers a relatively good prognosis for future children.

12 Interfamily mating increases the risk of the multiple-gene type of disorder reappearing to one out of four.

13 Some disorders associated with multiple-gene defects are:

  a Cleft lip (harelip). A congenital anomaly consisting of one or more clefts in the upper lip resulting from the failure in the embryo of the maxillary and median nasal processes to close. Treatment is surgical repair in infancy.

  b Cleft palate. A congenital defect characterized by a fissure in the midline of the palate, resulting from the failure of the two sides to fuse during embryonic development. The fissure may be complete, extending through both the hard and soft palates into the nasal cavities, or it may show any degree of incomplete or partial cleft. The condition, which occurs approximately once in every 2500 live births and affects females more than males, is often associated with a cleft in the upper lip. Together, these abnormalities are the most common of the craniofacial malformations, accounting for half of the total number of defects. Feeding is best accomplished with special feeding devices.

  Surgical repair of the defect is usually not begun until the first or second year of life and is usually performed in steps. Care of the child requires a team approach that includes a plastic surgeon, orthodontist, dentist, nurse, speech and hearing therapists, and social workers. Long-term, postoperative problems, including speech impairment and hearing loss, improper tooth development and alignment, chronic respiratory and ear infections, and varying levels of emotional and social maladjustment may be largely avoided by modern techniques and reconstructive surgery.

  c Combination of items *a* and *b*.

  d Anencephaly. Congenital absence of the brain and spinal cord, in which the cranium does not close and the vertebral canal remains a groove. Transmitted genetically, anencephaly is not compatible with life.

It can be detected early in gestation by amniotic fluid tap and analysis or by ultrasonography.

e **Spina bifida.** Congenital neural tube defect characterized by a developmental anomaly in the posterior vertebral arch. Spina bifida is relatively common, occurring approximately 10 to 20 times per 1000 births. It may occur with only a small deformed lamina separated by a midline gap, or it may be associated with the complete absence of laminae surrounding a large area. In cases where the separation is wide enough, contents of the spinal canal protrude posteriorly, and a myelomeningocele is evident. This more serious deformity is associated with gross deficits not normally manifested in spina bifida. Neurologic deficits do not usually accompany the anomalies involving only bony deformity. Direct signs and symptoms are rarely noted in spina bifida, which is frequently diagnosed accidentally during radiographic examinations required for other reasons. Spina bifida that does not involve herniation of the meninges or the contents of the spinal canal rarely requires treatment. Also called spinal dysrhaphia.

f **Myelomeningocele.** A developmental defect of the central nervous system in which a hernial sac containing a portion of the spinal cord, its meninges, and cerebrospinal fluid protrudes through a congenital cleft in the vertebral column. The condition is caused primarily by the failure of the neural tube to close during embryonic development, although in some instances it may result from the reopening of the tube because of an abnormal increase in cerebrospinal fluid pressure. Also called meningomyelocele.

OBSERVATIONS: The defect, which occurs in approximately two in every 1000 live births, is readily apparent and easily diagnosed at birth. Although the opening may be located at any point along the spinal column, the anomaly characteristically occurs in the lumbar, low thoracic, or sacral region and extends for three to six vertebral segments. The saclike structure may be covered with a thin layer of skin or with a fine membrane that can be easily ruptured, increasing the risk of meningeal infection. The severity of neurologic dysfunction is directly related to the amount of neural tissue involved, which can be roughly estimated by the degree of the transillumination of the mass. Usually the condition is accompanied by varying degrees of paralysis of the lower extremities, by musculoskeletal defects (such as clubfoot, flexion and joint deformities, or hip dysplasia), and by anal and bladder sphincter dysfunction, which can lead to serious genitourinary disorders. Hydrocephalus, frequently related to the Arnold-Chiari malformation, is the most common anomaly associated with myelomeningocele and occurs in approximately 90% of the cases in which the spinal lesion is located in the lumbosacral region. In most cases hydrocephalus is apparent at birth, although it may appear shortly afterward.

Supplementary diagnostic procedures include x-ray examinations of the spine, skull, and chest to determine the extent of the vertebral defect and the presence of other malformations in other organ systems, a computerized axial tomographic (CT) scan of the brain to establish the ventricular size and the presence of any structural congenital anomalies, and laboratory examinations, especially urine analysis, culture, blood urea nitrogen evaluation, and creatinine clearance determination.

INTERVENTION: Supportive care and surgery are the only treatments for myelomeningocele, and they require a multidisciplinary approach involving specialists from neurology, neurosurgery, urology, pediatrics, orthopedics, rehabilitation, and physical therapy, as well as intensive nursing care. Initial treatment involves prevention of infection and assessment of neurologic involvement.

Immediate surgical repair is essential if the defect is causing cerebrospinal fluid leakage. However, surgical intervention may not be appropriate if neurologic involvement is extreme, if the lesion is infected, or if associated problems such as hydrocephalus are severe. When surgical repair of the spinal defect is recommended, associated problems are managed by appropriate measures, including shunt procedures for correction of hydrocephalus; antibiotic therapy to reduce the incidence of meningitis, urinary tract infections, and pneumonia; casting, bracing, traction, and surgical techniques for correction of hip, knee, and foot deformities; and prevention and treatment of renal complications.

Although improved surgical techniques and other treatment modalities have significantly increased the survival rate, these procedures cannot alter the major physical disability and deformity, mental retardation, and chronic urinary tract and pulmonary infections that afflict these children for life, nor can they alter the financial and emotional burden on and within the family. Prognosis is determined by the severity of neurologic involvement and the number of associated anomalies. With proper care and long-term maintenance, most children can survive and do well. Early death is usually caused by central nervous system infection or by hydrocephalus, whereas mortality in later childhood is caused by urinary tract infection, renal failure, complications from shunt therapy, or pulmonary disease.

NURSING CONSIDERATIONS: Care of the child with a spinal defect entails both immediate and long-term nursing goals. Immediate care centers on the prevention of local infection and trauma by careful handling and positioning of the infant, applying sterile moist dressings to the membranous sac, avoiding fecal contamination and breakdown of sensitive skin areas, and maintaining warmth, proper nutrition, and adequate hydration and electrolyte balance. Gentle range of motion exercises are carried out to prevent or minimize hip and lower extremity deformity. An important function of the nurse is to involve the parents in the care of the infant as soon as adequate home care is arranged, including how to observe for signs of complications. The nurse also helps the parents in long-term management by planning activities appropriate to the developmental age and physical limitations of the child, by providing information for teaching all family members about the condition, and, if appropriate, by assisting with placement in schools that can accommodate the special needs of handicapped children.

g Variety of congenital cardiac anomalies. Any structural or functional abnormalities or defect of the heart or great vessels existing from birth. Congenital heart disease is a major cause of neonatal distress and is the most common cause of death in the newborn, other than problems related to prematurity. The incidence of congenital cardiovascular anomalies is 8 to 10 per 1000 live births, with the mortality greatest in the neonatal period. Approximately 90% of all deaths from congenital heart disease occur during the first year of life. Congenital heart defects may result from genetic causes, primarily single-gene mutations and chromosomal aberrations, or from environmental factors, such as maternal infection or exposure to radiation or noxious substances during pregnancy. Most defects are probably a result of some interaction between genetic and environmental factors that results in arrested embryonic development. Congenital heart anomalies are classified broadly according to the resulting alteration in circulation as either acyanotic, in which no unoxygenated blood mixes in the systemic system, or cyanotic, in which unoxygenated blood enters the systemic system. The general effects of cardiac malformations on cardiovascular functioning are increased cardiac workload, involving either systolic or diastolic overloading, increased pulmonary vascular resistance, inadequate systemic cardiac output, and decreased oxygen saturation from the shunting of unoxygenated blood directly into the systemic system.

The general physical symptoms of these pathophysiologic alterations are growth retardation, decreased exercise tolerance, recurrent respiratory infections, dyspnea, tachypnea, tachycardia, cyanosis, tissue hypoxia, and murmurs, all of which vary in severity depending on the type and degree of the defect.

Kinds of congenital cardiac anomalies include aortic stenosis, atrial septal defect, coarctation of the aorta, patent ductus arteriosus, pulmonic stenosis, Fallot's tetralogy, transposition of the great vessels, tricuspid atresia, truncus arteriosus, and ventricular septal defect.

h Clubfoot. A congenital deformity of the foot, sometimes resulting from intrauterine constriction and characterized by unilateral or bilateral deviation of the metatarsal bones of the forefoot. Of all clubfoot deformities, 95% are equinovarus, characterized by medial deviation and plantar flexion of the forefoot, but a few are calcaneovalgus, characterized by lateral deviation and dorsiflexion. Treatment depends on the extent and rigidity of the deformity. Splints and casts in infancy may produce complete correction; surgery in several steps may be necessary to achieve normal function.

i Congenital hip dislocation. A congenital orthopedic defect in which the head of the femur does not articulate with the acetabulum, owing to an abnormal shallowness of the acetabulum. Treatment consists of maintaining continuous abduction of the thigh so that the head of the femur presses into the center of the shallow cavity, causing it to deepen. It is also called congenital dysplasia of the hip and congenital subluxation of the hip.

j Idiopathic epilepsy. Epilepsy without a known cause. An idiopathic disease may have a recognizable pattern of signs and symptoms, and it may be curable, but its cause is not known. It may be a group of neurologic disorders characterized by recurrent episodes of convulsive seizures, sensory disturbances, abnormal behavior, loss of consciousness, or all of these. Common to all types of epilepsy is an uncontrolled electrical discharge from the nerve cells of the cerebral cortex. Although most epilepsy is of unknown cause, it may sometimes be associated with cerebral trauma, intracranial infection, brain tumor, vascular disturbances, intoxication, or chemical imbalance. Kinds of epilepsy include grand mal epilepsy, jacksonian epilepsy, petit mal epilepsy, and psychomotor epilepsy.

OBSERVATIONS: The frequency of attacks may range from several times a day to intervals of several years. In predisposed individuals, seizures may occur during sleep or after physical stimulation, such as by a flickering light or sudden loud sound. Emotional disturbances also may be significant trigger factors. Some seizures are preceded by an aura, but others have no warning symptoms. Most epileptic attacks are brief. They may be localized or general, with or without clonic movements, and are often followed by drowsiness or confusion. Diagnosis is made by observation of the pattern of seizures and abnormalities on an electroencephalogram.

INTERVENTION: The kind of epilepsy determines the selection of preventive medication. Correctable lesions and metabolic causes are eliminated when possible. During an attack the patient should be protected from injury without being severely restrained.

NURSING CONSIDERATIONS: A person observing an epileptic attack, in addition to protecting the patient from injury, should carefully note and accurately describe the sequence of seizure activity. The patient and family must be fully informed and counseled about the disorder, the importance of regularly taking prescribed medication, never discontinuing treatment without professional advice, toxic effects of

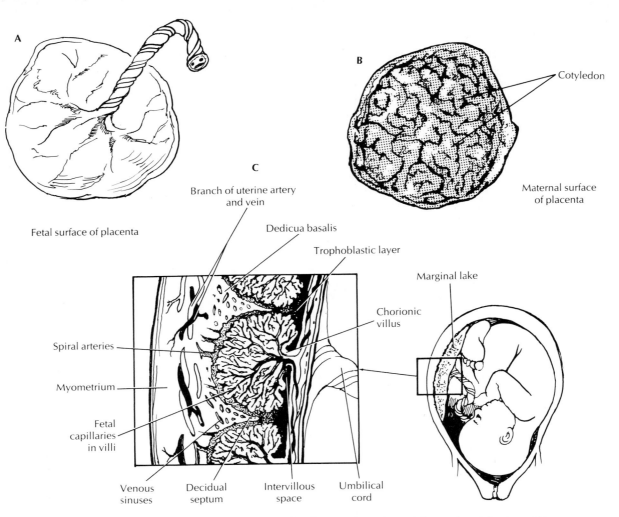

FIGURE 26-4 Normal placenta. (Reprinted with permission of Ross Laboratories, Columbus, OH 43216 from Clinical Educ. Aid # 12, June 1978.)

medication, wearing a medical identification tag, and continuing to live as normal a life as possible. Health professionals also have a responsibility to help improve the public's attitude toward epilepsy and to correct misunderstanding, which limits educational and occupational opportunities for patients with this diagnosis.

14 Some disorders seem to appear by pure chance and cannot be definitely linked to any specific cause. These are the *chromosomal abnormality defects*.

a This type of disorder is demonstrated by structural defects of the chromosome, an extra chromosome, or a deleted chromosome.

b Some examples are Down's syndrome (extra chromosome on 21st pair) and Turner's syndrome (absence or any partial presence of one of the X chromosomes in the female).

4.0 FETAL DEVELOPMENT OF THE CARDIOPULMONARY SYSTEM

4.1 The placenta

1 The placenta shape is round (the Latin meaning "flat cake") and weighs approximately one sixth (15%) of the fetus weight. Its size is about 6 to 8 inches in diam-

eter and about 1 inch thick. During pregnancy it occupies one third of the intrauterine surface.

2 The placenta is the point at which, in normal pregnancies, maternal and fetal circulation meet (Fig. 26-4, *A*, *B*, and *C*. See also Fig. 26-11). One side of the placenta is anchored into the uterine wall until labor. The other side is covered with a shiny surface called the amniotic membrane, with the umbilical cord centered. In some pregnancies abnormalities may occur, causing the placenta to be improperly located or partially or completely detached (prematurely) from the uterine wall (Fig. 26-5, *A* through *F*).

3 The placenta has 15 to 20 segments called cotyledons, each containing the chorionic villi and intervillous space—the site of blood exchange.

4 Chorionic villi are fingerlike structures that begin to develop within the first week. Each of these structures consists of a core of fetal capillaries covered by epithelial tissue. During growth the chorionic villi erode the uterine vessels and tissues, resulting in maternal blood surrounding the structures. These sites are called intervillous spaces. The intervillous space is the site of maternal and fetal circulation exchange. The blood does

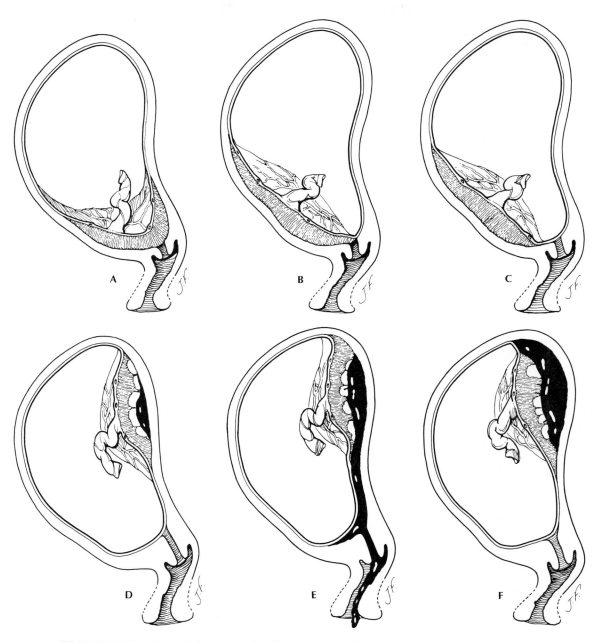

F I G U R E   2 6 - 5 A, Total placenta previa. Placenta completely covers internal os. **B,** Placenta previa marginalis (partial). Placenta partially covers internal cervical os. **C,** Placenta previa lateralis. Placenta lies just within the lower uterine segment. **D,** Abruptio placentae (partial). Premature separation of placenta with concealed bleeding. **E,** Abruptio placentae (partial). Premature separation of placenta with obvious bleeding. **F,** Abruptio placentae (complete). Complete premature separation of the placenta with concealed bleeding. (Reprinted with permission of Ross Laboratories, Columbus, OH 43216 from Clinical Educ. Aid # 12, June 1978.)

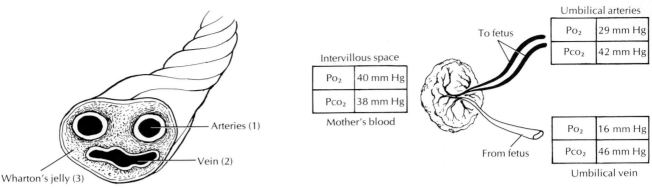

FIGURE 26-6 Cross-section of umbilical cord showing vein, arteries, and Wharton's jelly.

FIGURE 26-7 Placental gas exchange.

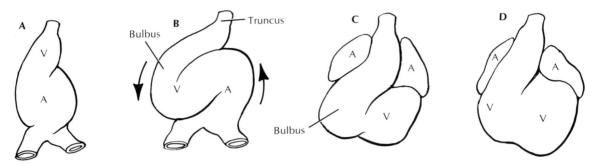

FIGURE 26-8 Early development of the heart. **A,** Early in the third week of gestation. **B,** Late in the third week of gestation. **C** and **D,** The four-chambered heart is formed between the fourth and eighth weeks of gestation.

not normally cross over, but provides an area for substance change.

5 The path of exchange from mother to fetus is through the epithelial layer of the chorionic villi, then the epithelial wall of the fetal capillary into the fetal blood.

6 The chorionic villi reduce in size but largely increase in number during the pregnancy to provide for increased fetal requirements for growth.

7 Maternal blood is provided to the intervillous space by spiral arterioles. At term, about 100 arteries provide blood to the placenta. Deoxygenated blood leaves the intervillous space by venous orifices adjacent to the spiral arteries. Intervillous space flow is by higher arterial pressure to a lower venous one. Spiral artery pressure is 70 to 80 mm Hg, whereas venous pressure is 8 mm Hg.

8 Fig. 26-5 (*A* through *F*) shows complications that can occur with the placenta.

4.2 The umbilical cord

1 The cross-sectional drawing on Fig. 26-6 shows:
  a Two thick-walled and muscular arteries *(1)*.
  b One vein that has thinner walls and is larger than the two arteries *(2)*.
  c A surrounding white gel called Wharton's jelly *(3)*.

2 Incoming blood from the umbilical arteries branches to each cotyledon. At the intervillous space, gas and nutritional exchange occur. Oxygenation of fetal blood,

as well as the exchange of carbon dioxide, occurs at the intervillous space (Fig. 26-7). The exchange site is normally 3.5 to 5.5 microns (μm) thick between the maternal and fetal blood.

4.3 Fetal circulation

To understand cardiac and pulmonary function, the reader must have a basic understanding of cardiac development and fetal circulation.

1 Before the third week of embryonic development, the embryo's needs are satisfied by simple diffusion. After the third week, the heart develops rapidly as a result of greatly increased growth and nutritional needs.

2 During the third week, the heart is composed of a single tube with two layers: the endocardium and the epimyocardidium (Fig. 26-8, *A*).

3 Growth continues rapidly, and the "heart" bends at its middle, with future cardiac features beginning to be recognizable (Fig. 26-8, *B*).

4 The four-chambered heart is formed between the fourth and eighth weeks (Fig. 26-8, *C* and *D*).

5 Internally, the simple heart's atria are formed and divided by the septum primum (Fig. 26-9, *A1*). The small hole left between the atria is called the foramen primum *(2)*.

6 Soon another opening appears in the septum primum, called the foramen secundum *(B3)*. As the septum primum continues to grow from the endocardial cushion

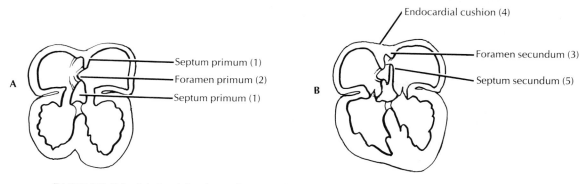

FIGURE 26-9 Atria of developing heart are divided by septum primum, which undergoes further development. (Reprinted with permission of Ross Laboratories, Columbus, OH 43216 from Clinical Educ. Aid # 12, June 1978.)

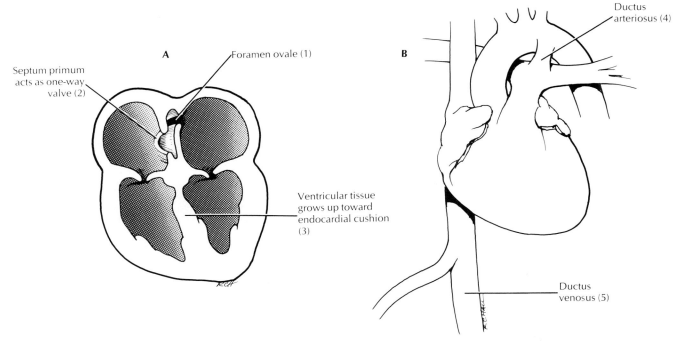

FIGURE 26-10 A, Development of septum secundum and foramen ovale. **B,** Ductus arteriosus: communication between the aorta and pulmonary artery.

(4), the foramen primum is obliterated, and only the opening between the atria is the foramen secundum.

7 A second septum begins to grow beside the septum primum *(5)* and is called the septum secundum.

The septum secundum lies to the right of the septum primum and grows downward from the top of the heart and upward from the endocardial cushion (Fig. 26-10, *A* and *B*). These two parts do not grow together but leave an opening called the *foramen ovale (1),* which permits blood flow between the atria.

8 The blood flow through the foramen ovale is one way, always going from right to left, because the septum primum acts as a one-way valve *(2).* This one-way flow provides for oxygenated blood from the mother to go to those fetal tissues needing the most oxygen.

9 The ventricles separate completely about a week after atrial septation. The floor of the ventricular tissue grows upward toward the endocardial cushion *(3).*

10 An important communication between the aorta and pulmonary artery is the *ductus arteriosus* (Fig. 26-10, *B4*).

11 The ductus arteriosus shunts blood away from the pulmonary system before birth. Together with the foramen ovale, the two fetal shunts prevent the lungs from being perfused before birth.

12 The freshly oxygenated blood arriving from the placenta is mixed with low oxygen-saturated blood returning from the gut and lower extremities at the *ductus venosus (5)* and the inferior vena cava.

13 Before going further into fetal circulation, the reader should note the following facts.

a The fetal blood flow has three normally occurring shunts:
  • The foramen ovale
  • The ductus arteriosus
  • The ductus venosus and inferior vena cava junction

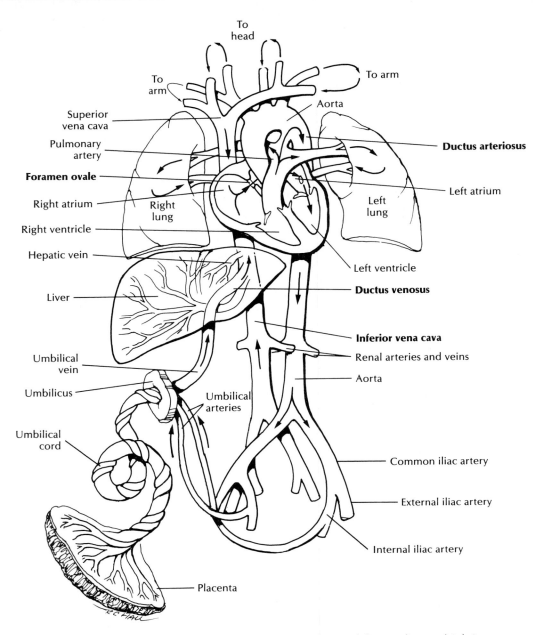

FIGURE 26-11 Fetal circulation showing blood flow from umbilicus to liver and inferior vena cava via the ductus venosus. (Reprinted with permission of Ross Laboratories, Columbus, OH 43216 from Clinical Educ. Aid # 1, June 1978.)

  b Fetal circulation utilizes placental circulation.
  c Only 3% to 7% of the fetal cardiac output flows into the fetal lungs.
14 Oxygenated blood from the chorionic villi flows through the umbilical vein, entering the fetus through the *umbilicus* (naval) (Fig. 26-11). Some blood goes to the liver, but the rest passes through the *ductus venosus* to the inferior vena cava.
15 Blood enters the heart through the inferior vena cava, and flow is divided by the natural opening between the two atria called the *foramen ovale.*
16 Some blood mixes with blood from the superior vena cava in the right atrium, creating a decreased oxygen tension (P_{O_2}) in the admixture. This admixture enters the right ventricle and then the pulmonary artery.
17 Some of this blood (3% to 7%) flows through the pulmonary vascular system, but the majority (93% to 97%) is shunted away through the ductus arteriosus to the descending aorta, continuing to the umbilical arteries to return to the placenta.
18 The reasons for this shunt occurrence follow.
  a High pulmonary vascular resistance in the fetus creates back pressure, and blood will flow along the path of least resistance.
  b The ductus arteriosus is large and fibrotic. It is approximately the same diameter as the aorta.

c The low P_{O_2} of the admixture causes the ductus arteriosus to dilate.

d The low P_{O_2} causes the pulmonary artery to constrict.

19 Although some blood flows to the right atrium, the major portion flows directly through the foramen ovale into the left atrium. At the left atrium the small amount of blood that passed through the pulmonary vasculature mixes with the major blood flow. This blood now enters the left ventricle to the ascending aorta, then to the aortic arch for distribution to the fetus.

20 At the moment of birth, critical physiologic changes begin to take place. Providing the lungs are mature and ready for gas exchange, the alveoli open and blood flow through the lungs increases (Fig. 26-12).

21 The increased pulmonary blood flow and resultant decreased pulmonary vascular resistance cause the left atrial pressure to increase.

22 As the left atrial pressure rises, the right atrial pressure falls. The foramen ovale, which has been permitting only right-to-left flow, is "pushed shut" by the new pressure differential.

23 With increasing oxygen saturation and the following pulmonary resistance changes, the ductus arteriosus constricts and this shunt is soon closed.

24 After the umbilical cord has been tied and cut, the arteries and veins used for moving fetal blood to the placenta are no longer of any use, and they deteriorate into ligaments. Likewise, the tissue forming the ductus arteriosus shrivels to form the ligamentum arteriosum.

4.4 Fetal blood and sampling

1 The hemoglobin of the fetal blood (HbF) differs in structure from adult hemoglobin. Refer to Module Four for a discussion of adult hemoglobin.

2 Fetal hemoglobin is capable of combining and dissociating oxygen at lower tensions than adult hemoglobin. This is probably because 2,3-diphosphoglycerate (2,3-DPG) does not normally bind to HbF.

3 The pH of fetal blood has been found to be the best correlating parameter in predicting fetal overall condition through birth. Normal fetal capillary pH is about 7.35. If it is found to be less than 7.20, this is indicative of fetal distress.

4 pH is an excellent prediction parameter because blood gases vary widely in range, but hypoxia results in anaerobic metabolism, producing lactic acidosis, and hypercapnia results in carbonic acidosis, both contributing to pH predicting the presence of one or both of these events.

5 The most common misleading event resulting in a false reading is acidosis of the maternal blood exchanging with the fetal blood. To differentiate this, an arterial blood gas (ABG) analysis is done from the mother's blood and compared with the fetal capillary blood gas. Sampling is done from capillary blood of the presenting part of the fetus, usually a scalp vein. In a high-risk infant, pH and other parameters are used to assess the need for interference with labor.

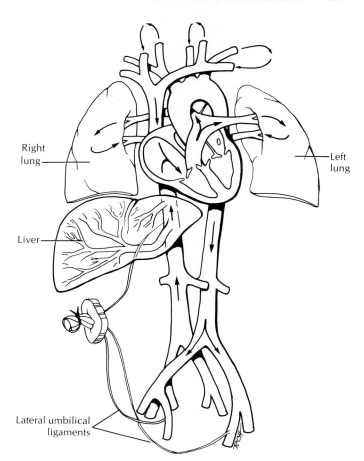

F I G U R E 2 6 - 1 2 Physiologic changes in circulation at the moment of birth.

4.5 Amniocentesis

1 Amniocentesis is the introduction of a needle into the amniotic cavity through the uterine and abdominal walls and withdrawing a sample of the fluid.

2 This sample can then be tested:

a For the severity of Rh incompatibility (erythroblastosis fetalis).

b For prediction of the presence of hyaline membrane disease (idiopathic respiratory distress syndrome, IRDS).

c To detect certain genetic disorders.

d To determine fetal age.

e For various other monitoring tests of the fetus.

3 Amniocentesis is a relatively safe procedure and can be performed as early as the twelfth week of gestation. Amniotic fluid testing for bilirubin is used to assess and plan therapy for Rh incompatibility (Fig. 26-13, *A, B,* and *C*).

a *Bilirubin* is a product of red cell breakdown and is abnormally high in the amniotic fluid of a fetus with Rh incompatibility.

b The bilirubin levels are plotted on a specific graph that shows regions of various levels of involvement in order that therapy can be planned.

c Results plotted in the *severe region* are indicative of the need for a fetal transfusion in the uterus or termination of the pregnancy.

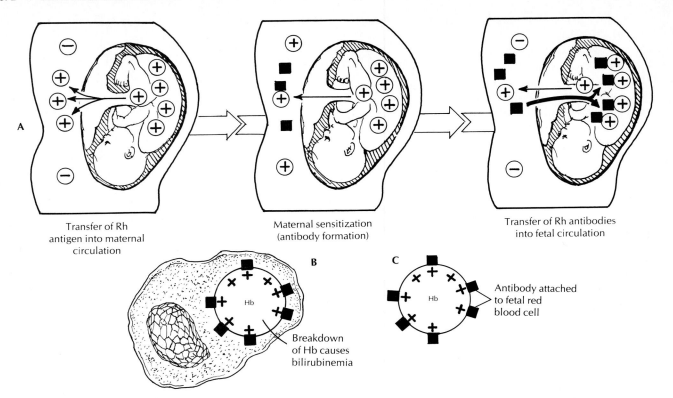

FIGURE 26-13 A, Rh incompatibility. **B** and **C,** Destruction of fetal red blood cell. (Reprinted with permission of Ross Laboratories, Columbus, OH 43216 from Clinical Educ. Aid # 12, June 1978.)

d If the results of testing fall in the *moderate region,* only frequent serial testing for monitoring the course is indicated.

e Results in the *mild region* indicate that no therapy is needed until after birth, when effective therapy will then be instituted.

f One often false positive determination is that hyperbilirubinemic mothers will have an abnormally high level in the amniotic fluid, but the fetus is not affected by erythroblastosis fetalis.

4 *Creatinine levels* are sometimes used in conjunction with other parameters to determine fetal age.

    a Creatinine is excreted from the fetal kidneys through the urine into the amniotic fluid.

    b The creatinine levels in the amniotic fluid increase with fetal age and in uncomplicated pregnancies carry a high degree of reliability of prediction of fetal age.

    c In complicated pregnancies, such as a toxemic mother or Rh incompatibility, the amniotic fluid creatinine levels may be elevated or decreased and thus lead to false fetal age predictions.

5 *Lecithin sphingomyelin (L/S) ratio* is a reliable test for fetal lung maturity.

    a Fluid from the fetal lung disperses into the amniotic fluid. The fluid contains surfactant, a polyphospholipid substance necessary for proper lung function after birth.

TABLE 26-1 Fetal being at stages of maturity

Gestation	L/S relationship
22-24 weeks	Lecithin concentrations are measurable and slightly higher than sphingomyelin concentrations. Sphingomyelin will remain at a fairly constant level, whereas lecithin concentrations will rise.
28-32 weeks	Lecithin levels will rise to 1²⁄₁₀ that of sphingomyelin or an L/S ratio of 1:1.2.
35 weeks	Lecithin level double that of a sphingomyelin (L/S ratio = 2), indicative of fetal lung maturity.

    b The determination of the ratio of two constituents of surfactant (lecithin and sphingomyelin) is used to determine fetal lung maturity (Table 26-1).

    c The graph in Fig. 26-14 shows that the lecithin *(solid line)* and the sphingomyelin *(dotted line)* ratio increases to 1.2 at 28 weeks and to 2 or more at 35 weeks. This increase predicts a low chance for the occurrence of postnatal hyaline membrane disease.

6 The presence of meconium, which is a thick, tarry substance present in the intestinal tract of the fetus, in amniotic fluid is indicative of fetal stress.

    a The postnatal complication known as *meconium aspiration* syndrome results from meconium being deposited deep in the fetal lung before birth.

    b The syndrome is often severe, requiring mechanical ventilation, and occasionally leads to death.

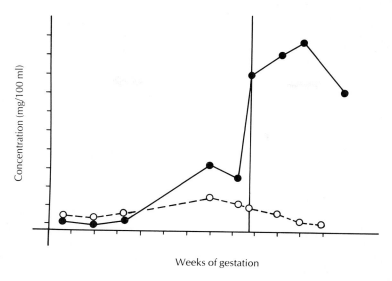

FIGURE 26-14 Levels of lecithin *(solid line)* and sphingomyelin *(dotted line)* in the amniotic fluid during fetal development.

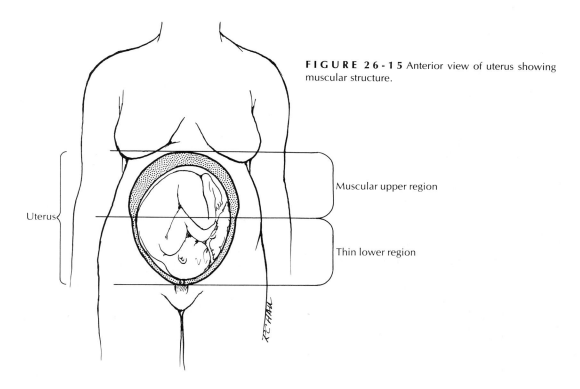

FIGURE 26-15 Anterior view of uterus showing muscular structure.

5.0 ANATOMIC AND PHYSIOLOGIC CHANGES OF THE CARDIOPULMONARY SYSTEM THAT OCCUR AT BIRTH

5.1 Normal labor and delivery

1 Labor is usually classified into three stages: (Figs. 26-15 and 26-16).

   a *First stage* begins with the initial dilation of the cervix and ends with the cervix completely dilated *(A)*.

   b *Second stage* begins with the expulsion of the fetus and ends with the birth of the infant *(B and C)*.

   c *Third stage* starts with placental expulsion and ends when the placenta is delivered (not shown).

2 The upper region of the uterus is more muscular than the lower region. This helps to propel the fetus toward the cervical canal (Fig. 26-15).

3 Before the onset of labor, the cervical canal is only a few millimeters across. At the completion of the *first stage,* it will dilate to about *10 centimeters* (cm). The cervical canal becomes wider and has thinner walls as a result of the cervix being pulled upward until it is part of the uterine wall. This is caused by repeated uterine *contractions.*

4 With the second stage, presentation of the fetus usually

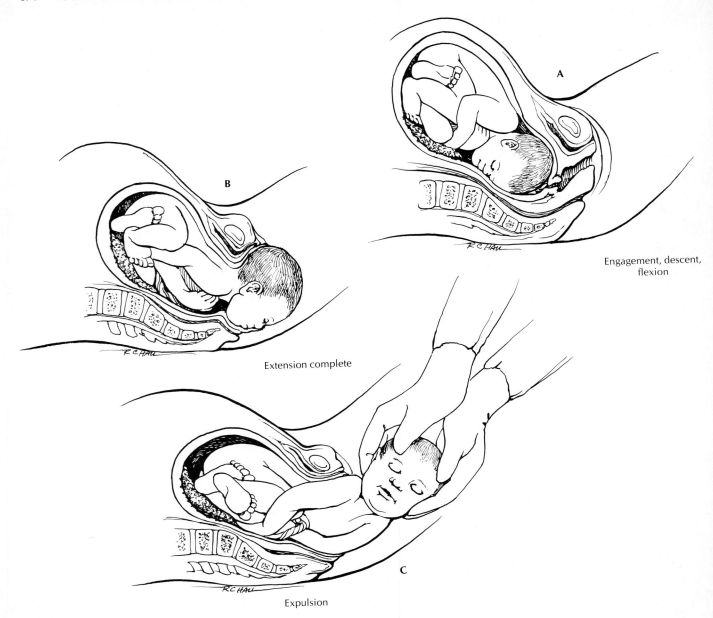

A

Engagement, descent, flexion

B

Extension complete

C

Expulsion

FIGURE 26-16 Cross section of uterus with fetus positioning for delivery (**A** through **C**). (Reprinted with permission of Ross Laboratories, Columbus, OH 43216 from Clinical Educ. Aid # 1, June 1978.)

begins after cervical dilation is complete. Uterine contractions and maternal abdominal muscle contractions against a fixed diaphragm (Valsalva's maneuver) begin to propel the fetus through the cervical canal.

a Normally the head will present first, face down.

b Next, the body of the fetus will rotate 90 degrees to accommodate the passage of the shoulders. The upper shoulder usually passes first, then the lower one.

c After the shoulders are through the cervical canal, the rest of the body is delivered rapidly.

d The cord is cut and clamped, leaving the remainder attached to the placenta.

e The *third stage* begins after the *birth* of the baby as uterine contractions continue to dislodge the placenta from the uterine wall.

• This stage is completed with expulsion of the placenta through the cervical canal.

5 *Examination* of a newborn infant will normally show skin that is thin, dry, and has visible veins; and there is often downy hair. If the infant cries, the skin flushes, and the veins of the head swell and throb.

a The head of the infant appears too big for the body. It may be temporarily malformed because of pressure at birth. There are two soft spots (fontanels) on the head. One is located above the brow; the other is close to the crown on the back of the head.

b The feet feel loose and wrinkled, attached to short legs that are drawn up against the body.

c The trunk is topped with a short neck with small sloping shoulders. The breasts are usually swollen. The abdomen, with the umbilical stump, is large and round.

d The pelvis and hips are slender and narrow; the genitals appear oversized for both sexes.

e The hands are normally held in a fist. The palms have fine lines; the wrist has deep creases, and the skin is loose fitting. The nails are very thin and dry.

f The neonate's face has pudgy cheeks, a broad flat nose, a receding chin, and an undersized lower jaw. The eyes appear dark blue with puffy lids. The ears are usually paper thin and flat against the head.

6 The fluid in fetal lungs differs from amniotic fluid by a lower protein concentration and is less viscous.

7 A term infant will have approximately 24 million alveoli. After 3 months this number will increase to approximately 77 million. The size of an alveolus of an infant is 50 μm in diameter, whereas the average adult size is 200 to 300 μm in diameter. The infant's is $\frac{1}{20}$ surface area for gas exchange of that of an adult. See Module Eight for a discussion of fetal lung development.

8 Recently it has been shown that the fetus has sporadic breathing patterns in utero and that there is tidal transfer of amniotic fluid. This fact is evidenced in part by the occasional presence of meconium in the infant's lungs. The infant's intrauterine breathing patterns have been detected as early as 13 weeks' gestation and vary in rate from 30 to 70/min.

5.2 Fetus-to-birth transition

1 Several important events occur in the lungs at birth.

a The movement of air by the lungs has to begin.

b This air has to overcome the fluid and physiologic resistance to lung expansion.

c The functional residual capacity (FRC) has to be established by some air remaining in the expanded lungs.

d The pulmonary vascular flow must drastically increase, and cardiac output must be redistributed.

2 No *single* factor has been identified to initiate air movement by the lungs.

a One factor that is being investigated is that intrauterine breathing patterns continue after birth. This idea still does not explain the first few forceful breaths shortly after birth.

b Asphyxia at birth is another possible initiator of air movement, and asphyxia is present to some extent in most normal births. A significant number of infants have an O_2 saturation of less than 10%; some have no measurable oxygen at all.

c The average carbon dioxide tension (P_{CO_2}) during birth is almost 60 mm Hg, decreasing the pH to

7.24, with a normal buffer base indicating respiratory acidosis.

d These changes (acidosis, hypercapnia, and hypoxia) activate the aortic and carotid chemoreceptors, causing nerve signals to be sent to the respiratory center in the medulla. Prolonged asphyxia, indicated by a decreased buffer base (metabolic acidosis), may provide the initial stimulation to begin air movement.

e It is thought that the decrease of the ambient temperature once the infant is extrauterine may initiate air movement. The intrauterine temperature is 37° C (98.6° F), whereas delivery rooms are in the 18° to 24° C (64° to 75° F) range. This rapid drop in ambient temperature activates dermal nerve endings, causing nerve signals to be sent to the respiratory center in the medulla and may explain the first few forceful respirations after birth. This response is similar to the gasp one makes when jumping into cold water.

f The continual decline of the newborn's core temperature (about 0.2° F/min) is believed to further stimulate breathing. However, accidental or intentional rapid cooling will cause respiratory depression because of cold stress.

g This idea is supported by experiments with lambs. When lambs are delivered into a saline bath heated to their normal intrauterine temperature instead of ambient temperature, the lambs failed to initiate respiratory movements.

h The normal tactile stimulation by handling during delivery is not believed to be a major factor in initiating respiration. Contrary to popular belief, slapping of the soles of the feet or buttocks has been found to be of little value in initiating breathing in a depressed infant.

3 The two most important factors of resistance to air entering the lungs are (a) alveolar surface tension and (b) the viscosity of fluid in the lungs.

a The small alveoli of a newborn have a greater tendency to collapse (Laplace's law) as a result of increased forces of surface tension. Surfactant in the alveoli reduces this surface tension.

b The main function of surfactant is to maintain residual expansion at end expiration after air has entered the alveoli. Without surfactant, alveolar collapse would occur (atelectasis).

4 For over 30 years scientists have known that fetal lungs *secrete a fluid separate from the amniotic fluid.* This lung fluid is a major resistance to air movement of the first few forceful breaths.

a Some of this fluid (30 to 40 ml) is ejected from the lungs as the chest is compressed, passing through the birth canal (vaginal squeeze). As the chest reexpands after it has passed through the canal, some air (7 to 42 ml) is pulled into the upper airway to replace the ejected fluid. Most of this fluid is removed across the alveoli-capillary membrane and by the lymph drainage.

b Experiments have shown an increased time for fluid removal with delivery by cesarean section rather than vaginal delivery.

5 After the first breath at the end of expiration, in normal infants, 40% of the full lung volume will remain, establishing the *functional residual capacity* (FRC).

a FRC is partially established by the first breath and will continue to increase until it reaches its maximum point about 3 hours after birth. Surfactant plays a significant part in establishing FRC.

b A high inspiratory pressure (60 to 80 cm H_2O) is required with the first breath to expand the lungs. With establishment of FRC, the second and succeeding breaths do not require this high pressure (i.e., each successive breath requires decreasing effort).

c In the absence of surfactant, FRC is not fully established, and each breath will continue to require a high opening pressure, increasing the work of breathing (a factor in idiopathic respiratory distress syndrome) and soon exhausting the infant.

6 There are critical changes that must occur in the cardiovascular system, coincidental with lung changes, to accommodate extrauterine life.

a Since the placental circulation is a low-resistance component of fetal systemic circulation, the clamping of the umbilical cord produces certain changes:

- The total intravascular area is significantly reduced (40% to 50%), which results in an increasing aortic blood pressure and a small decrease in venous pressures.

b As previously mentioned, fetal pulmonary vascular resistance is high, allowing only 3% to 7% of the cardiac output to perfuse the pulmonary capillaries. As the first few breaths enter the lungs, this resistance drops drastically (80% from fetal levels), and pulmonary blood flow increases five times more than the fetal perfusion levels. This phenomenon is believed to result from the elimination of fluid by compression of the arterioles and vasodilation from increasing O_2 tensions because of air entering the lungs.

c A gradual reduction in the infant's pulmonary vascular resistance will continue during the first 6 to 8 weeks after birth. The increased systemic resistance and pressure, along with the decreased pulmonary vascular resistance, cause blood flow similar to the adult circulatory flow.

d Now that this flow pattern is established, the normal fetal shunts begin to close. The foramen ovale is a flap of tissue that connects the right and left atria. It opens in only one direction, to the left atrium, and is governed by pressure gradients (one-way valve effect). Refer to Unit 4.3.

e In fetal circulation, pulmonary vascular resistance is high, producing a higher right atrial pressure than the left. This causes the foramen ovale to remain open.

f With the changeover from fetal to neonatal circulatory patterns, the left atrial pressure (systemic pressure) becomes higher than the right atrial pressure (venous pressure), causing functional closure of the foramen ovale.

g The *foramen ovale* will not automatically close for several months, since it is kept closed only by a higher pressure gradient. A sudden reversal of the pressure gradient (e.g., asphyxia) can cause the foramen ovale to reopen.

h The muscular *ductus arteriosus* can constrict to the point of total occlusion of the lumen. Constriction normally occurs as a response to increased O_2 tension levels after the initial breaths of the infant. The vasoconstriction response of the ductus to increased O_2 tensions is opposed by vasodilation response of the pulmonary artery to the same stimulus. This phenomenon creates the flow of least resistance through the pulmonary artery to the pulmonary vascular bed. It should be noted that any failure to increase O_2 tensions (e.g., IRDS) will cause the ductus to remain patent. Functional closure of the ductus usually occurs by 15 hours after birth, and anatomic closure (fibrosis) usually occurs within 3 weeks. As with the foramen ovale, functional closure of the ductus may reopen with decreased O_2 tensions; prematurity increases the chance of this occurrence.

i In the fetal circulation the *ductus venosus* is a connection between placenta, intestinal venous circulation, and the inferior vena cava. After birth, this channel has minimum blood flow through it, and within 3 to 7 days fibrotic anatomic closure of the ductus venosus will occur. The reason for this closure is not known at this time.

6.0 THE NEONATAL ENVIRONMENT, ISOLETTES, AND ASEPTIC PRINCIPLES OF THE NURSERY

6.1 Thermoregulation

1 Humans can maintain a narrow range for core (or deep) body temperature, regardless of changes in surrounding temperature. This characteristic is known as being *homothermic*.

2 The newborn infant reacts to surrounding temperature as a *poikilotherm* (e.g., a reptile). This is to say the infant's temperature changes in response to the surrounding temperature.

3 Thermoregulation is maintained by both heat loss and heat production. An imbalance of either will cause disturbances in the core temperature.

4 Fever is an example of these principles. When there is increased heat production in response to an initiating mechanism (infection, etc.) and heat production increases more than the mechanisms to promote heat loss (perspiration), the core temperature will rise.

5 Newborns, particularly premature and low birth weight term infants, have an imbalance in their thermoregulatory system. The newborn has adequate mechanisms of heat production, but heat *loss is far greater* than the levels of heat produced. The change from uterine to room temperature can be a hazard for newborns, especially small and sick ones.

6 The transfer of heat from the body to the surrounding area occurs through four principles of thermoexchange.

a *Convection*

- Convective transfer, in context of this discussion, means the loss of the infant's heat to the surrounding cooler air.
- Convective heat loss is increased when the surrounding air is flowing rapidly (draft).
- Infants should not be placed near air vents or drafty windows, as this promotes convective heat loss.

b *Radiation*

- Radiant transfer is a loss of the infant's heat to cooler surrounding solid objects that are *not* in direct contact with the infant (see Module Fourteen).
- An important principle of radiant heat transfer is that it is not related to the temperature of the surrounding air. To demonstrate this principle, observe the loss of heat by radiant transfer of an infant in a closed chamber, such as an Isolette.
- The closed Isolette does not allow for high air flows circulating through it, giving the impression that it is an adequately thermoregulated environment. However, if the closed Isolette were placed next to a drafty window, convection air currents would cool the walls of the Isolette. In spite of normal temperature readings of the air inside the Isolette, the heat transfer gradient by radiation from the child would be increased to the cooler Isolette walls.

c *Evaporation*

- Evaporative transfer is a loss of the infant's heat occurring during the vaporization of liquid on the infant's body surface (similar to perspiration in the adult, although infants do not noticeably perspire).
- Evaporative cooling occurs when an individual steps out of the water after a swim. Relative humidity influences the rate of vaporization (evaporation), as seen on days with a high relative humidity when water is slower to evaporate than on a day of low humidity.
- An infant is born covered with amniotic fluid. Unless the infant is dried promptly with warm dry towels, the evaporation of the fluid is enhanced by the dry, cool air in an air-conditioned delivery room. This rapid rate of evaporation promotes a rapid rate of heat loss from the infant.
- By the same principle, a newborn should not be bathed until body temperature is fully stablized in the normal range.

d *Conduction*

- Conductive transfer is a loss of the infant's heat to cooler solid objects that are in *direct* contact with the infant.
- Placing the naked infant on cold scales or on a cold x-ray cassette promotes conductive heat loss. This can be easily prevented by placing a diaper or receiving blanket between the infant and the cooler object.

6.2 Natural factors affecting heat loss

1 The body of the newborn is a factor in heat loss, especially in low weight and sick infants. As previously mentioned, the newborn has adequate heat production capability, the problem being heat loss in excess of production.

2 The major reason for this heat loss is the infant's body weight to body surface area relationship. When body surface area is relatively larger than body weight, heat transfer is increased.

3 A full-term newborn will have $\frac{1}{20}$ (5%) of an adult's weight and $\frac{1}{6}$ (15%) of an adult's body surface area. This large difference in body surface area to body weight provides a large surface for heat loss to the surrounding area.

4 Low birth weight infants have an increased difference in body surface area to body weight, increasing the surface area for heat loss even more. The heat loss in a term infant is four times greater than that of an adult, and a premature infant's is five times greater.

5 The reason term infants, and especially those weighing less than 2 kg, lose heat through the skin at a faster rate than adults is because of the decreased thickness of the fat tissues under the skin. This subcutaneous fat acts to insulate and decrease the heat loss gradient between core and skin temperature.

6 Sick infants have another problem that promotes heat loss. An infant usually has its arms and legs flexed and held close to the body. Flexed extremities help to minimize exposure of body surface area. A sick infant usually has poor muscle tone ("floppy baby") and cannot maintain this posture. This increases the body surface area, encouraging heat loss.

6.3 Cold stress

1 The newborn's response to heat loss is increasing its metabolic rate. This in turn increases O_2 consumption, and unless the FIO_2 is increased, hypoxia will occur. This is believed to result from pulmonary vasoconstriction secondary to norepinephrine release in response to heat loss.

2 Because of hypoxia, the breakdown conversion of glycogen to glucose is by anaerobic glycolysis. The anaerobic pathway uses glycogen 20 times faster than normal. This rapid rate of utilization depletes glycogen stores, resulting in hypoglycemia.

3 The anaerobic glycolysis itself causes an increase in lactic acid production. This metabolic acidosis will cause further pulmonary vasoconstriction, decreasing oxygenation even more.

4 In addition, it is believed that arterial oxygen tensions (Pao_2) of 45 mm Hg or less impair heat production in the infant. This *cold stress cycle*, if not interrupted, can easily become life threatening to an infant. This is especially true for low birth weight and sick infants.

5 One of the most important practices in the delivery room should be to dry and place the infant in a warm environment.

6 If there is need for resuscitation, the infant should be dried and placed under an open radiant warmer. This allows for maximum access to the infant while preventing cold stress.

7 Usually, term infants can maintain thermal balance in an open bassinet covered with a blanket. Caution must be taken to keep the room temperature about 24° C (75° F) and avoid placing the bassinet by drafts and air vents.

8 Sick infants and all low birth weight infants require a thermally controlled environment, usually an incubator or radiant warmer (see Module Fourteen).

6.4 Aseptic nursery principles

1 Advances in newborn care have required an increasing number of personnel to come in contact with the infant. Large newborn high-risk nurseries also admit patients from a large number of other hospitals. There is also a move to allow greater family participation in the intensive care area.

2 Many institutions have developed simple, but important, procedures to minimize infections in the nursery. The importance of *proper hand washing* cannot be overstressed. Failure to conduct proper hand washing and failure to wash hands between contact with different patients have been cited in numerous nursery infection outbreaks.

3 Most nurseries require an initial 2-minute wash above the elbows with antibacterial soap or an iodine preparation. A 15-second wash is required between patients.

4 Many nurseries require short-sleeve scrub dress and forbid jewelry on the hands and wrists in order to provide for ease of washing and to lessen the available places for bacteria to hide. Any person who holds an infant is usually required to wear a long-sleeved gown and to change to a new one before holding another infant. Parents can safely handle and visit their infant, provided they follow the same precautions as nursery personnel.

5 To prevent the spread to unaffected infants some nurseries are divided into an "infected" section for infants with diarrhea and certain infections.

6 All equipment that will come in contact with the infant can provide a pathway for infection. Nurseries vary in their equipment-cleaning technique. Most have a *bacteria survey program surveillance* and work closely with infectious disease control nurses and physicians to control outbreaks of infection. Autoclaving or ethylene oxide gas sterilization of all possible equipment will decrease the chance of transmitting infections.

7 Respiratory therapy equipment, because of its heat and moisture environments, offers a breeding ground for a number of gram-negative bacteria, commonly called "water bugs." The daily, and sometimes three times daily, changing of oxygen humidifiers and tubing, as

TABLE 26-2 The mother's history and possibility of infant's problem

Mother's history	Possible infant problem
1 Prematurity	
2 Diabetes	Hyaline membrane disease
3 Hemorrhage in the days before premature delivery	
4 Infection	
5 Premature rupture of membrane	Pneumonia
6 Prolonged labor	
7 Meconium-stained amniotic fluid	Meconium aspiration
8 Hydramnios (increased amniotic fluid)	Tracheoesophageal fistula, esophageal atresia
9 Excessive medication	CNS depression
10 Reserpine	Stuffy nose
11 Traumatic or breech birth	CNS hemorrhage, phrenic nerve paralysis
12 Fetal tachycardia or bradycardia	Asphyxia
13 Prolapsed cord or cord entanglement	Asphyxia
14 Heroin addiction	Fetal addiction
15 Alcohol addiction or heavy consumption	Fetal alcohol syndrome

well as the periodic discarding of humidifier water and replacement with sterile water, will greatly reduce the chance for bacteria to multiply. Most respiratory therapy equipment is sterilized in gluteraldehyde solutions or gassed with ethylene oxide.

7.0 NEONATAL AND MATERNAL HIGH-RISK FACTORS AND PRINCIPLES OF ASSESSMENT OF THE NEONATE

7.1 The high-risk infant

1 DEFINITION: The high-risk infant is any infant, regardless of length of gestation or birth weight, who will require, or is expected to require, special medical attention to survive. This medical attention may be required before, during, and after birth.

2 An accurate and complete history of the mother will often forewarn of conditions to be expected when the infant is born. Table 26-2 lists the history of the mother with the conditions to which her infant is susceptible.

3 Factors associated with high-risk labor are:
  a Prolonged labor
  b Delayed birth after membrane rupture
  c Beta streptococci, which can cause apnea problems
  d Placenta dislocation, rupture, etc.
  e Perinatal asphyxia (found usually in Apgar score less than 6)
  f Meconium-stained amniotic fluid
  g Mode of delivery
  h Medications

4 Common neonatal high-risk factors are:
  a A gestation period less than 37 weeks or greater than 42 weeks
  b Abnormal growth (quality and quantity)

TABLE 26-3 Clinical signs and related probable conditions

Signs in the infant	Probable associated conditions
1 Single umbilical artery	Congenital abnormalities
2 Other congenital abnormalities	Associated cardiopulmonary abnormalities
3 Scaphoid abdomen (boat-shaped)	Diaphragmatic hernia
4 Erb's palsy (a paralysis of the group of muscles of the shoulders and upper arms)	Phrenic nerve palsy
5 Cannot breathe with mouth closed	Choanal atresia, stuffy nose
6 Gasping with little air exchange	Upper airway obstruction
7 Overdistension of lungs	Aspiration, lobar emphysema, pneumothorax
8 Shift of apical pulse	Pneumothorax
9 Fever or rise in temperature in a constant temperature environment	Pneumonia
10 Shrill cry, hypertonia, or flaccid atonia	CNS disorder, trauma, poliomyelitis myatonia (lack of muscle tone)
11 Frothy blood from larynx	Pulmonary hemorrhage
12 Head extended in the absence of neurologic findings	Laryngeal obstruction, vascular ring
13 Choking after feedings	Tracheoesophageal fistula (TEF), pharyngeal incoordination

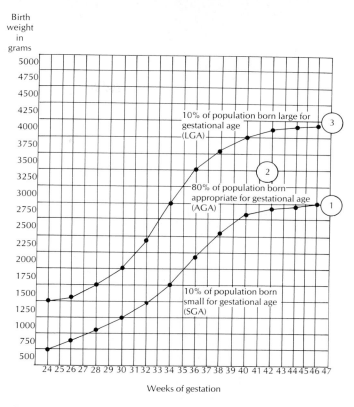

FIGURE 26-17 Birth weight compared to gestational age. Two S-shaped curves have been plotted by points on the graph, reflecting the percentile of the population who fall in various regions.

c Respiratory distress syndrome
d Hemolytic disease
e Infection
f Anomalies
g Drugs
h Surgery

5 Often observation of particular signs in the baby will give a clue to probable associated conditions (Table 26-3).

7.2 Birth weight and gestational age

1 Before 1961 infants who were born weighing less than 2500 grams (g) were considered premature, and those above 2500 g, *mature* at birth. In 1961 the World Health Organization made recommendations that infants be reclassified separately by both birth weight and gestational age.

2 Gestational age is calculated from the first day of the last menstrual period and classified as:

a *Premature:* an infant born before the end of 37 weeks' gestation.

b *Term:* an infant born between the beginning of 38 weeks' and the end of 41 weeks' gestation.

c *Postmature:* an infant born any time after the beginning of 42 weeks' gestation.

3 Birth weight is now compared to gestational age to assess the intrauterine growth status of the infant. Intrauterine growth is statistically correlated with the birth weight of infants of their particular period of gestation in the population. This information is graphically arranged, plotting gestational age against birth weight. S-shaped curves are plotted by points on the graph reflecting the percentile of the population who fall in various regions of the graph (Fig. 26-17).

a Those who fall below the 10% curve represent the 10% of the population who are born small for gestational age (SGA) *(1)*.

b Those who fall between the 10% and the 90% curves represent the 80% of the population who are born appropriate for gestational age (AGA) *(2)*.

c Those who fall above the 90% curve represent the 10% of the population who are born large for gestational age (LGA) *(3)*.

7.3 Risks related to gestational age and birth weight

1 The term "prematurity" was applied to any newborn infant weighing less than 2500 g, regardless of gestational age. This definition was put to disuse after much of the collected data showed many term infants were born weighing 2500 g. Today *prematurity* is simply defined as being born *before* 37 weeks' gestation.

2 Premature infants can survive at approximately 24 weeks of gestation and a body weight of approximately 500 grams (1 ¼ lbs). These occurrences are very rare because the infant is totally dependent on external assistance for life support and other environmental con-

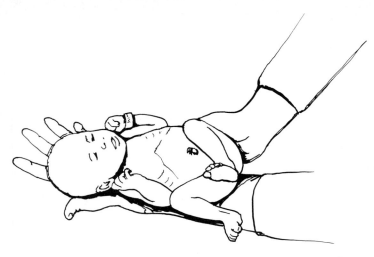

FIGURE 26-18 Relative size of premature newborn to adult hand. (Reprinted with permission of Ross Laboratories, Columbus, OH 43216 from Clinical Educ. Aid # 12, June 1978.)

TABLE 26-4 Comparison of infants (24 weeks to 40 weeks)

Weeks gestation	Height (inches)	Weight (lbs)
24	13	1¼
29	14½	2½
35	18½	5½
40	20	7

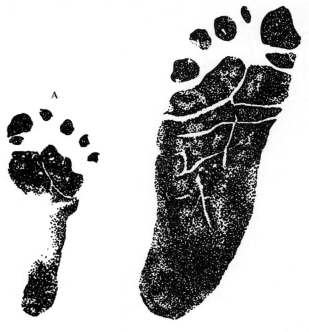

FIGURE 26-19 A, Actual size footprints of a premature infant, and **B,** full-term infant.

TABLE 26-5 Pathophysiology of retrolental fibroplasia

Stages of development	Action
Stage I	Dilation and tortuosity of retinal vessels; incompletely vascularized retina.
Stage II	Neovascularization; peripheral retinal clouding and hemorrhage; localized detachment.
Stage III	Peripheral retinal detachment; hemorrhage from newly formed vessels into vitreous body.
Stage IV	Moderate proliferation; hemispheric or circumferential retinal detachment, including half or more of the retina.
Stage V	Advanced proliferation; hemorrhage filling vitreous body; total retinal detachment.

trols. Table 26-4 presents a comparison of an infant's size and weight at 24 weeks to term.

Fig. 26-18 shows the relative size of a premature infant to an adult hand and Fig. 26-19 shows the actual size of a premature infant's footprint at 28 weeks (2 lbs, 10 oz) compared to that of a full-term infant (8 lbs 11 oz). Clearly, the development of neonatology as a speciality and the subsequent emergence of 420 Neonatal Intensive Care Units nationwide have been the primary factors in reducing premature infant mortality from more than 50% in the 1960s to less than 30% today.

3 In spite of the remarkable increase in survival it is generally agreed that 28 weeks' gestation is a break point. Extrauterine life is possible before 28 weeks, but only 5% of this group survive. Premature infants are known to be vulnerable to medical problems such as:

 a Periodic apnea
 b Pulmonary hemorrhage
 c Intracranial hemorrhage
 d Inability to ward off infection
 e Hyaline membrane disease
 f Fetal asphyxia

4 Premature infants are the largest group of newborns in whom retrolental fibroplasia (RLF) develops.

5 Retrolental fibroplasia is a complication of excessive O_2 therapy in which high arterial oxygen tensions (Pao_2 in excess of 100 mm Hg) causes the arteries of the retina to dilate and become tortuous, interrupting adequate blood flow to the retina. The results can range from no damage to partial damage and from vision impairment to complete detachment of the retina. Edema occurs in this area and the resultant scar tissue formation usually leads to blindness. For this reason, it is recommended that Pao_2 not exceed 80 mm Hg.

6 Koff, Eitzman, and Neu, in their recent text *Neonatal and Pediatric Respiratory Care,* described four stages to denote the pathophysiology of RLF (see Table 26-5).

7 In the early 1950s, the considered safe O_2 concentration that was administered to premature infants was limited to 40% FIo_2 and below. This was to eliminate retrolental fibroplasia, but it was noted a few years later that infants with hyaline membrane disease were dying at a higher rate because of insufficient O_2 administration.

8 The medical literature subsequently began to support

Scoring component	How component is tested	Score 0	Score 1	Score 2
Heart rate	Auscultation or count pulses at junction of umbilical cord and abdomen	Absent	Slow (below 100)	Over 100
Respiratory effort	Observation	Absent	Slow, irregular	Good
Muscle tone	Observation, resistance to straightening of extremities	Limp	Some flexion of extremities	Active motion
Reflex irritability	Flicking soles of feet/inserting catheter in nostril	No response	Cry/grimace	Vigorous cry, cough, sneeze
Color	Observation	Blue, pale	Body pink, hands and feet blue	Completely pink

F I G U R E   2 6 - 2 0 Components of Apgar scoring system used to assess the medical condition of a newborn at birth.

the idea that retrolental fibroplasia is the result of *excessive* Pao_2 rather than excessive FIo_2. Premature infants with lung diseases were then treated with O_2 concentrations greater than 40% when their survival required it.

9 The present safeguards against retrolental fibroplasia are to maintain Pao_2 in the 60 to 70 mm Hg range and to have a qualified ophthalmologist examine infants who weigh less than 2500 g and who receive O_2 therapy.

10 Common problems associated with infants who are born small for gestational age (SGA) are:
a Perinatal asphyxia
b Aspiration syndrome
c Hypoglycemia
d Heat loss
e Cerebral edema
f Polycythemia

11 The death rate for SGA infants is seven times higher than average for gestational age (AGA) infants at term. The survival rate of SGA infants is more than three times higher than AGA premature infants.

12 Large for gestational age (LGA) infants are those who fall above the 90th percentile of the gestational age to birth weight chart at any age. It is also correct to say any infant who weighs more than 4000 g at birth is LGA, regardless of gestational age. The largest known infant born weighed 29 pounds, 8 ounces, but lived only for 2 hours.

13 Diabetic mothers have a higher frequency of LGA births than do nondiabetic mothers (from 4 to 28 times higher), but nondiabetic mothers still contribute the majority of LGA infants.

14 LGA infants at term have a higher mortality rate than AGA term infants. This is largely a result of complications of vaginal delivery.

15 *Postmaturity* is being born after the 42nd week of gestation. Postmature infants may be AGA, but most are born wasted because of improper placental function.

Postmature infants compose 12% of all infants born. Mortality for postmature infants is higher than for those born at term—two to three times higher if they are born after 43 weeks. Three fourths of all postmature infant deaths occur during the stress of labor.

7.4 Infant assessment scoring systems

1 *Virginia Apgar*, in 1952, devised a widely used system to assess the medical condition of an infant at birth. The scoring was based on five components using Apgar's name as an acronym:
A—appearance (color)
P—pulse (heart rate)
G—grimace (reflex irritability)
A—activity (muscle tone)
R—respiration (respiratory effort)
Each component is usually evaluated at 1 and 5 minutes after birth and given a score of 0, 1, or 2 (Fig. 26-20).
a An Apgar score of 7 to 10 indicates a normal infant; no intervention is usually necessary.
b An Apgar score of 3 to 6 indicates a moderately depressed infant. Usual treatment is airway suctioning—bag and mask administration of 100% oxygen.
c An Apgar score of 0 to 2 indicates a severely depressed infant. The usual treatment is airway suctioning, intubation, and manual bagging with 100% oxygen. If heart rate is severely depressed or absent, external cardiac massage is indicated also.

2 The *Dubowitz scoring system* uses neurologic signs and physical development to assess gestational age. The test can be done any time before 5 days after birth. This information is useful in planning the management of sick infants.
a With the infant placed in specific positions, assessment is made of the infant's ability to flex and extend its muscles and the pliability of its joints. A numeric score is attached to specific levels of limb and joint movement.

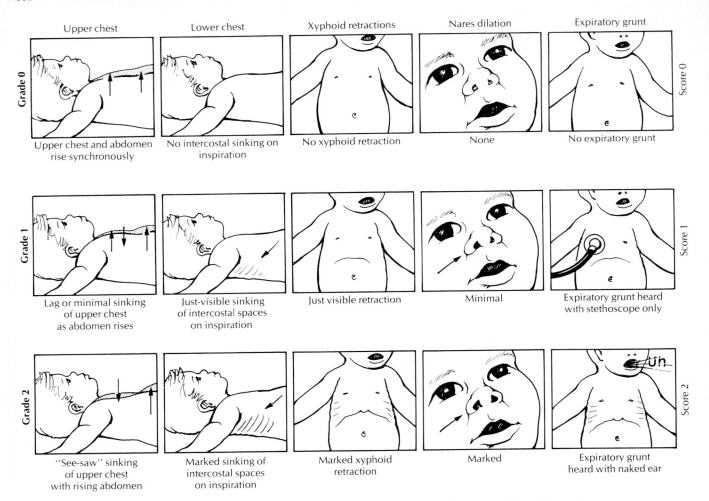

FIGURE 26-21 Components of the Silverman scoring system used to assess the breathing performance of premature infants.

b Physical development is also scored with such external indicators as ear development, genitals, and plantar creases.

c Refer to any standard pediatric nursing or intensive nursery care text for more details.

3 The *Silverman score* was developed for scoring the breathing performance of premature infants. The Silverman score is based on signs of respiratory distress. Unlike the Apgar, 0 is the best score, and 10 indicates severe distress (Fig. 26-21).

8.0 TREATMENT OF CARDIOPULMONARY DISORDERS OF THE NEONATE

8.1 Clinical signs of cardiac and pulmonary disease in the newborn

Cardiac and pulmonary diseases limit the life expectancy in a number of newborns. To decrease mortality, emphasis is being placed on the early recognition and proper management of cardiac and pulmonary diseases. Survival of a newborn with this type of disease is increasing with early recognition of the signs of distress in the cardiopulmonary system.

1 Cyanosis

a *Cyanosis* is a blue discoloration of the skin and/or the mucous membrane, depending on the type.

b Peripheral cyanosis (also known as acrocyanosis) is a blue discoloration of the extremities. It is caused by increased O_2 uptake from the blood slowed by vasoconstriction. A hypothermic environment or normally occurring high packed cell volume (hematocrit) is the usual cause. Peripheral cyanosis is not considered to be a pathologic finding.

c Central cyanosis is always considered a pathologic finding. It is a blue discoloration of not only the extremities (as in peripheral cyanosis) but also the mucous membranes of the mouth. Central cyanosis results from decreased O_2 levels in arterial blood, usually caused by cardiopulmonary disease.

2 Respiratory distress

a *Tachypnea* is usually defined as a respiratory rate greater than 60 breaths per minute (BPM) in a quiet infant.

b An irritable baby (hungry, etc.) may have a respiratory rate of 80, which will return to normal when the infant is quiet.

c *Retractions* indicate that the infant is using auxiliary muscles of respiration. They are usually signs of cardiac or pulmonary disorders. Retractions can be observed in the subcostal, intercostal, supraclavicular, and substernal regions.

d *Wheezing* is usually caused by edema around the small bronchi and bronchioles. It can also be caused by the constriction of smooth muscles in these regions. Epinephrine, administered subcutaneously, is used to distinguish between the two causes, as it often will relieve wheezing caused by smooth muscle constriction of the small bronchi and bronchioles.

e *Crackles* are usually caused by fluid collection in the alveoli and in the airways of the lower third of the tracheobronchial tree.

 • Wheezing and crackles caused by edema usually indicate pulmonary vascular engorgement resulting from cardiac or pulmonary disease.

f *Grunting* is a method of expiratory retardation of air flow to maintain alveolar patency by the created back pressure. Grunting helps to increase functional residual capacity, and the Pao_2 can increase 10 to 20 mm Hg by grunting. An expiratory sigh may also be noted. This functions, as does grunting, to increase oxygenation by the same method.

g *Nasal flaring* is usually indicative of air hunger from various causes. With the exception of pulmonary congestion secondary to severe failure of the left side of the heart, nasal flaring and grunting are not associated with cardiac pathology.

3 Systemic venous congestion

a The liver, in the circulatory pathway, is the organ nearest the heart. When cardiac output is not maintained secondary to failure of the right side of the heart, the backup of blood engorges the liver.

b *Hepatomegaly* is determined by palpation of the liver. It is usually measured below the right costal margin, in line with the right nipple. Normally the liver can be palpated about 2 cm below the costal margin. Palpation of the liver 3 cm or more below the costal margin is indicative of systemic venous congestion.

c *Peripheral edema* is not usually seen early in the course of heart disease in the neonate. Because the neonate is mainly in the prone position, edema occurs in the frontal and periorbital regions of the heart rather than in the lower extremities as with adults.

4 Cardiac distress

a Cardiac distress presents another group of signs:
 • Tachycardia
 • Cardiomegaly
 • Weak pulses

b The diseased heart will try to increase its cardiac output by increasing its rate. Heart rate, similar to respiratory rate, can be 160 to 180 BPM in a crying infant, but a heart rate greater than 140 in a quiet infant is usually associated with cardiopulmonary distress.

c *Cardiomegaly* (heart enlargement) is another compensatory mechanism of the heart to maintain cardiac output. Contractility of the heart is increased as the muscles of the heart increase in length, causing an increase in cardiac output. The increase occurs until the muscles are stretched beyond their physiologic limits, at which time heart failure will begin.

d One must use caution when determining cardiac size in a chest x-ray film. An infant can have a normal heart that occupies a large area of the thorax. It is generally agreed that a cardiac silhouette occupying more than 60% of the thoracic area is indicative of cardiomegaly.

e Weak pulses usually represent a decreased cardiac output resulting from decreased contractility of the heart.

8.2 Aspiration syndrome

1 *Aspiration* is a common cause of pulmonary problems in infants. Aspiration syndrome occurs in two forms: (a) the infant who aspirates amniotic or vaginal substances and (b) the infant who aspirates meconium.

2 Pathology

a If the aspiration occurs before birth, amniotic debris may enter the lungs.

b If the aspiration occurs after premature placental separation, maternal blood may enter the lungs.

c Aspiration of infected amniotic fluid or cervical mucus is a cause of postnatal pneumonia.

d Infants who have aspirated amniotic or vaginal substances without meconium do well and usually recover within 48 to 72 hours.

e The presence of meconium indicates that the infant possibly has had some type of asphyxia. The relationship between the presence of meconium and asphyxia is based on the increased activity of the intestine and relaxation of the anal sphincter muscle because of hypoxia.

f The presence of meconium in a healthy infant usually reflects transient hypoxia in the uterine state and is usually without significant pathology.

g Sometimes the fetus aspirates particles of meconium that are driven further into the tracheobronchial tree with the first few breaths or with positive pressure ventilatory assistance. This situation usually leads to a delayed course of respiratory distress.

3 Clinical findings

a The chest x-ray film shows patchy densities that are atelectatic areas produced by obstruction. The flattened diaphragm and wide-spaced ribs, indicating overdistension in spite of large areas of atelectasis, are usual findings.

b Arterial blood gases usually show hypercapnia and hypoxemia resulting from the large amount of shunting and the degree of diffusion impairment. A low pH is usually present because of respiratory acidosis and often metabolic acidosis from anaerobic metabolism.

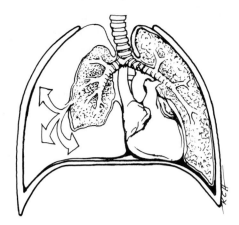

FIGURE 26-22 Spontaneous pneumothorax. Spontaneous lung rupture causing air from lung to fill intrapleural space and cause lung collapse.

c The infant may experience shock at birth and severe respiratory depression or bradycardia; it is usually "floppy" (no muscle tone). Ventilatory assistance is often necessary. Although pulmonary abnormalities usually resolve in 48 hours, they can last for a week.

4 Treatment

a Studies on tracheal suctioning of infants with meconium aspiration syndrome showed that infants who were suctioned have a considerable decrease in morbidity and mortality rates when compared to infants who are not suctioned. Unsuctioned infants have been found to require ventilatory assistance more frequently, and they have a higher incidence of pneumothorax and pneumomediastinum.

b The following items are considered standard treatment by most intensive care nurseries:
- Aspiration of the trachea
- Ventilatory assistance
- Humidified air and O_2 mixtures
- Thermoregulation
- Chest physical therapy
- Correction of metabolic acidosis
- Aspiration of swallowed meconium from the stomach

8.3 Pneumothorax

1 Pneumothorax as a result of barotrauma should be a prime suspect in any newborn respiratory distress. As previously mentioned, infants are exposed to a great variety of pressure changes in the lungs at and immediately after birth. One or two out of every hundred routine newborn chest x-ray studies show a pneumothorax without clinical signs and symptoms.

2 Pathology

a Pneumothorax can spontaneously occur in a partially expanded lung. The high distending pressures develop to open the unexpanded region and cause a spontaneous rupture in the unaffected regions (Fig. 26-22).

b Pneumothorax (extra alveolar air) can also occur as a complication of:

- Meconium aspiration
- Hyaline membrane disease
- Pneumonia
- Pulmonary hypoplasia
- Diaphragmatic hernia
- Excessively high positive pressure breathing

c Usually, the rupture at the alveoli results in interstitial emphysema, which leaks through the lung tissues into the mediastinum (pneumomediastinum) at the hilar region. This air will usually leak into the pleural space, but rarely into the pericardial space (pneumopericardium). Leaking of the ruptured alveoli directly into the pleural space does not occur as frequently as the listed processes. Occasionally air may leak into the peritoneal cavity. This condition is known as pneumoperitoneum.

3 Clinical findings

a Cyanosis, tachypnea, grunting, and nasal flaring are frequently associated with pneumothorax.

b One very important sign of pneumothorax is a shift in the point of maximal impulse (PMI), which is also called apical pulse. The PMI is normally found in the midclavicular line at the fifth intercostal space. A pneumothorax will cause a shift in the PMI away from the affected side. In the instances of bilateral pneumothorax, the PMI will usually have a downward shift.

c *Transillumination,* or placing a bright, cold light on a body region, is another method to aid in diagnosing pneumothorax. The pneumothorax will show up as an area of increased lucency (brightness) as compared to unaffected areas.

d Confirmation of a pneumothorax is accomplished by a chest x-ray study.

4 Treatment

a In the asymptomatic infant with a pneumothorax, observation and monitoring frequently for heart rate, respiratory rate, and color, along with frequent chest x-ray films, are all that is usually required.

b If the infant shows signs of distress, the methods of treatment vary from center to center, but all have the same goal—to evacuate the air from the pleural space.

c One method is to evacuate the pleural air with a needle and syringe attached to a three-way stopcock. An immediate chest x-ray film is taken and is then repeated 30 minutes to an hour later.

d If the pneumothorax remains resolved, observation and periodic chest x-ray studies are performed. If the pneumothorax is again present, a chest tube is inserted while the patient is given 100% oxygen, avoiding positive pressure breathing if possible. The chest tube is then attached to the proper source at 10 to 20 cm H_2O negative pressure. Improvement can be expected within 6 to 12 hours.

e Some clinicians suggest using 100% oxygen to aid in speeding up the reabsorption of pleural air by the lungs. It is reported that there is an increase in absorption six times faster with 100% O_2 administration. The complications of retrolental fibroplasia and bronchopulmonary dysplasia with this method must be taken into consideration and weighed against the benefit of using 100% oxygen.

8.4 Pneumonia

1 Pneumonia is the most common serious infectious condition for newborns. Pneumonia can be acquired in the intrauterine environment (congenital pneumonia) and in the extrauterine environment (nursery infection). Pneumonia may also result as a complication of meconium aspiration syndrome, hyaline membrane disease, and pulmonary hemorrhage. Viral pneumonias can also occur with herpes simplex, rhinovirus, *Enterovirus* species, rubella, cytomegalovirus, and influenza during epidemics.

2 Pathology

  a *Congenital* pneumonia is associated with:
  • Early membrane rupture
  • Prolonged labor
  • Maternal infections
  • Uncomplicated premature delivery

  b The most common pathogens are *Escherichia coli* and other enteric species and group B streptococci.

  c Symptoms are usually present *within* 48 hours after birth.

  d Within 24 hours after membrane rupture, 90% of the samples taken of amniotic fluid contain bacteria.

  e Premature infants have a higher risk of infection than term infants.

  f The onset of symptoms of *postnatal* pneumonia usually appears within 48 hours *after* birth.

  g The most common pathogens of postnatal pneumonia are *Pseudomonas aeruginosa,* penicillin-resistant staphylococci, and enteric organisms.

3 Clinical findings

  a The infant with congenital pneumonia is usually stillborn or born severely ill. The infant appears flaccid, pale, and cyanotic—often requiring resuscitation.

  b Respiration is usually slow to begin and often is not sufficient when initiated. Once respiration has been initiated, frequent episodes of apnea usually occur.

  c Tachypnea, poor feeding, or aspiration with feeding occurs. Because of vomiting and aspiration with feeding, the chest x-ray examination may show findings other than the usual aspiration picture, giving a clue to a preexisting pneumonia.

  d Prolonged hypothermia is usually found, especially in infants less than term.

  e The infected infant may have a fever, with term infants having fever more frequently than premature infants.

  f Occasionally, pulmonary edema and a descending liver herald the onset of heart failure in these infants.

  g White blood cell (WBC) count may be elevated. A WBC of less than 5000 or more than 15,000 per mm^3 is indicative of infection.

  h Crackles are sometimes present in the infant with pneumonia.

  i The chest x-ray examination is the most reliable method of detecting pneumonia.

4 Treatment

  a Intensive patient management and respiratory care

  b Proper thermoregulation

  c Fluid, electrolyte, and calorie maintenance

  d Medical aseptic technique

  e Identification of the pathogen and establishment of antibiotic therapy

  f Duration of antibiotic treatment is recommended for 2 weeks in gram-positive infections and 3 weeks in gram-negative infections.

8.5 Atelectasis

1 *Atelectasis* is the collapse of a lung or area of a lung, or the failure of these areas to properly expand.

2 Pathology

  a There are two main types of atelectasis:
  • *Primary* atelectasis. This type of atelectasis is caused by failure of lung area to mature and a weak breathing effort. A weak breathing effort can result from (1) respiratory muscle weakness, (2) chest wall being too soft and retracting with negative pressure, preventing proper lung expansion, (3) drug overdose, (4) respiratory center dysfunction or damage and breathing dysfunction resulting from other illnesses. Premature infants often have weak muscles of breathing, because they are not fully developed. They also have a softer chest wall than term infants.
  • *Secondary* atelectasis. This type of atelectasis is caused by (1) aspiration of amniotic substances, (2) mucous plugging, (3) inadequate levels of surfactant, and (4) congenital malformation of the airways.

3 Clinical findings

  a Primary atelectasis usually follows two clinical patterns. The affected infant will have persistent cyanosis with a weak breathing effort or periodic cyanosis with irregular breathing and occasional apnea.

  b In secondary atelectasis, the infant will have a rigorous breathing pattern. The affected infant may have apnea or may breathe normally at birth.

  c The chest x-ray study shows patchy areas of density that will sometimes increase because of weak breathing effort.

4 Treatment

  a In patients who have primary atelectasis, supportive measures are used to allow time for maturity or to correct other causes of a weak breathing effort. This support can range from oxygen and periodic "sighing" with a bag and mask to intubation and mechanical ventilation.

  b Obstructive atelectasis is treated with humidity, frequent turning, chest physical therapy, and suctioning.

c Congenital airway malformations and persistent areas that will not reexpand often require surgical correction.

8.6 Hyperinflated lung

1 Overdistension of the lungs or an area of the lungs occurs frequently in newborns. Overdistension (or hyperinflation) can affect the entire lung area or just a part of it.

2 Pathology

a *Ball-valve type.* This is an obstruction that permits air into the alveoli, but partially or completely blocks air leaving this area. This type of hyperinflation can be caused by:
- Mucus
- Meconium
- Exudates of various lung diseases
- Compression of the tracheobronchial tree by surrounding tissues (such as vascular ring, cyst, etc.)

b *Compensatory overdistension.* An area of the lung becomes hyperinflated to compensate for the loss of volume in another area of the lung. With a volume loss in an area of the lung, negative intrathoracic pressures increase. The increase in volume in the unaffected lung areas helps reduce the negative pressure. Compensatory overdistension can be caused by:
- Atelectasis
- Failure of a lung or lung area to fully develop (hypoplastic lung)
- Iatrogenic causes (e.g., an ET tube down too far that lodges in a bronchus)

  Hyperinflated lung syndrome can lead to interstitial emphysema, bullae and bleb formation, pneumothorax, and pneumomediastinum.

3 Clinical findings

a Hyperinflated lung syndrome can occur in premature and term infants. The onset of distress is at birth or immediately after. Tachypnea, retractions, nasal flaring, and grunting are usually present.

b The chest x-ray study usually shows a flattened diaphragm and hilar streaks. Blood gases show a slightly decreased pH and a slightly elevated P_{CO_2}.

4 Treatment. The goal of treatment is to remove obstructive material causing the problem. Turning, chest physical therapy, and suctioning aid in removing obstructive material. Extrapulmonary sources of compression of the tracheobronchial tree usually require surgical intervention.

8.7 Bronchopulmonary dysplasia

1 With the increased use of high O_2 concentrations and mechanical ventilation to support infants who have severe respiratory distress, bronchopulmonary dysplasia (BPD) is appearing more frequently. This complication of therapy carries a high mortality rate, and the few survivors usually have chronic lung disease for lengthy periods after the initial stages of the disease.

2 Pathology

a Bronchopulmonary dysplasia is a complication not only of high O_2 concentrations, as believed in the past, but it has also been associated with the presence of an endotracheal tube and positive pressure ventilation.

b Pathologic changes can include:
- Presence of hyaline membrane
- Dilation of lymphatics
- Alveolar collapse
- Squamous and ciliated cell sloughing
- Necrosis and repair of the alveolar lining
- The appearance of thick mucus
- Pulmonary fibrosis
- Bronchial hypertrophy
- Pulmonary artery hypertrophy
- Failure of the right side of the heart

c The thickening of alveolar walls and basement membranes, alveolar necrosis and repair, thick secretions, atelectasis, edema, and fibrosis cause a delay in O_2 diffusion between alveoli and the pulmonary capillary bed. This respiratory dysfunction makes prolonged O_2 support necessary in these patients, although oxygen has been cited as a causative factor in the disease.

3 Clinical findings

a Infants with BPD have a history of receiving high O_2 concentrations and mechanical ventilation for several days. The chest x-ray examination shows fine granular densities; the infant is ventilator-dependent, and small decreases in O_2 concentrations induce cyanosis. As the disease progresses, the chest film will show densities in all lung regions.

b After 2 to 3 weeks, some infants with BPD can be weaned from the ventilator, but many must remain on high O_2 concentrations, and they require mechanical ventilation to survive. Usually the chest x-ray study shows lacy interstitial cystic patterns at this time, along with the appearance of thick mucus secretions.

c Infants who have survived the disease for 4 weeks can usually be weaned from the ventilator, but must remain on O_2 support. Chest x-ray films show strands of density (fibrosis), wide intercostal spaces, and a flattened diaphragm (overinflation). Often, pulmonary hypertension, cor pulmonale, and failure of the right side of the heart will appear.

d If the infant is weaned from oxygen and discharged home, clinical (cyanotic spells) and radiographic (overinflated areas, fibrotic strands, atelectasis) signs will persist, with slow improvement over long periods of time.

4 Treatment

a When possible, prevention is the best treatment of BPD. The use of low-peak inspiratory pressures (less than 30 cm H_2O), continuous positive airway pressure (CPAP), or positive end expiratory pressure (PEEP) to allow adequate oxygenation at lower FI_{O_2}

for the shortest period of time possible has been shown to reduce the incidence of BPD.

  b For infants already afflicted with the disease, treatment is mainly supportive. Proper humidity, frequent chest physical therapy, positioning, and suctioning aid in the removal of thick secretions that frequently cause obstruction and consequent cyanosis and respiratory embarrassment.

  c Oxygen concentrations must be meticulously maintained and gradually (sometimes only by 1%) decreased as clinical and physiologic signs permit. The infant is usually weaned to a lower FIo_2 after several weeks, only to have an insult to the lungs, requiring FIo_2 to be returned to a higher-than-previous O_2 concentration. Even if the insult (obstructive mucous plug, aspiration, viral pneumonia, etc.) is of short duration, weaning the infant to the level of oxygen before the insult will require several weeks. This seesaw phenomenon from lower-to-higher-to-lower O_2 concentrations during the course of O_2 weaning is common in patients with BPD and a cause of frustration among those who provide supportive care.

  d In spite of prolonged and frustrating periods of supportive care, the overall outcome of patients who survive has been good. Many children, with proper posthospitalization care, "outgrow" the effects of the disease with minimum permanent damage.

8.8 Hyaline membrane disease

1 Hyaline membrane disease (HMD), respiratory distress syndrome (RDS), and idiopathic respiratory distress syndrome (IRDS) are all names for a severe respiratory disorder that occurs at, or shortly after, birth. The disease is found primarily in premature infants and in those with low birth weight. It is associated with low survival rate.

2 Pathology

  a Although other factors have been cited, surfactant deficiency is believed to be the causative *principal* factor of the disease. The concept is supported by the fact that term infants who have developed appropriate pathways to produce adequate surfactant, as shown by a lecithin/sphingomyelin (L/S) ratio equal to or greater than two, rarely develop HMD.

  b With the first breath that an infant takes in the presence of sufficient surfactant, functional residual capacity (FRC) is established. In the absence of adequate surfactant, FRC is not established, and each breath is as difficult as the first.

  c A number of infants with HMD have a small amount of surfactant present at birth and will breathe normally only to become distressed later, because surfactant production cannot be maintained.

  d Without adequate FRC and with the increased effort required to breathe, alveoli are not opened, and widespread atelectasis sets in. This atelectasis causes large right-to-left shunting of blood through the lung and fetal circulatory pathways, the foramen ovale,

and ductus arteriosus. This hypoperfusion of the lung results in hypoxia as well as metabolic and respiratory acidosis. Hypoxia and acidosis further impair pulmonary perfusion and create capillary and alveolar damage, increasing atelectasis even more.

3 Clinical findings

  a Signs and symptoms of HMD are:
  • Tachypnea and bradypnea in severely depressed infants
  • Grunting
  • Nasal flaring
  • Cyanosis on room air
  • Retractions
  • Decreased breath sounds
  • Pallor (not anemic type)
  • Flaccid or very decreased muscle tone
  • Apnea

  b The classic chest x-ray examination will show a "ground glass" appearance, although it is not always seen clearly in the course of the disease.

  c Arterial blood gases will show acidosis, hypoxia, and hypercapnia.

4 Treatment

  a Treatment is supportive until adequate surfactant production is established, usually within 3 to 5 days.

  b Adequate air and O_2 exchange must be established. CPAP is frequently used to establish an artificial FRC, decreasing atelectasis and work of breathing. If this fails to control hypoxia and hypercapnia, mechanical ventilation is indicated.

8.9 Diaphragmatic hernia

1 Diaphragmatic hernia is a congenital condition in which the abdominal organs herniate into the chest cavity through the diaphragm. This condition can be life threatening when too much lung area is compromised by abdominal organs in the chest (Fig. 26-23).

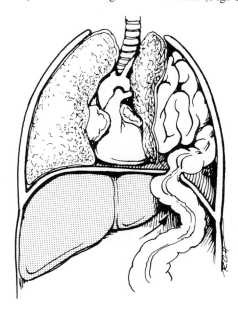

FIGURE 26-23 Diaphragmatic hernia showing abdominal contents pushed into lung area.

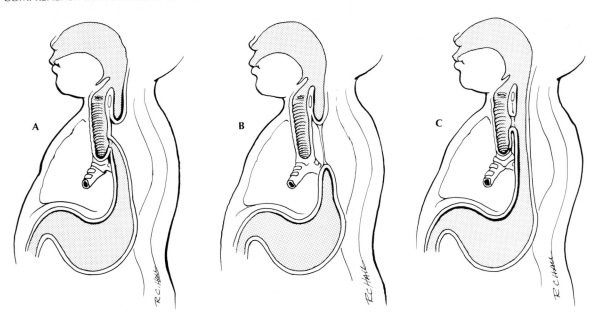

FIGURE 26-24 Forms of tracheoesophageal fistula (**A** through **C**).

2 Pathology

a A congenital defect in a region of the diaphragm allows both solid and hollow organs of the abdominal cavity to enter the chest cavity. The most common form is protrusion of the abdominal organs through posterolateral regions of the diaphragm. This region is called Bochdalek's foramen. Herniation of the diaphragm anteriorly behind the sternum (called Morgagni's foramen) and at the site at which the esophagus passes through the diaphragm (hiatus) occurs in fewer cases.

b Left-side herniation of the diaphragm occurs much more frequently than right-side herniation. In left-side herniation of the diaphragm, the stomach, spleen, and intestine can enter the chest cavity. In right-side herniation, the liver and intestine can enter the chest cavity.

3 Clinical findings

a The usual clue to the presence of diaphragmatic hernia is respiratory distress. The severity ranges from inability to establish respiration at birth to delayed but rapidly developing respiratory distress as intestinal gas expansion occurs.

b Displacement of the point of maximal impulse (PMI) is another finding. As with a pneumothorax, the PMI will be shifted away from the affected side.

c Diminished breath sounds and occasional bowel sounds are auscultated at the affected region. The chest x-ray examination is usually conclusive in the diagnosis. A lacy bowel gas pattern or uniform density of solid organs found in the chest often reveals the condition.

4 Treatment

a Prompt surgical correction and replacement of abdominal organs into their cavity is the only treatment.

b The mortality rate is high, with some infants never living long enough to have surgery.

8.10 Tracheoesophageal fistula

1 Tracheoesophageal fistula (TEF) is a congenital abnormality that commonly causes respiratory distress in newborns. There are several forms of this abnormality.

2 Pathology

a The most distinctive forms of TEF (Fig. 26-24) are:
  • Where the upper esophagus is a pouch (atresia) and the lower esophagus is connected to the trachea (fistula, *A*). This is the most common form of TEF.
  • Where there is a pouch and esophageal atresia, but no fistula between the esophagus and trachea *(B)*.
  • The H form, where the esophagus and trachea are normal, but a fistula connects them *(C)*.

b There are other forms of TEF, but they occur only rarely.

3 Clinical findings

a The most common signs are:
  • Constant pooling of nasal and pharyngeal secretions
  • Continuous or intermittent signs of respiratory distress
  • Choking with feedings
  • Repeated vomiting with or after feedings

b The abdomen may be distended because of gas accumulations from the tracheal fistula.

c The chest x-ray examination usually shows the pouch; it can easily be seen with contrast media or a radiolucent catheter. Persistent or recurring right upper lobe pneumonia or atelectasis is indicative of aspiration. Large amounts of gastrointestinal air are indicative of a fistula between the esophagus and trachea.

4 Treatment

  a Surgical correction of the abnormality is required in all forms.

  b Supportive care, until surgical correction is accomplished, is critical. A gastric feeding tube is usually used (if possible), and a constant suction placed in the pharynx is occasionally utilized to prevent secretions from entering the respiratory tract.

  c Surgical expertise in this area has been refined, but aspiration and its complications are the major cause of death in patients with TEF.

8.11 Choanal atresia

1 A choana is the normal funnel-shaped connection between the nose and the pharynx. Infants, being mandatory nose breathers early in life, can be distressed by atresia or stenosis in this area.

2 Pathology

  a A congenital malformation of bone or a membrane, causing partial or complete obstruction of one or both of the choana, may exist.

  b The complete obstruction (atresia) occludes the infant's airway and, unless the obstruction is treated, asphyxia will occur.

  c In partial obstruction (stenosis or unilateral atresia), overinflation and hypercapnia may occur.

3 Clinical findings

  a The first breath is usually through the mouth without problem, but the next attempts show a nonpatent airway by deep retractions and developing cyanosis.

  b The cause is usually found when a catheter or other probe fails to pass through the infant's nose. Often the nose will also have a large accumulation of thick secretions.

4 Treatment

  a If the obstructive cause is a membrane, its puncture will provide a patent airway.

  b Usually this is not possible, and an alternate airway must be established. An oropharyngeal airway will usually establish mouth breathing, but some infants will reestablish respiration only after intubation.

  c Surgical correction is usually necessary.

8.12 Transposition of the great arteries (Fig. 26-25)

1 Pathology. The aorta originates from the right ventricle and the pulmonary artery from the left ventricle. This causes the presence of two separate circulatory systems: one pulmonary and one systemic.

2 Pathophysiology

  a Deoxygenated blood entering the right atrium will flow into the right ventricle, but instead of entering the pulmonary artery for pulmonary circulation, it enters the aorta and circulates systemically.

  b Oxygenated blood entering the left atrium flows into the left ventricle but instead of entering the aorta and systemically circulating, it recirculates through the pulmonary artery and pulmonary vascular bed.

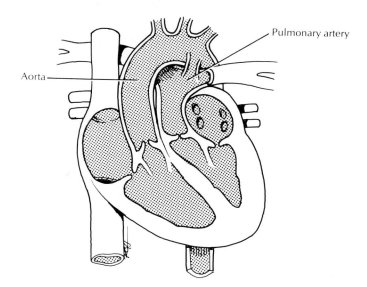

FIGURE 26-25 Transposition of the great arteries.

3 Clinical findings

  a A coexisting patent ductus arteriosus or a ventricular septal defect (VSD) allows survival for a few days by providing a means of arteriovenous admixture. This admixture causes the infant to have a mild-to-marked cyanosis. Marked cyanosis shortly after birth indicates the absence of adequate admixture, whereas infants with a large VSD will be only mildly cyanotic.

  b A murmur is not usually present. The chest x-ray examination shows cardiomegaly, especially right-side hypertrophy. Diagnosis is by cardiac catheterization and angiography.

4 Treatment

  a Initial management is to create a means of adequate admixture. This is done by the surgical creation of an atrial septal defect (Blalock-Hanlon operation) or by passing a catheter with a deflated balloon through the foramen ovale. The balloon is then inflated and, with a sudden jerk, the catheter is pulled back into the right atrium, rupturing the atrial septum (Rashkind balloon septostomy). This torn flap creates a shunt, allowing a bidirectional flow of blood at the atrial level.

  b Eventually, total corrective surgery is performed. One corrective surgery commonly used is the Mustard procedure. This involves creating a new atrial septum from the pericardium. This new atrial septum directs deoxygenated blood from the right atrium to the bicuspid (mitral) valve, the left ventricle, the transposed pulmonary artery, and into the pulmonary circulation. It also redirects oxygenated blood returning to the left atrium to the tricuspid valve, the right ventricle, the transposed aorta, and into systemic circulation.

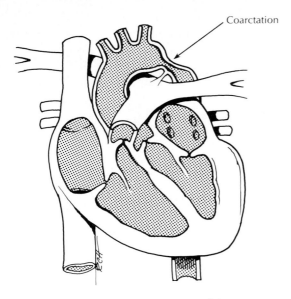

FIGURE 26-26 Coarctation of the aorta.

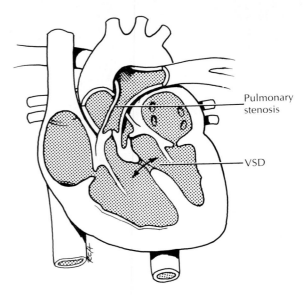

FIGURE 26-27 Fallot's tetralogy.

8.13 Coarctation of the aorta (Fig. 26-26)

1 Pathology
  a Coarctation of the aorta is an area of aortic stenosis past the subclavian artery where the ductus arteriosus joins the aorta. Although the stenosis is at the site of the ductus area, the terms "preductal" and "postductal" are often used to clarify the different groups.
  b The preductal group has a large blood shunt through the ductus arteriosus; it is associated with a high rate of mortality. The postductal group has a small blood shunt through the ductus arteriosus and a lower mortality rate.
2 Pathophysiology. The stenosis creates an elevated pressure in the ascending aorta and left ventricle. This hypertension can be severe enough to cause congestive heart failure.
3 Clinical findings. In the postductal group of coarctation, higher blood pressures and full pulses are usually found in upper extremities, with lower blood pressures and weaker pulses in the lower extremities. Patients may show signs of congestive heart failure, but the majority are asymptomatic.
4 Treatment
  a In young patients a trial of medical management of congestive heart failure is suggested first.
  b If this fails, surgical resection of the area of coarctation is required. The usual procedure is removal of the stenotic area and end-to-end reconnection (anastomosis) of the aorta without a graft.

8.14 Fallot's tetralogy (Fig. 26-27)

1 Pathology. Fallot's tetralogy is a group of four basic anatomic abnormalities:
  a A large ventricular septal defect (VSD)
  b Pulmonary stenosis
  c Right ventricular hypertrophy
  d Dextroposed aorta that receives blood from both ventricles

2 Pathophysiology. The pulmonary stenosis (pulmonary valve or pulmonary artery) causes an increase in the right ventricle and right ventricular hypertrophy. Deoxygenated blood flows through the VSD from the right ventricle into the left ventricle, creating an admixture systemically circulated.
3 Clinical findings
  a Cyanosis is the chief clinical finding. Its degree depends on the amount of pulmonary stenosis and size of the VSD.
  b Some infants are cyanotic at birth; others do not show cyanosis for months or even years. Once cyanosis develops, it becomes progressively worse. Digital clubbing may also appear.
4 Treatment. Severely cyanotic infants require immediate surgery to increase blood flow to the lungs, with complete corrective surgery once the child is older. Corrective surgery is to relieve pulmonary stenosis and closure of the VSD.

8.15 Ventricular septal defect (Fig. 26-28)

1 Pathology. A ventricular septal defect (VSD) is an opening between the ventricles that permits blood flow between them. The size of the defect can range from very small to the complete absence of the ventricular septum.
2 Pathophysiology. Because pressure is higher in the left ventricle than the right, a left-to-right shunt occurs through the defect.
3 Clinical findings
  a Patients with small defects are usually asymptomatic other than having a loud murmur, occasionally present with a thrill (a palpable murmur).
  b Patients with a medium VSD are also usually without symptoms other than faster onset of fatigue and a higher incidence of respiratory infections than others of their own age.

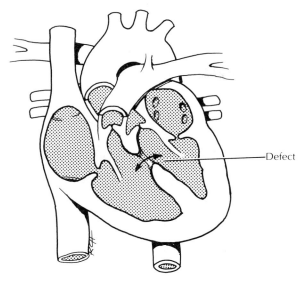

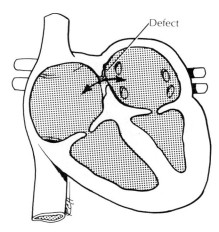

FIGURE 26-29 Atrial septal defect.

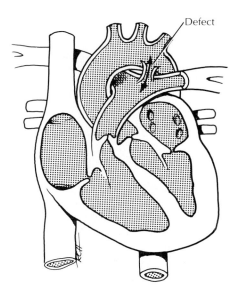

FIGURE 26-28 Ventricular septal defect.

c Patients with a large VSD usually show early congestive heart failure and are small for their age.

d Cardiac catheterization is diagnostic of the shunt size and degree of pulmonary involvement.

4 Treatment

a In asymptomatic patients, treatment is minimal, as most VSDs close spontaneously in the first 2 years of life.

b In patients with heart failure, the problem is managed medically before surgery. Surgical repair is by direct closure or a patch graft.

8.16 Atrial septal defect (Fig. 26-29)

1 Pathology. Atrial septal defect (ASD) is an opening between the atria that persists after birth.

2 Pathophysiology. There is a right-to-left shunt through the ASD as a result of the left atrial pressure being higher than the right. This causes an increase in pulmonary blood flow and increased work for the right side of the heart.

3 Clinical findings

a Most patients with ASD have few symptoms; those who do usually have respiratory symptoms.

b A pulmonary systolic ejection murmur is usually heard at the second left intercostal space and a diastolic murmur at the tricuspid area.

c The chest x-ray study shows right-sided heart and pulmonary artery hypertrophy with a relatively normal left side of heart.

d Cardiac catheterization confirms the diagnosis.

4 Treatment. Surgical correction is by direct closure or patch graft. This surgery is usually not indicated in infancy.

8.17 Patent ductus arteriosus (Fig. 26-30)

1 Pathology. The function and normal closure of the ductus arteriosus has been previously discussed. In some

FIGURE 26-30 Patent ductus arteriosus.

instances closure does not occur and results in a persistent patent ductus arteriosus (PDA).

2 Pathophysiology

a After birth, aortic pressure is higher than pulmonary artery pressure, creating a left-to-right shunt through the PDA.

b This increase in blood volume through the lungs creates increased work for the left heart.

3 Clinical findings

a Clinical findings are dependent on the size of the PDA and the volume of shunted blood.

b Although very young infants may develop congestive heart failure, most are asymptomatic, but they have a continuous murmur at the upper sternal border and under the left clavicle. Fatigability, slow growth, and frequent respiratory infections are sometimes seen.

c The chest x-ray study will usually show left ventricular and left atrial enlargement with a large aorta and pulmonary artery.

4 Treatment. Surgical correction by ligation of the ductus.

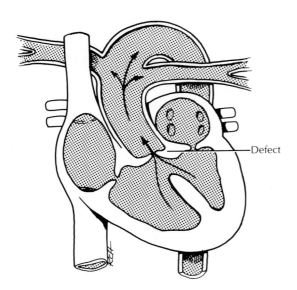

Defect

FIGURE 26-31 Truncus arteriosus. Retention of bulbar trunk, which receives blood directly from ventricles.

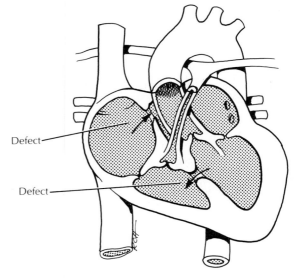

Defect

Defect

FIGURE 26-33 Tricuspid atresia. Small right ventricle and large left ventricle with diminished pulmonary circulation. Defect in septal walls causes mixing of oxygenated and unoxygenated blood.

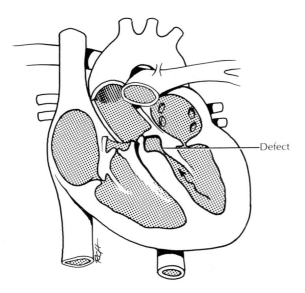

Defect

FIGURE 26-32 Subaortic stenosis. Fibrous ring below aortic valve decreases blood flow and increases work of ventricle.

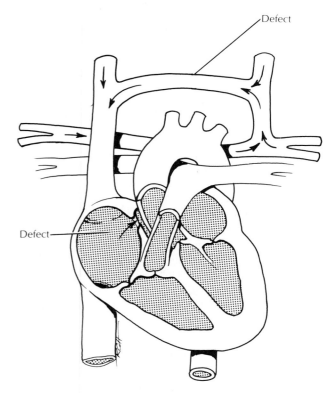

Defect

Defect

FIGURE 26-34 Anomalous venous return. Oxygenated blood from lungs is carried to right heart, resulting in mixing of oxygenated with unoxygenated blood.

8.18 Other congenital defects

1 Defects involving the aortic valve or the pulmonary valve caused by stenosis are also seen. Treatment is primarily surgical and a valvotomy is sometimes performed.

2 Other defects include:

  a Truncus arteriosus (Fig. 26-31)

  b Subaortic stenosis (Fig. 26-32)

  c Tricuspid atresia (Fig. 26-33)

  d Anomalous venous return (Fig. 26-34)

9.0 RESUSCITATION PRINCIPLES AND TECHNIQUES
9.1 Resuscitation of neonates, infants, and children

The principles and practice of cardiopulmonary resuscitation (CPR) are discussed in Module Twenty-Two. This section emphasizes CPR adaptation for infants and children. The protocol for CPR for infants and children is the same (A-B-C: airway, breathing, circulation, etc.) as for adults. With initial evaluation, airway patency and breathing effort are checked by placing the ear next to the infant's or child's nose and mouth) to feel the carotid pulse; the hand should be placed slightly below the left nipple to feel the apical beat. If the initial evaluation shows evidence of pulmonary or cardiopulmonary arrest, CPR should be initiated immediately, using basic principles with the following modifications:

1 *Airway*

  a Establishment of an airway in an infant or child is essentially the same as for adults. The infant's neck is so pliable that overextension may actually obstruct the airway. The small patient may be placed in a supine or slight head-down position.

  b Vomitus or foreign material may be cleared with a suctioning device or with the fingers, using caution with patients who have teeth. "Sweep" the material out. Do *not* push your fingers into the throat.

  c If endotracheal (ET) intubation is necessary to establish an effective airway, the American Hospital Association (AHA) and American Medical Association (AMA) recommend the sizes presented in Table 26-6.

  d Endotracheal tubes used on infants and small children are usually uncuffed because the cricoid cartilage is the narrowest part of the airway in this age-group.

  e An emergency rule of thumb for selecting ET tubes is to use a size that is approximately the same size as the patient's little finger.

  f Because of airway anatomy, a child from birth to 3 months is usually easier to intubate with the head flat on a surface or only *slightly* tilted back. After that, the airways assume a more adultlike anatomy, and the standard intubation position is used.

2 *Breathing*

  a For mouth-to-mouth breathing, the technique is slightly modified. For infants and small children, the entire mouth and nose are covered with the rescuer's

TABLE 26-6 Recommended size of tracheal tube and suction catheter

Age	Size (mm)	Suction catheter (French)
Premature	2.5	6
Newborn	3.0	6
6 months	3.5	8
18 months	4.0	8
3 years	4.5	8
5 years	5.0	10
6 years	5.5	10
8 years	6.0	10
12 years	6.5	10
16 years	7.0	10
Adult (female)	8.0-8.5	12
Adult (male)	8.5-9.0	14

mouth while short puffs from the rescuer's cheeks are administered once every 3 seconds.

  b If bag and mask ventilation is used, a gastric tube should be placed, if possible, with the stomach contents aspirated and the tube left open for air release. Pressures of 30 to 40 cm H_2O should be used for each breath.

  c Bag and mask ventilation is often used in the treatment of acute apnea, which is a common phenomenon occurring in infants. The approach is:

    • To first try stimulation; if the infant does not respond, begin bag and mask ventilation with 100% oxygen.

    – Effectiveness can be judged by color improvement and heart rate acceleration above 100 beats per minute (BPM)

    • In the event of failure of the heart rate to rise above 100 BPM after bagging for 1 minute:

    – Recheck the bag and mask mechanics.

    – Observe chest movement.

    – Listen for effective breath sounds.

      • Notify the attending physician. The patient may have to be intubated at this point.

3 *Circulation*

  a Cardiac compression for small children is performed with the heel of *one* hand. For small infants, the tips of the index and middle fingers are used (Fig. 26-35, *A* and *B*). An alternate method for small infants is to encircle the chest with the hands and compress the midsternum with both thumbs.

  b The site of compression should be midsternum because the ventricles lie higher in the chest. The risk of lacerating the liver is higher, as a result of the liver's high position being closer to the xiphoid and lower sternum.

  c The sternum of an infant should be depressed ½ to 1 inch, and for small children, 1 to 1½ inches. The compression rate is at least 100 per minute, with five compressions followed by one breath. A pause should be allowed after every fifth compression to

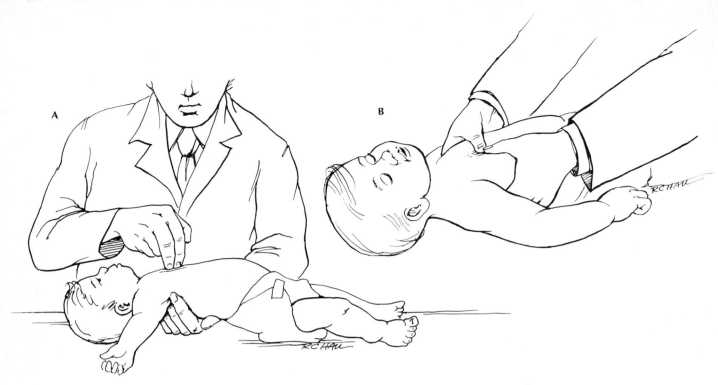

FIGURE 26-35 Proper use of hand(s) to perform compression on infants.

deliver the breath.

4 *Drugs*. The following is a list of drug dosages for infants and children:

  a Epinephrine: 0.1 ml/kg IV (of 1:10,000). (If only 1:1000 epinephrine is available, 1 ml of 1:10,000 can be made by using a graduated 1-ml syringe and drawing 0.9 ml of sterile water and 0.1 ml of 1:1000 epinephrine.)

  b Atropine: 0.01 to 0.02 mg/kg IV

  c Calcium chloride (10%): 0.2 ml/kg IV

  d Sodium bicarbonate: 1 ml (0.9 mEq)/kg (dilute 1:1 with sterile water)

  e Levarterenol bitartrate (Levophed):
    • Infants 1 mg/500 ml D5W
    • Children 2 mg/500 ml D5W
    • Titrate IV drip to desired effect

  f Lidocaine (Xylocaine):
    • Infants 0.5 mg/kg
    • Children 5 mg. Repeat dose until desired effect is obtained.
    • Isoproterenol HCl (Isuprel): IV drip 1 to 5 mg/500 ml D5W; titrate to desired effect.

  NOTE: Drugs are given only on the order or permission of a physician.

5 *ECG*. Electrocardiograms are conducted the same for children as for adults. Children do not often present the complex dysrhythmias that older patients do. They usually will have respiratory depression with sinus bradycardia, then go into respiratory arrest. If the respiratory arrest is not corrected, they will go into asystole.

6 *Defibrillation*. The anteroposterior paddle placement position is often easier to use with infants and small children because of their small chest size. The energy level usually recommended for use in patients under 50 kg is 3.5 to 6.0 watt-seconds per kg.

10.0 APPLICATIONS OF SYSTEMS FOR NEONATE AND PEDIATRIC PATIENTS
10.1 Continuous positive airway pressure and pediatric mechanical ventilation

1 Constant distending airway pressure (CDAP) in the form of positive end-expiratory pressure (PEEP) and continuous positive airway pressure (CPAP) has come into frequent use in neonatology and pediatrics since its successful use in the treatment of hyaline membrane disease (HMD) by G.A. Gregory (see Bibliography).

2 An issue of previous controversy was the difference between CPAP and PEEP. Initially CPAP was defined as positive airway pressure with spontaneous breathing, and PEEP was positive airway pressure with mechanical breathing.

  Currently CPAP describes a system that utilizes a high-pressure reservoir and a constant gas flow that exceeds the patient's peak inspiratory needs. This system may be used in conjunction with or without a mechanical ventilator and provides a positive airway pressure during inspiration and exhalation. A PEEP system utilizes an open-ended unpressurized reservoir. In order to obtain a gas flow the patient must drop the airway pressure from a preset positive end-expiratory level to below ambient.

  These mechanical differences are important because they can be translated to lung function. For example,

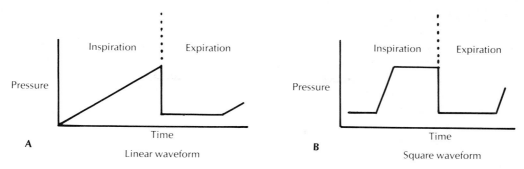

FIGURE 26-36 Square pressure waveform ventilation. Pressure sufficient to open collapsed alveoli is achieved early in the inspiratory phase and held at a constant level until expiration.

with PEEP the work of breathing is greater. This is because the patient must overcome the resistance of the breathing circuit and end level of positive pressure in order to create a pressure gradient for gas to flow.

a Physiologically this effort is translated as an increase in the work of breathing.

b In some patients this may be desirable; in others, hazardous.

c The point is that the practitioner must be aware of the potential.

3 Gregory's application of CPAP was with the use of a plastic chamber enclosing the infant's head. This has given way to newer forms of application that are not as inaccessible or bulky. One method is the use of special nasal prongs. Another is the placement of a nasotracheal tube with the tip in the pharynx. CPAP can also be applied to patients who are intubated or who have tracheostomy tubes.

4 When CPAP and/or PEEP is used with mechanical ventilation, most systems also incorporate an intermittent mandatory ventilation (IMV) mode. As was explained in Module Twenty-three, IMV was initially used as a method for weaning infants from mechanical ventilators. The principle of allowing an infant to breathe spontaneously from a reservoir with a controlled FIo_2 with preset intermittent mechanical positive pressure breaths was successful. Its application not only expedited the weaning process, but also resulted in lower mean intrapleural pressure and a lower incidence of barotrauma.

5 CPAP functions when used without IMV provide a constant flow of gas that elevates end-expired pressure above atmospheric levels and increases functional residual capacity (FRC). This type of system increases the potential for tension pressure thorax and other types of barotrauma.

6 A note of caution: Nasal CPAP and CPAP by nasopharyngeal tube may also cause gastric distension. This is easily relieved and controlled by placement of a gastric tube.

7 Since it has been discovered that bronchopulmonary dysplasia results from high pressure and high concentrations delivered by mechanical ventilation through an endotracheal tube, less hazardous protocols of mechanical ventilation have been established. Premature infants with hyaline membrane disease (HMD) were especially at risk to develop bronchopulmonary dysplasia (BPD) because of the aggressive ventilation management necessary to overcome the constant alveolar collapse.

8 The basis for pressure ventilation with HMD is that a pressure sufficient to open collapsed alveoli is achieved early in the inspiratory phase and held at a constant level until expiration. This is known as a *square pressure waveform* (Fig. 26-36, *A* and *B*). By maintaining peak pressure throughout most of the inspiratory phase, with the use of the "square wave," the alveoli remain open for gas exchange to occur longer *(B)*.

9 Use of the square pressure waveform allows ventilation at lower rates and lower pressures. A low rate of 20 to 30 breaths per minute (BPM) (low for an infant) is a good range, but higher rates may be necessary. Pressure settings below 30 cm H_2O are initially utilized, but some infants require a higher pressure. Pressures over 30 cm H_2O for prolonged periods of time have been associated with increased incidence of BPD.

10 In the late 1960s, physicians (primarily in Sweden) began to use reverse I:E ratios in mechanical ventilation. Because alveoli are opened to gas exchange for the majority of the inspiratory phase, it seemed logical to make the inspiratory phase longer. Not being able to lower rates to increase the inspiratory phase, the I:E was altered to shorten the expiratory phase. The complications of prolonged periods of positive pressure and short expiratory times (from the use of 2:1 or 3:1 ratios) that an adult patient would experience are not usually seen in the newborn. This results from the high elasticity of the newborn's lungs, creating a very short expiratory time (less than 1 second), as well as the "stiff tissue" or low compliance of the lungs, which does not usually allow positive pressure to impede venous return and which causes other complications.

11 Mechanically the use of reverse I:E ratios was replaced by high-frequency ventilation (HFV). Because this concept is fully explained in Module Twenty-three, it will suffice to point out that HFV has been successfully used in the treatment of infants who, for various reasons, did not favorably respond to more

conventional methods of mechanical ventilation.

a Most infants seem to respond best to cycling rates between 400 and 600 BPM, although success with rates at 1000 BPM or greater have been reported. Some HFV is capable of delivering rates faster than 2000 BPM. However, at rates greater than 2000 BPM, more problems are encountered with inadvertent PEEP and CO_2 retention, interference with mucociliary transport, and cardiovascular function. This requires the practitioner to be especially observant and responsive to the needs of these patients.

b Clearly HFV systems are not indicated for every patient needing mechanical ventilation.

c Like CPAP, PEEP, and IMV, clinical experience will be helpful to better identify the indications and contraindications for the use of HFV.

12 Even though not recommended practice in certain situations, it may become necessary to ventilate an infant or small child with a volume ventilator.

a In volume ventilators, gas compressibility and tubing elasticity cause some of the volume delivered by the ventilator to be "lost" in the circuit. This "lost volume" is known as *system (or mechanical) compliance,* and it plays a critical role when small tidal volumes are used.

An example of the significance of lost volume on the total volume follows:

Lost volume = Peak pressure × System compliance

Consider a volume ventilator with a system compliance of 3 ml/cm H_2O. A 150-kg adult is being ventilated at a tidal volume (V_T) of 10 ml/kg and develops a peak pressure of 25 cm H_2O. (See also Module Twenty-three.)

- Lost volume = Peak pressure × System compliance
  = 25 cm H_2O × 3 ml/cm H_2O
  = 75 ml

- V_T = Set volume − Lost volume
  V_T = 1500 − 75
  V_T = 1425 ml
  − 75 ml represents a 5% loss of volume delivered to this patient.

13 Now consider a 15 kg child being ventilated at a tidal volume of 10 ml/kg who develops a peak pressure of 25 cm H_2O.

a Lost volume = 25 × 3 = 75 ml

b V_T = 150 − 75 = 75 ml

- 75 ml represents a 50% loss of volume delivered to this patient.

14 As demonstrated by these two examples, anyone who works with small patients on volume ventilators must know how to calculate compliance loss. Aside from a volume loss standpoint, compliance calculation is often the only practical means of measuring the tidal volume. A 1-kg premature infant ventilated at 10 to 15 ml/kg will have a tidal volume of 10 to 15 ml, a volume below the levels of accurate measurement for many spirometers.

15 Compliance and tidal volume calculations can be performed by the following method:

a $\dfrac{\text{Set volume}}{\text{Occluded pressure}}$ = System compliance

b System compliance × Peak pressure = Lost volume

c Set volume − Lost volume = Tidal volume

16 To show how this method is used, take, for example, an 8-kg child who is to be placed on a Bennett MA-1 ventilator with a tidal volume of 8 to 10 ml/kg (64 to 80 ml).

a The ventilator is set to deliver a volume of 100 ml measured with a spirometer because knob markings are not precise enough. On the MA-1, a Wright respirometer measurement (or recalculation-readjustment) may have to be performed several times before a correct tidal volume is obtained.

b Next, the occluded pressure is obtained by placing the pressure limit knob at its maximum setting, occluding (completely obstructing) the circuit, and observing the pressure on the manometer when the ventilator cycles. In this example, say the occluded pressure was 33 cm H_2O.

c Next, the circuit is attached to the patient and, when stabilized, the peak pressure is noted. For our young patient, say it was 20 cm H_2O.

d After obtaining these measurements, the calculations are performed:

- Systems compliance = $\dfrac{100}{33}$ = 3.0 ml/cm H_2O

- Lost volume = 20 × 3.0 = 60 ml

- Tidal volume = 100 − 60 = 40 ml

e Our patient's tidal volume range should be 64 to 80 ml, so it is necessary to *increase the MA-1 volume setting.* This increase in volume will cause an increase in peak pressure and an increase in lost volume to the circuit. Systems compliance, being a linear function, will not have to be recalculated, but correction for lost volume will.

f We will increase the set volume to 150 ml (again using a spirometer). This causes the peak pressure to increase to 25 cm H_2O.

- Systems compliance = 3.0 ml/cm H_2O

- Lost volume = 25 × 3.0 = 75 ml

- Tidal volume − 150 − 75 = 75 ml

g The delivered volume (tidal volume) is now within the required range, and no further adjustments are necessary. In actual practice, however, the calculation-adjustment-recalculation-readjustment may have to be performed several times before a correct tidal volume is obtained.

17 As previously mentioned, systems compliance does not have to be recalculated because it is a linear function.

A linear function in this case means that when pressure and volume are plotted against one another, they form a straight line (linear) (Fig. 26-37).

18 Systems compliance does not have to be recalculated, *provided* there is no change in the circuit. The circuit will be altered if length or type of tubing is changed (e.g., permanent versus disposable tubing) and if the water level in the humidifier or nebulizer is not maintained at a constant level.

19 In our example, a child who weighed less than 18 pounds was ventilated with an adult volume ventilator. Not all adult volume ventilators are suitable for adaptation for small patients. The practitioner should be thoroughly aware of the limits of an adult volume ventilator before attempting to adapt it for pediatric use.

20 The reader is encouraged to review Module Twenty-three for details regarding specific infant and adult ventilators.

10.2 Newborn facilities and personnel

1 As was previously stated, the survival rate of premature infants has increased from approximately 50% in the 1960s to approximately 70% today. For example, in the 1960s hyaline membrane disease alone claimed 25,000 lives.

2 In the early 1970s, neonatology began to be recognized as a medical speciality and, in 1976, three levels of nurseries were identified by the March of Dimes in a publication titled *Towards Improving the Outcome of Pregnancy.*

3 In this publication, nurseries were catogorized as Levels I, II, or III on the basis of the sophistication of care available.

4 The Level I nursery provides routine care of the newborn and does not have the highly trained staff or life-support equipment necessary to care for long-term care infants.

5 The Level II nursery provides routine care plus intermediate life-support until long-term infants can be transferred.

6 The Level III nursery provides the highest level of care for the newborn. This level nursery has a full staff of specially trained personnel and the most current in life-support and environmental control equipment to maintain the newborn. A Level III nursery also has the capability of transporting and receiving newborns from other facilities.

7 Members of the transport team receive special training by the hospital and/or agency licensed to transport infants. Individuals serving on a transport team usually include a registered nurse, a registered respiratory therapist, and a physician.

8 The physician commonly is a neonatologist with special training or interest in transport services. This physician usually serves as the medical director for the team and is responsible for the overall training and performance of the team.

9 The medical director does not actually travel with the

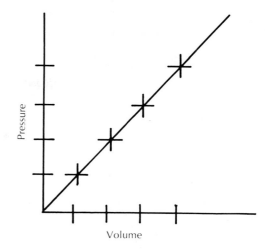

FIGURE 26-37 System compliance. Pressure and volume, when plotted against each other, form a straight line, showing that compliance is a linear function.

transport team, except in unusal circumstances warranting his or her expertise.

10 When the physician is not present, the transport team practices according to standing orders and/or by voice communication and telemetry with a medical base station.

10.3 Newborn and high-risk transport

1 Newborns may be transported from one facility to another via a land transportation vehicle (such as a van), by helicopter, or by fixed-wing aircraft.

2 When selecting a method of transportation, the following variables should be considered:

a *Distance.* Time is always an important consideration when relocating a critical patient from one care facility to another. This is especially true in premature infants who require a totally controlled environment along with life support. A rule of thumb is ground transport should be considered whenever distances are 80 miles or less one-way.

b *Availability of qualified transportation.* Even though distance is a primary consideration, one must be aware of the ability of the transport method to provide trained personnel and customized equipment and ability to gain easy access to the patient. For example, the distance to an airport in order to access a fixed wing aircraft plus the flying time may take as long or longer than transporting the patient over surface roads.

c *Equipment.* No matter which method of transport is selected, it is vital that the vehicle be equipped to continue the environmental and life-support requirements of the infant. In some cases this will require that the infant be transferred to equipment provided by the transport service or—ideally—the hospital will have transport equipment that is compatible with the transport vehicle. This vehicle should have the following equipment available:

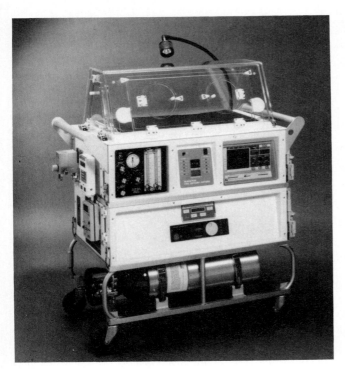

FIGURE 26-38 Typical infant transport chamber. (Courtesy International Biomedical, Inc, Houston, Tex.)

- Oxygen source adequate for the trip plus 2 hours
- Suction to meet the standards required by the American Heart Association (Module Twenty-two)
- Environmental chamber (transport unit) or ability to secure transport chamber from the hospital.
- Primary and back-up radios capable of communicating with medical base station(s)
- Room for the team to work with the infant during transport
- Adequate lighting, with back-up systems in the event of power failure
- Primary and back-up power sources to operate the infant's environmental chamber and monitors

    d *Physiologic effects on patient.* Transporting a patient is, at best, a trying procedure on an infant's system that is already stressed. If the patient is transported by land vehicle, the ride should be as smooth as possible, with no sudden movements that may jar the patient. If transportation is by air, then the practitioner must be aware of altitude-related problems. More specifically, as the altitude increases, any gas contained in a closed space will expand by more than one fourth of its initial volume. Even in pressurized aircraft, the cabin pressure is maintained at approximately 8000 feet. At this altitude, the cabin pressure will decrease from 760 mm Hg at sea level to approximately 565 mm Hg, or 26% of the sea level value. This change results in gas volume increases in the thorax, lungs, intestines, central nervous system, and other anatomic spaces, as well as

in equipment. In premature infants, even the slightest increase in gas volume may create pressures that can be hazardous.

10.4 Typical transport chamber (Fig. 26-38)

1 The following is one example of a high-risk infant transport chamber that can be used in a land vehicle, helicopter, or fixed wing aircraft.
2 This chamber, offered by Airborne Life Support Systems, incorporates the following features:
    a A double-wall transparent hood to prevent radiant heat loss and provide total visibility of infant
    b Adjustable heat controls and instruments that are highly visible and simple to operate
    c Audible and visual alarms for maximum safety
    d Humidity and oxygen support
    e Long-life internal power source (battery)
    f Lightweight self-contained transport base with built-in monitor, ventilator, and intravenous syringe pump capability

11.0 RESPIRATORY DISEASES OF OLDER INFANTS AND CHILDREN

11.1 Croup

1 Croup or laryngotracheobronchitis usually occurs in children between 6 months and 3 years of age. The disease is often a frightening experience for children and parents.
2 Pathology
    a Croup is mainly (85% of cases) a viral process associated with parainfluenza virus, adenovirus, and respiratory syncytial virus. Measles and influenza viruses have also been associated with croup. When caused by bacteria, *Haemophilus influenzae type B* is the usual causative agent.
    b The disorder infects the larynx, trachea, and bronchi; severity of symptoms is related to the degree of involvement of these various regions. The primary danger of croup is laryngeal obstruction and related complications.
3 Clinical findings
    a There is usually a history of the child's having had a cold or runny nose for several days before the onset of a barking cough, stridor, and retractions.
    b Fever, if present, is usually mild, and white blood cell count is usually below 15,000, mm^3.
    c As the disease process worsens, laryngeal obstruction is increased, as shown by increase in stridor and retractions, prolonged inspiratory and expiratory phases, and decreased breath sounds.
    d The patient may appear markedly apprehensive and short of breath. It is sometimes necessary to mildly sedate severe cases.
    e Cyanosis is a sign of severe, almost complete, obstruction of the larynx.
    f Airway x-ray examination shows obvious upper airway stenosis secondary to inflammation.

4 Treatment

  a Cool mist is very effective in reducing laryngeal edema. This is provided by croup tents in hospitals. Parents will often bring their child to the emergency room at night only to find the barking and stridor are gone. This results from the child's breathing the cool outside air en route to the hospital.

  b Racemic epinephrine has often been found effective in easing laryngeal swelling and can be used to control acute episodes. A common pediatric dosage is 0.05 ml (of 2.25% solution) diluted to 3.0 ml with normal saline.

  c Examples of commonly used dosages of racemic epinephrine are presented in Table 26-7.

  d The 1:1 solution (1.5 ml racemic epinephrine [RE] and 1.5 ml normal saline [NS]) is the strongest dosage given to patients weighing 30 kg and above. Treatments can be given up to every 30 minutes while cautiously checking heart rate.

  e In the event humidity and drug therapy are ineffective, an artificial airway may be necessary. This is accomplished by nasotracheal intubation or tracheostomy.

  f A word about around-the-clock treatments. Many medical writers insist that sleeping children and infants *never* be awakened to be given treatments. To do so will only increase the patient's apprehension and restlessness. This seems to be a reasonable and logical axiom.

11.2 Epiglottitis

1 This disease has a rapid acute onset, occurring mostly in the 3- to 7-year age-group. It is sometimes called supraglottic croup.

2 Pathology

  a The affected area is the epiglottis. Surrounding tissues of the larynx are not usually affected.

  b The most common cause of epiglottitis is *Haemophilus influenzae type B,* although other bacterial types have been found.

  c The supraglottic region will have a cherry red color because of inflammation. This inflammation causes difficulty in swallowing, as a result of swelling of the epiglottis. This swelling can rapidly worsen and obstruct the entire airway.

3 Clinical findings

  a The onset of symptoms is rapid. Younger patients show more involved respiratory distress and fever. Older ones may complain of a sore throat.

  b One prominent sign of epiglottitis is drooling or inability to swallow. The epiglottis can be visualized with a tongue blade to confirm the cherry red color of inflammation, but there is a risk of complete airway obstruction with stimulation of the region, especially if the child is apprehensive. Health care personnel should be prepared to immediately intubate or perform tracheotomy.

  c X-ray examination will show enlarged epiglottis, es-

TABLE 26-7 Common dosages of racemic epinephrine

Patient weight (kg)	Racemic epinephrine (ml)	Diluant (ml)	Total (ml)	Micrograms kg/minute
10	0.5	2.5	3.0	112.5
25	1.25	1.75	3.0	112.5
30	1.5	1.5	3.0	112.5

pecially a lateral film. White blood cell count is usually above 15,000 mm^3 and *H. influenzae* can usually be cultured from nasal and blood specimens.

4 Treatment

  a For mild-to-moderate cases the treatment is the same as for infantile croup.

  b The usual treatment of severe cases is an artificial airway. This is accomplished by tracheostomy or nasotracheal intubation by a competent experienced person (e.g., anesthesiologist) to reduce the incidence of further trauma.

  c Increased fluid intake (usually IV) and antibiotic therapy are usually instituted. The patient can usually be extubated in 2 to 3 days.

11.3 Bronchiolitis

1 In children, the area between the bronchi and respiratory units does not have much cartilage support. Until adolescence (the time of cartilage support development) inflammation in this region can cause considerable problems, especially smooth muscle constriction.

2 Pathology

  a The most common cause is the respiratory syncytial virus with bronchiolar obstruction and the primary lesion.

  b Bronchial obstruction from bronchial edema, mucus, or cellular debris may result in air trapping. Complete occlusion may result in absorption atelectasis, along with emphysema.

  c The decreased lumen resulting from thickening of the bronchial tissue increases the airway resistance.

  d Diffusion, especially of oxygen, is impaired because of scattered obstructed regions.

  e Respiratory failure and secondary bacterial infections are the main complications of the disease.

3 Clinical findings

  a A runny nose several days beforehand or viral illness in the family may be found. A low-grade fever, tachypnea, and tachycardia are usually seen.

  b Rales, cough, and wheezing are usually noted, along with dyspneic shallow breathing.

  c White blood cell count is usually normal. Chest x-ray films may be deceptively normal, but there is almost always hyperinflation and a flattened diaphragm seen especially well in a lateral film.

4 Treatment

  a Hydration is very important either by mouth or IV.

  b Oxygen should always be administered with adequate humidity, as the majority of patients with bronchiolitis are hypoxic. Mist is not usually therapeutic, other than humidifying the oxygen.

c Sometimes a trial of bronchodilators is helpful, but often it is not; the same is true for corticosteroids.

d Intubation and mechanical ventilation may be necessary.

e The disease usually lasts 7 to 10 days and has a low mortality rate and excellent prognosis.

11.4 Cystic fibrosis

1 Cystic fibrosis (CF, mucoviscidosis) is a mendelian recessive disorder (see Genetics) involving the exocrine glands of the body. It is a major cause of chronic lung disease and death in children. It was not clinically reported until 1936.

2 Pathology

a CF has three common findings, known as the triad of CF:
- Chronic pulmonary disease
- Pancreatic deficiency
- High sweat electrolyte concentration

b Chronic pulmonary disease begins as goblet cells increase in number and size, and hypersecretions of thick, tenacious mucus follow. This causes obstruction to occur, leading to overinflation, focal atelectasis, and a culture medium for bacterial growth (stagnant mucus). Further progress of the disease leads to tissue destruction, chronic bronchitis, bronchiectasis, fibrosis, abscesses, and repeated pneumonitis. Repeated secondary infections are usually *Staphylococcus aureus* and *Pseudomonas aeruginosa*. Over 90% of CF patients have pulmonary involvement, varying in the degree of severity. Pancreatic insufficiency is found in 80% of CF patients.

c Newborns may have normal pancreatic function at birth, but thick secretions beginning in the first few months cause dilation and eventual destruction of exocrine ducts. The fibrosis and fatty infiltration of the pancreas leads to the increased number and size of stools. The stool is foul-smelling and greasy, often giving family physicians a clue to the possibility of CF.

d There is often an increase in food consumption with a failure to gain weight. The pancreatic islets of Langerhans may not be affected until the latter phases of tissue destruction. This has been associated with the onset of diabetes mellitus.

e The excessive mucus production in the intestine causes a variety of obstructions. Meconium ileus is usually diagnostic of CF when present in a newborn. Approximately 10% of all CF infants are born with meconium ileus.

f Occasionally CF infants show excessive sweating. Sweat electrolyte levels are elevated from birth, believed to result from the failure of the sweat glands to reabsorb sodium, chloride, and potassium. Extreme exposure during hot weather can cause complications from excessive salt loss.

3 Clinical findings

a Abnormal sweat electrolyte
- The child may show excessive sweating, with salt buildup in the hair and a salty-tasting skin.
- The "Kiss Your Baby Week" program has been promoted by many CF organizations as a means of mass screening for CF.
- The induced sweat test for CF has about 98% reliability.

b Digestive
- A good appetite may or may not be present.
- Weight gain and physical growth are delayed. Skeletal maturation is slow to develop, resulting in small stature.
- Milk allergy in early infancy is present.
- The abdomen is often protuberant, and stools are loose, bulky, pale, greasy, and foul-smelling.
- Pancreatic insufficiency is present.
- Meconium ileus in the newborn is the earliest sign of CF; intestinal atresia may be present.

c Respiratory
- Physical abnormalities may include increased thoracic volume (barrel chest), digital clubbing, cyanosis, hyperresonance with percussion, pigeon breast, and intercostal retractions.
- Atelectasis, pneumothorax, and hemoptysis occur often.
- Paroxysmal cough, often severe enough to produce emesis, is a common finding.
- Chest x-ray studies usually show overinflation, scattered aeration, and hilar node enlargement.
- In the latter stages of the disease, hypoxemia, hypercapnia, and cor pulmonale are often seen.

d Treatment
- Diet is modified for adequate protein and reduction of fat intake. Powder or tablet pancreatic replacement with meals is necessary.
- Excessive salt loss can cause hypovolemic shock, which is usually treated with supplemental saline intake.
- Respiratory therapy is designed to mobilize secretions, aid in their removal, and control pulmonary infections.
- Acetylcysteine has found its most popular use in the treatment of CF. A recommended dose is 3.0 ml of 10% acetylcysteine, alternating with 3.0 ml of normal saline by aerosol four times a day (q.i.d.). The rationale for alternating acetylcysteine and normal saline is to reduce the incidence of hemoptysis and bronchial irritation.
- The aerosol given by updraft nebulizer is followed by chest physical therapy in *all* positions. The aerosol and physical therapy usually take 30 minutes to an hour, but are necessary to adequately remove secretions.
- Occasionally oxygen in the low-to-moderate range is necessary and should be monitored by arterial blood gas (ABG) analysis.

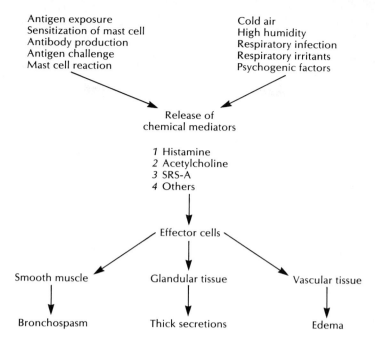

Antigen exposure
Sensitization of mast cell
Antibody production
Antigen challenge
Mast cell reaction

Cold air
High humidity
Respiratory infection
Respiratory irritants
Psychogenic factors

Release of
chemical mediators

1 Histamine
2 Acetylcholine
3 SRS-A
4 Others

Effector cells

Smooth muscle   Glandular tissue   Vascular tissue

Bronchospasm   Thick secretions   Edema

F I G U R E   2 6 - 3 9 Allergic response cycle.

- Prophylactic immunization for measles, pertussis, and influenza reduce the incidence of pulmonary infection. Measles can be especially dangerous to a CF patient.
- When a respiratory infection does occur, hospitalization is often necessary for IV antibiotics. Multiple antibiotics are sometimes used from 10 to 14 days of treatment, along with aerosol and physical therapy.

11.5 Asthma

1 Asthma is a reversible obstructive-restrictive airway disease that occurs in all ages, but most frequently in childhood and early adulthood. The term comes from a Greek word meaning "panting" and has been used to describe a number of pulmonary problems. The axiom that "all that wheezes is not asthma" remains true, and other wheezing disorders should be differentiated.

2 Pathology

a Allergic reaction is the most common form of asthma in pediatric patients. The IgE antibody, present in increased levels in atopic persons, is believed to be the primary mechanism. However, other mechanisms can also trigger an attack. On an insult from an allergen, IgE antibodies attach to mast cells of the tracheobronchial tree and react, causing mast cell damage.

b Mast cells are connective tissue cells that, after the IgE reaction, release histamine, acetycholine, and slow-reacting substances of anaphylaxis (SRS-A), Fig. 26-39 presents the allergic response cycle.

c The result of this release causes bronchial smooth muscle constriction, mucosal edema, and excessive thick bronchial secretions. These events lead to in-

creased airway resistance, small airway collapse, air trapping, obstruction by secretions, and severe disturbance in gas volume/volume flow of blood per unit of time $\dot{V}/\dot{Q}$.

d Asthma may also be triggered by:
- High humidity
- Cold weather exposure
- Exercise or physical stress
- Emotional stress
- Inhalation of irritating substances
- Infections

e Sensory fibers located in the upper and lower airways are stimulated by stress or irritation. As the impulses traveling along the vagus nerve reach the brainstem, a reflex output to vagal parasympathetic fibers returns to the lungs. This reflex causes bronchoconstriction and a release of mast cell substances, resulting in the same reaction as that of allergic asthma.

3 Clinical findings

a The usual onset is cough, tightness of the chest, wheezing, and dyspnea. The patient will usually be sitting upright, bending forward, and obviously struggling to breathe. Tachycardia is usually present. The patient is anxious and agitated.

b The chest is usually expanded (representing increased functional residual capacity [FRC] because of air trapping), accessory muscles are in use, and usually wheezing can be heard without a stethoscope. Expiratory time is increased significantly.

c Chest x-ray examination may be normal or show only overinflation. Occasionally thick mucous impactions may show up as small wedges moving to different areas on subsequent films as the patient expectorates old ones, and new ones form.

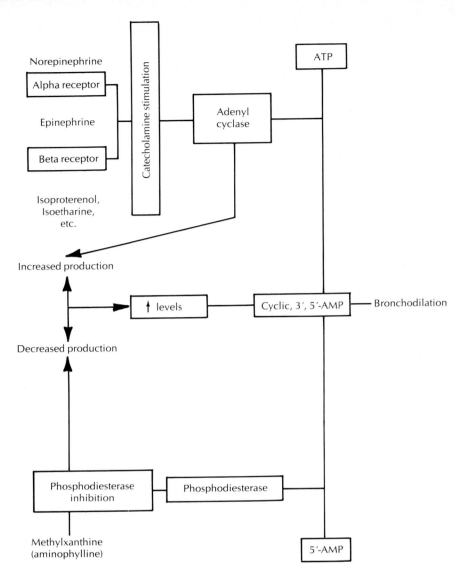

FIGURE 26-40 Two pharmacologic routes to obtain bronchodilation.

d Sputum is thick, white-to-clear, but occasionally yellow in status asthmaticus. Sputum may contain white spirals (Curschmann's spirals) and is so tenacious that sometimes a plug will be expectorated and retain the shape of the region of the tracheobronchial tree in which it was wedged (bronchial cast).

4 Treatment

a The beta-adrenergic theory describes two pharmacologic routes to obtain bronchodilation (Fig. 26-40).

- Adenylate cyclase catalyzes adenosine triophosphate (ATP) to cyclic 3',5'—adenosine monophosphate (3'-5'-cAMP). Catecholamine stimulation (epinephrine, isoetherine, isoproterenol, etc.) increases the level of adenylate cyclase, thus increasing the level of 3'-5'-cyclic AMP, causing bronchodilation.

- Phosphodiesterase breaks down 3',5'-cAMP to 5'-AMP. Methylxanthine inhibition (theophylline, aminophylline, etc.) decreases the level of phosphodiesterase, allowing a buildup of 3',5'-cyclic AMP.

- These two pathways explain the common use of IV aminophylline and topical bronchodilators like isoetherine.

b Increased levels of 3',5'-cyclic AMP cause smooth muscle relaxation and bronchodilation.

c The therapeutics used in asthma sometimes produce rapid relief, but at other times they are ineffective. Status asthmaticus is a term used to describe asthma that continues in spite of normal treatment and requires aggressive treatment to avoid possible life-threatening results.

d NOTE: One drug, cromolyn sodium (Disodium cromoglycate), has been shown to be effective in *preventing* attacks by blocking antigen-induced bronchial provocation responses (antigen challenges to the sensitized mast cells). Cromolyn sodium has *no* effect once an attack is under way.

e Initially patients with asthma should be placed on oxygen in low-to-medium levels, not only to overcome hypoxia but to prevent constriction of the pulmonary vascular bed, resulting from hypoxia.

f Subcutaneous epinephrine (1:1000) 0.2 to 0.5 ml is administered, usually repeated if necessary three times 15 to 30 minutes apart.

g ABG analysis can be obtained before treatment to establish a baseline for evaluation of therapy. Treatment of severe asthma should not be withheld only to establish baseline ABG values. Early and frequent ABGs are necessary to evaluate the extent of severity of the attack, as well as the effectiveness of the therapy. Asthmatic patients usually have decreased oxygen tension (Po_2) levels. Pco_2 levels are decreased in the early stages of the attack because of hyperventilation, and a normal or increased range Pco_2 is often a sign of severe ventilation impairment.

h Hydration is very important to aid in mobilization of the thick secretions. If increased oral hydration is not adequate, an IV at $1\frac{1}{2}$ times maintenance level is necessary. Hydration should begin in the early stages of treatment and be continued with the other therapeutic regimens.

i After epinephrine, aerosol bronchodilators should be administered, varying in frequency with the severity of the attack and effectiveness of the drug. The choice of drug and dosage varies. A common dose of isoetherine is 0.25 to 0.5 ml in 2.5 ml of normal saline, administered by updraft nebulizer. Initially three doses are given every 1 to 2 hours, carefully monitoring heart rate; then it is given on an occasional (p.r.n.) basis—as needed.

j IV aminophylline is the mainstay of asthmatic therapy, given from every 6 hours to a continuous infusion, depending on the severity of the attack.

k Sometimes corticosteroids are used to treat the attack, usually after routine measures have failed.

l Sometimes the patient does not respond to the usual regimen of therapy. The condition is known as status asthmaticus and is life threatening, requiring aggressive treatment. Indications of severity are as follows:
- General cyanosis
- Tachycardia
- Pulsus paradoxus
- Pao_2 less than 60 mm Hg
- $Paco_2$ greater than 40 mm Hg
- Poor response to bronchodilators
- Change in consciousness

m The patient should be in an intensive care unit (ICU) for monitoring and care should be provided by specially trained personnel.

n Intubation and mechanical ventilation may be necessary. Usually dyspnea is so severe the patient "fights the ventilator," rendering it ineffective. Thus the individual must be either sedated or paralyzed for effective mechanical ventilation.

o See Module Fifteen for further information on pharmaceutical agents.

BIBLIOGRAPHY

Air ambulance guidelines, U.S. Department of Transportation of the Highway Traffic Safety Administration and the Commission on Emergency Medical Services of the American Medical Association, Chicago, 1981, 2-9, 4-1.

Bell EF and Rios GR: A double wall incubator alters the partition of body heat loss of premature infants, Pediatrics 71:104 1983.

Bhat R et al: Colloid osmotic pressure in infants, with hyaline membrane disease, Chest 83:776, 1983.

Burton GG, Gee GN, and Hodgkin JE, editors: Respiratory care: a guide to clinical practice, Philadelphia, 1977, JB Lippincott Co.

Doyle H and Fried J: Reduction of circuit resistance in the Babybird ventilator, Respir Care 28:1143, 1983.

Epstein MF: Neonatal and pediatric respiratory care: an update on research, Respir Care 27:295, 1982.

Farrell PM and Wood RE: Epidemiology of hyaline membrane disease in the United States: analysis of national mortality statistics, Pediatrics 58:167, 1976.

Gregory GA et al: Treatment of the idiopathic respiratory distress syndrome with continuous positive airway pressure, N Engl J Med 284:1333, 1971.

Harpin VA and Rutter N: Humidification of incubators, Arch Dis Child 60:219, 1985.

Hislop AA, Wigglesunth BS, and De Sai R: Alveolar development in the human fetus and infant, Early Hum Dev 13:1, 1986.

Hodson WA: Development of the lung, New York, 1977, Marcel Dekker Inc.

Korones SB and Lancaster J: High-risk newborn infants: the basis for intensive nursing care, ed 3, St Louis, 1981, The CV Mosby Co.

Latham HC et al: Pediatric nursing, ed 3, St Louis, 1977, The CV Mosby Co.

Mosby's Medical & Nursing Dictionary, ed 3, St Louis, 1990, The CV Mosby Co.

O'Rourke PP: High frequency ventilation in the pediatric patient in 1983 Convention Lecture Series, American Scientific Products and American Association for Respiratory Therapy, Kansas City, 1983.

Pierson DJ: Persistent bronchopleural air leak during mechanical ventilation: a review, Respir Care 27:408, 1982.

Tanswell AK: Continuous distending pressure in the respiratory distress syndrome of the newborn: who, when, and why? Respir Care 27:257, 1982.

Personnel management and supervision

On completion of this module the reader will be able to:

1.1 Discuss basic concepts of management.

1.2 Explain the managerial grid.

1.3 Discuss the basic concepts of planning, organizing, coordinating, and controlling.

2.1 List the primary human motivational factors according to Maslow.

2.2 List job factors that are important motivators for employees.

3.1 Describe the concept of planning known as "management by objectives."

3.2 Define quality circles and point out the six-step process involved in their implementation.

3.3 Discuss the advantages of quality circles.

3.4 Discuss the disadvantages of quality circles.

3.5 Discribe theory Z management.

3.6 Discuss the advantages of using theory Z management.

3.7 Point out the disadvantages of using theory Z managment.

4.1 Schedule employees for optimum patient care and maximum employee satisfaction.

4.2 Explain and calculate real employee time, planning for vacation, holiday, and sick time.

4.3 Calculate the total number of employees necessary to staff a department with a specified number of employees per shift.

5.1 Draw and explain an organizational chart of a typical department, including a medical director, department manager, supervisors, and staff.

5.2 Explain the concept of span of control (management).

5.3 Identify the optimum and maximum number of employees who should work for one person (span of control).

5.4 Explain the concept of an employee having only one "boss."

6.1 Identify the major source of employee and management problems.

6.2 Describe an equitable grievance procedure.

6.3 Discuss the rights of an employee in a grievance procedure.

6.4 Describe a system of hiring, counseling, warning, suspension, and termination designed to be fair and equitable to both the employee and the hospital.

7.1 Describe the concept and techniques of active listening and its advantages.

7.2 Describe communication in the formal and informal organization.

7.3 Describe methods of communication that decrease the need for the informal organization.

8.1 Describe the use of job descriptions in managing a respiratory therapy department.

8.2 Describe the roles and responsibilities of the respiratory care practitioner as listed by the American Association for Respiratory Care (AARC) in "Delineation of the Roles and Functions of the Entry-Level Generalist Respiratory Therapy Practitioner" (Appendix A).

8.3 Discuss the role of the AARC Task Force on Professional Direction and the importance of its findings on the respiratory care profession.

9.1 Explain the role in patient care and hospital organization of a physician, nursing supervisor, and registered nurse.

10.1 Describe the concept of an exempt and a nonexempt employee.

10.2 Delineate the responsibilities of a department manager.

10.3 Describe the basic concepts of formulating procedures for departmental use.

10.4 Describe the legal liabilities of a department manager.

11.1 Describe evaluation by objectives.

11.2 Describe evaluation by the critical incident technique.

11.3 Demonstrate understanding of in-service education.

12.1 Define the terms "cognitive," "affective," and "psychomotor."

12.2 Develop long- and short-term educational objectives.

12.3 Complete an exercise on writing educational objectives.

12.4 Develop a plan for in-service education.

12.5 Complete an exercise on developing an educational plan.

12.6 Evaluate the effectiveness of an educational project.

12.7 Complete an exercise on evaluating the effectiveness of the educational program developed in Units 12.3 and 12.5.

13.1 Explain the standards set forth by the Joint Commission on Accreditation of Hospital Organizations (JCAHO) for the operation of respiratory care services in a hospital (Appendix B).

13.2 Evaluate a respiratory care department and hospital respiratory care services by JCAHO standards.

13.3 Formulate suggestions and alternative methods by which a department that does not meet JCAHO standards could come into compliance.

14.1 Explain the ten commandments of good organization.

15.1 Describe how PPS (DRGs) has affected respiratory care departments and practice budget planning and other administrative skills according to Procedures 27-1 through 27-13.

15.2 Show appreciation for the need to be prepared for job advancement by discussing what qualities usually result in promotion.

15.3 Discuss the applications of a well-written resumé and differentiate between two typical formats.

15.4 Point out what steps should be considered when preparing for a job interview and discuss typical questions asked by an interviewer.

1.0 CONCEPTS OF MODERN MANAGEMENT

1.1 Basic concepts of management

1 Modern management has been called *both* an art and a science. Many phases of management require formal study in order for an individual to become a better manager.

2 It has been said that competent respiratory therapists and technicians do not necessarily make competent managers or supervisors. However, all therapists and technicians should be aware of good management techniques and principles so that, should the opportunity arise, they will be able to make an informed choice about the desirability of a management position.

3 Management basically means *action,* and professional management is *purposeful* action. Action is controlled by *thought,* and much more thought is now required of allied health managers than has been the case in the past. Tomorrow's managers will have to understand not only respiratory care and hospital rules but also state and federal regulations that will have an impact on hospital reimbursement.

4 Good management consists of getting things done through other people. A good manager needs to understand:

a Planning—what to do?

b Organization of human resources—who should do it?

c Organization of physical resources—what resources are needed to do the job?

d Standards of performance—how well does it have to be done?

e Performance reviews and measurements—how well is it being done?

f Development and controls—what has to be done in order to get it done better?

g Rewards and incentives—what is it worth to get it done right?

5 Qualities that distinguish an inspired leader from a mediocre manager are:

a A sense of mission. A leader has a purpose in life that is not accomplished at the expense of other people.

b Use of consultative supervision. A leader uses participative management and appreciates the experience, knowledge, and creativity of other people.

c Intellectual maturity. A leader's mind is trained to change when new facts make change appropriate.

d Emotional stability. A leader shows very little conflict between personal philosophy and gain and the way that the job is carried out.

6 Other characteristics of leadership and good management are:

a The capacity to conceptualize—to be able to size up the situation.

b The capacity to communicate—to be able to share and receive information at many different levels within the organization.

c The capacity for self-confidence and security—to be able to act out of belief, not our need for approval from others.

d The capacity to command—to be able to apply knowledge in an organizational manner.

e The capacity for consistent action—to be able to respond in an effective manner when faced with unpleasant and/or unknown situations.

f The capacity for criticism—to be able to accept being wrong and to learn from mistakes.

g The capacity for a sound value system—to be able to live the kind of life and maintain the kind of values that elicit respect.

1.2 The management grid

Understanding the managerial grid will help explain management concepts.

1 The managerial grid is a diagrammatic illustration of the manager's concern for two areas—*productivity* and *people* (Fig. 27-1).

2 The horizontal axis indicates concern for production (task) while the vertical axis indicates concern for people.

3 Each is expressed as a nine-point maximum scale of concern. The number one in each instance represents

minimum concern. The nine stands for maximum concern.

4 The *9,1* manager (self-sufficient decision maker—*1*) believes that it is wasted time and energy to be concerned for employees' thoughts and actions. This individual does not believe that the quantity or quality of the task is affected by the employees' cognitive or affective inputs. He or she, as a manager, simply gives orders and expects them to be carried out, i.e., produce or perish. Results may be achieved through this style for a short time, but not for long. It motivates people to "beat the system" and cuts down their contribution to the organization.

5 The *1,9* manager ("nice guy" decision maker—*2*) feels the task is incidental to good morale within the work group. This style produces warmth and good fellowship at the expense of results.

NOTE: 9,1 and 1,9 styles of management are equally nonproductive in task accomplishment.

6 The *9,9* manager (integrated approach decision maker—*3*) believes that the task and the people are not mutually exclusive but that if either is neglected, the task will suffer. This participatory style of management is seen as the most productive. High standards are used to achieve rigorous organization goals through involvement, commitment, and the readiness to confront issues needing resolution.

7 The *5,5* manager (traditional or compromise decision maker—*4*) believes that the task comes first but that pushing people too hard will make them ineffective. This manager compromises between task and people and makes slow, gradual progress—much more slowly and less efficiently than it needs to be.

8 The *1,1* manager (default decision maker—*5*) believes that the task is impossible and that people are "no damn good." This individual is self-protective, always "goes by the book" so as not to draw unfavorable attention, and usually does just enough to get by and "stay out of trouble." Creative problem solving is foreign to this type of manager.

NOTE: A 9,1 type who manages a 1,1, type is usually very pleased because the 1,1 takes orders and does not cause trouble.

9 It is possible to apply all five styles to one person in a very effective manner, referred to as the *ideal fallback order* or:
  a 9,9 integrated approach
  b 5,5 compromise decision maker
  c 1,9 nice guy
  d 9,1 self-sufficient decision maker
  e 1,1 default decision maker

10 The manager who is in a conflict or problem-solving situation should try to solve it with a 9,9 style and, if that fails, fall back to a 5.5 compromise, etc.

11 The complete fallback method consists of the following sequence.
  a The 9,9 manager knows that creative, intelligent, well-intentioned people will naturally come into conflict. Out of this conflict will come productive, innovative answers, and feelings will not be hurt because the people involved have well-developed and secure egos.
  b However, if a 9,9 strategy does not work, a compromise between people and task is called for, and a shift is made to 5,5.
  c If neither *a* nor *b* works, there must be some information that is not out in the open. It may be of a sensitive nature and therefore a "nice guy" approach (1,9) is called for.
  d If all these approaches fail, the manager may now "get tough." The 9,1 style is based on pure responsibility, and the manager can tell employees to fulfill the task whether they want to or not.
  e If everything fails, a final fallback can be made to 1,1, and the matter can be referred to a higher authority.

1.3 Tasks of management

1 Tasks of management are often complex, difficult, and without clear solutions. Experts have developed a system of approaching management problems that aids the manager in formulating effective decisions and in guiding personnel to carry them out. The four basic parts of this formula are:
  a Planning
  b Organizing
  c Coordinating
  d Controlling

2 All tasks, if they are to reach a successful conclusion, must be planned. *Planning* involves several specific steps that the manager can adapt to his or her style.

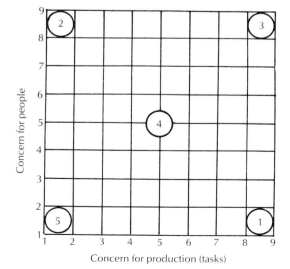

FIGURE 27-1 Managerial grid. (Modified from Blake R and Mouton J: The managerial grid, Houston, 1964, Gulf Publications.)

a Identify what you are going to achieve (goal setting).

b Identify where you are now in relation to that goal (assessment).

c Identify all methods available for achieving the goal.

d Consider all of the positive and negative aspects of each alternative, and select the optimum plan for your department.

e Complete the plan in as much detail as possible by setting a rigorous but realistic timetable for each step.

3 After planning, all of the resources of the department must be *organized* to carry out that plan.

a List the resources necessary for the completion of each phase of the task.

b Assess the resources of the department to meet these needs.

c Acquire any needed resources.

d Schedule resource availability to meet the needs of the plan.

4 *Coordination* is the phase of management in which the plan of action is put into play. If planning and organizing are properly and fully carried out, the job of coordination is primarily one of communicating ideas to the individuals who are expected to carry out the plan.

5 All programs, no matter how well planned, will need a measure of *control*. The reason is this: personnel are not machines, and occasionally an employee will need to be counseled or even terminated to prevent delaying the progress of the program or lowering morale through poor performance and behavior.

2.0 THE NEED AND TECHNIQUES FOR MOTIVATING PEOPLE

2.1 Motivation

1 Motivating people to complete a desired task is one of the most documented and least understood aspects of management. Much research has been done and many books written on the topic of motivation, and there is still great controversy over just what makes people want to do things.

2 Abraham Maslow, the American psychologist, proposed a theory that is now one of the best known and most widely received.

3 Maslow proposed that people are motivated by various factors in an ascending order, ranging from the most basic physical needs, such as food and shelter, to more sophisticated psychologic needs, such as self-growth and fulfillment of one's potential in life (Fig. 27-2).

4 Maslow further proposed that people would not be motivated by the next higher factor until the previous one had been fulfilled.

a Physical: food, water, shelter, air, sleep, sex

b Safety: an environment safe from physical or economic harm: a stable environment and one not likely to change radically. The individual does not have to control this environment, but must know that the person in control is someone trustworthy. Employees much prefer a consistent taskmaster who is in control

to a nice guy who exerts no managerial authority and attempts to be friends with everyone.

c Social: companionship, friendship, love, social acceptance

d Self-esteem: status, recognition from others, pride, self-respect, recognition of oneself as a superior performer

e Self-actualization: beyond the need for recognition or praise from others to a point of creating personal goals and behavior and generating self-recognition. Growth evolves in the difficult-to-define areas of:
 • Truth
 • Goodness
 • Beauty
 • Individuality
 • Perfection
 • Justice
 • Completion
 • Order
 • Simplicity
 • Self-sufficiency

5 The hierarchy in Fig. 27-2 is only a model and does not mean that the individual must follow a rigid pattern of behavior. There are many hidden factors between the levels.

a A person whose sole goal seems to center on self-esteem and the gaining of prestige, wealth, and status may, after closer examination, reveal a great need for love. The drive for esteem is merely a substitute for that love.

b Also, not all people can even strive for self-actualization. A person with a history of unemployment strives only for safety and security and to protect basic needs.

2.2 Job motivators

1 It is safe to say that no universal motivators exist. One person's needs are relative to background, current needs, and future aspirations. Nor is it necessary to fulfill a lower level need in order to work toward a higher one.

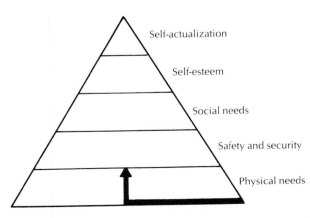

FIGURE 27-2 Human needs.

2 Variable factors influence motivation. These factors include oneself and one's environment.

    a Self-image is formed early in life and is reflected by dress, speech, actions, and habits. This image of self is fairly constant throughout life, and it gives others a means of predicting the individual's behavior.

    b On the job, one concern involving motivation is the person's perception of his or her degree of competence and ability to achieve. Early success generally leads to later successes by reinforcement. By the same manner, failure, whether real or imagined, destroys confidence and self-image and therefore achievement.

    c Achievement, or lack of it, molds the environment in which a person lives. People who develop power over their environment seem to be able to better cope with it by seemingly controlling it.

    d Once a person exercises control over his or her environment, a high degree of reward is expected and, when received, the person gains much self-confidence.

    e Conversely, a person who consistently fails (or feels as though he or she is failing) is led toward an environment image that is hostile and negative.

3 In order to motivate employees, managers must either *create felt needs* within the employee or offer a means of satisfying already existing needs.

4 Unfortunately, the most widely used incentive is money, yet evidence is overwhelming that mere money does *not* make good workers. However, money:

    a Can be exchanged for goods and services.

    b Can psychologically create security.

    c May symbolize achievement, success, power, or prestige.

5 The following types of people are most capable of responding to money as primary incentives:

    a People who feel they have high control over their environment and have high reward expectations.

    b People who feel they have high control over their environment and have low reward expectations.

6 The people in *5a* are usually in highly trained technical or professional fields. Their training in itself represents success. Money becomes a continuing symbol of success and achievement. Although those in *b* expect little, they feel as if they can control their environment. This second group responds to money not because of its status but because it shows continued ability to control the environment (successful managers usually fall into this second group).

7 The following two groups do *not* generally respond to money as a primary incentive because they do not think of themselves as having any power or control over their environment:

    a People who have little control over their environment and have high reward expectations.

    b People who have little control over their environment and have low reward expectations.

8 What do most employees want? Putting theory aside and dealing in practical terms, most employees desire:

    a A challenging job that offers the promise of achievement.

    b A chance to communicate—to feel a part of the decision-making process.

    c Responsibility and autonomy—to be able to make independent judgments.

    d Advancement and recognition—to have work that will lead to internal and external rewards.

    e Enjoyment of their work.

9 What makes employees unhappy? For the most part the inadequacy of certain factors is not directly related to performance of the job:

    a Wages and benefits (retirement, insurance).

    b Rest and coffee breaks.

    c Physical comfort (heat, air conditioning, lighting, environmental conditions).

    d Social contact.

    e Titles and seniority.

10 When do most employees become unhappy? When they no longer feel they have the opportunity for achievement, they become hypersensitive to their environment and begin to look for faults.

11 An in-depth study of employee maintenance (worker happiness) needs, outlined by M. Scott Myer*, highlighted the following needs:

    a Physical. Work layout, job demands, work rules, equipment, location, grounds, parking facilities, aesthetics, lunch facilities, noise, temperature, ventilation, lighting, rest rooms.

    b Social. Work groups, coffee groups, lunch groups, social groups, office parties, car pools, outings, sports, professional groups, interest groups.

    c Status. Job classification, title, furnishings, location, privileges, relationships, company status.

    d Orientation. Job instruction, work rules, group meetings, shop talk, newspapers, bulletins, handbooks, letters, bulletin boards, grapevine.

    e Security. Fairness, consistency, reassurance, friendliness, seniority rights, grievance procedure.

    f Economic. Wages and/or salary, automatic increases, profit sharing, social security, workmen's compensation insurance, unemployment compensation, retirement, paid leave, insurance, tuition, discounts.

12 Myer outlines employee motivational needs as the job, growth, achievement, responsibility, recognition, involvement, goal setting, planning, problem solving, work simplification, performance appraisal, delegation of authority, access to information, freedom to act, atmosphere of approval, merit increases, discretionary awards, profit sharing, utilized aptitudes, work itself, inventions, publications, company growth, promotions, transfers and rotations, education, and memberships.

---

*Who are your motivated workers? Harvard Business Review 42:86, Jan.-Feb. 1964.

13 Obviously, anyone who believes that all an employee wants from a job is a pay check simply does not understand management. One should keep in mind that no two employees are going to weigh any of the dozens of criteria listed here in the same way.

3.0 MANAGEMENT
3.1 Management by objectives

1 Management by objectives (MBO) is a goal-setting managerial technique that sets out specific objectives for an employee to accomplish in a specific period of time and to a specified standard. The objectives are typically set by the manager according to the needs of the organization and in consultation with the employee. At the end of the time period, the employee is evaluated as to the completion of the objectives set.

2 Sisk, in his text, *Management and Organization,* defines an *objective* as "the end point or goal toward which management directs its efforts." It is important to note that some people may interchangeably use the terms "goals" and "objectives." Others may define a goal as a long-term commitment that may or may not have a time of completion. An objective is usually a short-term commitment with a well-defined time frame and standard of completion set to accomplish a goal or goals.

3 Thus, stating an objective is also *stating a purpose* and, when applied to a business or professional service, becomes the organization's reason for being. Just as the objectives at the beginning of this module help plan the necessary study, so objectives in an organization help direct its services.

4 Sisk lists four major values of objectives.
   a Objectives provide direction. They identify the end point toward which all direct their efforts. Objectives aid not only the entire organization but each and every unit of the organization.
   b Objectives serve as motivators. Incentive plans, for example, are monetary rewards used to compensate earned objectives. Accomplishing objectives can be rewarded by many other factors (see Unit 2.2).
   c Objectives contribute to the management process. Easily and clearly understood objectives create a basis for the control process. Control is not possible when there are no goals against which progress can be measured.
   d Objectives are the basis for a management philosophy. When objectives have not been *formally* stated, the solutions of immediate emergencies become a series of short-term projects that lack cohesiveness. This short-term process is known as a *drive,* is often contradictory, and moves in different directions. For example, planning for the midwinter "croup season" after it has already started is a drive. Having a plan a year in advance for extraordinary workloads is an objective.

5 Respiratory care employees typically receive their ob-

jectives on a daily basis in the form of the patient care they are assigned, but certain employees may be assigned to long-term projects that may better lend themselves to goals. In the following example the manager has selected a goal, set a time limit, and charged the proper individual with its completion:
   a Goal. One year from this date, use of pulmonary function equipment will increase by 100%.
   b Responsibility for completion. Chief pulmonary function laboratory manager.

6 Responsible people like to know what is expected of them and thus enjoy a challenge (goal) and a time limit. Research has shown that people will adjust themselves to the time set. If no time is set, the goal will not be met.

7 In *no. 5b* the manager, in consultation with the pulmonary function laboratory manager, established a mutual goal. Now, together, they will formulate the plan for physician contact, public relations, etc., in order to reach this goal. The manager may have to agree to actively participate in the project and to give the laboratory manager extra free time for public relations work to achieve this goal.

8 The key to effective management by objectives is a *clear understanding of the goal* by both the manager and the employee and a *clear understanding of the time limit* and the *resources necessary to make achieving the goal a possibility*. Goals without resources are not realistic!

9 More information concerning management objectives is available from the public library. Refer to the works of Peter Drucker, Henry L. Sisk, George S. Odiorne, and Walter S. Wikstrom.

3.2 Quality circles (QC)

1 Quality circles are a Japanese industrial concept in which small groups of people who have similar interests and perform similar tasks meet together to discuss areas of mutual concern.

2 These areas are stated as objectives.

3 Different quality circles may be formed to address different areas. For example, one QC may focus on production, another on employee morale, and still another on quality control.

4 Quality circles that focus primarily on employee working conditions are sometimes referred to as quality of life circles.

5 Quality circles are held in a formal environment and usually involve a six-step process, such as the one shown in Fig. 27-3.

6 Participants must keep the stated objectives in mind as each step is completed.

7 Evaluation is conducted upon the completion of each step and after implementation, to determine the success or failure of the project.

3.3 Advantages of quality circles

1 The single largest contribution of quality circles is that they facilitate communication.

2 A second advantage is that they enable interested and responsible employees to become a part of the planning process.

3 A third advantage is that they frequently achieve the stated objectives.

3.4 Disadvantages of quality circles

1 Problems with quality circles include:

a They fail to achieve stated objectives.

b They are viewed primarily as a management tool and can lead to discontent of employees.

c Employees expect rewards for their participation.

d They may create jealousy among employees.

3.5 Theory Z management

1 Theory Z management is a human resource management style that incorporates worker participation in decisions.

2 It is a blend of Japanese management style with the more traditional American style.

3 The theory Z management applies one of three principles:

a *The intelligent worker model.* Workers will improve and manage their own production. Management's role is to motivate.

b *Family model.* The work group interrelates as a family. Employees are as loyal to the company as they are to their families. The company rewards them for this loyalty with lifetime employment, profit sharing, or other golden handcuff types of rewards.

c *One-for-all model.* The work group is more important than the individual. With this concept, pay is

based on seniority rather than individual merit for a given period of time, such as 20 years.

3.6 Advanatages of theory Z management

1 Employees virtually have a job for life.

2 Employees usually are cross-trained and allowed to work in different positions.

3 Employees feel they are a part of the decision-making process.

4 Less formal control is required of employees because of group peer pressure.

5 Employees tend to take pride in their work.

6 Employees tend to show concern for the whole person rather than just job skills.

3.7 Disadvantages of theory Z management

1 Innovation is suppressed because of peer pressure.

2 Competitiveness for success among workers is discouraged, causing the more assertive employees to leave.

3 It is not adaptive to small firms with limited resources.

4 It frequently results in complacency and false security, causing blind spots about the competition.

4.0 COORDINATING THE ACTIVITIES OF PEOPLE
4.1 Scheduling employees

1 Employee schedules are extremely important and should be considered as a primary task of management.

2 Scheduling for shift needs is a function of management planning. Planning is defined by Sisk as "the analysis of relevant information from the present and the past and an assessment of probable future development, so that a cause of action (plan) may be determined that enables the organization to meet its stated objectives."

3 Planning by objectives follows the scientific method very closely and consists of the following six steps:

a Statement of objective

b Statement of problem

c Designation of planning authority

d Collection and interpretation of data

e Formulation and testing of tentative plan

f Statement of final plan

4 Once a scheduling plan has been put into words, the following features need to be addressed.

a How comprehensive is the plan? How many people will it require to carry out the plan?

b How shall the duties be assigned? Effective plans require that specific duties be assigned to designated personnel.

c What control features are available? For example, time, budget, department structure, personnel designation, feedback, and department meetings should be considered.

d How flexible is the plan? Flexible means alternative courses of action. Changing internal and external conditions (e.g., turnover, patient load increases/decreases, sick time, overtime) requires that schedules be adjustable with minimum departmental disruption.

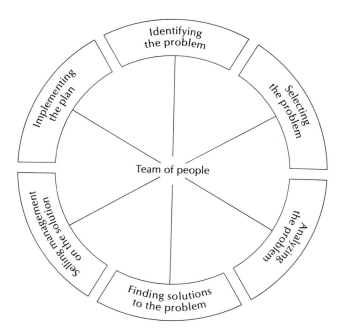

FIGURE 27-3 Quality circle process.

5 The following are general considerations to be addressed when scheduling personnel.

  a Schedules should be posted as soon before implementation as possible. This allows for employee long-range personal planning and reduces "call-ins" and "sick-outs."

  b Schedules should rarely, if ever, be changed after they have been distributed. In cases of emergency, the manager must make the decision to change the schedule and how it is to be changed. Having only one person responsible for schedule changes also reduces misunderstanding and contradictions.

  c Employees should have a way to communicate scheduling preferences or needs to the manager before the schedule is formulated.

  d Scheduling must be done in a fair and impartial manner.

6 A *sample technique* for figuring a personnel schedule follows.

  a Determine how many people are needed for each shift (morning, evening, and night) and what level of skill is needed for each. Let us use, for example, a department that requires certified respiratory therapy technicians (CRTT) on all shifts in the following numbers:

- 7:00 AM-3:00 PM,

              7 days × 4 individuals = 28 shifts

- 3:00 PM-11:00 PM,

              7 days × 3 individuals = 21 shifts

  11:00 PM-7:00 AM,

              7 days × 1 individual = <u> 7 shifts</u>

    TOTAL   56 shifts

  b Assuming each individual works 5 shifts per week (holidays, vacation, and sick leave will be considered later), the staff needed to fill this schedule will be:

    56 ÷ 5 = 11 technicians, plus 1

  c The one extra may be made up by:

- Overtime
- Utilizing an employee of higher classification: supervisor, registered therapist, etc.
- Leaving one shift per week short a person
- Hiring another full-time employee

4.2 Real employee time

1 Another factor involved in calculating total staff needed is time paid for but not worked. The three major categories consist of *vacation, holiday, and sick time*.

2 Each CRTT in our example would usually receive:

  a Two weeks vacation = 10 days

  b Seven holidays   = 7 days

  c Actual used sick days = <u> 6 days</u>

    TOTAL   23 days

  d 23 days × 11 employees = 253 shifts not worked.

3 One employee works 52 weeks × 5 days = 260 days

    Working days off   = <u> 23 days</u>

    REAL WORKING DAYS   237 days

4.3 Calculating employees needed

1 Assuming a staff of 12 CRTTs, the annual schedule is now *understaffed* according to the following calculation:

  a 56 shifts needed per week ×

           52 weeks = 2912 shifts needed per year

  b Less 12 employees ×

        237 shifts worked = <u>2844</u> shifts worked per year

  c Total understaffed   68 shifts per year

2 By taking into account the fact that sick leave is not scheduled, that hospital work is variable and often seasonal and that employees occasionally want some overtime, it might be best to leave the 68 shifts unstaffed.

3 On the other hand, personal experience with constant understaffing may dictate filling those unstaffed shifts.

4 It should be noted that many hospitals are moving towards a less traditional work week of four 10-hour days.

    A study published by Judy Newman, RRT, and Paul Grossi, BA, of Kettering Medical Center* showed that this type of staffing schedule was beneficial. Noted benefits included:

  a Increase in staff development time with no loss in productivity.

  b A rise in productivity.

  c Zero turnover in personnel.

  d A decrease in unscheduled absences.

  e Smoother shift transition.

  f A financial gain for the department with no decrease in the quality of care.

5.0 ORGANIZATIONAL STRUCTURE OF A HOSPITAL
5.1 Departmental organization

1 The *organizational chart* (Fig. 27-4) delineates proper channels of communication and authority in any department or business. The positions that are placed above another have the right to approve, disapprove, or, if necessary, override the decisions of those below them. Generally communication should never jump over a level, but follow the chart.

2 Fig. 27-4 shows the department head reporting directly to the hospital administration and to the medical director. The medical director can communicate directly with both the hospital administrators and the department manager. This situation of the department having two "bosses" works because the information transmitted to each is essentially different. One is primarily financial and administrative and the other primarily medical.

3 If the medical director were between the manager and hospital administration, as shown below, the manager would have to channel all administrative material through the medical director. Considering the time constraints of most physicians, this is an *undesirable situation*.

---

*Respir Care 27:1227, 1982.

Hospital administrator

↓

Medical director

↓

Department manager

4 In Fig. 27-4 three supervisors and an educational coordinator are under the department manager's authority. All of the manager's work not completed either personally or through his or her secretary should be finished by, or through the efforts of, these individuals.

5 If work is not being completed appropriately (to a standard) by a staff employee, the manager should hold the *supervisor* responsible. It is then the responsibility of the supervisor to handle the problem or face disciplinary action.

6 Staff members should not be separated by credentials or education because all staff report directly to the supervisor, not to one another according to rank.

5.2 Span of control (management)

1 *Span of control* refers to the number of individuals, departments, or areas under the control of one person.

2 Span of management has been suggested as a more accurate term because that individual is responsible for planning, organizing, and leading, as well as controlling.

3 Whatever it is called, the span between order and execution is dependent on the hierarchical levels discussed in Unit 5.1, and the number of levels determine the length of the lines of communication.

4 As the span is increased, the manager's lines are decreased, and, as the manager's span is decreased, lines of communication are increased.

5 Personnel theory generally supports a limited span for executives and managers because of the exponential increase in potential relationships that skyrocket past seven employees. The following potential relationship formula, developed by A. V. Graicunas, is presented in its simplest form.

a Manager M has three supervisors, A, B, and C, reporting to him.

b A *direct* relationship exists between M and A, M and B, and M and C.

c However, there are times when M talks to A with B or C present; therefore *group* relationships exist.

d In addition, *cross-relationships* exist between A and B and C without M.

e In total, there are:
- Three direct relationships
- Nine group relationships (*MAB, MBA, MAC, MCA, MBC, MCB, MABC, MCBA, MBAC*)
- Six cross-relationships (*AB, BA, AC, BC, CA, CB*) – or 18 *potential* interactions

f A fourth supervisor raises the potential to 44, a fifth to 100, and so on, according to the following list:

Number of supervisors	Potential relationships
6	222
7	490
8	1080
9	2376
10	5210, etc.

5.3 Ideal spans of control

1 Ideal spans of control range from three to ten employees, depending on the nature of the work and the background of the employees. Generally, the more routine the task, the larger the span of control may be.

2 When the span of control is too small, managers often become coercive and dictatorial. Often they have too much idle time that they spend interfering with their employees' work.

3 When the span of control is too large, the situation may become reversed. The manager is forced to rely on too many unsupervised individuals to do too much work without leadership or control.

4 A wise manager will rely heavily on supervisors and

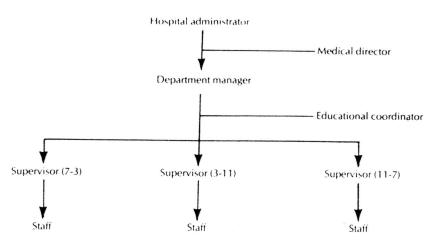

FIGURE 27-4 Organizational chart delineating proper channels of communication and authority in any department or business.

avoid interfering directly in the staff/supervisor relationship. A manager who has, in addition to other work, 12 employees reporting directly to him or her will not be able to do an adequate job in any area.

5.4 Concept of one "boss"

1 A fundamental rule of management is that an employee should have no more than one boss.
2 When an employee is asked to serve two people above him or her on the organizational chart, employee satisfaction, safety, and communication are all at risk, employee turnover rates increase with dissatisfaction, and frustration rises.
3 The following case illustrates this point.
  a Jane Smith was given 18 intermittent positive pressure breathing (IPPB) treatments to administer during an 8-hour shift. On counting them, she refused to do more than ten and threw eight back on the supervisor's desk. The supervisor took back the other ten treatments and suspended Smith without pay for 2 days for insubordination. This conformed to hospital and departmental policy.
  b Disregarding the hospital grievance procedure, Smith called the department manager, who in turn instructed the supervisor to do it Smith's way.
  c The supervisor resigned the following day.
  d Answer the following questions.
    • Who were Smith's two bosses?
    • Who was the most powerful?
    • Whom did Smith serve?
    • Could the supervisor have ever effectively supervised Smith again? Smith's associates?
    • How should the department manager have handled the problem?

6.0 PROBLEMS OF AND SOLUTIONS FOR EMPLOYEE RELATIONS

6.1 Major employee/management problems

1 The major source of employee/management problem is a *lack of communication,* both from management to employees and employees to management.
2 People want to know:
  a Policies
  b Procedures
  c What is expected of them
  d What they can expect from management
  e What the hospital is planning
  f The basic organizational structure of the hospital
3 People want to be able to communicate to the hospital administration their ideas to improve the hospital, their jobs, the product or service they produce, and their specific complaints about some phase of the hospital's operation.
4 Most people will accept a truthful explanation and see that a problem either must wait or perhaps cannot be solved. Communication usually ends bitterness, gossip, and unrest, even if the problem cannot be solved.

6.2 Grievance procedures

1 Communication is fostered by a formal structure, both for positive suggestions and for *grievances.*
2 Grievance procedures vary in their attempt to open and resolve conflict, but most follow a similar pattern. The essential factors are:
  a A quick and equitable resolution.
  b A process to allow appeal to an authority higher than only the department manager.
  c An appeal system that rigorously follows the organizational chart of the hospital.
  d Total fairness to all individuals involved.
  e Every step documented on a permanent record as well as verbally discussed in unemotional detail.
3 A sample grievance procedure follows.

Employee's action	*Management's action*
a Files grievance with immediate supervisor (written).	Must respond in writing within 10 days.
b If not satisfied, appeals to next organizational level.	Must respond in writing within 10 days.
c If not satisfied, may appeal to each higher manager up to a specified level, usually the administrator or the board of directors.	Each successive appeal must be responded to in writing within 10 days.
d The decision of the highest level is final and binding.	

6.3 Employee rights

An employee who feels that he or she has been unjustly or unfairly treated has the right to:
1 Present the grievance to supervisory personnel.
2 Be afforded confidential and equitable resolution of the grievance.
3 Be afforded an appeals procedure if the grievance is not resolved to his or her satisfaction.
4 Be afforded the opportunity to seek outside assistance (an attorney, governmental agency, or private agency) without fear of reprisal from the hospital.

6.4 Fair and equitable employee treatment

1 New employees should be required to read, discuss, and then sign a copy of the hospital policy manual. An employee who knows hospital policy and then deliberately breaks it creates his or her own problems.
2 The procedure by which an employee is counseled, suspended, and terminated must be written, approved by hospital administration, and made known to the employee.
3 Offenses that lead to the termination of employment are of two categories.
  a Extremely serious offenses. These offenses usually result in immediate termination. They usually include:
    • Unprofessional conduct leading to injury of either the patient's reputation or person
    • Stealing
    • Commission of a crime on hospital property

- Reporting to work under the influence of alcohol and/or drugs
- Possession of illegal drugs on hospital property
- Other offenses that seriously compromise the welfare of the patients or the hospital

b Lesser offenses. For lesser offenses, counseling the employee is appropriate to attempt to correct the problem before termination is necessary. Steps involved in investigating and processing lesser offenses include:

- Documenting the incident or incidents involved.
- Obtaining written statements of witnesses, if possible.
- Speaking with the employee privately, informing him or her that this is a *first* warning and advising corrective actions.
- Documenting the substance of the meeting and the date, asking the employee to sign that the meeting took place and that the summary is correct (not necessarily an agreement), and informing the employee of the next two steps of the procedure, including them in the documentation.
- On a *repeat* of the offense, the supervisor speaks with the employee as noted, advising him or her that this is a *second* warning and that he or she is suspended from employment for 3 days (variable) without pay. A *third* offense will result in termination. The supervisor documents the second meeting and asks the employee to sign the document.
- On a *third* offense, the employee is immediately terminated according to hospital procedure.

7.0 SKILLS INVOLVED IN GOOD COMMUNICATION
7.1 Active listening

1 Communication is a function of both verbal and nonverbal means of passing or relaying information.
2 One usually thinks of talking when communication is mentioned, but in dealing with employees, the most helpful form of communication is *active listening* on the part of the manager.
3 We all know people who are "easy to talk to." This is usually because those people are good listeners; they communicate to us that they are interested in what we have to say.
4 The active listener will use phrases during a conversation that
   a Are not judgmental.
   b Do not attempt to solve the problem for the primary speaker.
   c Indicate to the speaker that what he or she said was heard and understood.
5 The active listener can, with an attentive attitude and open posture, communicate interest in the speaker, even while maintaining silence.
6 Simple phrases such as "yes," "I see," "mm-hm," and affirmative nods of the head say to the speaker "Go on, I'm with you," or "I'm listening and following you."

7 *Restatement* of what the speaker has said involves a reflection of what was heard. The active listener communicates to the speaker: "I am listening very carefully, so carefully, in fact, that I can restate what you have said. I am helping you hear yourself through me."
   a Restatement may be very simple:
   - Speaker: "I felt very lonely."
   - Listener: "You were very lonely."
   b It may involve a significant part of what was said:
   - Speaker: "So both of these guys ganged up on me, and before I realized it, I was in the middle of a really heavy argument."
   - Listener: "They ganged up on you and pulled you into an argument."
   c Restatement may take the form of a summary:
   - Speaker: "I just couldn't tell her because we were never alone. I tried to tell her, but with all those people around, the words just wouldn't come."
   - Listener: "You couldn't get her alone long enough to tell her."
8 *Reflection* is an in-depth form of active listening that is often difficult to achieve. To *accurately* reflect the feeling and attitudes of the speaker requires deep empathic listening and understanding of the speaker's point of view, even when it is foreign to the listener's viewpoint.
9 Reflection is *not* interpretation or "psychoanalyzing." It simply brings to the surface and expresses in words those feelings and attitudes behind the speaker's words.
10 When reflecting, the listener must *not* guess or assume. The listener must voice what is behind the word content and bring it to the surface as the emotional content that has been present all the time, but unexpressed by the speaker. For example:
   a Speaker: "I was fired yesterday . . . big layoff . . . after all those years . . . don't know what to do." Listener: "After many years of steady employment, you are now jobless and feel completely lost."
   b Speaker: "It's so hard with her in the hospital, and there's nothing I can do about it." Listener: "It's really tough to feel so helpless."
   c Speaker: "If it had been Jim who had done that, Mr. Johnson wouldn't have done a thing. It's never been any different." Listener: "You feel like your supervisor has always discriminated against you, and you resent it."
11 Active listening can be one of the most valuable management tools for personnel communication. The active listener often has to initiate the conversation by keeping a watchful eye out for the subtle outward signs that people give to indicate that they are troubled or have something about which they would like to talk.
12 Active listening can be used in problem solving, disciplining, evaluating, planning, friendly conversation, and just about every other employer-employee situation, except information passing, in which the manager plays the active speaker role.

7.2 Communication in the formal and informal organization

1 The formal organization (Unit 5.1) is the planned authority and communication structure of the group.

2 The informal organization is the structure of communication that develops among the staff and often management, which does not follow planned structure, but rather develops according to the personalities of the individuals involved. The problem in Unit 5.4 is an example of this structure.

3 In this example, the employee holds more authority than the supervisor and communicates directly with the department head. In most organizations, the effect is not as obvious as in the example, yet it does exist, often as a primary tool of communication in which the formal channels of communication are not properly utilized.

7.3 Decreasing the informal organization

1 Simple techniques on the part of management can often reduce the need for and reduce the effectiveness of the informal organization. In the presence of very little organizational communication, rumor and gossip often take the place of facts and honesty.

2 Suggested techniques are:
  a Open communication:
    • Management to supervisors
    • Supervisors to employees
    • Administration to all employees
  b Recognize the employee's need to know
  c Practicing a policy of honesty
  d Practicing a policy of impartiality among employees
  e Respecting employees as individuals and professionals
  f Utilizing the formal structure for upward as well as downward communication.

3 The informal organization can be used either for or against the formal organization. The leader of the informal organization, often a staff employee, can be utilized by the manager as a communication tool with the ability to disseminate information to the entire staff. In this way the employee will develop a sense of self-worth and be an asset to the manager. Formal organizational lines, however, must not be crossed in this process. The supervisors must receive information before the staff or departmental structure and morale will suffer.

8.0 ROLE DELINEATIONS AND THE USE OF JOB DESCRIPTIONS

8.1 Job descriptions

1 The job description indicates what responsibilities and what authority are associated with a specific position. It should be narrow enough to accurately describe the position, but broad enough to allow for changes in responsibility and special tasks without exceeding its limits. Statements included in the job summary serve this purpose, such as " . . and all other tasks as assigned by the department manager," without attempting to cover all possible situations that might arise in an employee's job.

2 The job description is a communications tool that lets the employee know what is expected and protects both the employee and the hospital from arbitrary changes in the job.

3 The job description should contain information pertinent to the job and to the employee. In addition to listing the primary tasks of the employee in the job description and job summary section, it should indicate the immediate supervisor for that position, the physical and mental capabilities necessary for the position, and the professional qualifications needed to fill the position. Once a comprehensive job description has been completed, an effective personnel department can screen applicants and save the manager time in interviewing unqualified applicants.

8.2 Respiratory care entry-level practitioner roles and functions

1 In 1978 the American Association for Respiratory Therapy (AART), currently the American Association for Respiratory Care (AARC), completed a nationwide study called the "Delineation of the Roles and Functions of the Entry-Level Generalist Respiratory Therapy Practitioner." Portions of this study are reprinted at the end of Module Thirty as Appendix A. This study did not describe the job function of any specific existing level in respiratory therapy (e.g., technician or therapist). Instead, it inventoried the competencies expected of an individual should the respiratory care profession move toward a single-entry practitioner.

  a In 1979 the profession did begin to move toward a single-entry practitioner concept when the National Board for Respiratory Therapy, Inc. (now the National Board for Respiratory Care, Inc.—NBRC) began development of an Entry Level Examination.

  b Successful completion of this examination, required of all persons seeking credentials from the NBRC, resulted in a person becoming a certified respiratory therapy technician (CRTT).

  c The first examination was given on March 12, 1983, to over 5500 candidates.

2 Role delineation is useful because it does identify the gamut of tasks currently being performed by respiratory care personnel at the various professional levels. As such, it can be useful for identifying and assigning role functions to technicians, therapists, etc., within a hospital setting.

3 In addition to the Entry-Level Examination, the National Board for Respiratory Care, Inc. completed a new Written Registry Examination for the Advanced Respiratory Therapy Practitioner in 1984 and a Certification Examination for Entry Level Pulmonary Function Personnel in the same year.

4 The profession of respiratory care is rapidly changing from one of primarily on-the-job training, without receipt of credentials, to formal education of practitioners who earn at least one recognized certificate.

8.3 AARC Task Force on Professional Direction

1 In the spring of 1985, the American Association for Respiratory Care appointed a task force of respiratory care professionals, representing various areas of expertise, including clinicians, managers, administrators, and educators.

2 This group, known as the AARC Task Force on Professional Direction, was appointed with the understanding that it would not be political. It would exist for the primary purpose of identifying current levels of practice and projecting changes in patterns and scope of practice for respiratory care professionals in the future.

3 Its official mission statement was "The AARC will direct the respiratory care profession in its response to trends towards consolidation of appropriate and related ancillary services and to expedite the development of multiskilled respiratory care practitioners."

4 To accomplish its mission, the task force mailed *seven* surveys, from the spring of 1985 to the spring of 1988.

5 These surveys were mailed to:
   a Respiratory Care Department Managers.
   b Hospital Administrators of JCAHO-approved Respiratory Care Departments.
   c Medical Directors of JCAHO-approved Respiratory Care Departments.
   d Program Directors of AMA (CAHEA)-accredited Respiratory Therapist Educational Programs.
   e Program Directors of AMA (CAHEA)-accredited Respiratory Therapy Technician Educational Programs.
   f Respiratory Care Department Managers (follow-up survey).
   g Cardiovascular invasive and noninvasive survey to all department managers of JCAHO-accredited hospitals.

6 In each of the above surveys, the percentage and types of returns were statistically sufficient to draw valid conclusions.

7 Most significantly, it was concluded that:
   a Respiratory care services in hospitals provide more than just respiratory care as described by the AARC Scope of Practice for the respiratory care practitioner presented below:
   Respiratory Care Scope of Practice
   "Respiratory care is a health care occupation comprised of practitioners who, under physician supervision, are trained to actively participate in the care of patients, especially the monitoring and treatment of cardiopulmonary function. The practice of respiratory care encompasses activities in the areas of diagnosis, therapeutics, administration, and education. Diagnostic concerns include, but are not limited to: the obtaining of blood samples and therefrom the determination of acid-base status and the blood-gas values, and pulmonary function measurements. Therapeutic concerns include, but are not limited to, the application and monitoring of: (1) oxygen therapy; (2) ventilatory therapy; (3) artificial airway care; (4) bronchial hygiene therapy; (5) cardiopulmonary resuscitation; and (6) respiratory rehabilitation therapy."
   b Respiratory care personnel are, or need to be, multiskilled, with competencies in pulmonary function testing, cardiovascular testing, electroencephalography, extracorporeal circulation, hyperbaric therapy, health promotion, and multiple other areas.

8 The work of the task force has moved to a second stage, which involves sharing information with department managers and educators about the working role of the respiratory care practitioner and, in some cases, developing model projects for implementation and evaluation. For more information about the task force, the reader is encouraged to contact the American Association for Respiratory Care, Dallas, Texas.

9.0 ROLES OF OTHER HEALTH CARE PERSONNEL IN THE HOSPITAL

9.1 Intraprofessional relationships

1 Superimposed on the formal organization chart are the relationships that have been established between and among the professionals in the health care system.

2 The *physician* is the primary advocate and communicator for the patient. All procedures performed on the patient by the hospital are by the physician's orders only and by his or her permission. No one goes to the patient except by way of the physician.

3 The *nursing supervisor* is subordinate to the director of nursing and in charge of patient care in the area assigned to him or her for a specified period of time. In the absence of other hospital or nursing administrative personnel, the nursing supervisor is in charge of the *entire hospital,* including respiratory therapy.

4 The *registered nurse* is given charge of the patient's care in the physician's absence. The nurse is in charge of carrying out or supervising the completion of all ordered care and may, with the physician's permission, order a limited amount of care or medication. All personnel who treat the patient do so with the nurse's permission and authority as delegated by the physician. The nurse may stop or refuse therapy for the patient and remains at all times in authority over anyone treating the patient (except, of course, the physician).

10.0 ROLE AND SPECIAL CONSIDERATIONS OF BEING A DEPARTMENT MANAGER

10.1 Exempt and nonexempt employees

1 Certain employees, by virtue of their high salaries, professional positions, and/or the nature of their duties, are exempt from the minimum wage and overtime regulations of the Fair Labor Standards Act (FLSA) of 1938.

2 Exempt managers generally hold the power of hiring, promoting, and assigning duties to others and spend no more than 20% of their time in nonmanagerial tasks.

3 Nonexempt employees are covered by the FLSA and other acts that require, among other things, a certain minimum wage and time and one half pay for work over 40 hours per week.

10.2 Department manager responsibilities

1 The responsibilities of the respiratory care department manager are diverse, numerous, and often peculiar to each institution.

2 Functions that are common to most managers include:

  a Personnel administration, including evaluation

  b Policy formulation

  c Procedure formulation

  d Financial control of the department

  e Equipment purchase and maintenance

  f Auditing to ensure efficacy of therapy

  g Planning departmental goals

  h Organizing personnel and materials

  i Controlling the operation of the department

  j Communication to and from:

    • Hospital administration

    • Medical staff

    • Respiratory therapy supervisory staff

    • Respiratory therapy staff

    • Hospital personnel

  k Responsibility for patient care

10.3 Procedure formulation

1 Formulating procedures, including updating the procedures manual, is one of the most vital functions of the department head in terms of accreditation, liability, and proper departmental foundation. The actual format varies from institution to institution, although there are basic factors common to each procedure that should be followed.

2 Procedures should include who is allowed to perform each procedure. They should contain accurate and up-to-date instructions, delineating each and every step of the task to be performed.

3 The procedure should include:

  a Indications

  b Contraindications

  c Hazards

  d A systems approach to evaluating the effectiveness and/or the detrimental effects of therapy

  e Special equipment needed to perform the procedure

4 The procedures manual and any additions to or deletions from it must be read and studied by each employee and documented in permanent records in the department.

10.4 Liabilities of the department manager

A department manager has certain legal liabilities in terms of:

1 Procedures

  a The department manager is liable for procedures that do not meet minimum patient safety standards and that, through negligence, may cause injury to the patient.

  b The department manager is liable for malpractice, not only for his or her own patient care, but also for that of subordinates.

  c If it can be shown that the manager was negligent in placing an untrained or otherwise unqualified individual in a patient care situation and that, as a result, a patient was injured, the manager, as well as the hospital, may be held liable for damages.

  d Individuals who perform procedures on patients without their permission or against their wishes may be held criminally liable for assault, battery, and possibly even manslaughter.

2 Personnel. Department managers, as agents of the hospital, are responsible for carrying out policies of the hospital according to the law of the land, without discrinimation. The manager who willfully violates this law (as well as the hospital) may be held liable.

11.0 TECHNIQUES FOR EVALUATING PERSONNEL

11.1 Evaluation by objectives

1 Evaluation by objectives is an integral part of a manager's responsibilities and is a part of management by objectives, mentioned earlier in the module.

2 The benefits of employee evaluation by objectives include the following.

  a Employees know what is expected of them and if they are achieving their goals.

  b The manager knows what is expected of the employees.

  c The evaluation is objective rather than subjective, (i.e., facts rather than opinion).

  d Clear, concise communication is enhanced.

  e The employees' work is directed toward the fulfillment of the overall departmental goals.

  f An employee who is doing unsatisfactory work is quickly identified, counseled, suspended, or terminated on the basis of performance.

  g Employees are encouraged to have input into the development of goals and may add personal improvement goals to the manager's departmental goals.

3 General techniques consist of the following.

  a At the time goals are established, the manager meets individually with the employee to discuss the goals and the objectives of the organization. The manager lets the employee know how his or her contribution fits into the overall success of the department.

  b The employee agrees with the goals and signs a statement to that effect, as if it were a contract.

  c The employee retains a copy and establishes a plan for completion of the goals. The employee often will not have access to the resources of the department manager and so will need help in establishing a plan for completion. Interim dates, as well as a final date for completion and evaluation, should be set.

  d The employee's goals and progress should be evaluated on a set periodic schedule (e.g., once a month).

If it appears that goals and plans are not being met, the manager provides guidance.

e The manager evaluates employees firmly and fairly. If an employee is not meeting goals and is not firmly disciplined, departmental morale will deteriorate, and the system will collapse.

11.2 Evaluating by the critical incident technique

1 Lacking a specific evaluation-by-objectives plan, evaluation must become more of the manager's observation and opinion than the employee's meeting objectives.

2 One popular technique is the *critical incident technique (CIT)*. The evaluator forms an overall impression of the individual by detailing critical incidents during the year that the manager believes demonstrate charcteristics of the employee's overall performance. These records should be kept in a file and frequently updated with subsequent observations. The following represent some sample entries made by the employee's supervisor.

  a *Employee A* (6/19): After treatment rounds, employee *A* returned to the department to clean equipment and fill out patient charge forms. This was beyond the employee's assigned duties and was done without supervision.

  b *Employee B* (7/10): *Employee B* observed in therapy. Administered IPPB therapy of 4 minutes duration, did not solicit a patient cough, and charted very briefly.

3 CIT is effective because people rarely see their own faults and need specific incidents to prove the point.

  a An employee who is going to change must first believe there is a need for a change and be shown proof.

  b Employees who feel that their good working habits gain them nothing over the marginal or poor employee are shown that, in fact, they do.

  c While not as valuable as an effective objective system, CIT far exceeds the system used by most institutions: that of a once-a-year subjective opinion from the manager as to the employee's performance.

11.3 Introduction to in-service and educational planning

Every department manager, whether supervising two employees or 200, is responsible for seeing that some on-going form of in-service and continuing education is available. It is not only a professional responsibility to keep employees' skills at peak training levels, but an administrative and hospital accreditation requirement.

Naturally, programs will vary because of department size, budget, available staff, space, equipment, and time. The following unit is meant to serve only as an outline of an educational program.

12.0 DEVELOPING AND IMPLEMENTING IN-SERVICE EDUCATION PROGRAMS
12.1 Objectives: basic terms

Educational objectives are written to effect one of three types of changes in the learner.

1 Cognitive. The learner will know or understand something that he or she previously did not know or understand.

2 Affective. The learner will feel or be able to feel an emotion or attitude that he or she previously did not feel.

3 Psychomotor. The learner will be able to perform a task that he or she previously could not perform.

12.2 Long- and short-term educational objectives

1 Objectives for learning should be established before the program begins, and they should include both short- and long-range goals.

2 Objectives should be stated positively and describe what the learner will be able to do, know, or feel at the conclusion of the educational program.

3 EXAMPLE: Module Seven, Unit 1.0—Understanding the atmosphere and gases used for medical purposes (long-term).

  a Unit 1.1. Discuss the origin and composition of the earth's atmosphere (short-term).

  b Unit 1.2. Describe how oxygen is commercially manufactured (short-term).

  c Unit 1.3. Explain the physical and chemical properties of oxygen (short-term).

  d Unit 1.4. Identify other medical gases that are commercially produced and discuss their physical properties (short-term).

12.3 Exercise

The reader is encouraged to develop a set of long- and short-term objectives for teaching oxygen administration by nasal cannula or another topic of choice.

12.4 Developing an educational plan

1 Having developed objectives for the learner to achieve, the instructor must then develop an educational plan.

2 The plan should include, but not be limited to, the following:

  a Goals of the in-service or educational classes.

  b Prerequisites for entrance into the program.

  c A time schedule for completion of objectives.

  d The learning resources necessary (texts, films, etc.).

  e The physical resources necessary (classrooms, projectors).

  f An evaluation tool for in-progress and final evaluation of the learner (test).

  g A method, if desired, for a learner to repeat a section that was not satisfactorily completed on the initial trial.

12.5 Exercise

The reader is encouraged to develop and educational plan for the objectives from Unit 12.3.

12.6 Evaluating effectiveness of an educational project

1 Testing

  a Objective: short-answer questions in which the answer is either correct or incorrect. These questions may be multiple choice, multiple-multiple choice, or fill in the blank.

   b Subjective: essay-type tests that call for descriptive answers, which may be partially correct.

2 Clinical simulation

   a Techniques completed for evaluation in a simulated patient setting.

   b Written questions designed to simulate patient care decisions.

3 Learning reinforcement and retention. Both are increased by frequent testing for cognitive recall and psychomotor performance.

12.7 Exercise

1 The reader is encouraged to write test questions, including objective, subjective, and clinical simulation-type questions for Unit 12.3.

2 One example is to develop a performance evaluation record for the cognitive and psychomotor skills of Unit 12.3.

13.0 JUDGING THE ORGANIZATION AND OPERATION OF A RESPIRATORY CARE DEPARTMENT BASED ON THE STANDARDS SET BY THE JOINT COMMISSION FOR ACCREDITATION OF HOSPITAL ORGANIZATIONS (JCAHO)

13.1 JCAHO standards and interpetation*

1 The Joint Commission on Accreditation of Hospital Organizations that judges, evaluates, and accredits hospitals has written standards of care for respiratory care departments.

2 It is part of every manager's job to ensure that the care, personnel, and equipment of his or her department meet the standards of the JCAHO.

3 The reader is encouraged to carefully study the document on Respiratory Care Services (Appendix B).

13.2 Exercise

The reader is encouraged to visit a hospital department and to compare its operation to JCAHO standards.

13.3 Exercise

The reader should formulate suggestions and alternatives by which a department that does not meet JCAHO standards could come into compliance.

14.0 ATTAINING EFFECTIVE ORGANIZATION

14.1 The ten commandments of good organization (American Management Association)

1 Definite and clear-cut responsibilities should be assigned to each executive (supervisor) and employee.

2 Responsibility should always be coupled with corresponding authority.

3 No change should be made in the scope or responsibilities of a position without a definite understanding to that effect on the part of all persons concerned.

4 No executive (supervisor) or employee occupying a single position in the organization should be subject to definite orders from more than one source.

5 Orders should never be given to subordinates over the head of a responsible supervisor.

6 Criticisms of subordinates should, whenever possible, be made privately, and in no case should a subordinate be criticized in the presence of executives (supervisors) or employees of equal or lower rank.

7 No dispute or difference between executives (supervisors) or employees as to authority or responsibilities should be considered too trivial for prompt and careful adjudication.

8 Promotions, wage changes, and disciplinary action should always be approved by the executive (department manager) immediately superior to the one directly responsible.

9 No executive (supervisor) or employee should ever be required, or expected, to be at the same time an assistant to and critic of another.

10 Those executives, supervisors, or employees whose work is subject to regular inspection, should, whenever practicable, be given the assistance and facilities necessary to enable them to maintain an independent check of the quality of their work.

15.0 ADMINISTRATION

15.1 Budget planning and other administrative skills

1 Financial planning, as related to the preparation and administration of a departmental budget, is an important aspect of a manager's job. This process must involve the general areas of:

   a Personnel planning

   b Capital equipment needs

   c Task cost analysis

   d Revenue-to-cost analysis

   e In-serve education requirements

2 A discussion on budget planning would not be complete without commenting on the prospective per-case payment system for the Medicare program. This program was implemented October 1, 1983, as a part of the Tax Equity and Fiscal Responsibility Act of 1982.

   a This system replaced the retrospective cost-based reimbursement plan, which allowed hospitals to recover from Medicare most of what *they spent* for treatment of Medicare beneficiaries.

   b Under the Prospective Payment System (PPS) the hospital is paid a *specific* amount for each patient treated for a *particular diagnosis*, regardless of the number or types of hospital services rendered.

   c In order to implement this program the Health Care Financing Administration (HCFA) collected data from 1.4 million patient records at 325 hospitals.

---

*A new edition of this document was released in 1984. Its major difference is in the section on quality assurance. The reader is encouraged to contact the Joint Commission for Accreditation of Hospital Organizations for the most current documents.

- These data were used to develop 467 different treatment categories called diagnosis-related groups (DRGs).
    - DRGs have been expanded to 475 categories to include patients with tracheotomies and endotracheal tubes. A listing of DRGs for Diseases and Disorders of the Respiratory System is presented in Table 27-1.
3 Each DRG accounts for a patient's primary diagnosis, primary procedure, secondary procedure, age, and discharge status.
    - a After discharge, the hospital is reimbursed, on the basis of a nationally fixed rate for the diagnosis treated.
    - b The hospital that is able to treat a patient for less than the fixed DRG fee may retain the difference as an incentive (bonus).
    - c The federal government believes that this approach to medical funding will help to control health care costs, will establish the government as a prudent buyer of services, and will provide incentives for hospital management to "streamline" health care delivery without affecting the quality of care.
    - d Since its implementation, variations of the PPS have spread to private insurance carriers as a means of calculating reimbursement for health care services.
4 Under PPS, the respiratory therapy manager's job requires a great deal of organizational skills and ability to recognize innovative ways of providing quality care at a low cost, which will result in patients being discharged according to nationally acceptable lengths of stay for a DRG.
    - a Budgets will be based on contributions of the respiratory therapy department to each DRG treated by the hospital.
    - b Factors of concern that must be addressed by the department manager include:

- Standard of care rendered
- Quality of overall care
- Utilization of human and other resources
- Current case mix and case mix changes that will result in maximum benefits to the patient and hospital
- Productivity of personnel

5 One way in which a department manager may address these concerns is to thoroughly delineate the responsibility of respiratory care personnel to each DRG.
    - a This is a laborious task, although the AARC has available a Uniform Reporting Manual that has divided the responsibilities into over 400 tasks, each with a time value. Using this manual, it would be much easier for a manager to identify specific procedures, to assign labor costs, and to direct material costs, department overhead, and general allocated overhead.
    - b Once this is accomplished for all respiratory care procedures, then a manager will be able to accurately predict the costs for respiratory care for any given DRG utilizing the service.
    - c With this information the department manager will be able to justify budgets and to defend the monetary and patient care contributions of respiratory care compared to other services in the hospital.
6 Administrators will no longer view respiratory care as a revenue source unless it can be demonstrated that the contribution of this service plays an important role in helping the hospital provide quality care and retain monetary incentives under PPS.

Performance evaluation (Procedures 27-1 through 27-13) may be used as guidelines for the following activities:

- a Setting up a work schedule
- b Interview techniques
- c Justification of a new position

TABLE 27-1 Major diagnostic categories (MDC-4) and DRG codes for diseases and disorders of the respiratory system*

DRGs	diseases and disorders of the respiratory system		
075	Major chest procedures	089	Simple pneumonia and pleurisy age $\geq$ 70 and/or Dx 2
076	O.r. proc. on the resp. system except major chest with Dx 2	090	Simple pneumonia and pleurisy age 18-69 w/o Dx 2
077	O.r. proc on the resp. system except major chest w/o Dx 2	091	Simple pneumonia and pleurisy age 0-17
078	Pulmonary embolism	092	Interstitial lung disease age $\geq$ 70 and/or Dx 2
079	Respiratory infections and inflammations age $\geq$ 70 and/or Dx 2	093	Interstitial lung disease age <70 w/o Dx 2
		094	Pneumothorax age <70 and/or Dx 2
080	Respiratory infections and inflammations age 18-69 w/o Dx 2	095	Pneumothorax age <70 w/o Dx 2
		096	Bronchitis and asthma age $\geq$ 70 and/or Dx 2
081	Respiratory infections and inflammations age 0-17	097	Bronchitis and asthma age 18-69 w/o Dx 2
082	Respiratory neoplasma	098	Bronchitis and asthma age 0-17
083	Major chest trauma age $\leq$70 and/or Dx 2	099	Respiratory signs and symptoms age $\geq$ 70 and/or Dx 2
084	Major chest trauma age <70 w/o Dx 2	100	Respiratory signs and symptoms age <70 w/o Dx 2
085	Pleural effusion age $\leq$70 and/or Dx 2	101	Other respiratory diagnoses age $\geq$ 70 and/or Dx 2
086	Pleural effusion age <70 w/o Dx 2	102	Other respiratory diagnoses age >70
087	Pulmonary edema and respiratory failure	474	Mechanical ventilation with tracheostomy
088	Chronic obstructive pulmonary disease	475	Use of mechanical ventilation with tracheal intubation

*Modified from AARC, Daedalus Enterprises.

d Writing job descriptions

e Ordering equipment

f Formulating a budget

g Setting up an in-service education program

h New employee orientation

i Task cost analysis

j Evaluating equipment performance

k Evaluating personnel

l Organizing staff meetings

m Teaching respiratory therapy procedures

15.2 Job advancement

1 Most employees enter respiratory care with the ambition of moving up in the organization. Hard work, dedication to the job, and good patient care, combined with knowledge and ability to succeed, are usually recognized by increases in pay and opportunity for advancement.

2 This advancement may be within the current organization or with another employer.
Regardless of the employer, most promotions into leadership roles require special preparation by the candidate.

3 This preparation usually includes a current resumé and/or a job interview. Both of these requirements can be frightening to the unprepared candidate.

4 The purpose of this unit is to cover components of preparing an effective resumé and improving the responses that a candidate may give to questions usually asked in a job interview.

15.3 Writing a resumé

1 According to *Webster's New Collegiate Dictionary,** a resumé is a short account of one's career and qualifications prepared typically by an applicant for a position.

2 A resumé generally satisfies the following functions:

a It helps the applicant organize his or her education and experiences.

b It serves as a calling card to help the applicant get an appointment.

c It can serve as an agenda for the interview.

d It serves as a reminder to the employer after the interview is over.

3 There are many formats for resumés. However, regardless of the format chosen, there are certain fundamentals that should be applied.

a A resumé should be clear and concise (usually one page).

b It should be typed without error on a high-grade bond paper of a white, grey, bone, beige, or other soft, pleasant color.

---

*ed 9, 1988, Merriam Webster.

c Some people prefer to have their resumé typeset and printed for best clarity and professional appearance.

d The resumé should reflect the personal character of the person who wrote it. It may be a chronologic resumé or a skills resumé such as the ones shown in Figs. 27-5 and 27-6.

4 Items generally *not* included in a resumé because of legal restrictions include age, marital status, sex, race or ethnic origin, height, weight, dependents, or religion.

5 Remember, a resumé must convince the employer to contact the applicant for an interview. Take the time necessary to do a thorough and convincing job.

15.4 Preparing for the job interview

1 As previously stated, preparing for the job interview can be frightening for the first-time applicant and/or the applicant who is not well prepared.

2 It is important to remember that the interview begins the moment that an appointment is scheduled.

3 The applicant's puncutality, physical appearance, dress, speaking voice, mannerisms, courtesy, attitude, and general presentation all are evaluated.

4 For this reason, it is probably a good idea to role play the interview with someone who is in a similar job and level of responsibility as the potential interviewer.

5 In the role-playing session, have the interviewer prepare a list of questions that he or she feels may be asked during the actual interview.

6 Typical questions include:

a Are you familar with the job (position) you are applying for?

b Why did you pick this company?

c Why should we consider you for this position?

d How can you prove to me that you can handle this job?

e What education, special training, or experience has qualified you for this job?

f What are your future goals?

g What are your strengths and weaknesses?

h What level of salary and benefits are you expecting?

7 Be prepared to explain how you are uniquely qualified for the job.

8 Give examples of other situations in which you were successful.

9 Be prepared to tell the interviewer about yourself.

10 Find out as much as you can about the company and the interviewer before the meeting.

11 Observe the interviewer and take his or her cue to end the interview.

12 If it was not covered in the interview, ask when and how you will be contacted about the results of your application.

13 Thank the interviewer, and do not forget to follow the interview with a thank you letter.

Name: _____   Date: _____

Address: _____   Telephone: _____

Objective: *(Be as specific as possible)*

Education: (List all education back to high school with most recent first. Give year, name of
              school, years attended, date of graduation and degree or diploma earned.)

Experience: (List all related job experience beginning with most current. Give dates of
              employment, name of employer and brief explanation of experience.)

Honors/Awards: (List all honors and awards that would indicate your leadership ability, commu-
                nity service, and academic success.)

References: (State that references will be made available upon request.)

FIGURE 27-5 Typical chronologic resumé format.

Name: _____   Date: _____

Address: _____   Telephone: _____

Objective: (Be as specific as possible)

Skills: *Job Content Skills* - (List your theoretical and practical knowledge about administra-
           tive and clinical duties. Be sure your skills verify your ability to satisfy your stated
           objective.)

           Functional Skills - (List any skills that you may use at home that would indicate your
           ability to be as cross trained, eg., organized, manage budget, teach others, etc.)

           Adaptive Skills - (List personal traits that you have that will make you a better
           employee; eg, prompt, honest, loyal, cooperative, flexible to change etc.)

References: (State that references will be made available on request.)

FIGURE 27-6 Typical skills resumé format.

PROCEDURE 27-1

Setting up a work schedule

No.	Steps in performing the procedure
	The practitioner will demonstrate knowledge of setting up a work schedule.
1	Prepare a schedule 3-4 weeks in advance of need.
2	Gather institutional data:
	2.1 Shift times
	2.2 Wage and hour rules
	2.3 Specialized functions to be scheduled
	2.4 Amount of coverage needed
3	Gather personnel data:
	3.1 Number of people involved
	3.2 Holiday and vacation days
	3.3 Personal requests
4	Make a rough draft of a workable schedule.
5	Discuss the draft with shift supervisors for input as to any special needs.
6	Check the schedule:
	6.1 Be sure shifts overlap.
	6.2 See that all functions are continuously covered.
	6.3 See that lunch breaks are scheduled without interrupting job function.
7	Make a final draft.
8	Disseminate the schedule to the employees.

PROCEDURE 27-2

Personnel interview technique

No.	Steps in performing the procedure
	The practitioner will demonstrate knowledge of personnel interviewing techniques.
1	Prepare questions for prospective employee in advance.
2	Develop straightforward questions.
3	Put the applicant at ease.
4	Encourage the applicant to speak freely.
5	Allow spontaneous questions.
6	Ask about previous experience and education.
7	Ask for references.
8	Ask why applicant picked your institution.
9	Ask about applicant's expectations.
10	Explain the job requirements.
11	Explain peculiarities of the job.
12	Explain fringe benefits.
13	Tour the department.
14	Measure the applicant's knowledge of respiratory care.
15	Introduce the applicant to the medical director and other appropriate personnel.
16	Close the interview, usually with no definite answer.
17	Make notes after the interview is completed.
18	Prepare for follow-up after interview.

PROCEDURE 27-3

Justification of a new position

No.	Steps in performing the procedure
1	The practitioner will demonstrate ability to justify a new position.
	Collect all objective data possible to support the request:
	1.1 Work load increases
	1.2 New procedures being performed
	1.3 New services being rendered
	1.4 Increased quality of services
2	Write a job description for the new position.
3	Correlate the job function to objective data gathered in *no. 1* terms of need.
4	Write a description of how the new position will create more revenue or increased quality of service.
5	Write a cover letter to a fictitious supervisor justifying your need for this position.
6	CAUTION: Do *not* overstate the case and do *not* depend on emotional arguments; use only the facts at hand.

PROCEDURE 27-4

Writing a job description

No.	Steps in performing the procedure
	The practitioner will demonstrate ability to write a job description.
1	Assign a position title.
2	Write the position of the job into the structure of the department.
3	Define the objectives of the job.
4	Describe the tasks performed on the job (include any paperwork and special tasks).
5	List the major types of equipment used in the job.
6	Write a description of the conditions under which the job is accomplished.
7	List the percentage of time involved in different areas of the job in terms of a work day, week, month, and year.
8	State arrival and departure times, as well as any special time requirements.
9	List the educational and experimental prerequisites for the job.
10	Decide on pay scale:
	10.1 Base
	10.2 Benefits
11	Clear the job description with personnel office.

PROCEDURE 27-5

Ordering equipment

No.	Steps in performing the procedure
	The practitioner will demonstrate ability to order equipment.
1	Consider personnel and space implications of the new piece of equipment.
2	Consider any special support personnel/services.
3	Specify (precisely) the piece of equipment and method of delivery.
4	Research the latest prices and equipment numbers.
5	Compare competitive brands for price, function, and service.
6	Write a purchase order requisition.
7	Justify the need.
8	Identify and justify a source.
9	Provide vendor information to the purchasing agent.
10	Review the bid proposal.
11	Evaluate the bids.
12	Receive the equipment.
	12.1 Account for a complete order.
	12.2 Test for operation.
13	Identify equipment with appropriate marking.
14	Add the new equipment to the inventory sheet.

PROCEDURE 27-6

Formulating a budget

No.	Steps in performing the procedure
	The practitioner will demonstrate knowledge about formulating a budget.
1	Collect data and information on:
	1.1 Long-term goals
	1.2 New objectives
	1.3 Old objectives
	1.4 Number of procedures
	1.5 Growth curves
	1.6 Last year's budget
	1.7 New programs
	1.8 Construction
2	Analyze all needs according to the data provided in *no. 1:*
	2.1 Personnel
	2.2 Equipment
	2.3 Space
	2.4 Utilities
	2.5 Supplies
	2.6 Facilities
3	Establish priorities with explanation and justification:
	3.1 Essential
	3.2 Needed
	3.3 Nice-to-have
	3.4 Superfluous
4	Develop the budget in proper format.
5	Submit the budget to administration for consideration.

PROCEDURE 27-7

Setting up an in-service education program

No.	Steps in performing the procedure
	The practitioner will demonstrate knowledge of developing an in-service education program.
1	Identify the group to receive education.
2	List the objectives of the educational program.
3	Write an activity outline; (i.e., course outline, lesson plan, etc.).
4	Develop evaluation measurements; (i.e., pretest, posttest).
5	Locate resources:
	5.1 Printed materials
	5.2 Reliable speakers
	5.3 Space
	5.4 Instructional aids
6	Schedule a regular meeting place with appropriate audio-visual equipment.
7	Publicize the program to the appropriate people.
8	Reconfirm guest speakers a few days in advance of their presentations.
9	Accommodate a speaker's special requirements.
10	Evaluate the accomplishment of objectives for individual classes.
11	Evaluate the accomplishment of objectives listed in *no. 2.*
12	Have students evaluate the activity.
13	Improve the activity as needed to meet objectives.

PROCEDURE 27-8

New employee orientation

No.	Steps in performing the procedure
	The practitioner will demonstrate knowledge of new employee orientation.
1	Introduce yourself.
2	Explain the steps of orientation to the new employee.
3	Tour the department and the hospital.
4	Explain the duties of the position.
5	Introduce the new employee to the supervisor, department head, and medical director.
6	Complete all necessary paperwork.
7	Explain fringe benefits and personnel policies.
8	Review the hospital procedure manual.
9	Explain the work routine.
10	Assign employee to work with experienced personnel.
11	Answer any questions or refer employee to the appropriate person.
12	Supervise the initial work period of the new employee closely.
13	Evaluate the employee according to policy.
14	Advise the employee of his or her progress.

PROCEDURE 27-9

Task cost analysis of a procedure

No.	Steps in performing the procedure
1	The practitioner will demonstrate the ability to analyze the cost of a task. Analyze personnel costs, i.e., employee time used to: **1.1** Accomplish the procedure **1.2** Clean equipment or dispose of disposable equipment **1.3** Store equipment **1.4** Assemble equipment **1.5** Receive the order
2	Analyze equipment cost: **2.1** Usage cost of nondisposable equipment **2.2** Cleaning, maintenance, and storage **2.3** Cost of disposable items **2.4** Disposal cost **2.5** Storage of disposable items **2.6** Interest on delayed payments **2.7** Equipment rental charges **2.8** Utilities (oxygen, electricity, space, and water) **2.9** Peripheral equipment
3	Time/motion study of efficiency.
4	Calculate the totals.

PROCEDURE 27-10

Evaluating equipment performance

No.	Steps in performing the procedure
1	The practitioner will demonstrate the ability to evaluate equipment performance. Compare equipment performance to manufacturer's specifications.
2	Evaluate the equipment performance to safety standards.
3	Assess ability of the equipment to perform.
4	Compare the utilities available to the utilities necessary for equipment operation.
5	Compare the equipment size and functional characteristics to space and personnel available.
6	Project equipment longevity.
7	Evaluate maintenance procedures and maintenance costs.
8	Evaluate expense of operation.
9	Evaluate expense of purchase.
10	Collect and articulate the above data.
11	Compare all data to the operation and expense of other similar pieces of equipment.

PROCEDURE 27-11

Evaluating personnel

No.	Steps in performing the procedure
1	The practitioner will demonstrate the ability to evaluate personnel. Maintain accurate written personnel records.
2	Observe personnel behaviors.
3	Make notes on observed behaviors.
4	Discuss problems as they arise.
5	Collect written data and appropriate forms, and set up a meeting with the employee.
6	Fill out the evaluation form.
7	Meet with the individual and discuss the evaluation. Any extremely positive or negative impressions should have been discussed previously. The evaluation discussion should not be a surprise.
8	Discuss solutions to any problems.
9	Complete appropriate steps to initiate any reward or punitive action required as a result of evaluation.
10	Inform the employee of any changes in his or her status.
11	Have employee sign the evaluation form.
12	Make notes of the discussion and place in the personnel file of the employee.

PROCEDURE 27-12

Organizing staff meetings

No.	Steps in performing the procedure
1	The practitioner will demonstrate the ability to organize staff meetings. Develop a meeting format.
2	Prepare an agenda.
3	Prepare objectives.
4	Schedule a meeting place and a time that is reasonable.
5	Send out notification and agenda to employees in advance.
6	Inform employees of their expected level of participation in the meeting.
7	Maintain control of the meeting. Avoid getting involved in emotional discussions.
8	Evaluate the objectives and appropriately change the system to better meet the objectives.

PROCEDURE 27-13

Teaching a respiratory care procedure

No.	Steps in performing the procedure
	The practitioner will demonstrate the ability to teach a respiratory care procedure.
1	Identify the current knowledge and experience of the learner.
2	Point out the tasks or procedures to be taught.
3	Relate the instruction to the learner's experience or current needs.
4	Gather any equipment and materials to be presented.
5	Present the instruction in a logical manner (i.e., easiest to more difficult).
6	Explain the physiologic effects.
7	Explain the clinical applications.
8	Explain the indications, contraindications, and precautions.
9	Explain the psychomotor skills necessary and involve the learner in a demonstration—return demonstration session.
10	Explain the mechanical principles.
11	Provide supervised practice; observe and teach effective skills.
12	Review the procedure.
13	Evaluate knowledge and performance.

BIBLIOGRAPHY

American Association for Respiratory Therapy: Administrative standards for respiratory care services and personnel (official statement), Respir Care 28:1033, 1983.

American Hospital Association: American Hospital Association proposal: Medicare prospective fixed price payment to hospitals, Chicago, April 1982. The Association.

Bolles RN: What color is your parachute?—a practical manual for job-hunters and career changes, Berkeley, California, 1989, Ten Speed Press.

Burton GG, Gee GN, and Hodgkin JE: Respiratory care: a guide to clinical practice, Philadelphia, 1977, JB Lippincott Co.

Cooper RB: A linear programming model for determining efficient combinations of 8-, 10-, and 12-hour shifts, Respir Care 26:1105, 1981.

Cromwell J and Kanak J: The effects of prospective reimbursement programs on hospital adoption and service sharing, Health Care Financing Rev 4:67, 1982.

Federal Register, Part II, Department of Health and Human Services, Health Care Financing Administration: Medicare program; payment for physician services furnished in hospitals, skilled nursing facilities, and comprehensive outpatient rehabilitation facilities; combined billing; final rule, Baltimore, Sept 1983.

Finley JE: Using diagnosis related groups (DRGs) in hospital payment: the New Jersey experience, prepared for U.S. Congress, Office of Technology Assessment, 1983.

Joint Commission on Accreditation of Hospital Organizations: Chicago, 1989 Accreditation Manual for Hospitals.

Myer MS: Who are your motivated workers? Harvard Business Rev 42:86, Jan-Feb 1964.

Pangborn J and Kahl K: Cost control and productivity management, AARC Times 12:7, 1988.

Sullivan J: Task force update: diversification and manpower, AARC Times 12:10, 1988.

Technical Standards and Safety Committee of the American Association for Respiratory Therapy: Recommendations for respiratory therapy equipment processing, handling, and surveillance, Respir Care 22:922, 1977.

Critical care/ cardiorespiratory monitoring

On completion of this module the reader will be able to:

1.1 Show appreciation for the importance and the limitations of special care units by discussing their evolution, problems, and expense.

2.1 Point out the various types of invasive and noninvasive techniques most commonly used today for monitoring respiratory care.

3.1 Demonstrate a belief in the importance of having trained professionals as the most valuable patient monitor by explaining the philosophy of using experienced personnel as the first line for patient safety and care.

4.1 List and describe the various measurement techniques that are appropriate for providing information about patients receiving respiratory care.

4.2 Discuss the importance of the following variables when conducting a physical examination of a patient:
  1 Heart rate and blood pressure
  2 Respiratory rate
  3 Chest inspection and auscultation

4.3 Explain the significance of accurate measurement of a patient's body weight.

4.4 Point out the measurements used to assess urine and explain their importance to the patient's treatment.

4.5 Discriminate between the variables that can be detected by x-ray examination of the chest.

4.6 Discuss the fact that ECG tracings are of limited value in the early detection of respiratory problems.

4.7 Describe the variables that directly or indirectly influence the accuracy and usefulness of an arterial blood gas measurement.

4.8 Explain how the measurement of tidal volume, expired minute volume, and inspiratory force are useful measurements of a patient's ventilatory status.

4.9 Define and compare the causes of physiologic dead space.

4.10 Differentiate between dynamic and static compliance and explain how each is useful in determining a patients' ventilatory status.

4.11 Define physiologic shunt and explain the effect of such shunts on Pa_{O_2} and mixed venous oxygen tension ($P\bar{v}_{O_2}$).

4.12 Describe how capnography and mass spectrometry are used to monitor patients' ventilation and correlate each to a corresponding ABG measurement.

5.1 Discuss how computers are used in critical care medicine today.

5.2 Point out limitations of using the computer for critical care monitoring.

6.1 Show appreciation for the development of new monitoring techniques by discussing common sense questions that should be asked before new techniques are used.

6.2 Defend the concept that the monitoring of biologic variables has therapeutic worth in the care of patients and discuss biologic variables that should be monitored.

7.1 Discuss the variables that are measured under the general category of hemodynamic monitoring.

7.2 Point out and describe the different parts of a Swan-Ganz thermodilution catheter unit.

7.3 Explain the operating principle of a Swan-Ganz catheter and discuss causes of alterations of normal pulmonary artery and pulmonary capillary wedge pressures.

7.4 Discuss the technique and theory for indirect measurement of left atrial pressure.

7.5 Point out the possible hazards associated with hemodynamic catheterization procedures.

1.0 CRITICAL CARE/SPECIAL CARE UNITS

1.1 Evolution of special care units

1 In 1952, the first intensive care unit (ICU) was reportedly established in Scandinavia to care for patients of a polio epidemic. Thomas Petty, M.D., and his team were first to report on the essentials of a respiratory unit in this country in 1971.

2 Currently, virtually every hospital of 200 beds or more has an ICU special care area. It is estimated that this discipline of medicine accounts for approximately 15% of a hospital's associated health care costs.

3 Before the introduction of prospective payment reimbursement guidelines (DRGs), special care units were very popular, because the related expense was not a main concern and they afforded the ultimate in modern medical care.

4 In October 1983, the implementation of DRGs underscored the need for cost containment, especially in an intensive care unit, where the cost of providing care is 3.8 times more expensive than in a general care unit.

5 A study performed by a large, major medical center in 1987 reported that the hospital's average loss for Medicare patients who required more than 3 days of mechanical ventilation to be more than $23,000 per patient.

6 A problem with special care units has been overutilization of space with an underutilization of actual services. For example, a recent study demonstrated that 40% of medical intensive care unit (MICU) patients and 30% of surgical intensive care unit (SICU) patients were admitted exclusively for monitoring with no special care delivered.

7 This misuse of special care is expensive and financially a loss for the hospital.

8 One alternative to this misuse of special care beds is to make high-technology monitoring available to patients in other areas or as immediate-level care.

2.0 RESPIRATORY MONITORING CONCEPTS
2.1 Need for respiratory monitoring

1 Monitoring of respiratory care patients involves invasive and noninvasive techniques, such as those shown in the box above.

2 Respiratory emergencies are commonplace in the treatment of critical care patients. For example, Zuillich found 400 complications in the prospective analysis of 354 consecutive mechanically ventilated patients.

3 Respiratory monitoring increases one's ability to detect complications of mechanical ventilation (see Module 23).

4 It should complement the clinician's ability to assess a patient's status and progress by providing objective data.

5 Although use of hemodynamic monitoring procedures such as the Swan-Ganz catheter has been accepted in critical care since the late 1970s, few measurements of respiratory function are routinely performed.

The above are diagnostic techniques that are available to most well-staffed and well-equipped intensive care units with pulmonary function laboratories.

3.0 DIAGNOSTIC TECHNIQUES
3.1 Humans versus machines

1 The simplest and most valuable patient monitoring is intelligent observation by experienced personnel.

Monitoring procedures

NONINVASIVE

Physical examination
Electrical sensing with surface electrodes such as ECG and EEG
Impedance phlebography
Arterial tonometry
Gas sampling using skin surface probes
Radiologic examination
Bedside mass spectrometry
Expired-gas analysis

INVASIVE

IV injection and blood samples from capillaries and peripheral veins
Cutaneous needle electrodes for ECG and EEG
Rectal probe for temperature
Bladder catheter for renal function
Tissue oxygen probe
Intraarterial and venous gas tension and pH analysis

HIGHLY INVASIVE

Arterial catheter
Intracardiac probes
Transcardiac probes for pulmonary artery catheter for pressures and flows
Subarachnoid probes for pressure
Intracranial probes for CSF pressures and flows

---

2 In the evaluation of pulmonary competence over time, physical examination and radiologic examination continue to be of prime importance. As more technically sophisticated means come into use, there is a tendency to neglect fundamental techniques. The time has not yet arrived when it is safe to do so, and it probably never will. Newer techniques should supplement, not supplant, these basic methods.

4.0 ASSESSMENT MEASUREMENTS
4.1 Measurement techniques

Procedures and measurements that are most appropriate for the patient with respiratory failure and that directly or indirectly provide information about respiratory function in most critical care settings are shown in the box on the opposite page. Not all measurements listed are necessary for every patient treated for respiratory failure. The clinician should select tests providing information valuable for clinical decision-making.

4.2 Physical examination

1 Heart rate and blood pressure: Tachycardia is a nonspecific variable usually suggesting blood volume or flow deficits.

2 Usually, the faster the heart rate the greater the cardiac impairment and hypovolemia, but an increased heart rate is not a specific indicator and may result from fever, anxiety, stress, and other causes.

3 Bradycardia in the face of low cardiac output is ominous and suggests inadequate coronary blood flow or oxygenation.

Critical care bedside measurements

Physical examination
Body weight
Urine output, plasma and urine osmolality, specific gravity, osmolar and free water clearance
Radiologic examination
Electrocardiogram (ECG)
Hematocrit and hemoglobin
Arterial blood gases
Intraarterial monitoring
Tidal volume (TV); expired minute volume ($\dot{V}E$) and inspiratory force.
Physiologic dead space (VD) or the ratio of dead space ventilation to total ventilation (VD/VT)
Bedside measurements of lung mechanics, Pmax, Pstat, compliance (C), resistance (Rp)
Hemodynamic monitoring
Physiologic shunt ($\dot{Q}s/\dot{Q}t$) and oxygen delivery ($CaO_2 \cdot QT$)
Inspired and expired gas measurements

---

4 Blood pressure is usually measured with a sphygmomanometer or arterial catheter.

5 The sphygmomanometer is not applicable for situations in which continuous monitoring is required. Measurements from the arterial catheter are continuous but as with other invasive techniques can be associated with complications.

6 An arterial tonometer is now being developed that uses a force transducer to measure intraluminal arterial blood pressure externally.

7 The principle of the tonometric method is based on the relationship of arterial pressure to the displacement of a force-sensing transducer located over a superficial artery. Advantages of the method are that it provides nontraumatic, nonocclusive, and continuous monitoring of arterial blood pressure.

8 Present-day tonometer sensors are relatively sophisticated devices that use well-defined algorithms that detect lateral and vertical displacement with reasonable fidelity.

9 Problems yet to be solved include artifacts from motion and from calibration errors because of tissue variation. Development is needed in senor technology and physical mounting.

10 Respiratory rate: One of the earliest responses to a decrease in PaO_2 or a rise in $PaCO_2$ is an increase in respiratory rate.

11 The normal range of 10 to 16/min and a rate over 20/min should be viewed as suggesting potential trouble, particularly if there is a trend upward.

12 Rates over 30/min indicate severe respiratory distress and may produce severe hypocarbia.

13 A sudden increase in respiratory rate may be the first detectable sign of sepsis or a pulmonary embolus.

14 Recently, large carbohydrate loads in total parenteral nutrition have been shown to markedly increase carbon dioxide production ($\dot{V}CO_2$) and require a much higher minute ventilation to excrete the excess CO_2 (Fig. 28-1). This can be a significant source of physiologic stress, especially to the patient with chronic obstructive lung disease who is already hypercapneic.

15 Thus overfeeding may make weaning impossible and be manifested first by a rapid respiratory rate and dyspnea on a t-tube.

16 Two alternatives are available:
   a Decrease in the caloric load
   b Use of fat emulsions as a source of nonprotein calories, because they are associated with lesser degrees of $\dot{V}CO_2$ than isocaloric amounts of glucose

17 Chest inspection and auscultation: By observing chest movement, one can often get a general assessment of ventilatory adequacy.

18 Asymmetric movement of the chest or asymmetric breath sounds indicate unequal ventilation as may occur with right main stem bronchial intubation, atelectasis, or pneumothorax.

19 Aschronous motion of chest and abdomen is also an indicator of diaphragmatic fatigue (Fig. 28-2).

20 The presence of crackles, wheezes, and dullness on percussion are usually late signs of pulmonary disease. Nevertheless, physical examination is important in detecting chronic pulmonary disease preoperatively and detecting failure of ventilation and airway obstruction.

21 Auscultation may allow detection of an inadequately inflated cuff on an endotracheal or tracheostomy tube.

4.3 Body weight

1 An accurate record of daily weight is often the most important indicator of fluid balance.

2 Patients receiving only intravenous fluid usually lose 0.3 to 0.5 kg (0.6 to 1.1 lb) per day.

3 If weight loss is greater than this, it is excessive.

4 Unless a patient is receiving substantial intravenous or enteral alimentation, a stable weight or a weight gain indicates retention of water.

4.4 Urine analysis

1 Renal failure complicating respiratory failure leads to a synergistic effect on mortality.

2 In over 400 critically ill patients Sweet et al. found a mortality of 32% with respiratory failure alone, 44% in renal failure alone, and 65% with combined renal and respiratory failure.

3 A significant increase in the requirements of positive end expiratory pressure (PEEP) was found with combined renal-respiratory failure, compared with patients with respiratory failure alone.

4 Alterations in renal hemodynamics and tubular function occur in respiratory failure as a result of hypoxemia, acidosis, mechanical ventilation, and PEEP. Decreased urine output, decreased sodium excretion, and increased levels of antidiuretic hormone have been associated with mechanical ventilation and PEEP.

5 Other factors implicated in renal failure are hypovolemia, hypotension, sepsis, and nephrotoxic drugs.

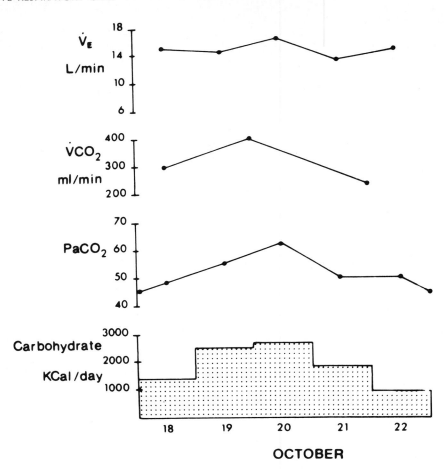

FIGURE 28-1 Gas exchange with changes in total parenteral nutrition. (Reproduced, with permission, from: Covelli HD et al, Respiratory failure precipitated by high carbohydrate loads. *Ann Intern Med.* 1981; 95:579-581.)

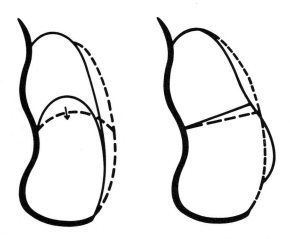

FIGURE 28-2 During normal inspiration, diaphragm descends *(left)*. Thorax and abdomen move outward synchronously. On expiration, chest and abdomen move inward synchronously. With synchronous breathing *(right)*, outward movement of abdomen occurs during expiration. Asynchronous breathing probably results from inefficient postion of diaphragm plus maximal use of accessory muscles of respiration. (From Bone RC: Treatment of respiratory failure due to advanced chronic obstructive lung disease, Arch Intern Med 140:1018-1021, Copyright 1980, American Medical Association.)

6 Renal failure in the critically ill patient can be classified into four types: prerenal azotemia, oliguric acute tubular necrosis, nonoligiuric acute tubular necrosis, and obstructive uropathy. (See also Module 4, Unit 35.5).

7 Patients with respiratory failure and prerenal azotremia have the greatest mortality compared with the other categories of renal failure despite a lower mean serum creatinine.

8 Respiratory failure combined with renal failure must be treated prophylactically or aggressively as they occur.

9 Urine output is a good indicator of renal perfusion.

10 Assessment of urine specific gravity is a good screening test of renal concentration ability.

11 Creatinine and BUN levels are traditionally used to monitor renal function, but other less frequently used tests may also be useful.

12 An early sign of relative hypovolemia may be a falling of urine sodium concentration or a rising urine osmolality. A urine sodium less concentration of than 10 to 20 mEq/L or a urine osmolality greater than 600 mOsm/L suggest hypovolemia.

13 Renal function can also be monitored by measurement of plasma (Posm) and urine (Uosm) osmolality as well as osmolar and free water clearance.

14 The $^{Uosm}/_{Posm}$ ratio is calculated and if greater than 1.7, the kidney has good concentrating ability.

15 The osmolar clearance (Cosm) is calculated according to the following equation:

$$Cosm = \frac{Uosm}{Posm} \times Urine\ output$$

16 The osmolar clearance reflects the rate of removal of solutes from plasma.

17 The normal osmolar clearance is 120 ml/hr and is decreased in renal failure.

18 Free water clearance is calculated by subtracting Cosm from the urine output. The free water clearance (C_{H_2O}) is negative (-125 to -100 ml/hr), and values close to zero precede renal failure.

19 Normal osmolality of body fluid is 275 to 295 mOsm/L of H_2O.

20 Plasma osmolality can be calculated by the following formula:

$$Plasma\ osmolality\ (mOsm/L) = 2\ Sodium\ mEq/L +$$
$$Glucose\ \frac{(mg/dl)}{18} + BUN\ \frac{(mg/dl)}{2.8}$$

An osmolality above 320 mOsm/L is poorly tolerated, and levels greater than 350 mOsm/L may be fatal.

21 Calculated in this way, the serum osmolality is normally 5 to 8 mOsm less than the measured osmolality.

22 This is called the *osmolar discriminant* and is caused by anions such as lactate or phosphate. The greater the osmolar discriminant, the greater is the lactate and the poorer is the patient's prognosis.

4.5 Radiologic examination

1 The chest x-ray examination may not reflect immediate changes. However, it is very useful in following the course of treatment, particularly with respiratory failure.

2 As positive end expiratory pressure (PEEP) is applied to patients with adult respiratory distress syndrome (ARDS), the chest x-ray examination may assist in evaluation of localized hyperinflation associated with unequal lung damage.

3 It is also useful for detecting certain complications such as atelectasis, pneumonia, and right mainstem bronchial intubation.

4 The chest x-ray film should be examined for position of the artificial airway, remembering that the tube may move in and out of a main bronchus with respiration or movement of the neck. For example, with flexion, a tube will move 2.4 cm toward the carina and with extension 2.4 cm away.

5 An especially important role of chest radiography is the recognition of pneumothorax from trauma, subclavian venous catheterization, or pulmonary barotrauma associated with localized lung hyperinflation.

6 The recognition of pneumothorax depends on the recognition of air separating the visceral and parenteral pleura. Usually a thin white line representing visceral pleura and a peripheral lucent space devoid of lung structures are seen.

7 When only supine films are available for interpretation, the diagnosis may be more difficult.

8 Two more recent findings for suspecting pneumothorax on a supine film include (a) an abrupt curvilinear change in density projected over the upper quadrant of the abdomen with increased radiolucency over the upper quadrant and (b) a deep lateral costophrenic angle on the involved side. After either finding, cross-table lateral or decubitus film should be made to confirm the diagnosis of pneumothorax.

4.6 Electrocardiogram (ECG)

1 Visual systems for detection of arrhythmias are an integral part of most monitoring systems. Computer programs are now available to detect arrhythmias with more accuracy and consistency than human observers can.

2 Arrhythmias are usually late manifestations of respiratory problems and should not be relied on to detect early events.

3 Approximately 10% of patients receiving postoperative care have serious arrhythmias.

4 About half of these arrhythmias are caused by usually undetected respiratory complications.

4.7 Arterial blood gases

1 Arterial blood gas levels are determined by the composition of alveolar gas and the ability of pulmonary capillary blood reach equilibrium with the alveolar gas (See also Module 8, Unit 8.0.)

2 The alveolar gas composition depends on composition of the inspired gas, the matching of ventilation and blood flow, and the composition of mixed venous blood.

3 Since mixed venous gases are related to cardiac output, nonpulmonary factors such as cardiac output also determine the values for arterial blood gases.

4 It is extremely important to be aware that nonpulmonary factors can cause significant hypoxemia to avoid a misinterpretation of a fall in Pao_2 in a sick patient as being caused by deterioration in lung function when it may instead signal deteriorating cardiovascular function.

5 The arterial oxygen tension divided by the alveolar oxygen tension is called the *a/A ratio*. This ratio is relatively stable with a varying FIo_2 unlike the classic alveolar-arterial gradient. Thus a useful index of changes in lung function is a change in the patient's oxygen concentration.

6 The normal a/A ratio is greater than 0.85.

7 The ratio can also be used to predict the new Pao_2 that will result from a change in inspired oxygen concentration.

8 Another nonpulmonary factor that can significantly affect gas exchange is the level of CO_2 production ($\dot{V}CO_2$). The amount of CO_2 produced by the body is a function of the metabolic rate and the substrate used as fuel.

9 The CO_2 production varies from 70% to 100% of the $\dot{V}O_2$ as the fuel is switched from fat to carbohydrate.

10 When caloric input exceeds metabolic needs, excess calories are converted to fat, which further increases CO_2 production.

11 Askanazi et al. have shown that hospitalized patients receiving hyperalimentation can increase their $\dot{V}CO_2$ much as 50% (see Fig. 28-1). To excrete this excess CO_2, an increased minute ventilation is needed, which might be impossible in a patient with COPD or might cause a failure to wean from mechanical ventilation.

12 Marked changes in PaO_2 in critically ill patients that may be missed by intermittent sampling occur during the administration of drugs, suctioning, and during changes in body position.

13 Continuous monitoring of PaO_2 by electrodes in the femoral, radial, and brachial arteries as well as in mixed venous blood in the pulmonary artery has been done. Obviously, these techniques will have the same problems as other invasive techniques, and further experience is needed before it can be concluded that such monitoring is indicated in the management of critically ill patients.

14 Because of the intermittent nature of blood gas measurement and the lag in reporting results, considerable effort has been directed to developing noninvasive methods of continuously monitoring blood and tissue gas values.

15 Pulse oximetry is the most widely used technique. Advances in oximeter technology have eliminated early problems with this technique and now allow accurate calibration and measurement of oxygen saturation. (See also Module 16, Unit 14.0).

16 A beam of light of appropriate wave length shines through the ear lobe or finger; change in transmittance is determined by oxyhemoglobin saturation. The disadvantages of the technique are that the sensor must be maintained in position on the ear lobe or finger, which may yield an inaccurate reading if the skin is deeply pigmented or if the cardiac output is low. Reproducibility in other situations has generally been good.

17 Pulse oximetry is most accurate in the steep portion of the oxyhemoglobin dissociation curve when changes in PaO_2 are accompanied by significant changes in oxygen saturation. This is not a major problem in monitoring the patient with respiratory failure, because the range of greatest clinical interest falls on the steep portion of the oxygen-hemoglobin dissociation curve where saturation is a sensitive index of oxygen tension.

18 Another approach that has proved effective in monitoring infants with respiratory failure is transcutaneous blood gas analysis. (See Module 8, Fig. 8-54 and 8-55).

19 Warming of the skin underneath an appropriate electrode increases blood flow to the skin out of proportion to its needs to eliminate heat. Thus capillary gas tensions present are minimally affected by tissue metabolism. (See also Module 8, Unit 19.0; and Module 16, Unit 14.0).

20 Under most circumstances, transcutaneous values in infants accurately reflect arterial blood gases.

21 Situations associated with changes in oxygen delivery to the skin (changes in cardiac output, blood volume, hematocrit, and acid base balance) may cause considerable differences between directly measured arterial gases and transcutaneous values.

22 In fact, in some adults monitored using continuous arterial PO_2 monitoring with an intraarterial electrode, transcutaneous PO_2 correlated better with changes in blood pressure than arterial PO_2.

23 In patients with leukocytosis and thrombocytosis, spurious hypoxemia can occur in arterial or mixed venous blood as a result of consumption of oxygen by leukocytes and platelets before laboratory analysis.

24 With extreme leukocytosis this can be as much as 72 mm Hg within the first 2 minutes after drawing the blood.

25 The spurious hypoxemia is obliterated by adding potassium cyanide and blunted by placing the blood on ice.

26 Since these patients often have respiratory complications, spurious hypoxemia must be differentiated from true hypoxemia to avoid unnecessary diagnostic and therapeutic procedures.

27 The most elegant evaluation of ventilation and perfusion relationship was developed by Wagner et al., who studied gas exchange with a multiple gas elimination technique.

28 With this technique the distribution of blood flow and ventilation is related to the ventilation-perfusion ratio ($\dot{V}a/\dot{Q}$) (Fig. 28-3).

29 True shunt is quantified and separated from units with low Va/Q ratios. Also, dead space is quantified and is separated from units with high Va/Q ratios.

30 This multicompartmental model of the lung, despite its complexity, has added insights not available from the traditional three-compartment analysis of Riley and Cournand. (Fig. 28-4).

4.8 Tidal volume, expired minute volume, and inspiratory force

1 Bedside spirometry is possible using either a waterless volume displacement spirometer or any of the variety of electronic spirometers that are readily available (see Module 24). Dry gas meters are also available to measure exhaled volumes. Two of the most practical and useful instruments for clinical work are the Wright and Drager respirometers (see Module 23).

2 Tachypneic ventilation with low tidal volumes (V_T) may divert too much volume to dead space ventilation and decrease alveolar ventilation.

3 The product of rate and V_T is minute volume ($\dot{V}E$), a useful measure of total ventilation.

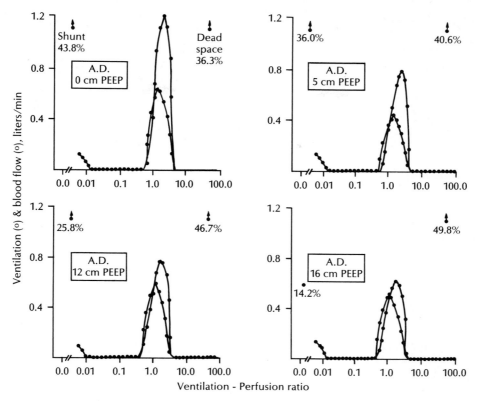

FIGURE 28-3 Ventilation-perfusion distribution in a patient with adult respiratory distress syndrome. The blood flow is divided between lung units that are well ventilated and those that are shunt. (From Dantzker DR: Gas exchange in the adult respiratory distress syndrome, Clinics Chest Med 3(1):57-62, 1982.)

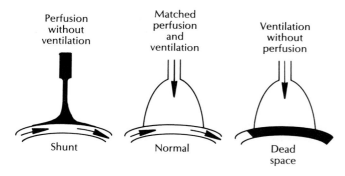

FIGURE 28-4 Hypoxemia in the adult respiratory distress syndrome (ARDS) results from intrapulmonary shunting. Shunting results from perfused but unventilated alveoli *(left)*. In ARDS many alveoli are also ventilated but not perfused, resulting in an increased physiologic dead space *(right)*. Both shunt and physiologic dead space may exceed 50% in severe ARDS. (From Bone RC: Treatment of severe hypoxemia due to the adult respiratory distress syndrome, Arch Intern Med 140:85-89, Copyright 1980, American Medical Association.)

4 High $\dot{V}E$ warns of severe hypocarbia, large dead space, and increased respiratory work, which may lead to exhaustion.

5 V_T greater than 5 ml/kg and vital capacity (VC) greater than 10 ml/kg are useful guidelines for ventilation capacity consistent with successful weaning from mechanical ventilation.

6 Measurement of $\dot{V}E$ and maximum inspiratory force (MIP) may also allow decisions regarding weaning from mechanical ventilation.

7 Sahn et al. showed that a resting $\dot{V}E$ of less than 10 L and ability to double the resting $\dot{V}E$ predict success in weaning.

8 A maximum inspiratory force (MIF) greater than minus 20 cm H_2O can also predict success.

4.9 Physiologic dead space (V_D)

1 Physiologic dead space (V_D) represents wasted ventilation and is the portion of V_T that does not particpate in gas exchange.

2 In healthy subjects, the V_D is approximately 150 ml at rest (about 20% to 30% of each tidal volume). This represents the anatomic dead space from the mouth, pharynx, larynx, trachea, bronchi, and bronchioles as well as the contribution of any alveoli that are overventilated relative to perfusion, which also contributes to V_D.

3 Positive-pressure ventilation alone can increase V_D.

4 In respiratory failure, the V_D is increased because of continued ventilation of alveoli whose perfusion is either absent or decreased.

5 Varieties of V_D and the expired CO_2 curve resulting from series and parallel dead space are possible (Fig. 28-5).

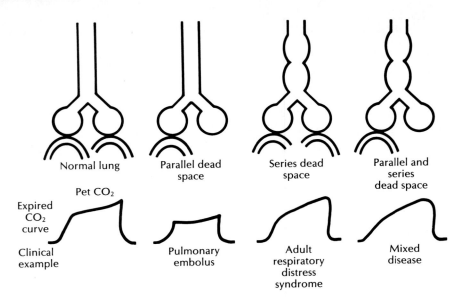

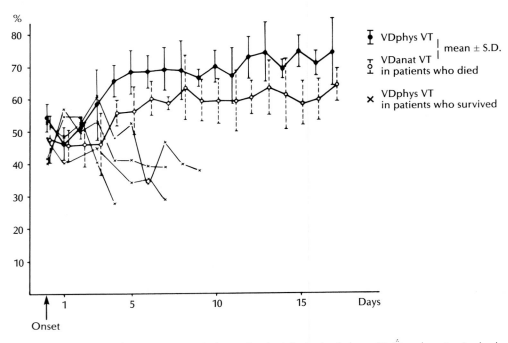

FIGURE 28-5 Physiologic dead space. Physiologic dead space can be increased by diseases causing ventilation that exceeds perfusion. Graphic representations of diseases producing increased dead space and the resulting expired carbon dioxide curve are shown. (From Bone RC, Monitoring Respiratory Function in the Patient with Acute Respiratory Distress Syndrome, in *Seminars in Respiratory Medicine*, Volume 2, Number 3, New York, 1981, Thieme Medical Publishers, Inc. Reprinted by permission.)

FIGURE 28-6 The time course of change in physiologic dead space ($V_D/\dot{F}$) and anatomic dead space V_D anat) to tidal volume (V_T) ratios in patients with adult respiratory distress syndrome. (From Shimada Y et al: Evaluation of the progress and prognosis of adult respiratory distress syndrome, simple respiratory physiologic measurement, Chest 76:180, 1979.)

6 The ratio of V_D to V_T (V_D/V_T) can be calculated by measurement of arterial and mixed expired CO_2 tension (PE_{CO_2}) by the Bohr equation:

$$V_D = PA_{O_2} - PE_{CO_2}$$
$$V_T = P_{CO_2} - PE_{CO_2}$$

7 The Enghoff modification of the Bohr equation is often used clinically:

$$V_D = Pa_{CO_2} - \frac{P\overline{E}_{CO_2}}{Pa_{CO_2}}$$

8 If the end tidal P_{CO_2} (PET_{CO_2}) is substituted for the Pa_{CO_2}, anatomic dead space can be calculated requiring only expired air.

9 Measurements made recently of V_D during respiratory failure from ARDS showed a striking relationship to survival (Fig. 28-6).

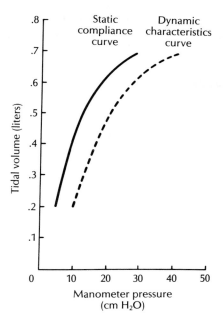

F I G U R E 2 8 - 7 Pressure-volume relationship. Pressure-volume measurements at different tidal volumes. These measurements are made from many breaths and differ from the compliance measurements made in the pulmonary function laboratory which are measured during a single breath. (From Bone RC, Monitoring Respiratory Function in the Patient with Acute Respiratory Distress Syndrome, in *Seminars in Respiratory Medicine*, Volume 2, Number 3, New York, 1981, Thieme Medical Publishers, Inc. Reprinted by permission.)

4.10 Bedside measurement of mechanics (see also Module 23)

1 If the pressure dial on a cycling ventilator is studied, one will note a rapid rise of airway pressure with a peak at the end of inspiration and a rapid fall to resting pressure during exhalation.

2 This peak pressure is the pressure required to overcome the elastic properties of the lung and chest wall and the flow-restrictive properties of the airway.

3 The volume delivered by the ventilator divided by the peak pressure is called dynamic characteristics, because it is actually an impedance measurement and includes compliance and resistance components.

4 If one momentarily occludes the outflow of the ventilator (by pinching the tubing to control the expiratory valve or dialing in "expiratory retard" or inspiratory hold), the pressure dial will show a momentary plateau at which no air is flowing.

5 The normal compliance of the lung and chest wall in the mechanically ventilated patient is about 70 ml/cm H_2O.

6 When the static compliance of the lung and chest wall is less than 25 ml/cm H_2O, as in severe respiratory failure, difficulties in weaning are common because of the high work of breathing.

7 The term *chest wall* includes all structures outside the lungs that move during breathing.

8 Pressure is measured from the anaeroid pressure gauge usually located on the panel of the ventilators; these are sufficiently accurate for clinical purposes.

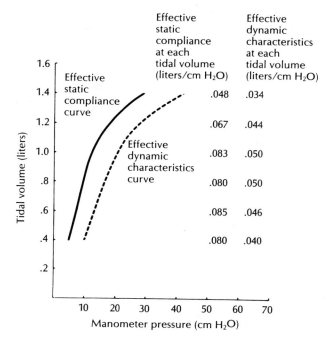

F I G U R E 2 8 - 8 Pressure-volume curves with static compliance and dynamic characteristics calculated at each tidal volume. (From Kirby RR: Monitoring the patient and ventilator during respiratory failure, part 2, bedside techniques, Curr Rev in Respir Therapy 1:139, 1979.)

9 This plateau presure divided by the tidal volume is the static compliance of the lungs and chest.

10 One can plot the peak and plateau pressure at a stable tidal volume at different time intervals and get an estimate of changes in the airways and lungs (Fig. 28-7).

11 If one ventilates the lung at various tidal volumes and records the peak and plateau pressure for each volume, dynamic and static curves can be quickly graphed; the former correlates with airway resistance and the latter is a measure of lung stiffness (Fig. 28-8).

12 The method is as follows:

  a Explain procedure when the patient is awake.

  b Ensure adequate tracheal tube cuff pressure during procedure to prevent leaks.

  c Dial in expiratory retard.

  d Select a series of settings to be used, such as 7, 10, 13, and 16 ml/kg body weight, or 400, 600, 800, 1,000 VT.

  e For each volume, record:
    • Spirometer volume
    • Peak airway pressure
    • Plateau pressure

When PEEP is being used, PEEP pressure must be subtracted from peak and plateau pressure before charting.

Static compliance =

$$\frac{\text{Spirometer volume} - \text{Tube expansion volume}}{\text{Plateau pressure} - \text{PEEP}}$$

  f Repeat this step for each volume setting selected.

  g If at any setting the pressure increases significantly, do not go to larger volumes, because pulmonary barotrauma could result.

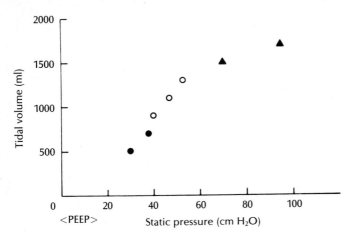

FIGURE 28-9 Static pressure-volume relationship of the lungs and thorax. Each observation represents the inflation hold manometer pressure of the ventilator on the horizontal axis, which relates to the tidal volume indicated on the vertical axis. Static compliance = Tidal volume/Inflation hold pressure − PEEP pressure. In this example PEEP pressure is 10 cm H_2O. Compliance for tidal volumes indicated by 0 = 25 ml/cm H_2O; 0 = 30 ml/cm H_2O. It can be seen that tidal volumes above this level are the tidal volumes producing "optimal compliance." (From Bone RC: Treatment of severe hypoxemia due to the acute respiratory distress syndrome, Arch Intern Med 140:85-89, Copyright 1980, American Medical Association.)

h Remove expiratory retard.

i Readjust cuff pressure.

j Carry out a complete ventilator check.

k Chart data on graph.

13 These measurements can be made at one volume and followed numerically, or an even simpler method of plotting measurements is to plot static and dynamic pressure at a constant tidal volume as graphing these pressures. This can be a useful and faster monitoring tool.

14 At higher tidal volumes and/or PEEP, a decreasing static compliance can signal lung hyperinflation.

15 The decrease in static compliance is most pronounced when high tidal volumes are combined with PEEP (Fig. 28-9).

16 The incidence of pulmonary barotrauma (pneumothorax, pneumomediastinum, and subcutaneous emphysema) can be decreased by using tidal volumes not associated with lung hyperinflation.

17 More information is available from inspection of the graphic measurement of the curves at multiple volumes. Fig. 28-10 shows that conditions affecting the

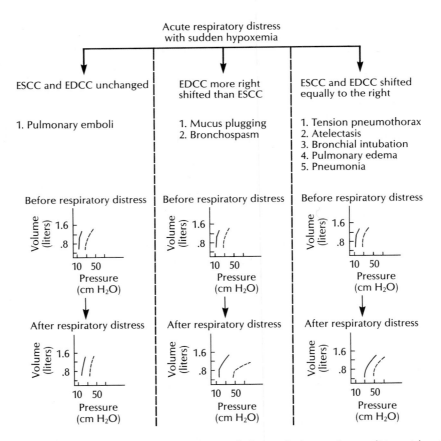

FIGURE 28-10 Pressure-volume measurements before and after respiratory distress taken from reference 2. ESCC is effective static compliance curve. EDCC is effective dynamic characteristics curve. (From Bone RC, Monitoring Respiratory Function in the Patient with Acute Respiratory Distress Syndrome, in *Seminars in Respiratory Medicine*, Volume 2, Number 3, New York, 1981, Thieme Medical Publishers, Inc. Reprinted by permission.)

airway will shift the dynamic curve to the right and flatten it (higher pressure per volume increase).

18 Those conditions producing increased lung or chest wall stiffness shift both the static and dynamic curve to the right and flatten both.

19 If the patient is hypoxemic and the compliance curves are unchanged, then pulmonary embolus should be suspected.

20 Two types of errors in these measurements are possible with unrelaxed respiratory muscles. If the patient is resisting mechanical ventilation ("fighting the ventilator"), the total pressure developed by the ventilator will be greater than that required to inflate the lungs of the relaxed patient.

21 Also, if the patient is actively inspiring, the pressure developed by the ventilator will be less than the total pressure required.

22 The factors that are clinically important in respiratory failure produce mechanical changes in lung function that can be detected by doing the above measurements. The advantage of the method is that it requires no special equipment, takes only a few minutes, and can be done routinely by the respiratory therapist.

23 The serial curves give warning of decreasing compliance and help separate airway from parenchymal disease.

24 Further, when the compliance decreases, hyperinflation is present.

25 The difference between peak (Pp) and static (Pst) pressure is the pressure used to overcome flow resistance.

26 If flow is measured, airway resistance (R_{aw}) can be calculated:

$$R_{aw} = \frac{Pp - Pst}{\dot{V}}$$

27 The flow is measured at end inspiration at the time of peak pressure (Fig. 28-11).

$$R_{aw} = (40 - 20)/2 = 10 \text{ cm H}_2\text{O/L/sec}$$

Alternatively, R_{aw} can be calculated at other points during inspiration. For example, the flow at 0.5 L/sec is corrected for static compliance, which equals the tidal volume divided by the static pressure minus PEEP. Thus:

$$Cst = 500/20 - 10 = 50 \text{ ml/cm H}_2\text{O}$$

28 Assuming a constant Cst, the elastic pressure component at a volume of 200 ml is 4 cm H_2O (200 ml − 50 ml/cm). The R_{aw} at 0.5 L/sec flow can then be calculated:

$$\frac{20 - \text{PEEP} - Pst}{\dot{V}}$$

$$R_{aw} = \frac{20 - 10 - 4}{0.5}$$

$$= 12 \text{ cm H}_2\text{O/L/sec}$$

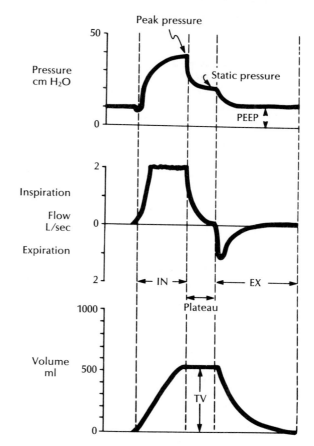

FIGURE 28-11 Monitoring pressure, flow, and volume in a patient requiring mechanical ventilation. (From Bone RC, Monitoring Respiratory Function in the Patient with Acute Respiratory Distress Syndrome, in *Seminars in Respiratory Medicine*, Volume 2, Number 3, New York, 1981, Thieme Medical Publishers, Inc. Reprinted by permission.)

29 In healthy subjects, R_{aw} ranges between 2 to 3 cm H_2O/L/sec.

30 When measured at flow rates of 1 L/sec, approximately 10% of R_{aw} is caused by turbulence.

31 With bronchospasm or inflamed airways, R_{aw} may be 10 times that seen in healthy individuals.

4.11 Physiologic shunt

1 One useful index of ventilation-perfusion inequality is the physiologic shunt (also called venous admixture, or wasted blood flow).

2 The shunt equation can be used in the following form:

$$\dot{Q}s/\dot{Q}t = Ci_{O_2} - \frac{Ca_{O_2}}{Ci_{O_2} - C\bar{v}_{O_2}}$$

Where $\dot{Q}s$ refers to physiologic shunt, $\dot{Q}t$ to total lung blood flow and Ci_{O_2}, Ca_{O_2}, and $C\bar{v}_{O_2}$ refer respectively to the oxygen content of ideal, arterial, and mixed venous blood.

3 The normal value is less than 5%.

4 If physiologic shunt is determined on other than an Fi_{O_2} of 1.0, hypoxemia caused by $\dot{V}t/\dot{Q}$ inequality contributes to shunt.

TABLE 28-1 Hemodynamic profile

	Unit	5 cm H$_2$O PEEP	10 cm H$_2$O PEEP	15 cm H$_2$O PEEP
Blood pressure	mm Hg	140/80	132/82	112/82
Pulse	Min	100	90	103
Wedge pressure	mm Hg	10	13	15
Pulmonary artery pressure	mm Hg	45/22	37/17	51/15
Cardiac output	L/min	5.9	5.8	4
Blood gases				
pH	3	7.3	7.39	7.32
Pa$_{CO_2}$	mm Hg	28	38	32
Pa$_{O_2}$	mm Hg	50	80	55
Sat	Percent	85	95	82
Hemoglobin	g	12	12	12
Urine	ml/hr	50	50	30
Oxygen delivery	ml O$_2$/min	847	933.4	544

5 Shunt is measured during 100% oxygen breathing, and overestimation of shunt may result if inadequate time is given to completely wash out N$_2$ from poorly ventilating alveoli.

6 On the other hand, prolonged breathing of 100% O$_2$ can increase Qs/Qt by increasing atelectasis.

7 Po$_2$ electrodes may underestimate the true Po$_2$ at high Po$_2$.

8 The magnitude of physicologic shunt is related to cardiac output. A decrease in flow or cardiac output will increase the effect of shunt on Pao$_2$.

9 On the other hand, increasing cardiac output by volume expansion or by pharmacological means may increase shunt in septic shock.

10 Thus the magnitude of shunt's effect on Pao$_2$ should be interpreted in relationship to cardiac output.

11 In the critically ill patient, arteriovenous oxygen difference is often estimated rather than measured. This frequently leads to considerable inaccuracy in the estimation of physiologic shunt. A clinical example of maximizing oxygen delivery is shown below.

Case study

A 24-year old woman with ARDS secondary to thrombotic thrombocytopenic purpura is treated with PEEP. The initial hemodynamic profile is shown in Table 28-1. The optimum level of PEEP is 10 cm H$_2$O, because it is associated with the best tissue oxygen delivery, which was 933.4 ml O$_2$/min. The calculation at 10 cm H$_2$O PEEP is shown below. Tissue delivery of oxygen = cardiac output × oxygen content of arterial blood:

$$CaO_2 - Hbn \text{ (g)} \times 1.39 \text{ ml } [O_2/g \text{ Hgb}] \times$$

$$[12 \times 1.39 \times 0.95] + 0.24 = 15.8 + 0.24 = 16.1$$

$$CO \cdot Cao_2 = \frac{5800 \text{ ml/min} \times 16.1 \text{ ml } O_2}{100 \text{ ml/blood}} = 933.4 \text{ ml } O_2/min$$

12 The *mixed venous oxygen tension* (P$\bar{v}O_2$) has gained popularity as an index of tissue oxygenation, a trend facilitated by the relative ease with which P$\bar{v}O_2$ measurements can be made from the pulmonary artery catheter.

13 At best, the P$\bar{v}O_2$ is a weighted mean of tissue oxygen because of variable flow rates and extraction in different organs.

14 Blood drawn from a central venous catheter is necessary.

15 A P$\bar{v}O_2$ <30 mm Hg is a sign of severe tissue hypoxia.

16 It is easy to draw a P$\bar{v}O_2$ whenever a Pao$_2$ is drawn, with a Swan-Ganz catheter in place (Fig. 28-12).

17 Experience has shown that P$\bar{v}O_2$ is an accurate measure of tissue oxygen in hemorrhagic and hypoxic shock but is falsely high with endotoxin shock because of arteriovenous shunting peripherally.

18 Others have shown that P$\bar{v}O_2$ at which lactate appeared was different for anemic and hypoxic hypoxia.

19 Danek et al. also have shown the P$\bar{v}O_2$ may not be quite as useful as previously assumed to estimate oxygen delivery during a PEEP trial.

20 When the patient is in a basal state with a constant oxygen consumption, cardiac output is inversely related to Cao$_2$ − C$\bar{v}O_2$, as shown by the Fick equation:

$$\dot{V}O_2 = (Cao_2) \times \dot{Q}T$$

21 With simultaneous measurement of PaO$_2$, P$\bar{v}O_2$ cardiac output, and hemoglobin, the oxygen consumption can be calculated.

22 Danek et al. showed that in patients with ARDS who are treated with PEEP, as oxygen delivery decreases, there is a decrease in oxygen consumption that may not be reflected by P$\bar{v}O_2$ or even Cao$_2$ − C$\bar{v}O_2$. Catheters are now available that continuously monitor mixed venous oxygen saturation.

4.12 Inspired and expired gas analysis

1 The analysis of expired air has definite appeal for monitoring because of its attributes of noninvasiveness and continuous availability. Both the respiratory mass spectrometer and new O$_2$ and CO$_2$ analyzers have made such measurements possible.

2 *Capnography* is the recording of carbon dioxide waveforms during the respiratory cycle. Capnography can be an important diagnostic tool.

3 The peak expired pressure of carbon dioxide is directly

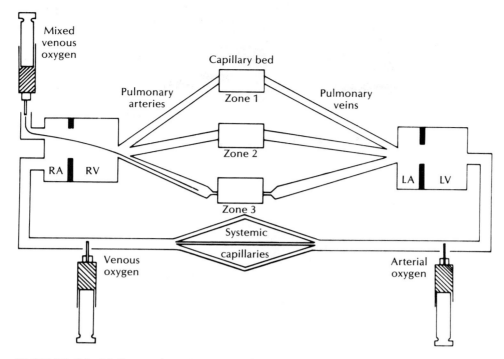

FIGURE 28-12 Oxygen determinations can be obtained from the arterial, peripheral venous, or mixed venous blood. Arterial blood provides essential information about lung function. In certain circumstances the Pa_{O_2} might increase despite a deterioration in oxygen delivery to tissue. For example, the application of PEEP in a relatively hypovolemic patient with ARDS might increase Pa_{O_2} but depress cardiac output. In this situation, the arterial mixed venous oxygen content difference increases, reflecting decreased cardiac output. Peripheral venous oxygen measurements are unreliable because they do not reflect changes from vital organs. $P\bar{v}_{O_2}$ gives important information about decreased tissue oxygenation despite improvement of arterial oxygenation. A $P\bar{v}_{O_2}$ of less than 20 mm Hg suggests critical impairment of oxygen delivery. $P\bar{v}_{O_2}$ is obtained from the pulmonary artery as shown in this example. Also, the flow directed pulmonary artery catheter is more likely to locate in better perfused lung regions (zone 2 or 3). In the supine patient, zone 3 is posterior and in the upright patient it is inferior. (From Bone RC: Treatment of severe hypoxemia due to the adult respiratory distress syndrome, Arch Intern Med 140:85-89, Copyright 1980, American Medical Association.)

related to the Pa_{CO_2}, which in turn is primarily dependent on CO_2 production, alveolar ventilation, and pulmonary capillary blood flow.

4 Monitoring expired carbon dioxide may be advantageous to ventilator management.

5 Alveolar ventilation ($\dot{V}A$) is inversely related to alveolar carbon dioxide tension (Pa_{CO_2}), as defined by the following equation:

$$VA = \frac{\dot{V}_{CO_2} \times 0.863}{Pa_{CO_2}} = \frac{V_{CO_2} \times 0.863}{PetCO_2}$$

6 With continuous measurement of the expired CO_2 waveforms, an end-tidal CO_2 concentration can be measured (Fig. 28-13).

7 The end-tidal CO_2 ($PetCO_2$) concentration has a relationship to Pa_{CO_2} and thus can serve as a readily available noninvasive estimate of the Pa_{CO_2}.

8 Thus, the $PetCO_2$ will be increased if alveolar ventilation is decreased or carbon dioxide production is increased.

9 Access to breath-by-breath $PetCO_2$ measurements allows a gradual change in Pa_{CO_2} during mechanical ventilation.

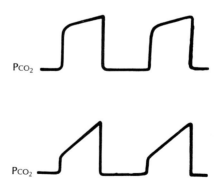

FIGURE 28-13 End-tidal carbon dioxide in normal lungs with ventilation-perfusion mismatching.

10 Nonintubated patients may be monitored continuously through placement of the mass spectrometer probe in an oxygen catheter placed in the posterior nasopharynx. This could be of help in monitoring the recent extubated patient.

11 Since Pet CO_2 has a rather consistent relationship to Pa_{CO_2}, access to $PetCO_2$ may decrease blood drawn to

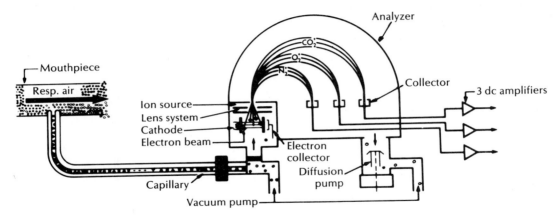

FIGURE 28-14 Magnetic sector mass spectrometer. (See text for description of operation.) (From Bone RC, Monitoring Respiratory Function in the Patient with Acute Respiratory Distress Syndrome, in *Seminars in Respiratory Medicine*, Volume 2, Number 3, New York, 1981, Thieme Medical Publishers, Inc. Reprinted by permission.)

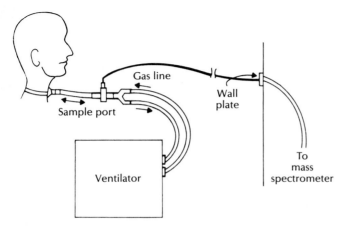

FIGURE 28-15 Mass spectrometer can be multiplexed to multiple patients in a time-sharing arrangement or devoted to a single patient. (From Bone RC, Monitoring Respiratory Function in the Patient with Acute Respiratory Distress Syndrome, in *Seminars in Respiratory Medicine*, Volume 2, Number 3, New York, 1981, Thieme Medical Publishers, Inc. Reprinted by permission.)

find the Pa_{CO_2} and should reduce much of the guesswork associated with ventilator adjustment.

12 Pet_{CO_2} can be monitored satisfactorily on a breath-by-breath basis with the infrared technique of the mass spectrometer.

13 The Pet_{CO_2} measurement corresponds closely to the Pa_{CO_2} in the normal subject at rest.

14 The Pet_{CO_2} is markedly dependent on tidal volume (at a constant Va).

15 Unfortunately, the presence of $\dot{V}A/\dot{Q}$ inequality and shunt in lung disease leads to a divergence of Pa_{CO_2} values.

16 As the distribution of $\dot{V}a/\dot{Q}$ abnormality increases the expired air is weighted by lungs units with a high Va/Q and dead space, and the arterial blood is weighted by lung regions with a low $\dot{V}a/\dot{Q}$ and shunt. This is managed by doing an initial measurement to establish the $Pa - Pet_{CO_2}$ difference.

17 *Mass spectrometry* is an analysis of the molecular components of a substance. A mass spectrometer is an instrument that determines components and component concentrations of a substance.

18 The type of mass spectrometer most commonly used to measure gases is the magnetic sector mass spectrometer (Fig. 28-14).

19 Gases O_2, CO_2, N_2 are ionized, separated according to their mass weight, and their concentrations are measured with respiratory mass spectrometers.

20 The mass spectrometer converts the gas into a beam of ions. The ion beam is then passed into a magnetic field, where the ions are deflected to a collector plate. Deflection is related to ion mass; the deposited ions give up an electrical charge whose current is proportional to the number of ions in the sample.

21 Assuming there are collectors present for all ions formed from the sample, the mass spectrometer will measure the concentration of each gas in the sample.

22 Inspired and expired oxygen are best measured by the mass spectrometer, because most other techniques of gas analysis have a slow response time.

23 However, some have found the hot ceramic oxygen polarograph electrode to respond rapidly enough for breath-by-breath measurements.

24 For computer-based calculations, a response time of 90% in 200 msec is adequate. Most mass spectrometers and carbon dioxide analyzers and some oxygen polarographs fulfill this requirement.

25 If a number of patients are to be monitored, the mass spectrometer may be more cost effective, since a single unit can be multiplexed to several beds (Fig. 28-15). The mass spectrometer also has a faster response time, requires a smaller sampling volume, and can detect a variety of gases.

26 In practice, most difficulties with spectrometer measurements have been primarily related to plugging of probe catheters with moisture and secretions, as well as other problems of gas sampling and instrument failure.

27 Routine measurement of functional residual capacity is difficult. Several systems have been devised to allow the measurement to be performed. The most popular is

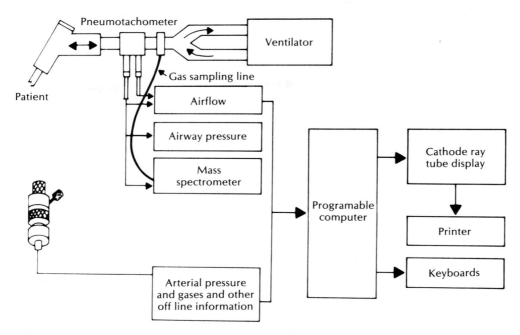

FIGURE 28-16 Respiratory monitoring system. Air flow, pressure and gas concentrations measured simultaneously. Calculations made by a computer using these signals and off-line information. (From Bone RC, Monitoring Respiratory Function in the Patient with Acute Respiratory Distress Syndrome, in *Seminars in Respiratory Medicine*, Volume 2, Number 3, New York, 1981, Thieme Medical Publishers, Inc. Reprinted by permission.)

a helium dilution technique using a *bag-in-box system*. However, no system is clinically practical as yet.

28 In a system in which information is desired from the mass spectrometer and simultaneous information from the flow and pressure signals, these signals will have to be matched in time. This may be difficult to solve, because gas flow will depend on viscosity and temperature, both of which might change.

29 Temperature change can result from use of heated humidifiers or because the patient is febrile or hypothermic. Also, there is about a 16% change in calibration between air and 100% oxygen.

30 Coupling of other pulmonary measurements, such as flow rate, volume, and airway pressure with mass spectrometry, has proved technically troublesome at present for on-line computation.

31 Other potential disadvantages at many institutions are the size of the mass spectrometer, its high initial cost, and the technical inability to measure carbon monoxide because of its molecular weight equivalency with nitrogen.

32 In general, many of the claimed capabilities of the respiratory mass spectrometer in the intensive care unit have not yet been substantiated. Literature describing clinical applications of mass spectrometry–based monitoring is largely anecdotal. At the present time mass spectrometry is best viewed as a research tool with potential clinical usefullness.

33 *On-line mechanics* is the measurement of gas flow and volume and forces causing such activity. The repiratory system behaves mechanically as a pump with flow-resistive components and volume-elastic components connected in series.

34 According to Newton's Third Law of Motion, to produce a volume change, opposing forces must be overcome. An increase in pressure at the mouth causes a flow of gas through the airways, which exhibits resistance to flow.

35 The pressure not dissipated in overcoming a airway resistance is dissipated by the volume-elastic component that is capable of deformation and volume change.

36 The pressure applied must overcome elastic forces (1/C) to produce a volume change (V), resistive forces (R) to produce flow ($\dot{V}$), and inertial forces (i) to produce acceleration ($\ddot{V}$).

37 These can be combined to form the equation of motion for the respiratory system:

$$P = (1/C \times V) + (R \times \dot{V}) + (I \times \ddot{V})$$

38 Changes resulting from inertia (I) are small and for clinical use can be ignored.

39 The measurement of the mechanical function of the lung requires the continuous recording of pressure and flow during the respiratory cycle (Fig. 28-16).

40 Flow is usually measured by a *pneumotachograph* from the differential pressure across a resistance ventilator (see Module 23).

41 Inspiratory and expiratory pneumotachographs are a part of some monitoring systems. With on-line pneumotachographs, expired volume measurements that include volume expended in expansion of the tubing are less of a problem.

42 However, pneumotachographs introduce an entirely new set of problems, ranging from incorrect information caused by mucous plugging of the pneumotacho-

graph to problems of calibration changes caused by changing gas concentrations.

43 Because of problems with constant measurements with the Fleish pneumotachograph, other flow measuring devices have been developed including the variable orifice flowmeter, ultrasonic flowmeter, and turbulent flowmeter.

44 These flowmeters are presently undergoing clinical trials, and their accuracy and durability are still to be determined.

45 Calibration of the pneumotachograph must be done frequently to avoid error. This can be accomplished with a 1 to 3 L syringe in line with a standard spirometer.

46 Since pneumotachographs are sensitive to temperature, humidity, and flow, they should be calibrated under clinical conditions for reliable results.

47 Flow rates should be linear over a range of 0 to 3 L/sec for ventilator patients.

48 Some patients with respiratory failure may have expiratory peak flow rates exceeding 5 L/sec, and appropriate pneumotachographs should be used in those patients.

49 In automated systems, airway pressure is measured by strain gauges (see Module 23). Reliable strain gauges are now available that provide a linear electrical output spanning a range of 0 to 200 cm H_2O.

50 A Fleish pneumotachograph with pressure and gas sampling lines leading to a mass spectrometer and computer allows simultaneous measurement of inspired and expired gases and mechanics. The system requires a pneumotachograph, mass spectrometer, and computer.

51 To measure lung compliance rather than lung and chest wall compliance, a measurement of transpulmonary pressure must be made.

52 This can be done by pressure measurements by an esophageal balloon or from the proximal port of a thermodilution Swan-Ganz catheter or a central venous catheter.

53 Esophageal balloons are now available that attach to standard nasogastric tubes.

54 Lung plus chest wall compliance as measured from airway pressure on the ventilator patient is affected by muscle contractions.

55 The direct measurement of pleural pressure thus adds both specificity and resolution but at the cost of instability and is not clinically practical. The static compliance curve plotted in the pulmonary physiology laboratory is measured from static measurements of total lung capacity. The plot of static transpulmonary pressure against lung volume is curvilinear; compliance is equal to the slope of the curve at a particular point.

56 Unless functional residual capacity is measured and the compliance curve is measured at multiple volumes on deflation from a single breath, static compliance in the intensive care unit is not equivalent to static compliance measured in the pulmonary function laboratory.

57 In the intensive care unit, lung volume is often unknown, and a decrease in compliance could be caused by a true increase in elastic recoil (e.g., pulmonary edema) of the same elastic recoil exerted on a small volume (e.g., atelectasis).

58 Regardless of the mechanism of decrease in compliance, the knowledge that it is decreased is important information and should not be ignored because of the lack of knowledge of absolute lung volume before and after atelectasis or pulmonary edema.

5.0 COMPUTERS IN CRITICAL CARE
5.1 Applications (See also Module 30)

Computers are increasingly being used in critical care medicine.

1 Currently, computers are used to:
 a Automate recordkeeping
 b Provide immediate feedback in certain critical care settings such as oxygen and ventilator adjustments, particularly PEEP trials
 c Monitor hemodynamic changes related to the ventilator and drug adjustments

2 Two examples of the concordance of modern technology and computer interfacing with patient care are exercise testing and sleep apnea monitoring.

3 Terminology is important in understanding computers (see the box on the opposite page). Computer-based monitoring systems allow the rapid computation of multiple physiologic variables and provide a trend analysis of changing variables.

4 A properly programmed computer-based system should assist in gathering, processing, and displaying pertinent information.

5 With this type of information, critical care personnel should be freed from repetitive duties and provided more time for patient contact and decision-making.

6 Analog signals are fed to a microcomputer after the signals are sorted and arranged in an order easily accepted by the computer by an electronic device called the *multiplexer*.

7 The minicomputer serves as a storage and processing unit and can be programmed to perform computations automatically.

8 The computer required for such computation is relatively expensive. The microcomputer is inexpensive enough to be dedicated to continuous respiratory monitoring.

9 This is an advance, since the time-sharing arrangement necessary for use of central computers is often a disadvantage to monitoring rapidly changing respiratory variables.

5.2 Limitations of the computer

1 Despite many advances in electronic, computer, and engineering technology, sophisticated monitoring of respiratory function in the critically ill patient has advanced slowly. Experience with mass spectrometry and on-line measurements of mechanics is largely anecdotal.

2 The usefulness of these tools depends on their ability to

Terminology commonly used in automated data handling

Analog input Electronic signal from a spirometer, gas analyzer, plethysmograph, or pneumotach.

A/D converter Analog-to-digital converter; changes electronic signals into computer language.

Byte Includes eight bits. A bit is a single character of data.

Computer Electronic device that is centrally located and is capable of performing high-speed calculations and assembling and storing information in a memory; computers can correlate and cross-reference by means of a logic or processor unit.

CRT (cathode ray tube) Video terminal that consists of a typewriter keyboard and viewing screen that allows the operator to manually supply information to the computer and to initiate and terminate procedures.

Hardware The physical equipment comprising the computer and memory.

Language System of symbols that allows a programmer to instruct the computer to perform a certain task.

Memory Electronic or mechanical device used to store data and programs; types of memory include magnetic core, floppy disk, magnetic tape, and tape cassettes; the amount of information that can be stored is described in bits, each of which approximates one character; memory size is usually classified in *K*, thousands of bits, or *mega*, millions of bits.

Microprocessor A single electronic component that is hardwired or contained on chips; microprocessors usually have fixed programs and can be built into testing systems to perform calculations, do some assembly, and have a limited storage or memory.

On-line Denotes a direct connection between the testing instrument and the computer.

Plotter Electromechanical device that converts digital outputs into tracings.

Printer Electromechanical device that reports data in hard-copy form on paper.

Peripherals Devices that allow communication with the computer and other devices such as terminals, printers, and plotters.

Real time Denotes direct user response by the compuer.

Shared time Denotes a computer with multiple users, working one at a time; the most sophisticated systems use a combination of real time and shared time modes.

Software All programs including those that control computer functions and those that process input data.

Word Specified number of bits.

---

provide information in a cost-effective and dependable fashion. Some automated monitors, such as the regulation of intravenous infusion rates based on heart rate or blood pressure, may decrease time expenditure by staff.

3 It is unlikely that respiratory monitoring will reach that stage of sophistication in the near future.

4 It is likely that mass spectrometry and continuous measurements of mechanics will take more rather than less staff time to analyze and interpret the new information. It will also require sophisticated bioengineering skills to keep the machinery functioning.

5 Personnel must be trained thoroughly in calibration, use, and maintenance of the new equipment. It is demoralizing to staff and hospital administration to purchase an expensive piece of machinery that is "down" most of the time. These considerations must be weighed before purchase of such a system.

6 Respiratory monitoring equipment will not function continuously without attention. It will function continuously with dedicated attention.

6.0 DEVELOPMENT OF NEW MONITORING TECHNIQUES

6.1 Practicality

1 Special scrutiny should be applied to two areas in assessing the potential value of new monitoring techniques.

2 The first question to be asked is, "Can this technique provide the information it claims in a reliable manner, under usual clinical conditions?" If a method is proved in the technical sense, we still must ask, "Of what value to patient management are the data produced?"

3 Few convincing data are available to answer these questions with regard to newer, more sophisticated respiratory monitoring methods. Economic considerations demand that resources not be devoted to gathering useless information, although some redundant information is valuable for detecting errors.

4 Possibly the most serious danger of adopting monitoring techniques uncritically is "drowning" clinicians in a flood of numbers.

5 The presentation of more data than can be assimilated can contribute to incorrect clinical decisions.

6 This factor is too often ignored in assessing the utility of new measurements.

7 Electronic computers have potential for alleviating some of these problems. They can perform much of the tedious work of analyzing large amounts of data and reducing it to a form useful for making decisions. For example, they can produce summaries that list only aberrant values, reduce long lists of numbers to graphic form, or display only data considered relevant according to some predetermined criterion.

8 Even though the availability of inexpensive, powerful microcomputers makes such applications feasible, little has been done in determining how they can best perform such clerical functions. Thus far, most effort has been devoted to overcoming difficulties associated with on-line data acquisition and solving various technical problems.

9 As the quantitative data generated in the intensive care unit increase, it will become increasingly important to have machines do what machines can do best to spare people for tasks that require uniquely human abilities.

6.2 Biologic variables that should be monitored

1 What biologic variables should be monitored? The answer to this question remains unclear, but the generally accepted therapeutic goal of maintaining biologic variables in the normal range is being questioned. For example, blood pressure and cardiac output can be restored to normal values after shock, yet the patient still dies.

2 Survivors often show supernormal values, reflecting their stress response to a critical illness and the subsequent metabolic and circulatory adjustment.

3 Bland et al. monitored the 20 most common variables in a series of 113 critically ill patients. For arterial pressure, heart rate, central venous pressure, and cardiac output, normal values were restored in 75% of the survivors and 76% of patients who died. They felt we may not have the right therapeutic goals or we may not be monitoring the right variables.

4 The ability of the most commonly monitored variables to predict outcome such as vital signs, heart rate, and hemoglobin were poor. Perfusion-related variables, which express the interrelationship of oxygen transport to red cell volume and flow were the predictors of outcome.

5 Perfusion-related variables reflecting the maldistribution of system circulation should get as much attention as variables reflecting maldistribution of the pulmonary circulation in future research.

7.0 HEMODYNAMIC MONITORING
7.1 Overview

1 Hemodynamic monitoring is the assessment of the patient's circulatory status.

2 It includes measurement of heart rate, intraarterial pressure, pulmonary pressure, pulmonary capillary wedge pressures, central venous pressure, cardiac output, and blood volume. It is used to monitor patients with cardiopulmonary complications and patients who are on life support devices, such as mechanical ventilation and hemodialysis.

3 Before 1970, direct assessment of left ventricular end-diastolic pressure was limited to studies conducted in the cardiac catheterization laboratory.

4 In 1970, H.J.C. Swan and W. Ganz et al. first reported in the *New England Journal of Medicine* on "Catheterization of the heart in man with the use of a flow-directed balloon tipped catheter."

5 Since that time all brands of balloon flotation pulmonary artery catheters have been commonly referred to as Swan-Ganz catheters, even though the name is a trademark for catheters manufactured by Edwards Laboratories.

7.2 Parts of the catheter unit

1 There are several variations to the balloon flotation pulmonary artery catheter originally described by Swan and Ganz et al.

2 The following is an explanation of the Swan-Ganz thermodilution catheter.

3 This catheter is a 7 Fr. Polyvinyl tube, 110 cm long, that encloses four individual and separate channels (lumens) (Fig. 28-17, *A* and *B*). These lumens all have external connectors (ports) that can be used to activate different functions of the catheter (Fig. 28-17, *A, 1-4*).

4 The distal lumen *(1)* is the largest and terminates at the tip of the inflation balloon (catheter). When the balloon is inflated, this opening lies in the pulmonary artery and is used to monitor PA, PAO, PCW pressures and to sample venous blood.

5 The balloon lumen *(2)* is used to inflate and deflate the balloon located about 1 cm from the end of the catheter. The balloon (cuff) *(3)* is made of thin latex rubber. When inflated it blocks blood flow but does not cover the tip of the catheter.

6 The thermistor lumen *(3)* ends in an opening located approximately 4 cm above the inflation balloon. This lumen contains thermistor wires for measuring blood temperature required when determining cardiac output by thermodilution technique.

7 The proximal (RA) lumen *(4)* is located 30 cm from the tip of the catheter. This opening rests in the right atrium of the heart. It measures right atrium (CVP) pressure.

8 The exposed end of the catheter when it is in place contains four external connectors attached to the following equipment (Fig. 28-17, *A*):
   a The thermistor lumen (port), when connected to a bedside cardiac output computer, measures temperature of blood flowing over the thermistor wires.
   b The *proximal lumen* (RA port), when connected to either a pressure transducer or manometer, monitors CVP or RA pressures and is used to infuse IV fluids.
   c The *distal lumen* (PA port), when connected to a pressure transducer and CRT, monitors continuous PA pressure, PAO, or wedge pressure with the balloon inflated.
   d The *balloon lumen* (port), when connected to a syringe, is used for inflation of the latex balloon with 1½ ml of air.

7.3 Principle of operation

1 The pulmonary artery catheter is inserted by a physician through the internal jugular, subclavian, antecubital, or femoral veins by percutaneous puncture or venotomy.

2 Before the catheter is advanced, the transmission tube must be connected, the stopcock opened, and the lumen irrigated. This will facilitate passage of the catheter and verification of location based on pressure tracings.

3 The catheter is advanced according to the following sequence by monitoring catheter tip pressures and viewing waveforms on a pressure monitor (Fig. 28-18):
   a The catheter is advanced into the superior vena cava and the balloon is inflated.

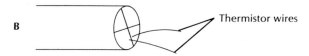

Cross section of tip of catheter showing 4 lumens

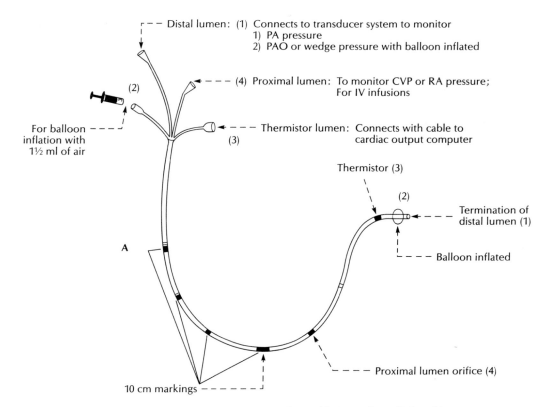

FIGURE 28-17 The Swan-Ganz thermodilution catheter (7 French).

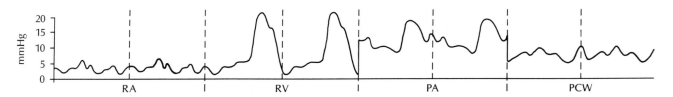

FIGURE 28-18 Pressure changes as the catheter moves through the right heart and wedges in the pulmonary capillary.

b The catheter is carried by blood through the right atrium and tricuspid valve into the right ventricle.

c From the right ventricle the catheter flows into the main pulmonary artery.

d Blood flow carries the catheter deeper into the pulmonary vessels until the inflated balloon becomes lodged against the walls. This is the *pulmonary capillary wedge position.*

e Pressure is recorded at this point as an indicator of left ventricular function.

4 Pressures should be recorded with the patient in the supine position unless this position is contraindicated.

5 Pressures should be read at the end of expiration.

6 A ventilator patient should have readings taken at end-expiration, since positive pressure ventilation increases intrathoracic pressure giving a falsely elevated reading.

7 Balloon inflation should be adjusted and a characteristic PA pressure tracing should be observed. Once this tracing is achieved, balloon inflation should be stopped to prevent overinflation and possible rupture.

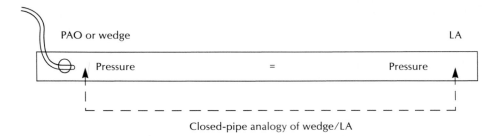

FIGURE 28-19 Analogy of wedge pressure measurement to closed tube. The relationship between PAO and LA pressures can be thought to be similar to a tube closed at both ends. Thus, if no flow exists through the tube, the pressures at each end must be the same.

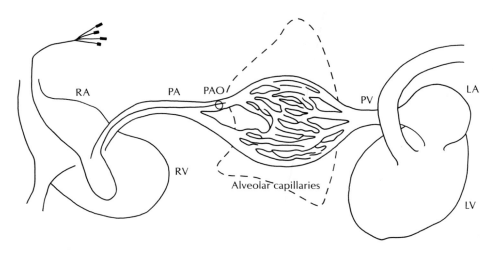

FIGURE 28-20 Schematic representation of catheter in the wedge position.

8 Normal mean pressures are:
  a Pulmonary artery (PAP)—12 to 18 mm Hg
  b Pulmonary artery occlusion or wedge (PAWP)—4 to 12 mm Hg
  c Central venous or right arterial pressure (CVP)—3 to 12 mm Hg
9 Conditions that may alter these pressures from normal care are presented in the box at the right.

7.4 Theory for indirect measurement of left atrial pressure

  1 The theory for use of the Swan-Ganz catheter to measure left atrial pressure is based on the physical concept that if a pipe is closed on both ends and flow is blocked, the pressures at each end must be the same (Fig. 28-19).
  2 Consequently, once the catheter balloon is in the wedged position, flow is blocked in the segment of the pulmonary artery.
  3 At this point the pressure sensing tip of the catheter is in direct continuity with the pulmonary capillaries, veins, and left atrium.
  4 Since pulmonary artery blood flow is blocked by the balloon, this closed system must reflect pressure throughout. Therefore pulmonary artery occlusion pressure reflects left atrial pressure (Fig. 28-20).

Causes of alterations of normal pressure	
INCREASES IN PAP	**INCREASES IN CVP OR RAP**
Pulmonary vascular resistance	Pulmonary congestion and edema
Chronic obstructive lung disease	Cardiac insufficiency and failure
Pulmonary congestion or edema	Tricuspid valve insufficiency
Pulmonary embolism	Cirrhosis of the liver
Acute pulmonary insufficiency	
Hypovolema	
INCREASES IN PAO OR PCWP	**DECREASES IN PAO OR PCWP**
Hypovolemia	Positive inotropic agents intended to improve myocardial contractility and left ventricular function
Pulmonary edema or congestion	
Cardiac insufficiency or failure	Hypovolemia/non-cardiac pulmonary edema
Mitral valve insufficiency	

7.5 Complications of catheterization

1 Any invasive procedure has potential hazards to the patient and catheterization is no exception.

2 These potential hazards include:

For arterial catheterization

a Ischemia

b Infections

c Vasospasm

d Aneurysm

e Ruptured balloon

For central venous catheterization

a Hematoma

b Pneumothorax

c Hemothorax and hemomediastinum

d Thrombosis

e Emboli

f Infections

g Malpositioned catheter

For pulmonary artery catheterization

a Infections

b Thrombi and infarcts

c Rupture of pulmonary artery

d Kinking of catheter

BIBLIOGRAPHY

Askanazi J et al: Nutrition for the patients with respiratory failure: glucose fat, Anesthesiology 54:373, 1981.

Askanazi J et al: Respiratory changes induced by the large glucose loads of parenteral nutrition, JAMA 243:1444, 1980.

Bahr DE and Clark KR: Continuous arterial tonometry in essential noninvasive monitoring in anesthesia. In Groverstein JS et al, editors: New York, 1980, Grune and Stratton Inc.

Blumenfeld W et al: On-line respiratory gas monitoring, Computers Biomed Res 6:139, 1973.

Bone RC: Diagnosis of causes for acute respiratory distress by pressure-volume curves, Chest 70:740, 1976.

Bone RC: Monitoring patients in acute respiratory failure, Respir Care 27:700, 1982.

Bone RC: Monitoring respiratory function in the patient with the adult respiratory distress syndrome. 2:140, 1981.

Bone RC: Treatment of respiratory failure due to advanced obstructive lung disease, Arch Intern Med 140:101, 1980.

Danek SI et al: The dependence of oxygen uptake on oxygen delivery in the adult respiratory distress syndrome, Am Rev Respir Dis 22:387, 1980.

Dantzker D: Abnormalities of oxygen transfer. In Bone RC, editor: Pulmonary disease reviews, New York, 1980, 1:1, John Wiley & Sons.

Downs JB and Douglas ME: Assessment of cardiac filling pressure occurring in continuous positive pressure ventilation, Crit Care Med 8:285, 1980.

Fallat RJ: Bedside testing and intensive care monitoring of pulmonary function in standards and controversies in pulmonary function testing, Calif Thorac Soc Ann Postgrad Course Jan 1980.

Fox MG, Brady JS, and Weintraub LR: Leukocyte larceny: a case of supreious hypoxemia, Am J Med 676:742, 1979.

Ganz W et al: A new technique for measurement of cardiac output by thermodilution in man, Am J Cardiol 27:392, 1971.

Gilbert F and Keightley JF: The arterial/alveolar oxygen tension ratio: an index of gas exchange applicable to varying inspired concentrations, Am Rev Respir Dis 109:142, 1974.

Goecbenjan G: Continous measurement of arterial PO_2—significance and indications in intensive care, Biotel Pat Monit 6:51, 1979.

Gordon R: The deep sulcus sign, Radiology 136:25, 1980.

Grossman W: Cardiac catheterization and angiography. Philadelphia, 1980, Lea & Febiger.

Ian EM, Heldman JJ, and Chen S: Coronary hemodynamics and oxygen utilization after hematocrit variations in hemorrhage, Am J Physiol 243:H325, 1980.

Jordan E et al: Venous admixture in human septic shock: comparative effects of blood volume expansion, dopamine infusion and isoproterenol infusion on mismatching of ventilation and pulmonary blood flow in peritonitis, Circulation 60:155, 1979.

Luterman A et al: Withdrawal from positive end-expiratory pressure, Surg 83:328, 1978.

Newell JC et al: Pulmonary pressure-volume relationships in traumatized man, J Surg Res 26:114, 1979.

Osborne JJ et al: Respiratory causes of "sudden unexplained arrhythmia" in post-thoracotomy patients, Surg 69:24, 1971.

Peabody JL et al: Clinical limitations and advantages of transcutaneous oxygen electrodes, Acta Anesth Scand (Suppl) 68:76, 1978.

Popovich J et al: Mass spectrometry, Respir Therap 10:50, 1980.

Ream AK: Systolic, diastolic, mean or pulse: which is the best measurement of arterial pressure? Noninvasive Monit IG, ref 3, pp 53, 1980.

Rhea JT, Sooenberg EV, McLoud the supine adult, Radiology 133:593, 1979.

Rothe CF and Kim KC: Measuring systolic arterial blood pressure: possible errors from extension tubes or disposable transducer domes, Crit Care Med 8:683, 1980.

Sahn SA and Lakshminarayan S: Bedside criteria for discontinuation of mechanical ventilation, Chest 63:1002, 1973.

Shimada Y et al: Evaluation of the progress and prognosis of adult respiratory distress syndrome: simple physiologic measurement, Chest 76:180, 1979.

Shoemaker WC and Czor LSC: Evaluation of the biological importance of various hemodynamic and oxygen transport variables, Crit Care Med 7:424, 1979.

Skillman JJ, Awwad HK, and Moore FD: Plasma protein kinetics of the early transcapillary refill after hemorrhage in man, Surg Gynecol Obstet 123:983, 1967.

Suwa K, Hedley-White J, and Bendexen HH: Circulation and physiological dead space changes on controlled ventilation of dogs, J Appl Physiol 231:1855, 1966.

Swan HTC, Ganz W, Forrester J, et al: Catheterization of the heart in man with use of a flow-directed balloon-tipped catheter, N Engl J Med 283:447, 1970.

Sweet SJ et al: Synergistic effect of acute renal failure and respiratory failure in the surgical intensive care unit, Ann J Surg 141:492, 1981.

Tremper KK et al: Transcutaneous oxygen monitoring during arrest and CPR, Crit Care Med :377, 1980.

Tremper KK, Waxman K, and Shoemaker WC: Effects of hypoxia and shock on transcutaneous PO_2 values in dogs. Crit Care Med 7:526, 1979.

Turney SZ, McAslan TC, and Cowley RA: The continuous measurement of pulmonary gas exchange and mechanics, Ann Thorac Surg 13:229, 1973.

Versmold HT et al: Limits of $tcPO_2$ monitoring in sick neonates: Relation to blood pressure, blood volume, peripheral blood flow and acid-base status, Acta Anesth Scand (Suppl) 68:88, 1978.

Wald A et al: A computer system for respiratory parameters, Computers Biomed Res 2:411, 1969.

Wagner PD: Diffusion and chemical reaction in pulmonary gas exchange, Physiol Rev 57:257, 1977.

Wagner PD, Saltzman HA, and West JB: Measurement of continuous distributions of ventilation-perfusion ratios: theory, J Appl Physiol 36:588, 1974.

Wagner PD and West JB: Effects of diffusion impairment on O_2 and CO_2 time courses in pulmonary capillaries, J Appl Physiol 33:62, 1972.

West JB and Wagner PD: Pulmonary gas exchange. In West JB, editor: Bioengineering aspects of the lung, New York, 1977, Miscel Dekkor.

Wilson RS: Monitoring the lung: mechanics and volume, Anesthesiology 45:135, 1976.

Zwillich CW et al: Complications of assistant ventilation, Am J Med 57:161, 1974.

Gerontology

On completion of this module the reader will be able to:

1.1 Define longevity.

1.2 Compare the number of persons 65 years of age and older of today to those who will be 65 in the year 2040.

1.3 Explain the significance of the statement that "the older population itself is getting older."

1.4 Point out the difference in the 65 to 74 age-group in 1989 to a similar group in 1900.

1.5 Compare the size of the 75- to 84-year-old age-group and the 85-year-old age-group of 1989 to 1900.

1.6 Point out the difference in life expectancy for a baby born in 1989 to one born in 1900.

1.7 Differentiate between the life expectancy of the male and female born today and in the year 2040.

2.1 Identify the different types of aging.

   1 Discuss the effect on an individual of the various types of aging.

2.2 Explain when aging begins.

2.3 List and differentiate six major theories of aging.

2.4 Show appreciation for the complexity of aging by discussing general principles that apply to the aging process and patient care.

2.5 Define senescence.

2.6 Point out physical, physiologic, and psychosocial changes that occur wtih senescence.

2.7 Discuss the concept of a rectangular society or squaring of the morbidity and mortality curve.

2.8 Explain how the heart changes anatomically with age.

2.9 Point out physiologic changes that occur as the heart and blood vessels age.

2.10 Discuss the effects of aging on blood vessels.

2.11 Discuss the effect of aging on the chest.

2.12 Explain how the lungs are structurally altered with age.

2.13 Differentiate the various functional changes that occur with the lung as it ages.

2.14 Point out and discuss the most frequently occurring respiratory conditions of the aged.

2.15 Summarize common disabilities of the elderly.

3.1 Describe the three major causes of institutionalization of the elderly.

3.2 Identify the number of women who are residents in nursing homes.

3.3 Explain the economic influence of the elderly on health care by identifying their impact on hospital census.

3.4 Show appreciation for the socioeconomic impact on the elderly of the cost of living on a fixed income by discussing general demographics of the elderly.

3.5 Define ADLs and distinguish which activity is the biggest problem to the elderly.

3.6 Point out the geographical locations most preferred by the elderly.

4.1 through **4.4** Differentiate the various alternatives for care of the elderly and discuss the one most popular with the elderly.

4.5 Discuss 18 questions that may be used to screen the efficiency and desirability of one nursing home over another.

4.6 Explain the function of a home health agency.

4.7 Point out different ways in which the elderly are cared for in foreign countries.

5.1 Show appreciation for the importance of allied health professionals in care of the elderly by discussing the numbers of health care workers nationwide.

5.2 Discuss how the nursing profession is responding to the increasing need for professionals trained in the care of the elderly.

5.3 Demonstrate belief in promoting geriatrics and gerontology by pointing out various activities that are being taken by professional groups to prepare for care of the elderly.

5.4 Discuss curriculum changes necessary to prepare practioners for caring for an aging population.

6.1 Explain why one health care discipline alone is not capable of meeting the needs of the elderly.

6.2 Discuss the growing role of respiratory care personnel in care of the elderly.

6.3 through **6.4** Differentiate between the role of the respiratory care practitioner in the hospital, home, and nursing home in care of the elderly.

6.5 Define and give the function of geriatric education centers (GECs), and list the GECs closest to your home.

Health care in America is among the best in the world. As a result, people are living longer. The question has become one of whether they are also living better.

Today over 1.4 million allied health professionals make up 63% of the total health care work force. Between the years 2020 and 2030, 75% of these health workers' time will be spent with elderly persons. The challenge has become one of preparing these workers to handle the special needs and to treat the unique disorders of this ever-increasing elderly population.

Respiratory care practitioners are important members of the health care team who will be required to service the needs of the elderly in the hospital and in alternative care settings.

Gerontology is the study of the aging process and its effects on the elderly.

Because of space limitations this module presents only a mosaic picture of the life and needs of the elderly. We hope that the reader will accept the challenge to learn more about the elderly and their care and become prepared to serve on the health teams of tomorrow that will be needed to serve this potentially large patient population.

1.0 AGING OF AMERICA

1.1 Longevity is the duration of life of an individual member of a particular species or population. Americans as a population are getting older.

1.2 The over-65 age-group is the fastest growing segment of the population today, totalling some 40 million persons. By the year 2040, when most of the baby boom generation have entered their elderly years, this age-group may number over 87 million, or 25% of the total U.S. population (Fig. 29-1).

Population 55 years and over by age: 1900-2050

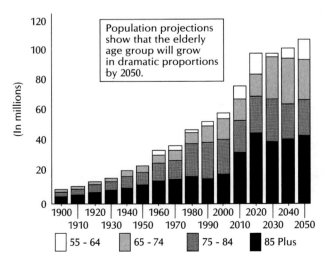

FIGURE 29-1 Growth of the U.S. population from 1990 to 2050. (Modified from U.S. Census of Population, 1890-1980 and projections of the United States: 1983-2050.)

1.3 Of equal significance is the fact that the older population itself is continuing to get older as more individuals reach 65.

1.4 For example, in 1989 the 65 to 74 age-group (17 million) was eight times larger than this age-group in 1900.

1.5 The 75- to 84-year-old group was 11 times larger than in 1900 (8.8 million), and the 85 and older age-group was 22 times larger (2.7 million).

1.6 What this means is that people are living longer. A baby born in 1989 is expected to live approximately 75 years, compared with approximately 50 years of age for a person born in 1900.

1.7 By the year 2040, American men are expected to live to 87 years (17 years longer than today), and the average women will live for 92 years, compared with a life expectancy of 78 years today.

2.0 BIOLOGY OF AGING

2.1 Aging is a complex process that involves:
  a Biologic aging—time-related changes in cells, tissues systems
  b Economic aging—changes in financial status
  c Psychologic aging—changes in behavior
  d Social aging—acquired social habits

2.2 Biologically, cells begin aging from the moment of birth. Most gerontologists agree that physically a human's peak years are during the early twenties, although some believe that they end with puberty.

2.3 There are six major theories as to why cells age and ultimately cease to function (die). These include, in no specific order:
  a The GENE theory: Cells are preprogrammed so that one or more genes become activated with age, causing the organism to ultimately die.
  b The PROGRAMMED theory: Similar to the gene theory in that evolution has preprogrammed humans to live for a certain length of time.
  c The FREE RADICAL theory: Noxious compounds called free radicals are released in the cell as a by-product of metabolism (more specifically, glycolysis). These free radicals react with other substances, especially unsaturated fats, to cause holes to occur in the cell membrane and damage to DNA. In young, healthy cells these free radicals are controlled by separation membranes and neutralizers called *scavengers*. As the cells age the separation membranes become less efficient and the ratio of free radicals to scavengers greater. This process continues until the damaged cells eventually die. The free radical theory of aging is plausible when one investigates the amount of lipofuscin in aged cells. Lipofuscin is a yellow-brown age pigment that accumulates in the cells of older animals. In the human heart this pigment increases at the rate of approximately 0.06% per year. Research has shown that one can reduce this rate of buildup by taking antioxidants (scavengers) such as vitamin E, or selenium.*

d The CROSS-LINKAGE theory: The accumulation of cross-linking compounds such as proteins causes the cells and structures to deteriorate.

e The CLINKER theory: Cellular metabolism causes waste products, much like the debris (clinkers) that is left as coal is burned. These waste products eventually accumulate to the point that normal cellular activity is interrupted.

f The ERROR theory: As cells age, random errors occur in the cells' DNA and transcription of the cells' genes. In time, these errors interfere with protein synthesis, the basis for all life.

2.4 Regardless of the theory of aging applied, the following principles apply to the aging process and patient care:

a Organs do not age simultaneously.

b A given organ does not age at the same rate in different individuals.

c Aging begins with birth and is most noticeable beginning between at 50 to 60 years.

d Conditions of the elderly usually involve multiorgan failure.

2.5 The aging process begins with embryologic development and progresses through maturation to senescence. Senescence is the final biologic stage in maturation when the degenerative phase of aging begins (50 to 55 years old).

2.6 The following changes occur with senescence:

a External appearance changes (e.g., stooped appearance, wrinkled skin, shuffling gate).

b Internal functions of all organs and systems change, including the senses (Table 29-1).

---

*For information on the relationship of diet and antioxidants to free radicals the reader is encouraged to study biochemistry texts or even books on diets by Roy L. Walford, M.D., Professor of Pathology, Schools of Medicine, University of California at Los Angeles.

c Psychomotor ability and ability to adjust to environment fails, resulting in falls and infections.

d Malnutrition results from loss of taste, teeth and poor diet.

e Social activity is decreased as a result of the death of friends.

f Mental health and memory may deteriorate.

2.7 Many gerontologists describe the elderly of today as the beginning of a rectangular society. In this society the morbidity and mortality curve is squared compared to previous generations. What this means is that modern adults will live healthier and more active lives until they actually "drop dead." Senescence is delayed, and the long months and years of sickness and debilitation that normally precede death are delayed until the organism suffers massive multiorgan failure and dies. This concept is presented graphically in Fig. 29-2.

Advances in medicine and changing life-styles with an emphasis on wellness contribute to the trend toward a longer and healthier life during the elderly years. Rather than attempt to cover all the changes that occur with the various body systems with aging this unit will focus on those that relate to the cardiopulmonary system.

2.8 *Anatomically*, the heart changes in the following ways:

a Increase in fat deposits

b Red healthy muscle turns brown and less efficient

c Cardiomegaly and hypertrophy common

d Endocardium thickens, becomes less elastic

e Heart valves thicken, become rigid and less functional

f The number and size of muscle fibers are decreased resulting in a less effective pump

2.9 *Physiologically*, the heart changes by:

a Decrease in cardiac output of 0.7% per year after age 20 (5.0 L/min to 3.5 L/min at 75 years)

b Cardiac index decreases 0.79% per year

c Decrease in heart rate between ages 60 and 84 years

TABLE 29-1 Effect of aging on the senses

Alteration in sensory function	Cause	Effect
Seeing	Lenses' failure to adjust Retinopathy glaucoma Cataracts Muscular degeneration causes light scatter, resulting in glare Sagging eyelids block light	Seventy percent of 11 million persons with uncorrectable visual impairment are 65 or older. More than 50% of legally blind persons are 65 or older. Over 40 million have cataracts. 37% have glaucoma.
Hearing	Long-term exposure to sound Effect of medications (aspirin)	More than 12 million persons 65 or older have some hearing loss. Deafness causes psychologic features of depression, confusion, inattentiveness, stress, and loss of communication skills.
Smelling	Decreased number of smell receptors; Alzheimer's disease destroys smell as well as memory	Loss of sense of smell leads to loss of appetite and malnutrition.
Tasting	Loss of nerve endings to sense, hot, cold, spices, sour, and so on	Inability to taste certain foods causes changes in eating habits and deficits in diets.
Touching	Skin becomes fragile and less sensitive; cells regenerate more slowly with eventual loss of function of nerve endings directly under the skin	Skin becomes dry, less elastic and leathery in appearance. Extremes of heat and cold to extremities may not be detected, resulting in injury from burn and/or frostbite.

NOTE: It has been shown that age has the least effect on touch, yet people fail to show as much affection to the elderly through touch compared with that given to younger people.

from 70 beats/min to 65 to 68 beats/min

  d ECG remains the same except as altered by pathologic conditions

2.10 Blood vessels become arteriosclerotic with thickening of walls and loss of resiliency. Yearly, arteriosclerosis and atherosclerosis cause the death of 9,320 people per 100,000 (9% of total population). It is important to note that changes in vascular systems are not uniform. For example, at age 75, cardiac output is only 65% of what it was at age 30. Cerebral blood flow is 80% of what it was at age 30.

2.11 Anatomically, the chest undergoes the following changes as a result of aging:

  a Kyphosis—curvature of the spine caused by changes in elderly persons' posture and muscle tone

  b Increased rigidity of the ribcage caused by loss of muscle and ineffective mechanics, combined with calcification of bones and rigidity and/or loss of cartilage resulting from arthritic changes

  c Increased rigidity of trachea and connecting airways caused by loss of muscle tone and pathologic conditions

  d Increased anteroposterior diameter and barrel chest appearance in patients with chronic obstructive lung disease

2.12 Structurally, aging causes the lungs to:

  a Decrease in weight as a result of loss of mass

  b Change color from yellowish-pink to grey with patches of dark pigmentation

  c Develop emphysema—loss of tissue elasticity and alveolar walls

  d Lose lung surface area by approximately 0.27 square meters or 2.9 square feet per year from age 30 to age 74

  e Have less efficient alveoli as a result of loss of collagen in relationship to elastin

  f Lose functional pulmonary capillaries as alveoli are destroyed

2.13 Possible functional effects of aging on the lungs are listed below:

  a Exhalation is more pronounced than inspiration.

  b Abnormal breathing patterns such as Cheyne-Stokes are more common.

  c Tidal volume remains unchanged.

  d V_D/V_T is increased from 20:25% at a rate of 2.4% every 10 years.

  e Minute volume remains unchanged, although efficiency is decreased.

  f Vital capacity is decreased 40% beginning with age 20 through 85 years.

  g Residual volume is increased.

  h Maximum ventilatory volume is decreased from 165 L/min at age 25 to 75 L/min at age 85. Fig. 29-3 shows the effect of aging on lung values compared to a 30-year-old.

  i $PaCO_2$ does not change with age, except with a related pathologic condition.

  j PaO_2 decreases with age from approximately 100 mm Hg at age 20 to 79 mm Hg at age 80.

2.14 Most frequently occurring respiratory conditions of the aged include*:

  a Emphysema

  b Interstitial fibrosis

  c Oxygen toxicity

  d Pulmonary embolism and infarction

  e Sleep disorders

---

*These conditions are explained in Module 8.

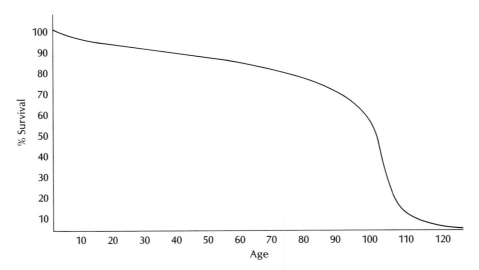

FIGURE 29-2 A great percentage of today's elderly are surviving to age 90+. As this approaches 100% at age 100, a rectangle will be graphically presented. (Adapted from Walford RL: 120-year diet, New York, 1986, Simon & Schuster.)

f Other diseases such as pneumonia and other infections that are not directly related to the aging process

2.15 A summary of common disabilities of the elderly by age is presented as Table 29-2.

3.0 MAJOR CAUSES OF INSTITUTIONALIZATION OF THE ELDERLY

3.1 The three major causes of institutionalization of the elderly are:

a The need for help with activities of daily living (ADL) (see 3.5)

b The prevalence of chronic conditions such as heart conditions, arthritis, and visual and hearing impairments

c Chronic mental illness, including depression, persistent paranoia, and senile dementia from Alzheimer's disease

3.2 Among the 1.2 million elderly residents in nursing homes in the United States, approximately 75% (900,000) are women.

3.3 In 1984, older persons accounted for 30% of all hospital stays and 41% of all care days in hospitals.

3.4 The socioeconomic and health care impact of these statistics are very significant when one considers that based on today's statistics and support services:

a Eighty-five percent of all elderly Americans are *not* insured or are insufficiently insured to provide for adequate health care.

b In 1988, 8.5 million elderly adults were living below the poverty level with over one-fifth of this population reported as poor or near poor.

c Based on longevity, more women than men will require assistance, especially in activities of daily living (ADLs) (see below). For example, in the 65 to 69 age-group, there are 81 men per 100 women, but in the 85 to 89 age group, there are only 43 men per 100 women.

3.5 ADLs relate to six personal care activities that younger persons take for granted. The following lists ADLs according to their most frequently reported degree of difficulty.

a Walking

b Bathing

c Transferring (getting in and out of bed and chairs)

d Toilet use

e Dressing

f Eating

3.6 Elderly Americans are on the move to desirable climate and living conditions. Fig. 29-4 shows the states most frequently chosen by the elderly.

4.0 CARING FOR THE ELDERLY
4.1 Alternatives for care of the elderly

American alternatives for care of the elderly who need assistance include home care, day care, nursing homes, and hospitals. Some of the socioeconomic costs of caring for the elderly were presented in Unit 1.0.

T A B L E   2 9 - 2 Common disabilities of the elderly

Disability	All ages (percent)	Age 65+ (percent)
Mental illness	26.4	2.4
Orthopedic impairments	20.9	7.9
Mental retardation	12.1	0.8
Visual impairment	9.1	45.4
Hearing impairment	6.1	24.8
Digestive disturbance	5.1	4.5
Extremity disorders	2.6	5.8
Respiratory conditions	0.8	0.6

From Rehabilitation Services Administration, 1979.

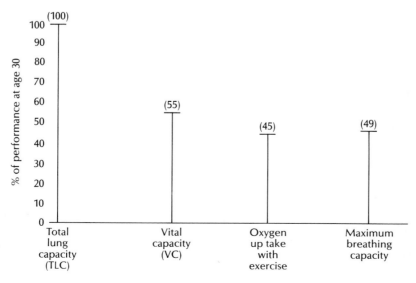

F I G U R E   2 9 - 3 Comparison of test results in elderly persons compared with persons who are age 30.

4.2 Home care

1 The elderly prefer to live in their own homes.

2 In 1985, San Francisco gerontologist Ethel Shances reported that only 5% of those 65 and older are in retirement homes or nursing homes.

3 More than 94% of those 85 and older still live in independent households.

4 For this reason, home care has become a popular alternative to institutionalization of the elderly. Home care is provided directly by home care companies who specialize in equipment and by home health agencies. Most home health agencies are nonprofit and are governed by strict state and federal guidelines.

5 In 1987, Americans spent over $9 billion on home care. By the year 2050 this figure may exceed $40 billion.

6 This cost, which seems exceedingly high, is reasonable when compared to hospital costs of $500 per day and nursing home fees of $27,000 to $30,000 annually to provide a similar level of care for the elderly patient.

7 Unfortunately, use and abuse of home care reimbursement has forced the federal government to issue very strict guidelines for reimbursement of patients on Medicare.

8 These guidelines change so frequently that the reader is encouraged to contact a local home care agency or home health agency for current information on reimbursement.

4.3 Day care

1 Day care agencies are available to care for the elderly during the day while the money earner(s) work.

2 Many of these agencies provide entertainment, useful classes, meals, and a healthy social environment for the elderly.

4.4 Nursing homes

1 The elderly fear nursing homes. For them it is the least desirable of all alternatives for their care.

2 On any given day approximately 5% of the elderly are residents of nursing homes, yet it is projected that 20% of the elderly will require nursing homes before death.

3 Because of longevity and economics, more women than men are residents.

4 In 1985, nearly 50% of nursing home residents paid for their own care.

5 The predominant reason for admission to nursing homes was the fact that the elderly lived alone and could not peform the ADLs needed for independent living as described earlier.

6 The elderly perceive nursing homes in general as places of mass neglect, where residents enter and lose their dignity as they are engulfed by the daily routine and the number of residents.

7 The following anonymous letter from a nursing home resident to a local newspaper is one example of how the elderly feel about nursing homes:

Hello! Is there anyone out there who will listen to me? How can I convince you that I am a prisoner? For the past five years I have not seen a park or the ocean or even just a few feet of grass. I am an 84-year-old woman, and the only crime I have committed is that I have an illness which is called chronic. I have severe arthritis and five years ago I broke my hip. While I was recuperating in the hospital I realized that I would need extra help at home. But there was no one. My son died 35 years ago and my husband 25 years ago. I have a few nieces and nephews who come to visit once in a while, but I couldn't ask them to take me in, and the few friends I still have are just getting by. So I wound up in a convalescent hospital. All kinds of people are thrown together here. I sit watch, day after day. As I look around this room, I see the pathetic ones (may be the lucky ones) who have lost their minds and the poor souls who should be out but nobody comes to get them, and the sick ones who are in pain. We are all locked up together.

I have been keeping in touch with the world through the newspaper, my one great luxury. For the last few years I have been reading about the changes in Medicare regulations. All I can see from these improvements is that nurses spend more time writing. For, after all, how do you regulate caring?

Most of the nurses' aides who work here are from other countries. Even those who can speak English don't have much in common with us. So they hurry to get their work done as quickly as possible. There are a few caring people who work here, but there are so many of us who are needy for that kind of honest attention.

A doctor comes to see me once a month. He spends three to five seconds with me and then a few more minutes writing in the chart or joking with the nurses. . . . I sometimes wonder how the aides feel when they work so hard for so little money and then

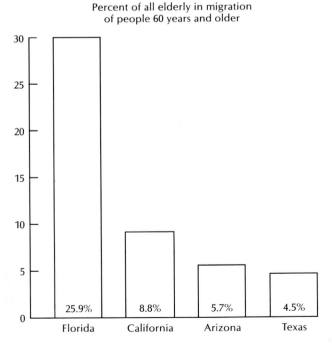

Percent of all elderly in migration of people 60 years and older

	Florida	California	Arizona	Texas
	25.9%	8.8%	5.7%	4.5%

FIGURE 29-4 The elderly's (age 60+) four most frequently chosen states for relocation, 1975 to 1980. (Adapted from American Demographics.)

see that the one who spends so little time is the one who is paid the most. . . . Most of the physicians who come here don't even pay attention to things like whether their patients' fingernails are trimmed or whether their body is foul smelling. . . . I hadn't had a bath in ten days . . . the aide wrote in the chart that she gave me a shower. Who would check or care? I would be labeled as a complainer or as losing my memory, and that would be worse.

As I write this, I keep wishing I were exaggerating. These last five years feel like the last five hundred of my life. . . . How can I tell you that for me growing old in America is an unbelievable, lonely nightmare?

I am writing this because many of you may live to be old like me, and then it will be too late. You too will be stuck here and wonder why nothing is being done, and you too will wonder if there is any justice in life.

Right now I pray every night that I may die in my sleep and get this nightmare of what someone has called life over with if it means living in this prison day after day.

– Anonymous letter to the *Los Angeles Times,* October 1979.

8 In spite of their perceived reputation, nursing homes are a needed option for care of the elderly, especially for those with dementia.

9 It is projected that at least an additional 1.2 million nursing home beds will be needed by the year 2050 to accommodate the increasing elderly population (Fig. 29-5).

4.5 Questions to ask in assessing nursing homes

The following list of questions may prove useful for potential users of nursing home services to ask before selecting a specific agency.

1 Is the facility licensed by the state to provide the level of care needed for the resident?

2 Will the nursing home provide a copy of its admission contract and patient care policies to study?

3 Is a statement of patients' rights available and posted in clear view?

4 Is the environment warm and friendly?

5 Are family and friends encouraged to visit?

6 Do residents look well cared for and happy?

7 Are residents dressed in street clothes?

8 Are residents allowed to decorate their own rooms?

9 What is the policy for calling a doctor as the need may arise?

10 Is the home safety-minded, with fire exits marked, an evacuation plan, smoke alarms, emergency lights, sprinklers, and so on?

11 Are special therapists available to assist residents?

12 How are residents, families, and friends encouraged to participate in the care?

13 Are interesting and educational activities planned?

14 Are outside trips planned?

15 Are toilet and other facilities available to accomodate the disabled?

16 What is the base monthly charge?

17 What services are included in the charge?

18 Are advance payments returned if the resident dies or leaves early?

4.6 Home health agencies

1 Home health agencies (also known as visiting nurses associations in some states) generally are federally and/or state funded agencies that provide for care of the elderly in the home.

2 The federal government has specific guidelines that must be followed for a home health agency to receive Medicare and Medicaid funds.

3 One requirement is that a health care team be available for care of the elderly. This team includes a physician, social workers, nurses, dietitians, physical and occupational therapists, and home health aides.

In most agencies, respiratory therapists are employed to assist in the care of patients who require respiratory care at home.

4.7 Other ways of caring for the elderly abroad

1 Foreign countries such as Sweden, Denmark, and Finland use alternative care plans that enable the elderly to live out their lives with dignity, security, and independence at home.

2 The Scandinavians use a system called *open old-age care.* Under this system the elderly are helped to live their mature years in their own homes.

3 To accomplish this, the government uses home helpers who are trained and paid to help the elderly at home. Tasks include shopping, housecleaning, cooking and assistance with ADLs that cannot be performed by the elderly.

4 Home workers are primarily young people who are trained and employed by each municipality. In some instances the more able-bodied elderly are also trained and used.

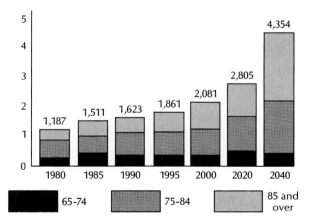

Nursing home population projections

FIGURE 29-5 Nursing home population projections to the year 2020. (Modified from Manton and Liu, The Future Growth of the Long-Term Care population: Based on the 1977 National Nursing Home Survey and the 1982 Long-Term Care Survey, March 1984.)

5 Day care centers are available to the elderly who are able to travel.

6 For those who must remain at home, elderly persons are provided with alarm devices that connect them to emergency care centers.

7 Many governments have taken positive steps to care for the elderly by providing trained personnel.

8 In the United States in 1987, there were approximately 66 home care workers per 100,000 people needing help, compared with 1500 per 100,000 in Sweden.

5.0 ROLE OF ALLIED HEALTH PERSONNEL IN CARE OF THE ELDERLY

5.1 Numbers of allied health workers

1 As was stated in the introduction to this module, over 1.4 million allied health workers representing over 63% of the total health care work force provide patient care nationwide.

2 Most of the 13 allied health professions recognized under the Allied Health Professions Educational Assistance Act of 1967 are taking steps to prepare for care of the expanded numbers of the elderly in the year 2000.

5.2 Allied health recruitment in nursing

1 Nursing is recruiting more students to enter the profession. Based on today's patient population, 1.7 million additional nurses will be needed by the year 2020.

2 Nursing programs are also adding geriatrics and gerontology to their curricula and preparing instructors at the advanced degree level.

Geriatrics is the branch of medicine that studies the problems of the aged, diagnosis, and treats the diseases and the conditions of the elderly. Gerontology is the study of the aging process, including socioeconomic impact.

5.3 Allied health areas requiring increases in workers

1 There are other areas in allied health care that will need additional specialists/practitioners as the population continues to age. They include the following:
a Audiology
b Dental hygiene
c Dietetics
d Occupational therapy
e Pharmacy
f Physical therapy
g Physician's assistant
h Respiratory therapy
i Social work

5.4 Curriculum changes

1 To educate these professionals, changes in curriculum are needed at the entry level to include courses on aging and at the upper levels to prepare educators and specialists.

2 Even though the curriculum will vary from school to school, it is generally agreed that practitioners, to obtain a certificate in gerontology, should complete courses in the following subject areas:
a Psychology of aging
b Biophysiologic aspects of aging
c Aging and social policy
d Sociology of aging
e Introduction to geriatrics and gerontology
f Common disorders and health maintenance of the elderly
g Pharmacokinetics of drugs used for the elderly
h Health promotion and disease prevention
i Socioeconomics of aging

6.0 ROLE OF RESPIRATORY CARE PRACTITIONERS IN CARE OF ELDERLY

6.1 Interdisciplinary approaches

1 Care of the elderly usually involves the treatment of multiple medical and psychologic conditions that cannot be served by a single discipline.

2 Gerontologists usually agree that the use of interdisciplinary and transdisciplinary teams is the most efficient and effective means of treating the elderly.

Transdisciplinary approach is a new concept that relates to a commitment by professionals from different disciplines to teach and practice health care principles across traditional disciplinary boundaries.

3 This team approach involves all allied health professionals and has the following advantages to the patient:
a Access to a broader range of knowledge, skills and experience
b Greater opportunity for preventive and educational services
c Better communication and coordination of efforts toward completion of a holistic care plan

6.2 Growth in respiratory care utilization

1 Since 1983, respiratory related hospital admissions have increased 45%. There has been a 55% increase in the utilization of respiratory care with 38% of all patient days attributed to care of patients 65 years or older.

6.3 In-hospital role

1 Evaluate, test, and treat patients as a member of a geriatric evaluation unit.

2 Serve as a consultant to a discharge planner or as a discharge planner.

3 Serve as cardiorespiratory technologists in the evaluation and testing of the elderly in hospital rehabilitation and wellness centers.

6.4 Outpatient role/home care

1 Work with patient care teams in the planning and coordinating of respiratory care services and equipment in the outpatient facility and home care setting.

2 Direct health services in health promotion and disease prevention programs.

3 Promote respiratory care education as a part of geriatric and gerontologic programs.

4 Serve as a consultant to freestanding clinics and other alternative care agencies such as nursing homes and home health agencies.

5 Promote programs and other educational activities on the care of the elderly.

6 Serve as a consultant to geriatric education centers, industry, and schools on care of the elderly.

6.5 Geriatric education centers (GEC)

1 The federal government, under Section 788 of the Public Health Service Act, established funding in 1983 to establish four centers nationwide to promote the study of geriatrics and gerontology and to disseminate this information to caregivers and the general public.

2 Since 1983, funding has been expanded to 33 centers nationwide. The local and national influence of these centers on the education and care of the elderly is important to all allied health practitioners.

3 Respiratory care personnel who wish to care for the elderly should contact a GEC and become involved with its programs. These GECs are also important centers for information and educational resources on aging. A list of geriatric education centers and contact persons is presented in Table 29-3.

T A B L E 2 9 - 3 Geriatric education center grants—fiscal year 1988
Division of Associated and Dental Health Professions BHPr, HRSA, PHS, DHHS
Budget Period: 10/01/88—09/30/89

Center name	Grantee	Program director Address/phone
PHS REGION I		
University of Connecticut Geriatric Education Center	University of Connecticut Farmington, Connecticut	Richard W. Besdine, M.D. Travelers Center on Aging University of Connecticut School of Medicine 263 Farmington Avenue Farmington, CT 06032 (203) 674-3959
Harvard Geriatric Education Center	Harvard Medical School Boston, Massachusetts	Benjamin Liptzin, M.D. Division on Aging 643 Huntington Avenue Boston, MA 02115 (617) 732-1463
PHS REGION II		
Western New York Geriatric Education Center	State University of New York at Buffalo Buffalo, New York	Evan Calkins, M.D. State Univ. of NY at Buffalo Beck Hall 3435 Main Street Buffalo, NY 14214 (716) 831-3176
Geriatric Education Center of University of Puerto Rico	University of Puerto Rico San Juan, Puerto Rico	Elizabeth Sanchez, Ph.D. University of Puerto Rico School of Medicine Medical Sciences Campus G.P.O. Box 5067 San Juan, PR 00936 (809) 751-2478
Hunter/Mt. Sinai Geriatric Education Center	Hunter College Jointly with Research Foundation of CUNY New York City, New York	Rose Dobrof, D.S.W. Brookdale Center on Aging of Hunter College, CUNY 425 East 25th Street New York, NY 10010 (212) 481-5142 or 4416

Continued.

TABLE 29-3 Geriatric education center grants—fiscal year 1988—cont'd

Center name	Grantee	Program director Address/phone
PHS REGION III		
Geriatric Education Center of Pennsylvania	Temple University Philadelphia, Pennsylvania	Bernice A. Parlak, M.S.W. Temple University Institute on Aging University Services Building Room 206 1601 North Broad Street Philadelphia, PA 19122 (215) 787-6831
Delaware Valley Geriatric Education Center	University of Pennsylvania Philadelphia, Pennsylvania	Laurence H. Beck, M.D. University of Pennsylvania Center for the Study on Aging 3906 Spruce Street/H1 Philadelphia, PA 19104 (215) 898-3163
Geriatric Education Center at Virgina Commonwealth University	Virginia Commonwealth University Richmond, Virginia	Iris A. Parham, Ph.D. Virginia Commonwealth Univ. Medical College of Virginia Gerontology Department P.O. Box 568—MCV Station Richmond, VA 23298-0001 (804) 786-1565
PHS REGION IV		
Geriatric Education Center at University of Alabama at Birmingham	University of Alabama at Birmingham Birmingham, Alabama	Glenn H. Hughes, Ph.D. U.A.B., Center for Aging Medical Towers Building, 732 University Station Birmingham, AL 35294 (205) 934-5619
Mississippi Geriatric Education Center	University of Mississippi Medical Center Jackson, Mississippi	Ames F. Tryon, D.D.S. University of Mississippi Medical Center 2500 North State Street Jackson, MS 39216 (601) 987-4795
Ohio Valley/Appalachia Regional Geriatric Education Center	University of Kentucky Lexington, Kentucky	William R. Markesbery, M.D. Sanders-Brown Center on Aging University of Kentucky Lexington, KY 40536-0230 (606) 233-6040
University of Florida Geriatric Education Center	University of Florida Gainesville, Florida	George Caranasos, M.D. Department of Medicine JHMC Box J-277 University of Florida Gainesville, FL 32610 (904) 376-1611x5027
University of South Florida Geriatric Education Center	University of South Florida Tampa, FLorida	Eric Pfeiffer, M.D. Suncoast Gerontology Center University of South Florida Medical Center, Box 50 112901 N. 30th Street Tampa, FL 33612 (813) 974-4355
Duke University Geriatric Education Center	Duke University Durham, North Carolina	Harvey J. Cohen, M.D. Duke University Medical Center Center for the Study of Aging and Human Development Box 3303 Durham, NC 27710 (919) 684-2248
Miami Area Geriatric Education Center	University of Miami Coral Gables, Florida	Edwin J. Olsen University of Miami Department of Psychiatry P.O Box 016960 (D-29) Miami, FL 33101 (305) 549-6327

TABLE 29-3 Geriatric education center grants—fiscal year 1988—cont'd

Center name	Grantee	Program director Address/phone
PHS REGION V		
Western Reserve Geriatric Education Center	Case Western Reserve University Cleveland, Ohio	Jerome Kowal, M.D. Department of Medicine CWRU School of Medicine Cleveland, OH 44106 (216) 368-5433
Midwest Geriatric Education Center	Marquette University Milwaukee, Wisconsin	Jesley Ruff, D.D.S Marquette University School of Dentistry 604 North 16th Street Room 202H Milwaukee, WI 53233 (414) 224-3712
Great Lakes Geriatric Education Center	Chicago College of Osteopathic Medicine Chicago, Illinois	Jerry Rodos, D.O. Chicago College of Osteopathic Medicine 5200 South Ellis Avenue Chicago, IL 60615 (312) 947-4393
Geriatric Education Center of Michigan	Michigan State University East Lansing, Michigan	James O'Brien, M.D. Family Practice B100 Clinical Center Michigan State University East Lansing, MI 48824 (517) 353-0770
Illinois Geriatric Education Center	University of Illinois Chicago, Illinois	Leopold G. Selker, Ph.D. University of Illinois at Chicago College of Associated Health Professions 808 S. Wood St.—Room 169 CME Chicago, IL 60612 (312) 996-8236
Minnesota Area Geriatric Education Center	University of Minnesota St. Paul, Minnesota	Robert L. Kane, M.D. University of Minnesota School of Public Health 420 Delaware St. S.E. A302 Mayo Bldg., Box 197 Minneapolis, MN 55104 (612) 624-6669
PHS REGION VI		
Texas Consortium of Geriatric Education Centers	Baylor College of Medicine Houston, Texas	Robert E. Roush, Ed.D., M.P.H. Baylor College of Medicine One Baylor Plaza, Room 134-A Houston, TX 77030 (713) 799-6470
South Texas Geriatric Education Center	University of Texas Health Science Center San Antonio, Texas	Michele Saunders, D.M.D. UTHSC at San Antonio Department of Dental Diagnostic Science 7703 Floyd Curl Drive San Antonio, TX 78284-7919 (512) 691-6961
New Mexico Geriatric Education Center	University of New Mexico Albuquerque, New Mexico	Mark Stratton, Pharm.D. New Mexico Geriatric Education Center Rm. 179 A, Nursing/Pharmacy Bldg. University of New Mexico Albuquerque, NM 87131 (505) 277-0911

Continued.

TABLE 29-3 Geriatric education center grants—fiscal year 1988—cont'd

Center name	Grantee	Program director Address/phone
PHS REGION VII		
Iowa Geriatric Education Center	University of Iowa Iowa City, Iowa	Ian M. Smith, M.D. Department of Internal Med. University of Iowa Hospitals Iowa City, IA 52242 (319) 356-2727
Creighton Regional Geriatric Education Center	Creighton University School of Medicine Omaha, Nebraska	Eugene Barone, M.D. Department of Family Practice Creighton University School of Medicine 601 North 30th Street Omaha, NE 68131 (402) 280-4175
PHS REGION VIII		
Intermountain West Geriatric Education Center	University of Utah Salt Lake City, Utah	Margaret Dimond, R.N., Ph.D. University of Utah College of Nursing 25 South Medical Drive Salt Lake City, UT 84112 (801) 581-8198
Dakota Plains Geriatric Education Center	University of North Dakota Grand Forks, North Dakota	Clayton E. Jensen, M.D. UND School of Medicine Department of Family Medicine 221 South Fourth Street Grand Forks, ND 58201 (701) 780-3200
PHS REGION IX		
Stanford Geriatric Education Center	Stanford University Stanford, California	William Fowkes, M.D. Division of Family Medicine Stanford University School of Medicine 703 Welch Road, Suite G-1 Stanford, CA 94304-1760 (415) 723-7063
Pacific Islands Geriatric Education Center	University of Hawaii at Manoa Honolulu, Hawaii	Madeleine Goodman, Ph.D. Pacific Islands Geriatric Education Center 347 N. Kuakini Street Honolulu, HI 96817 (808) 523-8461
California Geriatric Education Center	University of California Los Angeles, California	John Beck, M.D. University of California Department of Medicine Division of Geriatrics 32-144 CHS 10833 Le Conte Avenue Los Angeles, CA 90024 (213) 825-9640
San Diego Geriatric Education Center	University of California LaJolla, California	Joe Ramsdell, M.D. University of California School of Medicine Department of Medicine San Diego, CA 92103 (619) 543-6275
PHS REGION X		
Northwest Geriatric Education Center	University of Washington Seattle, Washington	Itamar B. Abrass, M.D. Institute on Aging 3953 Univ. Way, N.E., JM-20 University of Washington Seattle, WA 98195 (206) 545-7478

BIBLIOGRAPHY

Aging in the eighties: Functional limitations of individuals aged 65 years and older, NCHS Advance Data No. 133, National Center for Health Statistics, June 10, 1987.

Anderson KB and Kass DI: Certificate of need regulation of entry into home health care, Bureau of Economic, Federal Trade Commission, January 1986.

Bass DM and Noelker LS: The influence of family caregivers on elders' use of inhome services: an expanded conceptual framework, J Health Soc Behav 20:184, 1987.

Becker RG: The physician assistant in geriatric long-term care, Gerontologist 16(4):318, 1976.

Black box of home care quality: hearing before the Select Committee on Aging, US Congress, House Select Committee on Aging Publ No 96-606, US Government Printing Office, July 29, 1986.

Campion EW: Observations from the 1981 White House Conference on Aging, N Engl J Med 306:373, 1982.

Granick R, Simson S, and Wilson LB: Survey of curriculum content related to geriatrics in physical therapy education programs, JAPTA 67(2):234, 1987.

Greenwald NF: Educational activities related to geriatrics in physical therapy, Geritopics :9, Winter 1982.

Hughes SL et al: Impact of long-term home care on hospital and nursing home use and cost, Health Serv Res 22(1):43, 1987.

Kane R et al: The future need for geriatric manpower in the United States, N Engl J Med 302:1327, 1980.

National Center for Health Statistics: Health statistics on older persons, US, 1986 (Vital and Health Statistics, Series 3, No 25), DHHS, PHS Publ No 87-1409, US Government Printing Office, June 1987.

Public Law 99-129, signed October 22, 1985, Sec 223: Study of the role allied health personnel in health care delivery, US Government Printing Office, 1985.

Rowe JW, Grossman E, and Bond E: Special report: academic geriatrics in the year 2000, N Engl J Med 316(22):1426, 1987.

Selker G, editor: An aging society: implications for health care needs impacts on allied health practice and education—a report of the National Task Force on Gerontology and Geriatric Care Education in Allied Health, J Allied Health 16:4, 1987.

Selker LG: Health promotion/disease prevention for special population groups: special implications for special populations—the elderly, J Allied Health 15:(4):311, 1986.

Technology and aging in America: US Congress, Office of Technology Assessment Publ No OTA-BA-264, US Government Printing Office, June 1985.

Toward a national strategy for long-term care of the elderly, Institute of Medicine, National Academy of Sciences Pub. No IOM-85-05, National Academy Press, April 1986.

US Government Report on supply/demand of registered nurses, as presented by R McGibbin in May 1984, Kansas City, Mo., American Nurses Association, July 16, 1987.

Walford RL: The 120-year diet, New York, 1986, Simon & Schuster.

Third-generation microprocessor ventilators

Warren G. Sanborn

1.0 HISTORICAL TRENDS IN VENTILATION

1.1 The concept of first, second, and third-generation ventilators

1 First-generation devices began as simple, foot-operated air pumps (e.g., the Fell O'Dwyer apparatus introduced in 1888). Early in the 1900s, the operation of the air pump was mechanized. Monitoring was crude, perhaps only a pressure gauge. Alarming was minimal or nonexistent, and the only mode was continuous mandatory ventilation (CMV). The first generation can be thought of as having lasted from perhaps 1888 to 1970 (Fig. 30-1). America's most popular first generation ventilator was the MA-1, with approximately 28,000 units sold worldwide.

2 During the second generation, which lasted from approximately 1970 to 1980, functions such as intermittent positive pressure breathing (IPPB), intermittent mandatory ventilation (IMV), synchronous intermittent mandatory ventilation (SIMV), and continous positive airway pressure (CPAP) were added. Monitoring and alarming were improved, and manufacturers began to introduce ventilators designed around differing types of pneumatic systems: some were volume based and some pressure based. Some were electrically/electronically based, whereas others were fluidically based. All second-generation ventilators were based on analog designs; that is to say, none incorporated or were based on computers, which require digital-based designs. Fig. 30-2 shows the relationship between features and functions of second-generation ventilators and their approximate time correlation.

Later in this module, the terms analog and digital will be discussed in greater depth. For the moment, it will be sufficient to define analog in the context of continuous operation. Although ventilators are cyclic devices, once they begin to deliver a breath, their control is continuous with respect to time. the reproduction of music by a record player is an example of analog oper-

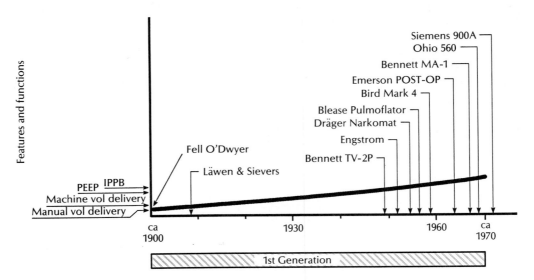

FIGURE 30-1 Growth of features and functions in first-generation ventilators. (Courtesy Puritan-Bennett Corp., Carlsbad, Calif.)

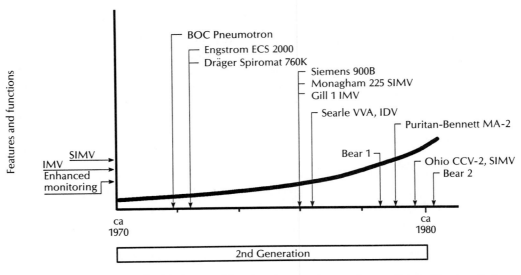

FIGURE 30-2 Growth of features and functions in second-generation ventilators. (Courtesy Puritan-Bennett Corp., Carlsbad, Calif.)

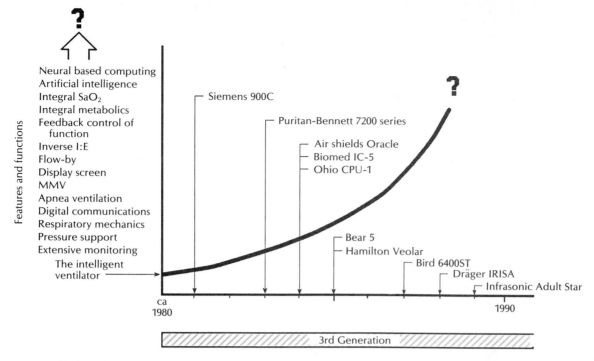

F I G U R E   3 0 - 3 Growth of features and functions in third-generation ventilators. (Courtesy Puritan-Bennett Corp., Carlsbad, Calif.)

ation. On the other hand, digital refers to discontinuous operation. Digital computers perform their "programs" one step at a time. When discrete events are performed very rapidly, they appear to be continuous. Thus a compact disk player is digital-based system, but we perceive it to be equivalent to the original (analog) event.

3 Beginning in 1980 (the approximate start of the third generation), computer-based ventilators came into use. The reasons for this transition will be discussed later. Some third-generation devices were based entirely on microprocessor control (e.g., Bear 5, Bird 6400ST, Hamilton Veolar and Amadeus, and 7200 series), whereas others had analog-based pneumatic systems with computer technology reserved for computation of data (e.g., Engstrom Erica) or digital communications (e.g. Siemens 900C). Fig. 30-3 shows the relationship between features and functions and time for third-generation ventilators. The remainder of this module will cover the reasons for this "explosion" of features and functions and the potential impact on respiratory care.

1.2 The apparent relationship between features and functions and time

1 When features and functions across all three generations of ventilators are combined and viewed against time, the result is seen in Fig. 30-4.

2 The rapid rate of increase of features and functions with time appears to have its origins in the early 1980s.

Throughout the 1960s and 1970s, the basic medical sciences such as physiology, immunology, biochemistry, biophysics, genetics, and molecular biology yielded a significant increase in the understanding of the human body. At the same time, computers and computer technology became more and more integrated with medicine.

3 Initially when new technologies emerge, they typically are confined to military and aerospace applications. (Remember that the first moon landing took place on July 20, 1969, the approximate transition point between the first- and second-generation ventilator.) Later, as costs are reduced, these new technologies can be applied to much more cost-sensitive sectors such as medicine. The first fully computer-controlled, commercial ventilator was introduced in 1983.

4 Fig. 30-5 illustrates a hypothetical relationship between medicine and technology. The leading force may be either medicine or technology, depending on time and personal viewpoint.

2.0 FACTORS DRIVING THE DESIGN OF MICROPROCESSOR-CONTROLLED VENTILATORS

The data shown in Fig. 30-3 and in 30-4 suggest that the dramatic increase in ventilator function began in the early 1980s. About this same time, computer-controlled (more appropriately stated, microprocessor-controlled) ventilators were introduced.

2.1 The origins of the commercialization of computer-controlled medical devices

1 What these data do not chronical is the availability of commercially priced, "high-powered," integrated circuits (microprocessors, memory, and so on), which entered the commercial market at the end of the 1970s.

2 The requisite events that lead to the expanded-function ventilator are suggested by Fig. 30-6. Once the sequence indicated by Fig. 30-6 was set into motion, the unknown factor became the receptiveness of the respiratory care community.

2.2 Reframing the ventilator concept

Not to be excluded from the event sequence illustrated was a conceptual reappraisal of ventilator function.

1 Framed in the context of a first-generation ventilator, the unspoken concept was simply "pump the good gas in and let the bad gas out."

2 For the second-generation ventilator, the unspoken concept built on that of first-generation ventilators but added enhanced control of the gas-delivery function with enough monitoring to ensure that gas delivery took place or an alarm sounded if gas delivery failed.

3 In concert with or perhaps because of the implications inherent in the scheme illustrated in Fig. 30-6, manufacturers and clinicians began to rethink the role and function of the ventilator. First- and second-generation thinking saw the ventilator as a mechanical substitute

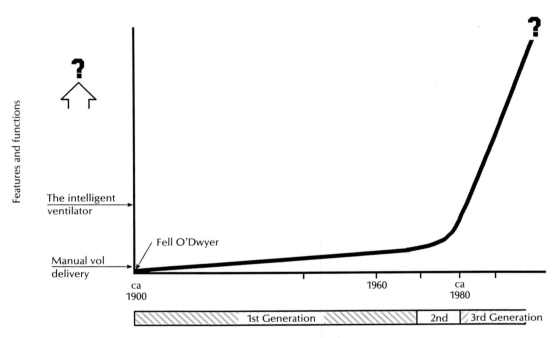

FIGURE 30-4 A broad view of features and functions against time. (Courtesy Puritan-Bennett Corp., Carlsbad, Calif.)

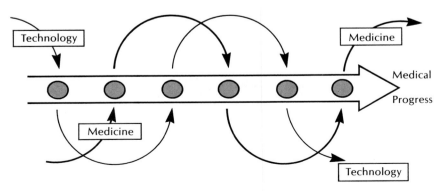

FIGURE 30-5 The interrelationship between advances in medicine and technology. (Courtesy Puritan-Bennett Corp., Carlsbad, Calif.)

for a compromised respiratory system. While this view is still true, it is too limiting. By studying Fig. 30-7, it can be appreciated that in the broadest context possible, the ventilator is a conduit for moving information into and out of the body. For example, a ventilator manages flows, volumes, pressures, temperatures, and gas composition—to name the most obvious. The manipulation of pressures and flow yields information about airway resistance; the manipulation of pressures and volumes yields information about compliance; and manipulation of O_2 consumed and CO_2 produced yields information about energy utilization. In quick order, the ventilator assumes the role of an information-capturing and -processing machine.

4 Once the concept of the ventilator as an information-capturing and -processing machine is recognized, there is an absolute requirement for the ventilator design to include microprocessor data-handling circuitry. An excellent example of this marriage is found in the Sie-

mens 900C. Although the 900C is unquestionably one of the most sophisticated analog-based ventilators on the market, it was introduced with the capability to send analog, but not digital, signals to a remote recording device. The 900C was not recognized as an information-processing machine until the mid-1980s, when Siemens introduced the 990 Servo Computer (digital communications) module. The configuration of the 900C is entirely understandable when it is recognized that the 900C evolved through the 900 and 900B designs—all of which were based on analog design principles.

5 The Puritan-Bennett 7200 Series Microprocessor Ventilator is an example of the fully computerized design. Having no computer-based predecessor, Puritan-Bennett chose to build the entire ventilator around a microprocessor-based system. As the need for new ventilator functions such as digital communications were identified, only minor changes were required.

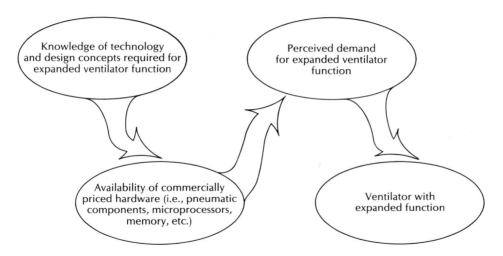

FIGURE 30-6 Requisite events leading to the expanded-function ventilator.

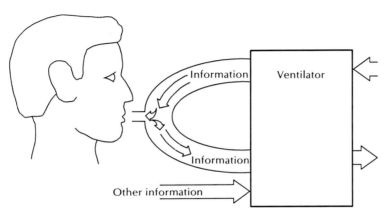

FIGURE 30-7 Information flow in a patient-ventilator system.

3.0 THE MEANING OF MICROPROCESSOR CONTROL: THE DESIGN MATRIX FOR THE UPGRADABLE VENTILATOR

This section will briefly explore the implications inherent in microprocessor-based systems and contrast them with analog-based systems.

3.1 Analog-based systems

1 In the context of this module, the term *analog* refers to continuous operation. A mercury-bulb thermometer is an analog system. At any point on the earth, temperature is a continually changing variable. Mercury in the bulb of the thermometer expands in direct proportion to the temperature. Hence the height of the mercury column bears a one-to-one relationship to the surrounding temperature. Once calibrated, the height of the column reads directly in degrees. The operation of an automobile by a driver is an example of analog control. The driver continually adjusts the position of the throttle to achieve a desired speed. Throttle position controls horsepower, which in turn controls the rotational velocity of the driving wheels. The result is the continual adjustment of the throttle position to achieve the speed desired by the driver.

2 Taking again the Siemens 900C as an example, all functions are continually controlled and all parameters are continually monitored. Functions like breath delivery may be cyclic, but once initiated, they are continually controlled.

3 The term analog carries no connotation of new or old, simple or complex. It may be true, however, that a simple system yields more easily to an analog design than to a digital design. For example, a portable device that measures voltage, current, or resistance (a multimeter) may be more cost effective when constructed with an analog design than with a digital design. For very complex systems, designers today turn to digital, microprocessor-based systems almost without exception. The reasons for this trend will be discussed later.

3.2 Digital-based systems

1 In the context of this module, the term *digital* refers to discontinuous operation. Just a few paragraphs back, there was an example of the analog measurement of temperature at some point on the earth. Since the local temperature cannot change more than a few degrees per hour, the relationship between temperature and the time of day could be known just as accurately by making periodic measurements instead of making a continuous measurement. Fig. 30-8 illustrates 24-hour temperature recordings commonly obtained for refrigerated rooms. Goods that require cold storage could be damaged if temperatures become too high. Such records are used to verify quality control. Disk A was made by an analog measuring device, whereas Disk B was made by a digital measuring device. Both temperature records can be said to convey the same information, given that the digital system samples the temperature more often than it can change and reverse its direction. If the digital sampling frequency is not properly chosen, a crucial event, for example a warming episode, perhaps caused by the refrigerator door being left open,

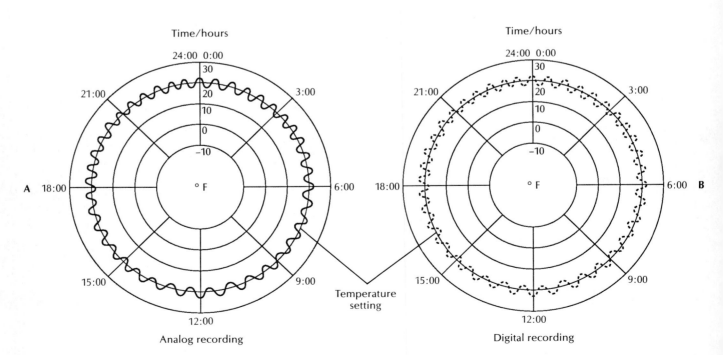

FIGURE 30-8 Examples of two 24-hour temperature records. **A,** Analog recording. **B,** Digital recording.

could occur and not be recorded. To better appreciate the digital technique, consider a compact disk recorder. The original music was an analog event. The digital recording system sampled and measured sound intensity periodically, at a very high frequency. The results of a digital recording system are encoded on the surface of the compact disk, which is available from a local music store. When the compact disk is placed in a compact disk player, the original musical event is recreated. To the extent that a listener could experience the original event and its recreation without discerning any differences, the two events could be said to be identical.

2 Communications technology today has advanced to the point at which virtually all systems are designed around the digital concept. It is interesting to reflect that neural communication and control within complex living organisms are handled digitally, and, insofar as science understands living systems today and the fossil remains of earlier life forms billions of years old, communication and control have always been "digital" events.

3 It is important to grasp the basic concepts of digital control. Because this module is about third-generation and beyond ventilators, a ventilator example is appropriate. First, it may be helpful to remember that third-generation ventilators are flow controllers. (Pressure is simply the result of flow into a closed system.)

4 Assume, now, that the task is to develop a control strategy that will yield a digital equivalent of a sine flow waveform. Fig. 30-9 illustrates the analog waveform to be digitally duplicated. Knowing the peak flow and inspiratory time is sufficient to mathematically specify the complete waveform. Consider as a first approximation a strategy that divides the inspiratory time into three equal intervals (a,b,c) as shown in Fig. 30-10. The flow valve will be off during interval a, on for b, and then off again for c. By making the amplitude of the "on pulse" sufficiently high, its volume can be made to equal the volume under the sine waveform. Even though the two tidal volumes are equal, the digital approximation is completely unacceptable. The ap-

parent solution to the exercise is to let the flow-pulse intervals become very small, as illustrated in Fig. 30-11. The next question is, how small is small? The answer will depend on many factors, such as the number of other sampling and controlling tasks, the maximum respiratory rate, the minimum tidal volume, and the maximum discrepancy between the analog waveform and the digital equivalent that can be accepted. When all considerations are addressed, the solution might be to use a faster microprocessor (more steps executed per unit time), or more than one microprocessor (one to handle control of the pneumatic system and one or more to handle other system functions such as the control panel, the display screen, and the processing of data). Designers consider these problems and make compromises between cost and performance.

5 Earlier in this module, a point was made about the absence of commercially successful, microprocessor-controlled ventilators before 1980. The situation then was something like the following. Powerful microprocessors were available (16 and 32 bit), but their cost was

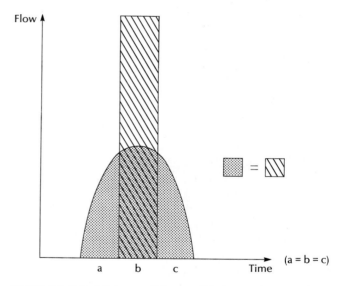

FIGURE 30-10 An unsatisfactory digital approximation of the sine waveform.

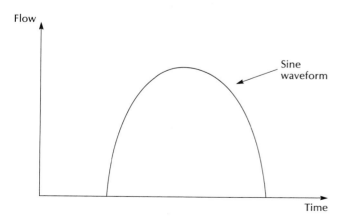

FIGURE 30-9 Sine waveform generated by a piston pump.

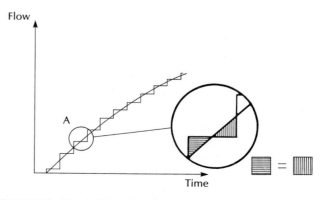

FIGURE 30-11 Example of a satisfactory digital approximation of the sine waveform.

prohibitively high for commercial applications. Less powerful microprocessors (4 and 8 bit) were available at commercially attractive prices, but even with multiple processor designs, predicted performance was unacceptable. Knowing that the commercial availability of the more powerful microprocessors lay just around the corner, manufacturers simply waited for these new integrated circuits. Thus, it was not a coincidence that the Puritan-Bennett 7200 Series Microprocessor Ventilator was introduced in the spring of 1983.

6 In summary, the terms analog and digital are not to be interpreted as inferior or superior. Excellent performance is possible using either design approach. As system complexity increases, however, the digital approach permits designers to solve some of the difficult sample and control problems in new, flexible, and cost-effective ways.

As digital circuitry decreases in price, it is possible to apply the digital approach to many of the designs which were previously well handled by the analog approach. From wrist watches to microwave ovens to compact disks, the digital-design approach is proving to be a cost-effective way to create analog-equivalent devices.

4.0 VENTILATOR DESIGN FROM A SYSTEMS VIEWPOINT

4.1 The impact of digital design on ventilator organization

1 While engineers always design their devices from a systems viewpoint, the digital approach seems to give greater emphasis to the specification of each subsystem.

2 First-generation ventilators were composed of three primary subsystems. First was the "heart" of any ventilator, the pneumatic subsystem. It could be based on a piston, a collapsible bag or bellows, or a flow controller. Second was the electronics subsystem, which provided low-level signals to switches, sensors, timing circuits, alarms, and lamp displays. Third was the electrical subsystem, which included the main power switch, power to the electric motors and heaters, and the power supply. In fluidically based ventilators, air power replaced electrical power.

3 Because second-generation ventilators were, in general, more sophisticated versions of their first-generation predecessors, there were few radical changes. In electrically powered ventilators, however, the electronics subsystem began to dominate. The Siemens 900 (a first-generation ventilator) and 900B (a second-generation ventilator) are interesting examples of a design that was from the outset based heavily on electronics and flow control.

4 With the exception of the Siemens 900C, which is an analog-based design and a logical extension of the earlier 900 and 900B models, all "full-range" third-generation ventilators are based on digital designs. While the total impact of this fundamental shift from analog to digital design has yet to be completely felt, some subsystems have grown in importance—most notably pneumatics and electronics—and, in recognition of the rapidly expanding information function, a digital communications subsystem has been added.

5 The next sections will identify and examine each subsystem and its impact on third-generation and beyond ventilators.

4.2 The microprocessor electronics subsystem (electronics and software)

1 At the heart of any microprocessor-based subsystem is the CPU (central processing unit, a term synonymous with microprocessor). The microprocessor is sometimes said to give a device "machine intelligence." As indicated in Fig. 30-12, three elements must be present before a machine becomes intelligent: sensors, CPU, and memory.

2 Microprocessors and other associated electronic circuitry, in combination with the software, are mutually dependent. It is convenient to define a term that identifies their unity; this term will be called *microprocessor electronics*.

3 Sensors measure what is happening within the operational boundaries of the ventilator. They measure parameters such as pressure, flow, temperature, and gas composition.

4 The CPU is sometimes referred to as the ventilator's "brain." While this analogy with a living organism has a certain charm, it is more accurate to think of the CPU as a statement executor, the statements residing in the software. Consider the simple example of making a glass of chocolate milk. The recipe is shown in Fig. 30-13.

a At the conclusion of step 12, there should be a glass of chocolate milk left on the sink.

b If the agent performing the mixing function is a person who already understands basic kitchen operations, no further instructions would be needed. On the other hand, the less the mixing agent knows about these common-place routines, the more explicit the instructions must be.

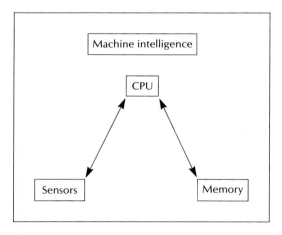

FIGURE 30-12 Requisite design elements necessary for machine intelligence.

5 Much of the success of today's personal computers is the result of "user friendly" software.

Although the chocolate milk exercise may appear simple, the example is at the root of microprocessor-based operation. The powerful software programs that are available for today's personal computers can be viewed as highly sophisticated, elaborate revisions of the chocolate milk algorithm.

Take, for example, one of today's word-processing software packages. Focus on a specific operation such as *delete paragraph*. Although the person performing the deletion action need only be familiar with the concept of deletion, the actual deletion of the paragraph requires a series of complex steps. This series of steps are said to be *transparent*, meaning that the software performs the actual operation.

6 What needs to be appreciated is that routines such as mixing a glass of chocolate milk or word processing or for that matter, running a ventilator, can be reduced to a set of discrete steps. Once an operation is reduced to a set of discrete steps, it can be executed by a microprocessor. Because all of the operational routines are reduced to a set of discrete operations, a microprocessor-based system can perform an impressive array of seemingly unrelated operations.

7 Consider what happens in a microprocessor-controlled device after the power is turned on. Most all such de-

vices perform what is called a power-on self-test, or POST. Because turning on the power is a unique event, a special POST routine becomes active and takes over. Before the device assumes normal operation, the POST routine causes the microprocessor first to check itself, then check all other electronic subsystems. In general, the operator waits and does nothing until POST either passes or fails. Pass generally leads to normal operation, whereas fail generally causes the display of an error code or message. Thus the successful completeion of the POST routine ensures that the device (a ventilator for the purpose of this module) meets the design criteria required for normal operation.

8 Many ventilators and other microprocessor-based devices also incorporate in their design an extended self-test. These routines can essentially be fully automated or at least semiautomated, meaning that the operator is required to perform certain tasks while the extended self-test runs. What formerly required a few to several hours can be accomplished in a few to several minutes.

9 Microprocessor-based devices are run by instruction sets called routines and subroutines. These instruction sets are called the software. Software resides in memory, of which there are two kinds: permanent, called programmable read only memory (PROM), and nonpermanent, called random access memory (RAM). As expected, the operational instructions reside in PROM, and temporary data, such as calculated parameters, reside in RAM.

10 Fig. 30-14 is a schematic representation of a microprocessor-based design. Whatever is happening within the boundaries of the ventilator and patient is monitored by sensors. Examples of sensors are temperature, O_2, flow, pressure, CO_2 and SaO_2. By reading the sensors, as directed by the software, the microprocessor is apprised of the status of the ventilator. By comparing the readings of several sensors within a logical framework, the microprocessor can determine whether the ventilator is operating within the bounds of normal performance. An illogical appraisal brings on an alarm. All of the software routines, as well as temporary calculations, are stored in memory. As the microprocessor samples each sensor under the direction of the software, outputs are calculated and displayed.

11 Within the general software are special instructions for ensuring that information, passing back and forth within the system, is meeting the design criteria. For lack of a better term, these operations that run while the ventilator is on are called *ongoing checks*. Ongoing checks, in combination with power-on self-test (POST) and extended self-testing, compose a powerful safety net system that cannot be duplicated in analog-based designs.

12 Sensors, so essential to aerospace technology, are relatively new to medical equipment. Although pressure gauges or manometers have appeared on ventilators for many years, they were only there to present informa-

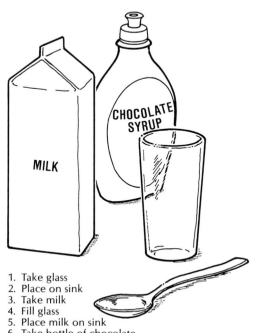

1. Take glass
2. Place on sink
3. Take milk
4. Fill glass
5. Place milk on sink
6. Take bottle of chocolate
7. Add 2 tablespoons
8. Place chocolate on sink
9. Take spoon
10. Place spoon in glass
11. Stir for 2 minutes
12. Place spoon on sink

F I G U R E   3 0 - 1 3 Recipe for mixing chocolate milk.

tion to the operator. The ventilator did not alter its performance if the value of some parameter was not what it should have been. The use of sensors to provide input to microprocessor electronics about actual performance is relatively new. The availability of cost-effective sensors is the cornerstone of third-generation ventilation. By reading each sensor on a schedule of every several milliseconds, microprocessor electronics can monitor actual performance and make corrections to bring actual performance in line with expected performance.

4.3 The pneumatic subsystem

1 The terms ventilator and pneumatic system are inseparable. Whatever else a ventilator may do, such as performing respiratory mechanics calculations or outputting digital information, the fundamental function of a ventilator is gas delivery. Therefore a ventilator cannot be more sophisticated than its pneumatic system.

2 During the relatively short history of the commercial ventilator, the number of uniquely different pneumatic systems can be counted on the fingers of one hand. With the exception of high-frequency ventilation, the primary function of a pneumatic system is that of managing the cyclic inflation and deflation of the lungs. Inflation generally results from the delivery of a preset volume of gas to the lungs or from pressurization of the lungs. Although the design of a "pure" pressure controller is theoretically possible, such a system would be impractical because of the dangerously high pressures required. All pressure controllers are more correctly classified as flow controllers. How the volume is delivered, either by a moving piston in a cylinder or by pressure collapsing a bag or bellows, or how flow is controlled, either by fluidics or by electromechanical valves, is less important than the fundamental technique—volume delivery or flow and pressure control.

3 Pure volume delivery systems (Fig. 30-15, *A*) are adequate for controlled or machine-cycled ventilation (the control feature of CMV), but they may burden the patient with a relatively high "trigger" work during assisted breathing. This was particularly true of second-generation ventilators. The high trigger work can be traced to the inertial constraints that limit the rate at which gas can be initially expelled from the gas-storage space. For the same reasons, flow shaping, as required for the generation of a square waveform, is not handled well by the pure, piston-based volume delivery system. NOTE: Very recent results with rolling seal pistons driven by linear motors suggest that volume displacement devices may soon rival the performance of flow-controlled devices. Those developments are of particular interest regarding the home-care ventilator.

4 The inherent flexibility afforded by flow-control valves operating either under analog control (e.g., Siemens 900C) or microprocessor electronics (digital) has induced all manufacturers of third-generation ventilators

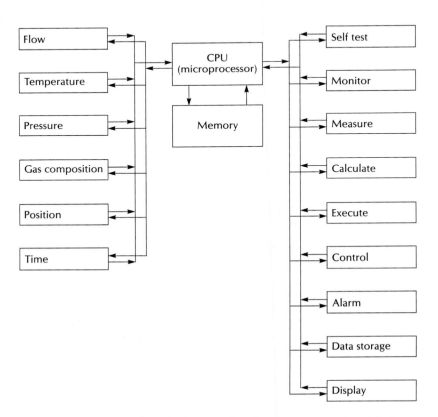

FIGURE 30-14 Schematic representation of a microprocessor-based design.

to adopt this design concept for their pneumatic systems.

5 Fig. 30-15, *B, C,* and *D,* illustrates variations of the flow-control concept. In these designs, pressure upstream of the flow-control valve is maintained constant at a moderately high value (perhaps between 10 and 15 psi) by a precision regulator. Flow is controlled by a rapidly adjustable orifice. Typically, flow can climb from zero to the maximum in less than 10 milliseconds. Flow controllers, therefore, mimic pure volume delivery systems. Waveform control is limited only by the designers' ability to specify the proper requirements.

6 Whether a flow controller requires an accumulator or plenum chamber is determined by the method of air and oxygen mixing and the flow characteristics of the gases supplied to the pneumatic system. If gas is mixed by a separate device, a blender, whether separate from or integral to the ventilator, the pneumatic system will consist of an accumulator and a single flow-control valve. Because blenders limit flow to a maximum of approximately 120 L/min, the accumulator stores mixed pressurized gas, which can be used to augment flow early in the breath (see Fig. 30-15, *B* and *C*).

7 An accumulator may also be used to augment flow early in the delivery of a breath, irrespective of the method of mixing air and oxygen. Siemens, with their 900 series ventilators, incorporated a spring-loaded reservoir bag in their pneumatic system. By giving the operator control of the "working pressure" within the bag, the peak flow and rate of flow out of the bag can be adjusted to suit the patient's individual needs. An inappropriate setting for the working pressure, however, can lead to flow oscillation during breath delivery.

8 If the pneumatic system is designed around two flow control valves (see Fig. 30-15, *D*), one for air and one for oxygen, the need for an accumulator may be eliminated. The flow control algorithms, however, are more complex, because air and oxygen are mixed as each breath is delivered.

9 Third-generation pneumatic systems, based around digitally controlled flow valves, seem ideally suited for the present and near future, because their response time is rapid enough to meet the expectations of a patient's inspiratory demands and because breath-delivery schemes can be changed merely by rewriting software.

4.4 The monitoring and alarming subsystem

1 Early ventilators incorporated a simple pressure manometer, which monitored pressure in the patient circuit. An operator watching the manometer could judge how well ventilation was proceeding; later, a fail-to-cycle alarm was added. As long as this alarm remained inactive, an operator could assume with some confidence that the ventilator was performing as set. Whether the settings are appropriate or inappropriate is today's question!

2 Monitoring and alarming by today's third-generation ventilators have progressed literally to the point of alarm. So much information is being monitored that practitioners may feel overwhelmed. The solution to

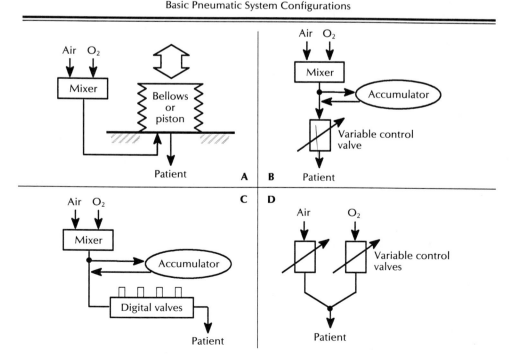

Basic Pneumatic System Configurations

FIGURE 30-15 Four basic configurations of pneumatic systems. (Courtesy Puritan-Bennett Corp., Carlsbad, Calif.)

the problem appears to lie with "smart" alarms and hierarchial enunciation. Through appropriately designed algorithms based on pattern recognition, monitoring and alarm strategies will assess the severity of the recognized problem and enunciate it with differing sounds and lights. Thus one enunciation pattern might mean "come immediately," while another might mean "come when time permits." It now appears that international regulatory bodies will set standards by which all manufacturers must abide.

4.5 The information subsystem

1 Fig. 30-7 conveys the idea that third-generation ventilators are becoming information machines. The more precision designed into the ventilator, the more accurate (and hence useful) the measured and calculated data.

2 The informational capacity of a ventilator stems from the fullest and most broad recognition of its life-support role. When third-generation ventilators became microprocessor controlled, the stage was set for information processing. Ventilatory support combined with information redefines the ventilator as a system rather than an isolated device.

3 Information processing and distribution appear to be moving through several distinct stages:

   a Simple monitoring by a direct-reading instrument, e.g., an airway pressure manometer.

   b Simple monitoring by a direct-reading instrument with settable mechanical limits, e.g., an airway pressure manometer with an adjustable, high-pressure relief.

   c Indirect monitoring by a sensor whose signal is read on a calibrated, universal type of gauge; e.g., monitoring airway pressure with an electromechanical sensor, the signal for which is displayed on a calibrated galvanometer and for which an over-range value causes the enunciation of audible and visual alarms.

   d Expansion of the previous scheme to include multiple parameters whose values are displayed in an alarm matrix; alarm enunciation is still on or off, with little differentiation between currently active and currently inactive but recently inactive alarms.

   e Expansion of the previous scheme with digital transmission of signals to a remote location, e.g., to a central station.

   f Expansion of the previous scheme with digital transmissions tied into a manufacturer-designed communications network.

   g Refinement of the previous scheme with differing devices linked into a universal type of network, e.g., the medical information bus (MIB).

4 At this writing, two of the schemes described above (i.e., 4.5, 3, e and f) are becoming more common in many hospitals, and work is progressing toward the adoption of the MIB concept (or its equivalent).

5 It appears that in the near future there will be a strong move toward hierarchial alarms. Signals from multiple sensors will be analyzed by decision-making algorithms to indicate, for example, that the patient and ventilator have become disconnected or that the setting for peak inspiratory flow is less than optimum. These signals can be sent to remote monitors by direct wiring or by telemetry. They could also be sent to hand-held devices that would identify the patient and the likely alarm problem.

6 Also in the early implementation phases are paperless management and data-capture systems. All procedures are entered into a bedside terminal or into a hand-held computer, later to be "up-loaded" into the departmental computer. Since the hospital information system has immediate access to these data, billing is automatic and error free. Also, the hand-held computer connects directly to the ventilator, capturing hourly or bihourly "snapshots" of all ventilator data. Such a paperless system is illustrated in Fig. 30-16.

7 Automatic operation of the ventilator, based on real-time analysis of multiple physiologic parameters, is all but certain. This should come as no surprise; "closed-loop" control of a ventilator (based on measurement of end-tidal CO_2) was successfully demonstrated in 1955. The Hamilton Veolar ventilator has a simple, closed-loop control algorithm that maintains a practitioner-set value for minute ventilation by adjusting pressure support. A more complex yet relatively simple closed-loop algorithm, based on the continuous sampling of both end-tidal CO_2 and SaO_2, may appear within a few years.

8 It is highly likely that the near future will see the fruition of closed-loop or quasi-closed-loop control based on highly complex and sophisticated analysis of multiple parameters.

   The technique, called the intelligent decision system approach, has been successfully applied to other areas in which closed-loop or quasi-closed-loop control was advantageous. Before closed-loop control becomes accepted, these so-called expert systems will rely on a quasi-closed-loop design. Here the clinician would be presented with recommendations for new ventilator settings, perhaps even with the reasons for the recommendations. The clinician then has the choice of accepting and acting on or rejecting the advice of the expert system. Simple two-parameter systems are already in the design and validation stages.

4.6 The operator interface subsystem

1 The term *operator interface* is another name for the control panel. Fig. 30-17 shows the control panel for an early Bennett (ca-1949) ventilator. Control for this and other similar ventilators is achieved by adjusting the various knobs, levers, cranks, and switches.

2 At least two fundamental aspects of the "control function" need to be addressed: first, the shape, size and configuration of the means of operation, and second, their spatial layout—where the means of control are

positioned on the panel. The disciplined study of human factors attempts to define the relationship between the human operator and the machine, thereby optimizing the ability of the operator to control the machine. Through the study of human factors, the engineer learns safe and effective ways to enable the operator to achieve control.

3 How control is achieved depends, by and large, on the technology of the day. When control is direct, that is, through the operator's direct action on the controlling device, the actions are limited to rotation and linear motion. Take, for example, the adjustment of tidal volume on the Emmerson ventilator shown in Fig. 30-18. Here a crank and jack screw physically adjust the stroke of the piston pump or volume generator. By today's standards, direct control may seem "old fashioned."

4 The operation of the Bear 5 is a good example of indirect control (Fig. 30-19). No action by the operator directly affects the function of the pneumatic subsystem. The valves that actually control flow are electromechanically actuated. The regulator that sets the level of PEEP is electromechanically actuated. Such indirect control predominates in a wide range of "high-tech" devices.

5 Once the means for safe and effective indirect control are achieved, the design of the operator interface can take many forms. Grouping the means of control by function lets the operator know where to look to observe specific data. The operator interface on the Puritan-Bennett 7200 Series ventilator system is an example of functional organization (Fig. 30-20). All operations that effect the control and operation of the ventilator are logically organized into common areas, which

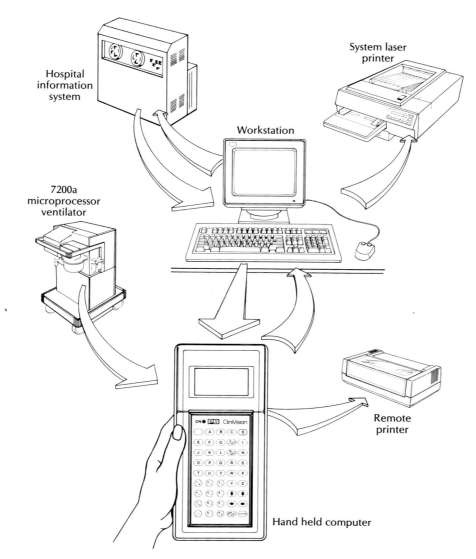

F I G U R E   3 0 - 1 6 Example of a paperless data management system. (Courtesy Puritan-Bennett Corp., Carlsbad, Calif.)

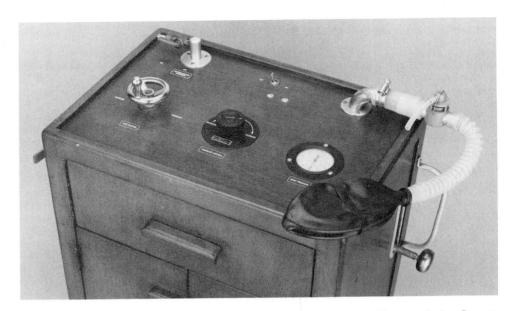

FIGURE 30-17 Control panel for an early-model Bennett respirator. (Courtesy Puritan-Bennett Corp., Carlsbad, Calif.)

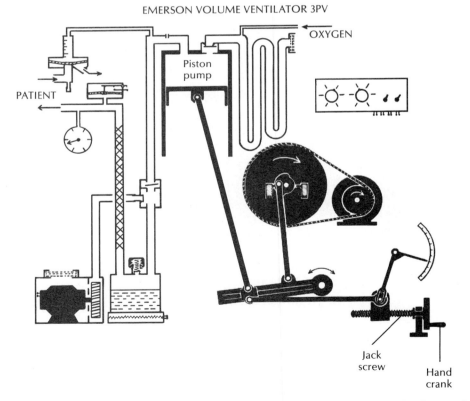

FIGURE 30-18 Control schematic for an Emerson 3PV ventilator. (Courtesy Blackwell Scientific Publications, London, England.)

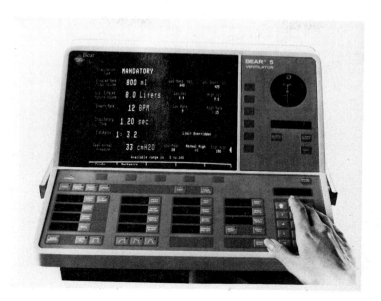

FIGURE 30-19 BEAR V control panel. Example of a design based completely on indirect control. (Courtesy Bear Medical Systems Inc, Riverside, Calif.)

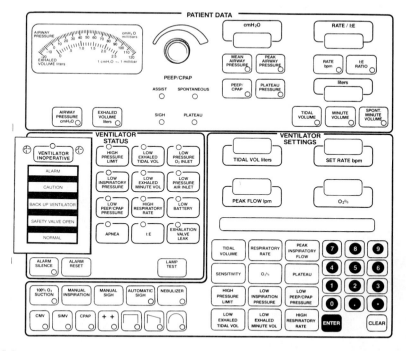

FIGURE 30-20 Control panel of a Puritan-Bennett 7200 Series Microprocessor ventilator. Example of the functional grouping of similar controls and informations. (Courtesy Puritan-Bennett Corp., Carlsbad, Calif.)

are outlined by a color-coded stripes. Those controls that govern what the ventilator does are grouped separately and are identifiably different from the controls that govern the limits within which patient and ventilator subsystem are expected to operate.

6 The means by which indirect adjustments are made takes two forms: knobs or keys. Before microprocessor control, most of the "either a or b" (i.e., on-off) operations were handled by a key, lever, or rotary switch, whereas most of the "adjustments to range" (e.g., 21% to 100% O_2 or 50 to 2000 ml tidal volume) were handled by knobs.

7 With the introduction of microprocessor control, all control operations can be handled either by knobs or keys. The concern here is more than one of aesthetics; the real issue is information and how it gets shared within and outside of the device.

8 Because of the growing importance of information in the medical setting, this aspect of design will be discussed further. As a simple example, consider the tidal volume control on the MA-1 (Fig. 30-21). This knob controls tidal volume indirectly. It can be rotated to any position between the limits of zero and 2200 ml. Once the knob is set and left alone, its setting becomes a piece of information. Because information was viewed rather narrowly when the MA-1 was manufactured, only two locations receive the tidal volume information: the front panel and the pneumatic system. A therapist who is completing a ventilator check must go to each ventilator, view the tidal volume knob, and the record its position (which is calibrated in units of volume). All first- and second-generation and some third-generation ventilators share this design. This type of knob-control can be "wired" to allow remote reading of its setting, but the process is costly and time consuming. Because of these limitations, analog knob-controls are rarely wired for remote reading.

9 With microprocessors comes greater variation in the means of control and the ability to share information outside of the device. Fig. 30-22 illustrates four means by which control may be effected. Example A is the same analog type of knob control just discussed. It has two limitations that must be considered. The first is cost and the second is the reverse flow of information. Consider the digital example, B, next because taking A and B together allows a more complete understanding of the problem. Knob B has no inherent position of its own, that is, its position does not define its setting. By rotating knob B counterclockwise or clockwise, microprocessor electronics cause the value of B (the setting of B) to decrease or increase. The actual information about the position of the "function controlled by B" resides not in the knob but in microprocessor electronics. The numeric (digital) display above knob B indicates the current value of B read from microprocessor electronics rather than from the position of B. Knob B can now be quite simple in design and therefore relatively inexpensive; information about the position or value of function B can be easily shared within or outside of the device; and most importantly (and distinctly different from knob A, function B can be changed from outside of the device. By placing the control of function B within microprocessor electronics, knob B becomes

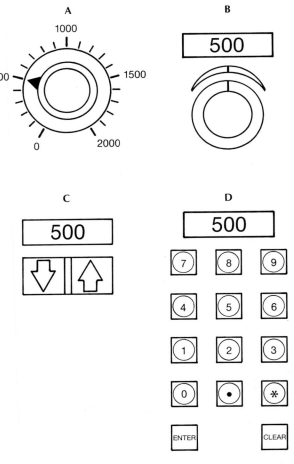

FIGURE 30-22 Four common types of indirect control.

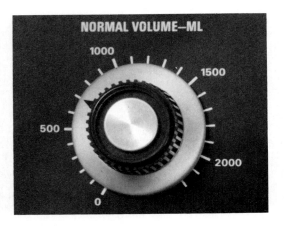

FIGURE 30-21 An example of indirect control. Volume control knob on Bennett MA1 ventilator. (Courtesy Puritan-Bennett Corp., Carlsbad, Calif.)

just one of several locations from which the command to change function *B* can originate.

10 While this difference between examples *A* and *B* may seem trivial, consider that most microprocessor-controlled devices can be tested automatically, after manufacture or repair, in a fraction of the time and cost compared to a conventional analog device. Because both algorithmic or closed-loop control and remote control require the type of function illustrated by knob *B* (and *C* and *D*), incorporating this feature into microprocessor-based designs lowers cost and reduces complexity.

11 Example *C* packages the decrease and increase (decrement and increment) actions of knob *B* in a key design. To reduce the value of function *C*, the operator presses the decrement key until the desired value is reached. Both examples *B* and *C*, however, lose the analog or position awareness that example *A* possesses. Once the rotational position of knob *A* is memorized, it can be rotated and the new position estimated by *feel*. No comparable interactive method has been developed for examples *B* and *C*.

12 Example *D* is a further variation on the separation of the control of a function and the means of control. Example *D* makes use of a numeric key pad from which the desired value of function *D* can be set. Thus, the numeric keypad offers the same advantages as examples *B* and *C*, but additionally permitting the direct setting of a desired value. The numeric keypad represents an additional cost over a digital knob and increment-decrement keys, but if many functions are to be set, as in the case of a ventilator, the numeric keypad may carry the lowest overall cost.

13 In recent years, designers have begun to make use of the "soft key" concept. Essential to this concept is a "configurable screen" like a video tube. Automatic teller machines employ this design. The actions of the column of keys on the side of the video tube are defined by the configuration of the video image. In other designs, the keys are "drawn" on the video screen. Placing a finger in the right box (pressing the right key) causes the stated function to execute. These designs have one feature in common: all control and action resides in microprocessor electronics. The keyboard, all of it, is defined by software, which can be changed at any time. The cost to change is measured in design time rather than in "hardware" cost.

14 Once the concept of a configurable design is accepted, the means for control and display become virtually limitless, (i.e., a software-defined layout). The entire control panel may be drawn on the video screen. A soft key or a "mouse" may be used to tell microprocessor electronics which function to change.

15 Consider another example: Inside the critical care unit (CCU) stands a new microprocessor-controlled ventilator. Except for a power switch and a few special keys, there is no control panel, at least when the power switch is off. Just below the screen is a handlelike lever that is designed to be grasped, each finger naturally comes to rest on a switch. The power being on, the screen is "lit" and set automatically to the default "page." Across the top of the screen are a series of message boxes. One reads "ventilator settings." Moving the lever toward this box causes a "cursor" to move toward the box. When the cursor hits the box, it highlights itself. Pressing one of the fingered switches causes the ventilator settings page (or menu) to appear. To change tidal volume, the handle is pressed in the direction that causes the cursor to "fly" to the tidal-volume box. When hit, the box highlights. A click of one of the fingered switches causes a vertical bar scale to appear beside the tidal volume box. The scaling of the bar matches that appropriate for adult ventilation, e.g., 300 to 3000 ml. The current setting for tidal volume being 600 ml, the bar is shaded up to the 600 ml mark. Sqeezing one of the fingered switches causes the tidal volume to increment, both the digital value and bar scale moving together. The new, desired value for tidal volume is 800 ml. As the bar and the digital value approach, then equal 800 ml, the switch is released. The click of a finger switch causes microprocessor electronics to accept the new value for tidal volume. The possibilities for such a control scheme are endless. Whether the advantages are real or only imaginary are not known at this moment. Such a design concept is certainly possible with today's technology. Only by experimentation and in-depth testing in the clinical setting will the advantages and disadvantages be revealed. Whatever the outcome, the ventilator of tomorrow will be controlled and operated in a manner different from that in use today.

4.7 The service and repair subsystem

1 While not a distinct and identifiable entity within the ventilator, software and hardware specially designed to facilitate service and repair will reside within the ventilator. What is beginning to emerge is a subsystem resembling the flight recorder carried by all commercial jet aircraft. Today's third-generation ventilators contain the rudiments of such a system, but a genuinely efficient and cost-effective design has not yet emerged. Liken the stage of development to the sound of two rocks striking one another compared to the sound of an orchestra. Current third-generation ventilators are closer to the "sound-of-two-rocks" end of the spectrum.

5.0 EXPECTED PERFORMANCE
5.1 Limits of the discussion

1 This module is not the place for a treatise on ventilator performance. It does seem appropriate, however, to discuss some of the solutions to the performance expectations voiced by the respiratory community.

2 While the lungs do perform some endocrine and enzymatic functions, their primary functions are the elimination of CO_2 from and oxygenation of the blood. The

execution of these functions carries two absolute re-quirements: blood must continually move through those areas of the lung that are supplied with a gas high in O_2 and low in CO_2. This statement of execution has been broadly formulated to encompass respiration at high atmospheric pressures, with He substituted for N_2, and by the nonphysiologic means of high-frequency ventilation. During normal breathing, the respiratory-muscle pump is responsible for maintaining the flow of gas into and out of the lungs. The fuel to power the respiratory muscle pump, oxygen, indirectly comes from the inspired gas; the direct source is oxyhemoglobin, replenished in the pulmonary circulation and pumped by the heart to the respiratory muscles.

3 In the context of this understanding, the ventilator, on the one hand, substitutes for or assists the respiratory-muscle pump. Stated another way, the ventilator fully or partially takes over a patient's work of breathing. On the other hand, the ventilator may be set up to promote more successful gas exchange when the lungs are fluid filled or when ventilation and perfusion are not well matched. Beyond the maintenance of optimum gas exchange and management of the work of breathing, there is little that the ventilator can do.

The following discussion focuses on those ventilator activities that most impact the work of breathing and gas exchange.

5.2 Gas delivery by the pneumatic subsystem

1 Although lingering confusion persists, there is one situation in which a ventilator-dependent patient (by definition any patient on a ventilator is ventilator dependent) does not expend work to breathe. This condition exists when the respiratory musles are not being caused to contract as a result of trains of nerve impulses conducted along their motor axons. Such a condition results from nerve or brain damage or through paralysis. In all other situations, the patient and ventilator compose a synergistic system. To analyze the work of breathing done by ventilator-dependent patients, one must consider two breathing patterns: mandatory (the ventilator defines the tidal volume, peak inspiratory flow, flow waveform, and triggering effort) and spontaneous (the ventilator defines only the triggering effort).

2 To gain a more thorough understanding of the patient-imitated mandatory breath, three elements that impact the work of breathing must be recognized. One must consider: (a) the trigger effort, which is a function of the set value of (pressure) sensitivity, (b) the set value of peak inspiratory flow, and (c) the set value for tidal volume.

   a While it is true that the work expended by the patient to trigger the mandatory breath may be a small fraction of the total work expended during the delivery of a breath, the trigger work can tire and frustrate the patient. Unsuccessful trigger efforts, in the sense that no mandatory breath follows the trigger effort,

lead to increasing levels of Pco_2 in the arterial blood. The increasing levels of CO_2 stimulate the respiratory center, resulting in more vigorous inspiratory efforts. With increasing vigor, triggering may be successful, but at the expense of further fatigue.

   b The second factor that may aggravate the work of breathing during delivery of the mandatory breath is a lower-than-optimum setting for the value of peak inspiratory flow. If the patient's respiratory center expects a higher inspiratory flow than that delivered by the ventilator, the patient "fights" the ventilator. The result is work unsuccessfully expended to increase the flow from the pneumatic subsystem. Even if the ventilator is designed to deliver incremental flow, generation of the supplemental flow requires additional work.

   c The third factor that can cause the patient to expend additional work is a lower-than-expected tidal volume. If the patient's respiratory system is expecting flow at the end of a too-low tidal volume, the patient momentarily fights for this nonexistent flow. The result is wasted work.

3 Even in a perfect situation in which inspiratory flow and tidal volume are well matched, contraction of the inspiratory muscles requires oxygen. As long as the patient continues to contract his or her inspiratory muscles, energy will be expended. The question to be addressed is how new breathing strategies can minimize rather than aggravate the inspiratory effort expended during a patient-initiated mandatory breath.

4 To minimize the patient's work during triggered, mandatory breaths, the ventilator should trigger easily and match the patient's expectations for inspiratory flow and tidal volume. Borrowing from the work-reducing concepts embodied in the continuous-flow strategy, Puritan-Bennett has introduced a feature called Flow-by. Functionally, Flow-by causes the ventilator's pneumatic subsystem to turn on with no more expenditure of energy than that required during the initial and early part of a continuous-flow supported breath. Once the ventilator's microprocessor electronics receive the signal to switch on the pneumatic substystem during Flow-by operation, a mandatory or spontaneous breath can follow.

5 While some very elegant mandatory breathing strategies have been developed to more optimally manage inspiratory flow and tidal volume, none has been incorporated into successful commercial designs, and none has been shown to clinically validate the theoretic implications. What may prove just as practical is "smart," patient-triggered (either by flow or pressure) pressure ventilation. In such a scheme, an algorithm manages both inspiratory pressure and time within prescribed boundaries to maintain a constant, or at least minimum, minute ventilation. The control algorithm would incorporate elements similar to Hamilton's MMV algorithm and Drager's pressure ventilation algorithm.

6 With regard to the spontaneous breath, the patient first

must trigger the pneumatic subsystem to turn on and then expend energy to expand the thoracic cavity, causing gas to move through the artificial airway, the airways of the lungs, and finally into the compliant lungs and chest wall. The continuous-flow breathing strategy essentially eliminates the trigger work but does nothing to lessen the work that must follow. Pressure support, as it is presently conceptualized, still requires trigger (pressure) work but provides for considerable latitude in the management of the bulk of the work of inspiration.

7 By flow-triggering pressure support, the practitioner would have near-optimum control of the whole of the spontaneous-breathing effort. Flow triggering is a new feature recently introduced by Puritan-Bennett. Instead of monitoring airway pressure, the ventilator monitors the flow of breathing gas into the patient's lungs while the patient circuit is open to the atmosphere (or PEEP) and supplied with a modest level of continuous gas flow (5 to 20 L/min). The distinctive feature of the flow-triggering concept is the open patient circuit, which is supplied with a low level of continuous flow. Some hybrid-type triggering systems are based on flow

"sucked" out of closed patient circuit. Data in the literature show that these systems require a level of trigger work comparable with that attending pressure triggering.

8 Practitioners who understand the function of the working pressure on the 900C know that its adjustment can be used to "tune" the early rate of flow into the patient's lungs. In practice, the working pressure acts as a flow-gain control. The lower the impedance into which the gas flows after leaving the patient Y, the higher can be the initial rate of flow without overshoot and flow and pressure oscillation. Fig. 30-23 illustrates a flow gain that is too aggressive relative to the impedance into which the gas is moving. Engineers talk about critically damped, overdamped, or underdamped gain functions. These three possibilities are illustrated in Fig. 30-24. For the overdamped curve, the gain is too low—the function reaches the target value significantly slower than the minimum time. On the other hand, the gain setting for the underdamped curve is too high. The feedback control algorithm cannot stop the function at the target value; it overshoots, then undershoots as the function oscillates about the target value. Literally, the function is out of control. The optimally damped curve illustrates the system response that results from a compromise between an aggressive rise time and minimal but acceptable oscillation. The curve rises rapidly to the target value, overshoots slightly, then is followed by a barely measurable undershoot. Thereafter the function stabilizes at the target value.

9 Only one third-generation microprocessor-controlled ventilator, the Evita/Irisa by Drager, currently offers the practitioner any control over the flow gain. As manufacturers move to exercise more control of the work of breathing, the practitioner will be given control of the flow-gain function. Direct control such as this will require the ability to see the flow or pressure

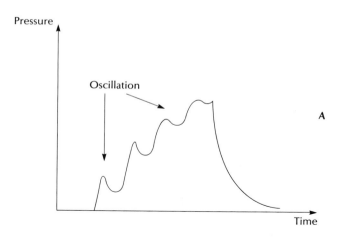

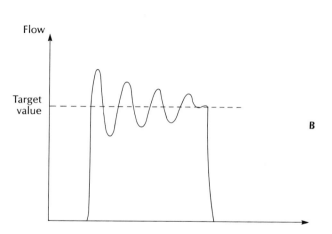

FIGURE 30-23 Examples of the effect of an overly aggressive flow delivery. **A,** The pressure-time trace. **B,** The flow-time trace.

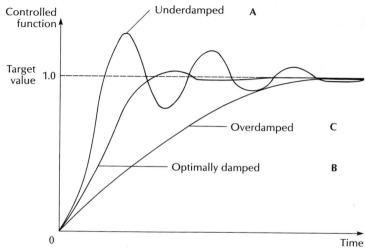

FIGURE 30-24 Examples of a time-dependent controlled function. **A,** Underdamped. **B,** Optimally damped. **C,** Overdamped.

waveform. A much more sophisticated approach would be for the practitioner to be able to select one of three choices: aggressive, moderate, or gentle. An algorithm would monitor flow, shifting the gain automatically to achieve some quantitative equivalence of aggressive, moderate, and gentle. Such a scheme would not require direct observation of the waveform.

5.3 Active control of the exhalation valve

1 The literature contains numerous studies of the whole range of exhalation valves found in first-, second-, and third-generation ventilators, as well as in continuous flow systems. While isolated and separate exhalation valves can be manufactured that exhibit the desirable characteristics of threshold restrictors, few valves integral to the ventilator show these qualities. These integral valves generally exhibit the properties of flow resistors. To incorporate the qualities of a threshold resistor in an integral exhalation valve, manufacturers of third-generation ventilators have begun to explore the use of active exhalation valves. Active means that the valve is opened fully early in exhalation by a mechanical actuation system when flow resistance is normally the highest, then is closed later when flows are lower. The active valve design, therefore, does not use the force of the exhalation flow to unseat the valve. The control algorithms must be quite sophisticated if resistance is to be minimized while control of PEEP or CPAP is maximized.

2 While the isolated exhalation valve has been the subject of modest study, little research has been devoted to the entire exhalation system, including the false airway, exhalation tube, condensate collection vial, filter, check valve, and flow sensor. There seems to be no consensus among the respiratory care community regarding the optimum resistance of the ideal exhalation system. In the 1970s some ventilator manufacturers offered exhalation valves that were based on the use of subatmospheric pressures (NEEP) to diminish the duration of exhalation. These systems came under attack because of their potential to collapse the small airways of the lung. In theory, a system can be designed that operates on the reverse principle of pressure support. With pressure reversed at the patient Y, a feedback-controlled negative pressure could be applied just distal to the exhalation valve. The system would quickly reduce and then maintain airway pressure at the Y to the baseline value. Such a system has the potential to reduce the exhalation interval by a substantial margin. Only bedside experience will show whether a feedback-controlled, negative pressure exhalation system is clinically useful and offers advantages over a conventionally designed system.

SUMMARY

From a foot-operated bellows no more complicated than an air pump used to inflate a basketball, the life support ICU ventilator has grown into a sophisticated, microprocessor-controlled system whose pneumatic subsystem possesses the flexibility to perform virtually any breathing pattern that can be defined. Early devices had a simple pressure gauge and no information processing capability; today's ICU ventilators capture and process virtually all of the information within the boundaries of the patient-ventilator system.

Given the power of "artificial intelligence," which appears to have great applicability in optimizing the life support function, the once-humble ventilator grows increasingly sophisticated as a focal device in the ICU. While the promise of some of today's newer concepts seems evident, considerable research and development will be required before these expectations are substantiated and actualized.

Delineation of the roles and functions of the entry-level generalist respiratory therapy practitioner*

I Participate in the formulation of the respiratory care plan.

A Select, review, and interpret written and graphic data from patient records and laboratory reports to include the following:

  1 Patient history
    a Smoking
    b Previous respiratory illnesses, therapy, and responses
    c Familial respiratory illnesses
    d Occupational characteristics
  2 Current admission respiratory care orders
  3 Progress notes, consultation reports, and remarks pertinent to patient's respiratory care
  4 Results of blood gas, electrolyte, hemoglobin, hematocrit, and white blood cell count analyses to determine the following:
    a Acid-base balance disturbances
    b Ventilatory sufficiency
    c Oxygen saturation of hemoglobin
    d Oxygen carrying capacity
    e Presence of infection
  5 Pulmonary function testing results
  6 Sputum culturing results
  7 Results of the following monitoring:
    a Ventilatory
    b Hemodynamic
    c Electrocardiac
    d Pleural drainage
    e Intake/output

B Inspect chest x-ray film(s) in order to identify the following:

  1 Presence and location of foreign objects to include:
    a Tracheostomy and/or endotracheal tubes
    b Transtracheal catheters
    c Chest tubes
    d Intravascular lines and catheters
    e Aspirated and penetrated objects
    f Implants
  2 Presence and/or serial positional changes of anatomic structures indicative of:
    a Pneumothorax
    b Atelectasis
    c Flail chest
    d Congenital defects
    e Hyperinflation
    f Diaphragmatic herniation
    g Congestive heart failure (CHF)
  3 Presence of and/or serial changes in densities indicative of:
    a Pneumothorax
    b Atelectasis
    c Pulmonary consolidation
    d Pulmonary congestion
    e Pleural fluid
  4 Techniques
    a Penetration
    b Contrast
    c Positions

C Solicit anecdotal information from other team members to include:

  1 Nonrespiratory care treatment/therapy schedules (physical/occupational therapy, medication administration, dietary, etc.)
  2 Patient attitude and state of consciousness
  3 Unusual or untoward patient conditions or responses to treatments

D Determine patient physical status by inspection of the following:

  1 General appearance (position, state of neatness, facial expressions, indications of dyspnea, presence and character of cough, diaphoresis, etc.)
  2 Respiratory status, indicated by:
    a Chest configurations to include:
      (1) Kyphosis and/or scoliosis
      (2) Pectus carinatum
      (3) Pectus excavatum
      (4) Hyperinflation
      (5) Obesity sufficient to impinge on ventilatory movement
    b Clubbing of the digits
    c Muscle wasting
    d Chest movements to include:
      (1) Accessory muscle activity, including active exhalation
      (2) Intercostal retractions
      (3) Asymmetric movement
    e Ventilatory patterns to include:

From American Association for Respiratory Care, 1720 Regal Row, Dallas, Tex. 75235

*Subproject I (HRA 231-75-0213)

(1) Tachypnea
(2) Bradypnea
(3) Hyperpnea
(4) Hypopnea
(5) Kussmaul
(6) Orthopnea
(7) Biot's
(8) Altered inspiratory to expiratory time ratios
(9) Cheyne-Stokes

3 Circulatory status as indicated by:

a Cyanosis

b Venous filling and/or peripheral edema indicative of abnormal volume and distribution of body fluids

4 Sputum, to include:

a Amount

b Texture/consistency

c Odor

d Color

e Hemoptysis

f *In vitro* response to mucolytic *versus* proteolytic agents

E Determine patient physical status by palpation of the following:

1 Peripheral pulses in the identification of:

a Cardiac rate

b Pulse strength

2 Chest movements to include:

a Accessory muscle activity

b Intercostal retractions

c Asymmetric movement

3 Tracheal deviation

4 Crepitance secondary to subcutaneous emphysema

5 Rhonchal fremitus indicating the presence of abnormal fluid (mucus, pus, edema) in the airways

6 Asymmetrically increased or decreased vocal fremitus

F Using chest auscultation, determine the presence of and/or serial changes in the following:

1 Asymmetric breath sounds

2 Increased or decreased breath sounds

3 Adventitious sounds to include rales, rhonchi, and wheezing

G Using percussion, determine the presence of and/or serial changes in asymmetric resonance of the chest.

H Through direct interview, assess patient's state of consciousness and willingness and ability to cooperate.

I Analyze data and information and classify the appropriateness of the respiratory care order as follows:

1 Appropriate for the patient's condition

2 Inappropriate because there is no indication that the patient requires respiratory care

3 Inappropriate because even though there is indication that the patient requires respiratory care, the therapy ordered might unnecessarily harm the patient

4 Inappropriate because even though there is indication that the patient requires respiratory care, the order is incomplete

J Recommend modification(s) in the respiratory care order when such order is determined inappropriate.

1 When order is inappropriate because there is no indication the patient requires respiratory care, recommend that the order be discontinued.

2 When order is inappropriate because even though there is indication that the patient requires respiratory care, the therapy ordered might unnecessarily harm the patient, discontinue the therapy and recommend technique(s) that match the indication.

3 When order is inappropriate because even though there is indication that the patient requires respiratory care, the order is incomplete, discontinue therapy and request a complete order recommending technique(s) that match the indication.

II Participate in the implementation of the respiratory care plan.

A Select and assemble therapeutic equipment and assure equipment function by testing before application to the patient, replacing nonfunctioning components.

1 Positive pressure ventilators

a Volume limited

b Pressure limited

2 PEEP circuits

3 IMV circuits

4 Incentive breathing devices

5 Dead-space breathing devices

6 Expiratory resistance devices

7 Aerosol generators

a Bernoulli-type

b Ultrasonic-type

c Babington-type

8 Aerosol patient attachments

9 Humidifiers

10 Medical gas delivery devices

a Low, controlled FIO_2

b Mid-range, variable FIO_2

c High, controlled FIO_2

11 Artificial airways

a Endotracheal

b Tracheostomy

c Pharyngeal

12 Chest physiotherapy devices

a Vibrators

b Percussors

B Assess the operation and assembly of patient monitors and therapeutic devices, correcting where malfunction exists.

1 Respiratory therapy equipment

2 Pleural drainage systems

3 Intravascular catheters and/or lines

4 Artificial airways

5 Cardiac and ventilatory monitors and attachments

C Protect patient from contamination.
  1 Confirm equipment cleanliness and disinfection and/or sterility.
  2 Employ aseptic procedures.
    a Isolation and reverse isolation procedures
    b Sterile gloving
    c Hand scrubbing
D Establish therapist/patient rapport.
  1 Elicit (conscious) patient confidences.
  2 Assess (conscious) patient anxiety toward therapy.
E Ensure (conscious) patient understanding of therapeutic goal(s) and technique(s).
  1 Assess patient's ability and willingness to understand.
  2 Modify communication to match patient's needs.
F Initiate and conduct therapeutic procedures, achieving one or a combination of the following outcomes:
  1 Bronchopulmonary secretion evacuation
    a Deep breathing
      (1) Positive pressure
        (a) IPPB
        (b) Bag/valve/mask
        (c) Expiratory resistance
      (2) Voluntary
        (a) Without accessory devices
        (b) Incentive device
        (c) Dead space
    b Pulmonary drainage
      (1) Positioning
      (2) Chest wall manipulation
        (a) Percussion
        (b) Vibration
        (c) Squeeze
        (d) Segmental compression
      (3) Controlled coughing
    c Drug administration
      (1) Aerosol inhalation
      (2) Tracheal instillation
      (3) Intravenous administration
    d Oral/pharyngeal/tracheal suctioning
  2 Artificial airway maintenance
    a Insertion
    b Anchoring
    c Repositioning
    d *In vivo* cleaning and disinfection of site and tube
    e Weaning
    f Removal
  3 Ventilatory support
    a Positive pressure ventilation
    b Negative pressure ventilation
    c Weaning
    d Helium/oxygen breathing
  4 Tissue oxygenation
    a Oxygen inhalation
    b Extracorporeal oxygenation
    c Hyperbaric administration

  5 Emergency resuscitation
G Assess patient's physical response to therapy by physiologic monitoring (see *I, D-G*)
H Assess patient attitudinal response to therapy.
I Modify and/or implement therapeutic technique(s) (not requiring physician's order) based on patient's response.
  1 Bronchopulmonary secretion evacuation (deep breathing, pulmonary drainage, drug administration, endotracheal suctioning)
    a Change the length of treatment time based on patient physiologic response.
    b Shorten the length of treatment time or decrease the number of treatments given in any period of time due to:
      (1) Patient attitudinal resistance
      (2) Presence and/or insistence of family or others
      (3) Interference of other scheduled therapies
      (4) Limited availability of time and/or personnel when other patients' therapeutic needs are greater
    c Increase or decrease the number of treatments given in any period of time based on patient physiologic response.
    d Discontinue therapy when patient response indicates that unnecessary harm is being done.
    e Initiate therapy without physician's order.
  2 IPPB
    a Adjust machine:
      (1) Pressure
      (2) Volume
      (3) Flow
      (4) Sensitivity
      (5) I:E ratio
    b Change type of ventilator.
    c Increase or decrease amount of dead space.
    d Add retard device or change resistance in such a device.
    e Change patient attachments (mask, mouthpiece, etc.).
    f Use oral airway.
  3 Bag/valve/mask
    a Increase or decrease volume delivered by adjusting pressure and flow.
  4 Expiratory resistance
    a Adjust amount of resistance.
  5 Incentive breathing device
    a Select device.
    b Increase or decrease incentive goal.
  6 Dead-space breathing
    a Select device.
    b Increase or decrease amount of dead space.
  7 Positioning for pulmonary drainage
    a Select position.
    b Determine duration in position.
  8 Chest wall manipulation (percussion, vibration, squeeze, segmental compression)

a Select technique to be used.

b Determine site on chest wall to apply technique.

9 Drug administration

 a Modify dosage/concentration.

 b Select administrative device.

 c Select solvent.

 d Select alternate drug.

10 Aerosol inhalation

 a Modify ventilatory pattern for deposition.

 b Modify patient position for deposition.

 c Select temperature of aerosol/carrier gas.

 d Add particle stabilizer.

11 Oral/pharyngeal/tracheal suctioning

 a Modify patient position.

 b Determine frequency.

 c Select catheter size and type.

 d Adjust vacuum.

 e Instill wetting agent.

 f Use oral or nasal airway.

 g Determine degree of cuff inflation on endotracheal or tracheostomy tube while suctioning.

12 Artificial airway maintenance

 a Select type.

 b Select length and diameter.

13 Positive pressure ventilation

 a Select/change equipment.

  (1) Pressure/flow waveform capabilities

  (2) Monitoring devices/alarms

  (3) Patient circuitry

  (4) Humidification device

 b Adjust ventilatory parameters (minute volume/tidal volume/rate, sigh ratio/volume, pressure limit, I:E ratio, sensitivity, assist/control) according to:

  (1) Blood gases

  (2) Blood pressure

  (3) Heart rate

  (4) Cardiac output

  (5) Fluid volume status (hypervolemia-hypovolemia)

  (6) Spontaneous ventilatory pattern

  (7) Pulmonary compliance

  (8) Patient psychologic dependence

 c Institute PEEP.

 d Increase or decrease dead space.

 e Add or adjust expiratory resistance.

 f Change machines according to prioritized patients' needs when limited machines are available.

14 Weaning

 a Determine patient readiness for weaning.

 b Select method and/or device.

 c Determine rate/volume adjustments when using IMV.

 d Determine time off of ventilator when not using IMV.

15 Helium/oxygen breathing

 a Select administration device.

 b Determine concentration.

 c Judge indication for use.

16 Tissue oxygenation

 a Determine desirable FIO_2 based on blood gases and/or patient condition.

 b Select administration device.

17 Emergency resuscitation

 a Determine when to initiate.

 b Intubate airway.

 c Start IV.

 d Administer drugs.

 e Defibrillate.

J Recommend modification(s) in respiratory care order based on patient response.

III Maintain records.

 A Select information and data for recording.

  1 Patient physical response to therapy

  2 Patient attitudinal response to therapy

  3 Fulfillment of therapeutic goal(s)

  4 Patient charges and credits

  5 Data for statistical reports

 B Question incongruous data.

 C Adhere to medicolegal standards and hospital methods for record keeping.

 D Employ standard terminology, symbols, acronyms, and abbreviations.

 E Perform and verify mathematical computations.

 F Ensure confidentiality of patient/hospital records.

IV Implement procedure and equipment quality control.

 A Assure equipment cleanliness and disinfection and/or sterility.

  1 Assure separation of contaminated and noncontaminated equipment.

  2 Disassemble and clean contaminated equipment.

  3 Disinfect equipment employing the following:

   a Liquid disinfectants

   b Pasteurization

  4 Prepare equipment for autoclave and/or ethylene oxide sterilization.

  5 Store clean and disinfected and/or sterilized equipment in a protected area, rotating stock to assure shortest shelf time.

 B Participate in bacteriologic surveillance.

  1 Collect specimens for bacteriologic culturing from equipment in storage and in use.

  2 Document results of bacteriologic surveillance.

  3 Interpret results of bacteriologic surveillance.

  4 Modify procedures for equipment handling, cleaning, disinfection, and sterilization based on results of bacteriologic surveillance.

 C Ensure equipment function through preventive maintanance and repair(s).

 D Adhere to departmental quality assurance policies and procedures.

  1 Document conformance to quality assurance standards.

2 Modify techniques and procedures to conform to quality assurance standards.

E Formulate quality assurance policies in response to advances in practice.

V Conduct diagnostic studies and procedures.

  A Select and prepare analyzing equipment.

  B Calibrate analyzing equipment.

  C Explain objective of diagnostic study to patient.

  D Explain procedure to patient.

  E Elicit cooperation from patient.

  F Obtain specimens for analysis.

  G Conduct procedure.

  H Obtain results.

  I Verify results.

  J Prepare data for interpretation.

VI Illustrate attitudes congruent with role as a therapist.

  A Operate a personal competency assurance program.

    1 Demonstrate attitude of scientific inquiry.

    2 Implement methods of self-appraisal and improvement.

    3 Recognize professional capabilities and limitations.

  B Be active in advancement of profession.

  C Respond with sensitivity, empathy, and responsiveness in communications with patient, family, and other care team members.

    1 Facilitate cooperative interaction with other health care team members.

    2 Apply knowledge of psychology of illness in patient interaction.

    3 Solicit feedback concerning communication skills.

    4 Provide feedback concerning communication skills.

    5 Respond to factors affecting communication.

    6 Modify approach based on persons involved in interactions.

    7 Strive to reconcile misunderstandings.

    8 Initiate communication as indicated.

  D Recognize primacy of patient welfare.

  E Apply current standards in ethical conduct.

  F Maintain mental and physical health.

Joint commission on accreditation of hospital organizations— respiratory care services

PRINCIPLE

Respiratory care services that meet the needs of patients as determined by the medical staff shall be available at all times.

Standard I

Respiratory care services that meet the needs of patients, as determined by the medical staff, are available at all times; are well organized, properly directed, and appropriately integrated with other units and departments of the hospital; and are staffed in a manner commensurate with the scope of services offered.

Interpretation. The relationship of the respiratory care department/service to other units and departments of the hospital shall be specified within the overall hospital organizational plan. The responsibility and accountability of the respiratory care department/service to the medical staff and hospital administration shall be defined.

Scope of services. The scope of the diagnostic and therapeutic respiratory care services provided to inpatients, ambulatory care patients, and home care patients shall be defined in writing. There shall be written guidelines for the transfer or referral of patients who require respiratory care services that are not provided by the hospital.

Pulmonary function studies and blood gas analysis capability shall be appropriate for the level of respiratory care services provided and shall be readily available to meet the needs of patients.

Hospitals providing any degree of respiratory care services, either from within the hospital or from an outside source, shall be evaluated for compliance with all applicable requirements of this section of the Manual. A hospital that provides continuous ventilatory support to patients shall comply with all requirements of this section of the Manual. A respiratory intensive care unit shall be evaluated for compliance with the requirements of this section and the Special Care Units section of this Manual.

Outside sources. When respiratory care services are provided to any extent from outside the hospital, the source(s) shall be approved by the medical staff through its designated mechanism, provide services whenever needed, meet all safety requirements, abide by all pertinent rules and regulations of the hospital and medical staff, document the quality control measures to be implemented, and meet all applicable requirements of this and related sections of the Manual.

Direction. Medical direction of the respiratory care department/service shall be provided by a physician member of the active medical staff who has special interest and knowledge in the diagnosis, treatment, and assessment of respiratory problems. Whenever possible, this physician should be qualified by special training and/or experience in the management of acute and chronic respiratory problems. The physician director shall designate a qualified physician member of the active medical staff to act in his absence. The physician director or his qualified designee shall be available to provide any required respiratory care consultation, particularly on patients receiving continuous ventilatory or oxygenation support. The physician director shall have the authority and responsibility for assuring that established policies are carried out; that overall direction in the provision of respiratory care services in the inpatient, ambulatory care, and home care settings is provided; and that a review and evaluation of the quality, safety, and appropriateness of respiratory care services is performed.

Staffing. Respiratory care services shall be provided by a sufficient number of qualified personnel under competent medical direction. When the scope of services warrants it, respiratory care services shall be supervised by a technical director who is registered or certified by the National Board for Respiratory Care, Inc., or has the documented equivalent education, training, and/or experience. The technical director's duties shall include responsibility for assuring the supervision of respiratory personnel in the performance of respiratory care and any designated related laboratory procedures; the care, maintenance, and disinfection or sterilization of all ventilatory equipment, accessories, and, as required, supplied; and the maintenance of appropriate records and reports. Additional responsibilities may be designated to the technical director by the physician providing medical direction for the respiratory care services.

Other qualified respiratory care personnel shall provide respiratory care services commensurate with their documented training, experience, and competence. Such per-

This is presented for concept. Yearly updates are available from the Joint Commission on Accreditation of Hospital Organizations, Chicago.

sonnel may include registered respiratory therapists or certified respiratory therapy technicians, or individuals with the documented equivalent in education, training, and/or experience; qualified cardiopulmonary technologists; and appropriately trained licensed nurses. This does not preclude the provision of respiratory care services by trainees or students supervised by qualified respiratory care personnel.

Personnel providing respiratory care services shall comply with all applicable federal, state, and local regulations.

The training of respiratory care students shall be carried out only in programs accredited by the appropriate professional educational organization. Individuals in student status shall be directly supervised by a qualified respiratory therapist or technician, particularly when engaged in patient care activities. When the hospital provides clinical facilities for the education and training provided by an outside program, the respective roles and responsibilities of the respiratory care department/service and the outside educational program shall be defined.

Standard II

Personnel are prepared for their responsibilities in the provision of respiratory care services through appropriate training and educational programs.

Interpretation. The education, training, and experience of personnel who provide respiratory care services shall be documented, and shall be related to each individual's level of participation in the provision of respiratory care services. A formal training program may be required as a prerequisite. Nonphysician respiratory care personnel shall perform patient procedures associated with a potential hazard, including arterial puncture for obtaining blood samples, only when authorized in writing by the physician director of the respiratory care department/service acting in accordance with medical staff policy. The director shall maintain documentation of the qualification of such personnel to perform these procedures. New personnel shall receive an orientation of sufficient duration and content to prepare them for their role in the provision of respiratory care services.

As appropriate, and before providing respiratory care services, individuals shall receive instruction and demonstrate competence in:

- Fundamentals of cardiopulmonary physiology, and of fluids and electrolytes.
- Recognition, interpretation, and recording of signs and symptoms of respiratory dysfunction and medication side effects, particularly those that require notification of a physician.
- Initiation and maintenance of cardiopulmonary resuscitation and other related life-support procedures.
- Prevention of contamination and of transfer of infection through appropriate aseptic techniques.
- Mechanics of ventilation and ventilator function.
- Principles of airway maintenance, including endotracheal and tracheostomy care.

- Effective and safe use of equipment for administering oxygen and other theapeutic gases, and for providing humidification nebulization, and medication.
- Pulmonary function testing and blood gas analysis (when such procedures are performed within the respiratory department/service).
- Methods that assist in the removal of secretions from the bronchial tree, such as hydration, breathing and coughing exercises, postural drainage, therapeutic percussion and vibration, and mechanical clearing of the airway through proper suctioning technique.
- Procedures and observations to be followed during and after extubation.
- Recognition of and attention to the psychologic and social needs of patients and their families.

All personnel providing respiratory care services shall participate in relevant in-service education programs. The director or his qualified designees shall contribute to the in-service education of respiratory care department/service personnel and other personnel who provide respiratory care services. In-service education shall include instruction in the safety and infection control requirements described elsewhere in this Manual. Cardiopulmonary resuscitation training for personnel performing respiratory care services shall be conducted as often as necessary, but not less than annually, except for individuals who can otherwise document their competence. Education programs for respiratory care services personnel shall be based, at least in part, on the findings from the review and evaluation of respiratory care services provided. Outside educational opportunities shall be provided as feasible, at least for supervisory personnel. The extent of participation in continuing education shall be documented, and shall be realistically related to the size of the staff and the scope and complexity of the respiratory care services provided.

Standard III

Respiratory care services are guided by written policies and procedures.

Interpretation. There shall be written policies and procedures specifying the scope and conduct of patient care to be rendered in the provision of respiratory care services. Such policies and procedures must be approved by the medical staff through its designated mechanism, and shall be reviewed at least annually, revised as necessary, dated to indicate the time of the last review, and enforced. The policies and procedures shall relate to at least the following:

- Specification as to who may perform specific procedures and provide instruction, under what circumstances, and under what degree of supervision. Such procedures include, but are not limited to, cardiopulmonary resuscitation; the obtaining of blood samples and their analysis; pulmonary function testing; therapeutic percussion and vibration; bronchopulmonary drainage; coughing and breathing exercises; mechanical ventilatory and oxygenation support for infants, children, and adults; and aerosol, humidification, and therapeutic gas administration.

- Assembly and sequential operation of equipment and accessories to implement therapeutic regimens.
- Steps to be taken in the event of adverse reactions, based on established criteria for the identification of undesirable side effects.
- Procurement, handling, storage, and dispensing of therapeutic gases.
- Pertinent safety practices, including the control of electrical, flammable, explosive, and mechanical hazards.
- Infection control measures to minimize the possibility of contamination and transfer of infection. This shall include changing equipment, accessories, and solutions according to an established schedule; and the methods of cleaning, disinfecting, and sterilizing reusable equipment.
- Administration of medications in accordance with the physician's order and the requirements of the Pharmaceutical Services section of this Manual.
- An established method of response to the absence of adequate, explicit instruction within the prescription for respiratory care services.

Standard IV

The respiratory care department/service has equipment and facilities to assure the safe, effective, and timely provision of respiratory care services to patients.

Interpretation. Sufficient space shall be provided for the respiratory care department/service to store, decontaminate, clean, disinfect or sterilize, maintain, and repair equipment; to store supplies; and to perform the administrative work related to the volume of services provided. There shall be sufficient space and equipment to perform any pulmonary function studies or blood gas analyses provided in the hospital. All requirements relating to the performance of pulmonary function studies or blood gas analyses must be met regardless of which hospital department is responsible for performing them.

All equipment shall be calibrated and operated according to the manufacturer's specification, and shall be periodically inspected and maintained according to an established schedule as part of the hospital's preventive maintenance program. A pin-index system, a diameter-index system, or another approved equivalent safety system shall be used with a therapeutic gas. Where piped-in gas supply systems are installed, an evaluation shall be made prior to use to assure identification of the gas and its delivery within an established safe pressure range. Oxygen analysis of the therapeutic gases delivered by the ventilators and aerosol units using the piped-in gas supply should be made at regular intervals and recorded. After cleaning and reassembling equipment delivering therapeutic gases to the patient, and prior to patient use, an assessment of the gas flow shall be made to assure that it is within established

safe limits. The temperature of inspired gas shall be measured at intervals that assure the temperature is not excessive, and shall be recorded. Ventilators used for continuous assistance or controlled breathing shall have operative alarm systems at all times.

Resuscitation, ventilatory, and oxygenation support equipment shall be available for patients of all sizes served by the hospital.

Standard V

Respiratory care services are provided to patients in accordance with a written prescription by the physician responsible for the patient and are documented in the patient's medical record.

Interpretation. The prescription for respiratory care shall specify the type, frequency, and duration of treatment, and, as appropriate, the type and dose of medication, the type of diluent, and the oxygen concentration. A written record of the prescription and any related respiratory consultation shall be maintained in the respiratory care department's/service's files, shall be incorporated into the patient's medical record, and shall include the diagnosis. When feasible, the goals or objectives of the respiratory therapy should also be stated in the medical record. All respiratory care services provided to a patient shall be documented in the patient's medical record, including the type of therapy, date and time of administration, effects of therapy, and any adverse reactions. The responsible physician shall document in the patient's medical record a timely, pertinent clinical evaluation of the overall results of respiratory therapy.

Prior to discharge of the patient, instructions appropriate to the respiratory problem should be given in all relevant aspects of pulmonary care. This may include instruction to the patient or the patient's family on postural drainage, therapeutic percussion, and other measures. The need for long-term oxygen therapy should be adequately documented in the medical records of patients discharged on such therapy. When appropriate, such need should be based on arterial blood gas results at rest and/or exercise.

Standard VI

As part of the hospital's quality assurance program, the quality and appropriateness of patient care provided by the respiratory care department/service are monitored and evaluated, and identified problems are resolved.

Interpretation. The physician director of the respiratory care department/service shall be responsible for assuring that a review and evaluation of the appropriateness and effectiveness of such services is accomplished in a timely manner, including respiratory care provided to inpatients, and, when applicable, to ambulatory care patients and home care patients. The review and evaluation shall be performed at least quarterly, and shall involve the use of the medical record and the use of pre-estalished criteria, including indications for use, effectiveness of treatment, and adverse effects requiring discontinuance of treatment. The review and evaluation shall include input from the medical staff and personnel of the respiratory care department/service. This review and evaluation should be performed within the overall hospital quality assurance pro-

gram. Particular attention shall be given to evaluation of the necessity for those respiratory care services having the highest utilization rate. The quality and appropriateness of respiratory care services provided by outside sources shall be included in the review and evaluation on the same regular basis.

Index

Entries referring to tables are denoted by a t following the page number. An *italic* number indicates an illustration.